To Wendy—

Thank you for your
dedication, support and
friendship on our long
friendship on Alzheimer therapeutics.
path to Warm regards,

Dennis

14 February, 2012

The Biology of
Alzheimer Disease

A subject collection from *Cold Spring Harbor Perspectives in Medicine*

OTHER SUBJECT COLLECTIONS FROM *COLD SPRING HARBOR PERSPECTIVES IN MEDICINE*

Angiogenesis: Biology and Pathology
HIV: From Biology to Prevention and Treatment

SUBJECT COLLECTIONS FROM *COLD SPRING HARBOR PERSPECTIVES IN BIOLOGY*

Extracellular Matrix Biology
Protein Homeostasis
Calcium Signaling
The Golgi
Germ Cells
The Mammary Gland as an Experimental Model
The Biology of Lipids: Trafficking, Regulation, and Function
Auxin Signaling: From Synthesis to Systems Biology
The Nucleus
Neuronal Guidance: The Biology of Brain Wiring
Cell Biology of Bacteria
Cell–Cell Junctions
Generation and Interpretation of Morphogen Gradients
Immunoreceptor Signaling
NF-κB: A Network Hub Controlling Immunity, Inflammation, and Cancer
Symmetry Breaking in Biology
The Origins of Life
The p53 Family

The Biology of
Alzheimer Disease

A subject collection from *Cold Spring Harbor Perspectives in Medicine*

EDITED BY

Dennis J. Selkoe

Harvard Medical School
Brigham and Women's Hospital

Eckhard Mandelkow

Max-Planck Unit for
Structural Molecular Biology

David M. Holtzman

Washington University
School of Medicine

COLD SPRING HARBOR LABORATORY PRESS
Cold Spring Harbor, New York • www.cshlpress.org

The Biology of Alzheimer Disease

A Subject Collection from *Cold Spring Harbor Perspectives in Medicine*
Articles online at www.perspectivesinmedicine.org

Executive Editor	Richard Sever
Managing Editor	Maria Smit
Production Editor	Diane Schubach
Project Manager	Barbara Acosta
Permissions Administrator	Carol Brown
Production Manager/Cover Designer	Denise Weiss
Publisher	John Inglis

Front cover artwork: Four self-portraits by the artist William Utermohlen, an American who lived in London, chronicle his experience with Alzheimer disease. Utermohlen was diagnosed at the age of 60; his powerful, emotionally complex depictions of the disease have garnered wide acclaim. The first in this series (*top left*) was painted in 1995, when he was diagnosed with the disease. The artist's wife, an art critic, has speculated that a growing awareness of cognitive decline may have contributed to the artist's depiction of himself behind windowpanes that resemble prison bars. The other pictures, which Utermohlen created over the course of the next 5 years, show a progressive loss of the ability to depict complex spatial relationships and provide evidence of growing perceptual difficulties. Soon after completing the last sketch, he ceased to work. (William Utermohlen's work reprinted with kind permission from Patricia Utermohlen and the Galerie Beckel Odille Boïcos, Paris.)

Library of Congress Cataloging-in-Publication Data

The biology of Alzheimer disease / edited by Dennis J. Selkoe, Eckhard Mandelkow, and David M. Holtzman.
    p. ; cm.
"A subject collection from Cold Spring Harbor perspectives in medicine"-- T.p. verso.
Includes bibliographical references and index.
ISBN 978-1-936113-44-6 (hardcover : alk. paper)
I. Selkoe, Dennis J. II. Holtzman, David M. (David Michael), 1961- III. Mandelkow, E. (Eckhard), 1943- IV. Cold Spring Harbor perspectives in medicine.
[DNLM: 1. Alzheimer Disease--physiopathology--Collected Works. WT 155]

LC classification not assigned
616.8'31--dc23
               2011030528

10 9 8 7 6 5 4 3 2 1

All Cold Spring Harbor Laboratory Press publications may be ordered directly from Cold Spring Harbor Laboratory Press, 500 Sunnyside Blvd., Woodbury, New York 11797-2924. Phone: 1-800-843-4388 in Continental U.S. and Canada. All other locations: (516) 422-4100. FAX: (516) 422-4097. E-mail: cshpress@cshl.edu. For a complete catalog of all Cold Spring Harbor Laboratory Press publications, visit our website at http://www.cshlpress.org.

Contents

Contents

Preface

Attempting to organize and review the extensive body of scientific literature on the biological basis of Alzheimer disease (AD) would seem to be a daunting task. The idea of preparing a book that does so comprehensively emerged from many discussions over the last decade about how this field of inquiry was progressing and how one might integrate the diversity of approaches and findings that it has generated. The editors of this volume took on the responsibility of identifying and sequencing the major topics to be covered and assembling a group of expert authors. As such, we are well aware that there are various ways such a huge body of research could be covered and that some topics will perforce receive more or less attention than others. The editors chose highly knowledgeable and scientifically active investigators in Alzheimer biology to contribute chapters on topics in which they have deep expertise. We are most grateful that virtually everyone invited to write for the book quickly agreed to participate, despite having very busy schedules. The diverse scientific viewpoints and collective wisdom of this talented group will, we hope, enable the volume to provide value to the broad biomedical community as it strives to achieve the intellectually fascinating and medically critical goal of solving AD.

The editors apologize in advance to those readers who may find missing elements or points of disagreement or overlap among the array of scientific findings reviewed here, and we recognize that no one volume can do full justice to this intense and rapidly advancing field. However, we would point out that, depending on its reception, this first comprehensive book reviewing the biological underpinnings of AD will be revised, updated, and thus improved within a few years. In this sense, we hope to have the opportunity to respond to issues we overlooked or covered insufficiently, given the space and time available to complete a project of this magnitude. It is likely that revised editions of this book—if they come to pass—will be even more detailed and compelling than this first effort. Nevertheless, we are hopeful that the multifaceted subjects covered here in considerable depth by distinguished authorities will prove useful to a broad audience of undergraduate, graduate, and medical students, postdoctoral fellows, junior and senior investigators, and, importantly, scientists and clinicians working outside the field of AD research.

Readers familiar with the Alzheimer field may notice that some chapters are coauthored by investigators who have had differing views of the topic under review or have sometimes been competitors. The editors purposely chose this path to encourage the synthesis of diverse perspectives and attempt to achieve clarity and common ground on unsettled issues. We are grateful to all of our chapter authors but particularly to those who at first pass found themselves facing the challenging task of melding disparate ideas and data.

We encourage readers not only to peruse chapters on topics that particularly intrigue—or confuse—them but also to read the first and last chapters of the book. Here, the editors have tried to step back from the wealth of details and convey a sense of what has motivated the global quest to understand the biology of AD, how sometimes competing concepts and lines of inquiry have proceeded, and, most importantly, where we believe this scientifically rich and therapeutically promising field is headed.

The editors thank Barbara Acosta, Richard Sever, and their colleagues at Cold Spring Harbor Laboratory Press for their excellent editorial and compositional efforts in putting this book together and their patience with the inevitable delays and minor crises that arise during such an ambitious undertaking. Each of the editors owes a very special thanks to past and current members of his respective laboratory and other local colleagues for innumerable discussions about the science of AD and how to think about its many unresolved questions. We also thank our gifted and dedicated administrative assistants who helped us in this work, especially Ms. Nicole Boucher (at BWH/HMS). One of us (D.J.S.) had the benefit of the careful bibliographical research, data analysis, and sage editorial advice of Marcia Podlisny, Ph.D., who had helped organize information relevant to this volume during an earlier effort some years ago. Finally, we are indebted to our families for their support and forbearance as we added the creation of this book to our already numerous responsibilities. We hope that the outcome will justify the collective efforts of the authors and editors and help illuminate the path toward scientifically well-grounded therapeutics that could ultimately prevent this common and devastating disorder.

DENNIS J. SELKOE
ECKHARD MANDELKOW
DAVID M. HOLTZMAN

Deciphering Alzheimer Disease

Dennis Selkoe[1], Eckhard Mandelkow[2], and David Holtzman[3]

[1]Center for Neurologic Diseases, Harvard Medical School and Brigham and Women's Hospital, Boston, Massachusetts 02115

[2]Max-Planck Unit for Structural Molecular Biology, Hamburg 22607, Germany; and DZNE, German Center for Neurodegenerative Diseases, and CAESAR Research Center, 53175 Bonn, Germany

[3]Department of Neurology, Washington University School of Medicine, St. Louis, Missouri 63110

Correspondence: dselkoe@rics.bwh.harvard.edu

Few diagnoses in modern medicine evoke greater apprehension and sadness than Alzheimer disease. Virtually unknown to the public just a generation ago, this protean disorder is now the subject of enormous concern on a personal level and represents a looming catastrophe for society. Most people in developed nations have encountered victims of the disease, often within their own families, and there is a palpable sense of urgency that something be done. Yet patients told that they have Alzheimer disease quickly learn that no proven disease-modifying treatment exists and that they are destined to experience the insidious loss of their most human qualities—memory, reasoning, abstraction, language, and emotional stability. Now, based on the power of reductionist biology, this bleak situation appears poised to change.

Breathtaking advances in our fundamental knowledge of molecular biology and cellular function during the last half-century have provided a platform on which thousands of scientists worldwide are building an understanding of how Alzheimer disease works. Like other new scientific subjects, research on Alzheimer disease has experienced its share of controversy and confusion. However, there are far more advances than setbacks, and many within the field believe that a rough consensus about how the disorder begins and evolves has emerged. The chapters in this book explore in depth many aspects of this complex syndrome and explain how molecular understanding is leading to novel therapeutic agents that may one day also be used to prevent the disorder.

THE MELDING OF BASIC AND APPLIED BIOLOGICAL RESEARCH

Most of us interested in science have grown up with the paradigm that there are two broad areas of scientific effort: "basic" and "applied." In biology, it is understood that many programs of experimentation seek to uncover the fundamental rules by which molecules are created, interact, and give rise to cellular and organismal function. On the other hand, there is great interest in pursuing a wide range of clues about how specific diseases begin, progress, and may ultimately be thwarted. However, in the last few decades, scientists have increasingly recognized that this paradigm constitutes an inaccurate dichotomy. Many investigators whose careers have focused on normal physiology are interested in the implications of their findings for the mechanisms of unsolved diseases. In turn, those who have intensively studied human disorders and cellular and animal models thereof have sometimes contributed novel and powerful insights into the normal functions of molecular and cellular systems. This blurring of the classical boundaries is not surprising and, indeed, is highly salutary for

Cite this article as *Cold Spring Harb Perspect Med* doi: 10.1101/cshperspect.a011460

both aspects of biological research. Scientists principally viewed as disease-oriented should strongly support more investment in so-called fundamental research, on which understanding of disease must be based, and traditionally "basic" scientists should be encouraged to extend their knowledge and methods directly into the mechanisms of the disorders that implicate the systems they are studying.

Research on the origins of Alzheimer disease and other age-related neurodegenerative disorders exemplifies this melding process. There is now an impressive list of genes and proteins, understanding of which emerged solely from an interest in Alzheimer disease. The amyloid β-protein precursor (APP), its homologous family members APLP-1 and APLP-2, the presenilins, and the β-secretases were all cloned within programs focused on elucidating Alzheimer disease. The discovery of presenilin (named after its role in the disease) as the first known intramembrane aspartyl protease and its function as a key signaling hub that processes many diverse receptors in multicellular organisms represents a signal contribution of Alzheimer research to protein biology. The recognition from studies of neurodegenerative diseases that certain neuronal proteins (e.g., tau, α-synuclein) that are normally soluble may undergo alternative folding and oligomerize to gain new functional properties has helped illustrate the inextricable relationship between normal and abnormal protein folding. These and numerous other examples in the field of human neurodegeneration underscore the relevance of disease-oriented research to normal biology. This recognition gives added excitement and urgency to delving ever deeper into the mechanisms of disease.

ALZHEIMER DISEASE AS A PROTOTYPE FOR THE MOLECULAR ELUCIDATION OF A COMPLEX, CHRONIC DISORDER OF THE HUMAN BRAIN

Not very long ago, disorders like Alzheimer, Parkinson, and Huntington diseases were often assigned to the backs of textbooks of medicine as mechanistically obscure and therapeutically intractable syndromes. However, advances in two areas, biochemical pathology and human genetics, have dramatically changed this situation over just two decades. For the first 60 years after the Bavarian psychiatrist Alois Alzheimer described his index patient in 1907 (Alzheimer 1907), virtually no progress in our understanding of the causes and mechanisms of the disorder occurred. Then, the seminal papers on the electron microscopy of Alzheimer cytopathology by Robert Terry and Michael Kidd in the mid-1960s piqued an upswing in scientific interest (Terry 1963; Kidd 1964). In 1968, Gary Blessed, Bernard Tomlinson, and Martin Roth published a key clinicopathological study that confirmed what some neuropathologists had long suspected: the neuropathology of many cases of common senile dementia was indistinguishable from that of Alzheimer disease (Blessed et al. 1968). The latter disorder had first been described in a woman who died at age 56 and had been thought of as a distinct "presenile" dementia. However, the 1968 study supported the concept that Alzheimer disease occurred along an age continuum, with relatively rare cases appearing before the 60s and the incidence rising steadily through the seventh to ninth decades and beyond.

This recognition of the shared neuropathological phenotype of cases regardless of age of onset soon led to a widespread awareness that Alzheimer disease, rather than being a rare presenile dementia, was a very common disorder. In 1976, Robert Katzman wrote a brief but influential piece that called attention to this fact and warned about an impending "epidemic" of cases as longevity rose in developed countries (Katzman 1976). In 1979, Jerome Stone and other lay Americans with affected family members organized the Alzheimer Association, headquartered in Chicago. This provided an enormous boost to public recognition of the disease and the personal and societal tragedy it represents. In the area of biochemical pathology, George Glenner first isolated and partially characterized the amyloid β-protein from the brains of patients who had died with Alzheimer disease or Down syndrome in 1984 (Glenner and Wong 1984a, b), and within two years, several laboratories had identified the microtubule-associated protein, tau, as the principal constituent of the neurofibrillary tangles (Brion et al. 1985; Grundke-Iqbal et al. 1986; Kosik et al. 1986; Nukina and Ihara 1986; Wood et al. 1986). The cloning of the amyloid β-protein precursor in 1987 and discoveries of its disease-causing mutations in 1990 and 1991 brought the field squarely into the era of molecular genetics and protein chemistry (Kang et al. 1987; Levy et al. 1990; Goate et al. 1991).

In this brief and incomplete overview of the emergence of modern Alzheimer research, one can sense the crescendo of public and scientific interest in the disorder. Today, hundreds of laboratories and clinics worldwide are intensely focused on applying many different approaches and techniques to characterize the Alzheimer phenotype at all levels and to search for opportunities to intervene. The array of observations, some seemingly contradictory, is daunting; it has become an enormous challenge to synthesize available findings into an accurate schema of how the disease starts, unfolds, and gradually devastates cognition, leading to the patient's premature death. In this book, some of the leading clinical and laboratory scientists who have contributed importantly to our emerging understanding of pathogenesis and treatment have come together to share their knowledge and perspectives. They represent a much larger global community of students of Alzheimer disease. Assuming that the rate of progress continues to accelerate, Alzheimer disease may become a salient example of the steady move from phenomenology to detailed molecular understanding in a disorder of the most advanced biological system we know, the human brain.

THE DRIVING FORCES THAT HAVE STIMULATED AD RESEARCH

The Quest for Scientific Clarity

As in all fields of scientific inquiry, by far the strongest force for progress on Alzheimer disease derives from the innate curiosity of the individuals who have chosen to study the topic.

Attempting to contribute to the unraveling of this very complicated riddle provides enormous stimulation to the intellect. We often find ourselves in the laboratory or the clinic at times when our friends and families expect us to put aside our work. The complexity of the problem and the diverse ways in which one might think about approaching it make for a fascinating adventure in biomedical research. In one sense, this may be surprising to colleagues in other medical fields, as Alzheimer disease and other brain degenerations have long been viewed with intense therapeutic nihilism. Why would one have wished to focus one's work on this (until recently) obscure and enigmatic syndrome?

One motivation arises from the fact that Alzheimer disease represents at its onset a remarkably pure and insidious impairment of intellect. To those who entered neuroscience because of a fascination with the mind–brain relationship, deciphering the origins of this syndrome provides a window into the anatomic and molecular substrates of clear, well-organized thinking and the subtle events that can perturb memory and reasoning. Inspired by the towering examples of nineteenth-century neuroscientists like Broca, Charcot, and Sherrington, who used neural deficits to elucidate normal nervous system function, investigators hope to help validate some of the emerging rules of normal memory and cognitive function by understanding which circuits and signaling pathways explain the earliest symptoms of Alzheimer disease. This relationship is illustrated not only by the molecular dissection of the disease in the laboratory but also by clinical approaches such as functional magnetic resonance imaging, in which one can examine in vivo the brain networks that become activated in abnormal ways when subjects destined to develop Alzheimer disease years later attempt to remember specific patterns such as face–name pairs.

In the last two decades, it has become apparent that Alzheimer disease involves changes in many overlapping molecular, cellular, and anatomical pathways. Students of the disease may choose to focus their work on neuropathology, protein folding, substrate-protease biochemistry, synaptic structure and function, signal transduction, cytoskeletal biology, inflammation, oxidative metabolism, neurotransmitter pharmacology, metal ion homeostasis, or behavioral phenotyping in murine models. In short, Alzheimer research touches upon virtually the entire range of biological inquiry. The breadth and heterogeneity of the field is evidenced by a bewildering array of findings, many seemingly unrelated, that appear in innumerable publications each month. Investigators generally tend to focus on a topic that is familiar to them and produce data that are often heralded as a critical insight into the mechanism of the disease. This experimental ferment provides intellectual stimulation but can also lead to confusion and controversy, with seemingly important observations not easily confirmed by other laboratories. Nevertheless, there has been a steady movement over the years toward mechanistic consensus, as discussed here.

The Personal Tragedy of Alzheimer Disease

For many who contribute to this field, a prime motivator for their work is a painful awareness of how Alzheimer disease and similar progressive dementias devastate the lives of victims and their families. Among chronic diseases, Alzheimer is particularly poignant in that it erodes the patient's intellectual and emotional life and often destroys the rewards of retirement that individuals have longingly anticipated throughout their working lives. There are few more painful experiences than to see a beloved parent or sibling slowly but inexorably become a person one can hardly recognize. In this sense, Alzheimer disease compounds its suffering by exacting enormous pressure and dislocation on the family of the victim.

An advantage of studying a highly prevalent disorder is that even those scientists who otherwise would have little occasion to witness the clinical syndrome first-hand are acquainted with patients harboring the disorder. The majority of researchers focused on Alzheimer disease globally are not clinicians caring for patients. However, the frequent linkage of these scientists to centers of clinical expertise,

coupled with active dissemination through professional and lay fora of what the Alzheimer phenotype is like, enables students of the problem at all levels to have an understanding of its clinical development and consequences. Those who interact professionally with patients and their loved ones and watch the disease unfold have a strong additional motivation for working on the problem beyond its scientific fascination. However, one does not need to be involved in patient care to feel the enormous desire to help these individuals. All of us engaged in this endeavor are inspired to contribute in ways large and small to the relief of suffering and, ultimately, to the prevention of this most common late-life dementia.

The Societal Crisis of Alzheimer Disease

As if the patient's personal burden were not sufficient motivation, the enormous public health impact of the rising prevalence of Alzheimer disease further focuses one's attention. Projections of the combined economic burden of medical care and lost productivity vary widely, but all of the estimates are alarmingly high. It is believed that the number of patients diagnosed with Alzheimer disease worldwide may rise from the current approximation of 20–25 million to perhaps three times that number by mid-century, assuming no meaningful disease-modifying intervention occurs. The scientific progress reviewed in this book makes that outcome increasingly unlikely, but many more cases will accrue before even optimistic predictions of early treatment and prevention show an impact on prevalence.

In the United States, the message that Alzheimer disease is a public health emergency has been brought forward most effectively by two entities: the National Institute on Aging (NIA) and the Alzheimer Association. Since its founding in 1974, the NIA has expended enormous effort to bring a message of urgency to both the scientific and lay communities. Among the several National Institutes of Health institutes that help fund aspects of Alzheimer research, the NIA serves as the principal funder of laboratory and clinical research nationally,

Cite this article as *Cold Spring Harb Perspect Med* doi: 10.1101/cshperspect.a011460

and it has sponsored countless initiatives, symposia, workshops, and calls to action that have dramatically moved the effort forward. Many investigators have been trained, nurtured, and enabled by the NIA's scientific leadership over almost four decades.

Another major breakthrough in the quest to defeat the disease came from the efforts of a few affected families around 1979–1980 to organize the lay public into a focused and effective force for raising public awareness, helping suffering patients in many ways, and gathering precious funds for research. The success of the Alzheimer Association, which now sponsors the largest and most impactful international scientific meetings on the disorder, cannot be overestimated. Indeed, the example of American families organizing in this way has spawned not only chapters in all of the states and many local communities, but also sister organizations in countries throughout the world. The NIA and the Alzheimer Association often work together to move the field forward, and the scientific community is deeply indebted to their unceasing efforts on behalf of the cause.

The Competition of Ideas and Findings: A Brief Perspective on "BAPtists versus TAUists"

To those working within the field and perhaps also to many outside of it, Alzheimer research has sometimes been viewed as unusually contentious. However, a measured examination of the trajectory of the field over the past three decades suggests that controversy arose in large part out of the newness of the topic and the initial need to focus on poorly defined phenomena of the phenotype: the imprecision of the concept of "senile dementia" and the presence of brains lesions (senile plaques and neurofibrillary tangles) that occurred in highly variable densities and patterns within the Alzheimer brain but also in seemingly unrelated disorders. The era of rigorous biological analysis of the disease arguably began in the 1960s and 1970s. In those early days, investigators started to apply electron microscopy, biochemistry, and immunohistochemistry in attempts to uncover the nature of the classical

morphological lesions and their local consequences. A growing focus on plaques and tangles as important phenomena of the disease was greeted with substantial skepticism, the argument being that the lesions Alzheimer described might well represent tombstones of a decades-long process and offer little insight into etiology.

Tissue deposits of amyloid, in particular, were well known to occur in certain systemic disorders of diverse cause, where they could arise as secondary reactions to more specific pathogenic events. The idea of "secondary amyloidosis" occurring in some hosts experiencing infectious, metabolic, or inflammatory disorders implied to some that the amyloid in Alzheimer disease might be an end-stage reaction with little pathogenic importance, the detritus of the process. This is a concern that is still voiced by some in the field, although the application of unbiased genetic approaches to familial Alzheimer disease has provided unequivocal evidence that at least some cases of the disorder are directly caused by dyshomeostasis of amyloid β-protein. Nonetheless, it remains a topic of debate as to whether these rare cases are closely related mechanistically to common "idiopathic" cases of Alzheimer disease. Because the two major lesions are composed of distinct proteins, tau in the case of the neurofibrillary tangles and amyloid β-protein in the case of amyloid plaques, the amusing aphorism that Alzheimer research is a kind of religious war between "BAPtists" and "TAUists" has even reached the lay public. However, the last few years have witnessed a palpable decrease in this tension, as inherited mutations in the APP or tau genes, mouse modeling of these genotypes, and careful analyses of the Alzheimer phenotype of Down syndrome have combined to clarify the order in which the two lesions arise in the disease. Several lines of evidence, all of which are reviewed in this book, suggest that the cerebral accumulation of amyloid β-protein precedes and helps drive the deposition of the tau protein in neuronal perikarya and their processes. This recognition does nothing to diminish the pathogenic importance of tau alteration and cytoskeletal impairment in Alzheimer disease. Indeed, recent studies suggest that the presence of the tau protein is necessary for expression of the downstream effects of amyloid β-protein on neurons.

Although it is interesting to attempt to assemble the myriad findings about the disease into a hypothetical sequence, one must bear in mind that dynamic information about the development of the process in Alzheimer patients themselves has been difficult to acquire. Almost certainly, many molecular and cellular changes occur virtually simultaneously and involve complex feedback loops, so that the evolution of the disorder is likely to be far less linear than current schemes propose. Nevertheless, the temporal ordering of events based on the latest available evidence can provide heuristic arguments for debate and pathogenic hypotheses that can be tested in animal models and later in human therapeutic trials. The rapid growth in fluid and imaging biomarker studies is particularly relevant to underpinning—or denying—the proposed cascades of pathogenesis.

THE KEY SCIENTIFIC QUESTIONS TO BE ADDRESSED: CAUSES, MECHANISMS, EFFECTS, AND THERAPIES

Because laboratory and clinical research on Alzheimer disease over the past four decades has involved so many approaches and findings, an attempt to incorporate these into one comprehensive text is an exercise marked by a degree of hubris. It is impossible to capture all of the complex observations and competing ideas that mark this field of inquiry. Nevertheless, the editors and authors of this book have attempted to cover the vast majority of the principal scientific topics that the Alzheimer research community concerns itself with today.

We begin with five chapters that cover the clinical, neuropsychological, neuropathological, imaging, and biomarker phenotypes of the disease (Blennow et al. 2011; Johnson et al. 2011; Serrano-Pozo et al. 2011; Tarweh

and Holtzman et al. 2011; Weintraub et al. 2011), including how these can be used to distinguish it from disorders that represent partial phenocopies. Next follows a chapter on the clues to causation and pathogenesis that arise from epidemiological studies of Alzheimer disease (Mayeux and Stern 2011). Then we embark upon an in-depth review of the latest ideas and findings on the biochemistry and molecular and cell biology of the processes that contribute to the development of the clinicopathological phenotype, including crucial insights that have arisen from human genetics (De Strooper et al. 2011; Goedert et al. 2011; Haass et al. 2011; Holtzman et al. 2011a; Ihara et al. 2011; LaFerla and Green 2011; Mandelkow and Mandeklow 2011; Masters and Selkoe 2011; Mucke and Selkoe 2011; Müller and Zheng 2011; Sagare et al. 2011; Saido and Leissring 2011; Tanzi 2011; Wyss-Coray and Rogers 2011). This detailed summary of the biology of the disorder represents the core of the book. We conclude with three chapters that discuss both existing treatments for Alzheimer disease and those that are currently in clinical trials or are expected to enter them before long (Aisen et al. 2011; Lee et al. 2011; Schenk et al. 2011). That therapeutic overview represents the promise of all of the multifaceted scientific efforts that the previous articles describe.

In the final chapter (Holtzman et al. 2011b), we speculate about how the expansive knowledge base may dramatically alter the way "Alzheimerology" is practiced within the next decade or two. We believe that the convergence of many scientific threads, particularly those from studies of fluid biomarkers and brain imaging, along with clinical genetics, should allow physicians to gauge risk with increasing accuracy and to monitor the development of the disease in its presymptomatic phase, before irreversible neuronal injury has occurred. The paradigm we describe emphasizes screening for the disorder in mid-life (perhaps earlier) and then offering a range of preventions intended to stave off—or permanently avoid—progressive cognitive decline. Our projections disclose a strong sense of optimism that emerges from extraordinary progress in deciphering the biology of Alzheimer disease during our lifetimes.

REFERENCES

*Reference is also in this collection.

* Aisen PS, Cummings JL, Schneider LS. 2011. Symptomatic and non-amyloid/tau-based pharmacologic treatment for Alzheimer disease. *Cold Spring Harb Perspect Med* doi: 10.1101/cshperspect.a006395.

Alzheimer A. 1907. Ueber eine eigenartige Erkrankung der Hirnrinde. *Centralblatt fur Nervenheilkunde und Psychiatrie* **30:** 177–179.

* Blennow K, Zetterberg H, Fagan AM. 2011. Fluid biomarkers in Alzheimer disease. *Cold Spring Harb Perspect Med* doi: 10.1101/cshperspect.a006221.

Blessed G, Tomlinson BE, Roth M. 1968. The association between quantitative measures of dementia and senile change in the cerebral grey matter of elderly subjects. *Br J Psychiat* **114:** 797–811.

Brion J, Passareiro E, Nunez J, Flament-Durand J. 1985. Mise en evidence immunologique de la protein tau au niveau des lesions de degenerescence neurofibrillaire de la maladie D'Alzheimer. *Arch Biol* **95:** 229–235.

* De Strooper B, Iwatsubo T, Wolfe MS. 2011. Presenilisn and γ-secretase: Structure, function, and role in Alzheimer disease. *Cold Spring Harb Perspect Med* doi: 10.1101/cshperspect.a006304.

Glenner GG, Wong CW. 1984a. Alzheimer's disease and Down's syndrome: Sharing of a unique cerebrovascular amyloid fibril protein. *Biochem Biophys Res Commun* **122:** 1131–1135.

Glenner GG, Wong CW. 1984b. Alzheimer's disease: Initial report of the purification and characterization of a novel cerebrovascular amyloid protein. *Biochem Biophys Res Commun* **120:** 885–890.

Goate A, Chartier-Harlin M-C, Mullan M, Brown J, Crawford F, Fidani L, Giuffra L, Haynes A, Irving N, James L, et al. 1991. Segregation of a missense mutation in the amyloid precursor protein gene with familial Alzheimer's disease. *Nature* **349:** 704–706.

* Goedert M, Ghetti B, Spillantini MG. 2011. Frontotemporal dementia: Implications for understanding Alzheimer disease. *Cold Spring Harb Perspect Med* doi: 10.1101/cshperspect.a006254.

Grundke-Iqbal I, Iqbal K, Quinlan M, Tung Y-C, Zaidi MS, Wisniewski HM. 1986. Microtubule-associated protein tau: A component of Alzheimer paired helical filaments. *J Biol Chem* **261:** 6084–6089.

* Haass C, Kaether C, Sisodia S, Thinakaran G. 2011. Trafficking and proteolytic processing of APP. *Cold Spring Harb Perspect Med* doi: 10.1101/cshperspect.a006270.

* Holtzman DM, Herz J, Bu G. 2011a. Apolipoprotein E and apolipoprotein E receptors: Normal biology and roles in Alzheimer disease. *Cold Spring Harb Perspect Med* doi: 10.1101/cshperspect.a006312.

* Holtzman DM, Mandelkow E, Selkoe DJ. 2011b. Alzheimer disease in 2020. *Cold Spring Harb Perspect Med* doi: 10.1101/cshperspect.a011585.

* Ihara Y, Morishima-Kawashima M, Nixon R. 2011. The ubiquitin–proteasome system and the autophagic–lysosomal system in Alzheimer disease. *Cold Spring Harb Perspect Med* doi: 10.1101/cshperspect.a006361.

* Johnson KA, Fox NC, Sperling RA, Klunk WE. 2011. Brain imaging in Alzheimer diseae. *Cold Spring Harb Perspect Med* doi: 10.1101/cshperspect.a006213.

Kang J, Lemaire H-G, Unterbeck A, Salbaum JM, Masters CL, Grzeschik K-H, Multhaup G, Beyreuther K, Muller-Hill B. 1987. The precursor of Alzheimer's disease amyloid A4 protein resembles a cell-surface receptor. *Nature* **325:** 733–736.

Katzman R. 1976. Editorial: The prevalence and malignancy of Alzheimer disease. A major killer. *Arch Neurol* **33:** 217–218.

Kidd M. 1964. Alzheimer's disease—An electron microscopical study. *Brain* **87:** 307–320.

Kosik KS, Joachim CL, Selkoe DJ. 1986. Microtubule-associated protein, tau, is a major antigenic component of paired helical filaments in Alzheimer's disease. *Proc Natl Acad Sci* **83:** 4044–4048.

* LaFerla F, Green KN. 2011. Animal models of Alzheimer disease. *Cold Spring Harb Perspect Med* doi: 10.1101/cshperspect.a006320.

* Lee V, Brunden KR, Hutton M, Trojanowski JQ. 2011. Developing therapeutic approaches to tau, selected kinases, and related neuronal protein targets. *Cold Spring Harb Perspect Med* doi: 10.1101/cshperspect.a006437.

Levy E, Carman MD, Fernandez-Madrid IJ, Power MD, Lieberburg I, van Duinen SG, Bots GTAM, Luyendijk W, Frangione B. 1990. Mutation of the Alzheimer's disease amyloid gene in hereditary cerebral hemorrhage, Dutch-type. *Science* **248:** 1124–1126.

* Mandelkow EM, Mandelkow E. 2011. Biochemistry and cell biology of tau protein in neurofibrillary degeneration. *Cold Spring Harb Perspect Med* doi: 10.1101/cshperspect.a006247.

* Masters CL, Selkoe DJ. 2011. Biochemistry of amyloid β-protein and amyloid deposits in Alzheimer disease. *Cold Spring Harb Perspect Med* doi: 10.1101/cshperspect.a006262.

* Mayeux R, Stern Y. 2011. Epidemiology of Alzheimer disease. *Cold Spring Harb Perspect Med* doi: 10.1101/cshperspect.a006239.

* Mucke L, Selkoe DJ. Neurotoxicity of amyloid β-protein: Synaptic networkdysfunction. *Cold Spring Harb Perspect Med* doi: 10.1101/cshperspect.a006338.

* Müller UC, Zheng H. 2011. Physiological functions of APP family proteins. *Cold Spring Harb Perspect Med* doi: 10.1101/cshperspect.a006288.

Nukina N, Ihara Y. 1986. One of the antigenic determinants of paired helical filaments is related to tau protein. *J Biochem* **99:** 1541–1544.

* Sagare AP, Bell RD, Zlokovic BV. 2011. Neutovascular dysfunction and faulty amyloid β-peptide clearance in Alzheimer disease. *Cold Spring Harb Perspect Med* doi: 10.1101/cshperspect.a011452.

* Saido T, Leissring MA. 2011. Proteolytic degradation of amyloid β-protein. *Cold Spring Harb Perspect Med* doi: 10.1101/cshperspect.a006379.

* Schenk D, Basi GS, Pangalos MN. 2011. Treatment strategies targeting amyloid β-protein. *Cold Spring Harb Perspect Med* doi: 10.1101/cshperspect.a006387.

* Serrano-Pozo A, Frosch MP, Masliah E, Hyman BT. 2011. Neuropathological alterations in Alzheimer disease. *Cold Spring Harb Perspect Med* doi: 10.1101/cshperspect.a006189.

* Tanzi RE. 2011. The genetics of Alzheimer disease. *Cold Spring Harb Perspect Med* doi: 10.1101/cshperspect.a006296.

* Tarawneh R, Holtzman DM. 2011. The clinical problem of symptomatic Alzheimer disease and mild cognitive impairment. *Cold Spring Harb Perspect Med* doi: 10.1101/cshperspect.a006148.

Terry RD. 1963. The fine structure of neurofibrillary tangles in Alzheimer's disease. *J Neuropathol Exp Neurol* **22:** 629–642.

* Weintraub S, Wicklund AH, Salmon DP. 2011. The neuropsychological profile of Alzheimer disease. *Cold Spring Harb Perspect Med* doi: 10.1101/cshperspect.a006171.

Wood JG, Mirra SS, Pollock NL, Binder LI. 1986. Neurofibrillary tangles of Alzheimer's disease share antigenic determinants with the axonal microtubule-associated protein tau. *Proc Natl Acad Sci* **83:** 4040–4043.

* Wyss-Coray T, Rogers J. 2011. Inflammation in Alzheimer disease—A brief review of the basic science and clinical literature. *Cold Spring Harb Perspect Med* doi: 10.1101/cshperspect.a006346.

Cite this article as *Cold Spring Harb Perspect Med* doi: 10.1101/cshperspect.a011460

The Clinical Problem of Symptomatic Alzheimer Disease and Mild Cognitive Impairment

Rawan Tarawneh[1,2,3] and David M. Holtzman[1,2,3]

[1]Department of Neurology, Washington University School of Medicine, St. Louis, St. Louis, Missouri 63110

[2]Hope Center for Neurological Disorders, Washington University School of Medicine, St. Louis, St. Louis, Missouri 63110

[3]The Knight Alzheimer's Disease Research Center, Washington University School of Medicine, St. Louis, St. Louis, Missouri 63110

Correspondence: holtzman@neuro.wustl.edu

Alzheimer disease (AD) is the most common cause of dementia in the elderly. Clinicopathological studies support the presence of a long preclinical phase of the disease, with the initial deposition of AD pathology estimated to begin approximately 10–15 years prior to the onset of clinical symptoms. The hallmark clinical phenotype of AD is a gradual and progressive decline in two or more cognitive domains, most commonly involving episodic memory and executive functions, that is sufficient to cause social or occupational impairment. Current diagnostic criteria can accurately identify AD in the majority of cases. As disease-modifying therapies are being developed, there is growing interest in the identification of individuals in the earliest symptomatic, as well as presymptomatic, stages of disease, because it is in this population that such therapies may have the greatest chance of success. The use of informant-based methods to establish cognitive and functional decline of an individual from previously attained levels of performance best allows for the identification of individuals in the very mildest stages of cognitive impairment.

Alzheimer disease (AD) is by far the most common cause of dementia in the United States, accounting for over 70% of dementia cases in individuals ≥ 70 years of age (Alzheimer's Association 2011). The incidence of AD increases exponentially with age, and doubles every 5 years after the age of 65 (Kukull et al. 2002).

Estimates from the Alzheimer's Association in 2011 indicate that over 5.4 million people in the United States have AD, including 5.2 million people 65 years of age or older. With the increasing age of the U.S. population, it is estimated that this number will increase by 50%—with over 7.7 million people in that age range affected by AD—by the year 2030, and will almost triple to 11–16 million by the year 2050. AD is the leading cause of nursing home placement, and a major economic health burden with costs estimated at $140 billion in healthcare, nursing home placement, and lost wages and productivity for family members and caregivers. In the absence of effective disease-modifying therapies or prevention strategies for AD, it is likely that the health, social, and economic burdens of AD will increase substantially in the next 10–20 years.

AD is the sixth-highest cause of death across all ages in the United States, and the fifth-highest cause of death for those 65 years of age or older (Alzheimer's Association 2011). Unlike most other major causes of mortality in the elderly, deaths from AD have continued to rise over the last decade; an increase of 66% in deaths owing to AD was reported in the period 2000–2008. As AD is often under-recognized as a cause of death, it is possible that increased mortality rates owing to AD may even be higher than previously reported.

Significant advances in our understanding of the clinical, psychometric, neuropathological, genetic, and biological characteristics of AD have been made since Alois Alzheimer presented the first case of "presenile dementia," later identified by Kraeplin as AD, in 1906 (Alzheimer et al. 1987). This article reviews the clinical presentation, diagnostic criteria, and differential diagnosis of AD with particular focus on its earliest symptomatic stages. Individuals with early stages of AD pathology are the most likely to benefit from disease-modifying therapies should they become available (Tarawneh and Holtzman 2009). Therefore, the ability of clinicians to accurately detect AD in the earliest symptomatic (or even presymptomatic) stages, and to reliably differentiate AD from other causes of dementia, will likely have major therapeutic and prognostic implications in the future.

HEALTHY COGNITIVE AGING

Several cognitive changes are associated with healthy nondemented aging. The speed of mental processing (Birren and Fisher 1995), simple and choice reaction times (Botwinick and Thompson 1968), and perception times (Walsh et al. 1979) are slowed in the elderly compared with their younger counterparts, and may represent the cognitive functions that most clearly decline with age. While these changes may result

in pervasive deficits in neuropsychological testing (Park et al. 1996), in the absence of a dementing illness, they do not appear to be functionally significant.

Short-term memory loss (exemplified by free recall of a list of words or stories; Gilbert and Levee 1971; Crook and West 1990), with relative preservation of immediate (Blum et al. 1970; Drachman and Leavitt 1972) and long-term memory (Luszcz and Bryan 1999) has been reported in healthy elderly as early as the sixth decade. Memory decline in early AD, as opposed to what occurs with normal aging, represents a consistent and progressive change from the individual's prior abilities, and often results in mild impairment in daily functions (Morris 1993). On the other hand, the "benign" forgetfulness of healthy aging is typically mild, inconsistent, and not associated with impairment in daily activities. In contrast to the amnestic-type memory impairment seen in AD, normal aging is associated with a retrieval deficit type of impairment that responds well to clues and multiple-choice questions (Farlow 2007).

Some decline in verbal fluency and difficulty with naming may begin to appear in the seventh or eighth decades, respectively (Albert et al. 1988). However, most language functions such as phonological characteristics, lexical decisions (Howard et al. 1981), and syntactic knowledge (Obler et al. 1985) remain intact with age. Sustained and selective attention is preserved well into the eighth or ninth decade (Albert 1994). Language difficulty beyond mild naming difficulty or marked attention deficits should alert to the possibility of an underlying pathology. A decline in working memory (i.e., the ability to simultaneously store and process information; Babcock and Salthouse 1990) and executive functions (Parkin and Walter 1992; Troyer et al. 1994) may be associated with normal aging. Insight, social engagement, and visuospatial functions are generally retained in healthy elderly (Farlow 2007).

It is a common notion that substantial cognitive changes may occur with healthy aging. However, some of the previous studies attributing cognitive changes to age may have been inadvertently contaminated by individuals with unrecognized mildly symptomatic or pre-symptomatic dementia (Howieson et al. 1993). Longitudinal studies of healthy elderly popula-tions who have been carefully assessed to avoid inclusion of those with underlying presympto-matic pathology generally demonstrate a largely flat trajectory with stable cognitive performance well into the ninth decade of life (Howieson et al. 1993; Rubin et al. 1998). The main clinical distinction between cognitive changes of aging and those of underlying dementia is that, in the absence of an underlying pathology, the cognitive changes of aging are benign and rela-tively static, whereas they are progressive and associated with functional impairment in de-mentia. Healthy elderly retain the ability to use compensatory strategies (e.g., keeping lists and calendars) and are capable of learning and adaption skills (e.g., as evidenced by practice effects on repeated neuropsychological testing and acclimation to the testing environment), which potentially contribute to their stable cog-nitive performance over time.

DEFINITION OF DEMENTIA

In general terms, dementia can be described as an acquired syndrome of impaired cognition produced by brain dysfunction. From a practi-cal perspective, dementia is characterized by a decline from a previously established level of cognitive and functional performance of an individual that is sufficient to interfere with daily activities. There are two commonly used sets of criteria for the clinical diagnosis of dementia. The National Institute on Neurolog-ical and Communicative Disorders and Stroke and the Alzheimer Disease and Related Disor-ders Association (NINCDS/ADRDA) criteria for AD describe a gradual and progressive decline in two or more cognitive domains that is confirmed by abnormalities on clinical and neuropsychological testing, and is associated with impairment in social or occupational functions (Table 1; McKhann et al. 1984). The *Diagnostic and Statistical Manual of Mental Disorders, Fourth Edition* (*DSM-IV*) criteria for dementia (Table 2; American Psychiatric

Association 1994, 2000) are comparable to those proposed by the NINCDS/ADRDA, and include insidious and progressive decline in memory and at least one more cognitive domain that results in social and occupational impairment.

DETECTION OF DEMENTIA

As described previously, the clinical diagnosis of dementia generally relies on the demonstration of measurable deficits in two or more cognitive domains. These deficits have traditionally been measured by the comparison of an individual's cognitive performance with that of a "norm" of nondemented individuals matched for age, gender, and education. This approach, there-fore, represents an interindividual comparison of psychometric performance and does not determine whether the impaired performance represents a decline for that individual from their previously attained level of cognitive per-formance. Inherent cultural, ethnic, and educa-tional biases in the test measures (Doraiswamy et al. 1995; Manly et al. 1998), and the insensi-tivity or "ceiling effect" of many measures for mild impairment, may limit the ability of neuropsychological testing to detect very early stages of dementia. Furthermore, because puta-tively normal samples are likely to be contami-nated by individuals with presymptomatic AD (Sliwinski et al. 1996), the cut-points may be too permissive and fail to capture some indi-viduals in the early stages of disease, further blurring the distinction between very mild impairment and healthy aging. By relying on intraindividual cognitive decline rather than interindividual comparisons of psychometric performance, it may be possible to identify individuals at even earlier stages of cognitive impairment.

ALZHEIMER DISEASE

The NINCDS/ADRDA criteria classify AD into "probable," "possible," or "definite" (Table 1; McKhann et al. 1984), and have been widely used in both clinical trials and research settings. The NINCDS/ADRDA criteria for "probable" AD and *DSM-IV* criteria both have acceptable

Table 1. National Institute of Neurological and Communicative Disorders and Stroke and the Alzheimer's Disease and Related Disorders Association criteria for Alzheimer disease

I. Criteria for the clinical diagnosis of *probable* Alzheimer disease

Dementia established by clinical examination and documented by the Mini-Mental State Examination, Blessed Dementia Scale, or some similar examination, and confirmed by neuropsychological tests

Deficits in two or more areas of cognition

Progressive worsening of memory and other cognitive functions

No disturbance of consciousness

Onset between ages 40 and 90, most often after age 65

Absence of systemic disorders or other brain diseases that could account for the dementia

II. A *probable* Alzheimer disease diagnosis is supported by

Progressive deterioration of specific cognitive functions such as language (aphasia), motor skills (apraxia), and perception (agnosia)

Impaired activities of daily living and altered patterns of behavior

Family history of similar disorders, particularly if confirmed neuropathologically

Laboratory results of normal lumbar puncture as evaluated by standard techniques

Normal pattern or nonspecific changes in EEG, such as increased slow-wave activity

Evidence of cerebral atrophy on computed tomography (CT) with progression documented by serial observation

III. Other clinical features consistent with the diagnosis of *probable* Alzheimer disease include

Plateaus in the course of progression of the illness

Associated symptoms of depression, insomnia, incontinence, delusions, illusions, hallucinations

Catastrophic verbal, emotional, or physical outbursts, sexual disorders, weight loss

Other neurologic abnormalities in some patients, especially with more advanced disease and including motor signs such as increased muscle tone, myoclonus, or gait disorders

Seizures in advanced disease

CT normal for age

IV. Features that make the diagnosis of *probable* Alzheimer disease uncertain or unlikely include

Sudden, apoplectic onset

Focal neurologic findings such as hemiparesis, sensory loss, visual field deficits, and incoordination early in the course of the illness

Seizures or gait disturbances at the onset or very early in the course of the illness

V. Criteria for *possible* Alzheimer disease may be made with

Dementia syndrome, in the absence of other neurologic, psychiatric, or systemic disorders sufficient to cause dementia, and in the presence of variations in onset, in the presentation, or in clinical course

Presence of second systemic or brain disorder sufficient to produce dementia, which is not considered to be the cause of the dementia

A single, gradually progressive severe cognitive deficit identified in the absence of other identifiable causes

VI. Criteria for diagnosis of *definite* Alzheimer disease are

The clinical criteria for probable Alzheimer disease

Histopathologic evidence obtained from a biopsy or autopsy

Clinical Diagnosis of AD: Report of the NINCDS-ADRDA Work Group under the auspices of the Department of Health and Human Services Task Force on Alzheimer's Disease. (Modified from KcKhann et al. 1984; reprinted, with permission, from Lippincott Williams & Wilkins © 1984.)

sensitivity (81%) and specificity (70%) for AD (Knopman et al. 2001), and are associated with neuropathological confirmation rates of 85% or greater (Berg et al. 1998).

As our knowledge of the clinical and biological aspects of AD has grown vastly over the last few decades, revisions to the 1984 criteria were recently proposed (McKhann et al. 2011). The focus of these revisions was to incorporate modern clinical, imaging, and laboratory assessments into the original criteria, with assurance of the flexibility of these criteria for

Table 2. Diagnostic and Statistical Manual of Mental Disorders

Multiple cognitive deficits
Criterion A
A1. Memory impairment
A2. One or more of the following:
    Aphasia (language disturbance)
    Apraxia (impaired motor activity)
    Agnosia (impaired recognition)
    Disturbed executive function
      (planning, organization, etc.)

Criterion B
Cognitive deficits in criteria A1 and A2 each cause
  impairment in social or occupational functioning
Are not due to a CNS disease
Are not due to a medical disorder
Do not occur solely during the course of delirium

Criterion C
Gradual and continued cognitive decline

Criterion D
Other systemic neurologic and psychiatric illnesses
  should be eliminated

Criterion E
Alzheimer disease should not be diagnosed in the
  presence of delirium

Data from the American Psychiatric Association 2000.

use by both general healthcare providers, who may not have access to neuropsychological testing, advanced imaging, or cerebrospinal fluid (CSF) testing, as well as specialized research investigators to whom such measures may be available.

Revisions to the core clinical criteria for "probable" AD include the description of dementia as a decline from an individual's previous level of functioning that is of sufficient degree to interfere with work or usual activities, the recognition of nonamnestic presentations of AD, and the acknowledgment of the distinguishing features of other causes of dementia that may be encountered in the elderly population. Additionally, the revised criteria suggest that, in individuals who meet clinical criteria for "probable" AD, biomarker evidence may increase the certainty that the basis of the clinical dementia syndrome is underlying AD pathology (referred to as "probable AD dementia with evidence of the AD pathophysiological process"). While biomarkers may assist in the diagnosis of AD in clinical trials and investigational studies, biomarker testing is not routinely recommended for the diagnosis of AD in the clinical setting (Knopman et al. 2001). Limitations include the lack of standardization of quantitative analyses across different centers, limited availability in community settings, and the need for further validation of diagnostic algorithms that incorporate biomarkers in the diagnosis of AD (McKhann et al. 2011).

In this context, the diagnosis of AD remains a fundamentally clinical diagnosis. Obtaining a detailed history from the patient *and* from a well-acquainted informant of the onset, course, progression, and characteristics of cognitive and functional decline is of primary importance. Other components of the clinical assessment include the mental state exam, a functional and behavioral assessment, general physical and neurological exam, and (optionally) neuropsychological testing. Risk factors should be determined, including previous vascular disease, hypertension, diabetes mellitus, lipid disorders, head trauma, and/or family history of dementia. Clinical features that distinguish AD from other dementia etiologies should be carefully sought. Concomitant medical, neurological, or psychiatric illness and the use of medications with possible effect on cognitive performance should be documented.

A wide variety of clinical measures are available for the evaluation of cognitive and behavioral performance of individuals with suspected dementia (Table 3). These measures provide useful information to aid in clinical diagnosis and monitoring of disease progression. In general, mental status testing includes level of alertness, attention, orientation, short-term and remote memory, language, visuospatial functioning, calculation, and executive functioning or judgment. The Mini-Mental State Exam (Folstein et al. 1975) and Clock Drawing (Brodaty and Moore 1997) are among the most widely used screening tools in clinical practice. Another brief instrument that may be useful to screen for dementia in the office consists of an informant questionnaire of eight items (Table 4; Galvin et al. 2005); however, its

Table 3. Selected clinical measures in evaluating patients suspected of dementia

Brief cognitive screening tests (bedside mental status examination)

Short Blessed Test (SBT)	Six-item weighted version of the Information–Memory–Concentration Test; usually completed in 5 min; good correlation with AD pathology
Mini-Mental Status Examination (MMSE)	Nineteen items measuring orientation, memory, concentration, language, and praxis; most widely used screening test
Seven-minute screen	Four tests (orientation, memory, clock drawing, and verbal fluency)
General Practitioner Assessment of Cognition (GPCOG)	A six-item screening test similar to the SBT, a clock drawing, and a five-item informant questionnaire
Clock Drawing	Single test measuring multiple cognitive domains; requires minimal training; multiple scoring systems with proven validity

Clinical staging instruments (global measures of dementia severity)

Clinical Dementia Rating (CDR)	Five-point ordinal scale; assesses cognitive ability by a structured informant interview and patient assessment in six domains with descriptors for each level of severity
Global Deterioration Scale (GDS)	Seven-point ordinal scale; has global descriptors for each level of severity
Cambridge Mental Disorders of the Elderly Examination	Five-point ordinal scale; assesses cognitive ability by a structured informant interview and patient testing; includes the Dementia Scale and the Mini-Mental Stage, and has global descriptors for each level of severity

Behavioral scales (noncognitive disturbances, e.g., affective disorders, personality or psychomotor changes, psychoses)

Geriatric Depression Scale (GDS)	Assesses 30 items (either self-rated or observer-rated) of depressive items in older adults
Agitation Inventory	A caregiver questionnaire that assesses the frequency of 29 behaviors in three categories: physically aggressive, physically nonaggressive, and verbally disruptive
Neuropsychiatric Inventory (NPI)	Assesses 10 behavioral disturbances for frequency and severity by an informant interview
Consortium to Establish a Registry for Alzheimer Disease (CERAD) Behavior Rating Scale for Dementia	Combination of items from other instruments; informant-based assessment of behavioral and psychiatric symptoms in patients with dementia

Modified from Morris et al. 2006.

diagnostic utility in clinical settings remains to be fully evaluated. Neuropsychological testing is not routinely required in clinical practice but may be helpful in delineating dementia profiles and monitoring cognitive decline in clinical trials. Most neuropsychological batteries for AD employ tests for episodic memory (e.g., delayed recall tasks) and executive function (e.g., attention-switching) among other cognitive domains.

The practice parameter guidelines of the American Academy of Neurology for the diagnosis of dementia recommend screening for hypothyroidism, vitamin B12 deficiency, and depression in the routine assessment of individuals with suspected dementia, as these comorbidities may potentially contribute to the cognitive impairment of AD (Knopman et al. 2001). Structural neuroimaging with noncontrast computed tomography (CT)

Table 4. AD8: Brief informant interview to differentiate aging and dementia: Report only a change caused by memory and thinking difficulties

Is there repetition of questions, stories, or statements?
Are appointments forgotten?
Is there poor judgment (e.g., buys inappropriate items, poor driving decisions)?
Is there difficulty with financial affairs (e.g., paying bills, balancing checkbook)?
Is there difficulty in learning or operating appliances (e.g., television remote control, microwave oven)?
Is the correct month or year forgotten?
Is there decreased interest in hobbies and usual activities?
Is there overall a problem with thinking and/or memory?

Data adapted from Galvin et al. 2005; reprinted, with permission, from Lippincott Williams & Wilkins © 2005.

or magnetic resonance imaging (MRI) to rule out undetected pathology (such as hydrocephalus, neoplasms, subdural hematoma, or cerebrovascular disease) should also be included in the initial assessment. ^{18}Fluoro-deoxyglucose–positron emission tomography (FDG-PET) may have promise as an adjunct to the clinical diagnosis of AD (Hoffman et al. 2000); however, further studies are needed to evaluate its diagnostic utility beyond that of a competent clinical diagnosis. In the particular cases when the differentiation between AD and frontotemporal dementia (FTD) on clinical grounds alone is problematic, the detection of bilateral frontal hypoperfusion with relative sparing of the posterior cortex using single-photon emission computed tomography (Tc^{99}-HMPAO-SPECT; Pickut et al. 1997) or hypometabolism of these regions on PET (Ishii et al. 1998) in FTD may assist in making the distinction. It is controversial whether the determination of the Apolipoprotein E (*APOE*) genotype in a patient with dementia improves diagnostic specificity to a sufficient degree to be clinically useful (Mayeux et al. 1998; Farlow 2007). Until disease-modifying treatments are available, there is currently no evidence to support the use of genetic analyses, CSF analyses, or other putative CSF biomarkers in the routine diagnosis of AD (Frank et al. 2003).

CLINICAL PHENOMENOLOGY OF AD

The core clinical features of AD include gradual and progressive decline in memory, executive function, and ability to perform daily activities. However, there is variability among individuals in age of onset, family history, and the appearance of noncognitive symptoms such as behavioral or motor abnormalities. Rates of disease progression and survival also vary considerably among different individuals.

Age is the most important risk factor for AD (Farlow 2007). The onset of clinical symptoms is uncommon before the age of 50, although rare cases in individuals in their twenties or thirties have been reported (Portet et al. 2003). The prevalence of AD increases with age from an estimated prevalence of 1%–2% of the population by the age of 65, to 15% by the age of 75, and 35%–50% by the age of 85 (Hebert et al. 2003). A positive family history is found in approximately 20% of the cases. Several genetic mutations have been identified in early-onset autosomal dominant familial AD, involving genes for amyloid precursor protein (*APP*), presenilin-1 (*PS-1*), and presenilin-2 (*PS-2*) (Waring and Rosenberg 2008). Together, these mutations cause less than 1% of all cases of AD (Blennow et al. 2006), and less than 10% of cases in individuals with a positive family history of AD who are under the age of 65.

Therefore, in most cases, AD is a sporadic, age-dependent, late-onset disease (Hebert et al. 2003). The major genetic risk associated with most cases of sporadic late-onset AD is conferred by a positive family history of dementia (Silverman et al. 1994) and by the *APOE* genotype (Saunders et al. 1993). The *APOE* ε4 allele is carried by 15%–20% of individuals and is associated with a higher risk of AD. Individuals who are homozygotes for *APOE* ε4 have a 50% risk of symptomatic AD in their mid to late 60s, whereas 50% of *APOE* ε4 heterozygotes develop symptomatic AD by their mid to late 70s (Saunders et al. 1993). The *APOE* ε4 genotype, however, does not seem to influence clinical disease progression following the onset of symptoms, and may have a differential effect in the early biological stages of disease.

Mortality is increased by 40% in AD (Ganguli et al. 2005), with cardiovascular, infectious, and respiratory causes of death being the most commonly reported. The median survival following a diagnosis of AD is 4 years for men and 6 years for women (Larson et al. 2004). In older adults, the presence of dementia as a predictor of mortality exceeds the risk of diabetes, heart disease, and other more common life-threatening illnesses by two- to threefold (Tschanz et al. 2004).

Initial Presentation (Very Mild and Mild AD)

Clinicopathological studies suggest the presence of a long preclinical phase of AD, with AD pathology estimated to begin a decade or longer prior to the onset of cognitive symptoms (Price and Morris 1999). Following the initial signs of cognitive impairment, patients progress at variable rates from the mildest to the most severe stages. In most cases, symptoms progress slowly in the very early stages so that several years of cognitive decline might occur before an individual with AD is brought to medical attention.

Significant impairment in short-term memory with inability to retain new information is the outstanding clinical feature on presentation in most individuals with AD. However, aphasic or visuoconstructional deficits may occasionally prevail. Characteristic reports of short-term memory loss by the informant include repetition of questions or statements, frequently misplacing items, and difficulty remembering the names of familiar people.

Working memory, long-term declarative memory, and implicit memory are affected to a much lesser degree than short-term declarative memory in AD (Forstl 2010). Individuals with early AD experience difficulties with executive functions such as planning and organizational skills, judgment and problem solving, and handling complicated tasks. More demanding house chores or financial transactions may be performed poorly or only with assistance.

There may be evidence of slight temporal or spatial disorientation including mild difficulty with time relationships, or the need for additional assistance in arriving at destinations. Spatial disorientation frequently causes problems with driving as individuals are less capable of estimating time and speed. Therefore, individuals with even mild AD should be carefully assessed for driving ability. Language impairment in early AD includes reduced verbal fluency, word-finding difficulty, hesitancy of speech, or circumlocution.

Subtle personality and behavioral changes (e.g., apathy, withdrawal, passivity, and reduced motivation) are seen in 25%–50% of the cases. Significant depressive symptoms and mood changes are reported in 20%–30% of cases with early-stage AD (Zubenko et al. 2003). Agitation, psychosis, and anxiety are not typically seen in these initial stages (Geldmacher 2009), and become increasingly more common with disease progression. Anosognosia, or unawareness of illness, is seen in 50% of individuals with AD. In many cases, this represents a domain-specific deficit in self-monitoring and should not be attributed to psychological denial (Geldmacher 2009).

Individuals with early AD usually appear normal to casual inspection and may be able to function independently outside the home, although they may require assistance with some activities.

Moderate and Severe AD

These stages are marked by progressive decline in cognitive functions resulting in more severe functional impairment and increasing dependence on others in activities of daily living. While some individuals with moderate AD may remain engaged in community affairs, individuals with severe AD have no pretense of independent function at home or in the community, and typically appear too ill to be taken to social functions outside the family home.

Individuals with moderate to severe AD have pronounced difficulty retaining new information. Newly learned material is rapidly lost or only fragments remain; individuals are often described by family as "living in the past." Disorientation becomes more marked and may occur in familiar environments, as individuals may be unable to recognize family members or close relatives. Individuals with moderate AD may continue to perform simple house chores (often with supervision); however, more complicated tasks are abandoned. Executive functions and logical reasoning significantly deteriorate at this stage.

Behavioral symptoms, when present, are more commonly seen in the advanced stages of AD. These include hallucinations, mostly of visual quality (Lauter 1968), delusions (including the "theft" of misplaced items or "infidelity" of spouse) and illusionary misidentification (Reisberg et al. 1996). Agitation with temper tantrums, verbal or physical aggression, disruption of sleep–wake cycles, anxiety, and aimless or restless activities such as wandering or hoarding are common at this stage (Devanand et al. 1997).

Almost all cognitive functions are lost in the severe stages of disease. Individuals are completely dependent on comprehensive nursing care. Language is reduced to simple phrases or even single words, although emotional receptiveness may be retained. Assistance with simple functions such as eating may be required, as even basic motor functions such as chewing and swallowing can be impaired. Double incontinence is common. Most patients are bedridden at this stage, and die of complications of aspiration, infection, or inanition.

NEUROLOGICAL EXAMINATION

The general physical and neurological exam may often remain normal throughout most of the course of AD. Extrapyramidal signs (e.g., bradykinesia, rigidity, and reduced facial expression) are seen in 30% of cases; however, rest tremor is rare (Scarmeas et al. 2004). Gait disturbances become more prominent with disease progression and are associated with a substantially higher risk for falls. Primitive reflexes, such as snout and grasp reactions, may also appear. Although only a small proportion of individuals with severe AD experience myoclonus and epileptic seizures, their incidence in AD is higher than that in the general population (Romanelli et al. 1990).

DIFFERENTIAL DIAGNOSIS

While AD accounts for the vast majority of dementia cases seen in clinical practice, clinical, psychometric, and neurologic findings that point to other causes should be carefully sought and evaluated. In a pathological study of 382 brains of individuals with dementia who were referred to the State of Florida Brain Bank, the vast majority (77%) had a pathological diagnosis of AD (Barker et al. 2002). Of these, 54% had "pure" AD pathology, whereas concomitant pathologies (e.g., Lewy body or vascular disease) were detected in the remainder. Additionally, AD pathology was present in most cases of dementia with Lewy bodies (DLB) (66%) and vascular dementia (77%) (Barker et al. 2002).

Vascular Dementia

Vascular dementia (VaD) is a heterogeneous phenotype that may result from a large spectrum of underlying vascular pathologies, types of vascular brain injury, and regional distribution of infarcts and hemorrhages (Chui and Nielsen-Brown 2007). No single neuropsychological profile is characteristic of VaD. However, abstraction, mental flexibility, information processing speed, and working memory are the domains most commonly involved (Desmond et al. 2000). Verbal memory, especially retention, tends to be better preserved in VaD than AD (Sachdev et al. 2004). Cognitive decline appears to be slower, whereas mortality rates are higher in VaD compared with AD (Chui and Nielsen-Brown 2007).

While several epidemiological surveys identify VaD as the second most common cause of dementia after AD (Fitzpatrick et al. 2004; Ravaglia et al. 2005; Chui and Nielsen-Brown 2007), VaD is probably overdiagnosed as a cause of dementia. It is estimated that less than 5% of dementia cases in the United States are caused by stroke alone (Barker et al. 2002). It is important, however, to recognize contributions of vascular pathology to dementia in AD; cerebrovascular lesions can precipitate the appearance of dementia in AD, or contribute to the cognitive impairment in the early stages. Vascular pathology is commonly observed in association with AD pathology (Barker et al. 2002), and cardiovascular risk factors are increasingly linked to a higher risk of AD in epidemiological studies (Casserly and Topol 2004).

Dementia with Lewy Bodies

DLB is perhaps the second most common cause of dementia after AD; as many as 40% of autopsied demented patients have sufficient cortical LBs to be diagnosed with DLB (Galvin et al. 2006; Tarawneh and Galvin 2007). In addition to dementia, DLB is characterized clinically by the presence of at least two of three core features: recurrent well-formed visual hallucinations (42%), spontaneous parkinsonism (55%), and cognitive fluctuations (15%–85%) (McKeith et al. 1996). Core features are usually apparent even when the dementia is mild. In the presence of one core feature, a diagnosis of "probable" DLB can be made if at least one suggestive feature, such as rapid eye movement (REM) sleep behavior disorder or neuroleptic sensitivity (McKeith et al. 1996), is also present.

Other features that may support the clinical diagnosis of DLB include repeated falls and syncope, transient (unexplained) loss of consciousness, autonomic dysfunction, depression, systematized delusions, and hallucinations in other modalities (McKeith et al. 1996). While these criteria have high diagnostic specificity for DLB, their diagnostic sensitivity is variable, and often low, even in specialized centers (Knopman et al. 2001). These criteria appear to be less useful in distinguishing the pure form of DLB (which is rare) from the more common form in which concomitant AD pathology is also present.

Compared with individuals with AD, individuals with DLB are more likely to be impaired on tests of psychomotor, executive, and visuoconstructive or visuoperceptual functions, and less likely to be impaired in verbal recall (Salmon et al. 1996), at the time of their initial evaluation (Stavitsky et al. 2006). Individuals with DLB are more likely to exhibit early psychiatric symptoms (e.g., hallucinations and delusions;

Weiner et al. 2003) and passive personality traits (diminished emotional responsiveness, apathy, and purposeless hyperactivity; Galvin et al. 2007) compared with individuals with AD.

Cognitive fluctuations (waxing and waning of arousal and cognition) may be difficult to reliably identify in DLB. Daytime drowsiness or lethargy, daytime sleep of 2 or more hours, staring episodes, and episodes of disorganized speech may help distinguish the fluctuations of DLB from AD (where patients may have "good" and "bad" days) and from nondemented aging (Ferman et al. 2004). REM behavior disorder is characterized by loss of normal muscle atonia during REM sleep associated with excessive activity while dreaming, and when present, may further help distinguish DLB from AD (Boeve et al. 2003).

Frontotemporal Lobar Degeneration

Frontotemporal lobar degeneration (FTLD) is a heterogeneous group of disorders characterized by progressive neurodegeneration in the frontal and anterior temporal regions (Brun 1987). FTLD typically presents between 45 and 65 years of age, and in this age group, has comparable prevalence to that of AD (Ratnavalli et al. 2002). FTLD accounts for up to 20% of all patients with degenerative dementias (Neary et al. 2000), and is associated with a positive family history in 40% of the cases (Viskontas and Miller 2007).

FTLD encompasses three subtypes: frontotemporal dementia, semantic dementia, and nonfluent aphasia (Neary et al. 1998). Different clinical, genetic, and neuropathologic features are seen among these subtypes (Viskontas and Miller 2007). In FTD (often referred to as "the behavioral variant of FTLD"), there is predominant involvement of the right frontal lobe, resulting in progressive behavioral and personality changes that disturb social conduct. Features include disinhibition, apathy, emotional blunting, lack of insight, disordered eating patterns, and executive dysfunction. Individuals with nonfluent aphasia have selective involvement of the left frontoinsular region, and present predominantly with hesitant nonfluent speech, agrammatism, phonological errors, and speech apraxia. Semantic dementia predominantly involves the anterior temporal lobe; individuals with predominant left temporal lobe involvement present with profound anomia and impaired word comprehension associated with progressive loss of conceptual knowledge of language, whereas individuals with predominantly right temporal lobe involvement present with deficits in empathy and knowledge about people's emotions, and may later progress to prosopagnosia and multimodality agnosia for objects.

While the clinical distinction between AD and fully expressed FTLD may not be difficult, this can be challenging in the mild stages of disease. Hypometabolism in the frontal lobes on PET (Ishii et al. 1998) and amyloid imaging using PET with Pittsburgh Compound B (PET-PIB) (Engler et al. 2008) may assist in the differentiation between FTLD and AD in these cases.

Medical and Psychiatric Disorders

Depression is a common diagnosis among elderly with cognitive complaints. In contrast to individuals with AD who often deny significant impairment, depression generally results in subjective, sometime pronounced, memory complaints with minor cognitive deficits in nondemented individuals (Powlishta et al. 2004). Deficits in attention and concentration are frequently reported (Gouras 2008). However, focal cognitive deficits such as aphasia or apraxia are not characteristic of depression, and should alert the clinician to an alternative diagnosis as the cause of the cognitive impairment.

The clinical distinction between depression and AD may sometimes be difficult. Some symptoms used to diagnose depression in the elderly (such as apathy, reduced motivation, loss of interest, and decreased energy) can be seen in AD. Moreover, AD and depression may overlap; depression was present in approximately 20% of individuals with early-stage AD in one study (Powlishta et al. 2004). There is no evidence that depression significantly worsens cognitive impairment beyond the effect of AD, or that depression alone can cause

dementia (Powlishta et al. 2004). Prospective studies suggest that individuals with depression and coexistent cognitive impairment are in fact highly likely to have an underlying dementia on follow-up (Alexopoulos et al. 1993; Visser et al. 2000).

Treatable medical conditions such as vitamin B12 deficiency and hypothyroidism are relatively common in the elderly; however, they are rarely the sole cause of dementia (Knopman et al. 2001). While these disorders may contribute to cognitive impairment in individuals with AD, treatment of the medical problem is unlikely to result in a significant cognitive benefit once AD is clinically established.

MILD COGNITIVE IMPAIRMENT

Mild cognitive impairment (MCI) has been proposed as a condition of impairment intermediate between what is considered "normal for aging" and that which is sufficient for a diagnosis of dementia or AD. The original criteria for MCI require the presence of a subjective memory complaint (preferably confirmed by a reliable collateral source) with objective evidence of memory impairment by cognitive testing in the setting of generally preserved activities of daily living. Impairment in memory is determined based on an individual's performance in reference to standardized neuropsychological data from age- and education-matched controls; performance below 1–1.5 standard deviations from "normal" is typically considered significant.

The utility of MCI criteria in identifying individuals as high risk for further cognitive decline and progression to AD (annual rate of 10%–15% in MCI compared with 1%–2% for nondemented elderly 80 years of age or less) was adopted by the American Academy of Neurology practice parameters for early detection of dementia and MCI in 2001. The concept of MCI has, however, evolved considerably over the years, leading to revisions to the diagnostic criteria (Petersen et al. 2009).

The original MCI criteria were designed to characterize the early stages of AD, and therefore focused on memory impairment (Petersen et al. 2001). However, our current knowledge indicates that not all MCI subjects progress to AD; some remain stable and others progress to non-AD dementias. Revisions to the criteria recognize impairment in nonmemory domains (e.g., attention, visuospatial function, executive function, and language) in the diagnosis of MCI (Winblad et al. 2004), resulting in the emergence of amnestic (including memory impairment) and nonamnestic (including nonmemory cognitive domains) MCI subtypes (Petersen 2004). Since recent studies indicate that individuals with MCI may experience some changes in everyday activities (e.g., financial capacity; Griffith et al. 2003), revisions to the criteria allow for some difficulty in performing daily functions that is not of a sufficient degree to impair these functions.

MCI criteria do not require the determination of an etiological basis for cognitive impairment. Some individuals who meet MCI criteria may be impaired because of incipient AD, incipient non-AD dementia, a potentially reversible disorder (e.g., depression or medication-induced cognitive dysfunction), or simply be at the lower end of normal (but stable) cognitive performance. While many individuals with MCI eventually progress to AD, others remain stable or progress to other forms of dementia, and a small proportion may actually improve. Thus, there is a considerable degree of heterogeneity in the MCI population. New research criteria for MCI that incorporate CSF biomarkers in the diagnostic algorithm may be particularly useful in the evaluation of the likelihood of a future diagnosis of AD versus non-AD dementia in individuals with nonamnestic MCI (McKhann et al. 2011).

There may be conceptual and practical limitations to the application of MCI criteria in clinical practice. For example, the diagnosis of amnestic MCI can be based solely on subjective memory complaints in the absence of collateral information. Studies suggest that self-reports of memory impairment are more likely to be associated with a diagnosis of depression than with a future diagnosis of dementia, and that verification of cognitive impairment by a collateral source improves the predictive ability

for progression to dementia (Carr et al. 2000). The distinction between "some difficulty" versus "impairment" in performing daily functions is arbitrary, and often depends on the judgment of the clinician and the availability and reliability of collateral information.

MCI criteria focus on objective testing of an individual's performance in reference to standardized norms derived from age- and education-matched controls to establish cognitive impairment (i.e., interindividual decline). However, based on our experience, the detection of cognitive decline from the premorbid level of functioning (i.e., intraindividual decline), through clinical evaluation and reports by a reliable collateral source, often allows an accurate diagnosis of AD to be made in individuals who meet criteria for MCI, or even in individuals who are insufficiently impaired to meet MCI criteria and often referred to as "pre-MCI." In one series, the clinical diagnosis of AD in individuals who met criteria for amnestic MCI, and who underwent autopsy, was confirmed by a neuropathological diagnosis of AD in 84% of the cases (Morris et al. 2001). Furthermore, amnestic MCI closely resembles the neurobiological phenotype of clinically diagnosed AD, although at a milder stage. Individuals with amnestic MCI and those clinically diagnosed with AD share several common features, including cognitive, behavioral, and psychometric performance (Feldman et al. 2004), as well as genetic (Dik et al. 2000), neuroimaging (Jack et al. 2004), and CSF (Pratico et al. 2002) biomarker characteristics. In the authors' opinion, informant-based methods that focus on intraindividual decline can accurately identify AD in a subset of individuals who meet criteria for amnestic MCI.

The ability of physicians to identify the earliest symptomatic stage of AD may have implications in counseling, prognosis, and therapeutic decision-making. Early detection may allow time for counseling regarding safety issues (e.g., driving), financial planning, advance directives, and home arrangements. Since disease-modifying therapies are most likely to be effective if administered in the early stages of disease, this population is the most likely to benefit from such therapies should they become available in the future.

CONCLUDING REMARKS

AD is the most common cause of dementia, and a leading cause of mortality and morbidity in the elderly. The identification of individuals in the earliest symptomatic (and presymptomatic) stages of the disease is important, because it is in this population that disease-modifying therapies may have the greatest chance of success. The NINCDS/ADRDA and *DSM-IV* criteria have good diagnostic accuracy for AD, and are widely used for the diagnosis of AD in clinical settings. Informant-based interviews that focus on establishing a decline in an individual's cognitive performance from previously attained levels of performance may allow for the identification of individuals with even very mild degrees of cognitive impairment.

ACKNOWLEDGMENTS

We acknowledge the contributions of Kim Lipsey and the Clinical Core of the Knight Alzheimer Disease Research Center.

REFERENCES

Albert M. 1994. Age-related changes in cognitive function. In *Clinical neurology of aging* (ed. Albert KJ). Oxford University Press, New York.

Albert MS, Heller HS, Milberg W. 1988. Changes in naming ability with age. *Psychol Aging* **3:** 173–178.

Alexopoulos GS, Meyers BS, Young RC, Mattis S, Kakuma T. 1993. The course of geriatric depression with "reversible dementia": A controlled study. *Am J Psychiat* **150:** 1693–1699.

Alzheimer A. 1987. Uber eine eigenartige Erkrankung der Hirnrinde. *Alzheimer Dis Assoc Disord* 7–8.

Alzheimer's Association. 2011. Alzheimer's disease facts and figures. *Alzheimer's Dementia* **7:** 20–21.

American Psychiatric Association. 1994. *Diagnostic and statistical manual of mental disorders*. American Psychiatric Association, Washington DC.

American Psychiatric Association. 2000. *Diagnostic and statistical manual of mental disorders, DSM-IV-TR*, 4th ed. American Psychiatric Association, Washington DC.

Babcock RL, Salthouse TA. 1990. Effects of increased processing demands on age differences in working memory. *Psychol Aging* **5:** 421–428.

Barker WW, Luis CA, Kashuba A, Luis M, Harwood DG, Loewenstein D, Waters C, Jimison P, Shepherd E, Sevush S, et al. 2002. Relative frequencies of Alzheimer disease, Lewy body, vascular and frontotemporal dementia, and hippocampal sclerosis in the State of Florida Brain Bank. *Alzheimer Dis Assoc Disord* **16:** 203–212.

Berg L, McKeel DW Jr, Miller JP, Storandt M, Rubin EH, Morris JC, Baty J, Coats M, Norton J, Goate AM, et al. 1998. Clinicopathologic studies in cognitively healthy aging and Alzheimer's disease: Relation of histologic markers to dementia severity, age, sex, and apolipoprotein E genotype. *Arch Neurol* **55:** 326–335.

Birren JE, Fisher LM. 1995. Aging and speed of behavior: Possible consequences for psychological functioning. *Annu Rev Psychol* **46:** 329–353.

Blennow K, de Leon MJ, Zetterberg H. 2006. Alzheimer's disease. *Lancet* **368:** 387–403.

Blum JE, Jarvik LF, Clark ET. 1970. Rate of change on selective tests of intelligence: A twenty-year longitudinal study of aging. *J Gerontol* **25:** 171–176.

Boeve BF, Silber MH, Parisi JE, Dickson DW, Ferman TJ, Benarroch EE, Schmeichel AM, Smith GE, Petersen RC, Ahlskog JE, et al. 2003. Synucleinopathy pathology and REM sleep behavior disorder plus dementia or parkinsonism. *Neurology* **61:** 40–45.

Botwinick J, Thompson LW. 1968. Age difference in reaction time: An artifact? *Gerontologist* **8:** 25–28.

Brodaty H, Moore CM. 1997. The Clock Drawing Test for dementia of the Alzheimer's type: A comparison of three scoring methods in a memory disorders clinic. *Int J Geriat Psychiat* **12:** 619–627.

Brun A. 1987. Frontal lobe degeneration of non-Alzheimer type. I. Neuropathology. *Arch Gerontol Geriatr* **6:** 193–208.

Carr DB, Gray S, Baty J, Morris JC. 2000. The value of informant versus individual's complaints of memory impairment in early dementia. *Neurology* **55:** 1724–1726.

Casserly I, Topol E. 2004. Convergence of atherosclerosis and Alzheimer's disease: Inflammation, cholesterol, and misfolded proteins. *Lancet* **363:** 1139–1146.

Chui H, Nielsen-Brown N. 2007. Vascular cognitive impairment. *Continuum Lifelong Learning Neurol* **13:** 109–143.

Crook TH, West RL. 1990. Name recall performance across the adult life-span. *Br J Psychol* **81:** 335–349.

Desmond DW, Moroney JT, Paik MC, Sano M, Mohr JP, Aboumatar S, Tseng CL, Chan S, Williams JB, Remien RH, et al. 2000. Frequency and clinical determinants of dementia after ischemic stroke. *Neurology* **54:** 1124–1131.

Devanand DP, Jacobs DM, Tang MX, Del Castillo-Castaneda C, Sano M, Marder K, Bell K, Bylsma FW, Brandt J, Albert M, et al. 1997. The course of psychopathologic features in mild to moderate Alzheimer disease. *Arch Gen Psychiat* **54:** 257–263.

Dik MG, Jonker C, Bouter LM, Geerlings MI, van Kamp GJ, Deeg DJ. 2000. APOE-epsilon4 is associated with memory decline in cognitively impaired elderly. *Neurology* **54:** 1492–1497.

Doraiswamy PM, Krishen A, Stallone F, Martin WL, Potts NL, Metz A, DeVeaugh-Geiss J. 1995. Cognitive performance on the Alzheimer's Disease Assessment Scale: Effect of education. *Neurology* **45:** 1980–1984.

Drachman DA, Leavitt J. 1972. Memory impairment in the aged: Storage versus retrieval deficit. *J Exp Psychol* **93:** 302–308.

Engler H, Santillo AF, Wang SX, Lindau M, Savitcheva I, Nordberg A, Lannfelt L, Langstrom B, Kilander L. 2008. In vivo amyloid imaging with PET in frontotemporal dementia. *Eur J Nucl Med Mol Imag* **35:** 100–106.

Farlow M. 2007. Alzheimer's disease. *Continuum Lifelong Learning Neurol* **13:** 39–68.

Feldman H, Scheltens P, Scarpini E, Hermann N, Mesenbrink P, Mancione L, Tekin S, Lane R, Ferris S. 2004. Behavioral symptoms in mild cognitive impairment. *Neurology* **62:** 1199–1201.

Ferman TJ, Smith GE, Boeve BF, Ivnik RJ, Petersen RC, Knopman D, Graff-Radford N, Parisi J, Dickson DW. 2004. DLB fluctuations: Specific features that reliably differentiate DLB from AD and normal aging. *Neurology* **62:** 181–187.

Fitzpatrick AL, Kuller LH, Ives DG, Lopez OL, Jagust W, Breitner JC, Jones B, Lyketsos C, Dulberg C. 2004. Incidence and prevalence of dementia in the Cardiovascular Health Study. *J Am Geriatr Soc* **52:** 195–204.

Folstein MF, Folstein SE, McHugh PR. 1975. "Mini-mental state." A practical method for grading the cognitive state of patients for the clinician. *J Psychiatr Res* **12:** 189–198.

Forstl H. 2010. What is Alzheimer's disease? In *Dementia* (ed. Ames D, O'Brien J, Burns A), p. 434. Hodder Education, London.

Frank RA, Galasko D, Hampel H, Hardy J, de Leon MJ, Mehta PD, Rogers J, Siemers E, Trojanowski JQ. 2003. Biological markers for therapeutic trials in Alzheimer's disease. Proceedings of the biological markers working group; NIA initiative on neuroimaging in Alzheimer's disease. *Neurobiol Aging* **24:** 521–536.

Galvin JE, Roe CM, Powlishta KK, Coats MA, Muich SJ, Grant E, Miller JP, Storandt M, Morris JC. 2005. The AD8: A brief informant interview to detect dementia. *Neurology* **65:** 559–564.

Galvin JE, Pollack J, Morris JC. 2006. Clinical phenotype of Parkinson disease dementia. *Neurology* **67:** 1605–1611.

Galvin JE, Malcom H, Johnson D, Morris JC. 2007. Personality traits distinguishing dementia with Lewy bodies from Alzheimer disease. *Neurology* **68:** 1895–1901.

Ganguli M, Dodge HH, Shen C, Pandav RS, DeKosky ST. 2005. Alzheimer disease and mortality: A 15-year epidemiological study. *Arch Neurol* **62:** 779–784.

Geldmacher D. 2009. Alzheimer disease. In *The American psychiatric publishing textbook of Alzheimer disease and other dementias* (ed. Weiner MF, Lipton AM), pp. 155–172. American Psychiatric Publishing, Arlington, VA.

Gilbert JG, Levee RF. 1971. Patterns of declining memory. *J Gerontol* **26:** 70–75.

Gouras GK. 2008. Dementia. In *Encyclopedia of neuroscience* (ed. Squire L), pp. 403–408. Elsevier, New York.

Griffith HR, Belue K, Sicola A, Krzywanski S, Zamrini E, Harrell L, Marson DC. 2003. Impaired financial abilities in mild cognitive impairment: A direct assessment approach. *Neurology* **60:** 449–457.

Hebert LE, Scherr PA, Bienias JL, Bennett DA, Evans DA. 2003. Alzheimer disease in the US population: Prevalence estimates using the 2000 census. *Arch Neurol* **60:** 1119–1122.

Hoffman JM, Welsh-Bohmer KA, Hanson M, Crain B, Hulette C, Earl N, Coleman RE. 2000. FDG PET imaging in patients with pathologically verified dementia. *J Nucl Med* **41:** 1920–1928.

Howard DV, McAndrews MP, Lasaga MI. 1981. Semantic priming of lexical decisions in young and old adults. *J Gerontol* **36:** 707–714.

Howieson DB, Holm LA, Kaye JA, Oken BS, Howieson J. 1993. Neurologic function in the optimally healthy oldest old. Neuropsychological evaluation. *Neurology* **43:** 1882–1886.

Ishii K, Sakamoto S, Sasaki M, Kitagaki H, Yamaji S, Hashimoto M, Imamura T, Shimomura T, Hirono N, Mori E. 1998. Cerebral glucose metabolism in patients with frontotemporal dementia. *J Nucl Med* **39:** 1875–1878.

Jack CR Jr, Shiung MM, Gunter JL, O'Brien PC, Weigand SD, Knopman DS, Boeve BF, Ivnik RJ, Smith GE, Cha RH, et al. 2004. Comparison of different MRI brain atrophy rate measures with clinical disease progression in AD. *Neurology* **62:** 591–600.

Knopman DS, DeKosky ST, Cummings JL, Chui H, Corey-Bloom J, Relkin N, Small GW, Miller B, Stevens JC. 2001. Practice parameter: Diagnosis of dementia (an evidence-based review). Report of the Quality Standards Subcommittee of the American Academy of Neurology. *Neurology* **56:** 1143–1153.

Kukull WA, Higdon R, Bowen JD, McCormick WC, Teri L, Schellenberg GD, van Belle G, Jolley L, Larson EB. 2002. Dementia and Alzheimer disease incidence: A prospective cohort study. *Arch Neurol* **59:** 1737–1746.

Larson EB, Shadlen MF, Wang L, McCormick WC, Bowen JD, Teri L, Kukull WA. 2004. Survival after initial diagnosis of Alzheimer disease. *Ann Intern Med* **140:** 501–509.

Lauter H. 1968. On the clinical study and psychopathology of Alzheimer's disease. Demonstration of 203 pathologically-anatomically verified cases. *Psychiatr Clin (Basel)* **1:** 85–108.

Luszcz MA, Bryan J. 1999. Toward understanding age-related memory loss in late adulthood. *Gerontology* **45:** 2–9.

Manly JJ, Jacobs DM, Sano M, Bell K, Merchant CA, Small SA, Stern Y. 1998. Cognitive test performance among nondemented elderly African Americans and whites. *Neurology* **50:** 1238–1245.

Mayeux R, Saunders AM, Shea S, Mirra S, Evans D, Roses AD, Hyman BT, Crain B, Tang MX, Phelps CH. 1998. Utility of the apolipoprotein E genotype in the diagnosis of Alzheimer's disease. Alzheimer's Disease Centers Consortium on Apolipoprotein E and Alzheimer's Disease. *New Engl J Med* **338:** 506–511.

McKeith IG, Galasko D, Kosaka K, Perry EK, Dickson DW, Hansen LA, Salmon DP, Lowe J, Mirra SS, Byrne EJ, et al. 1996. Consensus guidelines for the clinical and pathologic diagnosis of dementia with Lewy bodies (DLB): Report of the consortium on DLB international workshop. *Neurology* **47:** 1113–1124.

McKhann G, Drachman D, Folstein M, Katzman R, Price D, Stadlan EM. 1984. Clinical diagnosis of Alzheimer's disease: Report of the NINCDS-ADRDA Work Group under the auspices of Department of Health and Human Services Task Force on Alzheimer's Disease. *Neurology* **34**: 939–944.

McKhann GM, Knopman DS, Chertkow H, Hyman BT, Jack CR, Kawas CH, Klunk WE, Koroshetz WJ, Manly JJ, Mayeux R, et al. 2011. The diagnosis of dementia due to Alzheimer's disease: Recommendations from the National Institute on Aging-Alzheimer's Association workgroups on diagnostic guidelines for Alzheimer's disease. *Alzheimer's Dement* **7**: 263–269.

Morris JC. 1993. The Clinical Dementia Rating (CDR): Current version and scoring rules. *Neurology* **43**: 2412–2414.

Morris JC, Storandt M, Miller JP, McKeel DW, Price JL, Rubin EH, Berg L. 2001. Mild cognitive impairment represents early-stage Alzheimer disease. *Arch Neurol* **58**: 397–405.

Morris JC, Galvin JE, Holtzman DM. 2006. *Handbook of dementing illnesses*, 2nd ed. Taylor and Francis, New York.

Neary D, Snowden JS, Gustafson L, Passant U, Stuss D, Black S, Freedman M, Kertesz A, Robert PH, Albert M, et al. 1998. Frontotemporal lobar degeneration: A consensus on clinical diagnostic criteria. *Neurology* **51**: 1546–1554.

Neary D, Snowden JS, Mann DM. 2000. Classification and description of frontotemporal dementias. *Ann NY Acad Sci* **920**: 46–51.

Obler LK, Nicholas M, Albert ML, Woodward S. 1985. On comprehension across the adult lifespan. *Cortex* **21**: 273–280.

Park DC, Smith AD, Lautenschlager G, Earles JL, Frieske D, Zwahr M, Gaines CL. 1996. Mediators of long-term memory performance across the life span. *Psychol Aging* **11**: 621–637.

Parkin AJ, Walter BM. 1992. Recollective experience, normal aging, and frontal dysfunction. *Psychol Aging* **7**: 290–298.

Petersen RC. 2004. Mild cognitive impairment as a diagnostic entity. *J Intern Med* **256**: 183–194.

Petersen RC, Doody R, Kurz A, Mohs RC, Morris JC, Rabins PV, Ritchie K, Rossor M, Thal L, Winblad B. 2001. Current concepts in mild cognitive impairment. *Arch Neurol* **58**: 1985–1992.

Petersen RC, Roberts RO, Knopman DS, Boeve BF, Geda YE, Ivnik RJ, Smith GE, Jack CR Jr. 2009. Mild cognitive impairment: Ten years later. *Arch Neurol* **66**: 1447–1455.

Pickut BA, Saerens J, Marien P, Borggreve F, Goeman J, Vandevivere J, Vervaet A, Dierckx R, de Deyn PP. 1997. Discriminative use of SPECT in frontal lobe-type dementia versus (senile) dementia of the Alzheimer's type. *J Nucl Med* **38**: 929–934.

Portet F, Dauvilliers Y, Campion D, Raux G, Hauw JJ, Lyon-Caen O, Camu W, Touchon J. 2003. Very early onset AD with a de novo mutation in the presenilin 1 gene (Met 233 Leu). *Neurology* **61**: 1136–1137.

Powlishta KK, Storandt M, Mandernach TA, Hogan E, Grant EA, Morris JC. 2004. Absence of effect of depression on cognitive performance in early-stage Alzheimer disease. *Arch Neurol* **61**: 1265–1268.

Pratico D, Clark CM, Liun F, Rokach J, Lee VY, Trojanowski JQ. 2002. Increase of brain oxidative stress in mild cognitive impairment: A possible predictor of Alzheimer disease. *Arch Neurol* **59**: 972–976.

Price JL, Morris JC. 1999. Tangles and plaques in nondemented aging and "preclinical" Alzheimer's disease. *Ann Neurol* **45**: 358–368.

Ratnavalli E, Brayne C, Dawson K, Hodges JR. 2002. The prevalence of frontotemporal dementia. *Neurology* **58**: 1615–1621.

Ravaglia G, Forti P, Maioli F, Martelli M, Servadei L, Brunetti N, Dalmonte E, Bianchin M, Mariani E. 2005. Incidence and etiology of dementia in a large elderly Italian population. *Neurology* **64**: 1525–1530.

Reisberg B, Auer SR, Monteiro I, Boksay I, Sclan SG. 1996. Behavioral disturbances of dementia: An overview of phenomenology and methodologic concerns. *Int Psychogeriatr* **8**: 169–180; discussion 181–182.

Romanelli MF, Morris JC, Ashkin K, Coben LA. 1990. Advanced Alzheimer's disease is a risk factor for late-onset seizures. *Arch Neurol* **47**: 847–850.

Rubin EH, Storandt M, Miller JP, Kinscherf DA, Grant EA, Morris JC, Berg L. 1998. A prospective study of cognitive function and onset of dementia in cognitively healthy elders. *Arch Neurol* **55**: 395–401.

Sachdev PS, Brodaty H, Valenzuela MJ, Lorentz L, Looi JC, Wen W, Zagami AS. 2004. The neuropsychological profile of vascular cognitive impairment in stroke and TIA patients. *Neurology* **62**: 912–919.

Salmon DP, Galasko D, Hansen LA, Masliah E, Butters N, Thal LJ, Katzman R. 1996. Neuropsychological deficits associated with diffuse Lewy body disease. *Brain Cogn* **31**: 148–165.

Saunders AM, Strittmatter WJ, Schmechel D, George-Hyslop PH, Pericak-Vance MA, Joo SH, Rosi BL, Gusella JF, Crapper-MacLachlan DR, Alberts MJ, et al. 1993. Association of apolipoprotein E allele epsilon 4 with late-onset familial and sporadic Alzheimer's disease. *Neurology* **43**: 1467–1472.

Scarmeas N, Hadjigeorgiou GM, Papadimitriou A, Dubois B, Sarazin M, Brandt J, Albert M, Marder K, Bell K, Honig LS, et al. 2004. Motor signs during the course of Alzheimer disease. *Neurology* **63**: 975–982.

Silverman JM, Raiford K, Edland S, Fillenbaum G, Morris JC, Clark CM, Kukull W, Heyman A. 1994. The Consortium to Establish a Registry for Alzheimer's Disease (CERAD). Part VI. Family history assessment: A multicenter study of first-degree relatives of Alzheimer's disease probands and nondemented spouse controls. *Neurology* **44**: 1253–1259.

Sliwinski M, Lipton RB, Buschke H, Stewart W. 1996. The effects of preclinical dementia on estimates of normal cognitive functioning in aging. *J Gerontol B Psychol Sci Soc Sci* **51**.

Stavitsky K, Brickman AM, Scarmeas N, Torgan RL, Tang MX, Albert M, Brandt J, Blacker D, Stern Y. 2006. The progression of cognition, psychiatric symptoms, and functional abilities in dementia with Lewy bodies and Alzheimer disease. *Arch Neurol* **63**: 1450–1456.

Tarawneh R, Galvin JE. 2007. Distinguishing Lewy body dementias from Alzheimer's disease. *Expert Rev Neurother* **7**: 1499–1516.

Tarawneh R, Holtzman DM. 2009. Critical issues for successful immunotherapy in Alzheimer's disease: Development of biomarkers and methods for early detection and intervention. *CNS Neurol Disord Drug Targets* **8:** 144–159.

Troyer AK, Graves RE, Cullum CM. 1994. Executive functioning as a mediator of the relationship between age and episodic memory in healthy aging. *Aging Cogn* **1:** 45–53.

Tschanz JT, Corcoran C, Skoog I, Khachaturian AS, Herrick J, Hayden KM, Welsh-Bohmer KA, Calvert T, Norton MC, Zandi P, et al. 2004. Dementia: The leading predictor of death in a defined elderly population: The Cache County Study. *Neurology* **62:** 1156–1162.

Viskontas I, Miller B. 2007. Frontotemporal dementia. *Continuum Lifelong Learning Neurol* **13:** 87–108.

Visser PJ, Verhey FR, Ponds RW, Kester A, Jolles J. 2000. Distinction between preclinical Alzheimer's disease and depression. *J Am Geriatr Soc* **48:** 479–484.

Walsh DA, Williams MV, Hertzog CK. 1979. Age-related differences in two stages of central perceptual processes: The effects of short duration targets and criterion differences. *J Gerontol* **34:** 234–241.

Waring SC, Rosenberg RN. 2008. Genome-wide association studies in Alzheimer disease. *Arch Neurol* **65:** 329–334.

Weiner MF, Hynan LS, Parikh B, Zaki N, White CL 3rd, Bigio EH, Lipton AM, Martin-Cook K, Svetlik DA, Cullum CM, et al. 2003. Can Alzheimer's disease and dementias with Lewy bodies be distinguished clinically? *J Geriatr Psychiat Neurol* **16:** 245–250.

Winblad B, Palmer K, Kivipelto M, Jelic V, Fratiglioni L, Wahlund LO, Nordberg A, Backman L, Albert M, Almkvist O, Arai, et al. 2004. Mild cognitive impairment– beyond controversies, towards a consensus: Report of the International Working Group on Mild Cognitive Impairment. *J Intern Med* **256:** 240–246.

Zubenko GS, Zubenko WN, McPherson S, Spoor E, Marin DB, Farlow MR, Smith GE, Geda YE, Cummings JL, Petersen RC, et al. 2003. A collaborative study of the emergence and clinical features of the major depressive syndrome of Alzheimer's disease. *Am J Psychiat* **160:** 857–866.

Cite this article as *Cold Spring Harb Perspect Med* doi: 10.1101/cshperspect.a006148

The Neuropsychological Profile of Alzheimer Disease

Sandra Weintraub[1], Alissa H. Wicklund[1], and David P. Salmon[2]

[1]Cognitive Neurology and Alzheimer's Disease Center (CNADC), Northwestern University
 Feinberg School of Medicine, Chicago, Illinois 60611

[2]Department of Neurosciences, University of California San Diego, La Jolla, California 92093-0662

Correspondence: sweintraub@northwestern.edu

Neuropsychological assessment has featured prominently over the past 30 years in the characterization of dementia associated with Alzheimer disease (AD). Clinical neuropsychological methods have identified the earliest, most definitive cognitive and behavioral symptoms of illness, contributing to the identification, staging, and tracking of disease. With increasing public awareness of dementia, disease detection has moved to earlier stages of illness, at a time when deficits are both behaviorally and pathologically selective. For reasons that are not well understood, early AD pathology frequently targets large-scale neuroanatomical networks for episodic memory before other networks that subserve language, attention, executive functions, and visuospatial abilities. This chapter reviews the pathognomonic neuropsychological features of AD dementia and how these differ from "normal," age-related cognitive decline and from other neurodegenerative diseases that cause dementia, including cortical Lewy body disease, frontotemporal lobar degeneration, and cerebrovascular disease.

Over the past 30 years, neuropsychological assessment has featured centrally in characterizing the dementia associated with Alzheimer disease (AD), identifying the most salient and earliest cognitive and behavioral symptoms and contributing to the staging and tracking of disease (Flicker et al. 1984; Morris et al. 1989; Storandt and Hill 1989; Storandt 1991; Welsh et al. 1991, 1992; Locascio et al. 1995; Albert 1996; Storandt et al. 1998; see also Salmon and Bondi 2009). As research has increasingly focused on earlier stages of illness, it has become clear that biological markers of AD can precede cognitive and behavioral symptoms by years. It has also become clear that the early symptoms of AD represent the selective targeting by disease of specific, "large-scale" neuroanatomical networks, with clinical deficits consistent with the anatomical locus of impact (Weintraub and Mesulam 1993, 1996, 2009; Seeley et al. 2009). In the usual case, AD pathology is initially selective for limbic regions that subserve episodic memory, which leads to a circumscribed memory deficit in the early stages of the disease (Braak and Braak 1991; Jack et al. 1997; de Toledo-Morrell et al. 2000). It is only as pathology progresses to other neocortical regions over time

(Braak and Braak 1996a,b; Braak et al. 1999; Jack et al. 2000) that additional cognitive symptoms emerge and the full dementia syndrome becomes apparent.

These discoveries have prompted a revision of the established research diagnostic criteria for AD dementia that had served so well since 1984 (McKhann et al. 1984). The new criteria define not only the dementia of AD (McKhann et al. 2011) but also incorporate a fuller spectrum of cognitive aging, including an intermediate stage of mild cognitive impairment (MCI) that precedes the dementia (Albert et al. 2011). A third, even earlier, stage of "preclinical AD" has also been identified (Sperling et al. 2011). This prodromal period is characterized by the presence of biomarkers, such as brain amyloid deposition and CSF tau and amyloid, that can be detected in vivo in asymptomatic individuals years before the onset of cognitive decline (Perrin et al. 2009; Sperling et al. 2009; Jack et al. 2010). At present, the recommended use of biomarkers to detect AD applies mainly to research. Thus, neuropsychological assessment continues to provide reliable symptom markers of AD that are critical for early diagnosis. The present article describes the profile of neuropsychological deficits associated with the dementia of AD and contrasts it with cognitive changes that occur in "normal" aging and in other forms of neurodegenerative disease that cause dementia.

NEUROPSYCHOLOGICAL DEFICITS IN ALZHEIMER DISEASE

Episodic Memory

The earliest neurofibrillary changes that are part of the pathology of AD usually occur in medial temporal lobe structures (e.g., hippocampus, entorhinal cortex; see Braak and Braak 1991), interrupting the neural network critical for episodic memory function. Thus, it is not surprising that a deficit in the ability to learn and remember new information (i.e., anterograde amnesia) is the clinical hallmark of AD pathology. However, the amyloid pathology that likely occurs years prior to the onset of

symptoms (Morris et al. 1996; Reiman et al. 1996; Moonis et al. 2005; Mintun et al. 2006; Becker et al. 2010; De Meyer et al. 2010) is not particularly abundant in medial temporal lobe, but instead in the regions comprising the "default mode network" (Buckner et al. 2005; Sperling et al. 2009). These changes in the default mode network, comprised of a set of functionally interconnected cortical areas (posterior cingulate, inferior parietal lobule, lateral temporal neocortex, ventromedial and dorsomedial prefrontal cortex) that project heavily to medial temporal lobe structures (Buckner et al. 2008), presage cell death in the hippocampus by years.

Numerous studies have shown that patients with AD are impaired on episodic memory tests that use a variety of cognitive procedures (e.g., free recall, recognition, paired-associate learning) across virtually all modalities (e.g., auditory, visual, olfaction) (for review, see Salmon 2000). Evidence from many of these studies suggests that the episodic memory deficit of AD patients is due in large part to ineffective consolidation or storage of new information. Early studies that characterized the episodic memory deficit in AD used word list learning tasks such as those from the Consortium to Establish a Registry for Alzheimer Disease (CERAD) (Welsh et al. 1991) and the California Verbal Learning Test (CVLT) (Delis et al. 1991). These studies consistently showed that AD patients rapidly forget information over time and are equally impaired (relative to age-matched controls) on recognition and free recall components of the tasks. This pattern of performance is consistent with impaired consolidation rather than ineffective retrieval of new information (Delis et al. 1991).

Indices of rapid forgetting have important clinical utility for the early detection and differential diagnosis of AD. Welsh and colleagues (1991), for example, found that the amount of information recalled after a 10-min delay on the CERAD word list learning task differentiated very early AD patients from healthy elderly controls with better than 90% accuracy. This measure was superior in this regard to other measures derived from this task, including immediate recall on each of three learning trials, recognition memory score, and the number of intrusion errors produced throughout the test. Other studies have shown that measures of rapid forgetting can differentiate mildly demented AD patients from healthy elderly controls with ~85%–90% accuracy (Flicker et al. 1984; Butters et al. 1988; Knopman and Ryberg 1989; Morris et al. 1991; Welsh et al. 1991; Tröster et al. 1993). Additional mechanisms contributing to episodic memory impairment in AD include increased sensitivity to interference due to decreased inhibitory processes leading to the production of intrusion errors (Fuld et al. 1982; Jacobs et al. 1990; Delis et al. 1991), and defective use of semantic information to bolster encoding (see Martin et al. 1985; Dalla Barba and Wong 1995; Dalla Barba and Goldblum 1996).

A number of prospective longitudinal studies of cognitive function in nondemented older adults have shown that a subtle decline in episodic memory often occurs before the emergence of the obvious cognitive and behavioral changes required for a clinical diagnosis of AD (Bondi et al. 1994; Jacobs et al. 1995; Linn et al. 1995; Grober and Kawas 1997; Howieson et al. 1997; Small et al. 2000; Backman et al. 2001; Kawas et al. 2003). Some of these studies suggest that memory performance may be poor, but stable, a number of years before the development of the dementia syndrome, and then declines rapidly in the period immediately preceding the AD dementia diagnosis. Small et al. (2000) and Backman et al. (2001), for example, found that episodic memory was mildly impaired 6 yr before dementia onset, but changed little over the next 3 yr. Chen et al. (2001) and Lange et al. (2002) showed a significant and steady decline in episodic memory on delayed recall conditions of word list and story memory tests beginning ~3 yr before the dementia diagnosis in individuals who were either initially asymptomatic or met criteria for MCI at enrollment in these longitudinal studies. Taken together, these studies suggest that an abrupt decline in memory in an elderly individual might better predict the imminent onset of dementia than poor but stable memory ability. These and similar findings led to the development of formal criteria for amnestic MCI (see Petersen et al. 2001), a predementia condition in elderly individuals, which is characterized by subjective and objective memory impairment that occurs in the face of relatively preserved general cognition and functional abilities (for reviews, see Collie and Maruff 2000; Albert and Blacker 2006).

Language and Semantic Knowledge

Mildly demented patients with AD are often impaired on tests of object naming (Bayles and Tomoeda 1983; Martin and Fedio 1983; Bowles et al. 1987; Hodges et al. 1991), verbal fluency (Martin and Fedio 1983; Butters et al. 1987; Monsch et al. 1992), and semantic categorization (Aronoff et al. 2006). The underlying nature of these deficits has been debated (see Nebes 1989) but there is evidence that they reflect deterioration in the structure and content of semantic memory (i.e., general knowledge of facts, concepts, and the meanings of words) that supports language. Knowledge for particular items or concepts and the associations between them may be disrupted as the neuropathology of AD encroaches upon the temporal, frontal, and parietal association cortices in which they are thought to be diffusely stored (for review, see Hodges and Patterson 1995).

Evidence for a deterioration of semantic memory in AD comes from several studies that probed for knowledge of particular concepts across different modes of access and output (e.g., fluency, confrontation naming, sorting, word-to-picture matching, and definition generation). These studies assume that loss of knowledge, as opposed to impaired retrieval of intact knowledge, would lead to consistency of performance across items (Chertkow and Bub 1990; Hodges et al. 1992). For example, if a patient has lost the concept of "horse," they should not be able to name a picture of a horse, generate "horse" on a verbal fluency test, sort horse into its proper category as a domestic animal, and so on. The results of these studies showed that patients with AD were significantly impaired on all measures of semantic memory and, when a particular stimulus item was missed (or correctly identified) in one task, it was likely to be missed (or correctly identified) in other tasks that accessed the same information in a different way.

Loss of knowledge of the attributes and associations that define a particular semantic category is also thought to reduce the ability of patients with AD to efficiently generate words from a small and highly related set of exemplars during tests of verbal fluency. Thus, patients with AD are more impaired on category fluency (e.g., generating lists of animals) than letter fluency (e.g., generating words beginning with a specific letter) (Butters et al. 1987; Monsch et al. 1992; Henry et al. 2004, 2005). The fact that patients with AD are more impaired on the fluency task that places greater demands on the integrity of semantic memory is consistent with the notion that they have a deterioration in the structure and organization of semantic memory rather than a general inability to retrieve or access semantic knowledge (see also Rohrer et al. 1995, 1999).

Executive Functions, Working Memory, and Attention

Deficits in "executive functions" responsible for the mental manipulation of information, concept formation, problem solving, and cue-directed behavior occur early in the course of AD and are often evident in the MCI stage (Perry and Hodges 1999; Chen et al. 2001). Executive function deficits in addition to difficulties with delayed memory recall predict subsequent progression to AD dementia (Albert 1996). Reduced ability to mentally manipulate information may be a particularly early feature based on a well-controlled study showing that very mildly demented AD patients were significantly impaired relative to cognitively normal controls on tests that required set shifting, self-monitoring, or sequencing, but not on tests that required cue-directed attention or verbal problem solving (Lefleche and Albert 1995). A number of other studies have similarly shown that

AD patients are impaired on difficult problem-solving tests that require mental manipulation such as the Tower of London puzzle (Lange et al. 1995), the modified Wisconsin Card Sorting Task (Bondi et al. 1993), tests of relational integration (Waltz et al. 2004), and other tests of executive functions such as the Porteus Maze Task, Part B of the Trail-Making Test, and the Raven Progressive Matrices (Grady et al. 1988). These deficits in executive functioning have been hypothesized to reflect AD pathology, especially neurofibrillary tangle burden, in prefrontal cortex. This regional prefrontal cortex pathology is particularly pronounced in a subset of AD patients who present early on with predominant executive dysfunction (Johnson et al. 1999; Waltz et al. 2004). This again highlights the impact of anatomical specificity of pathology on the disruption of distinct neocortical networks.

The deficit in mental manipulation exhibited by patients with AD may also be expressed on tests of working memory. "Working memory" refers to a processing system whereby information that is the immediate focus of attention is temporarily held in a limited-capacity, language- or visually-based, immediate memory buffer while being manipulated by a "central executive" (Baddeley 2003). Studies indicate that the working memory deficit of patients with AD is initially mild and primarily involves disruption of the central executive with relative sparing of immediate memory (Baddeley et al. 1991; Collette et al. 1999). It is not until later stages of AD that all aspects of the working memory system become compromised (Baddeley et al. 1991; Collette et al. 1999). Consistent with this model, mildly demented AD patients are often impaired on complex attention tasks that are dependent upon the effective allocation of attentional resources (e.g., dual-processing tasks) or that require efficient disengagement and shifting of attention (for reviews, see Parasuraman and Haxby 1993; Perry and Hodges 1999). In contrast, the ability to focus and sustain attention is usually only affected in later stages of the disease. This is apparent in the essentially normal performance of mildly demented AD patients on tests of immediate attention span compared with supraspan tests (Cherry et al. 2002).

Visuospatial Abilities

Patients with AD often exhibit deficits in visuospatial abilities at some point in the course of the disease (for review, see Cronin-Golomb and Amick 2001). It has also been suggested that visuospatial deficits may occur early, even in preclinical stages (Johnson et al. 2009). Changes in visuospatial function are apparent on visuoconstructional tasks and tasks that require visuoperceptual abilities and visual orientation. The visuoperceptual deficit exhibited by patients with AD may arise, in part, from the loss of effective interaction between distinct and relatively intact cortical information processing systems (Morrison et al. 1991). Studies have shown, for example, that when AD patients perform a visual search task to quickly identify targets on the basis of the conjunction of two or more features that are processed in different cortical regions (e.g., color and shape), they have disproportionately greater response times compared to controls than when required to identify targets solely on the basis of a single feature (Treisman 1996; Foster et al. 1999). Subsequent studies showed that this deficit in "feature-binding" (Treisman 1996; Foster et al. 1999) could not be attributed to the different attentional demands inherent in conjunction versus single-feature visual search tasks (Tales et al. 2002) A similar deficit was observed by Festa and colleagues (2005) on a task that required corticocortical integration of motion and color information which is processed in distinct dorsal (motion) and ventral (color) cortical visual information processing "streams."

Deficits in visual information processing and in selective and divided attention are observed in the course of normal aging but are exacerbated in individuals with AD (Parasuraman et al. 1995, 2000; Greenwood and Parasuraman 1997; Greenwood et al. 1997; Parasuraman and Greenwood 1998). In addition, visual motion detection has been shown to decline in some individuals with MCI, and more so in those with a diagnosis of AD

dementia, suggesting that this symptom may constitute an independent marker of those likely to have AD pathology (Mapstone 2003). The narrowing of the window of visuospatial attention has been demonstrated with the Useful Field of View (UFOV) paradigm in which reaction time to peripheral visual targets is measured in the presence of various levels of distracting visual stimuli (Ball et al. 1988). Older individuals react more slowly to peripheral stimuli compared to younger controls, and patients with AD show an even greater impairment. These deficits may account for the increased incidence of car crashes in patients with AD dementia (Rizzo et al. 1997; Ball and Owsley 2003).

Although rare, AD can initially present with relatively circumscribed posterior cortical atrophy (PCA), with dementia dominated by higher order visual dysfunction (see Caine 2004). Despite relatively preserved memory functions, intact language, and preserved judgment and insight, patients with the clinical syndrome of PCA usually have prominent visual agnosia, constructional apraxia, and exhibit some or all of the features of Balint's syndrome including optic ataxia, gaze apraxia, and simultanagnosia. They may also exhibit components of Gerstmann's syndrome including acalculia, right–left disorientation, finger agnosia, and agraphia. A visual field defect, decreased visual attention, impaired color perception, or decreased contrast sensitivity may also occur (Della Sala et al. 1996).

The clinical syndrome of PCA is usually associated with AD pathology but may also occur in the presence of neuropathological changes of cortical Lewy body disease or Creutzfeld–Jakob disease. Neuropathologic examination reveals disproportionate atrophy and pathologic lesions in the occipital cortex and posterior parietal cortex (Hof et al. 1997; Renner et al. 2004). Studies using positron emission tomography (PET) have shown particular involvement of the dorsal visual stream (Nestor et al. 2003). In the case of PCA due to AD, neurofibrillary tangles and neuritic plaques in the posterior cortical regions are qualitatively identical to those in typical AD (Hof et al. 1997).

The disproportionately posterior cortical distribution of AD pathology in PCA has recently been shown in living patients using PET imaging with Pittsburgh compound-B ($[^{11}C]$-PIB), an agent that binds to β amyloid in the brain (Tenovuo et al. 2008).

DISTINGUISHING ALZHEIMER DISEASE FROM OTHER CAUSES OF DEMENTIA

Although AD is the leading cause of dementia in the elderly, dementia can arise from a wide variety of etiologically and neuropathologically distinct disorders that give rise to somewhat different patterns of cognitive impairment. Knowledge of these differences might lead to better understanding of the neurobiological basis of normal and abnormal cognition and have important implications for differential diagnosis. Increasingly, AD pathology has been identified following a distribution other than the canonical temporal–limbic trajectory. Progressive visuospatial deficits, executive dysfunction, and aphasia syndromes have been described in association with AD pathology (Hof et al. 1993; Johnson et al. 1999; Mesulam 2008). Clinical criteria have shown diagnostic accuracy for AD (Dubois et al. 2007), but lack specificity in differentiating AD from other dementia syndromes. The lack of differentiation is due, in part, to the fact that, although memory impairment is a hallmark of AD, it may also occur with other neurodegenerative diseases. The remaining sections will review similarities and differences between the cognitive deficits of AD and those of other age-related causes of dementia: dementia with Lewy bodies (DLB), frontotemporal lobar degeneration (FTLD), and vascular dementia (VaD).

Alzheimer Disease versus Dementia with Lewy Bodies

DLB is a clinicopathologic condition characterized by cell loss and the presence of Lewy bodies (α-synuclein positive intracytoplasmic neuronal inclusion bodies) in subcortical regions affected in Parkinson's disease and diffusely distributed throughout the limbic system and neocortex. In most cases, AD pathology also occurs in the same general distribution as in "pure" AD (Ince et al. 1998). The dementia syndrome of DLB is similar to that of AD and the two disorders are often clinically confused during life (e.g., Hansen et al. 1990; Merdes et al. 2003). However, mild spontaneous motor features of Parkinsonism (e.g., bradykinesia, rigidity, and masked facies, but without a resting tremor), recurrent and well-formed visual hallucinations, and fluctuating cognition with pronounced variations in attention or alertness occur more frequently in patients with DLB than in those with pure AD (for review, see McKeith et al. 2005).

There are subtle differences in the patterns of neuropsychological deficits associated with DLB and AD. Studies comparing clinically diagnosed or autopsy-diagnosed patient groups on batteries of neuropsychological tests suggest that visuospatial, attention, and executive function deficits are more pronounced in DLB than AD (at the same stage of global dementia severity), whereas memory impairment is more pronounced and may be qualitatively different in AD compared to DLB (Hansen et al. 1990; Johnson et al. 2005; Kraybill et al. 2005; Ferman et al. 2006; Guidi et al. 2006; Stavitsky et al. 2006). These studies also suggest that the severity of the visuospatial deficit may be the most salient difference between patients with AD and patients with DLB, perhaps because of significant occipital cortex dysfunction only in the latter group. Studies using PET or SPECT neuroimaging have shown that patients with DLB have hypometabolism and decreased blood flow in primary visual and visual association cortex that is not evident in AD (Minoshima et al. 2001). They also have unique occipital cortex pathology that includes white matter spongiform change with coexisting gliosis (Higuchi et al. 2000), and in some cases deposition of Lewy bodies (e.g., Gomez-Tortosa et al. 2000).

The prominence of the visuospatial deficits in DLB has important clinical utility. In one study, for example, the presence of visual hallucinations was the best positive predictor (positive predictive value: 83%) of DLB (vs. AD) at autopsy, whereas lack of visuospatial impairment was the best negative predictor (negative predictive value: 90%) (Tiraboschi et al. 2006). In another study, Hamilton and colleagues (2008) showed that poor baseline performance on visuospatial tests, but not tests of other cognitive abilities, was strongly associated with a rapid rate of global cognitive decline over the subsequent two years in patients with DLB but not in those with AD. Thus, early severe visuospatial deficits may identify DLB patients who face a particularly malignant disease course.

The memory deficit of patients with DLB is generally less severe than that of patients with AD and may reflect a qualitative difference in the processes affected. This was shown in a study that directly compared the performance of patients with autopsy-confirmed DLB (all with concomitant AD pathology) or with pure AD on the CVLT and the WMS-R logical memory test (Hamilton et al. 2004). Although the two groups were equally impaired in their ability to learn new verbal information on these tests, the DLB patients exhibited better retention and better recognition memory than patients with pure AD. The better retention and recognition memory of the DLB patients suggests that a deficit in retrieval plays a greater role in their memory impairment than in that of patients with AD.

Alzheimer Disease versus Frontotemporal Lobar Degeneration

FTLD encompasses a class of neurodegenerative diseases that share an affinity for the frontal and temporal lobes of the brain and are marked by distinctive neuropathologic features. The dementia syndromes associated with FTLD are characterized by the absence of true amnesia in the early stages. Instead, they can be divided into two broad categories: a language-based dementia referred to as primary progressive aphasia (PPA) (Mesulam 1982, 2001, 2003), and a dementia in which changes in social cognition, behavior and personality mark the earliest stages, known as behavioral variant frontotemporal dementia (bvFTD) (Rascovsky et al. 2007a, 2011).

The earliest characterization of a dementia marked by significant personality changes was initially called "frontal lobe dementia" and shown to be related to Pick's disease (i.e., neocortical deposition of Pick bodies) and to nonspecific neuropathology designated as "frontal lobe degeneration of non-Alzheimer type" (Brun 1987; Gustafson 1987). Subsequent classification led to the delineation of three syndromes, namely, frontotemporal dementia, progressive nonfluent aphasia, and semantic dementia (Neary et al. 1994, 1998; Neary and Snowden 1996). However, rapid accumulation of information on the neuroimaging and neuropathologic features of these non-AD dementias over the past decade has necessitated further revision of the clinical and neuropathologic diagnostic criteria, which are likely to continue to evolve.

Beginning about 20 years ago, neuropathologic entities associated with FTLD syndromes were designated as either a form of tauopathy or as "dementia lacking distinctive histopathology" (Knopman et al. 1990). As clinical, pathological, and molecular characterization was enhanced over subsequent years, new discoveries led to an increase in the number of pathologic diagnoses that now fall under the rubric of FTLD. At present, the neuropathologic diagnosis is based on the molecular nature of intraneuronal inclusions, which include tarDNA binding protein (TDP-43), fused-in-sarcoma protein (FUS), entities characterized by different molecular forms of tau, and a smaller class of as yet uncharacterized entities (Mackenzie et al. 2010). Genetic mutations in tau, progranulin, valosin-containing protein (VCP) (Watts et al. 2004), and CHMP2B (Skibinski et al. 2005; Holm et al. 2007) have been associated with frontotemporal dementia syndromes. Neuroimaging studies have shown that left perisylvian language regions show the most marked structural changes and salient hypometabolism in patients with PPA (Sonty et al. 2003; Gorno-Tempini et al. 2004), whereas bilateral frontal and anterior temporal atrophy and hypometabolism characterize bvFTD (Whitwell et al. 2004, 2009; Knopman et al. 2009). These patterns are distinct from the well-known medial temporal lobe atrophy (Jack et al. 1997) and bilateral tem-poroparietal hypometabolism (Foster et al. 1983) associated with typical AD dementia.

Primary Progressive Aphasia

There has been growing interest in PPA since the modern-day description of six patients with "slowly progressive aphasia" (Mesulam 1982). Three variants have been defined, each with a distinctive clinical, neuroanatomic, and neuro-pathologic profile (Mesulam et al. 2008, 2009; Gorno-Tempini et al. 2011). Nonfluent/agram-matic PPA (PPA-G), is characterized by deficits in grammatical features of language with or without nonfluent speech output. PPA-G has been associated predominantly with FTLD-tau-opathy (Mesulam et al. 2008; Grossman 2010). Semantic variant PPA (PPA-S) is characterized by fluent speech production and single word comprehension deficits. PPA-S is mainly associ-ated with the pathology of TDP-43 proteinop-athy (Mesulam et al. 2008). PPA-S overlaps with semantic dementia, a disorder in which there are visual processing deficits in addition to aphasia (see Hodges and Patterson 2007). A third variant, logopenic PPA (PPA-L), is characterized by hesitant, grammatically correct speech and spared language comprehension (Gorno-Tempini et al. 2004; Mesulam et al. 2009). PPA-L is most often associated with AD pathology disproportionately distributed in language-related cortical areas (Mesulam et al. 2008). Patients with a familial form of PPA due to a progranulin mutation have been reported to have disproportionate TDP-43 pathology in language-related areas in the left cerebral hemisphere (Gliebus et al. 2009).

As mentioned earlier, anomia and reduced word list generation are features of AD that may be indicative of a more general dissolution of semantic processing. In contrast, anomia and verbal fluency deficits in PPA can occur without associated semantic loss. Early language deficits in PPA also include agrammatism, phono-logical sequencing deficits, and paraphasias in speech. In typical AD these types of language deficits occur only in advanced stages of disease in which patients may develop frank aphasia

against a background of more widespread cog-nitive dysfunction (Bayles 1982). A greater def-icit in naming verbs than naming nouns is associated with nonfluent, agrammatic forms of PPA (Hillis et al. 2004). Verb processing deficits can also occur in AD, but the deficits are linked to impaired processing of the se-mantic rather than the syntactic information carried by verbs (Grossman et al. 1996; Kim and Thompson 2004).

Neuropsychological studies that directly compared patients with clinically diagnosed PPA, bvFTD, and AD have shown that those with PPA have relatively preserved reasoning and episodic memory compared with the other two groups (Wicklund et al. 2004, 2006). Fur-thermore, functional ability reflected in activ-ities of daily living (ADL) is better preserved in patients with PPA than in the other two groups when duration of illness is controlled (Wicklund et al. 2007). Perhaps this occurs because the rel-ative preservation of episodic memory and judg-ment in patients with PPA is less detrimental to complex ADL than aphasia, at least initially. Lan-guage deficits are most prominent in PPA early in the course of illness, but also develop and wor-sen in patients with bvFTD. Language deficits have a more indolent course in AD than in PPA or bvFTD (Blair et al. 2007).

Behavioral Variant Frontotemporal Dementia

The behavioral variant of FTD usually begins insidiously with personality and behavioral changes such as inappropriate social conduct, inertia and apathy, disinhibition, perseverative behavior, loss of insight, hyperorality, and decreased speech output (for reviews, see Miller et al. 1997; Snowden et al. 2001; Rascovsky et al. 2007a; Rabinovici et al. 2008; Caycedo et al. 2009). These changes are followed by cognitive deficits which include alterations in judgment, problem solving, concept formation, and exec-utive functions, often with relative sparing of visuospatial abilities and episodic memory. BvFTD and probable AD can be difficult to dis-tinguish during life because of overlap in symp-toms, but it has been suggested that AD is more often associated with constructional deficits than bvFTD. Although recent attempts to differentiate bvFTD and AD on the basis of the nature and severity of behavioral symptoms has met with some success (e.g., Barber et al. 1995, 2000; Miller et al. 1997; Mendez et al. 1998; Bozeat et al. 2000; Kertesz et al. 2000), behavior-based methods are only partially effective and might be improved by considering other aspects of the disorders. This has led some researchers to investigate the possibility that differences in the patterns of cognitive deficits associated with bvFTD and AD might aid in differential diagnosis (Elfgren et al. 1994; Binetti et al. 1996; Mendez et al. 1996; Pachana et al. 1996; Thomas-Anterion et al. 2000; Rascovsky et al. 2002; Kramer et al. 2003). Revised criteria for the clinical diagnosis of bvFTD have recently been validated against pathologically verified FLTD (Rascovsky et al. 2011), which may improve diagnostic accuracy.

Particularly compelling are retrospective studies that have shown a double dissociation in which mildly to moderately demented patients with autopsy-confirmed FTLD are more impaired than those with autopsy-confirmed AD on tests sensitive to frontal lobe dysfunction (e.g., word generation tasks), but less impaired on tests of memory and visuospatial abilities sensitive to dysfunction of medial temporal and parietal association cortices (e.g., Rascovsky et al. 2002; Grossman et al. 2007). In one study, Rascovsky and colleagues (2002) used multivariate analysis of covariance to show that FTLD patients performed significantly worse than AD patients on word generation tasks that are sensitive to frontal lobe dysfunction (particularly letter fluency), but significantly better on tests of memory (i.e., Mattis Dementia Rating Scale [DRS] Memory subscale) and visuospatial abilities (i.e., WAIS Block Design and Clock Drawing tests), which are sensitive to dysfunction of medial temporal and parietal association cortices, respectively. A logistic regression model using scores from letter fluency, the Mattis DRS memory subscale, and the Block Design test correctly classified 91% of AD patients and 77% of FTLD patients. A follow-up study (Rascovsky et al. 2007b) that compared the performance

of autopsy-confirmed FTLD and AD patients on letter and semantic category fluency tasks showed that FTLD patients performed worse than AD patients overall and showed similar impairment in letter and semantic category fluency, whereas AD patients showed greater impairment in semantic fluency than letter fluency. A measure of the disparity between letter and semantic fluency (the Semantic Index) correctly classified 26 of 32 AD patients (82%) and 12 of 16 FTLD patients (75%). Interestingly, the few misclassified FTLD subjects all had clinical presentations of PPA. When these cases were excluded, a dissociation was apparent with letter worse than semantic fluency for the FTLD patients and semantic worse than letter fluency for the AD patients. In addition, the Semantic Index now correctly classified 90% of FTD and AD patients. These unique patterns of fluency deficits may be indicative of differences in the relative contribution of frontal lobe–mediated retrieval deficits and temporal lobe–mediated semantic deficits in FTLD and AD, respectively.

Taken together, the results of these studies indicate that distinct cognitive profiles are associated with FTLD and AD and suggest that they might aid in differentiating between the two diseases. This conclusion is supported by several other studies using clinically diagnosed patients that found similar levels of discriminability when differentiating FTD from AD on the basis of tests of executive function, visuospatial abilities, and episodic memory (Elfgren et al. 1994; Gregory et al. 1997; Lipton et al. 2005; Libon et al. 2007). These differences are robust enough to be detected with relatively brief dementia-screening instruments that tap multiple cognitive functions (Mathuranath et al. 2000; Bier et al. 2004; Slachevsky et al. 2004).

Alzheimer Disease versus Vascular Dementia

VaD refers to a cumulative decline in cognitive functioning secondary to multiple or strategically placed infarctions, ischemic injury, or hemorrhagic lesions (for review, see Wetzel and Kramer 2008). Research diagnostic criteria for VaD require that multiple cognitive deficits occur in the presence of focal neurological signs and symptoms and/or laboratory (e.g., CT or MRI scan) evidence of cerebrovascular disease that is thought to be etiologically related to the cognitive impairment (Chui et al. 1992; Roman et al. 1993). A relationship between dementia and cerebrovascular disease is often indicated if the onset of dementia occurs within several months of a recognized stroke, there is an abrupt deterioration in cognitive functioning, or the course of cognitive deterioration is fluctuating or stepwise. The clinical and neuropathologic presentation of VaD is quite heterogeneous and can include multi-infarct dementia (MID) associated with multiple large cortical infarctions, dementia due to strategically placed infarction, and subcortical ischemic vascular dementia due to subcortical small vessel disease that results in multiple lacunar strokes, leukoaraiosis, or diffuse white matter pathology (Hodges and Graham 2001).

Neuropsychological studies largely show that patients with VaD are more impaired than those with AD on tests of executive functions, whereas patients with AD are more impaired than those with VaD on tests of episodic memory (particularly delayed recall) (Desmond et al. 1999; Graham et al. 2004; Reed et al. 2007). Executive dysfunction is often the most prominent deficit in VaD, perhaps because white matter pathology (particularly in subcortical ischemic vascular dementia) interrupts fronto-subcortical networks that mediate this aspect of cognition. Consistent with this possibility, Price et al. (2005) showed that VaD patients with significant white matter abnormality on imaging exhibited greater executive dysfunction and visuoconstructional impairment than memory and language impairment (see also Mathias and Burke 2009, for review).

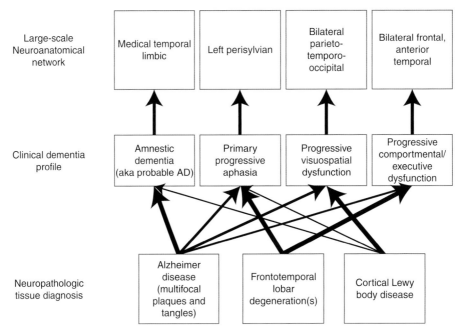

Figure 1. The neuropsychological profiles of dementia reflect the impact of disease on distinctive neuroanatomic networks associated with complex cognitive domains. For example, prominent amnesia is associated with medial temporal dysfunction, whereas aphasia is a consequence of left perisylvian dysfunction. The relationship between clinical symptoms and underlying neuropathology, however, is less straightforward, as indicated by the multiple neuropathologic diagnoses associated with the various clinical dementia syndromes. The thickness of the lines connecting the clinical and neuropathologic levels represents the strength of associations between them (Mesulam 2000).

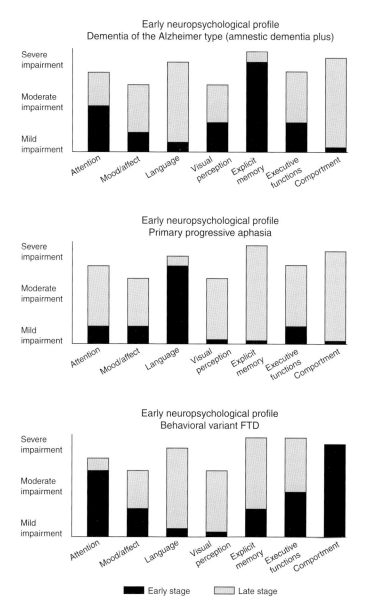

Figure 2. Three graphs, each schematically representing early- and late-stage cognitive/behavioral profiles of three neuropsychologically distinct dementia syndromes. The height of the bars represents the level of impairment: mild, moderate, or severe. In late stages of any dementia syndrome (represented by gray bars) cognitive functions are similarly impaired in an undifferentiated manner and it is difficult to pinpoint one single domain that characterizes the syndrome. However, in early stages, represented by black bars, it is possible to differentiate among domains that are unimpaired or mildly impaired and those that are distinctly abnormal. The most typical early cognitive profile of dementia of the Alzheimer type is one of a prominent amnesia with additional cognitive deficits ("plus"; *top* graph); in primary progressive aphasia, the early stages are marked by salient language deficits in relative isolation (*middle* graph); in behavioral variant frontotemporal dementia, the most salient findings in early stages are in the domains of comportment and executive functions (*bottom* graph).

Unfortunately, cognitive measures appear to be limited in their ability to effectively discriminate between VaD and AD (Mathias and Burke 2009). When neuropsychological profiles were compared in patients with autopsy-confirmed VaD or AD, only 45% of VaD patients exhibited a profile with more prominent executive dysfunction than memory impairment, and 71% of AD patients exhibited a profile with memory impairment more prominent than executive dysfunction (Reed et al. 2007). Studies based on clinically diagnosed groups are even more likely to be inconclusive because of the overlap in the pathology of AD and VaD. Schneider and colleagues (2007), for example, found that 38% of 50 demented patients who came to autopsy had pathological AD plus infarctions, whereas 30% had AD pathology alone. Vascular pathology increased the odds of dementia and exacerbated memory dysfunction in those with AD.

CONCLUSIONS

Neuropsychology has contributed importantly to the characterization of the dementia associated with the neuropathology of AD, its differentiation from cognitive changes accompanying normal aging, and its distinction from dementias associated with other types of neuropathology. The neuropsychological study of AD has advanced our understanding of other diseases that cause dementia, including cortical Lewy body disease, cerebrovascular disease, and FTLD. The very earliest neuropsychological symptoms of a dementia reflect the neuroanatomical systems that bear the load of the associated pathology but the relationship between the symptoms and underlying disease is less obvious (Fig. 1). Amnestic dementia has the highest likelihood of being associated with AD pathology, but early aphasia, progressive visuospatial deficits, and changes in personality can also be associated with AD neuropathology. As dementia progresses from early to late stages, symptom domain boundaries become blurred and distinctive profiles are difficult to discern (Fig. 2). Thus, neuropsychological profiles are most informative in early stages. The development

of fluid and neuroimaging biomarkers will no doubt improve diagnosis and ultimately be used to measure treatment effects. However, neuropsychological characterization remains essential to understanding the individual patient's deficits so that nonpharmacologic interventions can be appropriately applied and so that patient and caregiver educational materials are appropriately targeted (Weintraub and Morhardt 2005).

ACKNOWLEDGMENTS

The authors wish to acknowledge the following grants: AG13854 (Northwestern Alzheimer's Disease Core Center) and AG05131 (University of California San Diego Alzheimer's Disease Research Center), both from the National Institute on Aging.

REFERENCES

Albert MS. 1996. Cognitive and neurobiologic markers of early Alzheimer disease. *Proc Natl Acad Sci* **93:** 13547–13551.

Albert MS, Blacker D. 2006. Mild cognitive impairment and dementia. *Annu Rev Clin Psychol* **2:** 379–388.

Albert MS, Dekosky ST, Dickson D, Dubois B, Feldman HH, Fox NC, Gamst A, Holtzman DM, Jagust WJ, Petersen RC, et al. 2011. The diagnosis of mild cognitive impairment due to Alzheimer's disease: Recommendations from the National Institute on Aging-Alzheimer's Association workgroups on diagnostic guidelines for Alzheimer's disease. *Alzheimers Dement* **7:** 270–279.

Aronoff JM, Gonnerman LM, Almor A, Arunachalam S, Kempler D, Andersen ES. 2006. Information content versus relational knowledge: Semantic deficits in patients with Alzheimer's disease. *Neuropsychologia* **44:** 21–35.

Backman L, Small BJ, Fratiglioni L. 2001. Stability of the preclinical episodic memory deficit in Alzheimer's disease. *Brain* **124:** 96–102.

Baddeley A. 2003. Working memory: Looking back and looking forward. *Nat Rev Neurosci* **4:** 829–839.

Baddeley AD, Bressi S, Della Sala S, Logie R, Spinnler H. 1991. The decline of working memory in Alzheimer's disease. A longitudinal study. *Brain* **114:** 2521–2542.

Ball K, Owsley C. 2003. Driving competence: It's not a matter of age. *J Am Geriatr Soc* **51:** 1499–1501.

Ball KK, Beard BL, Roenker DL, Miller RL, Griggs DS. 1988. Age and visual search: Expanding the useful field of view. *J Opt Soc Am A* **5:** 2210–2219.

Barber R, Snowden JS, Craufurd D. 1995. Frontotemporal dementia and Alzheimer's disease: Retrospective differentiation using information from informants. *J Neurol Neurosurg Psychiatry* **59**: 61–70.

Barber PA, Varma AR, Lloyd JJ, Haworth B, Snowden JS, Neary D. 2000. The electroencephalogram in dementia with Lewy bodies. *Acta Neurol Scand* **101**: 53–56.

Bayles KA. 1982. Language function in senile dementia. *Brain Lang* **16**: 265–280.

Bayles KA, Tomoeda CK. 1983. Confrontation naming impairment in dementia. *Brain Lang* **19**: 98–114.

Becker JA, Hedden T, Carmasin J, Maye J, Rentz DM, Putcha D, Fischl B, Greve DN, Marshall GA, Salloway S, et al. 2010. Amyloid-β associated cortical thinning in clinically normal elderly. *Ann Neurol* **69**: 1032–1042.

Bier JC, Ventura M, Donckels V, Van Eyll E, Claes T, Slama H, Fery P, Vokaer M, Pandolfo M. 2004. Is the Addenbrooke's cognitive examination effective to detect fronto-temporal dementia? *J Neurol* **251**: 428–431.

Binetti G, Cappa SF, Magni E, Padovani A, Bianchetti A, Trabucchi M. 1996. Disorders of visual and spatial perception in the early stage of Alzheimer's disease. *Ann NY Acad Sci* **777**: 221–225.

Blair M, Marczinski CA, Davis-Faroque N, Kertesz A. 2007. A longitudinal study of language decline in Alzheimer's disease and frontotemporal dementia. *J Int Neuropsychol Soc* **13**: 237–245.

Bondi MW, Monsch AU, Butters N, Salmon DP, Paulsen JS. 1993. Utility of a modified version of the Wisconsin Card Sorting Test in the detection of dementia of the Alzheimer type. *Clin Neuropsychol* **7**: 161–170.

Bondi MW, Monsch AU, Galasko D, Butters N, Salmon DP, Delis DC. 1994. Preclinical cognitive markers of dementia of the Alzheimer type. *Neuropsychology* **8**: 374–384.

Bowles NL, Obler LK, Albert ML. 1987. Naming errors in healthy aging and dementia of the Alzheimer type. *Cortex* **23**: 519–524.

Bozeat S, Gregory CA, Ralph MA, Hodges JR. 2000. Which neuropsychiatric and behavioural features distinguish frontal and temporal variants of frontotemporal dementia from Alzheimer's disease? *J Neurol Neurosurg Psychiatry* **69**: 178–186.

Braak H, Braak E. 1991. Neuropathological staging of Alzheimer-related changes. *Acta Neuropathol (Berl)* **82**: 239–259.

Braak H, Braak E. 1996a. Development of Alzheimer-related neurofibrillary changes in the neocortex inversely recapitulates cortical myelogenesis. *Acta Neuropathol (Berl)* **92**: 197–201.

Braak H, Braak E. 1996b. Evolution of the neuropathology of Alzheimer's disease. *Acta Neurol Scand Suppl* **165**: 3–12.

Braak E, Arai K, Braak H. 1999. Cerebellar involvement in Pick's disease: Affliction of mossy fibers, monodendritic brush cells, and dentate projection neurons. *Exp Neurol* **159**: 153–163.

Brun A. 1987. Frontal lobe degeneration of non-Alzheimer type. I. Neuropathology. *Arch Gerontol Geriatr* **6**: 193–208.

Buckner RL, Snyder AZ, Shannon BJ, LaRossa G, Sachs R, Fotenos AF, Sheline YI, Klunk WE, Mathis CA, Morris JC, et al. 2005. Molecular, structural, and functional characterization of Alzheimer's disease: Evidence for a re-lationship between default activity, amyloid, and memory. *J Neurosci* **25**: 7709–7717.

Buckner RL, Andrews-Hanna JR, Schacter DL. 2008. The brain's default network: Anatomy, function, and relevance to disease. *Ann NY Acad Sci* **1124**: 1–38.

Butters N, Granholm E, Salmon DP, Grant I, Wolfe J. 1987. Episodic and semantic memory: A comparison of amnesic and demented patients. *J Clin Exp Neuropsychol* **9**: 479–497.

Butters N, Salmon DP, Cullum CM, Cairns P, Troster AI, Jacobs D, Moss M, Cermak LS. 1988. Differentiation of amnesic and demented patients with the Wechsler memory scale—Revised. *Clin Neuropsychol* **2**: 133–148.

Caine D. 2004. Posterior cortical atrophy: A review of the literature. *Neurocase* **10**: 382–385.

Caycedo AM, Miller B, Kramer J, Rascovsky K. 2009. Early features in frontotemporal dementia. *Curr Alzheimer Res* **6**: 337–340.

Chen P, Ratcliff G, Belle SH, Cauley JA, DeKosky ST, Ganguli M. 2001. Patterns of cognitive decline in presymptomatic Alzheimer disease: A prospective community study. *Arch Gen Psychiatry* **58**: 853–858.

Cherry BJ, Buckwalter JG, Henderson VW. 2002. Better preservation of memory span relative to supraspan immediate recall in Alzheimer's disease. *Neuropsychologia* **40**: 846–852.

Chertkow H, Bub D. 1990. Semantic memory loss in dementia of Alzheimer's type. What do various measures measure? *Brain* **113**: 397–417.

Chui HC, Victoroff JI, Margolin D, Jagust W, Shankle R, Katzman R. 1992. Criteria for the diagnosis of ischemic vascular dementia proposed by the State of California Alzheimer's Disease Diagnostic and Treatment Centers. *Neurology* **42**: 473–480.

Collette F, Van der Linden M, Bechet S, Salmon E. 1999. Phonological loop and central executive functioning in Alzheimer's disease. *Neuropsychologia* **37**: 905–918.

Collie A, Maruff P. 2000. The neuropsychology of preclinical Alzheimer's disease and mild cognitive impairment. *Neurosci Biobehav Rev* **24**: 365–374.

Cronin-Golomb A, Amick M. 2001. Spatial abilities in aging, Alzheimer's disease, and Parkinson's disease. In *Handbook of neuropsychology, vol. 6: Aging and dementia*, 2nd ed. (ed. Boller F, Cappa S), pp. 119–143. Elsevier, Amsterdam.

Dalla Barba G, Goldblum MC. 1996. The influence of semantic encoding on recognition memory in Alzheimer's disease. *Neuropsychologia* **34**: 1181–1186.

Dalla Barba G, Wong C. 1995. Encoding specificity and intrusion in Alzheimer's disease and amnesia. *Brain Cogn* **27**: 1–16.

Delis DC, Massman PJ, Butters N, Salmon DP, Cermak LS, Kramer JH. 1991. Profiles of demented and amnesic patients on the California verbal learning test: Implications for the assessment of memory disorders. *Psychol Assessment* **3**: 19–26.

Della Sala S, Spinnler H, Trivelli C. 1996. Slowly progressive impairment of spatial exploration and visual perception. *Neurocase* **2**: 299–323.

De Meyer G, Shapiro F, Vanderstichele H, Vanmechelen E, Engelborghs S, De Deyn PP, Coart E, Hansson O,

Minthon L, Zetterberg H, et al. 2010. Diagnosis-independent Alzheimer disease biomarker signature in cognitively normal elderly people. *Arch Neurol* **67:** 949–956.

Desmond DW, Erkinjuntti T, Sano M, Cummings JL, Bowler JV, Pasquier F, Moroney JT, Ferris SH, Stern Y, Sachdev PS, et al. 1999. The cognitive syndrome of vascular dementia: Implications for clinical trials. *Alzheimer Dis Assoc Disord* **13** (Suppl 3)**:** S21–S29.

de Toledo-Morrell L, Goncharova I, Dickerson B, Wilson RS, Bennett DA. 2000. From healthy aging to early Alzheimer's disease: In vivo detection of entorhinal cortex atrophy. *Ann NY Acad Sci* **911:** 240–253.

Dubois B, Feldman HH, Jacova C, Dekosky ST, Barberger-Gateau P, Cummings J, Delacourte A, Galasko D, Gauthier S, Jicha G, et al. 2007. Research criteria for the diagnosis of Alzheimer's disease: Revising the NINCDS-ADRDA criteria. *Lancet Neurol* **6:** 734–746.

Elfgren C, Brun A, Gustafson L, Johanson A, Minthon L, Passant U, Risberg J. 1994. Neuropsychological tests as discriminators between dementia of Alzheimer's type and frontotemporal dementia. *Int J Geriatr Psychiatry* **9:** 635–642.

Ferman TJ, Smith GE, Boeve BF, Graff-Radford NR, Lucas JA, Knopman DS, Petersen RC, Ivnik RJ, Wszolek Z, Uitti R, et al. 2006. Neuropsychological differentiation of dementia with Lewy bodies from normal aging and Alzheimer's disease. *Clin Neuropsychol* **20:** 623–636.

Festa EK, Insler RZ, Salmon DP, Paxton J, Hamilton JM, Heindel WC. 2005. Neocortical disconnectivity disrupts sensory integration in Alzheimer's disease. *Neuropsychology* **19:** 728–738.

Flicker C, Bartus RT, Crook TH, Ferris SH. 1984. Effects of aging and dementia upon recent visuospatial memory. *Neurobiol Aging* **5:** 275–283.

Foster NL, Chase TN, Fedio P, Patronas NJ, Brooks RA, Di Chiro G. 1983. Alzheimer's disease: Focal cortical changes shown by positron emission tomography. *Neurology* **33:** 961–965.

Foster JK, Behrmann M, Stuss DT. 1999. Visual attention deficits in Alzheimer's disease: Simple versus conjoined feature search. *Neuropsychology* **13:** 223–245.

Fuld PA, Katzman R, Davies P, Terry RD. 1982. Intrusions as a sign of Alzheimer dementia: Chemical and pathological verification. *Ann Neurol* **11:** 155–159.

Gliebus G, Bigio E, Caplan D, Mesulam M, Geula C. 2009. Phenotypically concordant TDP-43 neuroanatomy in the PPA3 family with progranulin mutation. *Soc Neurosci Abstr Online.* 434437/L431.

Gomez-Tortosa E, Irizarry MC, Gomez-Isla T, Hyman BT. 2000. Clinical and neuropathological correlates of dementia with Lewy bodies. *Ann NY Acad Sci* **920:** 9–15.

Gorno-Tempini ML, Dronkers NF, Rankin KP, Ogar JM, Phengrasamy L, Rosen HJ, Johnson JK, Weiner MW, Miller BL. 2004. Cognition and anatomy in three variants of primary progressive aphasia. *Ann Neurol* **55:** 335–346.

Gorno-Tempini ML, Hillis AE, Weintraub S, Kertesz A, Mendez M, Cappa SF, Ogar JM, Rohrer JD, Black S, Boeve BF, et al. 2011. Classification of primary progressive aphasia and its variants. *Neurology* **76:** 1006–1014.

Grady CL, Haxby JV, Horwitz B, Sundaram M, Berg G, Schapiro M, Friedland RP, Rapoport SI. 1988. Longitudinal study of the early neuropsychological and cerebral metabolic changes in dementia of the Alzheimer type. *J Clin Exp Neuropsychol* **10:** 576–596.

Graham NL, Emery T, Hodges JR. 2004. Distinctive cognitive profiles in Alzheimer's disease and subcortical vascular dementia. *J Neurol Neurosurg Psychiatry* **75:** 61–71.

Greenwood PM, Parasuraman R. 1997. Attention in aging and Alzheimer's disease: Behavior and neural systems. In *Attention, development, and psychopathology* (ed. Burback JA, Enns JT, et al.), pp. 288–317. Guildford Press, New York.

Greenwood PM, Parasuraman R, Alexander GE. 1997. Controlling the focus of spatial attention during visual search: Effects of advanced aging and Alzheimer disease. *Neuropsychology* **11:** 3–12.

Gregory CA, Orrell M, Sahakian B, Hodges JR. 1997. Can frontotemporal dementia and Alzheimer's disease be differentiated using a brief battery of tests? *Int J Geriatr Psychiatry* **12:** 375–383.

Grober E, Kawas C. 1997. Learning and retention in preclinical and early Alzheimer's disease. *Psychol Aging* **12:** 183–188.

Grossman M. 2010. Primary progressive aphasia: Clinicopathological correlations. *Nat Rev Neurol* **6:** 88–97.

Grossman M, Mickanin J, Onishi K, Hughes E. 1996. Verb comprehension deficits in probable Alzheimer's disease. *Brain Lang* **53:** 369–389.

Grossman M, Libon DJ, Forman MS, Massimo L, Wood E, Moore P, Anderson C, Farmer J, Chatterjee A, Clark CM, et al. 2007. Distinct antemortem profiles in patients with pathologically defined frontotemporal dementia. *Arch Neurol* **64:** 1601–1609.

Guidi M, Paciaroni L, Paolini S, De Padova S, Scarpino O. 2006. Differences and similarities in the neuropsychological profile of dementia with Lewy bodies and Alzheimer's disease in the early stage. *J Neurol Sci* **248:** 120–123.

Gustafson L. 1987. Frontal lobe degeneration of non-Alzheimer type. II. Clinical picture and differential diagnosis. *Arch Gerontol Geriatr* **6:** 209–223.

Hamilton JM, Salmon DP, Galasko D, Delis DC, Hansen LA, Masliah E, Thomas RG, Thal LJ. 2004. A comparison of episodic memory deficits in neuropathologically-confirmed dementia with Lewy bodies and Alzheimer's disease. *J Int Neuropsychol Soc* **10:** 689–697.

Hamilton JM, Salmon DP, Galasko D, Raman R, Emond J, Hansen LA, Masliah E, Thal LJ. 2008. Visuospatial deficits predict rate of cognitive decline in autopsy-verified dementia with Lewy bodies. *Neuropsychology* **22:** 729–737.

Hansen L, Salmon D, Galasko D, Masliah E, Katzman R, DeTeresa R, Thal L, Pay MM, Hofstetter R, Klauber M, et al. 1990. The Lewy body variant of Alzheimer's disease: A clinical and pathologic entity. *Neurology* **40:** 1–8.

Henry JD, Crawford JR, Phillips LH. 2004. Verbal fluency performance in dementia of the Alzheimer's type: A meta-analysis. *Neuropsychologia* **42:** 1212–1222.

Henry JD, Crawford JR, Phillips LH. 2005. A meta-analytic review of verbal fluency deficits in Huntington's disease. *Neuropsychology* **19:** 243–252.

Higuchi M, Tashiro M, Arai H, Okamura N, Hara S, Higuchi S, Itoh M, Shin RW, Trojanowski JQ, Sasaki H. 2000. Glucose hypometabolism and neuropathological correlates in brains of dementia with Lewy bodies. *Exp Neurol* **162:** 247–256.

Hillis AE, Oh S, Ken L. 2004. Deterioration of naming nouns versus verbs in primary progressive aphasia. *Ann Neurol* **55:** 268–275.

Hodges JR, Graham NL. 2001. Vascular dementias. In *Early onset dementia: A multidisciplinary approach* (ed. Hodges JR), pp. 319–337. Oxford University Press, Oxford.

Hodges JR, Patterson K. 1995. Is semantic memory consistently impaired early in the course of Alzheimer's disease? Neuroanatomical and diagnostic implications. *Neuropsychologia* **33:** 441–459.

Hodges JR, Patterson K. 2007. Semantic dementia: A unique clinicopathological syndrome. *Lancet Neurol* **6:** 1004–1014.

Hodges JR, Salmon DP, Butters N. 1991. The nature of the naming deficit in Alzheimer's and Huntington's disease. *Brain* **114:** 1547–1558.

Hodges JR, Salmon DP, Butters N. 1992. Semantic memory impairment in Alzheimer's disease: Failure of access or degraded knowledge? *Neuropsychologia* **30:** 301–314.

Hof PR, Archin N, Osmand AP, Dougherty JH, Wells C, Bouras C, Morrison JH. 1993. Posterior cortical atrophy in Alzheimer's disease: Analysis of a new case and re-evaluation of a historical report. *Acta Neuropathol* **86:** 215–223.

Hof PR, Vogt BA, Bouras C, Morrison JH. 1997. Atypical form of Alzheimer's disease with prominent posterior cortical atrophy: A review of lesion distribution and circuit disconnection in cortical visual pathways. *Vision Res* **37:** 3609–3625.

Holm IE, Englund E, Mackenzie IR, Johannsen P, Isaacs AM. 2007. A reassessment of the neuropathology of frontotemporal dementia linked to chromosome 3. *J Neuropathol Exp Neurol* **66:** 884–891.

Howieson DB, Dame A, Camicioli R, Sexton G, Payami H, Kaye JA. 1997. Cognitive markers preceding Alzheimer's dementia in the healthy oldest old. *J Am Geriatr Soc* **45:** 584–589.

Ince PG, Perry EK, Morris CM. 1998. Dementia with Lewy bodies. A distinct non-Alzheimer dementia syndrome? *Brain Pathol* **8:** 299–324.

Jack CR Jr, Petersen RC, Xu YC, Waring SC, O'Brien PC, Tangalos EG, Smith GE, Ivnik RJ, Kokmen E. 1997. Medial temporal atrophy on MRI in normal aging and very mild Alzheimer's disease. *Neurology* **49:** 786–794.

Jack CR Jr, Petersen RC, Xu Y, O'Brien PC, Smith GE, Ivnik RJ, Boeve BF, Tangalos EG, Kokmen E. 2000. Rates of hippocampal atrophy correlate with change in clinical status in aging and AD. *Neurology* **55:** 484–489.

Jack CR Jr, Knopman DS, Jagust WJ, Shaw LM, Aisen PS, Weiner MW, Petersen RC, Trojanowski JQ. 2010. Hypothetical model of dynamic biomarkers of the Alzheimer's pathological cascade. *Lancet Neurol* **9:** 119–128.

Jacobs D, Salmon DP, Tröster AI, Butters N. 1990. Intrusion errors in the figural memory of patients with Alzheimer's and Huntington's disease. *Arch Clin Neuropsychol* **5:** 49–57.

Jacobs DM, Sano M, Dooneief G, Marder K, Bell KL, Stern Y. 1995. Neuropsychological detection and characterization of preclinical Alzheimer's disease [comment]. *Neurology* **45:** 957–962.

Johnson JK, Head E, Kim R, Starr A, Cotman CW. 1999. Clinical and pathological evidence for a frontal variant of Alzheimer disease. *Arch Neurol* **56:** 1233–1239.

Johnson DK, Morris JC, Galvin JE. 2005. Verbal and visuospatial deficits in dementia with Lewy bodies. *Neurology* **65:** 1232–1238.

Johnson DK, Storandt M, Morris JC, Galvin JE. 2009. Longitudinal study of the transition from healthy aging to Alzheimer disease. *Arch Neurol* **66:** 1254–1259.

Kawas CH, Corrada MM, Brookmeyer R, Morrison A, Resnick SM, Zonderman AB, Arenberg D. 2003. Visual memory predicts Alzheimer's disease more than a decade before diagnosis. *Neurology* **60:** 1089–1093.

Kertesz A, Nadkarni N, Davidson W, Thomas AW. 2000. The Frontal Behavioral Inventory in the differential diagnosis of frontotemporal dementia. *J Int Neuropsychol Soc* **6:** 460–468.

Kim M, Thompson CK. 2004. Verb deficits in Alzheimer's disease and agrammatism: Implications for lexical organization. *Brain Lang* **88:** 1–20.

Knopman DS, Ryberg S. 1989. A verbal memory test with high predictive accuracy for dementia of the Alzheimer type. *Arch Neurol* **46:** 141–145.

Knopman DS, Mastri AR, Frey WH 2nd, Sung JH, Rustan T. 1990. Dementia lacking distinctive histologic features: A common non-Alzheimer degenerative dementia. *Neurology* **40:** 251–256.

Knopman DS, Jack CR Jr, Kramer JH, Boeve BF, Caselli RJ, Graff-Radford NR, Mendez MF, Miller BL, Mercaldo ND. 2009. Brain and ventricular volumetric changes in frontotemporal lobar degeneration over 1 year. *Neurology* **72:** 1843–1849.

Kramer JH, Jurik J, Sha SJ, Rankin KP, Rosen HJ, Johnson JK, Miller BL. 2003. Distinctive neuropsychological patterns in frontotemporal dementia, semantic dementia, and Alzheimer disease. *Cogn Behav Neurol* **16:** 211–218.

Kraybill ML, Larson EB, Tsuang DW, Teri L, McCormick WC, Bowen JD, Kukull WA, Leverenz JB, Cherrier MM. 2005. Cognitive differences in dementia patients with autopsy-verified AD, Lewy body pathology, or both. *Neurology* **64:** 2069–2073.

Lange KW, Sahakian BJ, Quinn NP, Marsden CD, Robbins TW. 1995. Comparison of executive and visuospatial memory function in Huntington's disease and dementia of Alzheimer type matched for degree of dementia. *J Neurol Neurosurg Psych* **58:** 598–606.

Lange KL, Bondi MW, Salmon DP, Galasko D, Delis DC, Thomas RG, Thal LJ. 2002. Decline in verbal memory during preclinical Alzheimer's disease: Examination of the effect of APOE genotype. *J Int Neuropsychol Soc* **8:** 943–955.

Lefleche G, Albert MS. 1995. Executive function deficits in mild Alzheimer's disease. *Neuropsychology* **9:** 313–320.

Libon DJ, Xie SX, Moore P, Farmer J, Antani S, McCawley G, Cross K, Grossman M. 2007. Patterns of neuropsychological impairment in frontotemporal dementia. *Neurology* **68:** 369–375.

Linn RT, Wolf PA, Bachman DL, Knoefel JE, Cobb JL, Belanger AJ, Kaplan EF, D'Agostino RB. 1995. The "pre-clinical phase" of probable Alzheimer's disease. A 13-year prospective study of the Framingham cohort. *Arch Neurol* **52:** 485–490.

Lipton AM, Ohman KA, Womack KB, Hynan LS, Ninman ET, Lacritz LH. 2005. Subscores of the FAB differentiate frontotemporal lobar degeneration from AD. *Neurology* **65:** 726–731.

Locascio JJ, Growdon JH, Corkin S. 1995. Cognitive test performance in detecting, staging, and tracking Alzheimer's disease. *Arch Neurol* **52:** 1087–1099.

Mackenzie IR, Neumann M, Bigio EH, Cairns NJ, Alafuzoff I, Kril J, Kovacs GG, Ghetti B, Halliday G, Holm IE, et al. 2010. Nomenclature and nosology for neuropathologic subtypes of frontotemporal lobar degeneration: An update. *Acta Neuropathol* **119:** 1–4.

Mapstone M, Steffenella TM, Duffy CJ. 2003. A visuospatial variant of mild cognitive impairment: getting lost between aging and AD. *Neurology* **60:** 802–808.

Martin A, Fedio P. 1983. Word production and comprehension in Alzheimer's disease: The breakdown of semantic knowledge. *Brain Lang* **19:** 124–141.

Martin A, Brouwers P, Cox C, Fedio P. 1985. On the nature of the verbal memory deficit in Alzheimer's disease. *Brain Lang* **25:** 323–341.

Mathias JL, Burke J. 2009. Cognitive functioning in Alzheimer's and vascular dementia: A meta-analysis. *Neuropsychology* **23:** 411–423.

Mathuranath PS, Nestor PJ, Berrios GE, Rakowicz W, Hodges JR. 2000. A brief cognitive test battery to differentiate Alzheimer's disease and frontotemporal dementia. *Neurology* **55:** 1613–1620.

McKeith IG, Dickson DW, Lowe J, Emre M, O'Brien JT, Feldman H, Cummings J, Duda JE, Lippa C, Perry EK, et al. 2005. Diagnosis and management of dementia with Lewy bodies: Third report of the DLB Consortium. *Neurology* **65:** 1863–1872.

McKhann G, Drachman D, Folstein M, Katzman R, Price D, Stadlan E. 1984. Clinical diagnosis of Alzheimer's disease: Report of the NINCDS-ADRDA Work Group under the auspices of Department of Health and Human Services Task Force on Alzheimer's Disease. *Neurology* **34:** 939–944.

McKhann GM, Knopman DS, Chertkow H, Hyman BT, Jack CR Jr, Kawas CH, Klunk WE, Koroshetz WJ, Manly JJ, Mayeux R, et al. 2011. The diagnosis of dementia due to Alzheimer's disease: Recommendations from the National Institute on Aging–Alzheimer's Association workgroups on diagnostic guidelines for Alzheimer's disease. *Alzheimers Dement* **7:** 263–269.

Mendez MF, Cherrier M, Perryman KM, Pachana N, Miller BL, Cummings JL. 1996. Frontotemporal dementia versus Alzheimer's disease: Differential cognitive features. *Neurology* **47:** 1189–1194.

Mendez MF, Perryman KM, Miller BL, Cummings JL. 1998. Behavioral differences between frontotemporal dementia and Alzheimer's disease: A comparison on the BEHAVE-AD rating scale. *Int Psychogeriatr* **10:** 155–162.

Merdes AR, Hansen LA, Jeste DV, Galasko D, Hofstetter CR, Ho GJ, Thal LJ, Corey-Bloom J. 2003. Influence of Alzheimer pathology on clinical diagnostic accuracy in dementia with Lewy bodies. *Neurology* **60:** 1586–1590.

Mesulam M. 1982. Slowly progressive aphasia without generalized dementia. *Ann Neurol* **11:** 592–598.

Mesulam M-M. 2000. Aging, Alzheimer's disease, and dementia: Clinical and neurobiological perspectives. In *Principles of cognitive and behavioral neurology*, 2nd ed. (ed. Mesulam M-M), pp. 439–522. Oxford University Press, New York.

Mesulam M. 2001. Primary progressive aphasia. *Ann Neurol* **49:** 425–432.

Mesulam M. 2003. Primary progressive aphasia—A language-based dementia. *N Engl J Med* **349:** 1535–1542.

Mesulam M. 2008. Primary progressive aphasia pathology. *Ann Neurol* **63:** 124–125.

Mesulam M, Wicklund A, Johnson N, Rogalski E, Leger GC, Rademaker A, Weintraub S, Bigio EH. 2008. Alzheimer and frontotemporal pathology in subsets of primary progressive aphasia. *Ann Neurol* **63:** 709–719.

Mesulam M, Wieneke C, Rogalski E, Cobia D, Thompson CK, Weintraub S. 2009. Quantitative template for subtyping primary progressive aphasia. *Arch Neurol* **66:** 1545–1551.

Miller BL, Ikonte C, Ponton M, Levy M, Boone K, Darby A, Berman N, Mena I, Cummings JL. 1997. A study of the Lund–Manchester research criteria for frontotemporal dementia: Clinical and single-photon emission CT correlations. *Neurology* **48:** 937–942.

Minoshima S, Foster NL, Sima AA, Frey KA, Albin RL, Kuhl DE. 2001. Alzheimer's disease versus dementia with Lewy bodies: Cerebral metabolic distinction with autopsy confirmation. *Ann Neurol* **50:** 358–365.

Mintun MA, Larossa GN, Sheline YI, Dence CS, Lee SY, Mach RH, Klunk WE, Mathis CA, DeKosky ST, Morris JC. 2006. [11C]PIB in a nondemented population: Potential antecedent marker of Alzheimer disease. *Neurology* **67:** 446–452.

Monsch AU, Bondi MW, Butters N, Salmon DP, Katzman R, Thal LJ. 1992. Comparisons of verbal fluency tasks in the detection of dementia of the Alzheimer type. *Arch Neurol* **49:** 1253–1258.

Moonis M, Swearer JM, Dayaw MP, St George-Hyslop P, Rogaeva E, Kawarai T, Pollen DA. 2005. Familial Alzheimer disease: Decreases in CSF Aβ42 levels precede cognitive decline. *Neurology* **65:** 323–325.

Morris JC, Heyman A, Mohs RC, Hughes JP, van Belle G, Fillenbaum G, Mellits ED, Clark C. 1989. The Consortium to Establish a Registry for Alzheimer's Disease (CERAD). Part I. Clinical and neuropsychological assessment of Alzheimer's disease. *Neurology* **39:** 1159–1165.

Morris JC, Storandt M, McKeel DW Jr, Rubin EH, Price JL, Grant EA, Berg L. 1996. Cerebral amyloid deposition and diffuse plaques in "normal" aging: Evidence for presymptomatic and very mild Alzheimer's disease. *Neurology* **46:** 707–719.

Morrison JH, Hof PR, Bouras C. 1991. An anatomic substrate for visual disconnection in Alzheimer's disease. *Ann NY Acad Sci* **640:** 36–43.

Neary D, Snowden J. 1996. Fronto-temporal dementia: Nosology, neuropsychology, and neuropathology. *Brain Cogn* **31:** 176–187.

Neary D, Brun A, Englund B, Gustafson L, Passant U, Mann DMA, Snowden JS. 1994. Clinical and neuropathological criteria for frontotemporal dementia. *J Neurol Neurosurg Psychiatry* **57:** 416–418.

Neary D, Snowden JS, Gustafson L, Passant U, Stuss D, Black S, Freedman M, Kertesz A, Robert PH, Albert M, et al. 1998. Frontotemporal lobar degeneration: A consensus on clinical diagnostic criteria. *Neurology* **51:** 1546–1554.

Nebes RD. 1989. Semantic memory in Alzheimer's disease. *Psychol Bull* **106:** 377–394.

Nestor PJ, Caine D, Fryer TD, Clarke J, Hodges JR. 2003. The topography of metabolic deficits in posterior cortical atrophy (the visual variant of Alzheimer's disease) with FDG-PET. *J Neurol Neurosurg Psychiatry* **74:** 1521–1529.

Pachana NA, Boone KB, Miller BL, Cummings JL, Berman N. 1996. Comparison of neuropsychological functioning in Alzheimer's disease and frontotemporal dementia. *J Int Neuropsychol Soc* **2:** 505–510.

Parasuraman R, Greenwood PM. 1998. Selective attention in aging and dementia. In *The attentive brain* (ed. Parasuraman R), pp. 461–487. MIT Press, Cambridge, MA.

Parasuraman R, Haxby JV. 1993. Attention and brain function in Alzheimer's disease: A review. *Neuropsychology* **7:** 242–272.

Parasuraman R, Greenwood PM, Alexander GE. 1995. Selective impairment of spatial attention during visual search in Alzheimer's disease. *Neuroreport* **6:** 1861–1864.

Parasuraman R, Greenwood PM, Alexander GE. 2000. Alzheimer disease constricts the dynamic range of spatial attention in visual search. *Neuropsychologia* **38:** 1126–1135.

Perrin RJ, Fagan AM, Holtzman DM. 2009. Multimodal techniques for diagnosis and prognosis of Alzheimer's disease. *Nature* **461:** 916–922.

Perry RJ, Hodges JR. 1999. Attention and executive deficits in Alzheimer's disease. A critical review. *Brain* **122:** 383–404.

Petersen RC, Doody R, Kurz A, Mohs RC, Morris JC, Rabins PV, Ritchie K, Rossor M, Thal L, Winblad B. 2001. Current concepts in mild cognitive impairment. *Arch Neurol* **58:** 1985–1992.

Price CC, Jefferson AL, Merino JG, Heilman KM, Libon DJ. 2005. Subcortical vascular dementia: Integrating neuropsychological and neuroradiologic data. *Neurology* **65:** 376–382.

Rabinovici GD, Rascovsky K, Miller BL. 2008. Frontotemporal lobar degeneration: Clinical and pathologic overview. *Handb Clin Neurol* **89:** 343–364.

Rascovsky K, Salmon DP, Ho GJ, Galasko D, Peavy GM, Hansen LA, Thal LJ. 2002. Cognitive profiles differ in autopsy-confirmed frontotemporal dementia and AD. *Neurology* **58:** 1801–1808.

Rascovsky K, Hodges JR, Kipps CM, Johnson JK, Seeley WW, Mendez MF, Knopman D, Kertesz A, Mesulam M, Salmon DP, et al. 2007a. Diagnostic criteria for the behavioral variant of frontotemporal dementia (bvFTD): Current limitations and future directions. *Alzheimer Dis Assoc Disord* **21**.

Rascovsky K, Salmon DP, Hansen LA, Thal LJ, Galasko D. 2007b. Disparate letter and semantic category fluency

deficits in autopsy-confirmed frontotemporal dementia and Alzheimer's disease. *Neuropsychology* **21:** 20–30.

Rascovsky K, Hodges JR, Knopman D, Mendez MF, Kramer JH, Neuhaus J, van Swieten JC, Seelaar H, Dopper EGP, Onyike CU, et al. 2011. Sensitivity of revised diagnostic criteria for the behavioral variant of frontotemporal dementia. *Brain* **134:** 2456–2477.

Reed BR, Mungas DM, Kramer JH, Ellis W, Vinters HV, Zarow C, Jagust WJ, Chui HC. 2007. Profiles of neuropsychological impairment in autopsy-defined Alzheimer's disease and cerebrovascular disease. *Brain* **130:** 731–739.

Reiman EM, Caselli RJ, Yun LS, Chen K, Bandy D, Minoshima S, Thibodeau SN, Osborne D. 1996. Preclinical evidence of Alzheimer's disease in persons homozygous for the epsilon 4 allele for apolipoprotein E [see comments]. *New Engl J Med* **334:** 752–758.

Renner JA, Burns JM, Hou CE, McKeel DW Jr, Storandt M, Morris JC. 2004. Progressive posterior cortical dysfunction: A clinicopathologic series. *Neurology* **63:** 1175–1180.

Rizzo M, Reinach S, McGehee D, Dawson J. 1997. Simulated car crashes and crash predictors in drivers with Alzheimer disease. *Arch Neurol* **54:** 545–551.

Rohrer D, Wixted JT, Salmon DP, Butters N. 1995. Retrieval from semantic memory and its implications for Alzheimer's disease. *J Exp Psychol Learn Mem Cogn* **21:** 1127–1139.

Rohrer D, Salmon DP, Wixted JT, Paulsen JS. 1999. The disparate effects of Alzheimer's disease and Huntington's disease on semantic memory. *Neuropsychology* **13:** 381–388.

Roman GC, Tatemichi TK, Erkinjuntti T, Cummings JL, Masdeu JC, Garcia JH, Amaducci L, Orgogozo JM, Brun A, Hofman A, et al. 1993. Vascular dementia: Diagnostic criteria for research studies. Report of the NINDS-AIREN International Workshop. *Neurology* **43:** 250–260.

Salmon DP. 2000. Disorders of memory in Alzheimer's disease. In *Handbook of neuropsychology, vol. 2: Memory and its disorders*, 2nd ed. (ed. Cermak LS), pp. 155–195. Elsevier, Amsterdam.

Salmon DP, Bondi MW. 2009. Neuropsychological assessment of dementia. *Annu Rev Psychol* **60:** 257–282.

Schneider JA, Arvanitakis Z, Bang W, Bennett DA. 2007. Mixed brain pathologies account for most dementia cases in community-dwelling older persons. *Neurology* **69:** 2197–2204.

Seeley WW, Crawford RK, Zhou J, Miller BL, Greicius MD. 2009. Neurodegenerative diseases target large-scale human brain networks. *Neuron* **62:** 42–52.

Skibinski G, Parkinson NJ, Brown JM, Chakrabarti L, Lloyd SL, Hummerich H, Nielsen JE, Hodges JR, Spillantini MG, Thusgaard T, et al. 2005. Mutations in the endosomal ESCRTIII-complex subunit CHMP2B in frontotemporal dementia. *Nat Genet* **37:** 806–808.

Slachevsky A, Villalpando JM, Sarazin M, Hahn-Barma V, Pillon B, Dubois B. 2004. Frontal assessment battery and differential diagnosis of frontotemporal dementia and Alzheimer disease. *Arch Neurol* **61:** 1104–1107.

Small BJ, Fratiglioni L, Viitanen M, Winblad B, Backman L. 2000. The course of cognitive impairment in preclinical

Alzheimer disease: Three- and 6-year follow-up of a population-based sample. *Arch Neurol* **57:** 839–844.

Snowden JS, Bathgate D, Varma A, Blackshaw A, Gibbons ZC, Neary D. 2001. Distinct behavioural profiles in frontotemporal dementia and semantic dementia. *J Neurol Neurosurg Psychiatry* **70:** 323–332.

Sonty SP, Mesulam M, Thompson CK, Johnson NA, Weintraub S, Parrish TB, Gitelman DR. 2003. Primary progressive aphasia: PPA and the language network. *Ann Neurol* **53:** 35–49.

Sperling RA, Laviolette PS, O'Keefe K, O'Brien J, Rentz DM, Pihlajamaki M, Marshall G, Hyman BT, Selkoe DJ, Hedden T, et al. 2009. Amyloid deposition is associated with impaired default network function in older persons without dementia. *Neuron* **63:** 178–188.

Sperling RA, Aisen PS, Beckett LA, Bennett DA, Craft S, Fagan AM, Iwatsubo T, Jack CR Jr, Kaye J, Montine TJ, et al. 2011. Toward defining the preclinical stages of Alzheimer's disease: Recommendations from the National Institute on Aging–Alzheimer's Association workgroups on diagnostic guidelines for Alzheimer's disease. *Alzheimers Dement* **7:** 280–292.

Stavitsky K, Brickman AM, Scarmeas N, Torgan RL, Tang MX, Albert M, Brandt J, Blacker D, Stern Y. 2006. The progression of cognition, psychiatric symptoms, and functional abilities in dementia with Lewy bodies and Alzheimer disease. *Arch Neurol* **63:** 1450–1456.

Storandt M. 1991. Neuropsychological assessment in Alzheimer's disease. *Exp Aging Res* **17:** 100–101.

Storandt M, Hill RD. 1989. Very mild senile dementia of the Alzheimer type. II. Psychometric test performance. *Arch Neurol* **46:** 383–386.

Storandt M, Kaskie B, Von Dras DD. 1998. Temporal memory for remote events in healthy aging and dementia. *Psychol Aging* **13:** 4–7.

Tales A, Butler SR, Fossey J, Gilchrist ID, Jones RW, Troscianko T. 2002. Visual search in Alzheimer's disease: A deficiency in processing conjunctions of features. *Neuropsychologia* **40:** 1849–1857.

Tenovuo O, Kemppainen N, Aalto S, Nagren K, Rinne JO. 2008. Posterior cortical atrophy: A rare form of dementia with in vivo evidence of amyloid-β accumulation. *J Alzheimers Dis* **15:** 351–355.

Thomas-Anterion C, Jacquin K, Laurent B. 2000. Differential mechanisms of impairment of remote memory in Alzheimer's and frontotemporal dementia. *Dement Geriatr Cogn Disord* **11:** 100–106.

Tiraboschi P, Salmon DP, Hansen LA, Hofstetter RC, Thal LJ, Corey-Bloom J. 2006. What best differentiates Lewy body from Alzheimer's disease in early-stage dementia? *Brain* **129:** 729–735.

Treisman A. 1996. The binding problem. *Curr Opin Neurobiol* **6:** 171–178.

Troster AI, Butters N, Salmon DP, Cullum CM, Jacobs D, Brandt J, White RF. 1993. The diagnostic utility of savings scores: Differentiating Alzheimer's and Huntington's diseases with the logical memory and visual reproduction tests. *J Clin Exp Neuropsychol* **15:** 773–788.

Waltz JA, Knowlton BJ, Holyoak KJ, Boone KB, Back-Madruga C, McPherson S, Masterman D, Chow T, Cummings JL, Miller BL. 2004. Relational integration and executive function in Alzheimer's disease. *Neuropsychology* **18:** 296–305.

Watts GD, Wymer J, Kovach MJ, Mehta SG, Mumm S, Darvish D, Pestronk A, Whyte MP, Kimonis VE. 2004. Inclusion body myopathy associated with Paget disease of bone and frontotemporal dementia is caused by mutant valosin-containing protein. *Nat Genet* **36:** 377–381.

Weintraub S, Mesulam M. 1993. Four neuropsychological profiles of dementia. In *Handbook of neuropsychology* (ed. Boller F, Grafman J). Elsevier, Amsterdam.

Weintraub S, Mesulam M-M. 1996. From neuronal networks to dementia: Four clinical profiles. In *La demence: Pourquoi?* (ed. Fôret F, Christen Y, Boller F), pp. 75–97. Foundation Nationale de Gerontologie, Paris.

Weintraub S, Mesulam M. 2009. With or without FUS, it is the anatomy that dictates the dementia phenotype. *Brain* **132:** 2906–2908.

Weintraub S, Morhardt DJ. 2005. Treatment, education and resources for non Alzheimer dementia: One size does not fit all. *Alzheimer's Care Q* **July/September:** 201–214.

Welsh K, Butters N, Hughes J, Mohs R, Heyman A. 1991. Detection of abnormal memory decline in mild cases of Alzheimer's disease using CERAD neuropsychological measures. *Arch Neurol* **48:** 278–281.

Welsh KA, Butters N, Hughes JP, Mohs RC, Heyman A. 1992. Detection and staging of dementia in Alzheimer's disease. Use of the neuropsychological measures developed for the Consortium to Establish a Registry for Alzheimer's Disease. *Arch Neurol* **49:** 448–452.

Wetzel ME, Kramer JH. 2008. The neuropsychology of vascular dementia. In *Handbook of clinical neurology* (ed. Goldenberg G, Miller B), pp. 567–583. Elsevier, New York.

Whitwell JL, Anderson VM, Scahill RI, Rossor MN, Fox NC. 2004. Longitudinal patterns of regional change on volumetric MRI in frontotemporal lobar degeneration. *Dement Geriatr Cogn Disord* **17:** 307–310.

Whitwell JL, Przybelski SA, Weigand SD, Ivnik RJ, Vemuri P, Gunter JL, Senjem ML, Shiung MM, Boeve BF, Knopman DS, et al. 2009. Distinct anatomical subtypes of the behavioural variant of frontotemporal dementia: A cluster analysis study. *Brain* **132:** 2932–2946.

Wicklund AH, Johnson N, Weintraub S. 2004. Preservation of reasoning in primary progressive aphasia: Further differentiation from Alzheimer's disease and the behavioral presentation of frontotemporal dementia. *J Clin Exp Neuropsychol* **26:** 347–355.

Wicklund AH, Johnson N, Rademaker A, Weitner BB, Weintraub S. 2006. Word list versus story memory in Alzheimer disease and frontotemporal dementia. *Alzheimer Dis Assoc Disord* **20:** 86–92.

Wicklund AH, Johnson N, Rademaker A, Weitner BB, Weintraub S. 2007. Profiles of decline in activities of daily living in non-Alzheimer dementia. *Alzheimer Dis Assoc Disord* **21:** 8–13.

Neuropathological Alterations in Alzheimer Disease

Alberto Serrano-Pozo[1], Matthew P. Frosch[1,2], Eliezer Masliah[3], and Bradley T. Hyman[1]

[1]Alzheimer Research Unit of the MassGeneral Institute for Neurodegenerative Disease, Department of Neurology of the Massachusetts General Hospital, and Harvard Medical School, Charlestown, Massachusetts 02129-4404

[2]C.S. Kubik Laboratory for Neuropathology, Massachusetts General Hospital, Boston, Massachusetts 02114

[3]Department of Neuroscience and Department of Pathology, University of California-San Diego School of Medicine, La Jolla, California 92093-0624

Correspondence: bhyman@partners.org

The neuropathological hallmarks of Alzheimer disease (AD) include "positive" lesions such as amyloid plaques and cerebral amyloid angiopathy, neurofibrillary tangles, and glial responses, and "negative" lesions such as neuronal and synaptic loss. Despite their inherently cross-sectional nature, postmortem studies have enabled the staging of the progression of both amyloid and tangle pathologies, and, consequently, the development of diagnostic criteria that are now used worldwide. In addition, clinicopathological correlation studies have been crucial to generate hypotheses about the pathophysiology of the disease, by establishing that there is a continuum between "normal" aging and AD dementia, and that the amyloid plaque build-up occurs primarily before the onset of cognitive deficits, while neurofibrillary tangles, neuron loss, and particularly synaptic loss, parallel the progression of cognitive decline. Importantly, these cross-sectional neuropathological data have been largely validated by longitudinal in vivo studies using modern imaging biomarkers such as amyloid PET and volumetric MRI.

The neuropathological changes of Alzheimer disease (AD) brain include both positive and negative features. Classical positive lesions consist of abundant amyloid plaques and neurofibrillary tangles, neuropil threads, and dystrophic neurites containing hyperphosphorylated tau (see Box 1 for glossary) (Terry et al. 1994; Mandelkow and Mandelkow 1998; Trojanowski and Lee 2000; Iqbal and Grundke-Iqbal 2002; Crews and Masliah 2010), that are accompanied by astrogliosis (Beach et al. 1989; Itagaki et al. 1989), and microglial cell activation (Rogers et al. 1988; Itagaki et al. 1989; Masliah et al. 1991). Congophilic amyloid angiopathy is a frequent concurrent feature. Unique lesions, found primarily in the hippocampal formation, include Hirano bodies and granulovacuolar degeneration. In addition to these positive lesions, characteristic losses of neurons, neuropil, and synaptic elements are core negative features of AD (Scheff et al. 1990, 2006, 2007; DeKosky and Scheff 1990;

Terry et al. 1991; Masliah et al. 1993b; Scheff and Price 1993, 1994; Gomez-Isla et al. 1996, 1997; Knowles et al. 1999). Each of these lesions has a characteristic distribution, with plaques found throughout the cortical mantle, and tangles primarily in limbic and association cortices (Arnold et al. 1991; Braak and Braak 1991; Thal et al. 2002). The hierarchical pattern of neurofibrillary degeneration among brain regions is so consistent that a staging scheme based on early lesions in the entorhinal/perirhinal cortex, then hippocampal Ammon subfields, then association cortex, and finally primary neocortex is well accepted as part of the 1997 NIA-Reagan diagnostic criteria (NIA-RI Consensus 1997). Neuronal loss and synapse loss largely parallel tangle formation, although whether tangles are causative of neuronal loss or synaptic loss remains uncertain (Gómez-Isla et al. 1997; Iqbal and Grundke-Iqbal 2002; Bussière et al. 2003; Hof et al. 2003; Yoshiyama et al. 2007; Spires-Jones et al. 2008; de Calignon et al. 2009, 2010; Kimura et al. 2010).

BOX 1. Glossary

Amyloid plaques: extracellular deposits of amyloid β abundant in the cortex of AD patients. Amyloid plaques are commonly classified in diffuse and dense-core based on their morphology and positive or negative staining with Thioflavin-S or Congo Red.

Dense-core plaques: fibrillar amyloid deposits with compact core that stains with Thioflavin-S and Congo Red. Dense-core plaques are typically surrounded by dystrophic neurites (neuritic plaques), reactive astrocytes and activated microglial cells, and associated with synaptic loss. A semi-quantitative score of neuritic plaques is used for the pathological diagnosis of AD because their presence is generally associated with the presence of cognitive impairment.

Diffuse plaques: amorphous amyloid deposits with ill-defined contours that are Congo Red and Thioflavin S negative. Diffuse plaques are usually nonneuritic and not associated with glial responses or synaptic loss. This plaque type is not considered for the pathological diagnosis of AD because it is a relatively common finding in the brain of cognitively intact elderly people.

Cerebral amyloid angiopathy (CAA): deposits of amyloid β in the tunica media of leptomeningeal arteries and cortical capillaries, small arterioles and medium-size arteries, particularly in posterior areas of the brain. Some degree of CAA, usually mild, is present in ≈80% of AD patients. If severe, CAA can weaken the vessel wall and cause life-threatening lobar hemorrhages.

Amyloid β: a 40 or 42 amino acid peptide derived from amyloid precursor protein (APP) after its sequential cleavage by β- and γ-secretases. Its physiological role is likely related to the modulation of synaptic activity although still controversial. In AD Aβ accumulates forming intermediate soluble oligomers that are synaptotoxic as well as insoluble β-sheet pleated amyloid fibrils that are the main constituent of dense-core plaques (mainly Aβ42) and cerebral amyloid angiopathy (primarily Aβ40).

Neurofibrillary tangles (NFTs): intraneuronal aggregates of hyperphosphorylated and misfolded tau that become extraneuronal ("ghost" tangles) when tangle-bearing neurons die. NFTs have a stereotypical spatiotemporal progression that correlates with the severity of the cognitive decline. In fact, a topographic staging of NFTs (Braak and Braak 1991) is used for the pathological diagnosis of AD.

Neuropil threads: axonal and dendritic segments containing aggregated and hyperphosphorylated tau that invariably accompany neurofibrillary tangles in AD.

Tau: a microtubule-associated protein normally located to the axon, where it physiologically facilitates the axonal transport by binding and stabilizing the mictrotubules. In AD, tau is translocated to the somatodendritc compartment and undergoes hyperphosphorylation, misfolding, and aggregation, giving rise to neurofibrillary tangles and neuropil threads.

Although all these neuropathological characteristics are useful diagnostic markers, the cognitive impairment in patients with AD is closely associated with the progressive degeneration of the limbic system (Arnold et al. 1991; Klucken et al. 2003), neocortical regions (Terry et al. 1981), and the basal forebrain (Teipel et al. 2005). This neurodegenerative process is characterized by early damage to the synapses (Masliah and Terry 1993, 1994; Masliah 2000; Crews and Masliah 2010) with retrograde degeneration of the axons and eventual atrophy of the dendritic tree (Coleman and Perry 2002; Higuchi et al. 2002; Grutzendler et al. 2007; Perlson et al. 2010) and perikaryon (Hyman et al. 1986; Lippa et al. 1992). Indeed, the loss of synapses in the neocortex and limbic system is the best correlate of the cognitive impairment in patients with AD (DeKosky and Scheff 1990; Terry et al. 1991; DeKosky et al. 1996).

In addition to the lesions detected by classical histopathological stains, including silver stains for tangles and plaques or immunostaining and quantitative analysis (or quantitative EM) for synaptic alterations, several lines of investigation now support the view that increased levels of soluble amyloid-β_{1-42} (Aβ) oligomers, might lead to synaptic damage and neurodegeneration (Lambert et al. 1998; Klein et al. 2001; Klein 2002; Walsh et al. 2002; Walsh and Selkoe 2004; Glabe 2005; Lesne et al. 2006; Townsend et al. 2006; Lacor et al. 2007). In experimental models, it has been shown that transsynaptic delivery of Aβ, for example from the entorhinal cortex to the molecular layer of the dentate gyrus, promotes neurodegeneration characterized by synapse loss (Harris et al. 2010a) and alterations to calbindin-positive neurons (Palop et al. 2003). This is accompanied by circuitry dysfunction and aberrant innervation of the hippocampus by NPY-positive fibers among others (Harris et al. 2010b; Palop et al. 2011). The Aβ oligomers secreted by cultured neurons inhibit long-term potentiation (LTP), damage spines and interfere with activity-regulated cytoskeleton associated protein (Arc) distribution (Klein et al. 2001; Walsh and Selkoe 2004; Townsend

et al. 2006; Selkoe 2008). Together, these studies indicate that Aβ oligomers ranging in size from 2 to 12 subunits might be responsible for the synaptic damage and memory deficits in AD (Lacor et al. 2007). Similar neurotoxic Aβ oligomers found in vitro and in APP transgenic models have been also identified in the CSF (Klyubin et al. 2008) and in the brains of patients with AD (Shankar et al. 2008; McDonald et al. 2010; Pham et al. 2010). These studies have shown that Aβ oligomers progressively accumulate in the brains of AD patients, although their relationship to the severity of the cognitive impairment remains uncertain.

In summary, in recent years, the concept of neurodegeneration in AD has been expanded from the idea of general neuronal loss and astrogliosis to include earlier alterations such as synaptic and dendritic injury and disturbances in the process of adult neurogenesis (Jin et al. 2004; Li et al. 2008; Crews et al. 2010), circuitry dysfunction, and aberrant innervation. All of these factors are important targets to consider when developing neuroprotective treatments for AD.

MACROSCOPIC FEATURES

Although the gross visual examination of the AD brain is not diagnostic, a typical symmetric pattern of cortical atrophy predominantly affecting the medial temporal lobes and relatively sparing the primary motor, sensory, and visual cortices, is considered strongly suggestive of AD being the condition underlying the patient's dementia. As a result of this pattern of cortical thinning, the lateral ventricules, particularly their temporal horns, can appear prominently dilated (ex vacuo hydrocephalus). This pattern is stereotypic and can be recognized early in the clinical course of the disease by MRI scan (Dickerson et al. 2009, 2011). Cerebrovascular disease, usually in the form of small vessel occlusive disease caused by chronic hypertension and other vascular risk factors, is a condition that frequently accompanies aging in general and also AD in particular. Thus, it is relatively common to find some cortical microinfarcts, lacunar infarcts in the basal ganglia, and demyelination of the periventricular white matter. The presence of cortical petechial microbleeds or even evident lobar hemorrhages, particularly in the posterior parietal and occipital lobes, should lead to the suspicion of a concurrent severe cerebral amyloid angiopathy. Unless there is a concomitant Parkinson's disease or dementia with Lewy bodies, the substantia nigra shows a normal coloration; in contrast, the locus coeruleus is affected in the early stages of AD (Braak and Del Tredici 2011).

MICROSCOPIC FEATURES

Neurofibrillary Tangles

Composition

The neurofibrillary tangles (NFTs) were first described by Alois Alzheimer in his original autopsy case report as intraneuronal filamentous inclusions within the perikaryal region of pyramidal neurons. Ultrastructural studies on AD brain specimens revealed that NFTs are primarily made of paired helical filaments (PHFs), that is, fibrils of $\approx$10 nm in diameter that form pairs with a helical tridimensional conformation at a regular periodicity of $\approx$65 nm (Kidd 1963, 1964; Wisniewski et al. 1976). A small proportion of fibrils within the NFTs do not form pairs, but give the appearance of straight filaments without the periodicity of PHFs (Crowther 1991). Occasional hybrid filaments, with a sharp transition between a paired helical segment and a straight segment, have also been described within NFTs (Crowther 1991). Recently, modern high-resolution molecular microscopy techniques have revealed the presence of twisted ribbon-like assemblies of tau fibrils in vitro, thus challenging the PHF concept (Wegmann et al. 2010). Regardless of the morphology of their structural units, the major constituent of NFTs was found to be the microtubule-associated protein tau, which is aberrantly misfolded and abnormally hyperphosphorylated. Invariably accompanying NFTs are the neuropil threads, which are thought to

result from the breakdown of dendrites and axons of the tangle-bearing neurons.

Morphological Characteristics

The NFTs are argyrophilic and can be shown by silver impregnation methods such as the Gallyas technique (Braak and Braak 1991). An alternative method to examine NFTs is their staining with fluorescent dyes such as Thioflavin-S, which recognize the β-sheet pleated structure of the paired helical filaments (Arnold et al. 1991), or by immunostaining with anti-tau antibodies (Fig. 1). Three morphological stages have been distinguished: (1) Pre-NFTs or diffuse NFTs are defined by a diffuse, sometimes punctate, tau staining within the cytoplasm of otherwise normal-looking neurons, with well-preserved dendrites and a centered nucleus; (2) Mature or fibrillar intraneuronal NFTs (iNFTs) consist of cytoplasmic filamentous aggregates of tau that displace the nucleus toward the periphery of the soma and often extend to distorted-appearing dendrites and to the proximal segment of the axon; (3) extraneuronal "ghost" NFTs (eNFTs) result from the death of the tangle-bearing neurons and are identifiable by the absence of nucleus and stainable cytoplasm (Su et al. 1993; Braak et al. 1994; Augustinack et al. 2002). Both silver and Thioflavin-S stains, as well as some phosphotau antibodies such as AT8 and PHF1, preferentially identify the iNFTs and the eNFTs (Braak et al. 1994; Augustinack et al. 2002). By contrast, other phosphoepitopes (e.g., pThr153, pSer262, pThr231) and a certain conformational epitope recognized by the antibodies MC1 and Alz50 also recognize pre-NFTs, suggesting that the misfolding of the tau molecule and its phosphorylation in certain sites represent an early step prior to tau aggregation (Carmel et al. 1996; Weaver et al. 2000; Augustinack et al. 2002). Interestingly, the immunoreactivity for a caspase-cleaved form of tau with a faster rate of fibrillization than the full length molecule in vitro colocalize with Alz50 immunoreactivity in pre-NFTs, suggesting that the caspase-mediated cleavage of the carboxy-terminal region of the tau molecule is

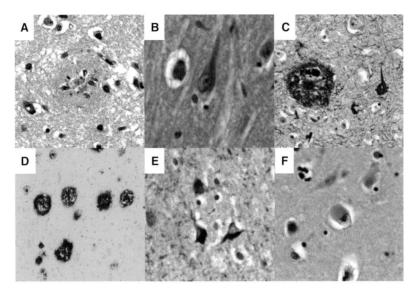

Figure 1. Photomicrographs of the core pathological lesions observed in Alzheimer and Lewy body diseases. (A) Plaque evident on routine H&E stained section of frontal cortex; (B) tangle in a hippocampal pyramidal neuron on routine H&E stained section; (C) silver stain highlights both a plaque and a tangle; (D) immunohistochemistry against Aβ highlights plaques; (E) immunohistochemistry against tau highlights tangles; (F) a cortical Lewy body can be seen in a layer V neuron on a routine H&E stained section of frontal cortex.

also a necessary step prior to further aggregation (Guillozet-Bongaarts et al. 2005).

Topographical Distribution

The spatiotemporal pattern of progression of NFTs (and neuropil threads in parallel) is rather stereotypical and predictable (Arnold et al. 1991; Braak and Braak 1991; Braak et al. 2006). Briefly, the neurofibrillary degeneration starts in the allocortex of the medial temporal lobe (entorhinal cortex and hippocampus) and spreads to the associative isocortex, relatively sparing the primary sensory, motor, and visual areas. In their clinicopathological study, Braak and Braak distinguished six stages that can be summarized in three: entorhinal, limbic, and isocortical (Fig. 2). The first NFTs consistently appear in the transentorhinal (perirhinal) region (stage I) along with the entorhinal cortex proper, followed by the CA1 region of the hippocampus (stage II). Next, NFTs develop and accumulate in limbic structures such as the subiculum of the hippocampal formation (stage III) and the amygdala, thalamus, and

claustrum (stage IV). Finally, NFTs spread to all isocortical areas (isocortical stage), with the associative areas being affected prior and more severely (stage V) than the primary sensory, motor, and visual areas (stage VI). A severe involvement of striatum and substantia nigra can occur during the late isocortical stage. Of note, this neurofibrillary degeneration follows a laminar pattern affecting preferentially the stellate neurons of layer II, the superficial portion of layer III, and the large multipolar neurons of layer IV within the entorhinal cortex; the stratum pyramidale of CA1 and subiculum within the hippocampal formation, and the pyramidal neurons of layers III and V within the isocortical areas (Hyman et al. 1984; Arnold et al. 1991; Braak and Braak 1991).

Clinicopathological Correlations

Multiple clinicopathological studies from different groups have established that the amount and distribution of NFTs correlate with the severity and the duration of dementia (Arriagada et al. 1992a; Bierer et al. 1995; Gómez-Isla et al.

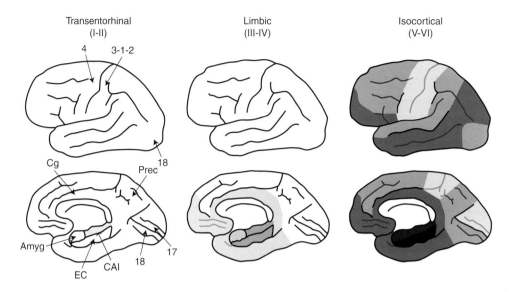

Figure 2. Spatiotemporal pattern of neurofibrillary degeneration. Shading indicates the distribution of NFTs with darker colors representing increasing densities. Amyg, amygdala; EC, entorhinal cortex; CA1, cornus ammonis 1 hippocampal subfield; Cg, cingulate cortex; Prec, precuneus; 4, primary motor cortex; 3-1-2, primary sensory cortex; 17, primary visual cortex; 18, associative visual cortex (data based on Arnold et al. 1991; Braak and Braak 1991; Arrigada et al. 1992a,b; Braak et al. 1994).

1997; Giannakopoulos et al. 2003; Ingelsson et al. 2004). Moreover, the selective rather than widespread topographical distribution of NFTs described above matches with the hierarchical neuropsychological profile typical of the AD-type dementia syndrome. The prominent initial impairment of episodic memory characteristic of AD is explained by the isolation of the medial temporal lobe structures from the association isocortex and the subcortical nuclei because of the ongoing massive neurofibrillary degeneration. Next, the involvement of multimodal high-order association isocortical areas accounts for the progressive impairment of additional cognitive domains, including executive dysfunction (prefrontal cortex), apraxias (parietal cortex), visuospatial navigation deficits (occipitoparietal cortex), visuoperceptive deficits (occipitotemporal cortex), and semantic memory (anterior temporal cortex), giving rise to the full-blown dementia syndrome. By contrast, the late involvement of primary motor, sensory, and visual isocortical areas explains the sparing of motor, sensory, and

primary visual functions (Hyman et al. 1984; Arnold et al. 1991; Braak and Braak 1991). However, as discussed below, whether NFT formation is a necessary precursor of the neuronal death in AD or represents a protective response of damaged neurons (and thus more of a surrogate marker of the ongoing pathological process) is still controversial.

Amyloid Plaques

Composition

The senile plaques described by Alois Alzheimer in his original case report result from the abnormal extracellular accumulation and deposition of the amyloid-β peptide (Aβ) with 40 or 42 amino acids (Aβ40 and Aβ42), two normal byproducts of the metabolism of the amyloid precursor protein (APP) after its sequential cleavage by the enzymes β- and γ-secretases in neurons. Because of its higher rate of fibrillization and insolubility, Aβ42 is more abundant than Aβ40 within the plaques.

Morphological Characteristics

Attempts to understand the evolution of the amyloid plaque after its formation based on morphological criteria gave rise to a number of terms, including "primitive," "classical," and "burn-out" plaques. However, a more practical and widely used morphological classification distinguishes only two types of amyloid plaques–diffuse versus dense-core plaques–based on their staining with dyes specific for the β-pleated sheet conformation such as Congo Red and Thioflavin-S. This simpler categorization is relevant to the disease because, unlike diffuse Thioflavin-S negative plaques, Thioflavin-S positive dense-core plaques are associated with deleterious effects on the surrounding neuropil including increased neurite curvature and dystrophic neurites, synaptic loss, neuron loss, and recruitment and activation of both astrocytes and microglial cells (Itagaki et al. 1989; Masliah et al. 1990, 1994; Pike et al. 1995; Knowles et al. 1999; Urbanc et al. 2002; Vehmas et al. 2003). Indeed, diffuse amyloid plaques are commonly present in the brains of cognitively intact elderly people, whereas dense-core plaques, particularly those with neuritic dystrophies, are most often found in patients with AD dementia. However, the pathological boundaries between normal aging and AD dementia are not clear-cut and, as we will further discuss below, many cognitively normal elderly people have substantial amyloid burden in their brains.

Electron microscopy studies revealed that the ultrastructure of dense-core plaques is comprised of a central mass of extracelullar filaments that radially extend toward the periphery, where they are intermingled with neuronal, astrocytic, and microglial processes. These neuronal processes, known as dystrophic neurites, often contain packets of paired helical filaments, as well as abundant abnormal mitochondria and dense bodies of probable mitochondrial and lysosomal origin (Kidd 1964; Hirai et al. 2001; Fiala et al. 2007). Plaque-associated neuritic dystrophies represent the most notorious evidence of Aβ-induced neurotoxicity and feature many of the pathophysiological processes downstream Aβ. Their origin can be axonal or dendritic and their morphology can be either elongated and distorted or bulbous (Su et al. 1993). They can be argyrophylic (Fig. 1C) and Thioflavin-S positive because of the aggregation of β-sheet pleated tau fibrils, which can also be shown with many phosphotau and conformation-specific tau antibodies (Su et al. 1993, 1994, 1996). Interestingly, dystrophic neurites can also be immunoreactive for APP (Cras et al. 1991; Su et al. 1998). Cytoskeletal abnormalities in dystrophic neurites explain their immunoreactivity for neurofilament proteins (Su et al. 1996, 1998; Dickson et al. 1999; Knowles et al. 1999). These cytoskeletal abnormalities can lead to a disruption of the normal axonal transport and, indeed, a subset of dystrophic neurites are positive for mitochondrial porin and chromogranin-A because of the abnormal accumulation of mitochondria and large synaptic vesicles, respectively (Dickson et al. 1999; Woodhouse et al. 2006a; Pérez-Gracia et al. 2008). Moreover, some axonal dystrophic neurites contain either cholinergic, glutamatergic, or gabaergic markers, suggesting a plaque-induced aberrant sprouting (Benzing et al. 1993; Ferrer et al. 1993; Masliah et al. 2003; Bell et al. 2007). Finally, dystrophic neurites can be displayed with immunohistochemical studies for ubiquitin and lysosomal proteins, indicating that there is a compensatory attempt to degrade and clear the abnormal accumulation of proteins and organelles (Dickson et al. 1990; Barrachina et al. 2006). A less-evident expression of the plaque-induced neuritic changes is the increase in the curvature of neurites located in the proximity of dense-core plaques (Knowles et al. 1999).

Topographic Distribution

Unlike NFTs, amyloid plaques accumulate mainly in the isocortex. Although the spatiotemporal pattern of progression of amyloid deposition is far less predictable than that of NFTs, in general the allocortex (including entorhinal cortex and hippocampal formation), the basal ganglia, relevant nuclei of the brainstem, and the cerebellum, are involved to a lesser extent and later than the associative iso-cortex. The dissociation between amyloid and NFT burdens in the medial temporal lobe is particularly noticeable. Among the isocortical areas, likewise NFTs, primary sensory, motor, and visual areas tend to be less affected as compared to association multimodal areas. (Arnold et al. 1991; Braak and Braak 1991). Despite this poorer predictability of the progression of amyloid deposition, two staging systems have been proposed. Braak and Braak distinguished three stages: (1) Stage A, with amyloid deposits mainly found in the basal portions of the frontal, temporal, and occipital lobes; (2) Stage B, with all isocortical association areas affected while the hippocampal formation is only mildly involved, and the primary sensory, motor, and visual cortices are devoid of amyloid; and (3) Stage C, characterized by the deposition of amyloid in these primary isocortical areas and, in some cases, the appearance of amyloid deposits in the molecular layer of the cerebellum and subcortical nuclei such as striatum, thalamus, hypothalamus, subthalamic nucleus, and red nucleus (Braak and Braak 1991). Thal et al. proposed a descendent progression of amyloid deposition in five stages: (1) Stage 1

or isocortical; (2) Stage 2, with additional allocortical deposits (entorhinal cortex, hippo-campal formation, amygdala, insular, and cingulated cortices); (3) Stage 3, with additional involvement of subcortical nuclei including striatum, basal forebrain cholinergic nuclei, thalamus and hypothalamus, and white matter; (4) Stage 4, characterized by the involvement of brainstem structures, including red nucleus, substantia nigra, reticular formation of the medulla oblongata, superior and inferior colliculi; and (5) Stage 5, with additional amyloid deposits in the pons (reticular formation, raphe nuclei, locus ceruleus) and the molecular layer of the cerebellum (Thal et al. 2002). These five Thal stages can be summarized in three: stage 1 or isocortical; stage 2, allo-cortical or limbic, and stage 3 or subcortical (Fig. 3).

Amyloid deposits usually involve the six layers of the isocortex, although layers I and VI are usually relatively more spared than layers II-V (Arnold et al. 1991; Braak and Braak 1991). However, in advanced cases it is frequent to observe band-like diffuse amyloid deposits in the subpial surface of the cortex and even a few amyloid deposits in the white matter close to its transition with the cortical layer VI.

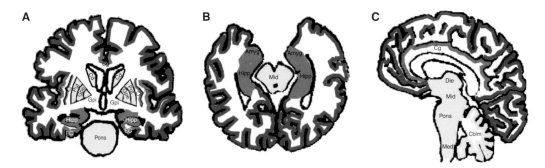

Figure 3. Spatiotemporal pattern of amyloid plaque deposition according to Thal et al. (2002). Coronal (*A*), axial (*B*), and sagittal (*C*) views of the brain. The five Thal stages of amyloid deposition are here summarized in three stages. Amyloid deposits accumulate first in isocortical areas (stage 1 or isocortical, in red), followed by limbic and allocortical structures (stage 2 or limbic, in orange), and in a later stage, by subcortical structures including basal ganglia, selected nuclei in diencephalon and brainstem, and the cerebellar cortex (stage 3 or subcortical, in yellow). Amyg, amygdala; EC, entorhinal cortex; Hipp, hippocampus; Cg, cingulate cortex; Cd, caudate nucleus; Put, putamen; Gpe, globus pallidus externus; Gpi, globus pallidus internus; Cl, claustrum; Ins, insular cortex; Die, diencephalon; Mid, midbrain; Med, medulla oblongata; Cblm, cerebellum.

Clinicopathological Correlations

Clinicopathological studies have established that the amyloid burden (either total amyloid plaques, dense-core plaques or only neuritic plaques) does not correlate with the severity or the duration of dementia (Arriagada et al. 1992a, Hyman et al. 1993; Bierer et al. 1995; Gómez-Isla et al. 1997; Giannakopoulos et al. 2003; Ingelsson et al. 2004). Indeed, in a region of early amyloid deposition such as the temporal associative isocortex, the amyloid burden reaches a plateau early after the onset of the cognitive symptoms or even in the preclinical phase of the disease (Ingelsson et al. 2004; Serrano-Pozo et al. 2011) and not even the size of the plaques grows significantly with the progression of the disease (Hyman et al. 1993). However, it is possible that the amount of amyloid measured over the entire cortical mantle does increase during the clinical course of the disease as the distribution of amyloid deposits "spread" following the above stages. Preliminary data from longitudinal amyloid PET imaging studies in living patients have recently supported this possibility (Jack et al. 2009).

Cerebral Amyloid Angiopathy

Composition

The amyloid-β peptide not only deposits in the brain parenchyma in the form of amyloid plaques but also in the vessel walls in the form of cerebral amyloid angiopathy (CAA). Indeed, the more insoluble and aggregation-prone Aβ42 peptide tends to accumulate in the core of senile plaques, while the more soluble Aβ40 peptide is the major constituent of CAA, accumulating mainly in the interstitium between the smooth muscle cells of the tunica media. Although CAA can also appear in isolation (pure CAA), it is more common in the context of AD, with ≈80% of AD patients showing some degree, usually mild, of CAA at autopsy,

Morphological Characteristics

The same methods described for the examination of amyloid plaques are valid for CAA, that is Thioflavin-S or Congo red staining or immunohistochemical studies with anti-Aβ antibodies. A morphological staging system has been implemented to describe the severity of CAA within a single vessel: grade 0 or absence of staining; grade 1 or congophilic rim around an otherwise nomal-appearance vessel; grade 2 or complete replacement of the tunica media by congophilic material; grade 3 or cracking of $\geq 50\%$ of the circumference of the vessel, giving a "vessel-within-vessel" or "double-barrel" appearance; and grade 4 or fibrinoid necrosis of the vessel wall, often accompanied by additional amyloid deposits in the surrounding neuropil ("dyshoric" changes) (Greenberg and Vonsattel 1997). In this severe stage, Prussian blue (Perl's) staining is useful to show hemosiderin-laden macrophages in the parenchyma surrounding CAA-affected vessels, indicative of chronic microbleeds.

Topographic Distribution

CAA usually affects cortical capillaries, small arterioles and middle-size arteries as well as leptomeningeal arteries, whereas venules, veins, and white-matter arteries are rarely involved. For unknown reasons, posterior parietal and occipital areas are usually more prominently affected than frontal and temporal lobes, and within the same area, leptomeningeal arteries usually show more severe CAA than cortical arteries. A semiquantitative scoring system has been proposed to characterize the severity of CAA within a region of the cortex: 0 = no Thioflavin-S-stained leptomeningeal or cortical vessels; 1 = scattered positivity in either leptomeningeal or cortical vessels; 2 = strong circumferential positivity in at least some vessels either leptomeningeal or cortical; 3 = widespread circumferential staining in many leptomeningeal and cortical vessels, and 4 = presence of "dyshoric" perivascular amyloid deposits in addition to score 3. A global severity score can be obtained by averaging the scores from several regions (Olichney et al. 2000).

Clinicopathological Correlations

According to the Boston criteria, CAA should be suspected after one or multiple major symptomatic lobar hemorrhages in an elderly patient

(Knudsen et al. 2001). But in the context of AD, unless it becomes symptomatic because of this hemorrhagic complication, CAA is usually diagnosed at autopsy. However, three independent postmortem longitudinal studies have revealed that the otherwise apparently asymptomatic CAA can also be a synergistic contributor to cognitive decline in AD (MRC CFAS 2001; Pfeifer et al. 2002; Greenberg et al, 2004; Arvanitakis et al. 2011).

Granuovacuolar Degeneration and Hirano Bodies

Granulovacuolar degeneration (GVD) and Hirano bodies are two poorly understood lesions present in the cytoplasm of hippocampal pyramidal neurons of AD patients. Although they are increasingly observed with aging in cognitively intact elderly people, these two lesions are more severe and frequent in age-matched AD patients. (Ball 1978; Xu et al. 1992).

GVD consists of the accumulation of large double-membrane bodies. Their origin and significance are uncertain. Early immunohistochemical studies reported immunoreactivity of GVD bodies for cytoskeletal proteins including tubulin, neurofilament proteins and tau (Kahn et al. 1985; Price et al. 1986; Dickson et al. 1987; Bondareff et al. 1991; Mena et al. 1992; Ikegami et al. 1996). Because GVD bodies are also positive for some tau kinases, a role in tangle formation has been proposed (Ghoshal et al. 1999; Leroy et al. 2002; Kannanayakal et al. 2006). Other authors have postulated a role in the apoptotic cell death because of their immunoreactivity for activated caspase-3 (Selznick et al. 1999; Stadelmann et al. 1999; Su et al. 2002). More recent studies have suggested that these bodies might derive from the endoplasmic reticulum and represent the stress granules that feature the unfolded protein response, because they are positive for several stress kinases (Zhu et al. 2001; Lagalwar et al. 2007; Thakur et al. 2007; Hoozemans et al. 2009). Finally, based on their positivity for ubiquitin and autophagic markers, it has been proposed that these granules are late-stage autophagic vacuoles (Okamoto et al. 1991;

Barrachina et al. 2006; Yamazaki et al. 2010; Funk et al. 2011).

Hirano bodies are eosinophilic rod-like cytoplasmic inclusions relatively common in the stratum lacunosum of the hippocampal CA1 region in the elderly. However, in AD patients the number of Hirano bodies is abnormally high and they are translocated to the neurons of the stratum pyramidale (Gibson and Tomlison 1977). Although the significance of Hirano bodies in AD is not completely understood, they are recognized by antibodies against tau, neurofilament proteins, actin, and other cytoskeletal proteins (Goldman 1983; Galloway et al. 1987a,b; Schmidt et al. 1989; Maciver and Harrington 1995; Rossiter et al. 2000). Other immunoreactivities associated with Hirano bodies are inducible nitric oxide synthase (Lee et al. 1999), advanced glycation endproducts (Münch et al. 1998), and the carboxy-terminal fragments of APP (Muñoz et al. 1993).

Glial Responses

Reactive astrocytes and activated microglial cells are commonly associated to dense-core amyloid plaques, indicating that amyloid-β is a major trigger of this glial response (Itagaki et al. 1989; Pike et al. 1995; Vehmas et al. 2003). However, we have recently observed a linear increase in reactive astrocytes and activated microglial cells through the entire disease course despite an early plateau in amyloid deposition in the temporal associative isocortex. Indeed, we found a highly significant positive correlation between both astrocytosis and microgliosis and NFT burden but not between both reactive glial cell types and amyloid burden, suggesting that glial responses are also related to neurofibrillary degeneration (Ingelsson et al. 2004; Serrano-Pozo et al. 2011).

Neuronal Loss

Neuronal loss is the main pathological substrate of cortical atrophy and, although usually evident in sections stained with hematoxylin and eosin, it can be more readily shown with a Nissl staining or a NeuN immunohistochemistry. Nissl staining (for example with cresyl violet) reveals the negatively charged ribosomic RNA present in the ribosomes of the rough endoplasmic reticulum (Nissl substance or granules), giving a dark blue appearance to the perinuclear region of neurons. By contrast, NeuN is a neuronal-specific nuclear antigen, although NeuN immunohistochemistry also stains the perinuclear region and some proximal processes of neurons.

The regional and laminar pattern of neuronal loss matches that of NFTs, but, importantly, within the same region neuronal loss exceeds the numbers of NFTs, so that it is a better correlate of cognitive deficits than the number of NFTs (Gómez-Isla et al. 1996, 1997). Indeed, quantitative stereology-based studies of neurons, iNFTs and eNFTs have concluded that iNFTs can last for up to two decades and that neurons bearing iNFTs might still be viable as evidenced by their positive Nissl staining (Bussiére et al. 2003; Hof et al. 2003). This dissociation between the extent of neuronal loss and that of NFTs suggests that there are least two mechanisms of neuronal death in AD: one affecting tangle-bearing neurons, that will lead to the appearance of ghost extracellular tangles, and another affecting tangle-free neurons. Although the mechanisms of neuronal death in AD are beyond the scope of this article, it will be noted that postmortem studies on apoptosis have yielded controversial results, with some studies showing a widespread distribution of apoptotic markers (Troncoso et al. 1996; Su et al. 2001), while others have only reported a scattered distribution (Selznick et al. 1999; Woodhouse et al. 2006b).

Synapse Loss

Besides neuronal loss, synapse loss is another contributor to the cortical atrophy of the AD brain. Synapse loss in AD was shown with immunohistochemical studies using antibodies against pre- or postsynaptic proteins—typically the presynaptic protein synaptophysin—and with electron microscopy studies.

The spatiotemporal and laminar pattern of synapse loss matches that of neuron loss. Synaptic loss is not only caused by neuronal loss but can exceed the existing neuronal loss within a particular cortical area. This indicates that synapse loss predates neuronal loss and that the remaining neurons become less well connected to their synaptic partners than expected just by the number of viable neurons surviving in a particular circuit. Likely this is why synaptic density is the best correlate of cognitive decline in AD (DeKosky and Scheff 1990; Scheff et al. 1990, 1993, 2007; Terry et al. 1991; Masliah et al. 1994; Ingelsson et al. 2004). Interestingly, an inverse correlation has been observed between synaptic density and the size of remaining synapses as measured by the length of the postsynaptic density. This enlargement of remaining synapses has been interpreted as a compensatory response, rather than as selective loss of small synapses (DeKosky and Scheff 1990; Scheff et al. 1990; Scheff and Price 1993).

CRITERIA FOR THE PATHOLOGICAL DIAGNOSIS OF ALZHEIMER DISEASE

Of all pathological features described above, amyloid plaques and NFTs are the most characteristic of AD and, understandably, the criteria for the pathological diagnosis of AD rely on their amount and/or distribution.

The first pathological criteria for the diagnosis of AD were based on the highest density of total amyloid plaques (both diffuse and neuritic) in any cortical field, adjusted for age so that the older the patient at death, the greater the density required for diagnosis (Khachaturian 1985). The presence of NFTs was not required and diffuse plaques—relatively frequent in nondemented elderly people—had the same consideration as neuritic plaques. Although meritorious, these criteria were soon abandoned because, despite a very high sensitivity to diagnose AD dementia, they lacked sufficient specificity (Geddes et al. 1997). In 1991, the Consortium to Establish a Registry for Alzheimer Disease (CERAD) proposed more specific diagnostic criteria by emphasizing the importance of neuritic plaques over diffuse plaques (Mirra et al. 1991, 1997). CERAD criteria use a semiquantitative score of the density of neuritic plaques in the most severely affected region of the isocortex (frontal, temporal, or parietal) and the patient's age at death to obtain an age-related plaque score. This score is then integrated with clinical information regarding the presence or absence of dementia to establish one of three levels of certainty that dementia is explained by the AD pathological changes: possible, probable, and definite. A diagnosis of AD is made if the criteria for probable or definite AD are met. Although higher than that of Khachaturian criteria, the specificity of CERAD criteria proved to be still insufficient because they did not incorporate the scoring of the severity of NFTs (Geddes et al. 1997). By contrast, the use of Braak and Braak staging of NFTs alone—with the isocortical stages V and VI as criteria of definite AD—showed a high specificity at the expense of a low sensitivity (Geddes et al. 1997).

Current pathological criteria for AD were defined in 1997 by a workshop of the National Institute of Aging and the Reagan Institute. The NIA-RI consensus recommendations combine the CERAD semiquantitative score of neuritic plaques and the Braak and Braak staging of NFTs to distinguish three probabilistic diagnostic categories: (1) high likelihood, if there are frequent neuritic plaques (CERAD definite) and abundant isocortical NFTs (Braak stage V/VI); (2) intermediate likelihood, if there are moderate neuritic plaques (CERAD probable) and NFTs are restricted to limbic regions (Braak III/IV), and (3) low likelihood, if there are infrequent neuritic plaques (CERAD possible) and NFTs are restricted to the entorhinal cortex and/or hippocampus (Braak I/II). A diagnosis of AD is made when the criteria for intermediate or high likelihood of AD are met and the patient had a clinical history of dementia (NIA-RI Consensus 1997). Because experience has revealed infrequent cases with many AD pathological lesions but no or few cognitive symptoms (and vice versa) and these circumstances were not addressed by the NIA-RI consensus workgroup, these diagnostic criteria are currently under review.

Both CERAD and NIA-RI criteria also incorporated the assessment of other pathologies, particularly vascular and Lewy body diseases, already recognizing the high prevalence of mixed pathologies underlying dementia in elderly people, a circumstance well documented by more recent longitudinal community-based clinicopathological studies (MRC CFAS 2001; Schneider et al. 2007). Thus, in many practical instances, the CERAD criteria for "possible AD" and the NIA-RI criteria for "intermediate probability of AD" are not only based on a moderate amount and distribution of AD pathology but also on the coexistence of vascular or Lewy body pathology with sufficient severity to contribute to the patient's dementia.

NEUROPATHOLOGY OF MILD COGNITIVE IMPAIRMENT AND EARLY ALZHEIMER DISEASE

Clinicopathological correlation studies have taught us that at the moment of the clinical diagnosis, patients with AD-type dementia often already have a Braak stage V or VI of neurofibrillary degeneration and a substantial and widespread synaptic and neuronal loss. To anticipate the clinical diagnosis of AD before the stage of full-blown dementia, a new clinical construct was needed. Petersen et al. proposed the concept of "mild cognitive impairment" (MCI) as a new diagnostic entity for the transition between normal aging and AD dementia. Patients with MCI have already some cognitive complaints that are detectable with the appropriate cognitive tests and represent a decline from a previous higher baseline level but that, unlike the definition of dementia, do not interfere with their activities of daily life. Importantly, MCI patients have an increased risk of developing dementia, which has been reported between 10% and 15% per year (Petersen et al. 1999, 2001; Petersen 2004).

Autopsy studies on MCI patients are scarce but they have reproducibly found a stage of AD pathology intermediate between cognitively intact subjects and demented patients, particularly regarding neurofibrillary degeneration, that is consistent with the idea of a transition phase between normal aging and definite AD (Jicha et al. 2006; Markesbery et al. 2006; Petersen et al. 2006; Schneider et al. 2009). Specifically, MCI patients usually have a moderate number of neuritic plaques and a limbic stage of NFTs (Braak stage III or IV), fitting into the NIA-RI category of intermediate likelihood of AD (sufficient to cause dementia) and providing a pathological validation for this clinical construct. Along the same lines, patients with a Clinical Dementia Rating score of 0.5 (equivalent to MCI or very mild AD) have already a ≈30% of neuron loss in the entorhinal cortex compared to cognitively intact controls (CDR = 0), but still no evident neuronal loss in the superior temporal sulcus (Gómez-Isla et al. 1996, 1997). Moreover, electron microscopy studies have shown that MCI patients also have an intermediate number of synapses between nondemented controls and mild AD patients in the hippocampus, further indicating that many individuals with the clinical symptoms of MCI have early AD (Scheff et al. 2006, 2007). Of note, a paradoxical, presumably compensatory, up-regulation in the density of presynaptic glutamatergic boutons has been reported in the frontal cortex of MCI patients compared to nondemented controls and mild AD patients (Bell et al. 2007).

Although AD was the most common pathological diagnosis underlying MCI in the above case series, it should be noted that there was a high degree of pathological heterogeneity underlying the clinical diagnosis of MCI, with vascular disease, Lewy body disease, argyrophilic grain disease, and hippocampal sclerosis as major concurrent or alternative pathologies (Jicha et al. 2006; Petersen et al. 2006; Schneider et al. 2009). In addition, in the largest study a high proportion (up to 25%) of MCI patients had no pathology at autopsy (Schneider et al. 2009). Finally, no significant pathological differences have been observed between the amnestic and the nonamnestic subtypes of MCI nor in their pathological outcome after conversion to dementia (Jicha et al. 2006; Schneider et al. 2009).

ALZHEIMER NEUROPATHOLOGY IN "NORMAL AGING"

Longitudinal prospective clinicopathological studies in nondemented elderly people have revealed that up to 45% of nondemented elderly

would meet the NIA-RI criteria for AD had they been demented, usually the intermediate likelihood category of these criteria, and rarely the high likelihood category (Schmitt et al. 2000; Knopman et al. 2003; Bennet et al. 2006; Price et al. 2009; Schneider et al. 2009). Moreover, the pattern of regional distribution of pathological changes in nondemented controls matches that of AD patients (Arriagada et al. 1992b). Thus, mounting evidence from clinicopathological studies support the view that AD is a continuous spectrum between asymptomatic lesions in cognitively normal elderly and dementia, with MCI as a transition phase between these two ends.

The apparent dissociation between AD pathology and cognitive status in some elderly people is remarkable because these so-called "high-pathology nondemented controls" or "individuals with asymptomatic AD" seem to be resilient to the neurotoxic effects of amyloid plaques and NFTs and to contradict the aforementioned positive correlation between NFT burden and cognitive decline. Understanding the biochemical and morphological substrates of this resilience to cognitive decline in the presence of abundant AD pathology might be crucial to discover new therapeutic targets for the disease. As expected from the highly significant clinicopathological correlations of synaptic and neuronal loss in AD, high-pathology controls have preserved synaptophysin levels compared to AD patients with a similar burden of plaques and NFTs (Lue et al. 1996), and they do not seem to have significant neuronal loss, not even in vulnerable regions such as the entorhinal cortex and the hippocampus (Price et al. 2001; West et al. 2004). Moreover, they have lower levels of neuroinflammatory markers than pathology-matched AD patients (Lue et al. 1996). This resistance to AD pathology has also been related to a nucleolar, nuclear, and cell body hypertrophy of the hippocampal and cortical neurons, suggestive of a compensatory metabolic activation to face the neurotoxic effects of AD lesions (Riudavets et al. 2007; Iacono et al. 2008). In keeping with these pathological reports, a MRI-neuropathological correlation study revealed larger brain and hippocampal volumes in high-pathology controls than in pathology-matched demented patients, further supporting the preservation of both neurons and synapses (Erten-Lyons et al. 2009).

OVERLAP OF AD WITH LEWY BODY DISEASE

Alzheimer disease and Parkinson's disease (PD) are the leading causes of dementia and movement disorders in the aging population. It is estimated that over 10 million people live with these devastating neurological conditions in the United States. It is estimated that over 10 million people live with these devastating neurological conditions in the United States, and that this country alone will see a 50% annual increase of AD and PD by the year 2025 (Herbert et al. 2001).

PD and AD are two distinct clinicopathological entities. While in AD, abnormal accumulation of misfolded Aβ protein in the neocortex and limbic system is thought to be responsible for the neurodegenerative pathology (Selkoe 1990; Sisodia and Price 1995), intracellular accumulation of α-synuclein has been centrally implicated in the pathogenesis of PD (Spillantini et al. 1997; Hashimoto et al. 1998; Trojanowski and Lee 1998). In AD, Aβ protein accumulates in the intracellular (LaFerla et al. 1995; Skovronsky et al. 1998) and extracellular space, leading to the formation of plaques, whereas intracellular polymerization of phosphorylated cytoskeletal molecules such as tau results in the formation of neurofibrillary tangles (Greenberg and Davies 1990; Lee et al. 2001). In PD, intracellular accumulation of α-synuclein—an abundant synaptic terminal protein (Iwai et al. 1995)—results in the formation of characteristic inclusions called Lewy bodies (LBs) (Fig. 1F) (Spillantini et al. 1997; Wakabayashi et al. 1997; Takeda et al. 1998). The new consortium criteria for the classification of Lewy body diseases (LBD) recognizes two clinical entities, the first denominated dementia with LBs (DLB) and the second PD dementia (PDD) (McKeith et al. 1996; Aarsland et al. 2004; Burn 2006; McKeith 2006; Lippa et al. 2007). While in patients with

DLB, the clinical presentation is of dementia followed by parkinsonism, in patients with PDD the initial signs are of parkinsonism followed by dementia (Litvan et al. 1998; Janvin et al. 2006; McKeith 2006). Interestingly, the brains of patients with DLB and PDD display very similar pathology, with the exception that recent studies have shown extensive deposition of Aβ and α-synuclein in the striatum and hippocampus in DLB compared to only α-synuclein in PDD cases (Duda et al. 2002; Jellinger and Attems 2006). Because of the implications for the management and treatment of parkinsonism and dementia in patients with PD and DLB, loss of dopaminergic neurons in the midbrain (Dickson et al. 1994; Tsuboi and Dickson 2005) and cholinergic cells in the nucleus basalis of Meynert have been characterized in detail (Perry et al. 1978; Hansen et al. 1990). Although the severity of the neuronal loss within these subcortical regions might explain some of the neurological deficits in patients with PD and DLB, the neuronal populations responsible for the more complex cognitive and psychiatric alterations have not been completely characterized. Abnormal accumulation of α-synuclein in the CA2-3 region of the hippocampus (Harding and Halliday 2001; Bertrand et al. 2004), insula, amygdala and cingulate cortex has been shown to be an important neuropathological feature (Dickson et al. 1994; Spillantini et al. 1997; Trojanowski et al. 1998; Aarsland et al. 2004).

Remarkably, despite being initially considered distinct clinicopathological conditions, several studies have now confirmed that the clinical features and the pathology of AD and PD can overlap (McKeith 2000, 2006; Lippa et al. 2007). Approximately 25% of all patients with AD develop parkinsonism, and about 50% of all cases of PD develop AD-type dementia after 65 years of age (Hansen et al. 1990). Moreover, 70% of patients with sporadic AD display the formation of α-synuclein-positive LB-like inclusions in the amygdala and limbic structures (Lippa et al. 1998; Trojanowski et al. 1998; Hamilton 2000). Similarly, in patients with familial AD (FAD) and Down syndrome, LB-like pathology and parkinsonism have been reported (Lippa et al. 1999). Last, as mentioned above, the single most important neuropathological finding that distinguishes PDD from DLB is the presence of Aβ deposits in the striatum (Duda et al. 2002) and in the hippocampus (Masliah et al. 1993a).

A number of studies provide extensive support for an interaction between pathogenic pathways in AD and LBD and argue against a coincidental concurrence of both disorders (i.e., merely because of their high prevalence in the elderly). FAD cases with presenilin mutations that present with significant LB pathology strongly support an interaction between Aβ and α-synuclein (Rosenberg 2005; Snider et al. 2005; Leverenz et al. 2006). Although plaques, tangles and LBs are useful neuropathological and diagnostic markers of these disorders, the initial injury that results in the cognitive and movement alterations is likely the damage of the synaptic terminals in selected circuitries (DeKosky and Scheff 1990; Masliah and Terry 1993; Masliah et al. 1994, 2001a, Klucken et al. 2003). Several lines of investigation support the notion that oligomeric forms of Aβ and α-synuclein, rather than the polymers and fibrils associated with plaques and LBs, accumulate in the neuronal membranes and lead to the characteristic synaptic pathology (Lambert et al. 1998; Conway et al. 2000; Lashuel et al. 2002; Haass and Selkoe 2007; Kramer and Schulz-Schaeffer 2007; Koffie et al. 2009; Scott et al. 2010). Some studies have shown that underlying interactions between α-synuclein and Aβ play a fundamental role in the pathogenesis of LBD (Lippa et al. 1998; Hashimoto et al. 2000; Masliah et al. 2001b, Pletnikova et al. 2005). Specifically, Aβ promotes the oligomerization and toxic conversion of α-synuclein (Masliah et al. 2001b; Mandal et al. 2006), Aβ exacerbates the deficits associated with α-synuclein accumulation, Aβ and α-synuclein colocalize in membrane and caveolar fractions, and Aβ stabilizes α-synuclein multimers that might form channel-like structures in the membrane (Tsigelny et al. 2007, 2008). Both lysosomal leakage (Nixon and Cataldo 2006) and oxidative stress (Smith et al. 1996) appear to be involved in the process of neurotoxicity and

pathological interactions between Aβ and α-synuclein (Rockenstein et al. 2005).

Therefore, it is possible that the combined effects of α-synuclein and Aβ might lead to synaptic damage and selective degeneration of neurons in the neocortical, limbic, and subcortical regions. A more precise mapping of the neuronal populations affected in these regions is needed to understand the cellular basis for the characteristic cognitive dysfunction in PDD and DLB and to develop new treatments for these conditions.

CONCLUSIONS

Classical neuropathological lesions including senile amyloid plaques and neurofibrillary tangles define AD but they likely represent the "tip of the iceberg" of the pathological alterations that cause the cognitive decline associated with AD. Indeed, the development of new biomarkers and imaging tools has made evident that these neuropathological stigmata of AD begin to accumulate a decade or more prior to a clinical diagnosis of dementia. Synaptic loss, plasticity changes, neuronal loss, and the presence of soluble microscopic oligomeric forms of Aβ and even of tau, likely contribute to the progressive neural system failure that occurs over decades. An understanding of this natural history of the disease is critical to design primary or secondary prevention strategies to halt the disease progression before the damage to the neural system becomes irreversible.

ACKNOWLEDGMENTS

This work was funded by the National Institutes of Health grants AG5131, AG18840, AG22074, NS057096, and AG10435 (to E.M.), and P50AG05134 and AG08487 (to B.T.H. and M.P.F.). A.S.P. was supported with a Research Fellowship from Fundación Alfonso Martín Escudero (Madrid, Spain).

REFERENCES

Aarsland D, Ballard CG, Halliday G. 2004. Are Parkinson's disease with dementia and dementia with Lewy bodies the same entity? *J Geriatr Psychiatry Neurol* **17:** 137–145.

Arnold SE, Hyman BT, Flory J, Damasio AR, Van Hoesen GW. 1991. The topographical and neuroanatomical distribution of neurofibrillary tangles and neuritic plaques in the cerebral cortex of patients with Alzheimer's disease. *Cereb Cortex* **1**: 103–116.

Arriagada PV, Growdon JH, Hedley-Whyte ET, Hyman BT. 1992a. Neurofibrillary tangles but not senile plaques parallel duration and severity of Alzheimer's disease. *Neurology* **42**: 631–639.

Arriagada PV, Marzloff K, Hyman BT. 1992b. Distribution of Alzheimer-type pathologic changes in non-demented elderly individuals matches the pattern in Alzheimer's disease. *Neurology* **42**: 1681–1688.

Arvanitakis Z, Leurgans SE, Wang Z, Wilson RS, Bennet DA, Schneider JA. 2011. Cerebral amyloid angiopathy pathology and cognitive domains in older persons. *Ann Neurol* **69**: 320–327.

Augustinack JC, Schneider A, Mandelkow EM, Hyman BT. 2002. Specific tau-phosphorylation sites correlate with severity of neuronal cytopathology in Alzheimer's disease. *Acta Neuropathol* **103**: 26–35.

Ball MJ, Nuttal K. 1978. Topographic distribution of neurofibrillary tangles and granulovacuoles in hippocampal cortex of aging and demented patients. A quantitative study. *Acta Neuropathol* **42**: 73–80.

Barrachina M, Maes T, Buesa C, Ferrer I. 2006. Lysosome-associated membrane protein 1 (LAMP-1) in Alzheimer's disease. *Neuropathol Appl Neurobiol* **32**: 505–516.

Beach T, Walker R, McGeer E. 1989. Patterns of gliosis in Alzheimer's disease and aging cerebrum. *Glia* **2**: 420–436.

Bell KFS, Bennet DA, Cuello AC. 2007. Paradoxical upregulation of glutamatergic presynaptic boutons during mild cognitive impairment. *J Neurosci* **27**: 10810–10817.

Bennet DA, Schneider JA, Arvanitakis Z, Kelly JF, Aggarwal NT, Shah RC, Wilson RS. 2006. Neuropathology of older persons without cognitive impairment from two community-based studies. *Neurology* **66**: 1837–1844.

Benzing WC, Ikonomovic MD, Brady DR, Mufson EJ, Armstrong DM. 1993. Evidence that transmitter-containing dystrophic neurites precede paired helical filament and Alz-50 formation within senile plaques in the amygdala of nondemented elderly and patients with Alzheimer's disease. *J Comp Neurol* **334**: 176–191.

Bertrand E, Lechowicz W, Szpak GM, Lewandowska E, Dymecki J, Wierzba-Bobrowicz T. 2004. Limbic neuropathology in idiopathic Parkinson's disease with concomitant dementia. *Folia Neuropathol* **42**: 141–150.

Bierer LM, Hof PR, Purohit DP, Carlin L, Schneider J, Davis KL, Perl DP. 1995. Neocortical neurofibrillary tangles correlate with dementia severity in Alzheimer's disease. *Arch Neurol* **52**: 81–88.

Bondareff W, Wischik CM, Novak M, Roth M. 1991. Sequestration of tau by granulovacuolar degeneration in Alzheimer's disease. *Am J Pathol* **139**: 641–647.

Braak H, Braak E. 1991. Neuropathological stageing of Alzheimer-related changes. *Acta Neuropathol* **82**: 239–259.

Braak H, Del Tredici K. 2011. The pathological process underlying Alzheimer's disease in individuals under thirty. *Acta Neuropathol* **121**: 171–181.

Braak E, Braak H, Mandelkow EM. 1994. A sequence of cytoskeleton changes related to the formation of neurofibrillary tangles and neuropil threads. *Acta Neuropathol* **87**: 554–567.

Braak H, Alafuzoff I, Arzberger T, Kretzschmanr H, Del Tredici K. 2006. Staging of Alzheimer disease-associated neurofibrillary pathology using paraffin sections and immunhistochemistry. *Acta Neuropathol* **112**: 389–404.

Burn DJ. 2006. Parkinson's disease dementia: What's in a Lewy body? *J Neural Transm Suppl* **70**: 361–365.

Bussière T, Gold G, Kövari E, Giannakopoulos P, Bouras C, Perl DP, Morrison JH, Hof PR. 2003. Stereologic analysis of neurofibrillary tangle formation in prefrontal cortex area 9 in aging and Alzheimer's disease. *Neuroscience* **117**: 577–592.

Carmel G, Mager EM, Binder LI, Kuret J. 1996. The structural basis of monoclonal antibody Alz50's selectivity for Alzheimer's disease pathology. *J Biol Chem* **271**: 32789–32795.

Coleman MP, Perry VH. 2002. Axon pathology in neurological disease: A neglected therapeutic target. *Trends Neurosci* **25**: 532–537.

Conway KA, Lee SJ, Rochet JC, Ding TT, Williamson RE, Lansbury PT Jr. 2000. Acceleration of oligomerization, not fibrillization, is a shared property of both α-synuclein mutations linked to early-onset Parkinson's disease: Implications for pathogenesis and therapy. *Proc Natl Acad Sci* **97**: 571–576.

Cras P, Kawai M, Lowery D, Gonzalez-DeWhitt P, Greenberg B, Perry G. 1991. Senile plaque neurites in Alzheimer disease accumulate amyloid precursor protein. *Proc Natl Acad Sci* **88**: 7552–7556.

Crews L, Masliah E. 2010. Molecular mechanisms of neurodegeneration in Alzheimer's disease. *Hum Mol Genet* **19**: R12–R20.

Crews L, Rockenstein E, Masliah E. 2010. APP transgenic modeling of Alzheimer's disease: Mechanisms of neurodegeneration and aberrant neurogenesis. *Brain Struct Funct* **214**: 111–126.

Crowther RA. 1991. Straight and paired helical filaments in Alzheimer disease have a common structural unit. *Proc Natl Acad Sci* **88**: 2288–2292.

de Calignon A, Spires-Jones TL, Pitstick R, Carlson GA, Hyman BT. 2009. Tangle-bearing neurons survive despite disruption of membrane integrity in a mouse model of tauopathy. *J Neuropathol Exp Neurol* **68**: 757–761.

de Calignon A, Fox LM, Pitstick R, Carlson GA, Bacskai BJ, Spires-Jones TL, Hyman BT. 2010. Caspase activation precedes and leads to tangles. *Nature* **464**: 1201–1204.

DeKosky ST, Scheff SW. 1990. Synapse loss in frontal cortex biopsies in Alzheimer's disease: Correlation with cognitive severity. *Ann Neurol* **27**: 457–464.

DeKosky ST, Scheff SW, Styren SD. 1996. Structural correlates of cognition in dementia: Quantification and assessment of synapse change. *Neurodegeneration* **5**: 417–421.

Dickerson BC, Bakkour A, Salat DH, Feczko E, Pacheco J, Greve DN, Grodstein F, Wright CI, Blacker D, Rosas HD, et al. 2009. The cortical signature of Alzheimer's disease: Regionally specific cortical thinning relates to symptom severity in very mild to mild AD dementia and is detectable in asymptomatic amyloid-positive individuals. *Cereb Cortex* **19**: 497–510.

Dickerson BC, Stoub TR, Shah RC, Sperling RA, Killiany RJ, Albert MS, Hyman BT, Blacker D, Detoledo-Morrell L. 2011. Alzheimer-signature MRI biomarker predicts AD dementia in cognitively normal adults. *Neurology* **76:** 1395–1402.

Dickson DW, Ksiezak-Reding H, Davies P, Yen SH. 1987. A monoclonal antibody that recognizes a phosphorylated epitope in Alzheimer neurofibrillary tangles, neurofilaments and tau proteins immunostains granulovacuolar degeneration. *Acta Neuropathol* **73:** 254–258.

Dickson DW, Wertkin A, Mattiace LA, Fier E, Kress Y, Davies P, Yen SH. 1990. Ubiquitin immunoelectron microscopy of dystrophic neurites in cerebellar senile plaques of Alzheimer's disease. *Acta Neuropathol* **79:** 486–493.

Dickson DW, Schmidt ML, Lee VM, Zhao ML, Yen SH, Trojanowski JQ. 1994. Immunoreactivity profile of hippocampal CA2/3 neurites in diffuse Lewy body disease. *Acta Neuropathol* **87:** 269–276.

Dickson TC, King CE, McCormack GH, Vickers JC. 1999. Neurochemical diversity of dystrophic neurites in the early and late stages of Alzheimer's disease. *Exp Neurol* **1:** 100–110.

Duda JE, Giasson BI, Mabon ME, Lee VM, Trojanowski JQ. 2002. Novel antibodies to synuclein show abundant striatal pathology in Lewy body diseases. *Ann Neurol* **52:** 205–210.

Duda JE, Giasson B, Lee V-M, Trojanowski JQ. 2003. Is the initial insult in Parkinson's disease and Dementia with Lewy bodies a neuritic dystrophy? *Ann NY Acad Sci* **991:** 295.

Erten-Lyons D, Woltjer RL, Dodge H, Nixon R, Vorobik R, Calvert JF, Leahy M, Montine T, Kaye J. 2009. Factors associated with resistance to dementia despite high Alzheimer disease pathology. *Neurology* **72:** 354–360.

Ferrer I, Zújar MJ, Rivera R, Soria M, Vidal A, Casas R. 1993. Parvalbumin-immunoreactive dystrophic neurites and aberrant sprouts in the cerebral cortex of patients with Alzheimer's disease. *Neurosci Lett* **158:** 163–166.

Fiala JC, Feinberg M, Peters A, Barbas H. 2007. Mitochondrial degeneration in dystrophic neurites of senile plaques may lead to extracellular deposition of fine filaments. *Brain Struct Funct* **212:** 195–207.

Funk KE, Mrak RE, Kuret J. 2011. Granulovacuolar degeneration bodies of Alzheimer's disease resemble late-stage autophagic organelles. *Neuropathol Appl Neurobiol* **37:** 295–306.

Galloway PG. Perry G, Gambetti P. 1987a. Hirano bodies filaments contain actin and actin-associated proteins. *J Neuropathol Exp Neurol* **46:** 185–199.

Galloway PG, Perry G, Gambetti P. 1987b. Hirano bodies contain tau protein. *Brain Res* **403:** 337–340.

Geddes JW, Tekirian TL, Soultanian NS, Ashford JW, Davis DG, Markesbery WR. 1997. Comparison of neuropathologic criteria for the diagnosis of Alzheimer's disease. *Neurobiol Aging* **18:** S99–S105.

Ghoshal N, Smiley JF, DeMaggio AJ, Hoekstra MF, Cochran EJ, Binder LI, Kuret J. 1999. A new molecular link between fibrillar and granulovacuolar lesions of Alzheimer's disease. *Am J Pathol* **155:** 1163–1172.

Giannakopoulos P, Herrmann FR, Bussière T, Bouras C, Kövari E, Perl DP, Morrison JH, Gold G, Hof PR. 2003.

Tangle and neuron numbers, but not amyloid load, predict cognitive status in Alzheimer's disease. *Neurology* **60:** 1495–1500.

Gibson PH, Tomlison BE. 1977. Numbers of Hirano bodies in the hippocampus of normal and demented people with Alzheimer's disease. *J Neurol Sci* **33:** 199–206.

Glabe CC. 2005. Amyloid accumulation and pathogensis of Alzheimer's disease: Significance of monomeric, oligomeric and fibrillar Aβ. *Subcell Biochem* **38:** 167–177.

Goldman JE. 1983. The association of actin with Hirano bodies. *J Neuropathol Exp Neurol* **42:** 146–152.

Gómez-Isla T, Price JL, McKeel DW Jr, Morris JC, Growdon JH, Hyman BT. 1996. Profound loss of layer II entorhinal cortex neurons occurs in very mild Alzheimer's disease. *J Neurosci* **16:** 4491–4500.

Gómez-Isla T, Hollister R, West H, Mui S, Growdon JH, Petersen RC, Parisi JE, Hyman BT. 1997. Neuronal loss correlates with but exceeds neurofibrillary tangles in Alzheimer's disease. *Ann Neurol* **41:** 17–24.

Greenberg SG, Davies P. 1990. A preparation of Alzheimer paired helical filaments that displays distinct tau proteins by polyacrylamide gel electrophoresis. *Proc Natl Acad Sci* **87:** 5827–5831.

Greenberg SM, Vonsattel JPG. 1997. Diagnosis of cerebral amyloid angiopathy: Sensitivity and specificity of cortical biopsy. *Stroke* **28:** 1418–1422.

Greenberg SM, Gurol ME, Rosand J, Smith EE. 2004. Amyloid angiopathy-related vascular cognitive impairment. *Stroke* **35:** 2616–2619.

Grutzendler J, Helmin K, Tsai J, Gan WB. 2007. Various dendritic abnormalities are associated with fibrillar amyloid deposits in Alzheimer's disease. *Ann NY Acad Sci* **1097:** 30–39.

Guillozet AL, Weintraub S, Mash DC, Mesulam MM. 2003. Neurofibrillary tangles, amyloid, and memory in aging and mild cognitive impairment. *Arch Neurol* **60:** 729–736.

Guillozet-Bongaarts AL, García-Sierra F, Reynolds MR, Horowitz PM, Fu Y, Wang T, Cahill ME, Bigio EH, Berry RW, Binder LI. 2005. Tau truncation during neurofibrillary tangle evolution in Alzheimer's disease. *Neurobiol Aging* **26:** 1015–1022.

Haass C, Selkoe DJ. 2007. Soluble protein oligomers in neurodegeneration: Lessons from the Alzheimer's amyloid β-peptide. *Nat Rev Mol Cell Biol* **8:** 101–112.

Hamilton RL. 2000. Lewy bodies in Alzheimer's disease: A neuropathological review of 145 cases using α-synuclein immunohistochemistry. *Brain Pathol* **10:** 378–384.

Hansen L, Salmon D, Galasko D, Masliah E, Katzman R, DeTeresa R, Thal L, Pay MM, Hofstetter R, Klauber M, et al. 1990. The Lewy body variant of Alzheimer's disease: A clinical and pathologic entity. *Neurology* **40:** 1–8.

Harding AJ, Halliday GM. 2001. Cortical Lewy body pathology in the diagnosis of dementia. *Acta Neuropathol* **102:** 355–363.

Harris JA, Devidze N, Verret L, Ho K, Halabisky B, Thwin MT, Kim D, Hamto P, Lo I, Yu GQ, et al. 2010a. Transsynaptic progression of amyloid-β-induced neuronal dysfunction within the entorhinal-hippocampal network. *Neuron* **68:** 428–441.

Harris JA, Devidze N, Halabisky B, Lo I, Thwin MT, Yu GQ, Bredesen DE, Masliah E, Mucke L. 2010b. Many neuronal and behavioral impairments in transgenic mouse models of Alzheimer's disease are independent of caspase cleavage of the amyloid precursor protein. *J Neurosci* **30**: 372–381.

Hashimoto M, Hernandez-Ruiz S, Hsu L, Sisk A, Xia Y, Takeda A, Sundsmo M, Masliah E. 1998. Human recombinant NACP/α-synuclein is aggregated and fibrillated in vitro: Relevance for Lewy body disease. *Brain Res* **799**: 301–306.

Hashimoto M, Takenouchi T, Mallory M, Masliah E, Takeda A. 2000. The role of NAC in amyloidogenesis in Alzheimer's disease. *Am J Pathol* **156**: 734–736.

Hebert LE, Beckett LA, Scherr PA, Evans DA. 2001. Annual incidence of Alzheimer disease in the United States projected to the years 2000 through 2050. *Alzheimer Dis Assoc Disord* **15**: 169–173.

Higuchi M, Lee VM, Trojanowski JQ. 2002. Tau and axonopathy in neurodegenerative disorders. *Neuromolecular Med* **2**: 131–150.

Hirai K, Aliev G, Nunomura A, Fujioka H, Russell RL, Atwood CS, Johnson AB, Kress Y, Vinters HV, Tabaton M, et al. 2001. Mitochondrial abnormalities in Alzheimer's disease. *J Neurosci* **21**: 3017–3023.

Hof PR, Bussière T, Gold G, Kövari E, Giannakopoulos P, Bouras C, Perl DP, Morrison JH. 2003. Stereologic evidence for persistence of viable neurons in layer II of the entorhinal cortex and the CA1 field in Alzheimer disease. *J Neuropathol Exp Neurol* **62**: 55–67.

Hoozemans JJ, van Haastert ES, Nijholt DA, Rozemuller AJ, Eikelenboom P, Scheper W. 2009. The unfolded protein response is activated in pretangle neurons in Alzheimer's disease hippocampus. *Am J Pathol* **174**: 1241–1251.

Hyman BT, Van Hoesen GW, Damasio AR, Barnes CL. 1984. Alzheimer's disease: Cell-specific pathology isolates the hippocampal formation. *Science* **225**: 1168–1170.

Hyman BT, Van Hoesen GW, Kromer LJ, Damasio AR. 1986. Perforant pathway changes in the memory impairment of Alzheimer's disease. *Ann Neurol* **20**: 472–481.

Hyman BT, Marzloff K, Arriagada PV. 1993. The lack of accumulation of senile plaques or amyloid burden in Alzheimer's disease suggests a balance between amyloid deposition and resolution. *J Neuropathol Exp Neurol* **52**: 594–600.

Iacono D, O'Brien R, Resnick SM, Zonderman AB, Pletnikova O, Rudow G, An Y, West MJ, Crain B, Troncoso JC. 2008. Neuronal hypertrophy in asymptomatic Alzheimer disease. *J Neuropathol Exp Neurol* **67**: 578–589.

Ikegami K, Kimura T, Katsuragi S, Ono T, Yamamoto H, Miyamoto E, Miyakawa T. 1996. Immunohistochemical examination of phophorylated tau in granulovacuolar degeneration granules. *Psychiatry Clin Neurosci* **50**: 137–140.

Ingelsson M, Fukumoto H, Newell KL, Growdon JH, Hedley-Whyte ET, Frosch MP, Albert MS, Hyman BT, Irizarry MC. 2004. Early Aβ accumulation and progressive synaptic loss, gliosis, and tangle formation in AD brain. *Neurology* **62**: 925–931.

Iqbal K, Grundke-Iqbal I. 2002. Neurofibrillary pathology leads to synaptic loss and not the other way around in Alzheimer disease. *J Alzheimers Dis* **4**: 235–238.

Itagaki S, McGeer PL, Akiyama H, Zhu S, Selkoe D. 1989. Relationship of microglia and astrocytes to amyloid deposits of Alzheimer disease. *J Neuroimmunol* **24**: 173–182.

Iwai A, Masliah E, Yoshimoto M, Ge N, Flanagan L, de Silva HA, Kittel A, Saitoh T. 1995. The precursor protein of non-Aβ component of Alzheimer's disease amyloid is a presynaptic protein of the central nervous system. *Neuron* **14**: 467–475.

Jack CR Jr, Lowe VJ, Weigand SD, Wiste HJ, Senjem ML, Knopman DS, Shiung MM, Gunter JL, Boeve BF, Kemp BJ, et al. 2009. Serial PIB and MRI in normal, mild cognitive impairment and Alzheimer's disease: Implications for sequence of pathological events in Alzheimer's disease. *Brain* **132**: 1355–1365.

Janvin CC, Larsen JP, Salmon DP, Galasko D, Hugdahl K, Aarsland D. 2006. Cognitive profiles of individual patients with Parkinson's disease and dementia: Comparison with dementia with Lewy bodies and Alzheimer's disease. *Mov Disord* **21**: 337–342.

Jellinger KA, Attems J. 2006. Does striatal pathology distinguish Parkinson disease with dementia and dementia with Lewy bodies? *Acta Neuropathol* **112**: 253–260.

Jicha GA, Parisi JE, Dickson DW, Johnson K, Cha R, Ivnik RJ, Tangalos EG, Boeve BF, Knopman DS, Braak H, et al. 2006. Neuropathologic outcome of mild cognitive impairment following progression to clinical dementia. *Arch Neurol* **63**: 674–681.

Jin K, Peel AL, Mao XO, Xie L, Cottrell BA, Henshall DC, Greenberg DA. 2004. Increased hippocampal neurogenesis in Alzheimer's disease. *Proc Natl Acad Sci* **101**: 343–347.

Kahn J, Anderton BH, Probst A, Ulrich J, Esiri MM. 1985. Immunohistological study of granulovacuolar degeneration sing monoclonal antibodies to neurofilaments. *J Neurol Neurosurg Psychiatry* **48**: 924–926.

Kannanayakal TJ, Tao H, Vandre DD, Kuret J. 2006. Casein kinase-1 isoforms differentially associate with neurofibrillary and granulovauoclar degeneration lesions. *Acta Neuropathol* **111**: 413–421.

Khachaturian ZS. 1985. Diagnosis of Alzheimer's disease. *Arch Neurol* **42**: 1092–1105.

Kidd M. 1963. Paired helical filaments in electron microscopy of Alzheimer's disease. *Nature* **197**: 192–193.

Kidd M. 1964. Alzheimer's disease: An electron microscopy study. *Brain* **87**: 307–320.

Kimura T, Fukuda T, Sahara N, Yamashita S, Murayama M, Mirozoki T, Yoshiike Y, Lee B, Sotiropoulos I, Maeda S, et al. 2010. Aggregation of detergent-insoluble tau is involved in neuronal loss but not in synaptic loss. *J Biol Chem* **285**: 38692–38699.

Klein WL. 2002. Aβ toxicity in Alzheimer's disease: Globular oligomers (ADDLs) as new vaccine and drug targets. *Neurochem Int* **41**: 345–352.

Klein WL, Krafft GA, Finch CE. 2001. Targeting small Aβ oligomers: The solution to an Alzheimer's disease conundrum? *Trends Neurosci* **24**: 219–224.

Klucken J, McLean PJ, Gomez-Tortosa E, Ingelsson M, Hyman BT. 2003. Neuritic alterations and neural system dysfunction in Alzheimer's disease and dementia with Lewy bodies. *Neurochem Res* **28**: 1683–1691.

Klyubin I, Betts V, Welzel AT, Blennow K, Zetterberg H, Wallin A, Lemere CA, Cullen WK, Peng Y, Wisniewski T, et al. 2008. Amyloid β protein dimer-containing human CSF disrupts synaptic plasticity: Prevention by systemic passive immunization. *J Neurosci* **28:** 4231–4237.

Knopman DS, Parisi JE, Salviati A, Floriach-Robert M, Boeve BF, Ivnik RJ, Smith GE, Dickson DW, Johnson KA, Petersen LE, et al. 2003. Neuropathology of cognitively normal elderly. *J Neuropathol Exp Neurol* **62:** 1087–1095.

Knowles RB, Wyart C, Buldyrev SV, Cruz L, Urbanc B, Hasselmo ME, Stanley HE, Hyman BT. 1999. Plaque-induced neurite abnormalities: implications for disruption of neural networks in Alzheimer's disease. *Proc Natl Acad Sci* **96:** 5274–5279.

Knudsen KA, Rosand J, Karluk D, Greenberg SM. 2001. Clinical diagnosis of cerebral amyloid angiopathy: Validation of the Boston criteria. *Neurology* **56:** 537–539.

Koffie RM, Meyer-Luehmann M, Hashimoto T, Adams KW, Mielke ML, Garcia-Alloza M, Micheva KD, Smith SJ, Kim ML, Lee VM, et al. 2009. Oligomeric amyloid β associates with postsynaptic densities and correlates with excitatory synapse loss near senile plaques. *Proc Natl Acad Sci* **106:** 4012–4017.

Kramer ML, Schulz-Schaeffer WJ. 2007. Presynaptic α-synuclein aggregates, not Lewy bodies, cause neurodegeneration in dementia with Lewy bodies. *J Neurosci* **27:** 1405–1410.

Lacor PN, Buniel MC, Furlow PW, Clemente AS, Velasco PT, Wood M, Viola KL, Klein WL. 2007. Aβ oligomer-induced aberrations in synapse composition, shape, and density provide a molecular basis for loss of connectivity in Alzheimer's disease. *J Neurosci* **27:** 796–807.

LaFerla F, Tinkle B, Bieberich C, Haudenschild C, Jay G. 1995. The Alzheimer's Aβ peptide induces neurodegeneration and apoptotic cell death in transgenic mice. *Nat Genet* **9:** 21–30.

Lagalwar S, Berry RW, Binder LI. 2007. Regulation of hippocampal phospho-SAPK/JNK granules in Alzheimer's disease and tauopathies to granulovacuolar degeneration bodies. *Acta Neuropathol* **113:** 63–73.

Lambert MP, Barlow AK, Chromy BA, Edwards C, Freed R, Liosatos M, Morgan TE, Rozovsky I, Trommer B, Viola KL, et al. 1998. Diffusible, nonfibrillar ligands derived from Aβ1–42 are potent central nervous system neurotoxins. *Proc Natl Acad Sci* **95:** 6448–6453.

Lashuel HA, Petre BM, Wall J, Simon M, Nowak RJ, Walz T, Lansbury PT Jr. 2002. α-synuclein, especially the Parkinson's disease-associated mutants, forms pore-like annular and tubular protofibrils. *J Mol Biol* **322:** 1089–1102.

Lee SC, Zhao ML, Hirano A, Dickson DW. 1999. Inducible nitric oxide synthase immunoreactivity in the Alzheimer disease hippocampus: Association with Hirano bodies, neurofibrillary tangles, and senile plaques. *J Neuropathol Exp Neurol* **58:** 1163–1169.

Lee VM, Goedert M, Trojanowski JQ. 2001. Neurodegenerative tauopathies. *Annu Rev Neurosci* **24:** 1121–1159.

Leroy K, Boutajangout A, Authelet M, Woodgett JR, Anderton BH, Brion JP. 2002. The active form of glycogen synthase kinase-3β is associated with granulovacuolar degeneration in neurons in Alzheimer's disease. *Acta Neuropathol* **103:** 91–99.

Lesne S, Koh MT, Kotilinek L, Kayed R, Glabe CG, Yang A, Gallagher M, Ashe KH. 2006. A specific amyloid-β protein assembly in the brain impairs memory. *Nature* **440:** 352–357.

Leverenz JB, Fishel MA, Peskind ER, Montine TJ, Nochlin D, Steinbart E, Raskind MA, Schellenberg GD, Bird TD, Tsuang D. 2006. Lewy body pathology in familial Alzheimer disease: Evidence for disease- and mutation-specific pathologic phenotype. *Arch Neurol* **63:** 370–376.

Li B, Yamamori H, Tatebayashi Y, Shafit-Zagardo B, Tanimukai H, Chen S, Iqbal K, Grundke-Iqbal I. 2008. Failure of neuronal maturation in Alzheimer disease dentate gyrus. *J Neuropathol Exp Neurol* **67:** 78–84.

Lippa CF, Hamos JE, Pulaski-Salo D, DeGennaro LJ, Drachman DA. 1992. Alzheimer's disease and aging: Effects on perforant pathway perikarya and synapses. *Neurobiol Aging* **13:** 405–411.

Lippa CF, Fujiwara H, Mann DM, Giasson B, Baba M, Schmidt ML, Nee LE, O'Connell B, Pollen DA, St George-Hyslop P, et al. 1998. Lewy bodies contain altered α-synuclein in brains of many familial Alzheimer's disease patients with mutations in presenilin and amyloid precursor protein genes. *Am J Pathol* **153:** 1365–1370.

Lippa CF, Schmidt ML, Lee VM, Trojanowski JQ. 1999. Antibodies to α-synuclein detect Lewy bodies in many Down's syndrome brains with Alzheimer's disease. *Ann Neurol* **45:** 353–357.

Lippa CF, Duda JE, Grossman M, Hurtig HI, Aarsland D, Boeve BF, Brooks DJ, Dickson DW, Dubois B, Emre M, et al. 2007. DLB and PDD boundary issues: Diagnosis, treatment, molecular pathology, and biomarkers. *Neurology* **68:** 812–819.

Litvan I, MacIntyre A, Goetz CG, Wenning GK, Jellinger K, Verny M, Bartko JJ, Jankovic J, McKee A, Brandel JP, et al. 1998. Accuracy of the clinical diagnoses of Lewy body disease, Parkinson disease, and dementia with Lewy bodies: A clinicopathologic study. *Arch Neurol* **55:** 969–978.

Lue LF, Brachova L, Civin WH, Rogers J. 1996. Inflammation, Aβ deposition, and neurofibrillary tangle formation as correlates of Alzheimer's disease neurodegeneration. *J Neuropathol Exp Neurol* **55:** 1083–1088.

Maciver SK, Harrington CR. 1995. Two actin binding proteins, actin depolymerizing factor and cofilin, are associated with Hirano bodies. *Neuroreport* **6:** 1985–1988.

Mandal PK, Pettegrew JW, Masliah E, Hamilton RL, Mandal R. 2006. Interaction between Aβ peptide and α synuclein: Molecular mechanisms in overlapping pathology of Alzheimer's and Parkinson's in dementia with Lewy body disease. *Neurochem Res* **31:** 1153–1162.

Mandelkow EM, Mandelkow E. 1998. Tau in Alzheimer's disease. *Trends Cell Biol* **8:** 425–427.

Markesbery WR, Schmitt FA, Kryscio RJ, Davis DG, Smith CD, Wekstein DR. 2006. Neuropathologic substrate of mild cognitive impairment. *Arch Neurol* **63:** 38–46.

Masliah E. 2000. The role of synaptic proteins in Alzheimer's disease. *Ann NY Acad Sci* **924:** 68–75.

Masliah E, Terry R. 1993. The role of synaptic proteins in the pathogenesis of disorders of the central nervous system. *Brain Pathol* **3:** 77–85.

Masliah E, Terry R. 1994. The role of synaptic pathology in the mechanisms of dementia in Alzheimer's disease. *Clin Neurosci* **1:** 192–198.

Masliah E, Terry RD, Mallory M, Alford M, Hansen LA. 1990. Diffuse plaques do not accentuate synapse loss in Alzheimer's disease. *Am J Pathol* **137:** 1293–1297.

Masliah E, Mallory M, Hansen L, Alford M, Albright T, Terry R, Shapiro P, Sundsmo M, Saitoh T. 1991. Immunoreactivity of CD45, a protein phosphotyrosine phosphatase, in Alzheimer disease. *Acta Neuropathol* **83:** 12–20.

Masliah E, Mallory M, DeTeresa R, Alford M, Hansen L. 1993a. Differing patterns of aberrant neuronal sprouting in Alzheimer's disease with and without Lewy bodies. *Brain Res* **617:** 258–266.

Masliah E, Mallory M, Hansen L, DeTeresa R, Terry RD. 1993b. Quantitative synaptic alterations in the human neocortex during normal aging. *Neurology* **43:** 192–197.

Masliah E, Mallory M, Hansen L, DeTeresa R, Alford M, Terry R. 1994. Synaptic and neuritic alterations during the progression of Alzheimer's disease. *Neurosci Lett* **174:** 67–72.

Masliah E, Mallory M, Alford M, DeTeresa R, Hansen LA, McKeel DW Jr, Morris JC. 2001a. Altered expression of synaptic proteins occurs early during progression of Alzheimer's disease. *Neurology* **56:**127–129.

Masliah E, Rockenstein E, Veinbergs I, Sagara Y, Mallory M, Hashimoto M, Mucke L. 2001b. β-amyloid peptides enhance α-synuclein accumulation and neuronal deficits in a transgenic mouse model linking Alzheimer's disease and Parkinson's disease. *Proc Natl Acad Sci* **98:** 12245–12250.

Masliah E, Alford M, Adame A, Rockenstein E, Galasko D, Salmon D, Hansen LA, Thal LJ. 2003. Aβ1–42 promotes cholinergic sprouting in patients with AD and Lewy body variant of AD. *Neurology* **61:** 206–211.

McDonald JM, Savva GM, Brayne C, Welzel AT, Forster G, Shankar GM, Selkoe DJ, Ince PG, Walsh DM. 2010. The presence of sodium dodecyl sulphate-stable Aβ dimers is strongly associated with Alzheimer-type dementia. *Brain* **133:** 1328–1341.

McKeith IG. 2000. Spectrum of Parkinson's disease, Parkinson's dementia, and Lewy body dementia. *Neurol Clin* **18:** 865–902.

McKeith IG. 2006. Consensus guidelines for the clinical and pathologic diagnosis of dementia with Lewy bodies (DLB): Report of the Consortium on DLB International Workshop. *J Alzheimers Dis* **9:** 417–423.

McKeith IG, Galasko D, Kosaka K, Perry EK, Dickson DW, Hansen LA, Salmon DP, Lowe J, Mirra SS, Byrne EJ, et al. 1996. Consensus guidelines for the clinical and pathologic diagnosis of dementia with Lewy bodies (DLB): Report of the consortium on DLB international workshop. *Neurology* **47:** 1113–1124.

McKeith IG, Dickson DW, Lowe J, Emre M, O'Brien JT, Feldman H, Cummings J, Duda JE, Lippa C, Perry EK, et al. 2005. Diagnosis and management of dementia with Lewy bodies: Third report of the DLB consortium. *Neurology* **65:** 1863–1872.

Mena R, Robitaille Y, Cuello AC. 1992. New patterns of intraneuronal accumulation of the microtubular binding domain of tau in granulovacuolar degeneration. *J Geriatr Psychiatry Neurol* **5:** 132–141.

Mirra SS, Heyman A, McKeel D, Sumi SM, Crain BJ, Brownlee LM, Vogel FS, Hughes JP, van Belle G, Berg L. 1991. The Consortium to Establish a Registry for Alzheimer's Disease (CERAD). Part II. Standardization of the neuropathological assessment of Alzheimer's disease. *Neurology* **41:** 479–486.

Mirra SS, Gearing M, Nash F. 1997. Neuropathological assessment of Alzheimer's disease. *Neurology* **49:** S14–S16.

Münch G, Cunningham AM, Riederer P, Braak E. 1998. Advance glycation endproducts are associated with Hirano bodies in Alzheimer's disease. *Brain Res* **796:** 307–310.

Muñoz DG, Wang D, Greenberg BD. 1993. Hirano bodies accumulate C-terminal sequences of β-amyloid precursor protein (β-APP) epitopes. *J Neuropathol Exp Neurol* **52:** 14–21.

Neuropathology Group of the Medical Research Council Cognitive Function and Aging Study (MRC CFAS). 2001. Pathological correlates of late-onset dementia in a multicenter community-based population in England and Wales. *Lancet* **357:** 169–175.

Nixon RA, Cataldo AM. 2006. Lysosomal system pathways: Genes to neurodegeneration in Alzheimer's disease. *J Alzheimers Dis* **9:** 277–289.

Okamoto K, Hirai S, Iizuka T, Yanagisawa T, Watanabe M. 1991. Reexamination of granulovacuolar degeneration. *Acta Neuropathol* **82:** 340–345.

Olichney JM, Hansen LA, Hoffstetter CR, Lee JH, Katzman R, Thal LJ. 2000. Association between severe cerebral amyloid angiopathy and cerebrovascular lesions in Alzheimer disease is not a spurious one attributable to apolipoprotein E4. *Arch Neurol* **57:** 869–874.

Palop JJ, Jones B, Kekonius L, Chin J, Yu GQ, Raber J, Masliah E, Mucke L. 2003. Neuronal depletion of calcium-dependent proteins in the dentate gyrus is tightly linked to Alzheimer's disease-related cognitive deficits. *Proc Natl Acad Sci* **100:** 9572–9577.

Palop JJ, Mucke L, Roberson ED. 2011. Quantifying biomarkers of cognitive dysfunction and neuronal network hyperexcitability in mouse models of Alzheimer's disease: Depletion of calcium-dependent proteins and inhibitory hippocampal remodeling. *Methods Mol Biol* **670:** 245–262.

Pérez-Gracia E, Torrejón-Escribano B, Ferrer I. 2008. Dystrophic neurites of senile plaques in Alzheimer's disease are deficient in cytochrome c oxidase. *Acta Neuropathol* **116:** 261–268.

Perlson E, Maday S, Fu MM, Moughamian AJ, Holzbaur EL. 2010. Retrograde axonal transport: Pathways to cell death? *Trends Neurosci* **33:** 335–344

Perry EK, Tomlinson BE, Blessed G, Bergmann K, Gibson PH, Perry RH. 1978. Correlation of cholinergic abnormalities with senile plaques and mental test scores in senile dementia. *Br Med J* **2:** 1457–1459.

Petersen RC. 2004. Mild cognitive impairment as a diagnostic entity. *J Intern Med* **256:** 183–194.

Petersen RC, Smith GE, Waring SC, Ivnik RJ, Tangalos EG, Kokmen E. 1999. Mild cognitive impairment: Clinical characterization and outcome. *Arch Neurol* **56:** 303–308.

Cite this article as *Cold Spring Harb Perspect Med* doi: 10.1101/cshperspect.a006189

Petersen RC, Doody R, Kurz A, Mohs RC, Morris JC, Rabins PV, Ritchie K, Rossor M, Thal L, Winblad B. 2001. Current concepts in mild cognitive impairment. *Arch Neurol* **58:** 1985–1992

Petersen RC, Parisi JE, Dickson DW, Johnson KA, Knopman DS, Boeve BF, Jicha GA, Ivnik RJ, Smith GE, Tangalos EG, et al. 2006. Neuropathologic features of amnestic mild cognitive impairment. *Arch Neurol* **63:** 665–672.

Pfeifer LA, White LR, Ross GW, Petrovich H, Launer LJ. 2002. Cerebral amyloid angiopathy and cognitive function: The HAAS autopsy study. *Neurology* **58:** 1629–1634.

Pham E, Crews L, Ubhi K, Hansen L, Adame A, Cartier A, Salmon D, Galasko D, Michael S, Savas JN, et al. 2010. Progressive accumulation of amyloid-β oligomers in Alzheimer's disease and in amyloid precursor protein transgenic mice is accompanied by selective alterations in synaptic scaffold proteins. *FEBS J* **277:** 3051–3067.

Pike CJ, Cummings BJ, Cotman CW. 1995. Early association of reactive astrocytes with senile plaques in Alzheimer's disease. *Exp Neurol* **132:** 172–179.

Pletnikova O, West N, Lee MK, Rudow GL, Skolasky RL, Dawson TM, Marsh L, Troncoso JC. 2005. Aβ deposition is associated with enhanced cortical α-synuclein lesions in Lewy body diseases. *Neurobiol Aging* **26:** 1183–1192.

Price DL, Altschuler RJ, Struble RG, Casanova MF, Cork LC, Murphy DB. 1986. Sequestration of tubulin in neurons in Alzheimer's disease. *Brain Res* **385:** 305–310.

Price JL, Ko AI, Wade MJ, Tsou SK, McKeel DW, Morris JC. 2001. Neuron number in the entorhinal cortex and CA1 in preclinical Alzheimer disease. *Arch Neurol* **58:** 1395–1402.

Price JL, McKeel DW Jr, Buckles VD, Roe CM, Xiong C, Grundman M, Hansen LA, Petersen RC, Parisi JE, Dickson DW, et al. 2009. Neuropathology of nondemented aging: Presumptive evidence for preclinical Alzheimer disease. *Neurobiol Aging* **30:** 1026–1036.

Riudavets MA, Iacono D, Resnick SM, O'Brien R, Zonderman AB, Martin LJ, Rudow G, Pletnikova O, Troncoso JC. 2007. Resistance to Alzheimer's pathology is associated with nuclear hypertrophy in neurons. *Neurobiol Aging* **28:** 1484–1492.

Rockenstein E, Schwach G, Ingolic E, Adame A, Crews L, Mante M, Pfragner R, Schreiner E, Windisch M, Masliah E. 2005. Lysosomal pathology associated with alpha-synuclein accumulation in transgenic models using an eGFP fusion protein. *J Neurosci Res* **80:** 247–259.

Rogers J, Luber-Narod J, Styren S, Civin W. 1988. Expression of immune system-associated antigens by cells of the human central nervous system: Relationship to the pathology of Alzheimer's disease. *Neurobiol Aging* **9:** 339–349.

Rosenberg RN. 2005. New presenilin 1 mutation with Alzheimer disease and Lewy bodies. *Arch Neurol* **62:** 1808.

Rossiter JP, Anderson LL, Yang F, Cole GM. 2000. Caspase-cleaved actin (fractin) immunolabeling of Hirano bodies. *Neuropathol Appl Neurobiol* **26:** 342–346.

Scheff SW, Price DA. 1993. Synapse loss in the temporal lobe in Alzheimer's disease. *Ann Neurol* **33:** 190–199.

Scheff SW, DeKosky ST, Price DA. 1990. Quantitative assessment of cortical synaptic density in Alzheimer's disease. *Neurobiol Aging* **11:** 29–37.

Scheff SW, Price DA, Schmitt FA, Mufson EJ. 2006. Hippocampal synaptic loss in early Alzheimer's disease and mild cognitive impairment. *Neurobiol Aging* **27:** 1372–1384.

Scheff SW, Price DA, Schmitt FA, DeKosky ST, Mufson EJ. 2007. Synaptic alterations in CA1 in mild Alzheimer disease and mild cognitive impairment. *Neurology* **68:** 1501–1508.

Schmidt ML, Lee VM, Trojanowski JQ. 1989. Analyses of epitopes shared by Hirano bodies and neurofilament proteins in normal and Alzheimer's disease hippocampus. *Lab Invest* **60:** 513–522.

Schmitt FA, Davis DG, Wekstein DR, Smith CD, Ashford JW, Markesbery WR. 2000. "Preclinical" AD revisited. Neuropathology of cognitively normal older adults. *Neurology* **55:** 370–376.

Schneider JA, Arvanitakis Z, Bang W, Bennet DA. 2007. Mixed brain pathologies account for most dementia cases in community-dwelling older persons. *Neurology* **69:** 2197–2204.

Schneider JA, Arvanitakis Z, Leurgans SE, Bennet DA. 2009. The neuropathology of probable Alzheimer's disease and mild cognitive impairment. *Ann Neurol* **66:** 200–208.

Scott DA, Tabarean I, Tang Y, Cartier A, Masliah E, Roy S. 2010. A pathologic cascade leading to synaptic dysfunction in α-synuclein-induced neurodegeneration. *J Neurosci* **30:** 8083–8095.

Selkoe D. 1989. Amyloid β protein precursor and the pathogenesis of Alzheimer's disease. *Cell* **58:** 611–612.

Selkoe D. 1990. Amyloid β-protein deposition as a seminal pathogenic event in AD: An hypothesis. *Neurobiol Aging* **11:** 299.

Selkoe D. 1993. Physiological production of the β-amyloid protein and the mechanisms of Alzheimer's disease. *Trends Neurosci* **16:** 403–409.

Selkoe DJ. 2008. Soluble oligomers of the amyloid β-protein impair synaptic plasticity and behavior. *Behav Brain Res* **192:** 106–113.

Selznick LA, Holtzman DM, Han BH, Gökden M, Srinivasan AN, Johnson EM Jr, Roth KA. 1999. In situ immunodetection of neuronal caspase-3 activation in Alzheimer disease. *J Neuropathol Exp Neurol* **58:** 1020–1026.

Serrano-Pozo A, Mielke ML, Gómez-Isla E, Betensky RA, Growdon JH, Frosch MP, Hyman BT. 2011. Reactive glia not only associates with plaques but also parallels tangles in Alzheimer's disease. *Am J Pathol* **179.** doi: 10.1016/j.ajpath.2011.05.047.

Shankar GM, Li S, Mehta TH, García-Munoz A, Shepardson NE, Smith I, Brett FM, Farrell MA, Rowan MJ, Lemere CA, et al. 2008. Amyloid-beta protein dimers isolated directly from Alzheimer's brains impair synaptic plasticity and memory. *Nat Med* **14:** 837–842.

Sisodia SS, Price DL. 1995. Role of the β-amyloid protein in Alzheimer's disease. *FASEB J* **9:** 366–370.

Skovronsky DM, Doms RW, Lee VM-Y. 1998. Detection of a novel intraneuronal pool of insoluble amyloid β-protein that accumulates with time in culture. *J Cell Biol* **141:** 1031–1039.

Smith MA, Perry G, Richey PL, Sayre LM, Anderson VE, Beal MF, Kowall N. 1996. Oxidative damage in Alzheimer's. *Nature* **382:** 120–121.

Snider BJ, Norton J, Coats MA, Chakraverty S, Hou CE, Jervis R, Lendon CL, Goate AM, McKeel DW Jr, Morris JC. 2005. Novel presenilin 1 mutation (S170F) causing Alzheimer disease with Lewy bodies in the third decade of life. *Arch Neurol* **62:** 1821–1830.

Spillantini M, Schmidt M, Lee V-Y, Trojanowski J, Jakes R, Goedert M. 1997. α-Synuclein in Lewy bodies. *Nature* **388:** 839–840.

Spires-Jones TL, de Calignon A, Matsui T, Zehr C, Pitstick R, Wu HY, Osetek JD, Jones PB, Bacskai BJ, Feany MB, et al. 2007. In vivo imaging reveals dissociation between caspase activation and acute neuronal death in tangle-bearing neurons. *J Neurosci* **28:** 862–867.

Stadelmann C, Deckwerth TL, Srinivasan A, Bancher C, Brück W, Jellinger K, Lassmann H. 1999. Activation of caspase-3 in single neurons and autophagic vacuoles of granulovacuolar degeneration in Alzheimer's disease. Evidence for apoptotic cell death. *Am J Pathol* **155:** 1459–1466.

Su JH, Cummings BJ, Cotman CW. 1993. Identification and distribution of axonal dystrophic neurites in Alzheimer's disease. *Brain Res* **625:** 228–237.

Su JH, Cummings BJ, Cotman CW. 1994. Subpopulations of dystrophic neuritis in Alzheimer's brain with distinct immunocytochemical and argentophilic characteristics. *Brain Res* **637:** 37–44.

Su JH, Cummings BJ, Cotman CW. 1996. Plaque biogenesis in brain aging and Alzheimer's disease. I. Progressive changes in phosphorylation states of paired helical filaments and neurofilaments. *Brain Res* **739:** 79–87.

Su JH, Cummings BJ, Cotman CW. 1998. Plaque biogenesis in brain aging and Alzheimer's disease. II. Progressive transformation and developmental sequence of dystrophic neurites. *Acta Neuropathol* **96:** 463–471.

Su JH, Zhao M, Anderson AJ, Srinivasan A, Cotman CW. 2001. Activated-caspase-3 expression in Alzheimer's and aged control brain: Correlation with Alzheimer pathology. *Brain Res* **898:** 350–357.

Su JH, Kesslak JP, Head E, Cotman CW. 2002. Caspase-cleaved amyloid precursor protein and activated caspase-3 are co-localized in the granules of granulovacuolar degeneration in Alzheimer's disease and Down's syndrome brain. *Acta Neuropathol* **104:** 1–6.

Takeda A, Mallory M, Sundsmo M, Honer W, Hansen L, Masliah E. 1998. Abnormal accumulation of NACP/α-synuclein in neurodegenerative disorders. *Am J Pathol* **152:** 367–372.

Teipel SJ, Flatz WH, Heinsen H, Bokde AL, Schoenberg SO, Stockel S, Dietrich O, Reiser MF, Moller HJ, Hampel H. 2005. Measurement of basal forebrain atrophy in Alzheimer's disease using MRI. *Brain* **128:** 2626–2644.

Terry R, Peck A, DeTeresa R, Schechter R, Horoupian D. 1981. Some morphometric aspects of the brain in senile dementia of the Alzheimer type. *Ann Neurol* **10:** 184–192.

Terry RD, Masliah E, Salmon DP, Butters N, DeTeresa R, Hill R, Hansen LA, Katzman R. 1991. Physical basis of cognitive alterations in Alzheimer's disease: Synapse loss is the major correlate of cognitive impairment. *Ann Neurol* **30:** 572–580.

Terry R, Hansen L, Masliah E. 1994. Structural basis of the cognitive alterations in Alzheimer disease. In *Alzheimer disease* (ed. R. Terry, R. Katzman), pp. 179–196. Raven, New York.

Thakur A, Wang X, Siedlak SL, Perry G, Smith MA, Zhu X. 2007. c-Jun phosphorylation in Alzheimer disease. *J Neurosci Res* **85:** 1668–1673.

Thal DR, Rüb U, Orantes M, Braak H. 2002. Phases of Aβ-deposition in the human brain and its relevance for the development of AD. *Neurology* **58:** 1791–1800.

The National Institute of Aging, and Reagan Institute working group on the diagnostic criteria for the neuropathological assessment of Alzheimer's disease. 1997. Consensus recommendations for the postmortem diagnosis of Alzheimer's disease. *Neurobiol Aging* **18:** S1–S2.

Townsend M, Shankar GM, Mehta T, Walsh DM, Selkoe DJ. 2006. Effects of secreted oligomers of amyloid β-protein on hippocampal synaptic plasticity: A potent role for trimers. *J Physiol* **572:** 477–492.

Trojanowski JQ, Lee VM. 1998. Aggregation of neurofilament and α-synuclein proteins in Lewy bodies: Implications for the pathogenesis of Parkinson disease and Lewy body dementia. *Arch Neurol* **55:** 151–152.

Trojanowski JQ, Lee VM. 2000. "Fatal attractions" of proteins. A comprehensive hypothetical mechanism underlying Alzheimer's disease and other neurodegenerative disorders. *Ann NY Acad Sci* **924:** 62–67.

Trojanowski JQ, Goedert M, Iwatsubo T, Lee VM. 1998. Fatal attractions: Abnormal protein aggregation and neuron death in Parkinson's disease and Lewy body dementia. *Cell Death Differ* **5:** 832–837.

Troncoso JC, Sukhov RR, Kawas CH, Koliatsos VE. 1996. In situ labeling of dying cortical neurons in normal aging and in Alzheimer's disease: Correlations with senile plaques and disease progression. *J Neuropathol Exp Neurol* **55:** 1134–1142.

Tsigelny IF, Bar-On P, Sharikov Y, Crews L, Hashimoto M, Miller MA, Keller SH, Platoshyn O, Yuan JX, Masliah E. 2007. Dynamics of α-synuclein aggregation and inhibition of pore-like oligomer development by β-synuclein. *FEBS J* **274:** 1862–1877.

Tsigelny IF, Crews L, Desplats P, Shaked GM, Sharikov Y, Mizuno H, Spencer B, Rockenstein E, Trejo M, Platoshyn O, et al. 2008. Mechanisms of hybrid oligomer formation in the pathogenesis of combined Alzheimer's and Parkinson's diseases. *PLoS One* **3:** e3135.

Tsuboi Y, Dickson DW. 2005. Dementia with Lewy bodies and Parkinson's disease with dementia: Are they different? *Parkinsonism Relat Disord* **11:** S47–S51.

Uboga NV, Price JL. 2000. Formation of diffuse and fibrillar tangles in aging and early Alzheimer's disease. *Neurobiol Aging* **21:** 1–10.

Urbanc B, Cruz L, Le R, Sanders J, Hsiao-Ashe K, Stanley HE, Irizarry MC, Hyman BT. 2002. Neurotoxic effects of thioflavin S-positive amyloid deposits in transgenic mice and Alzheimer's disease. *Proc Natl Acad Sci* **99:** 13990–13995.

Vehmas AK, Kawas CH, Stewart WF, Troncoso JC. 2003. Immune reactive cells in senile plaques and cognitive decline in Alzheimer's disease. *Neurobiol Aging* **24:** 321–331.

Wakabayashi K, Matsumoto K, Takayama K, Yoshimoto M, Takahashi H. 1997. NACP, a presynaptic protein, immunoreactivity in Lewy bodies in Parkinson's disease. *Neurosci Lett* **239:** 45–48.

Walsh DM, Selkoe DJ. 2004. Oligomers on the brain: The emerging role of soluble protein aggregates in neurodegeneration. *Protein Pept Lett* **11:** 213–228.

Walsh DM, Klyubin I, Fadeeva JV, Cullen WK, Anwyl R, Wolfe MS, Rowan MJ, Selkoe DJ. 2002. Naturally secreted oligomers of amyloid β protein potently inhibit hippocampal long-term potentiation in vivo. *Nature* **416:** 535–539.

Weaver CL, Espinoza M, Kress Y, Davies P. 2000. Conformational change as one of the earliest alterations of tau in Alzheimer's disease. *Neurobiol Aging* **21:** 719–727.

Wegmann S, Jung YJ, Chinnathambi S, Mandelkow EM, Mandelkow E, Muller DJ. 2010. Human tau isoforms assemble into ribbon-like fibrils that display polymorphic structure and stability. *J Biol Chem* **285:** 27302–27313.

West MJ, Kawas CH, Stewart WF, Rudow GL, Troncoso JC. 2004. Hippocampal neurons in pre-clinical Alzheimer's disease. *Neurobiol Aging* **25:** 1205–1212.

Wisniewski HM, Narang HK, Terry RD. 1976. Neurofibrillary tangles of paired helical filaments. *J Neurol Sci* **27:** 173–181.

Woodhouse A, Vickers JC, Dickson TC. 2006a. Cytoplasmic cytochrome c immunolabeling in dystrophic neurites in Alzheimer's disease. *Acta Neuropathol* **112:** 429–437.

Woodhouse A, Dickson TC, West AK, McLean CA, Vickers JC. 2006b. No difference in expression of apoptosis-related proteins and apoptotic morphology in control, pathologically aged and Alzheimer's disease cases. *Neurobiol Dis* **22:** 323–333.

Xu M, Shibayama H, Kobayashi H, Yamada K, Ishihara R, Zhao P, Takeuchi T, Yoshida K, Inagaki T, Nokura K. 1992. Granulovacuolar degeneration in the hippocampal cortex of aging and demented patients: A quantitative study. *Acta Neuropathol* **85:** 1–9.

Yamazaki Y, Takahashi T, Hiji M, Kurashige T, Izumi Y, Yamawaki T, Matsumoto M. 2010. Immunopositivity for ESCRT-III subunit CHMP2B in granulovacuolar degeneration of neurons in the Alzheimer's disease hippocampus. *Neurosci Lett* **477:** 86–90.

Yoshiyama Y, Higucho M, Zhang B, Huang SM, Iwata N, Saido TC, Maeda J, Suhara T, Trojanowski JQ, Lee VM. 2007. Synapse loss and microglial activation precede tangles in a P301S tauopathy mouse model. *J Neuron* **53:** 337–351.

Zhu X, Raina AK, Rottkamp CA, Aliev G, Perry G, Boux H, Smith MA. 2001. Activation and redistribution of c-jun N-terminal kinase/stress activated protein kinase in degenerating neurons in Alzheimer's disease. *J Neurochem* **76:** 435–441.

Brain Imaging in Alzheimer Disease

Keith A. Johnson[1], Nick C. Fox[2], Reisa A. Sperling[3], and William E. Klunk[4]

[1]Departments of Radiology and Neurology, Massachusetts General Hospital, Brigham and Women's Hospital, Harvard Medical School, Boston, Massachusetts 02114

[2]Dementia Research Centre, UCL Institute of Neurology, University College, London WCIN 3AR, United Kingdom

[3]Center for Alzheimer Research and Treatment, Brigham and Women's Hospital, Massachusetts General Hospital, Harvard Medical School, Boston, Massachusetts 02115

[4]Departments of Psychiatry and Neurology, University of Pittsburgh School of Medicine, Pittsburgh, Pennsylvania 15213

Correspondence: klunkwe@upmc.edu

Imaging has played a variety of roles in the study of Alzheimer disease (AD) over the past four decades. Initially, computed tomography (CT) and then magnetic resonance imaging (MRI) were used diagnostically to rule out other causes of dementia. More recently, a variety of imaging modalities including structural and functional MRI and positron emission tomography (PET) studies of cerebral metabolism with fluoro-deoxy-D-glucose (FDG) and amyloid tracers such as Pittsburgh Compound-B (PiB) have shown characteristic changes in the brains of patients with AD, and in prodromal and even presymptomatic states that can help rule-in the AD pathophysiological process. No one imaging modality can serve all purposes as each have unique strengths and weaknesses. These modalities and their particular utilities are discussed in this article. The challenge for the future will be to combine imaging biomarkers to most efficiently facilitate diagnosis, disease staging, and, most importantly, development of effective disease-modifying therapies.

THE CHANGING ROLES AND SCOPE OF NEUROIMAGING IN ALZHEIMER DISEASE

There has been a transformation in the part played by neuroimaging in Alzheimer disease (AD) research and practice in the last decades. Diagnostically, imaging has moved from a minor exclusionary role to a central position. In research, imaging is helping address many of the scientific questions outlined in Selkow et al. (2011): providing insights into the effects of AD and its temporal and spatial evolution. Furthermore, imaging is an established tool in drug discovery, increasingly required in therapeutic trials as part of inclusion criteria, as a safety marker, and as an outcome measure.

Concomitantly the potential of brain imaging has expanded rapidly with new modalities and novel ways of acquiring images and of analysing them. This article cannot be comprehensive. Instead, it addresses broad categories of structural, functional, and molecular imaging in AD. The specific modalities included are magnetic resonance imaging (MRI; both structural and functional) and positron emission tomography (PET; for assessment of both cerebral metabolism and amyloid). These modalities have different strengths and limitations and as a result have different and often complementary roles and scope.

Imaging in the Diagnosis and Prognosis of AD

The uncertainty inherent in a clinical diagnosis of AD has driven a search for diagnostic imaging markers. A definitive diagnosis still requires histopathological confirmation and the inaccessibility of the brain means imaging has a key role as a "window on the brain." Historically, imaging—first computed tomography (CT) and then MRI—was used only to exclude potentially surgically treatable causes of cognitive decline. Now its position in diagnosis also includes providing positive support for a clinical diagnosis of AD in symptomatic individuals by identifying characteristic patterns (signatures) of structural and functional cerebral alterations. We can now also visualize the specific molecular pathology of the disease—amyloid deposits—with amyloid imaging. Alongside this increasing specificity for AD, imaging also contributes to differential diagnosis in practice by identifying alternative and/or contributory pathologies. Imaging is central to identifying vascular and non-AD degenerative pathologies and has helped in the recognition of the prevalence of mixed pathology in dementia.

In the setting of mild cognitive impairment (MCI) (Petersen 2004), the determination of underlying pathology carries immediate prognostic importance. Only a fraction of patients with MCI progress to clinical AD over 5–10 years (Petersen et al. 1999; Ritchie et al. 2001; Visser et al. 2006) and a recent meta-analysis concluded that most people with MCI will not progress to dementia even after 10 years of follow-up (Mitchell and Shiri-Feshki 2009). Two community-based studies have shown over one-third of patients diagnosed with MCI at baseline may eventually return to normal cognition (Larrieu et al. 2002; Ganguli

et al. 2004). Obviously, it would be of great value to be able to predict which MCI subjects were destined to progress to a clinical diagnosis of AD. This is true even in the absence of disease-modifying treatments, but will be especially critical when disease-modifying treatments become available.

Looking to the future, imaging has helped establish that there is a long preclinical and presymptomatic period where the pathological effects of AD are detectable. Although more data are needed, imaging is starting to provide prognostic information at this early preclinical stage. The need for an earlier and more certain diagnosis will only increase as disease-modifying therapies are identified. This will be particularly true if, as expected, these therapies work best (or only) when initiated at the preclinical stage.

Understanding the Biology of AD

Importantly, imaging has a major role to play in improving our understanding of this disease (or diseases). Uniquely, imaging is able to delineate in life the location within the brain of the effects of AD. Together with this topographical information imaging can quantify multiple different aspects of AD pathology and assess how they relate to each other and how they change over time. The clinical correlations of these changes and their relationships to other biomarkers and to prognosis can be studied. Ultimately the role of imaging in improving our understanding of the biology of AD underpins all its applications and is a theme that runs through the following sections of this article.

STRUCTURAL MRI IN AD

Basics of Structural MRI as Applied to AD

MRI utilizes the fact that protons have angular momentum which is polarized in a magnetic field. This means that a pulse of radiofrequency can alter the energy state of protons and, when the pulse is turned off, the protons will, on returning to their energy stage, emit a radiofrequency signal. By a combination of different gradients and pulses, "sequences" can be designed to be sensitive to different tissue characteristics. In broad terms structural MRI in AD can be divided into assessing atrophy (or volumes) and changes in tissue characteristics which cause signal alterations on certain sequences such as white matter hyperintensities on T2-weighted MRI as a result of vascular damage. A number of MR sequences that are sensitive to microstructural change (e.g., magnetization transfer or diffusion) have shown alterations in AD. These sequences are already important research tools; however, they have not yet found a place in routine clinical practice in AD and they will not be considered further here.

Utility of Structural MRI in the Study of AD

Atrophy in AD

Progressive cerebral atrophy is a characteristic feature of neurodegeneration that can be visualized in life with MRI (best with T1-weighted volumetric sequences; see Fig. 1). The major contributors to atrophy are thought to be

dendritic and neuronal losses. Studies of regional (e.g., hippocampal) MRI volumes have shown these are closely related to neuronal counts at autopsy (Bobinski et al. 2000; Gosche et al. 2002; Jack et al. 2002). The pattern of loss differs between diseases reflecting selective neuronal vulnerability and/or regional disease expression. AD is characterized by an insidious onset and inexorable progression of atrophy that is first manifest in the medial temporal lobe (Scahill et al. 2002). The entorhinal cortex is typically the earliest site of atrophy, closely followed by the hippocampus, amygdala, and parahippocampus (Lehericy et al. 1994; Chan et al. 2001; Dickerson et al. 2001; Killiany et al. 2002). Other structures within the limbic lobe such as the posterior cingulate are also affected early on. These losses then spread to involve the temporal neocortex and then all neocortical association areas usually in a symmetrical fashion. This sequence of progression of atrophy on MRI most closely fits histopathological studies that have derived stages for the spread of neurofibrillary tangles (Braak and Braak 1991).

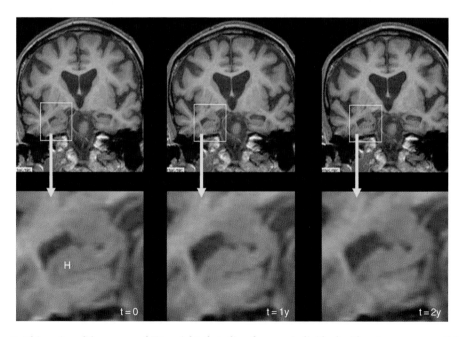

Figure 1. This series of three coronal T1-weighted studies, from an individual with autopsy-proven Alzheimer disease (AD), were each acquired ∼1 yr apart and show progressive hippocampal (H) atrophy as the individual progressed from memory complaints (*left* column, t = 0) to MCI (*center*, t = 1y) and on to fulfill criteria for AD.

Nonetheless, a significant minority of AD cases have atypical presentations and in these cases the pattern of atrophy accords with clinical phenotype: with language presentations particularly having left temporal atrophy and visual variants having posterior cortical atrophy.

It is increasingly clear that by the time a typical AD patient comes to diagnosis atrophy is well established. Even in mildly affected individuals (e.g., mean MMSE of $\sim24/30$) entorhinal volumes are already reduced by $\sim20-30\%$ and hippocampal volumes by $\sim15-25\%$ (Chan et al. 2001; Dickerson et al. 2001; Schuff et al. 2009). Because rates of hippocampal atrophy in mild AD are $\sim3-5\%$ per year (Barnes et al. 2009) this suggests that there must have been a period of several years before diagnosis where medial temporal lobe atrophy was already in process. Longitudinal MRI studies of individuals who are initially asymptomatic but who subsequently develop AD support this suggestion and find that hippocampal volumes are already reduced by about 10% 3 years before receiving a diagnosis of dementia due to AD and that rates of hippocampal atrophy increase gradually some 5 years before diagnosis. By the time a clinical diagnosis is made, atrophy is also quite widespread with whole brain volumes down by $\sim6\%$; rates of loss having gradually accelerated (at $\sim0.3\%/\mathrm{yr}^2$) in the 2–4 years up to a diagnosis (Chan et al. 2003; Ridha et al. 2006; Jack et al. 2008b).

Assessment of medial temporal atrophy on MRI has been shown to have positive predictive value for AD. Visual assessment differentiates mild AD from normal aging with a sensitivity and specificity of $\sim80-85\%$ (Scheltens et al. 1992; Duara et al. 2008; Burton et al. 2009). Differentiating MCI subjects who will progress to AD in the near future from those who will not is a more difficult task: Medial temporal atrophy on MRI is still a very significant predictor of progression with sensitivity and specificity of $\sim50-70\%$ for distinguishing individuals who will progress to AD from those who will not (Korf et al. 2004; DeCarli et al. 2007). For these reasons medial temporal lobe atrophy now forms one of the biomarkers of AD included in proposed criteria for diagnosing

(prodromal) AD at a pre-dementia stage (Dubois et al. 2007). The severity of hippocampal atrophy tends to be greater in AD than in dementia with Lewy bodies (DLB) or vascular dementia (VaD)—when matched for clinical severity. Nonetheless, hippocampal atrophy is a feature of DLB and VaD, and in frontotemporal dementia (FTD) can be more severe anteriorly than in AD (Barber et al. 2000; Chan et al. 2001; McKeith et al. 2005; Burton et al. 2009). The differential diagnosis of AD therefore needs to take into account the overall pattern of imaging (and other) features of these dementias: for instance, focal frontal/temporal lobar atrophy on MRI would point to a diagnosis of FTD, whereas marked signal changes in white matter may suggest VaD (Chan et al. 2001; Scheltens et al. 2002; Likeman et al. 2005; Rabinovici et al. 2007; Frisoni et al. 2010). The overall pattern of atrophy is used in clinical practice and there is interest in automated pattern classification of MRI to predict AD at an early stage and to distinguish it from other dementias (Kloppel et al. 2008; Misra et al. 2009; Vemuri et al. 2009).

Measuring Progression in AD with Structural MRI

The fact that pathologically increased cerebral atrophy starts early (even presymptomatically), continues relentlessly, at least until individuals are severely affected, and correlates with clinical decline has led to atrophy on MRI being suggested as a marker of disease progression and a potential outcome measure in trials. The amount, distribution, and rate of cerebral atrophy are all closely correlated with cognitive deficits (Hua et al. 2008; Ridha et al. 2008; Cardenas et al. 2009; Fox et al. 1999b). In the absence of an intervention cerebral volume loss in AD has clear, direct, and profound negative clinical consequences. Epidemiological-autopsy studies of individuals with and without dementia showed that, whereas plaques, tangles, and atrophy are all associated with dementia, atrophy was the factor that most strongly correlated with dementia at all ages (Savva et al. 2009). It appears that histopathological hallmarks of AD are markers of disease process whereas the clinical state is captured by the extent of neurodegeneration—for which atrophy may be considered an in vivo measure. Rates of regional and/or global atrophy on MRI have as a result been proposed as outcome measures in trials seeking to show a disease-modification effect in AD; the motivation for this is the potentially increased power to detect a disease-slowing effect. Sample size calculations based on natural history studies would support this with only ~20% as many patients being expected to be needed for the same effect using MRI measures than if clinical scales were used (Fox et al. 2000; Jack et al. 2008a; Ridha et al. 2008; Schuff et al. 2009). Rates of hippocampal and whole brain atrophy on MRI have to date been the most widely included imaging measures in trials; however, other MRI measures show promise, including cortical thickness or composites of change (Lerch et al. 2005; Hua et al. 2008; Jack et al. 2008a; Vemuri et al. 2009). The validation of this approach, however, awaits the discovery of disease-modifying therapies particularly as therapies may have an effect on progression of volume loss through mechanisms other than reduced rates of neuronal loss (e.g., hydration, inflammatory, and anti-inflammatory effects) (Fox et al. 2005a). It is likely that multiple imaging and fluid biomarkers will be included in trials that seek to understand as well as measure effects on disease progression.

Availability and Utility of Structural MRI

An obvious strength of MRI is its availability. A testament to its value in diagnosis in dementia is the fact that European and U.S. guidelines recommend that all subjects with cognitive decline undergo structural imaging (MRI or CT) and that it is part of proposed diagnostic criteria for AD and for other dementias (Waldemar et al. 2000; Knopman et al. 2001; McKeith et al. 2005; Dubois et al. 2007). In most centers, MRI is regarded as an essential investigation in dementia—a marker of its utility. Although not as rapid as CT, a typical high-resolution volumetric sequence can be acquired in 5–10

min and more basic sequences in considerably less time. MRI is safe and as it does not involve ionizing radiation individuals can be imaged serially without concerns about carcinogenicity. MRI offers a range of different sequences that can probe different tissue characteristics providing multiple clinical and research measures in the same session. Atrophy as an outcome measure has strengths over clinical measures because it is not subject to practice effects or (realistically) to floor or ceiling effects, and it theoretically has a greater ability to detect disease slowing. MRI measures of atrophy reflect cumulative neuronal damage which in turn is directly responsible for clinical state. When compared with other imaging markers (and other biomarkers) cerebral atrophy has, as a strength, its strong correlation with cognitive decline.

Limitations of Structural MRI in AD

Structural MRI lacks molecular specificity. It cannot directly detect the histopathological hallmarks of AD (amyloid plaques or neurofibrillary tangles) and as such it is downstream from the molecular pathology. Cerebral atrophy is a nonspecific result of neuronal damage and, whereas certain patterns of loss are characteristic of different diseases, they are not entirely specific. Atrophy patterns overlap with other diseases and unusual forms of AD have atypical patterns of atrophy too. In more severely affected individuals and those with claustrophobia, MRI may not be tolerated whereas a rapid CT scan may be more feasible. In terms of measuring progression, volume changes on MRI may be produced by factors other than the progression of neuronal loss and as such assessment of disease modification may be obscured, at least in the short term, by such spurious effects. As the name implies, structural MRI cannot assess function; this is provided with increasing sophistication by functional MRI and PET.

Overall the availability, ease of use, and multiple applications of structural MRI in AD mean it will play a central role in research and practice for some years to come. Increasingly, the other (complementary) modalities described in this article will address the weaknesses of MRI.

FUNCTIONAL MRI IN AD

Basics of Functional MRI as Applied to AD

Functional MRI (fMRI) is being increasingly used to probe the functional integrity of brain networks supporting memory and other cognitive domains in aging and early AD. fMRI is a noninvasive imaging technique which provides an indirect measure of neuronal activity, inferred from measuring changes in blood oxygen level–dependent (BOLD) MR signal (Ogawa et al. 1990; Kwong et al. 1992). Whereas fluoro-deoxy-D-glucose (FDG)-PET is thought to be primarily a measure of synaptic activity, BOLD fMRI is considered to reflect the integrated synaptic activity of neurons via MRI signal changes because of changes in blood flow, blood volume, and the blood oxyhemoglobin/deoxyhemoglobin ratio (Logothetis et al. 2001). fMRI can be acquired during cognitive tasks, typically comparing one condition (e.g., encoding new information) to a control condition (e.g., viewing familiar information or visual fixation on a cross-hair), or during the resting state to investigate the functional connectivity (fc-MRI) within specific brain networks. Fc-MRI techniques examine the correlation between the intrinsic oscillations or time course of BOLD signal between brain regions (Fox et al. 2005b), and have clearly documented the organization of the brain into multiple large-scale brain networks (Damoiseaux et al. 2006; Vincent et al. 2006). Both task-related and resting fMRI techniques have the potential to detect early brain dysfunction related to AD, and to monitor therapeutic response over relatively short time periods; however, the use of fMRI in aging, MCI, and AD populations thus far has been limited to a relatively small number of research groups.

Utility of Functional MRI in the Study of AD

Much of the early fMRI work in MCI and AD used episodic memory tasks, and was focused on the pattern of fMRI activation in hippocampus and related structures in the medial temporal lobe. In patients with clinically diagnosed AD, the results have been quite consistent, showing decreased hippocampal activity during the encoding of new information (Small et al. 1999; Rombouts et al. 2000; Kato et al. 2001; Gron et al. 2002; Machulda et al. 2003; Sperling et al. 2003; Remy et al. 2004; Golby et al. 2005; Hamalainen et al. 2007). Several studies have reported increased prefrontal cortical activity in AD patients (Grady et al. 2003; Sperling et al. 2003; Sole-Padulles et al. 2009), suggesting that other networks may increase activity as an attempted compensatory mechanism during hippocampal failure.

A relatively small number of fMRI studies have been published in subjects at risk for AD, including MCI subjects and genetic at-risk individuals yielding somewhat discrepant findings. Several studies have reported decreased mesial temporal lobe (MTL) activation in MCI (Small et al. 1999; Machulda et al. 2003; Johnson et al. 2006; Petrella et al. 2006) and genetic at-risk subjects (Smith et al. 1999; Lind et al. 2006a,b; Trivedi et al. 2006; Borghesani et al. 2007; Mondadori et al. 2007; Ringman et al. 2010). Interestingly, several fMRI studies have reported evidence of *increased* MTL activity in at-risk subjects, particularly among very mild MCI subjects (Dickerson et al. 2004, 2005; Celone et al. 2006; Hamalainen et al. 2006; Heun et al. 2007; Kircher et al. 2007; Lenzi et al. 2009), and cognitively intact individuals with genetic risk for AD (Bookheimer et al. 2000; Smith et al. 2002; Wishart et al. 2004; Bondi et al. 2005; Fleisher et al. 2005; Han et al. 2007; Filippini et al. 2009). It is likely that these discrepant results are related to specific paradigm demands, stage of impairment, and behavioral performance. A common feature of the studies reporting evidence of increased fMRI activity is that the at-risk subjects were able to perform the fMRI tasks reasonably well. In particular, the event-related fMRI studies have found that hyperactivity was observed specifically during successful memory trials, which suggested that hyperactivity might represent a compensatory mechanism in the setting of early AD pathology (Dickerson and Sperling 2008; Sperling et al. 2009).

Cross-sectional studies suggest that the hyperactivity may be present only at early stages of MCI, followed by a loss of activation in late stages of MCI, similar to the pattern seen in AD patients (Celone et al. 2006). Longitudinal studies furthermore suggest that the presence of hyperactivity at baseline is a predictor of rapid cognitive decline (Bookheimer et al. 2000; Dickerson et al. 2004; Miller et al. 2008a), and loss of hippocampal function on serial fMRI (O'Brien et al. 2010). The mechanistic underpinnings of MTL hyperactivation remain unclear; however, these new longitudinal data suggest that hyperactivity may be a marker of impending neuronal failure. This phenomena may reflect cholinergic or other neurotransmitter up-regulation (DeKosky et al. 2002), aberrant sprouting of cholinergic fibers (Masliah et al. 2003), inefficiency in synaptic transmission (Stern et al. 2004), increased calcium influx, and evidence of excitotoxicity (Palop et al. 2007; Busche et al. 2008).

Converging data suggest that memory function is subserved by a network of brain regions, which includes not only the MTL system, but also a set of cortical regions, including the precuneus, posterior cingulate, lateral parietal, lateral temporal, and medial prefrontal regions, collectively known as the "default network" which typically deactivate during memory encoding and other cognitively demanding tasks focused on the processing of external stimuli (Raichle et al. 2001; Buckner et al. 2008). Recent studies have also suggested that the default network shows markedly abnormal responses during memory tasks in clinical AD patients and in subjects at risk for AD (Lustig and Buckner 2004; Celone et al. 2006; Petrella et al. 2007a; Pihlajamaki et al. 2008, 2009). Interestingly, it is the same default network regions that typically show beneficial deactivations in healthy subjects, particularly, the posterior cingulate/precuneus (Daselaar et al. 2004; Miller et al. 2008b), which tend to manifest a paradoxical increase in fMRI activity (or loss of normal default network deactivation) in both at-risk groups and clinical AD patients (Petrella et al. 2007b; Pihlajamaki et al. 2008; Fleisher et al. 2009; Sperling et al. 2010).

There has been a recent emphasis on BOLD fMRI techniques to study spontaneous brain activity and the interregional correlations during the resting state. These studies have clearly documented the organization of the brain into multiple large-scale brain networks (Damoiseaux et al. 2006; Vincent et al. 2007). Interestingly, both independent component analyses and "seed-based" connectivity techniques have shown the robust intrinsic connectivity between the posteromedial nodes of the default network, in particular the posterior cingulate/precuneus, with the hippocampus. Multiple groups have confirmed impaired intrinsic functional connectivity in the default network during the resting state in MCI and AD (Greicius et al. 2004; Rombouts et al. 2005, 2009; Sorg et al. 2007; Bai et al. 2008; Koch et al. 2010) over and above more general age-related disruption of large-scale networks (Andrews-Hanna et al. 2007; Damoiseaux et al. 2008). One recent study suggests that these resting fMRI techniques may be more readily applied to at-risk clinical populations than task fMRI (Fleisher et al. 2009). Fc-MRI may be particularly advantageous for use in clinical trials, as no special equipment is required, subjects do not have to be able to perform a cognitive task, and a resting run could be added to the end of a safety or volumetric MRI protocol. Additional longitudinal work is needed to determine if longitudinal changes in fc-MRI will parallel clinical decline.

Interestingly, the default network regions showing aberrant task-related fMRI activity and dysconnectivity in MCI and AD also overlap the anatomy of regions with the highest amyloid burden in AD patients (Fig. 2; Klunk et al. 2004; Buckner et al. 2005, 2009; Sperling et al. 2009). Several recent studies in cognitively normal older individuals with evidence of amyloid deposition on PET imaging have shown evidence of disrupted default network activity during memory tasks and at rest (Hedden et al. 2009; Sheline et al. 2009; Sperling et al. 2009), suggesting these markers may be particularly useful to track response to antiamyloid therapies in preclinical trials.

fMRI, either during cognitive paradigms or during resting state, may hold the greatest potential for the evaluation of novel pharmacological strategies to treat AD. Several studies in

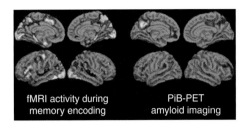

fMRI activity during
memory encoding

PiB-PET
amyloid imaging

Figure 2. (*Left*) Group map of fMRI activity showing regions that increase activity (yellow/red) or decrease (blue) activity during successful encoding. (*Right*) Group map of 11C-PiB retention in a group of non-demented older individuals. Note the anatomic overlap of PiB retention to default network (regions in blue on *left*).

healthy young and older subjects suggest that fMRI can detect acute pharmacological effects on memory networks (Thiel et al. 2001; Sperling et al. 2002; Kukolja et al. 2009). To date, only a few small fMRI studies have shown enhanced brain activation after acute or prolonged treatment with cholinesterase inhibitors in MCI and AD, although these studies were not conducted as typical double-blind, placebo-controlled trials (Rombouts et al. 2002; Goekoop et al. 2004; Saykin et al. 2004; Shanks et al. 2007; Bokde et al. 2009; Venneri et al. 2009). fMRI is now being incorporated into a small number of investigator-initiated add-on studies to ongoing Phase II and Phase III trials, which should provide some valuable information regarding the potential utility of these techniques in clinical trials.

Limitations of fMRI in AD

There are multiple challenges in performing longitudinal fMRI studies in patients with neurodegenerative dementias. It is likely that fMRI will remain quite problematic in examining patients with more severe cognitive impairment, as these techniques are very sensitive to head motion. If the patients are not able to adequately perform the cognitive task, one of the major advantages of task fMRI activation studies is lost. Resting state fMRI may be more feasible in more severely impaired patients.

It is critical to complete further validation experiments. BOLD fMRI response is known

to be variable across subjects, and very few studies examining the reproducibility of fMRI activation in older and cognitively impaired subjects have been published to date (Clement and Belleville 2009; Putcha et al. 2010). Longitudinal functional imaging studies are needed to track the evolution of alterations in the fMRI activation pattern over the course of the cognitive continuum from preclinical to prodromal to clinical AD. It is also important to evaluate the contribution of structural atrophy to changes observed with functional imaging techniques in neurodegenerative diseases. Finally, longitudinal multimodality studies, including structural MRI, fMRI, and FDG-PET and PET amyloid imaging techniques, are needed to understand the relationship between these markers, and the relative value of these techniques in tracking change along the clinical continuum of AD (Jack et al. 2010).

FLUORODEOXYGLUCOSE (FDG) PET IN AD

Basics of FDG PET as Applied to AD

Brain FDG PET primarily indicates synaptic activity. Because the brain relies almost exclusively on glucose as its source of energy, the glucose analog FDG is a suitable indicator of brain metabolism and, when labeled with Fluorine-18 (half-life 110 min) is conveniently detected with PET. The brain's energy budget is overwhelmingly devoted to the maintenance of intrinsic, resting (task-independent) activity, which in cortex is largely maintained by glutamaturgic synaptic signaling (Sibson et al. 1997). FDG uptake strongly correlates at autopsy with levels of the synaptic vesicle protein synaptophysin (Rocher et al. 2003). Hence, FDG PET is widely accepted to be a valid biomarker of overall brain metabolism to which ionic gradient maintenance for synaptic activity is the principal contributor (Schwartz et al. 1979; Magistretti 2006). In this context, a single, specific AD-related alteration in FDG metabolism has not been identified and therefore the FDG-PET abnormalities described below are assumed to be the net result of some combination of processes putatively involved in the pathogenesis of AD including, but not limited to, expression of specific genes, mitochondrial dysfunction, oxidative stress, deranged plasticity, excitotoxicity, glial activation and inflammation, synapse loss, and cell death.

Utility of FDG PET in the Study of AD

The Pattern of FDG Hypometabolism Is an Endophenotype of AD

A substantial body of work over many years has identified a FDG-PET endophenotype of AD (Fig. 3)—that is, a characteristic or signature ensemble of limbic and association regions that are typically hypometabolic in clinically established AD patients (Foster et al. 1983; Reiman et al. 1996; Minoshima et al. 1997; De Santi et al. 2001). The anatomy of the AD signature includes posterior midline cortices of the parietal (precuneus) and posterior cingulate gyri, the inferior parietal lobule, posterolateral portions of the temporal lobe, as well as the hippocampus and medial temporal cortices. Metabolic deficits in AD gradually worsen throughout the course of the disease. Bilateral asymmetry is common at early stages, more

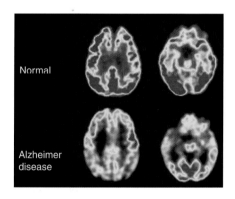

Figure 3. Transaxial FDG-PET images of a normal control subject and a patient with mild AD. Note severe hypometabolism (yellow and blue cortical regions) in association and limbic cortex. These are the typically involved brain regions that define the FDG endophenotype of AD. They include posteriomedial parietal (precuneus), lateral parietal, lateral temporal, and medial temporal lobes. This pattern slowly worsens in parallel with symptoms and is well correlated at autopsy with AD pathologic diagnosis.

advanced disease usually involves prefrontal association areas, and in due course even primary cortices may be affected. Interestingly, the regions initially hypometabolic in AD are anatomically and functionally interconnected and form part of the large-scale distributed brain network known as the default mode network (Raichle et al. 2001). We now know in addition that these regions are highly vulnerable to amyloid-β (Aβ) deposition (Klunk et al. 2004; Buckner et al. 2005).

Less severe or consistent hypometabolism has been identified in MCI patients, some of whom were found on follow-up examination to have converted to AD (Arnaiz et al. 2001; de Leon et al. 2001; Jagust et al. 2002, 2007; Chetelat et al. 2003; Caselli et al. 2008; Langbaum et al. 2009; Landau et al. 2010). Differences in FDG between MCI and normal aging have not typically been large, but the control groups in most of these studies were likely contaminated with a number of individuals who, although clinically normal, were amyloid positive (see below) and possibly in earlier phases of preclinical AD. FDG hypometabolism parallels cognitive function along the trajectory of normal, preclinical, prodromal, and established AD (Minoshima et al. 1997; Furst et al. 2010); however, higher levels of brain and cognitive reserve are well known to attenuate the strength of these correlations and highly intelligent AD patients can be clinically mild, but severely hypometabolic (Stern et al. 1992; Alexander et al. 1997). Coexisting vascular disorders, including ischemia, amyloid angiopathy, and micro-hemorrhage, potentially confound the relation of FDG to clinical phenotype, but the classic AD FDG pattern is well correlated with histopathologic diagnosis of AD at autopsy (Hoffman et al. 2000; Jagust et al. 2007).

FDG Hypometabolism Is Related to Other AD Biomarkers and to Genes

The association between amyloid deposition and brain function in AD has been studied with FDG PET. Longitudinal data has shown that, once the stage of established AD is reached, amyloid deposition in most regions has plateaued (Engler et al. 2006; Jack et al. 2009), but FDG continues to decline along with cognitive function (Engler et al. 2006). Several groups have observed high amyloid deposition in parietal regions to be associated with co-localized FDG hypometabolism, possibly indicating a local toxicity (Klunk et al. 2004; Engler et al. 2006; Edison et al. 2007; Cohen et al. 2009). In other groups, this association was not statistically significant, possibly because the amyloid burden in these patients was already at its plateau (Kadir et al. 2008; Furst et al. 2010). An important clue to this relationship could lie in the observation that the relation is consistently weaker in frontal regions, where some of the highest amyloid burdens are found (Klunk et al. 2004; Edison et al. 2007). Interestingly, amyloid-positive MCI patients in one study had preserved FDG metabolism that was *positively* correlated with extensive Pittsburgh Compound-B (PiB) retention, possibly suggesting a mediating role for metabolism, perhaps either as a brain reserve factor or as an accelerant of deposition (Cohen et al. 2009). Additional longitudinal data will be required to clarify these relationships, but clearly FDG metabolism appears to be changing as amyloid is accumulating. It is possible that FDG data could signal an intermediate stage between the initiating pathologic event and the subsequent development of synaptic failure and neurodegeneration (Cohen et al. 2009).

Brain volume loss is also observed in AD hypometabolic areas, but the FDG findings have generally survived MRI-based corrections for cortical atrophy (Meltzer et al. 1996; Ibanez et al. 1998; Jagust et al. 2006; Cohen et al. 2009; Lowe et al. 2009; Rabinovici et al. 2010), suggesting that volume loss and function loss are separable phenomena in AD. Both domains of data are reported to have predictive power: FDG hypometabolism that predicts ultimate development of AD occurs before impairment (de Leon et al. 2001; Jagust et al. 2006) and brain volume loss has also been reported in cognitively normal individuals who go on to develop AD (Fox et al. 1999a; Jack et al. 2004). Systematic comparison of two imaging biomarkers requires caution because of rapidly evolving

technology. For example, recently developed methods for subject-specific MRI segmentation have revealed subtle cortical thinning in a distribution similar to that seen with FDG (Walhovd et al. 2009; Karow et al. 2010). A continuing challenge is presented by the fact that FDG-PET data inherently contains volume information, and PET-based partial volume correction (e.g., with deconvolution [Tohka and Reilhac 2008]), may eventually be useful to disentangle FDG retention and structural loss.

Initial reports associating FDG hypometabolism and AD-related CSF measures have varied, likely due in part to image and fluid sample processing differences. FDG was associated with low CSF Aβ and increased CSF tau in amyloid-positive clinically normal older individuals (Petrie et al. 2009), but with CSF Aβ and not tau in an Alzheimer's Disease Neuroimaging Initiative (ADNI) study of AD, MCI, and controls, adjusted for diagnosis (Jagust et al. 2009).

Carriers of the apolipoprotein-E (APOE) ε4 allele have a higher risk of developing AD, and the classic AD pattern of hypometabolism described above is seen in cognitively normal APOE ε4 carriers (Reiman et al. 1996, 2005). A relationship of this FDG pattern to serum cholesterol and to an aggregate cholesterol-related genetic score in middle age has also been reported (Reiman et al. 2008, 2010). Maternal history of dementia has recently been related both to increased PiB retention and to FDG hypometabolism in AD-related areas among asymptomatic individuals (Mosconi et al. 2009, 2010).

FDG PET Is a Valid AD Biomarker

Over the course of three decades of investigation, FDG PET has emerged as a robust marker of brain dysfunction in AD. Its principal value is twofold: first, clinical utility has been documented when confounding conditions (e.g., DLB or frontotemporal lobar degeneration [FTLD]), are in question. Thus, when frontotemporal rather than temporoparietal hypometabolism is prominent, a clinically uncertain AD diagnosis may be changed to FTLD (Foster et al. 2007); when prominent occipital hypometabolism is found in addition to temporoparietal, the data are highly suggestive of DLB (Albin et al. 1996; Mosconi et al. 2008).

Second, FDG has emerged as a robust biomarker of neurodegeneration with which hypometabolism can be observed to precede the appearance of cognitive symptoms and to predict the rate of progressive cognitive decline in individuals who are later found to have progressed to AD (de Leon et al. 2001; Jagust et al. 2006). FDG hypometabolism is also predictive of the rate of memory decline in APOE ε4 carriers with mild memory loss over 2 years (Small et al. 2000). Most importantly for AD treatment research, a recent analysis of ADNI FDG data found that AD and MCI groups each showed progression of AD-like hypometabolism over 1 year that paralleled changes in a standard clinical endpoint, the clinical dementia rating scale (CDR) sum-of-boxes (Chen et al. 2010). These authors calculated that the use of FDG PET in clinical trials of AD therapy could reduce sample sizes by approximately one order of magnitude.

The Limitations of FDG PET in AD

FDG PET is relatively expensive and, like all PET techniques, has more limited availability, although its use in oncology has dramatically increased availability in the USA over the past decade. It requires intravenous access and involves exposure to radioactivity, although at levels well below significant known risk. Brain FDG retention is a nonspecific indicator of metabolism that can be deranged for a variety of reasons (e.g., ischemia or inflammation) and may in certain individuals be irrelevant or only indirectly related to any AD-related process.

AMYLOID PET IN AD

Basics of Amyloid PET as It Is Applied to AD

An important "first principle" of amyloid imaging in the context of AD is that amyloid PET is intended first and foremost as an in vivo surrogate for Aβ pathology, and not necessarily as a surrogate for clinical diagnosis. As discussed below, there are diagnostic applications of amyloid imaging, but these share the same strengths and limitations as postmortem determinations of Aβ content. Another important principle of amyloid imaging is that the substrate for all currently known Aβ tracers is fibrillar Aβ in a beta-sheet conformation (Ikonomovic et al. 2008). When speaking of the binding substrates of amyloid tracers, it is preferable to think in terms of fibrillar and nonfibrillar Aβ rather than visual descriptions of plaques as fleecy, amorphous, diffuse, compact, cored, neuritic, etc., because there can be varying amounts of fibrillar Aβ in any of these plaque types. Compact, cored, and neuritic plaques typically have large amounts of fibrillar amyloid and fleecy and amorphous plaque deposits typically have very little (particularly in the cerebellum). However, diffuse plaques are not a precisely defined term and can have widely varying amounts of fibrillar Aβ from case to case. Along similar lines, cerebrovascular amyloid typically has a high degree of fibrillar Aβ and appears to be a very good substrate for amyloid tracer binding (Bacskai et al. 2007; Johnson et al. 2007; Lockhart et al. 2007; Ikonomovic et al. 2008). Increasing recognition has been given to the toxicity of oligomeric species of Aβ and this is described in Mucke and Selkow (2011). Although it is possible that currently available amyloid tracers could bind to oligomers of Aβ in a beta-sheet conformation once they reach a necessary size (probably at least a trimer or tetramer), the in vivo signal of amyloid tracers is not directly representative of these species because of their low concentration relative to insoluble Aβ fibrils. However, there may be a relationship between the amyloid PET signal and oligomer concentration based on the existence of an equilibrium between monomers, oligomers, and fibrillar Aβ. Although claims have been made that some tracers can image neurofibrillary tangles, there have been no validation studies in this regard. To the contrary, there is evidence that some amyloid tracers do not bind neurofibrillary pathology (Klunk et al. 2003; Ikonomovic et al. 2008).

K.A. Johnson et al.

With regard to specific amyloid imaging agents, this review will discuss "amyloid tracers" in general, while acknowledging that most of the statements are derived from data on the most widely evaluated PET tracer, PiB (Klunk et al. 2004). At the time of writing, there have been one or two, small published studies using each of the fluorine-18-labelled tracers, [F-18]florbetaben (18F-BAY94-9172 or AV-1; Rowe et al. 2008), [F-18]florbetapir (AV-45; Wong et al. 2010; Clark et al. 2011) and [F-18]flutemetamol (3′F-PiB or GE-067; Nelissen et al. 2009; Vandenberghe et al. 2010) in AD patients. Although the PiB PET findings may ultimately be found to extend to these F-18-labeled tracers as well, this cannot be assumed until appropriate studies have been repeated with each individual tracer or until pharmacological equivalency to PiB has been established by direct comparison in the same subjects.

Utility of Amyloid PET in the Study of AD

The obvious strength of amyloid imaging is that it has allowed the determination of brain Aβ content to be moved from the pathology laboratory into the clinic. Amyloid imaging can detect cerebral β-amyloidosis and appears specific for this type of amyloid pathology, giving negative signals in pathologically confirmed cases of prion amyloid (Villemagne et al. 2009), pathologically confirmed pure α-synucleinopathy (Burack et al. 2010), as well as in apparently pure cases of tauopathy in semantic dementia (Drzezga et al. 2008).

In the setting of clinical dementia, particularly in clinically atypical presentations, this has important diagnostic utility. Reviewing recent publications from 15 research groups who have performed amyloid PET on clinically diagnosed AD patients, 96% of AD patients were amyloid positive (Fig. 4; Kemppainen et al. 2006; Aizenstein et al. 2008; Edison et al. 2008; Shin et al. 2008; Drzezga et al. 2009; Hedden et al. 2009; Lowe et al. 2009; Maetzler et al. 2009; Wolk et al. 2009; Devanand et al. 2010; Forsberg et al. 2010; Jagust et al. 2010; Rabinovici et al. 2010; Roe et al. 2010; Rowe et al. 2010; Tolboom et al. 2010). One assumption is that amyloid-negative demented patients diagnosed as AD have been given an incorrect diagnosis. Another possibility is that amyloid imaging was simply not sensitive enough in some patients and these patients would become amyloid positive over time. One follow-up of three amyloid-negative subjects initially diagnosed as AD (Klunk et al. 2004), has shown that all three subjects have remained amyloid negative for 5 years (Kadir et al. 2010), suggesting that sensitivity was not the issue and that these patients are not likely to have AD as the cause of their cognitive deficits. On the other side of the coin are amyloid-positive patients who have been diagnosed with a dementia other than AD. In the case of FTD, it has been assumed that patients who present with a

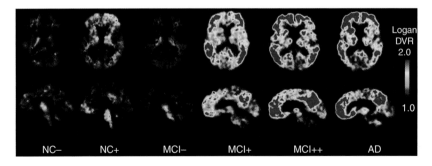

Figure 4. PiB PET Images of normal control, MCI, and AD subjects showing a range of amyloid-β deposition. Most controls show no evidence of amyloid-β deposition (NC−), but a substantial portion (~25%) do (NC+). Most patients with MCI show moderate (MCI+) or severe amyloid-β deposition (MCI++), but as many as 40%–50% show no evidence of amyloid-β pathology (MCI−). The vast majority of clinically diagnosed AD patients show heavy amyloid-β deposition (AD).

Cite this article as *Cold Spring Harb Perspect Med* doi: 10.1101/cshperspect.a006213

clinical FTD syndrome but have AD-like amy-loid PET scans are really atypical presentations of AD (Rabinovici et al. 2007, 2008; Engler et al. 2008), but pathological verification remains to be done. These patients will be particularly important to identify when there are effective treatments for AD directed at Aβ deposition.

In the setting of MCI, combined data from nine amyloid PET studies show that 161 of 272 MCI patients were amyloid positive (59%) (Fig. 4; Forsberg et al. 2008; Koivunen et al. 2008; Lowe et al. 2009; Okello et al. 2009; Tolboom et al. 2009; Wolk et al. 2009; Devanand et al. 2010; Jagust et al. 2010; Rowe et al. 2010). Five of these studies included longitudinal clinical follow-up for 1–3 years on 155 MCI patients and showed that 57 of these 155 progressed to clinical AD (37%) and 53 of these 57 were amyloid positive at baseline (93%); only four of 54 amyloid-negative MCI patients progressed to clinical AD in these studies (7%) (Forsberg et al. 2008; Koivunen et al. 2008; Okello et al. 2009; Wolk et al. 2009; Jagust et al. 2010).

The most substantial contribution of amyloid imaging may come in the setting of the cognitively normal elderly. It is at this clinically "invisible" stage that detection of underlying cerebral β-amyloidosis (the sine qua non of AD pathology) may give us the greatest insights into the very beginnings of this disease. Furthermore, it may be at this asymptomatic stage that our chances are greatest of discovering truly effective treatments. In a series of studies from 13 sites, 155 of 651 (24%) of cognitively normal controls showed evidence of cerebral Aβ deposition (Fig. 4; Kemppainen et al. 2006; Mintun et al. 2006; Edison et al. 2008; Shin et al. 2008; Hedden et al. 2009; Lowe et al. 2009; Maetzler et al. 2009; Wolk et al. 2009; Devanand et al. 2010; Jagust et al. 2010; Rabinovici et al. 2010; Roe et al. 2010; Rowe et al. 2010; Tolboom et al. 2010). In most cases, the degree of amyloid deposition was fairly easy to distinguish from that typically seen in AD (Aizenstein et al. 2008), but this is not always the case. The prevalence of amyloid positivity is related closely to age and apolipoprotein-E allele status (Morris

et al. 2010; Rowe et al. 2010). Although some subtle cognitive effects of PET amyloid positivity may be discernable in this population (Rentz et al. 2010), in most cases the overriding conclusion is that there is no tight, direct relationship between amyloid PET and cognition at these earliest stages of Aβ deposition. As discussed above, other protective or vulnerability factors must be invoked to fully explain the connection between early PET amyloid positivity and cognitive impairment. It is possible that the failure to directly assess oligomeric Aβ concentration could preclude the demonstration of amyloid PET-related cognitive effects, but vulnerability factors (such as subclinical cerebrovascular disease) and brain/cognitive reserve factors are likely to play a role as well (Kemppainen et al. 2008; Roe et al. 2008, 2010; Cohen et al. 2009; Rentz et al. 2010).

In Blennow et al. (2011), CSF biomarkers are discussed. There is clearly a large overlap in the information available from CSF Aβ42 levels and amyloid PET, but each technique has its advantages and limitations (see below). The advantages of amyloid PET center around the regional information and in the continuously variable nature of the biological changes. The latter refers to the fact that decreases in CSF Aβ42 appear to occur early (at least as early as changes in amyloid PET) and precipitously—achieving its final level very early in the course of the pathophysiological spectrum of AD—probably presymptomatically (Blennow and Hampel 2003; Hansson et al. 2006; Fagan et al. 2007, 2009). That is, the change in CSF appears to be a step-function and longitudinal studies have not shown a progressive decrease in CSF Aβ42 over time (Buchhave et al. 2009). This is not surprising given that typical concentrations of Aβ found in insoluble deposits in AD cortex are approximately 5000 μg/L ($\sim$1 μM), while typical CSF Aβ42 concentrations are around 0.5 μg/L—or 0.01% of insoluble cortical Aβ. Thus, it is not surprising that relatively little cortical Aβ would need to deposit before a new equilibrium would be established with CSF. This has an important implication for clinical trials: As an outcome measure, CSF Aβ42 is not likely to normalize until the vast majority of cortical Aβ deposits are removed. Thus, CSF Aβ42 and amyloid PET are likely to be equivalent as screening tools for clinical trials, but the more dynamic nature of amyloid PET and the fact that amyloid tracer retention correlates directly with Aβ load (Ikonomovic et al. 2008) makes this a more suitable outcome measure when the goal is to detect changes in brain Aβ load. In support of this statement, the ability of amyloid PET to show an amyloid-lowering effect of passive immunotherapy in humans has already been reported (Rinne et al. 2010).

A unique strength of amyloid PET across the entire clinical spectrum is the regionally specific nature of the quantitative data. Although we often reduce imaging data to a single number (e.g., mean cortical retention), we must remember that a strength of any imaging technique is the wealth of regional information that is supplied. Although amyloid PET can quantify amyloid load throughout the brain, it is not clear what pool of brain Aβ is represented by changes in CSF Aβ. One study has suggested that CSF Aβ is most tightly correlated with amyloid retention in brain regions adjacent to CSF spaces (Grimmer et al. 2009).

The Limitations of Amyloid PET in AD

Major deterrents to the widespread use of amyloid PET remain cost and availability. Availability has been improved by the development of F-18-labeled agents that can be distributed to PET scanners not associated with a cyclotron. Cost remains an issue, especially where CSF measurement of Aβ42 can provide very similar information when the question is simply the presence or absence of brain Aβ deposition. Being an early event in the pathogenesis of AD, amyloid PET is not a good surrogate marker of progression during the clinical stage of the disease (Engler et al. 2006; Kadir et al. 2010). This role is filled much better by structural MRI and FDG PET (Jack et al. 2010). Similarly, amyloid imaging gives much more of a binary diagnostic readout than techniques such as MRI and FDG PET. That is, amyloid imaging has a certain specificity for the pathology of AD, but when that pathology is absent, a negative amyloid PET scan will be identical regardless of the non-AD etiology of the dementia. In contrast, MRI and FDG PET may give an indication of a frontotemporal or vascular pathology when an amyloid PET scan would be ambiguously negative in both cases. The threshold of sensitivity of amyloid PET has yet to be precisely determined, but it is clear that some level of amyloid deposition is histologically detectable prior to the in vivo signal becoming "positive" (Cairns et al. 2009).

SUMMARY

State-of-the-(Imaging)-Art

In this chapter we briefly reviewed the most commonly used imaging technologies: structural and functional MRI and FDG and amyloid PET. Other MRI techniques such as diffusion tensor imaging (DTI) and associated tractography technologies, arterial spin labeling measures of cerebral blood flow and PET tracers targeted at the cholinergic system, microglial activation and other tracers in development are also contributing to our basic understanding of AD. A particularly exciting pursuit is PET ligands targeting the other major AD pathologic hallmark, the neurofibrillary tangle. Biomarkers of tau have been a particular challenge because of the need to target binding to something other than the β-sheet fibril dominated by Aβ deposits and the relatively smaller total mass of tau deposits, but steady progress is being made to achieve sufficient ligand affinity and selectivity. It should be clear from the above discussions that no single imaging technique can provide all of the answers. Fortunately, the strengths and weakness of the available imaging technologies are largely complementary. This has led to a variety of "multi-modal" imaging studies in which several techniques are simultaneously or sequentially applied to the same subjects for the same period of time. These direct comparisons have contributed greatly to our understanding of AD and the strengths and limitations of each technique.

Looking to the Future: The Role of Imaging in the Treatment of AD

The search for therapies that can modify the course of AD—to slow, delay, or prevent it—is clearly our most important challenge. That search has in turn led to a search for imaging markers that can be used as outcomes in drug discovery and trials. The value of any imaging technology will ultimately be determined by its contribution to meeting the challenge of finding and using effective therapies. This value includes contributions toward diagnosis. The large variability, intrinsic to clinical outcomes in AD, means that studies relying purely on clinical measures are necessarily large and consequently very costly. Using clinical outcomes to power studies to establish meaningful disease-slowing effects may require complicated designs and thousands of subjects. A major aim in academia and industry has been to find biomarkers that could identify disease-slowing effects earlier and/or with significantly fewer subjects exposed to treatment. Imaging is being increasingly incorporated into trial designs to measure the effects of a therapy on fibrillary amyloid (with amyloid imaging) on atrophy (with MRI) and on metabolism (PET and fMRI).

As increasingly biologically active therapies are studied, so too have side effects increased. Imaging is emerging as a means of detecting potential adverse effects that can initially be clinically silent or go unrecognized because of a patient's level of cognitive impairment and confusion (Salloway et al. 2009). Particularly with more biologically active therapies, regular monitoring, or so-called safety scans, are now a prerequisite in such trials.

The recognition that it may be necessary to intervene at a very early stage to effect disease modification has led to interest in "prevention" studies. Preclinical intervention studies, almost by definition, are difficult to power on clinical outcomes. Imaging and other biomarkers are likely to be needed to select subjects for these studies and to provide outcome measures that can assess whether therapies are having a disease-modifying effect that could potentially translate into a delay in clinical onset.

REFERENCES

*Reference is also in this collection.

Aizenstein HJ, Nebes RD, Saxton JA, Price JC, Mathis CA, Tsopelas ND, Ziolko SK, James JA, Snitz BE, Houck PR, et al. 2008. Frequent amyloid deposition without significant cognitive impairment among the elderly. *Arch Neurol* **65:** 1509–1517.

Albin RL, Minoshima S, D'Amato CJ, Frey KA, Kuhl DA, Sima AA. 1996. Fluoro-deoxyglucose positron emission tomography in diffuse Lewy body disease. *Neurology* **47:** 462–466.

Alexander GE, Furey ML, Grady CL, Pietrini P, Brady DR, Mentis MJ, Schapiro MB. 1997. Association of premorbid intellectual function with cerebral metabolism in Alzheimer's disease: Implications for the cognitive reserve hypothesis. *Am J Psychiatry* **154:** 165–172.

Andrews-Hanna JR, Snyder AZ, Vincent JL, Lustig C, Head D, Raichle ME, Buckner RL. 2007. Disruption of large-scale brain systems in advanced aging. *Neuron* **56:** 924–935.

Arnaiz E, Jelic V, Almkvist O, Wahlund LO, Winblad B, Valind S, Nordberg A. 2001. Impaired cerebral glucose metabolism and cognitive functioning predict deterioration in mild cognitive impairment. *Neuroreport* **12:** 851–855.

Bacskai BJ, Frosch MP, Freeman SH, Raymond SB, Augustinack JC, Johnson KA, Irizarry MC, Klunk WE, Mathis CA, Dekosky ST, et al. 2007. Molecular imaging with Pittsburgh Compound B confirmed at autopsy: A case report. *Arch Neurol* **64:** 431–434.

Bai F, Zhang Z, Yu H, Shi Y, Yuan Y, Zhu W, Zhang X, Qian Y. 2008. Default-mode network activity distinguishes amnestic type mild cognitive impairment from healthy aging: A combined structural and resting-state functional MRI study. *Neurosci Lett* **438:** 111–115.

Barber R, Ballard C, McKeith IG, Gholkar A, O'Brien JT. 2000. MRI volumetric study of dementia with Lewy bodies: A comparison with AD and vascular dementia. *Neurology* **54:** 1304–1309.

Barnes J, Bartlett JW, van de Pol LA, Loy CT, Scahill RI, Frost C, Thompson P, Fox NC. 2009. A meta-analysis of hippocampal atrophy rates in Alzheimer's disease. *Neurobiol Aging* **30:** 1711–1723.

Blennow K, Hampel H. 2003. CSF markers for incipient Alzheimer's disease. *Lancet Neurol* **2:** 605–613.

* Blennow K, Zetterberg H, Fagan AM. 2011. Fluid biomarkers in Alzheimer disease. *Cold Spring Harb Perspect Med* doi: 10.1101/cshperspect.a006221.

Bobinski M, de Leon MJ, Wegiel J, Desanti S, Convit A, Saint Louis LA, Rusinek H, Wisniewski HM. 2000. The histological validation of post mortem magnetic resonance imaging-determined hippocampal volume in Alzheimer's disease. *Neuroscience* **95:** 721–725.

Bokde AL, Karmann M, Teipel SJ, Born C, Lieb M, Reiser MF, Moller HJ, Hampel H. 2009. Decreased activation along the dorsal visual pathway after a 3-month treatment with galantamine in mild Alzheimer disease: A functional magnetic resonance imaging study. *J Clin Psychopharmacol* **29:** 147–156.

Bondi MW, Houston WS, Eyler LT, Brown GG. 2005. fMRI evidence of compensatory mechanisms in older adults at genetic risk for Alzheimer disease. *Neurology* **64:** 501–508.

Bookheimer SY, Strojwas MH, Cohen MS, Saunders AM, Pericak-Vance MA, Mazziotta JC, Small GW. 2000. Patterns of brain activation in people at risk for Alzheimer's disease. *New Engl J Med* **343:** 450–456.

Borghesani PR, Johnson LC, Shelton AL, Peskind ER, Aylward EH, Schellenberg GD, Cherrier MM. 2007. Altered medial temporal lobe responses during visuospatial encoding in healthy APOE*4 carriers. *Neurobiol Aging* **29:** 981–991.

Braak H, Braak E. 1991. Neuropathological staging of Alzheimer-related changes. *Acta Neuropathol (Berl)* **82:** 239–259.

Buchhave P, Blennow K, Zetterberg H, Stomrud E, Londos E, Andreasen N, Minthon L, Hansson O. 2009. Longitudinal study of CSF biomarkers in patients with Alzheimer's disease. *PLoS One* **4:** e6294.

Buckner RL, Snyder AZ, Shannon BJ, LaRossa G, Sachs R, Fotenos AF, Sheline YI, Klunk WE, Mathis CA, Morris JC, et al. 2005. Molecular, structural, and functional characterization of Alzheimer's disease: Evidence for a relationship between default activity, amyloid, and memory. *J Neurosci* **25:** 7709–7717.

Buckner RL, Andrews-Hanna JR, Schacter DL. 2008. The brain's default network: Anatomy, function, and relevance to disease. *Ann NY Acad Sci* **1124:** 1–38.

Buckner RL, Sepulcre J, Talukdar T, Krienen FM, Liu H, Hedden T, Andrews-Hanna JR, Sperling RA, Johnson KA. 2009. Cortical hubs revealed by intrinsic functional connectivity: Mapping, assessment of stability, and relation to Alzheimer's disease. *J Neurosci* **29:** 1860–1873.

Burack MA, Hartlein J, Flores HP, Taylor-Reinwald L, Perlmutter JS, Cairns NJ. 2010. In vivo amyloid imaging in autopsy-confirmed Parkinson disease with dementia. *Neurology* **74:** 77–84.

Burton EJ, Barber R, Mukaetova-Ladinska EB, Robson J, Perry RH, Jaros E, Kalaria RN, O'Brien JT. 2009. Medial temporal lobe atrophy on MRI differentiates Alzheimer's disease from dementia with Lewy bodies and vascular cognitive impairment: A prospective study with pathological verification of diagnosis. *Brain* **132:** 195–203.

Busche MA, Eichhoff G, Adelsberger H, Abramowski D, Wiederhold KH, Haass C, Staufenbiel M, Konnerth A, Garaschuk O. 2008. Clusters of hyperactive neurons near amyloid plaques in a mouse model of Alzheimer's disease. *Science* **321:** 1686–1689.

Cairns NJ, Ikonomovic MD, Benzinger T, Storandt M, Fagan AM, Shah A, Schmidt RE, Perry A, Reinwald LT, Carter D, et al. 2009. Absence of Pittsburgh Compound B detection of cerebral amyloid β in a patient with clinical, cognitive, and cerebrospinal fluid markers of Alzheimer disease. *Arch Neurol* **66:** 1557–1562.

Cardenas VA, Chao LL, Studholme C, Yaffe K, Miller BL, Madison C, Buckley ST, Mungas D, Schuff N, Weiner MW. 2009. Brain atrophy associated with baseline and longitudinal measures of cognition. *Neurobiol Aging* **32:** 572–580.

Caselli RJ, Chen K, Lee W, Alexander GE, Reiman EM. 2008. Correlating cerebral hypometabolism with future memory decline in subsequent converters to amnestic pre-mild cognitive impairment. *Arch Neurol* **65:** 1231–1236.

Celone KA, Calhoun VD, Dickerson BC, Atri A, Chua EF, Miller SL, DePeau K, Rentz DM, Selkoe DJ, Blacker D, et al. 2006. Alterations in memory networks in mild cognitive impairment and Alzheimer's disease: An independent component analysis. *J Neurosci* **26:** 10222–10231.

Chan D, Fox NC, Scahill RI, Crum WR, Whitwell JL, Leschziner G, Rossor AM, Stevens JM, Cipolotti L, Rossor MN. 2001. Patterns of temporal lobe atrophy in semantic dementia and Alzheimer's disease. *Ann Neurol* **49:** 433–442.

Chan D, Janssen JC, Whitwell JL, Watt HC, Jenkins R, Frost C, Rossor MN, Fox NC. 2003. Change in rates of cerebral atrophy over time in early-onset Alzheimer's disease: Longitudinal MRI study. *Lancet* **362:** 1121–1122.

Chen K, Langbaum JB, Fleisher AS, Ayutyanont N, Reschke C, Lee W, Liu X, Bandy D, Alexander GE, Thompson PM, et al. 2010. Twelve-month metabolic declines in probable Alzheimer's disease and amnestic mild cognitive impairment assessed using an empirically pre-defined statistical region-of-interest: Findings from the Alzheimer's Disease Neuroimaging Initiative. *Neuroimage* **51:** 654–664.

Chetelat G, Desgranges B, de la Sayette V, Viader F, Eustache F, Baron JC. 2003. Mild cognitive impairment: Can FDG-PET predict who is to rapidly convert to Alzheimer's disease? *Neurology* **60:** 1374–1377.

Clark CM, Schneider JA, Bedell BJ, Beach TG, Bilker WB, Mintun MA, Pontecorvo MJ, Hefti F, Carpenter AP, Flitter ML, et al. 2011. AV45-A07 Study Group. Use of florbetapir-PET for imaging β-amyloid pathology. *J Am Med Assoc* **305:** 275–283. Erratum in: *J Am Med Assoc* **305:** 1096.

Clement F, Belleville S. 2009. Test-retest reliability of fMRI verbal episodic memory paradigms in healthy older adults and in persons with mild cognitive impairment. *Hum Brain Mapp* **30:** 4033–4047.

Cohen AD, Price JC, Weissfeld LA, James J, Rosario BL, Bi W, Nebes RD, Saxton JA, Snitz BE, Aizenstein HA, et al. 2009. Basal cerebral metabolism may modulate the cognitive effects of Ab in mild cognitive impairment: An example of brain reserve. *J Neurosci* **29:** 14770–14778.

Damoiseaux JS, Rombouts SA, Barkhof F, Scheltens P, Stam CJ, Smith SM, Beckmann CF. 2006. Consistent resting-state networks across healthy subjects. *Proc Natl Acad Sci* **103:** 13848–13853.

Damoiseaux JS, Beckmann CF, Arigita EJ, Barkhof F, Scheltens P, Stam CJ, Smith SM, Rombouts SA. 2008. Reduced resting-state brain activity in the "default network" in normal aging. *Cereb Cortex* **18:** 1856–1864.

Daselaar SM, Prince SE, Cabeza R. 2004. When less means more: Deactivations during encoding that predict subsequent memory. *Neuroimage* **23:** 921–927.

DeCarli C, Frisoni GB, Clark CM, Harvey D, Grundman M, Petersen RC, Thal LJ, Jin S, Jack CR Jr, Scheltens P. 2007. Qualitative estimates of medial temporal atrophy as a predictor of progression from mild cognitive impairment to dementia. *Arch Neurol* **64:** 108–115.

DeKosky ST, Ikonomovic MD, Styren SD, Beckett L, Wisniewski S, Bennett DA, Cochran EJ, Kordower JH, Mufson EJ. 2002. Upregulation of choline acetyltransferase activity in hippocampus and frontal cortex of elderly subjects with mild cognitive impairment. *Ann Neurol* **51:** 145–155.

de Leon MJ, Convit A, Wolf OT, Tarshish CY, DeSanti S, Rusinek H, Tsui W, Kandil E, Scherer AJ, Roche A, et al. 2001. Prediction of cognitive decline in normal elderly subjects with 2-[(18)F]fluoro-2-deoxy-D-glucose/poitron-emission tomography (FDG/PET). *Proc Natl Acad Sci* **98:** 10966–10971.

De Santi S, de Leon MJ, Rusinek H, Convit A, Tarshish CY, Roche A, Tsui WH, Kandil E, Boppana M, Daisley K, et al. 2001. Hippocampal formation glucose metabolism and volume losses in MCI and AD. *Neurobiol Aging* **22:** 529–539.

Devanand DP, Mikhno A, Pelton GH, Cuasay K, Pradhaban G, Kumar JS, Upton N, Lai R, Gunn RN, Libri V, et al. 2010. Pittsburgh Compound B (11C-PIB) and Fluorodeoxyglucose (18F-FDG) PET in patients with Alzheimer disease, mild cognitive impairment, and healthy controls. *J Geriatr Psychiatry Neurol* **23:** 185–198.

Dickerson BC, Sperling RA. 2008. Functional abnormalities of the medial temporal lobe memory system in mild cognitive impairment and Alzheimer's disease: Insights from functional MRI studies. *Neuropsychologia* **46:** 1624–1635.

Dickerson BC, Goncharova I, Sullivan MP, Forchetti C, Wilson RS, Bennett DA, Beckett LA, deToledo-Morrell L. 2001. MRI-derived entorhinal and hippocampal atrophy in incipient and very mild Alzheimer disease. *Neurobiol Aging* **22:** 747–754.

Dickerson BC, Salat DH, Bates JF, Atiya M, Killiany RJ, Greve DN, Dale AM, Stern CE, Blacker D, Albert MS, et al. 2004. Medial temporal lobe function and structure in mild cognitive impairment. *Ann Neurol* **56:** 27–35.

Dickerson BC, Salat D, Greve D, Chua E, Rand-Giovannetti E, Rentz D, Bertram L, Mullin K, Tanzi R, Blacker D, et al. 2005. Increased hippocampal activation in mild cognitive impairment compared to normal aging and AD. *Neurology* **65:** 404–411.

Drzezga A, Grimmer T, Henriksen G, Stangier I, Perneczky R, Diehl-Schmid J, Mathis CA, Klunk WE, Price J, Dekosky S, et al. 2008. Imaging of amyloid plaques and cerebral glucose metabolism in semantic dementia and Alzheimer's disease. *Neuroimage* **39:** 619–633.

Drzezga A, Grimmer T, Henriksen G, Muhlau M, Perneczky R, Miederer I, Praus C, Sorg C, Wohlschlager A, Riemenschneider M, et al. 2009. Effect of APOE genotype on amyloid plaque load and gray matter volume in Alzheimer disease. *Neurology* **72:** 1487–1494.

Duara R, Loewenstein DA, Potter E, Appel J, Greig MT, Urs R, Shen Q, Raj A, Small B, Barker W, et al. 2008. Medial temporal lobe atrophy on MRI scans and the diagnosis of Alzheimer disease. *Neurology* **71:** 1986–1992.

Dubois B, Feldman HH, Jacova C, Dekosky ST, Barberger-Gateau P, Cummings J, Delacourte A, Galasko D, Gauthier S, Jicha G, et al. 2007. Research criteria for the diagnosis of Alzheimer's disease: Revising the NINCDS-ADRDA criteria. *Lancet Neurol* **6:** 734–746.

Edison P, Archer HA, Hinz R, Hammers A, Pavese N, Tai YF, Hotton G, Cutler D, Fox N, Kennedy A, et al. 2007. Amyloid, hypometabolism, and cognition in Alzheimer disease: An [11C]PIB and [18F]FDG PET study. *Neurology* **68:** 501–508.

Edison P, Archer HA, Gerhard A, Hinz R, Pavese N, Turkheimer FE, Hammers A, Tai YF, Fox N, Kennedy A, et al. 2008. Microglia, amyloid, and cognition in Alzheimer's disease: An [11C](R)PK11195-PET and [11C]PIB-PET study. *Neurobiol Dis* **32:** 412–419.

Engler H, Forsberg A, Almkvist O, Blomquist G, Larsson E, Savitcheva I, Wall A, Ringheim A, Langstrom B, Nordberg A. 2006. Two-year follow-up of amyloid deposition in patients with Alzheimer's disease. *Brain* **129:** 2856–2866.

Engler H, Santillo AF, Wang SX, Lindau M, Savitcheva I, Nordberg A, Lannfelt L, Langstrom B, Kilander L. 2008. In vivo amyloid imaging with PET in frontotemporal dementia. *Eur J Nucl Med Mol Imaging* **35:** 100–106.

Fagan AM, Roe CM, Xiong C, Mintun MA, Morris JC, Holtzman DM. 2007. Cerebrospinal fluid tau/β-amyloid$_{42}$ ratio as a prediction of cognitive decline in nondemented older adults. *Arch Neurol* **64:** 343–349.

Fagan AM, Mintun MA, Shah AR, Aldea P, Roe CM, Mach RH, Marcus D, Morris JC, Holtzman DM. 2009. Cerebrospinal fluid tau and ptau$_{181}$ increase with cortical amyloid deposition in cognitively normal individuals: Implications for future clinical trials of Alzheimer's disease. *EMBO Mol Med* **1:** 371–380.

Filippini N, MacIntosh BJ, Hough MG, Goodwin GM, Frisoni GB, Smith SM, Matthews PM, Beckmann CF, Mackay CE. 2009. Distinct patterns of brain activity in young carriers of the APOE-ε4 allele. *Proc Natl Acad Sci* **106:** 7209–7214.

Fleisher AS, Houston WS, Eyler LT, Frye S, Jenkins C, Thal LJ, Bondi MW. 2005. Identification of Alzheimer disease risk by functional magnetic resonance imaging. *Arch Neurol* **62:** 1881–1888.

Fleisher AS, Sherzai A, Taylor C, Langbaum JB, Chen K, Buxton RB. 2009. Resting-state BOLD networks versus task-associated functional MRI for distinguishing Alzheimer's disease risk groups. *Neuroimage* **47:** 1678–1690.

Forsberg A, Engler H, Almkvist O, Blomquist G, Hagman G, Wall A, Ringheim A, Langstrom B, Nordberg A. 2008. PET imaging of amyloid deposition in patients with mild cognitive impairment. *Neurobiol Aging* **29:** 1456–1465.

Forsberg A, Almkvist O, Engler H, Wall A, Langstrom B, Nordberg A. 2010. High PIB retention in Alzheimer's disease is an early event with complex relationship with CSF biomarkers and functional parameters. *Curr Alzheimer Res* **7:** 56–66.

Foster NL, Chase TN, Fedio P, Patronas NJ, Brooks RA, Di Chiro G. 1983. Alzheimer's disease: Focal cortical changes shown by positron emission tomography. *Neurology* **33:** 961–965.

Foster NL, Heidebrink JL, Clark CM, Jagust WJ, Arnold SE, Barbas NR, DeCarli CS, Turner RS, Koeppe RA, Higdon R, et al. 2007. FDG-PET improves accuracy in distinguishing frontotemporal dementia and Alzheimer's disease. *Brain* **130:** 2616–2635.

Fox NC, Warrington EK, Rossor MN. 1999a. Serial magnetic resonance imaging of cerebral atrophy in preclinical Alzheimer's disease. *Lancet* **353:** 2125.

Fox NC, Scahill RI, Crum WR, Rossor MN. 1999b. Correlation between rates of brain atrophy and cognitive decline in AD. *Neurology* **52:** 1687–1689.

Fox NC, Cousens S, Scahill R, Harvey RJ, Rossor MN. 2000. Using serial registered brain magnetic resonance imaging to measure disease progression in Alzheimer disease: Power calculations and estimates of sample size to detect treatment effects. *Arch Neurol* **57:** 339–344.

Fox NC, Black RS, Gilman S, Rossor MN, Griffith SG, Jenkins L, Koller M. 2005a. Effects of Aβ immunization (AN1792) on MRI measures of cerebral volume in Alzheimer disease. *Neurology* **64:** 1563–1572.

Fox MD, Snyder AZ, Vincent JL, Corbetta M, Van Essen DC, Raichle ME. 2005b. The human brain is intrinsically organized into dynamic, anticorrelated functional networks. *Proc Natl Acad Sci* **102:** 9673–9678.

Frisoni GB, Fox NC, Jack CR Jr, Scheltens P, Thompson PM. 2010. The clinical use of structural MRI in Alzheimer disease. *Nat Rev Neurol* **6:** 67–77.

Furst AJ, Rabinovici GD, Rostomian AH, Steed T, Alkalay A, Racine C, Miller BL, Jagust WJ. 2010. Cognition, glucose metabolism and amyloid burden in Alzheimer's disease. *Neurobiol Aging* (in press). doi: 10.1016/j.neurobiolaging.2010.03.011.

Ganguli M, Dodge HH, Shen C, DeKosky ST. 2004. Mild cognitive impairment, amnestic type: an epidemiologic study. *Neurology* **63:** 115–121.

Goekoop R, Rombouts SA, Jonker C, Hibbel A, Knol DL, Truyen L, Barkhof F, Scheltens P. 2004. Challenging the cholinergic system in mild cognitive impairment: A pharmacological fMRI study. *Neuroimage* **23:** 1450–1459.

Golby A, Silverberg G, Race E, Gabrieli S, O'Shea J, Knierim K, Stebbins G, Gabrieli J. 2005. Memory encoding in Alzheimer's disease: An fMRI study of explicit and implicit memory. *Brain* **128:** 773–787.

Gosche KM, Mortimer JA, Smith CD, Markesbery WR, Snowdon DA. 2002. Hippocampal volume as an index of Alzheimer neuropathology: Findings from the Nun Study. *Neurology* **58:** 1476–1482.

Grady CL, McIntosh AR, Beig S, Keightley ML, Burian H, Black SE. 2003. Evidence from functional neuroimaging of a compensatory prefrontal network in Alzheimer's disease. *J Neurosci* **23:** 986–993.

Greicius MD, Srivastava G, Reiss AL, Menon V. 2004. Default-mode network activity distinguishes Alzheimer's disease from healthy aging: Evidence from functional MRI. *Proc Natl Acad Sci* **101:** 4637–4642.

Grimmer T, Riemenschneider M, Forstl H, Henriksen G, Klunk WE, Mathis CA, Shiga T, Wester HJ, Kurz A, Drzezga A. 2009. Beta amyloid in Alzheimer's Disease: Increased deposition in brain is reflected in reduced concentration in cerebrospinal fluid. *Biol Psychiatry* **65:** 927–934.

Gron G, Bittner D, Schmitz B, Wunderlich AP, Riepe MW. 2002. Subjective memory complaints: Objective neural markers in patients with Alzheimer's disease and major depressive disorder. *Ann Neurol* **51:** 491–498.

Hamalainen A, Pihlajamaki M, Tanila H, Hanninen T, Niskanen E, Tervo S, Karjalainen PA, Vanninen RL, Soininen H. 2006. Increased fMRI responses during encoding in mild cognitive impairment. *Neurobiol Aging* **28:** 1889–1903.

Hamalainen A, Pihlajamaki M, Tanila H, Hanninen T, Niskanen E, Tervo S, Karjalainen PA, Vanninen RL, Soininen H. 2007. Increased fMRI responses during

encoding in mild cognitive impairment. *Neurobiol Aging* **28:** 1889–1903.

Han SD, Houston WS, Jak AJ, Eyler LT, Nagel BJ, Fleisher AS, Brown GG, Corey-Bloom J, Salmon DP, Thal LJ, et al. 2007. Verbal paired-associate learning by APOE genotype in non-demented older adults: fMRI evidence of a right hemispheric compensatory response. *Neurobiol Aging* **28:** 238–247.

Hansson O, Zetterberg H, Buchhave P, Londos E, Blennow K, Minthon L. 2006. Association between CSF biomarkers and incipient Alzheimer's disease in patients with mild cognitive impairment: A follow-up study. *Lancet Neurol* **5:** 228–234.

Hedden T, Van Dijk KR, Becker JA, Mehta A, Sperling RA, Johnson KA, Buckner RL. 2009. Disruption of functional connectivity in clinically normal older adults harboring amyloid burden. *J Neurosci* **29:** 12686–12694.

Heun R, Freymann K, Erb M, Leube DT, Jessen F, Kircher TT, Grodd W. 2007. Mild cognitive impairment (MCI) and actual retrieval performance affect cerebral activation in the elderly. *Neurobiol Aging* **28:** 404–413.

Hoffman JM, Welsh-Bohmer KA, Hanson M, Crain B, Hulette C, Earl N, Coleman RE. 2000. FDG PET imaging in patients with pathologically verified dementia. *J Nucl Med* **41:** 1920–1928.

Hua X, Leow AD, Parikshak N, Lee S, Chiang MC, Toga AW, Jack CR Jr, Weiner MW, Thompson PM. 2008. Tensor-based morphometry as a neuroimaging biomarker for Alzheimer's disease: An MRI study of 676 AD, MCI, and normal subjects. *Neuroimage* **43:** 458–469.

Ibanez V, Pietrini P, Alexander GE, Furey ML, Teichberg D, Rajapakse JC, Rapoport SI, Schapiro MB, Horwitz B. 1998. Regional glucose metabolic abnormalities are not the result of atrophy in Alzheimer's disease. *Neurology* **50:** 1585–1593.

Ikonomovic MD, Klunk WE, Abrahamson EE, Mathis CA, Price JC, Tsopelas ND, Lopresti BJ, Ziolko S, Bi W, Paljug WR, et al. 2008. Post-mortem correlates of in vivo PiB-PET amyloid imaging in a typical case of Alzheimer's disease. *Brain* **131:** 1630–1645.

Jack CR Jr, Dickson DW, Parisi JE, Xu YC, Cha RH, O'Brien PC, Edland SD, Smith GE, Boeve BF, Tangalos EG, et al. 2002. Antemortem MRI findings correlate with hippocampal neuropathology in typical aging and dementia. *Neurology* **58:** 750–757.

Jack CR Jr, Shiung MM, Gunter JL, O'Brien PC, Weigand SD, Knopman DS, Boeve BF, Ivnik RJ, Smith GE, Cha RH, et al. 2004. Comparison of different MRI brain atrophy rate measures with clinical disease progression in AD. *Neurology* **62:** 591–600.

Jack CR Jr, Petersen RC, Grundman M, Jin S, Gamst A, Ward CP, Sencakova D, Doody RS, Thal LJ. 2008a. Longitudinal MRI findings from the vitamin E and donepezil treatment study for MCI. *Neurobiol Aging* **29:** 1285–1295.

Jack CR Jr, Weigand SD, Shiung MM, Przybelski SA, O'Brien PC, Gunter JL, Knopman DS, Boeve BF, Smith GE, Petersen RC. 2008b. Atrophy rates accelerate in amnestic mild cognitive impairment. *Neurology* **70:** 1740–1752.

Jack CR Jr, Lowe VJ, Weigand SD, Wiste HJ, Senjem ML, Knopman DS, Shiung MM, Gunter JL, Boeve BF, Kemp BJ, et al. 2009. Serial PIB and MRI in normal, mild cognitive impairment and Alzheimer's disease: Implications for sequence of pathological events in Alzheimer's disease. *Brain* **132:** 1355–1365.

Jack CR Jr, Knopman DS, Jagust WJ, Shaw LM, Aisen PS, Weiner MW, Petersen RC, Trojanowski JQ. 2010. Hypothetical model of dynamic biomarkers of the Alzheimer's pathological cascade. *Lancet Neurol* **9:** 119–128.

Jagust WJ, Eberling JL, Wu CC, Finkbeiner A, Mungas D, Valk PE, Haan MN. 2002. Brain function and cognition in a community sample of elderly Latinos. *Neurology* **59:** 378–383.

Jagust W, Gitcho A, Sun F, Kuczynski B, Mungas D, Haan M. 2006. Brain imaging evidence of preclinical Alzheimer's disease in normal aging. *Ann Neurol* **59:** 673–681.

Jagust W, Reed B, Mungas D, Ellis W, Decarli C. 2007. What does fluorodeoxyglucose PET imaging add to a clinical diagnosis of dementia? *Neurology* **69:** 871–877.

Jagust WJ, Landau SM, Shaw LM, Trojanowski JQ, Koeppe RA, Reiman EM, Foster NL, Petersen RC, Weiner MW, Price JC, et al. 2009. Relationships between biomarkers in aging and dementia. *Neurology* **73:** 1193–1199.

Jagust WJ, Bandy D, Chen K, Foster NL, Landau SM, Mathis CA, Price JC, Reiman EM, Skovronsky D, Koeppe RA. 2010. The Alzheimer's Disease neuroimaging initiative positron emission tomography core. *Alzheimers Dement* **6:** 221–229.

Johnson SC, Schmitz TW, Moritz CH, Meyerand ME, Rowley HA, Alexander AL, Hansen KW, Gleason CE, Carlsson CM, Ries ML, et al. 2006. Activation of brain regions vulnerable to Alzheimer's disease: The effect of mild cognitive impairment. *Neurobiol Aging* **27:** 1604–1612.

Johnson KA, Gregas M, Becker JA, Kinnecom C, Salat DH, Moran EK, Smith EE, Rosand J, Rentz DM, Klunk WE, et al. 2007. Imaging of amyloid burden and distribution in cerebral amyloid angiopathy. *Ann Neurol* **62:** 229–234.

Kadir A, Andreasen N, Almkvist O, Wall A, Forsberg A, Engler H, Hagman G, Larksater M, Winblad B, Zetterberg H, et al. 2008. Effect of phenserine treatment on brain functional activity and amyloid in Alzheimer's disease. *Ann Neurol* **63:** 621–631.

Kadir A, Almkvist O, Forsberg A, Wall A, Engler H, Langstrom B, Nordberg A. 2010. Dynamic changes in PET amyloid and FDG imaging at different stages of Alzheimer's disease. *Neurobiol Aging* (in press). doi: 10.1016/j.neurobiolaging.2010.06.015.

Karow DS, McEvoy LK, Fennema-Notestine C, Hagler DJ Jr, Jennings RG, Brewer JB, Hoh CK, Dale AM. 2010. Relative capability of MR imaging and FDG PET to depict changes associated with prodromal and early Alzheimer disease. *Radiology* **256:** 932–942.

Kato T, Knopman D, Liu H. 2001. Dissociation of regional activation in mild AD during visual encoding: A functional MRI study. *Neurology* **57:** 812–816.

Kemppainen NM, Aalto S, Wilson IA, Nagren K, Helin S, Bruck A, Oikonen V, Kailajarvi M, Scheinin M, Viitanen M, et al. 2006. Voxel-based analysis of PET amyloid ligand [11C]PIB uptake in Alzheimer disease. *Neurology* **67:** 1575–1580.

Kemppainen NM, Aalto S, Karrasch M, Nagren K, Savisto N, Oikonen V, Viitanen M, Parkkola R, Rinne JO. 2008. Cognitive reserve hypothesis: Pittsburgh Compound B and fluorodeoxyglucose positron emission tomography in

relation to education in mild Alzheimer's disease. *Ann Neurol* **63:** 112–118.

Killiany RJ, Hyman BT, Gomez-Isla T, Moss MB, Kikinis R, Jolesz F, Tanzi R, Jones K, Albert MS. 2002. MRI measures of entorhinal cortex vs hippocampus in preclinical AD. *Neurology* **58:** 1188–1196.

Kircher TT, Weis S, Freymann K, Erb M, Jessen F, Grodd W, Heun R, Leube DT. 2007. Hippocampal activation in patients with mild cognitive impairment is necessary for successful memory encoding. *J Neurol Neurosurg Psychiatry* **78:** 812–818.

Kloppel S, Stonnington CM, Chu C, Draganski B, Scahill RI, Rohrer JD, Fox NC, Jack CR Jr, Ashburner J, Frackowiak RS. 2008. Automatic classification of MR scans in Alzheimer's disease. *Brain* **131:** 681–689.

Klunk WE, Wang Y, Huang GF, Debnath ML, Holt DP, Shao L, Hamilton RL, Ikonomovic MD, DeKosky ST, Mathis CA. 2003. The binding of 2-(4′-methylaminophenyl)-benzothiazole to postmortem brain homogenates is dominated by the amyloid component. *J Neurosci* **23:** 2086–2092.

Klunk WE, Engler H, Nordberg A, Wang Y, Blomqvist G, Holt DP, Bergström M, Savitcheva I, Huang GF, Estrada S, et al. 2004. Imaging brain amyloid in Alzheimer's disease with Pittsburgh Compound-B. *Ann Neurol* **55:** 306–319.

Knopman DS, DeKosky ST, Cummings JL, Chui H, Corey-Bloom J, Relkin N, Small GW, Miller B, Stevens JC. 2001. Practice parameter: Diagnosis of dementia (an evidence-based review). Report of the quality standards subcommittee of the American Academy of Neurology. *Neurology* **56:** 1143–1153.

Koch W, Teipel S, Mueller S, Benninghoff J, Wagner M, Bokde AL, Hampel H, Coates U, Reiser M, Meindl T. 2010. Diagnostic power of default mode network resting state fMRI in the detection of Alzheimer's disease. *Neurobiol Aging* (in press). doi: 10.1016/j.neurobiolaging2010.04.013.

Koivunen J, Pirttila T, Kemppainen N, Aalto S, Herukka SK, Jauhianen AM, Hanninen T, Hallikainen M, Nagren K, Rinne JO, et al. 2008. PET amyloid ligand [11C]PIB uptake and cerebrospinal fluid β-amyloid in mild cognitive impairment. *Dement Geriatr Cogn Disord* **26:** 378–383.

Korf ES, Wahlund LO, Visser PJ, Scheltens P. 2004. Medial temporal lobe atrophy on MRI predicts dementia in patients with mild cognitive impairment. *Neurology* **63:** 94–100.

Kukolja J, Thiel CM, Fink GR. 2009. Cholinergic stimulation enhances neural activity associated with encoding but reduces neural activity associated with retrieval in humans. *J Neurosci* **29:** 8119–8128.

Kwong KK, Belliveau JW, Chesler DA, Goldberg IE, Weisskoff RM, Poncelet BP, Kennedy DN, Hoppel BE, Cohen MS, Turner R, et al. 1992. Dynamic magnetic resonance imaging of human brain activity during primary sensory stimulation. *Proc Natl Acad Sci* **89:** 5675–5679.

Landau SM, Harvey D, Madison CM, Reiman EM, Foster NL, Aisen PS, Petersen RC, Shaw LM, Trojanowski JQ, Jack CR Jr, et al. 2010. Comparing predictors of conversion and decline in mild cognitive impairment. *Neurology* **75:** 230–238.

Langbaum JB, Chen K, Lee W, Reschke C, Bandy D, Fleisher AS, Alexander GE, Foster NL, Weiner MW, Koeppe RA, et al. 2009. Categorical and correlational analyses of baseline fluorodeoxyglucose positron emission tomography images from the Alzheimer's Disease Neuroimaging Initiative (ADNI). *Neuroimage* **45:** 1107–1116.

Larrieu S, Letenneur L, Orgogozo JM, Fabrigoule C, Amieva H, Le Carret N, Barberger-Gateau P, Dartigues JF. 2002. Incidence and outcome of mild cognitive impairment in a population-based prospective cohort. *Neurology* **59:** 1594–1599.

Lehericy S, Baulac M, Chiras J, Pierot L, Martin N, Pillon B, Deweer B, Dubois B, Marsault C. 1994. Amygdalohippocampal MR volume measurements in the early stages of Alzheimer disease. *Am J Neuroradiol* **15:** 929–937.

Lenzi D, Serra L, Perri R, Pantano P, Lenzi GL, Paulesu E, Caltagirone C, Bozzali M, Macaluso E. 2009. Single domain amnestic MCI: A multiple cognitive domains fMRI investigation. *Neurobiol Aging* **32:** 1542–1557.

Lerch JP, Pruessner JC, Zijdenbos A, Hampel H, Teipel SJ, Evans AC. 2005. Focal decline of cortical thickness in Alzheimer's disease identified by computational neuroanatomy. *Cereb Cortex* **15:** 995–1001.

Likeman M, Anderson VM, Stevens JM, Waldman AD, Godbolt AK, Frost C, Rossor MN, Fox NC. 2005. Visual assessment of atrophy on magnetic resonance imaging in the diagnosis of pathologically confirmed young-onset dementias. *Arch Neurol* **62:** 1410–1415.

Lind J, Ingvar M, Persson J, Sleegers K, Van Broeckhoven C, Adolfsson R, Nilsson LG, Nyberg L. 2006a. Parietal cortex activation predicts memory decline in apolipoprotein E-ε4 carriers. *Neuroreport* **17:** 1683–1686.

Lind J, Larsson A, Persson J, Ingvar M, Nilsson LG, Backman L, Adolfsson R, Cruts M, Sleegers K, Van Broeckhoven C, et al. 2006b. Reduced hippocampal volume in non-demented carriers of the apolipoprotein E ε4: Relation to chronological age and recognition memory. *Neurosci Lett* **396:** 23–27.

Lockhart A, Lamb JR, Osredkar T, Sue LI, Joyce JN, Ye L, Libri V, Leppert D, Beach TG. 2007. PIB is a non-specific imaging marker of amyloid-β (Aβ) peptide-related cerebral amyloidosis. *Brain* **130:** 2607–2615.

Logothetis NK, Pauls J, Augath M, Trinath T, Oeltermann A. 2001. Neurophysiological investigation of the basis of the fMRI signal. *Nature* **412:** 150–157.

Lowe VJ, Kemp BJ, Jack CR Jr, Senjem M, Weigand S, Shiung M, Smith G, Knopman D, Boeve B, Mullan B, et al. 2009. Comparison of 18F-FDG and PiB PET in cognitive impairment. *J Nucl Med* **50:** 878–886.

Lustig C, Buckner RL. 2004. Preserved neural correlates of priming in old age and dementia. *Neuron* **42:** 865–875.

Machulda MM, Ward HA, Borowski B, Gunter JL, Cha RH, O'Brien PC, Petersen RC, Boeve BF, Knopman D, Tang-Wai DF, et al. 2003. Comparison of memory fMRI response among normal, MCI, and Alzheimer's patients. *Neurology* **61:** 500–506.

Maetzler W, Liepelt I, Reimold M, Reischl G, Solbach C, Becker C, Schulte C, Leyhe T, Keller S, Melms A, et al. 2009. Cortical PIB binding in Lewy body disease is associated with Alzheimer-like characteristics. *Neurobiol Dis* **34:** 107–112.

Magistretti PJ. 2006. Neuron-glia metabolic coupling and plasticity. *J Exp Biol* **209:** 2304–2311.

Masliah E, Alford M, Adame A, Rockenstein E, Galasko D, Salmon D, Hansen LA, Thal LJ. 2003. Aβ1–42 promotes cholinergic sprouting in patients with AD and Lewy body variant of AD. *Neurology* **61:** 206–211.

McKeith IG, Dickson DW, Lowe J, Emre M, O'Brien JT, Feldman H, Cummings J, Duda JE, Lippa C, Perry EK, et al. 2005. Diagnosis and management of dementia with Lewy bodies: Third report of the DLB Consortium. *Neurology* **65:** 1863–1872.

Meltzer CC, Zubieta JK, Brandt J, Tune LE, Mayberg HS, Frost JJ. 1996. Regional hypometabolism in Alzheimer's disease as measured by positron emission tomography after correction for effects of partial volume averaging. *Neurology* **47:** 454–461.

Miller SL, Fenstermacher E, Bates J, Blacker D, Sperling RA, Dickerson BC. 2008a. Hippocampal activation in adults with mild cognitive impairment predicts subsequent cognitive decline. *J Neurol Neurosurg Psychiatry* **79:** 630–635.

Miller SL, Celone K, DePeau K, Diamond E, Dickerson BC, Rentz D, Pihlajamaki M, Sperling RA. 2008b. Age-related memory impairment associated with loss of parietal deactivation but preserved hippocampal activation. *Proc Natl Acad Sci* **105:** 2181–2186.

Minoshima S, Giordani B, Berent S, Frey KA, Foster NL, Kuhl DE. 1997. Metabolic reduction in the posterior cingulate cortex in very early Alzheimer's disease. *Ann Neurol* **42:** 85–94.

Mintun MA, Larossa GN, Sheline YI, Dence CS, Lee SY, Mach RH, Klunk WE, Mathis CA, DeKosky ST, Morris JC, et al. 2006. [11C]PIB in a nondemented population: Potential antecedent marker of Alzheimer disease. *Neurology* **67:** 446–52.

Misra C, Fan Y, Davatzikos C. 2009. Baseline and longitudinal patterns of brain atrophy in MCI patients, and their use in prediction of short-term conversion to AD: Results from ADNI. *Neuroimage* **44:** 1415–1422.

Mitchell AJ, Shiri-Feshki M. 2009. Rate of progression of mild cognitive impairment to dementia—Meta-analysis of 41 robust inception cohort studies. *Acta Psychiatr Scand* **119:** 252–265.

Mondadori CR, de Quervain DJ, Buchmann A, Mustovic H, Wollmer MA, Schmidt CF, Boesiger P, Hock C, Nitsch RM, Papassotiropoulos A, et al. 2007. Better memory and neural efficiency in young apolipoprotein E ε4 carriers. *Cereb Cortex* **17:** 1934–1947.

Morris JC, Roe CM, Xiong C, Fagan AM, Goate AM, Holtzman DM, Mintun MA. 2010. APOE predicts amyloid-β but not tau Alzheimer pathology in cognitively normal aging. *Ann Neurol* **67:** 122–131.

Mosconi L, Tsui WH, Herholz K, Pupi A, Drzezga A, Lucignani G, Reiman EM, Holthoff V, Kalbe E, Sorbi S, et al. 2008. Multicenter standardized 18F-FDG PET diagnosis of mild cognitive impairment, Alzheimer's disease, and other dementias. *J Nucl Med* **49:** 390–398.

Mosconi L, Mistur R, Switalski R, Brys M, Glodzik L, Rich K, Pirraglia E, Tsui W, De Santi S, de Leon MJ. 2009. Declining brain glucose metabolism in normal individuals with a maternal history of Alzheimer disease. *Neurology* **72:** 513–520.

Mosconi L, Rinne JO, Tsui WH, Berti V, Li Y, Wang H, Murray J, Scheinin N, Nagren K, Williams S, et al. 2010. Increased fibrillar amyloid-β burden in normal individuals with a family history of late-onset Alzheimer's. *Proc Natl Acad Sci* **107:** 5949–5954.

* Mucke L, Selkoe DJ. 2011. Neurotoxicity of amyloid β–protein: Synaptic and network dysfunction. *Cold Spring Harb Perspect Med* doi: 10.1101/cshperspect.a006338.

Nelissen N, Van Laere K, Thurfjell L, Owenius R, Vandenbulcke M, Koole M, Bormans G, Brooks DJ, Vandenberghe R. 2009. Phase 1 study of the Pittsburgh Compound B derivative 18F-Flutemetamol in healthy volunteers and patients with probable Alzheimer disease. *J Nucl Med* **50:** 1251–1259.

O'Brien JL, O'Keefe KM, LaViolette PS, DeLuca AN, Blacker D, Dickerson BC, Sperling RA. 2010. Longitudinal fMRI in elderly reveals loss of hippocampal activation with clinical decline. *Neurology* **74:** 1969–1976.

Ogawa S, Lee TM, Nayak AS, Glynn P. 1990. Oxygenation-sensitive contrast in magnetic resonance image of rodent brain at high magnetic fields. *Magn Reson Med* **14:** 68–78.

Okello A, Koivunen J, Edison P, Archer HA, Turkheimer FE, Nagren K, Bullock R, Walker Z, Kennedy A, Fox NC, et al. 2009. Conversion of amyloid positive and negative MCI to AD over 3 years: An 11C-PIB PET study. *Neurology* **73:** 754–760.

Palop JJ, Chin J, Roberson ED, Wang J, Thwin MT, Bien-Ly N, Yoo J, Ho KO, Yu GQ, Kreitzer A, et al. 2007. Aberrant excitatory neuronal activity and compensatory remodeling of inhibitory hippocampal circuits in mouse models of Alzheimer's disease. *Neuron* **55:** 697–711.

Petersen RC. 2004. Mild cognitive impairment as a diagnostic entity. *J Intern Med* **256:** 183–194.

Petersen RC, Smith GE, Waring SC, Ivnik RJ, Tangalos E, Kokmen E. 1999. Mild cognitive impairment. Clinical characterization and outcome. *Arch Neurol* **56:** 303–308.

Petrella J, Krishnan S, Slavin M, Tran T-T, Murty L, Doraiswamy P. 2006. Mild cognitive impairment: Evaluation with 4-T functional MR imaging. *Radiology* **240:** 177–186.

Petrella JR, Prince SE, Wang L, Hellegers C, Doraiswamy PM. 2007a. Prognostic value of posteromedial cortex deactivation in mild cognitive impairment. *PLoS One* **2:** e1104.

Petrella JR, Wang L, Krishnan S, Slavin MJ, Prince SE, Tran TT, Doraiswamy PM. 2007b. Cortical deactivation in mild cognitive impairment: High-field-strength functional MR imaging. *Radiology* **245:** 224–235.

Petrie EC, Cross DJ, Galasko D, Schellenberg GD, Raskind MA, Peskind ER, Minoshima S. 2009. Preclinical evidence of Alzheimer changes: Convergent cerebrospinal fluid biomarker and fluorodeoxyglucose positron emission tomography findings. *Arch Neurol* **66:** 632–637.

Pihlajamaki M, Depeau KM, Blacker D, Sperling RA. 2008. Impaired medial temporal repetition suppression is related to failure of parietal deactivation in Alzheimer disease. *Am J Geriatr Psychiatry* **16:** 283–292.

Pihlajamaki M, O'Keefe KM, Bertram L, Tanzi R, Dickerson B, Blacker D, Albert M, Sperling R. 2009. Evidence of altered posteromedial cortical fMRI activity in subjects at risk for Alzheimer disease. *Alzheimer Dis Assoc Disord* **24:** 28–36.

Putcha D, O'Keefe K, LaViolette P, O'Brien J, Greve D, Rentz D, Locascio JJ, Atri A, Sperling R. 2010. Reliability of fMRI associative encoding memory paradigm in nondemented elderly adults. *Human Brain Mapping* (in press). doi: 10.1002/hbm.21166.

Rabinovici GD, Furst AJ, O'Neil JP, Racine CA, Mormino EC, Baker SL, Chetty S, Patel P, Pagliaro TA, Klunk WE, et al. 2007. ^{11}C-PIB PET imaging in Alzheimer disease and frontotemporal lobar degeneration. *Neurology* **68:** 1205–1212.

Rabinovici GD, Jagust WJ, Furst AJ, Ogar JM, Racine CA, Mormino EC, O'Neil JP, Lal RA, Dronkers NF, Miller BL, et al. 2008. Aβ amyloid and glucose metabolism in three variants of primary progressive aphasia. *Ann Neurol* **64:** 388–401.

Rabinovici GD, Furst AJ, Alkalay A, Racine CA, O'Neil JP, Janabi M, Baker SL, Agarwal N, Bonasera SJ, Mormino EC, et al. 2010. Increased metabolic vulnerability in early-onset Alzheimer's disease is not related to amyloid burden. *Brain* **133:** 512–528.

Raichle ME, MacLeod AM, Snyder AZ, Powers WJ, Gusnard DA, Shulman GL. 2001. A default mode of brain function. *Proc Natl Acad Sci* **98:** 676–682.

Reiman EM, Caselli RJ, Yun LS, Chen K, Bandy D, Minoshima S, Thibodeau SN, Osborne D. 1996. Preclinical evidence of Alzheimer's disease in persons homozygous for the ε4 allele for apolipoprotein E. *New Engl J Med* **334:** 752–758.

Reiman EM, Chen K, Alexander GE, Caselli RJ, Bandy D, Osborne D, Saunders AM, Hardy J. 2005. Correlations between apolipoprotein E ε4 gene dose and brain-imaging measurements of regional hypometabolism. *Proc Natl Acad Sci* **102:** 8299–8302.

Reiman EM, Chen K, Caselli RJ, Alexander GE, Bandy D, Adamson JL, Lee W, Cannon A, Stephan EA, Stephan DA, et al. 2008. Cholesterol-related genetic risk scores are associated with hypometabolism in Alzheimer's-affected brain regions. *Neuroimage* **40:** 1214–1221.

Reiman EM, Chen K, Langbaum JB, Lee W, Reschke C, Bandy D, Alexander GE, Caselli RJ. 2010. Higher serum total cholesterol levels in late middle age are associated with glucose hypometabolism in brain regions affected by Alzheimer's disease and normal aging. *Neuroimage* **49:** 169–176.

Remy F, Mirrashed F, Campbell B, Richter W. 2004. Mental calculation impairment in Alzheimer's disease: A functional magnetic resonance imaging study. *Neurosci Lett* **358:** 25–28.

Rentz DM, Locascio JJ, Becker JA, Moran EK, Eng E, Buckner RL, Sperling RA, Johnson KA. 2010. Cognition, reserve, and amyloid deposition in normal aging. *Ann Neurol* **67:** 353–364.

Ridha BH, Barnes J, Bartlett JW, Godbolt A, Pepple T, Rossor MN, Fox NC. 2006. Tracking atrophy progression in familial Alzheimer's disease: A serial MRI study. *Lancet Neurol* **5:** 828–834.

Ridha BH, Anderson VM, Barnes J, Boyes RG, Price SL, Rossor MN, Whitwell JL, Jenkins L, Black RS, Grundman M, et al. 2008. Volumetric MRI and cognitive measures in Alzheimer disease: Comparison of markers of progression. *J Neurol* **255:** 567–574.

Ringman JM, Medina LD, Braskie M, Rodriguez-Agudelo Y, Geschwind DH, Macias-Islas MA, Cummings JL, Bookheimer S. 2010. Effects of risk genes on BOLD activation in presymptomatic carriers of familial Alzheimer's disease mutations during a novelty encoding task. *Cereb Cortex* **21**: 877–883.

Rinne JO, Brooks DJ, Rossor MN, Fox NC, Bullock R, Klunk WE, Mathis CA, Blennow K, Barakos J, Okello AA, et al. 2010. (11)C-PiB PET assessment of change in fibrillar amyloid-β load in patients with Alzheimer's disease treated with bapineuzumab: A phase 2, double-blind, placebo-controlled, ascending-dose study. *Lancet Neurol* **9**: 363–372.

Ritchie K, Artero S, Touchon J. 2001. Classification criteria for mild cognitive impairment: A population-based validation study. *Neurology* **56**: 37–42.

Rocher AB, Chapon F, Blaizot X, Baron JC, Chavoix C. 2003. Resting-state brain glucose utilization as measured by PET is directly related to regional synaptophysin levels: A study in baboons. *Neuroimage* **20**: 1894–1898.

Roe CM, Mintun MA, D'Angelo G, Xiong C, Grant EA, Morris JC. 2008. Alzheimer disease and cognitive reserve: Variation of education effect with carbon 11-labeled Pittsburgh Compound B uptake. *Arch Neurol* **65**: 1467–1471.

Roe CM, Mintun MA, Ghoshal N, Williams MM, Grant EA, Marcus DS, Morris JC. 2010. Alzheimer disease identification using amyloid imaging and reserve variables: Proof of concept. *Neurology* **75**: 42–48.

Rombouts SA, Barkhof F, Veltman DJ, Machielsen WC, Witter MP, Bierlaagh MA, Lazeron RH, Valk J, Scheltens P. 2000. Functional MR imaging in Alzheimer's disease during memory encoding. *Am J Neuroradiol* **21**: 1869–1875.

Rombouts SA, Barkhof F, Van Meel CS, Scheltens P. 2002. Alterations in brain activation during cholinergic enhancement with rivastigmine in Alzheimer's disease. *J Neurol Neurosurg Psychiatry* **73**: 665–671.

Rombouts SA, Barkhof F, Goekoop R, Stam CJ, Scheltens P. 2005. Altered resting state networks in mild cognitive impairment and mild Alzheimer's disease: An fMRI study. *Hum Brain Mapp* **26**: 231–239.

Rombouts SA, Damoiseaux JS, Goekoop R, Barkhof F, Scheltens P, Smith SM, Beckmann CF. 2009. Model-free group analysis shows altered BOLD FMRI networks in dementia. *Hum Brain Mapp* **30**: 256–266.

Rowe CC, Ackerman U, Browne W, Mulligan R, Pike KL, O'Keefe G, Tochon-Danguy H, Chan G, Berlangieri SU, Jones G, et al. 2008. Imaging of amyloid-β in Alzheimer's disease with (18)F-BAY94–9172, a novel PET tracer: Proof of mechanism. *Lancet Neurol* **7**: 129–135.

Rowe CC, Ellis KA, Rimajova M, Bourgeat P, Pike KE, Jones G, Fripp J, Tochon-Danguy H, Morandeau L, O'Keefe G, et al. 2010. Amyloid imaging results from the Australian imaging, biomarkers and lifestyle (AIBL) study of aging. *Neurobiol Aging* **31**: 1275–1283.

Salloway S, Sperling R, Gilman S, Fox NC, Blennow K, Raskind M, Sabbagh M, Honig LS, Doody R, van Dyck CH, et al. 2009. A phase 2 multiple ascending dose trial of bapineuzumab in mild to moderate Alzheimer disease. *Neurology* **73**: 2061–2070.

Savva GM, Wharton SB, Ince PG, Forster G, Matthews FE, Brayne C. 2009. Age, neuropathology, and dementia. *New Engl J Med* **360**: 2302–2309.

Saykin AJ, Wishart HA, Rabin LA, Flashman LA, McHugh TL, Mamourian AC, Santulli RB. 2004. Cholinergic enhancement of frontal lobe activity in mild cognitive impairment. *Brain* **127**: 1574–1583.

Scahill RI, Schott JM, Stevens JM, Rossor MN, Fox NC. 2002. Mapping the evolution of regional atrophy in Alzheimer's disease: Unbiased analysis of fluid-registered serial MRI. *Proc Natl Acad Sci* **99**: 4703–4707.

Scheltens P, Leys D, Barkhof F, Huglo D, Weinstein HC, Vermersch P, Kuiper M, Steinling M, Wolters EC, Valk J. 1992. Atrophy of medial temporal lobes on MRI in "probable" Alzheimer's disease and normal ageing: Diagnostic value and neuropsychological correlates. *J Neurol Neurosurg Psychiatry* **55**: 967–972.

Scheltens P, Fox N, Barkhof F, De Carli C. 2002. Structural magnetic resonance imaging in the practical assessment of dementia: Beyond exclusion. *Lancet Neurol* **1**: 13–21.

Schuff N, Woerner N, Boreta L, Kornfield T, Shaw LM, Trojanowski JQ, Thompson PM, Jack CR Jr, Weiner MW. 2009. MRI of hippocampal volume loss in early Alzheimer's disease in relation to ApoE genotype and biomarkers. *Brain* **132**: 1067–1077.

Schwartz WJ, Smith CB, Davidsen L, Savaki H, Sokoloff L, Mata M, Fink DJ, Gainer H. 1979. Metabolic mapping of functional activity in the hypothalamo-neurohypophysial system of the rat. *Science* **205**: 723–725.

* Selkoe D, Mandelkow E, Holtzman D. 2011. Deciphering Alzheimer disease. *Cold Spring Harb Perspect Med* doi: 10.1101/cshperspect.a011460.

Shanks MF, McGeown WJ, Forbes-McKay KE, Waiter GD, Ries M, Venneri A. 2007. Regional brain activity after prolonged cholinergic enhancement in early Alzheimer's disease. *Magn Reson Imaging* **25**: 848–859.

Sheline YI, Raichle ME, Snyder AZ, Morris JC, Head D, Wang S, Mintun MA. 2009. Amyloid plaques disrupt resting state default mode network connectivity in cognitively normal elderly. *Biol Psychiatry* **67**: 587–587.

Shin J, Lee SY, Kim SH, Kim YB, Cho SJ. 2008. Multitracer PET imaging of amyloid plaques and neurofibrillary tangles in Alzheimer's disease. *Neuroimage* **43**: 236–244.

Sibson NR, Dhankhar A, Mason GF, Behar KL, Rothman DL, Shulman RG. 1997. In vivo 13C NMR measurements of cerebral glutamine synthesis as evidence for glutamate-glutamine cycling. *Proc Natl Acad Sci* **94**: 2699–2704.

Small SA, Perera GM, DeLaPaz R, Mayeux R, Stern Y. 1999. Differential regional dysfunction of the hippocampal formation among elderly with memory decline and Alzheimer's disease. *Ann Neurol* **45**: 466–472.

Small GW, Ercoli LM, Silverman DH, Huang SC, Komo S, Bookheimer SY, Lavretsky H, Miller K, Siddarth P, Rasgon NL, et al. 2000. Cerebral metabolic and cognitive decline in persons at genetic risk for Alzheimer's disease. *Proc Natl Acad Sci* **97**: 6037–6042.

Smith CD, Andersen AH, Kryscio RJ, Schmitt FA, Kindy MS, Blonder LX, Avison MJ. 1999. Altered brain activation in cognitively intact individuals at high risk for Alzheimer's disease. *Neurology* **53**: 1391–1396.

Smith CD, Andersen AH, Kryscio RJ, Schmitt FA, Kindy MS, Blonder LX, Avison MJ. 2002. Women at risk for AD show increased parietal activation during a fluency task. *Neurology* **58:** 1197–1202.

Sole-Padulles C, Bartres-Faz D, Junque C, Vendrell P, Rami L, Clemente IC, Bosch B, Villar A, Bargallo N, Jurado MA, et al. 2009. Brain structure and function related to cognitive reserve variables in normal aging, mild cognitive impairment and Alzheimer's disease. *Neurobiol Aging* **30:** 1114–1124.

Sorg C, Riedl V, Muhlau M, Calhoun VD, Eichele T, Laer L, Drzezga A, Forstl H, Kurz A, Zimmer C, et al. 2007. Selective changes of resting-state networks in individuals at risk for Alzheimer's disease. *Proc Natl Acad Sci* **104:** 18760–18765.

Sperling RA, Greve D, Dale A, Killiany R, Rosen B, Holmes J, Rosas HD, Cocchiarella A, Firth P, Lake S, et al. 2002. fMRI detection of pharmacologically induced memory impairment. *Proc Natl Acad Sci* **99:** 455–460.

Sperling R, Bates J, Chua E, Cocchiarella A, Schacter DL, Rosen B, Albert M. 2003. fMRI studies of associative encoding in young and elderly controls and mild AD patients. *J Neurol Neurosurg Psychiatry* **74:** 44–50.

Sperling RA, Laviolette PS, O'Keefe K, O'Brien J, Rentz DM, Pihlajamaki M, Marshall G, Hyman BT, Selkoe DJ, Hedden T, et al. 2009. Amyloid deposition is associated with impaired default network function in older persons without dementia. *Neuron* **63:** 178–188.

Sperling RA, Dickerson BC, Pihlajamaki M, Vannini P, LaViolette PS, Vitolo OV, Hedden T, Becker JA, Rentz DM, Selkoe DJ, et al. 2010. Functional alterations in memory networks in early Alzheimer's disease. *Neuromolecular Med* **12:** 27–43.

Stern Y, Alexander GE, Prohovnik I, Mayeux R. 1992. Inverse relationship between education and parietotemporal perfusion deficit in Alzheimer's disease. *Ann Neurol* **32:** 371–375.

Stern EA, Bacskai BJ, Hickey GA, Attenello FJ, Lombardo JA, Hyman BT. 2004. Cortical synaptic integration in vivo is disrupted by amyloid-β plaques. *J Neurosci* **24:** 4535–4540.

Thiel CM, Henson RN, Morris JS, Friston KJ, Dolan RJ. 2001. Pharmacological modulation of behavioral and neuronal correlates of repetition priming. *J Neurosci* **21:** 6846–6852.

Tohka J, Reilhac A. 2008. Deconvolution-based partial volume correction in Raclopride-PET and Monte Carlo comparison to MR-based method. *Neuroimage* **39:** 1570–1584.

Tolboom N, van der Flier WM, Yaqub M, Boellaard R, Verwey NA, Blankenstein MA, Windhorst AD, Scheltens P, Lammertsma AA, van Berckel BN. 2009. Relationship of cerebrospinal fluid markers to 11C-PiB and 18F-FDDNP binding. *J Nucl Med* **50:** 1464–1470.

Tolboom N, van der Flier WM, Boverhoff J, Yaqub M, Wattjes MP, Raijmakers PG, Barkhof F, Scheltens P, Herholz K, Lammertsma AA, et al. 2010. Molecular imaging in the diagnosis of Alzheimer's disease: Visual assessment of [11C]PIB and [18F]FDDNP PET images. *J Neurol Neurosurg Psychiatry* **81:** 882–884.

Trivedi MA, Schmitz TW, Ries ML, Torgerson BM, Sager MA, Hermann BP, Asthana S, Johnson SC. 2006. Reduced hippocampal activation during episodic encoding in middle-aged individuals at genetic risk of Alzheimer's disease: A cross-sectional study. *BMC Med* **4:** 1.

Vandenberghe R, Van Laere K, Ivanoiu A, Salmon E, Bastin C, Triau E, Hasselbalch S, Law I, Andersen A, Korner A, et al. 2010. (18)F-flutemetamol amyloid imaging in Alzheimer disease and mild cognitive impairment: A phase 2 trial. *Ann Neurol* **68:** 319–329.

Vemuri P, Wiste HJ, Weigand SD, Shaw LM, Trojanowski JQ, Weiner MW, Knopman DS, Petersen RC, Jack CR Jr. 2009. MRI and CSF biomarkers in normal, MCI, and AD subjects: Predicting future clinical change. *Neurology* **73:** 294–301.

Venneri A, McGeown WJ, Shanks MF. 2009. Responders to ChEI treatment of Alzheimer's disease show restitution of normal regional cortical activation. *Curr Alzheimer Res* **6:** 97–111.

Villemagne VL, McLean CA, Reardon K, Boyd A, Lewis V, Klug G, Jones G, Baxendale D, Masters CL, Rowe CC, et al. 2009. 11C-PiB PET studies in typical sporadic Creutzfeldt–Jakob disease. *J Neurol Neurosurg Psychiatry* **80:** 998–1001.

Vincent JL, Snyder AZ, Fox MD, Shannon BJ, Andrews JR, Raichle ME, Buckner RL. 2006. Coherent spontaneous activity identifies a hippocampal-parietal memory network. *J Neurophysiol* **96:** 3517–3531.

Vincent JL, Patel GH, Fox MD, Snyder AZ, Baker JT, Van Essen DC, Zempel JM, Snyder LH, Corbetta M, Raichle ME. 2007. Intrinsic functional architecture in the anaesthetized monkey brain. *Nature* **447:** 83–86.

Visser PJ, Kester A, Jolles J, Verhey F. 2006. Ten-year risk of dementia in subjects with mild cognitive impairment. *Neurology* **67:** 1201–1207.

Waldemar G, Dubois B, Emre M, Scheltens P, Tariska P, Rossor M. 2000. Diagnosis and management of Alzheimer's disease and other disorders associated with dementia. The role of neurologists in Europe. European Federation of Neurological Societies. *Eur J Neurol* **7:** 133–144.

Walhovd KB, Fjell AM, Amlien I, Grambaite R, Stenset V, Bjornerud A, Reinvang I, Gjerstad L, Cappelen T, Due-Tonnessen P, et al. 2009. Multimodal imaging in mild cognitive impairment: Metabolism, morphometry and diffusion of the temporal-parietal memory network. *Neuroimage* **45:** 215–223.

Wishart HA, Saykin AJ, McDonald BC, Mamourian AC, Flashman LA, Schuschu KR, Ryan KA, Fadul CE, Kasper LH. 2004. Brain activation patterns associated with working memory in relapsing-remitting MS. *Neurology* **62:** 234–238.

Wolk DA, Price JC, Saxton JA, Snitz BE, James JA, Lopez OL, Aizenstein HJ, Cohen AD, Weissfeld LA, Mathis CA, et al. 2009. Amyloid imaging in mild cognitive impairment subtypes. *Ann Neurol* **65:** 557–568.

Wong DF, Rosenberg PB, Zhou Y, Kumar A, Raymont V, Ravert HT, Dannals RF, Nandi A, Brasic JR, Ye W, et al. 2010. In vivo imaging of amyloid deposition in Alzheimer disease using the radioligand 18F-AV-45 (flobetapir F 18). *J Nucl Med* **51:** 913–920.

Fluid Biomarkers in Alzheimer Disease

Kaj Blennow[1], Henrik Zetterberg[1], and Anne M. Fagan[2]

[1]Clinical Neurochemistry Laboratory, Institute of Neuroscience and Physiology, Department of Psychiatry and Neurochemistry, The Sahlgrenska Academy at University of Gothenburg, Sahlgrenska University Hospital, Mölndal, SE-431 80 Mölndal, Sweden

[2]Department of Neurology, The Charles F. and Joanne Knight Alzheimer's Disease Research Center, Hope Center for Neurological Disorders, Washington University School of Medicine, St. Louis, Missouri 63110

Correspondence: kaj.blennow@neuro.gu.se

Research progress has provided detailed understanding of the molecular pathogenesis of Alzheimer disease (AD). This knowledge has been translated into new drug candidates with putative disease-modifying effects, which are now being tested in clinical trials. The promise of effective therapy has created a great need for biomarkers able to detect AD in the predementia phase, because drugs will probably be effective only if neurodegeneration is not too advanced. In this chapter, cerebrospinal fluid (CSF) and plasma biomarkers are reviewed. The core CSF biomarkers total tau (T-tau), phosphorylated tau (P-tau) and the 42 amino acid form of β-amyloid (Aβ42) reflect AD pathology, and have high diagnostic accuracy to diagnose AD with dementia and prodromal AD in mild cognitive impairment cases. The rationale for the use of CSF biomarkers to identify and monitor the mechanism of action of new drug candidates is also outlined in this chapter.

In 1906, Alois Alzheimer presented the first case of the disease that was to bear his name, Alzheimer disease (AD). Alzheimer described the "miliary bodies" (plaques) and "dense bundles of fibrils" (tangles) which we today know are the hallmarks of the disease. In 1985, researchers succeeded in purifying plaque cores and amyloid angiopathy, and the 4 kD β-amyloid (Aβ) peptide was identified as the main component (Glenner and Wong 1984; Masters et al. 1985). This breakthrough paved the way for the cloning of the amyloid precursor protein (APP) gene (Kang et al. 1987). Almost at the same time, it was shown that tangles are composed of abnormally hyperphosphorylated tau protein (Grundke-Iqbal et al. 1986). These important achievements marked the start of modern AD research.

Today, detailed knowledge is available about APP metabolism and Aβ generation and on tau protein homeostasis. Largely based on the mutations found in familial AD (FAD), Aβ has been proposed as the driving force in the disease process. In line with this, the "amyloid cascade hypothesis" for AD (Hardy and Selkoe 2002) posits that an imbalance between the production and clearance of Aβ is the initiating event in disease pathogenesis, ultimately leading to neuronal degeneration and dementia. This research progress has been translated into novel treatment strategies with disease-modifying potential. A large number of anti-Aβ drug candidates, such as those used in Aβ immunotherapy, secretase inhibitors, and Aβ aggregation inhibitors, are in various phases of clinical treatment trials (Blennow et al. 2006). It should be noted, however, that the amyloid cascade hypothesis has not been proven with certainty in late-onset AD, the most common form of the disease.

Disease-modifying drugs will probably be most effective in the earlier stages of the disease, before plaque and tangle load and neurodegeneration become too severe (Das et al. 2001; Levites et al. 2006; Garcia-Alloza et al. 2009). Thus, these treatments should be administered in the predementia stage, or even in presymptomatic individuals. Further, in order for treatments to be labeled as "disease-modifying," they must show a beneficial effect on cognition, as well as evidence that the drug does indeed affect the central disease processes and hallmark neuropathology (Siemers 2009). These challenges have created a need for biomarkers that reflect core elements of the disease process, to serve as diagnostic aids and as tools to identify and monitor the biochemical mechanism of action of the drug. In this chapter, we review the development of candidate biomarkers of AD from cerebrospinal fluid (CSF) and plasma. We focus on established biomarkers, those that have been evaluated in several studies by different research groups, and we discuss their implementation in clinical routine and their potential role in clinical trials.

FLUID BIOMARKERS AND THE BRAIN

Biomarkers are objective measures of a biological or pathogenic process that can be used to evaluate disease risk or prognosis, to guide clinical diagnosis, or to monitor therapeutic interventions (Blennow et al. 2010). The CSF is in direct contact with the extracellular space of the brain, and biochemical changes in the brain are therefore reflected in the CSF. The CSF is thus the optimal source for AD biomarkers.

Since Aβ42 and tau have been shown to be the primary protein components of amyloid

plaques and neurofibrillary tangles, respectively, the levels of these proteins in CSF have been assessed as potential biomarkers of these pathologic features (Fig. 1). Levels of Aβ42 in postmortem ventricular CSF have been shown to correlate with plaque load at autopsy (Strozyk et al. 2003). Similar results have been reported in antemortem lumbar CSF, with low levels correlating with postmortem plaque load (Tapiola et al. 2009). The development of Aβ ligands suitable for positron emission tomography (PET) has enabled direct visualization of fibrillar Aβ load in the brain in living individuals. Studies have consistently found a relationship between in vivo amyloid load as assessed by Pittsburgh Compound B (PIB)-PET binding and CSF Aβ42, with higher [11C]PIB binding correlating with lower CSF Aβ42 levels (Fagan et al. 2006; Forsberg et al. 2008; Grimmer et al. 2009; Tolboom et al. 2009). A similar relationship has been found between CSF Aβ42 and binding of [18F]FDDNP, a PET ligand believed to label both plaques and tangles (Tolboom et al. 2009). These results support the idea that CSF Aβ42 is a measure of fibrillar Aβ42 and plaque load in the brain. The most widely accepted explanation for the reduced CSF level of Aβ42 in AD is that the aggregation of Aβ into plaques (and thus retention in the brain parenchyma) results in less Aβ being available to diffuse into the CSF.

Evidence that CSF total tau (T-tau) reflects the intensity of the neuronal and axonal damage and degeneration has come from several types of studies (Fig. 1). CSF T-tau increases markedly and transiently in acute disorders such as stroke and brain trauma, and the magnitude of the increase positively correlates with the size of the damaged tissue and negatively correlates with clinical outcome (Hesse et al. 2001; Ost et al. 2006; Zetterberg et al. 2006). The degree of increase in CSF T-tau in chronic neurodegenerative disorders is highest in disorders with the most rapid neuronal degeneration, such as Creutzfeldt–Jakob disease (Otto et al. 1997). High CSF T-tau is also associated with a faster progression from mild cognitive impairment (MCI) to AD (Blom et al. 2009), and a more rapid cognitive decline and higher mortality in

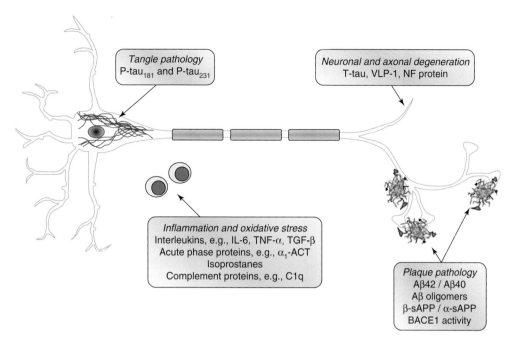

Figure 1. Schematic drawing of a neuron with intracellular neurofibrillary tangles and three neuritic plaques, together with two lymphocytes. Candidate cerebrospinal fluid biomarkers for different pathogenic processes are given.

AD cases (Samgard et al. 2009; Wallin et al. 2009). However, one study found that CSF T-tau correlates with postmortem tangle load (Tapiola et al. 2009), suggesting that the release of tau specifically from degenerating tangle-bearing neurons may contribute to the CSF level of T-tau. Consistent with this idea, binding of ^{18F}FDDNP, an agent that is reported to label both plaques and tangles, positively correlates with CSF T-tau levels (Tolboom et al. 2009).

It is logical to postulate that phosphorylated tau (P-tau) in CSF reflects the phosphorylation state of the tau protein in the central nervous system (CNS; Fig. 1). Positive correlations between CSF levels of P-tau$_{181}$ and P-tau$_{231}$ (tau phosphorylated at residues 181 and 231, respectively) and neocortical tangle pathology at autopsy have been reported (Buerger et al. 2006; Tapiola et al. 2009). High CSF P-tau181 is also associated with a faster progression from MCI to AD (Blom et al. 2009), and a more rapid cognitive decline in AD cases

(Samgard et al. 2009), as well as those with very mild AD dementia (Snider et al. 2009). These findings support the hypothesis that the CSF level of P-tau reflects the phosphorylation state of tau and the formation of tangles in the brain.

FLUID BIOMARKERS FOR AD DIAGNOSIS

β-Amyloid Isoforms

The discovery that β-amyloid (Aβ) is produced during normal cell metabolism and is secreted into the CSF served as the basis for Aβ biomarker development (Seubert et al. 1992). The subsequent finding that Aβ42 is the most abundant species in plaques made it logical to develop assays for this Aβ isoform (Jarrett et al. 1993). CSF Aβ42 in AD is decreased to approximately 50% of control levels, as has been shown using several different enzyme-linked immunosorbent assay (ELISA) methods (Sunderland et al. 2003; Blennow 2004).

Tau Protein

There are several isoforms of the tau protein in CSF, and the molecule has numerous phosphorylation sites (Portelius et al. 2008). The most commonly used ELISA method for T-tau is based on monoclonal antibodies that detect all isoforms of tau independently of phosphorylation state (Blennow et al. 1995). Numerous studies have used this assay, and consistently report a marked increase of CSF T-tau in AD to around 300% of control levels (Sunderland et al. 2003; Blennow 2004).

Phosphorylated Tau Protein

The most commonly used ELISA methods for P-tau in CSF use antibodies that are specific for phosphorylation at either threonine 181 (P-Tau181) or threonine 231 (P-Tau231; Kohnken et al. 2000; Vanmechelen et al. 2000). Studies using these assays have consistently found a marked increase in CSF P-tau in AD (Blennow 2004). Research that compared these P-tau assays directly found a very high correlation between the methods and similar diagnostic performances (Hampel et al. 2004).

Combination of Tau and Aβ as Biomarkers

Several studies have shown that the diagnostic accuracy for the combination of CSF T-tau, P-tau and Aβ42 is higher than for any biomarker alone (Galasko et al. 1998; Reimenschneider et al. 2002; Maddalena et al. 2003; Zetterberg et al. 2003; Hansson et al. 2006). A logical strategy, therefore, was to develop a multiparameter assay for simultaneous quantification of these CSF biomarkers, based on the Luminex™ xMAP technology (Olsson et al. 2005). This assay has been used in several recent large multicenter studies on CSF biomarkers, and its diagnostic performance has been good (Hansson et al. 2006; Lewczuk et al. 2008; Mattsson et al. 2009; Shaw et al. 2009). The measured values for CSF levels of the biomarkers differ between the Luminex technique and the ELISA methods (Olsson et al. 2005; Lewczuk et al. 2008). There are likely to be several reasons for this, including differences in the

pairs of antibodies selected, the method for coupling antibodies to beads, the method of coating plates, differences in the calibrators, and differences in the incubation conditions. Correction factors have been used to convert results from one technique to the other, allowing the results to be compared (Olsson et al. 2005; Mattsson et al. 2009).

DIAGNOSTIC PERFORMANCE OF FLUID BIOMARKERS

AD with Dementia

Numerous studies have found a marked increase in CSF T-tau and P-tau, together with a marked decrease in Aβ42, in AD cases with dementia. These measurements can be used to discriminate patients with AD from the nondemented aged with a sensitivity and specificity that both lie above 80% (Blennow and Hampel 2003; Blennow 2004). CSF levels of these markers are normal in several important differential diagnoses, such as depression and Parkinson disease (Blennow 2004). Combined analyses of these biomarkers give a better diagnostic performance than any biomarker alone (Galasko et al. 1998; Maddalena et al. 2003; Hansson et al. 2006; Mattsson et al. 2009). CSF P-tau, in particular, aids in the differentiation of AD from other dementias, such as frontotemporal dementia and Lewy body dementia (Hampel et al. 2004), but the diagnostic performance of CSF biomarkers to discriminate AD from other dementias is not optimal. There are several reasons for this. First, most studies of CSF biomarkers are based on clinically diagnosed cases, which introduces a relatively large percentage of misdiagnosis (Blennow 2005; Forman et al. 2006). Second, a significant percentage of the nondemented elderly have enough plaques and tangles to warrant a neuropathological diagnosis of AD (Snowdon 1997; Price and Morris 1999). Third, there is a large overlap in pathology between AD and other dementias, such as Lewy body dementia and vascular dementia (Jellinger 1996; Kotzbauer et al. 2001; Schneider et al. 2009). This overlap in pathology essentially precludes the possibility of finding any biomarkers that have close to 100% sensitivity and specificity for AD.

Autopsy-Verified AD

Several studies have examined the diagnostic performance of CSF biomarkers in patient series in which diagnosis can subsequently be confirmed by autopsy. CSF biomarkers have high sensitivity and specificity in discriminating AD from both the cognitively normal elderly and from patients with other dementias, such as frontotemporal dementia, Lewy body dementia and vascular dementia (Clark et al. 2003; Sunderland et al. 2003; Bian et al. 2008; Koopman et al. 2009; Shaw et al. 2009). CSF biomarkers have thus been validated in patient series with a neuropathological follow-up, showing similar or better discriminatory power than in patient series with clinical diagnoses only.

Prodromal AD

Cerebrospinal fluid biomarkers also have a high predictive value in identifying prodromal AD in MCI cases (Blennow and Hampel 2003). A recent study with an extended clinical follow-up period showed that the combination of all three core CSF biomarkers (T-tau, P-tau, and Aβ42) had a sensitivity of 95% for the identification of prodromal AD in MCI (Hansson et al. 2006). These CSF markers have also been shown to predict the rate of cognitive decline in patients with MCI/very mild AD dementia (Snider et al. 2009). A high predictive value has also been verified in large multicenter studies, including the ADNI study (Shaw et al. 2009), the DESCRIPA study (Visser et al. 2009), and the Swedish Brain Power project (Mattsson et al. 2009). These results demonstrate that CSF biomarkers may be valuable clinical diagnostic tools to identify MCI cases with prodromal AD.

Preclinical AD

Preclinical AD denotes cognitively normal individuals harboring early AD pathology, not severe enough to cause cognitive symptoms.

Some studies have examined whether CSF biomarkers are useful in the preclinical stage to identify patients who will subsequently develop AD dementia. Two population-based studies found a significant reduction in CSF Aβ42 in cognitively normal elderly who later developed AD, whereas there was no significant change in CSF T-tau or P-tau (Skoog et al. 2003; Gustafson et al. 2007). A recent clinical study also found that CSF Aβ42, but not T-tau and P-tau, predicts cognitive decline in the healthy elderly (Stomrud et al. 2007). Four independent studies have identified the CSF tau/Aβ42 ratio (but not these markers individually) as a strong predictor of future cognitive decline (within a few years) in nondemented elders (Fagan et al. 2007; Li et al. 2007; Craig-Schapiro et al. 2010; Tarawneh et al. 2011), similar to its ability to predict AD dementia in MCI cohorts (Hansson et al. 2006). Asymptomatic carriers of FAD mutations also have low CSF Aβ42 (Moonis et al. 2005), and high T-tau and P-tau (Ringman et al. 2008). These results extend earlier animal data suggesting that the amyloidogenic process is upstream of tau pathology in AD (Gotz et al. 2001; Lewis et al. 2001). Consistent with this idea, two recent studies reported an association between low CSF Aβ42 levels and brain atrophy in cognitively normal elders (Fagan et al. 2009a; Fjell et al. 2010), whereas CSF tau and ptau181 levels were associated with atrophy in early-stage MCI/AD (Fagan et al. 2009a). These biomarker observations suggest that Aβ aggregation and deposition (as evidenced by reduced CSF Aβ42) are associated with brain atrophy in the preclinical phase of the disease, whereas changes in CSF tau and accelerated brain atrophy are later events in the disease that occur with or just prior to cognitive decline and subsequent clinical progression (Fig. 2). Additional studies are required to confirm these findings.

A recent large study showed that cognitively normal elderly who are positive for PIB-PET (indicating the presence of brain amyloid) have low levels of CSF Aβ42 (Fagan et al. 2009b), confirming results from an earlier, smaller study (Fagan et al. 2006). However, in this larger cohort, CSF Aβ42 was found to also be low in a small subset of PIB-negative

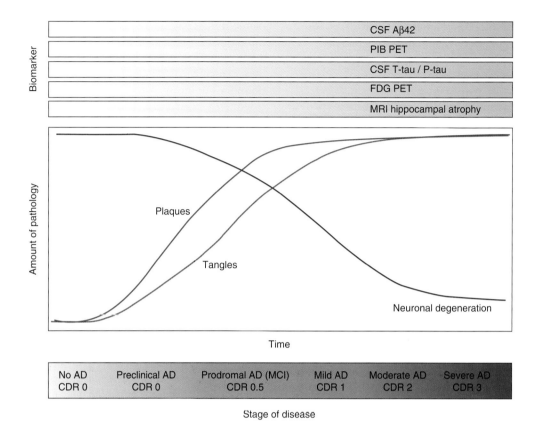

Figure 2. Hypothetical model of the temporal evolution of biomarkers for Alzheimer disease (AD) (*top*) in relation to pathogenic processes in the brain (*middle*) and clinical stage of the disease (*bottom*).

individuals (Fagan et al. 2009b). This finding suggests that low CSF Aβ42 may serve as a harbinger of future amyloid deposition in the preclinical period. Longitudinal PIB follow-up in these individuals will be required to test this hypothesis. Alternatively, low CSF Aβ42 in the absence of PIB positivity may be an indicator of Aβ aggregation in diffuse (PIB-negative) plaques or the accumulation of oligomeric species of Aβ within brain parenchyma prior to substantial fibrillar (PIB-positive) Aβ deposition, or may simply reflect the low end of the normal spectrum of CSF Aβ42 levels. In support of the first alternative hypothesis, one of the PIB-negative individuals with low CSF Aβ42 came to autopsy and was found to have widespread diffuse, but minimal fibrillar, plaque deposits, suggesting that low CSF Aβ42 may mark diffuse plaques in addition to fibrillar

plaques (Cairns et al. 2009). Regardless of the underlying biological mechanism(s), these results suggest that CSF Aβ42 is a marker of AD plaque pathology very early in the disease process (prior to cognitive symptoms). However, it remains to be determined whether CSF Aβ42 levels will allow the prediction of prodromal AD in individual cases. Also, although these data offer important insights into the normal pathophysiology of the disease, the use of biomarkers to predict AD in the asymptomatic elderly is not warranted until registered drugs are available that offer a distinct disease-modifying effect combined with few side-effects. However, such biomarkers may be very useful in the immediate future for the design and evaluation of prevention trials by allowing one to enroll individuals who are still cognitively normal but are in the preclinical stage of the disease and, importantly, are within a few years of developing cognitive symptoms.

NOVEL FLUID BIOMARKERS FOR AD

There are numerous publications describing candidate CSF biomarkers other than $A\beta$ and tau, but initial promising results have most often not been reproduced (Table 1). Here, we review novel biomarkers that have shown promise in two independent studies, and shown a reasonable sensitivity and specificity for AD. We also discuss some candidate biomarkers specifically related to $A\beta$ and APP metabolism.

sAPPβ and sAPPα

During APP processing, the large amino-terminal domains of APP, sAPPα, and sAPPβ, are secreted into the extracellular space and eventually reach the CSF. In sporadic AD and MCI, CSF levels of both sAPPα and sAPPβ are unaltered or slightly increased (Olsson et al. 2003; Zetterberg et al. 2008; Lewczuk et al. 2010). Although there is no consistent change in sAPP levels in AD, these CSF biomarkers may be valuable tools in treatment trials to monitor an effect on APP processing.

BACE1

The major β-secretase responsible for $A\beta$ generation is β-site APP-cleaving enzyme 1 (BACE1). BACE1 expression and enzymatic activity are both increased in postmortem brains of patients with AD (Fukumoto et al. 2002; Yang et al. 2003). BACE1 can be measured in CSF, and its concentration and activity increase in AD, preferentially in MCI cases with prodromal AD (Holsinger et al. 2004; Zhong et al. 2007; Zetterberg et al. 2008). These results suggest that up-regulation of BACE1 is an early pathogenic event in AD.

Aβ Oligomers

Aggregation of soluble $A\beta$ to form insoluble fibrillar aggregates in plaques has long been regarded as the central pathogenic event in AD. However, recent results suggest that soluble $A\beta$ oligomers inhibit long-term potentiation, the proposed biological substrate of memory, thereby playing a role in AD pathogenesis (Walsh and Selkoe 2007). Measurement of $A\beta$ oligomers in CSF may thus be an important core biomarker for AD. Some preliminary studies on $A\beta$ oligomers in CSF have been published. Using monoclonal antibodies for $A\beta$ oligomers in an assay with PCR-based signal amplification, one study reported a marked increase in AD autopsy CSF (Georganopoulou et al. 2005). Flow cytometric results also suggest that $A\beta$ oligomers are present in CSF, but no information on the diagnostic utility of this assay has been presented (Santos et al. 2007). A weak band migrating at the size expected for $A\beta$ dimers appears in CSF immunoprecipitation experiments, utilizing an anti-$A\beta$ antibody followed by SDS–PAGE and immunoblotting, but there is no clear correlation with AD (Klyubin et al. 2008). Immunoassays in which a monocloncal antibody is used for capture, and the same, biotinylated, antibody is used for detection, may be used to quantify protein aggregates, because monomers will not be detected since the epitope is already occupied by the capture antibody. Using ELISA methods based on this principle, higher CSF levels of $A\beta$ oligomers were found in AD (Fukumoto et al. 2010). These promising results call for further studies, and need to be replicated in larger independent patient materials. It seems clear that although $A\beta$ oligomers arc an attractive AD biomarker candidate, the level of such oligomers is very low compared with that of $A\beta$ monomers. Further, the identity of signals measured using different techniques must be verified by mass spectrometry.

Other Aβ Isoforms

$A\beta40$ is the most abundant $A\beta$ isoform in CSF (Portelius et al. 2006a). Although there is no major change in the level of CSF $A\beta40$ in AD, and $A\beta40$ levels do not correlate with amyloid load as evidenced by PIB binding (Fagan et al. 2006, 2009b), there is a marked decrease in the ratio of CSF $A\beta42/A\beta40$ in AD and MCI, which is more pronounced than the reduction in CSF

Table 1. Fluid biomarkers for Alzheimer disease related to β-amyloid and tau pathology and neuronal degeneration

Pathogenic process	Biomarker	Methodology	Change in AD	Stage of evaluation	Comment
APP/Aβ metabolism and plaque pathology	CSF Aβ42 and Aβ40	Commercially available in several different immunoassay formats. Assay characteristics and confounding factors well established	Approximately 50% reduction in CSF Aβ42 in AD with dementia and prodromal AD. CSF Aβ42/Aβ40 ratio may give slightly higher accuracy than Aβ42 alone	Consistent results from numerous publications	CSF Aβ42 is the central CSF biomarker for Aβ metabolism. CSF Aβ42 correlates with amyloid load measured by PIB-PET
	Plasma Aβ42 and Aβ40	Commercially available in several different immunoassay formats	No consistent change in AD. Large overlap with healthy elderly	Consistent results from numerous publications	Plasma Aβ42 and Aβ40 has no diagnostic value for AD. May be valuable in clinical trials
	CSF Aβ16	Immunoprecipitation combined with MALDI-TOF mass spectrometry	Increase in CSF Aβ16 in AD	Preliminary data. Needs verification using standard immunoassays	Analysis of the Aβ isoform pattern, including Aβ16, may be of value in clinical trials on secretase inhibitors
	CSF Aβ oligomers	Specialized techniques, e.g., Bio-barcode PCR assay, western blot, or high-sensitivity ELISA	Increased level or increased frequency of Aβ oligomers in AD	Preliminary data. Needs verification using standard immunoassays	The nature (dimers, trimers, dodecamers, high MW species) of Aβ oligomers in CSF has to be determined
	CSF APP isoforms (sAPPα, sAPPβ)	Commercial assays available	No change or slight increase in AD with large overlap with healthy elderly	Needs further evaluation	APP isoforms are not diagnostically useful, but may be valuable in clinical trials on, e.g., BACE1 inhibitors
	CSF BACE1 activity	Different research assays used in different publications	Increase in AD with dementia and prodromal AD	Data based on publications using different methods	The diagnostic value needs further evaluation. BACE1 activity may be useful in clinical trials on, e.g., BACE1 inhibitors
	Brain Aβ turnover	Infusion of labeled leucine and continuous CSF sampling; immunoprecipitation, tryptic digestion and mass spectrometry measurement of total Aβ	First study shows a decreased Aβ turnover	Needs further evaluation	May be valuable to gauge Aβ production and clearance in clinical drug trials

Cite this article as *Cold Spring Harb Perspect Med* doi: 10.1101/cshperspect.a006221

Category	Biomarker	Assay	Change	Evidence	Comment
Tau phosphorylation and tangle pathology	CSF P-tau181	Commercially available in different immunoassay formats. Assay characteristics and confounding factors well established	Increase in AD with dementia and prodromal AD	Consistent results from numerous publications	CSF P-tau is the central CSF biomarker for tau phosphorylation state. May be valuable as a downstream biomarker in anti-Aβ treatment trials
	CSF P-tau231	Commercial assay not available	Increase in AD with dementia and prodromal AD	Consistent results from numerous publications	CSF P-tau is the central CSF biomarker for tau phosphorylation state. May be valuable as a downstream biomarker in anti-Aβ treatment trials
Neuronal and axonal degeneration	CSF T-tau	Commercially available in different immunoassay formats. Assay characteristics and confounding factors well established	Increase in AD with dementia and prodromal AD	Consistent results from numerous publications	CSF T-tau is the central CSF biomarker to monitor the intensity of neuronal and axonal degeneration in treatment trials
	CSF VILIP-1	Single (research) assay	Increase in AD	Needs further evaluation	CSF VLP-1 levels correlate with CSF T-tau. May be a valuable complementary biomarker for axonal degeneration
	CSF NF proteins	Different (research) assays using in different publications	Normal in AD. High CSF NF proteins in disorders with subcortical pathology, e.g., VaD and NPH, and in FTD	Consistent results from numerous publications	CSF NF proteins may be valuable to differentiate AD from frontotemporal dementia and subcortical dementia disorders

Abbreviations: AD, Alzheimer disease; BACE1, β-site APP-cleaving enzyme 1; CSF, cerebrospinal fluid; FTD, frontotemporal dementia; NF, neurofilament; NPH, normal pressure hydrocephalus; PET, positron emission tomography; PIB, Pittsburgh compound B; P-tau, phosphorylated tau; T-tau, total tau; VaD, vascular dementia; VILIP-1, visinin-like protein 1.

Aβ42 alone (Mehta et al. 2000; Hansson et al. 2007a). Apart from Aβ42 and Aβ40, other carboxy-terminally truncated Aβ peptides can be identified in CSF, including Aβ37, Aβ38, and Aβ39 (Lewczuk et al. 2003). The CSF level of Aβ38 has been reported to be higher in AD, together with a decrease in the level of Aβ42 (Lewczuk et al. 2003; Schoonenboom et al. 2005), suggesting that the Aβ42/Aβ38 ratio may be used to improve diagnostic accuracy. The ratio of Aβ38/Aβ42 has also been shown to positively correlate with PIB binding in non-demented cohorts (Fagan et al. 2009b), with an association that is slightly stronger than CSF Aβ42 alone.

Several shorter carboxy-terminally truncated Aβ isoforms in CSF have also been identified and quantified by immunoprecipitation with an anti-Aβ monoclonal antibody and Matrix-assisted laser desorption/ionization time-of-flight (MALDI-TOF) mass spectrometry (Portelius et al. 2006a). An increase in CSF Aβ1−16 is found in AD together with the expected decrease in Aβ1−42 (Portelius et al. 2006b, 2010). Data from experimental studies show that the shorter Aβ isoforms Aβ1−14, Aβ1−15, and Aβ1−16 are produced by a novel pathway for APP processing involving the concerted action of β- and α-secretase, whereas the longer isoforms, from Aβ1−17 and up to Aβ1−42, are produced in the γ-secretase pathway (Portelius et al. 2009).

Neuronal and Synaptic Degeneration

Neuronal and synaptic proteins may prove valuable as CSF biomarkers because they provide information about cognitive function and disease progression. For example, visinin-like protein 1 (VILIP-1) is a highly expressed neuronal calcium sensor protein that was identified by gene array analyses designed to search for brain-specific protein biomarkers (Laterza et al. 2006). CSF VLP-1 increased markedly in AD in a clinical study, with a diagnostic performance similar to that of CSF tau and Aβ (Lee et al. 2008). CSF levels of VLP-1 were higher in APOE ε4-positive cases, and correlated with Mini-Mental State Examination (MMSE)

scores. A recent study of VILIP-1 showed that the ratio of VILIP-1/Aβ42 was as good or better than tau/Aβ42 in predicting progression from cognitively normal to very mild dementia (Tarawneh et al. 2011).

Neurofilament (NF) proteins are structural components of the neuronal axons. The expression of such proteins is particularly high in large myelinated axons (Friede and Samorajski 1970). Accordingly, high CSF levels of NF proteins are found in disorders with subcortical pathology, such as vascular dementia and normal-pressure hydrocephalus (Sjogren et al. 2001a; Agren-Wilson et al. 2007). CSF levels are also high in frontotemporal dementia, whereas they are normal in most cases of AD (Sjogren et al. 2000). CSF NF proteins may thus be valuable for differentiation between AD, frontotemporal dementia, and subcortical dementia disorders.

Clinicopathologic studies have demonstrated that synaptic density is the variable that best correlates with cognitive performance (Terry et al. 1991). Thus, one might predict that synaptic proteins would be the class of biomarkers most tightly linked to cognition. Several pre- and postsynaptic proteins have been identified in CSF using a procedure based on protein precipitation followed by liquid-phase isoelectric focusing and western blotting. These proteins include rab3a, synaptotagmin, growth-associated protein (GAP-43), synaptosomal-associated protein (SNAP-25), and neurogranin (Davidsson et al. 1999). An immunoassay for GAP-43 showed that CSF levels are higher in AD patients than in controls and patients with frontotemporal dementia (Sjogren et al. 2001b). There are also positive correlations between CSF GAP-43 and T-tau, supporting the idea that both biomarkers reflect axonal and synaptic degeneration.

Inflammation and Oxidative Stress

Neuroinflammation, in the way of glial activation (especially in the vicinity of amyloid plaques), is a robust but nonspecific feature of AD. A number of reports published in the 1990s and early 2000s describe alterations in the levels of various inflammatory and signaling molecules, as well as markers of oxidative stress (e.g., α1-antichymotrypsin, isoprostane, the interleukins, TNFα, interferon-γ, complement C1q, and TGF-β) in AD CSF (Zetterberg et al. 2004; Craig-Schapiro et al. 2009). However, results have been very inconsistent, probably owing to methodological differences (e.g., in the procedures for CSF collection and processing, assay differences, and criteria used for subject ascertainment), prevalence of comorbidities in the studied cohorts, and methods of diagnosis. Unbiased proteomics methods have more recently been used to identify molecules that differ between AD and control CSF (and serum and plasma). These studies have consistently identified a plethora of inflammatory markers that differ in abundance between clinical groups (Castano et al. 2006; Finehout et al. 2007). However, even in these unbiased screens, the direction of reported difference in abundance has not been consistent. Despite this, one astrocyte marker, YKL-40, discovered in an unbiased proteomic screen, has recently been validated in a large cohort of cognitively normal and AD subjects to be increased in AD and to predict clinical worsening from cognitively normal to very mild dementia (Craig-Shapiro et al. 2010). The recent availability of commercial multiplexed assays should permit analysis of a large panel of inflammatory and signaling molecules in large-scale studies. It is conceivable (and probable) that adding markers of neuroinflammation to the other CSF markers (such as Aβ42, tau, and P-tau) will further strengthen diagnostic and prognostic capability (Hu et al. 2010).

AD pathogenesis also includes free radical–mediated injury to neurons. Lipid peroxidation is an important consequence of such damage, and it generates many products, including F2-isoprostanes. These molecules may serve as biomarkers for this pathogenic process. CSF F2-isoprostane levels have been reported to be increased in AD (Montine et al. 2007). Recent studies also show an increase in F2-isoprostanes in MCI cases with prodromal AD (Brys et al. 2009a) and in asymptomatic carriers of FAD mutations (Ringman et al. 2008). In contrast, studies on F2-isoprostanes in plasma have reported conflicting results, probably because the contribution of brain-derived F2-isoprostanes to plasma is clouded by the much larger contribution of peripherally derived F2-isoprostanes (Montine et al. 2007).

SILK Technology

Recently a new in vivo technique, known as Stable Isotope Labeling Kinetics (SILK), has been developed to measure the production and clearance rates of CNS proteins in humans (Figure 3). In this technique, a stable (nonradioactive) isotope–labeled amino acid (e.g., $^{13}C_6$-leucine) is administered intravenously and becomes incorporated into newly synthesized proteins. CSF (and plasma) can then be sampled over time via intrathecal and intravenous catheters, respectively. Using mass spectrometry to compare the amounts of labeled versus unlabeled proteins over time, very precise synthesis, clearance, and dose–response curves can be developed. This technique was first applied to determine the synthesis and clearance rates of Aβ in the CNS (Bateman et al. 2006). The fractional production and clearance rates of Aβ in vivo was found to be extremely rapid (7.6% per hr and 8.3% per hr, respectively), with absolute concentrations in the CSF varying widely between sampling times. This technique was used more recently in a randomized, double-blind, placebo-controlled study to demonstrate the pharmacokinetic/pharmacodynamic relationship between an Aβ synthesis inhibitor and the absolute rate of CNS Aβ synthesis (Bateman et al. 2009). In addition, this method identified slower fractional Aβ clearance with no change in fractional Aβ synthesis in late-onset AD versus age-matched controls (Mawuenyega et al. 2010). Since this technique automatically labels all newly synthesized proteins, its potential lies in the fact that it allows for the evaluation of other proteins relevant to AD, other neurodegenerative diseases, and the metabolism of multiple biomarkers simultaneously. As such, this technology may uncover robust fluid biomarkers that will be useful for assessing disease risk, improving AD diagnosis and prognosis,

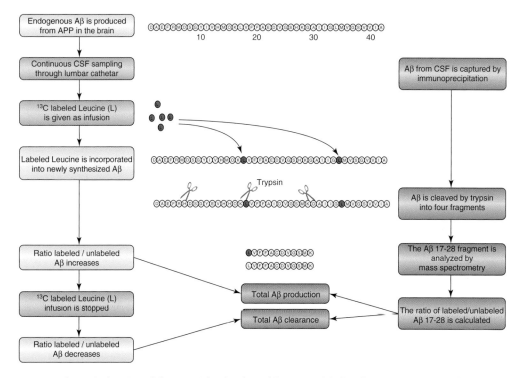

Figure 3. Schematic drawing of the principles for the stable isotope labeling kinetics technology for measuring the production and clearance of total β-amyloid (Aβ) in the brain.

tracking disease progression, and evaluating treatment efficacy.

Plasma Biomarkers

Efforts to find reliable biomarkers for AD in peripheral blood have had little success. Several candidate blood biomarkers have been proposed, but have been difficult to verify in independent studies. In this review we focus on plasma Aβ, which is the most extensively examined peripheral biomarker for AD. We also review some explorative pilot studies with promising results.

Many studies have examined plasma Aβ as a biomarker for AD, but the findings are contradictory. Some groups report slightly higher plasma levels of either Aβ42 or Aβ40 in AD, although with a broad overlap between patients and controls, whereas most studies find no change (Irizarry 2004). Studies examining the value of plasma Aβ in predicting AD in the cognitively normal elderly also show a very broad

overlap in plasma Aβ42 and Aβ40 levels. Some studies report that high plasma Aβ42, or a high Aβ42/Aβ40 ratio, is a risk indicator for future AD, whereas others report the opposite (Mayeux et al. 2003; Pomara et al. 2005; van Oijen et al. 2006; Graff-Radford et al. 2007). These discouraging results are probably due to the fact that the majority of plasma Aβ is derived from peripheral tissues, and does not reflect brain Aβ turnover or metabolism (Mehta et al. 2000). This is consistent with a lack of correlation between plasma Aβ species and brain amyloid load as determined by PIB binding (Fagan et al. 2006, 2009b). It is possible, however, that the hydrophobic nature of Aβ causes it to bind to plasma proteins, which may result in epitope masking and other analytical interferences (Kuo et al. 1999).

There are some recent reports that present promising novel blood biomarkers for AD. Combined multivariate analysis of 18 plasma signaling and inflammatory proteins was found to identify AD patients and predict future AD, with high accuracy, in MCI patients (Ray et al. 2007). This protein panel was identified after screening a large number of known proteins using a filter-based protein array. Further independent studies are needed to verify if this panel is the optimal combination of plasma biomarkers, as well as to determine their diagnostic value. Another study using explorative proteomics technology identified AD-associated changes in the plasma levels of complement factor H and α2-macroglobulin (Hye et al. 2006). This finding was replicated using semiquantitative immunoblotting techniques. A significant change was also reported in the ratio of the microcirculation regulating factor midregional pro-atrial natriuretic peptide to carboxy-terminal endothelin-1 precursor fragment, both of which regulate microcirculation, in plasma from AD patients (Buerger et al. 2009). If replicated in independent studies using immunoassay techniques suitable for routine diagnostic laboratories, these types of plasma protein panels may serve as useful screening tests for AD.

FLUID BIOMARKERS IN CLINICAL TRIALS

In addition to their potential as tools for clinical diagnosis, CSF biomarkers may be valuable in drug development in at least four different ways. These uses are as diagnostic markers for the enrichment of AD cases, for patient stratification, as safety markers, and as detectors and monitors of biochemical drug effects (Table 2).

Improved Diagnosis/Enrichment of AD Cases

Diagnosing early AD is a great challenge for clinicians because MCI cases only have a mild disturbance in episodic memory and executive dysfunction, whereas other specific symptoms are lacking or are vague and indistinct. The only clinical method available to determine which MCI patients have prodromal AD is an extended follow-up period. Indeed, even at specialized academic centers, the accuracy of the clinical diagnosis of AD in cases that have been followed clinically for several years can be relatively low, with sensitivity and specificity figures of 70–80% (Knopman et al. 2001).

These figures are considerably lower in patients with early AD (Visser et al. 2005) and in primary care settings (Ganguli et al. 2004). Assessment of cognitive changes within individuals over a number of years (as determined with semistructured interviews with the patient and a reliable collateral source who knows the patient well, such as a spouse or adult child), can increase diagnostic accuracy (Storandt et al. 2006). However, this laborious approach is probably not feasible in primary care settings.

Clinical MCI trials of cholinesterase inhibitors, in which having a reduced conversion rate to AD was used as a clinical endpoint, have failed to find any significant benefit of the drugs (Raschetti et al. 2007). These trials have recruited unselected MCI cases, meaning that approximately half of the cases do not have prodromal AD, and thus will not convert. This may have adversely affected the possibility of detecting any positive clinical effect of the drug (Cummings et al. 2007). Addition of positive CSF biomarkers as inclusion criteria in MCI and even prevention trials will increase the proportion of subjects with underlying AD pathology and thereby increase the possibility of detecting a positive effect of the drug.

Stratification of AD Cases Based on Biomarker Data

It is well established that AD is a heterogeneous disorder, at both the clinical and neuropathological levels (Blennow et al. 2006). It is quite possible that the effects of proposed disease-modifying drugs will differ between subgroups of AD patients with respect to degree of plaque and tangle pathology (as evidenced by biomarkers) or genetic determinants. As an example, passive immunization was reported to differ both in treatment effect and side-effects between *APOE* ε4 carriers and noncarriers (Salloway et al. 2009).

Since CSF biomarkers reflect the central pathogenic processes in AD, they may be used in post-hoc analyses to stratify the patient cohort in clinical trials. For example, one could postulate that a patient subgroup with a certain biomarker trait, such as low CSF Aβ42

Table 2. Use of fluid biomarkers in Alzheimer disease clinical trials

Application	Rationale	Time point for use	Comment
Enrichment of AD cases	CSF biomarkers may be valuable in clinical trials on early AD or MCI, to improve the diagnostic accuracy and enrich the patient sample with genuine AD cases	Baseline evaluation of CSF biomarkers in cases eligible for the trial	High T-tau and P-tau and low Aβ42 are indicative of AD
Post-hoc patient stratification	AD cases with biomarker evidence of a clear disturbance in the Aβ metabolism may have a more clear-cut effect of anti-Aβ disease-modifying drugs	Post-hoc stratification of AD cases based on baseline CSF biomarker data	CSF Aβ42 may be valuable to stratify AD cases enrolled in a trial on an anti-Aβ disease-modifying drug candidate CSF P-tau may be valuable to stratify AD cases enrolled in a trial on a drug targeting tau phosphorylation and tangle pathology
Safety monitoring	CSF biomarkers may, together with MRI scans, be used to identify cases with meningoencephalitis or vasogenic edema in Aβ immunotherapy clinical trials	Baseline evaluation CSF biomarkers to allow comparison with a CSF sample taken in the case of an adverse event	CSF cell count, IgG/IgM index, and IgG/IgM oligoclonal bands are standard measures to identify and monitor an inflammatory process, such as meningoencephalitis, within the CNS CSF/serum albumin ratio is the standard measure to identify and monitor a disturbance in the blood–brain barrier causing cerebral edema
Monitoring of drug activity on pathogenic processes	CSF biomarkers may provide information that the drug has an effect on a specific pathogenic process directly in patients with AD	Evaluation of CSF biomarkers in samples taken at baseline compared with samples taken at time points during the trial, including the last week of the trial	Primary CSF biomarkers for APP/Aβ metabolism (e.g., Aβ42, sAPPβ, BACE1 activity, and Aβ turnover) may give biochemical evidence for the specific effect of an anti-Aβ drug candidate. Downstream CSF biomarkers (e.g., P-tau and T-tau) may give biochemical evidence for downstream effects on tangle pathology and axonal degeneration of an anti-Aβ drug candidate

Abbreviations: AD, Alzheimer disease; APP, amyloid precursor protein; CSF, cerebrospinal fluid; MCI, mild cognitive impairment; T-tau, total tau; P-tau, phosphorylated tau.

indicating plaque pathology, will show a better effect of anti-Aβ disease-modifying drugs than a subgroup with normal CSF Aβ42 levels.

Safety Monitoring

Trials of the new type of disease-modifying treatments have been hampered by side-effects including meningoencephalitis, which was observed in a subset of cases in the AN-1792

trial on active Aβ immunotherapy, and vasogenic edema, which was observed in the AAB-001 trial of passive immunotherapy (Orgogozo et al. 2003; Salloway et al. 2009). CSF analysis is the standard method to diagnose both encephalitis and blood–brain barrier damage associated with disorders that cause edema (Tibbling et al. 1977; Andersson et al. 1994). It is also possible to use the baseline CSF sample to initially identify and exclude cases with chronic infectious or inflammatory CNS disorders that may mimic AD, such as neuroborreliosis (Andreason et al. 2010). The inclusion of such cases in a clinical trial might result in the erroneous conclusion that a side-effect, such as encephalitis, has occurred. Further, if a baseline CSF sample is taken for comparison before active therapy is initiated, it can be used to identify even minor inflammatory activation within the CNS that is due to side-effects of the drug, thus permitting safety monitoring in clinical trials. Lastly, biomarkers may also be valuable in demonstrating the absence of side-effects, such as immune activation, in longitudinal CSF samples during treatment.

Monitoring the Biochemical Effect of a Drug

The effects of disease-modifying anti-Aβ drugs on plaque pathology are commonly evaluated in AD transgenic mice, but these animal models have had a low predictive power for treatment success in patients with sporadic AD (Blennow et al. 2006). To bridge the gap between animal studies and large clinical trials, evidence for a true effect on AD pathogenesis directly in man would help in selecting the most promising drug candidates.

In slowly progressive disorders such as AD, evaluation of the clinical effect of a drug using rating scales requires large patient materials and extended treatment periods. For drugs with a symptomatic effect, such as cholinesterase inhibitors, an early improvement in cognitive function is expected. In contrast, a disease-modifying drug cannot be expected to have an early effect on symptoms, but will instead lead to a less pronounced decline in cognitive function over years. Thus, the number of patients needed to detect a disease-modifying effect on cognition is probably larger, and the treatment period longer, than for a symptom-modifying drug.

Biomarkers used to identify and monitor the biochemical effect of drugs are known as "theragnostic markers" (Blennow et al. 2010). Such markers may be used to identify and monitor both the specific effect of a drug on its intended target and its effect on downstream pathogenic events. A trial that uses

such markers would probably require relatively small amounts of patient materials and short treatment periods. Such a strategy may be particularly suitable for making a go/no-go decision for large and expensive phase II or III clinical trials. This approach is feasible given results from longitudinal studies demonstrating low intra-individual variability of CSF T-tau, P-tau, and Aβ42 levels over time (Blennow et al. 2007; Zetterberg et al. 2007). Some of these biomarkers might also serve as substitutes (proxies) for clinical endpoints. However, full-scale clinical trials will be required to determine whether this is possible. Lastly, for regulatory purposes, a claim for a disease-modifying effect can only be made when a drug has been proven to have both an effect on cognition and biomarker evidence of an effect on the central pathogenic processes (Siemers 2009; Vellas 2009). To date, there are only preliminary reports suggesting that CSF biomarkers may be useful as theragnostic markers. Importantly, drug candidates with no proven effect on the molecular pathogenesis of AD, such as cholinesterase inhibitors and lithium, have no effect on AD CSF core biomarkers (Blennow et al. 2007; Hampel et al. 2009). Nevertheless, data from animal studies show that treatment with γ-secretase inhibitors results in a reduction of cortical, CSF, and plasma levels of Aβ (Lanz et al. 2004; Anderson et al. 2005). Similarly, treatment in monkeys with a BACE1 inhibitor results in a reduction in CSF Aβ42, Aβ40, and sAPPβ levels (Sankaranarayanan et al. 2009). In AD cases, it is uncertain how CSF Aβ may respond to treatment with efficacious anti-Aβ drugs. In a phase IIa study of the Aβ clearance-enhancing compound PBT2, a significant dose-dependent reduction in CSF Aβ42 levels during treatment was observed (Lannfelt et al. 2008). Results from a clinical study on the amyloid-targeting drug phenserine also suggest that CSF Aβ levels as a biomarker may be valuable for evaluating treatment effects (Kadir et al. 2008). However, in the interrupted phase IIa AN1792 trial, no significant effect was found on CSF Aβ42, despite a decrease toward normal levels of the downstream biomarker T-tau (Gilman et al. 2005). A clinical study of γ-secretase inhibitor treatment also failed to find any effect on CSF Aβ42 levels (Fleisher et al. 2008). Nevertheless, this drug has a clear inhibitory effect on the Aβ production rate, as can be seen when evaluating its effect by measuring the isotope-labeled Aβ ratio in CSF; a clear inhibitory effect on the rate of Aβ production was observed (Bateman et al. 2009). Several other clinical trials of disease-modifying drug candidates that include biomarkers as endpoints are currently ongoing. These trials will provide further evidence of whether biomarkers will be useful as proof-of-concept tools for the mechanism of action of the drug, and as surrogate markers to predict clinical outcome.

FLUID BIOMARKERS AS ENDOPHENOTYPES IN GENETIC STUDIES

Just as CSF biomarker data from well-characterized, longitudinally followed cohorts may be used to guide diagnosis and estimate prognosis, it can also be used to identify genetic markers that are associated with AD risk. Compared with typical genetic studies of AD that rely on less precise clinical diagnoses, genetic studies based on quantitative endophenotype data can provide more power. In support of this approach, recent studies have shown that elevated CSF T-tau and P-tau levels are associated with single nucleotide polymorphisms in the *MAPT* gene (from which tau protein is produced; Kauwe et al. 2008). Likewise, CSF Aβ levels have been found to associate with polymorphisms in several genes (Kauwe et al. 2009). In this way, by "converting" endophenotype data derived from fluid biomarkers to novel genetic biomarkers, it may be possible to identify *individuals* at greater risk of developing AD and, in the near future, provide treatment options prior to the development of any AD pathology.

FUTURE PERSPECTIVES

Overlapping Pathology Influences Diagnostic Biomarker Accuracy

Currently available biomarkers are not perfect in diagnostic accuracy. However, except for technical shortcomings with the biomarkers,

there are several fundamental reasons for why a 100% sensitive and specific biomarker for AD is an unreachable goal. First, most biomarker studies are based on clinically diagnosed cases, which introduces a relatively large percentage of misdiagnosis (Forman et al. 2006; Engelborghs et al. 2008). Second, a significant percentage of nondemented elderly have enough plaques and tangles to warrant a neuropathological diagnosis of AD (Snowdon 1997; Price and Morris 1999). Third, there is a large overlap in pathology between AD and other dementias, such as Lewy body dementia and vascular dementia (Jellinger 1996; Kotzbauer et al. 2001; Schneider et al. 2009). This overlap in pathology essentially precludes the possibility of finding biomarkers that have close to 100% sensitivity and specificity for AD. One way out of this catch 22-like situation might be to reconsider the terminology. Instead of using the term "AD biomarkers," we could acknowledge that the biomarkers reflect distinct pathogenic or pathologic processes, for example, amyloid retention in the brain and degeneration of nonmyelinated cortical axons. These changes, especially in combination, are frequently seen in AD but may also be present in other neurodegenerative disorders, especially in isolation.

Combination of Multiple Biomarker Modalities

It is logical to suppose that the combination of CSF biomarkers with both structural (CT/MRI) and functional (SPECT/PET) brain imaging will increase the diagnostic accuracy as compared with the use of one biomarker alone. However, only a few studies to date have directly examined this issue. Positive CSF biomarkers combined with either CT or MRI measurements of medial temporal lobe atrophy have been found to increase the accuracy of an AD diagnosis (Schoonenboom et al. 2008; Zhang et al. 2008; Brys et al. 2009b). A recent study also showed that the combination of positive CSF biomarkers with the degree of structural AD-like abnormalities as shown by MRI improved prediction of the conversion from amnestic MCI to AD better than either biomarker alone

Cite this article as *Cold Spring Harb Perspect Med* doi: 10.1101/cshperspect.a006221

(Vemuri et al. 2009). Similarly, combining positive CSF biomarkers with an evaluation of regional cerebral blood flow using either the 133Xe method or SPECT has been shown to improve the accuracy of a prodromal AD diagnosis above that achieved with either biomarker alone (Okamura et al. 2002; Hansson et al. 2007b). Further, although no study has examined the added diagnostic value of PIB-PET and CSF biomarkers, there is a strict negative correlation between the degree of PIB binding as seen in PET images and the CSF level of Aβ42 (Fagan et al. 2006, 2009b; Forsberg et al. 2008; Grimmer et al. 2009). The relationship between PIB binding and the tau/Aβ42 and ptau/Aβ ratios is even stronger than for Aβ42 alone (Fagan et al. 2011). Large multicenter studies are needed to further define the added diagnostic value of combining multiple biomarker modalities. Such studies will also provide information on the optimal brain region to evaluate for atrophy by MRI or Aβ load by PET. Complementary data are also needed to evaluate whether new high-resolution MRI scanners and newly developed amyloid ligands, such as AZD2184 and AV-45, will improve diagnostic sensitivity and specificity (Choi et al. 2009; Nyberg et al. 2009).

Novel Research Criteria for AD

The current clinical diagnostic criteria for AD were outlined more than 25 years ago by the National Institute of Neurological and Communicative Disorders and Stroke and the Alzheimer Disease and Related Disorders (NINCDS-ADRDA) Work Group. They depend largely on the exclusion of causes other than AD for dementia (McKhann et al. 1984). These criteria state that a diagnosis of AD cannot be made until the patient has dementia, which is defined as "cognitive symptoms severe enough to interfere with social or occupational activities." The DSM-IV and ICD-10 criteria, which are used for routine diagnosis, also require that a patient demonstrate dementia before a diagnosis of AD is possible (WHO 1992; American Psychiatric Association 2000). If the new disease-modifying drugs prove to be effective

and become clinically available, these present criteria will hinder patients in the early stages of the disease, certainly in the preclinical stage, from receiving effective therapy.

For this reason, new criteria for different stages of AD have recently been suggested (Dubois et al. 2007; Albert et al. 2011; McKhann et al. 2011; Sperling et al. 2011). These criteria have been constructed to permit a diagnosis of AD in earlier stages of the disease, and are centered on the clinical identification of episodic memory impairment together with one or more abnormal biomarkers, including MRI, PET, and CSF markers. More detailed guidelines are needed to establish how the use of biomarkers can be implemented in the diagnostic procedure for early AD to be used in clinical practice. For example, details are needed regarding the scale that should be applied to measure memory impairment, which assays and cutoffs to use for CSF biomarkers, which brain region (whole brain, hippocampus, or entorhinal cortex) to use to evaluate brain atrophy by MRI, which amyloid ligand to use, and which brain region to use to evaluate brain Aβ load by PET. Studies on these issues are just beginning to emerge (Frisoni et al. 2009). Biomarker assays also need to be standardized between laboratories and centers to allow for general implementation of cutoff points in the diagnostic algorithms. As a first step in this direction, a global quality control program for CSF biomarkers was recently launched. This program also covers practical details on lumbar puncture and CSF sample processing (Blennow et al. 2010). Results from the first two rounds in this quality control program have recently been presented.

CONCLUSION

There is an enormous amount of literature showing good or excellent diagnostic performance of several biomarkers reflecting different facets of the disease process in AD. We have unprecedented possibilities to be able to phenotype our patients. Now is the time to develop the biomarker-based research criteria proposed by Dubois et al. (2007), into a detailed, practical and feasible diagnostic algorithm that will be applicable in clinics worldwide. It is easy to predict that this will be a challenging process. The proposed algorithm would need evaluation in a longitudinal clinical multicenter study to assess its diagnostic accuracy against postconversion clinical dementia diagnoses and, whenever possible, neuropathological findings before general implementation in the clinic.

REFERENCES

Agren-Wilsson A, Lekman A, Sjoberg W, Rosengren L, Blennow K, Bergenheim AT, Malm J. 2007. CSF biomarkers in the evaluation of idiopathic normal pressure hydrocephalus. *Acta Neurol Scand* **116:** 333–339.

Albert MS, Dekosky ST, Dickson D, Dubois B, Feldman HH, Fox NC, Gamst A, Holtzman DM, Jagust WJ, Petersen RC, et al. 2011. The diagnosis of mild cognitive impairment due to Alzheimer's disease: Recommendations from the National Institute on Aging—Alzheimer's Association workgroups on diagnostic guidelines for Alzheimer's disease. *Alzheimer's Dement* **7:** 270–279.

American Psychiatric Association. 2000. *Diagnostic and statistical manual of mental disorders (IV-TR)*, 4th ed. American Psychiatric Association, Washington, DC.

Anderson JJ, Holtz G, Baskin PP, Turner M, Rowe B, Wang B, Kounnas MZ, Lamb BT, Barten D, Felsenstein K, et al. 2005. Reductions in β-amyloid concentrations in vivo by the γ-secretase inhibitors BMS-289948 and BMS-299897. *Biochem Pharmacol* **69:** 689–698.

Andersson M, Alvarez-Cermeño J, Bernardi G, Cogato I, Fredman P, Frederiksen J, Fredrikson S, Gallo P, Grimaldi LM, Grønning M, et al. 1994. Cerebrospinal fluid in the diagnosis of multiple sclerosis: A consensus report. *J Neurol Neurosurg Psychiat* **57:** 897–902.

Andreasen N, Blennow K, Zetterberg H. 2010. Neuroinflammation screening in immunotherapy trials against Alzheimer's disease. *Int J Alzheimers Dis* **2010:** 638379.

Bateman RJ, Munsell LY, Morris JC, Swarm R, Yarasheski KE, Holtzman DM. 2006. Human amyloid-β synthesis and clearance rates as measured in cerebrospinal fluid in vivo. *Nat Med* **12:** 856–861.

Bateman RJ, Siemers ER, Mawuenyega KG, Wen G, Browning KR, Sigurdson WC, Yarasheski KE, Friedrich SW, Demattos RB, May PC, et al. 2009. A γ-secretase inhibitor decreases amyloid-β production in the central nervous system. *Ann Neurol* **66:** 48–54.

Bian H, Van Swieten JC, Leight S, Massimo L, Wood E, Forman M, Moore P, de Koning I, CLark CM, Rosso S, et al. 2008. CSF biomarkers in frontotemporal lobar degeneration with known pathology. *Neurology* **70:** 1827–1835.

Blennow K. 2004. Cerebrospinal fluid protein biomarkers for Alzheimer's disease. *NeuroRx* **1:** 213–225.

Blennow K. 2005. CSF biomarkers for Alzheimer's disease: Use in early diagnosis and evaluation of drug treatment. *Expert Rev Mol Diagn* **5:** 661–672.

Blennow K, Hampel H. 2003. CSF markers for incipient Alzheimer's disease. *Lancet Neurol* **2:** 605–613.

Blennow K, Wallin A, Agren H, Spenger C, Siegfried J, Vanmechelen E. 1995. Tau protein in cerebrospinal fluid: A biochemical marker for axonal degeneration in Alzheimer disease? *Mol Chem Neuropathol* **26:** 231–245.

Blennow K, de Leon MJ, Zetterberg H. 2006. Alzheimer's disease. *Lancet* **368:** 387–403.

Blennow K, Zetterberg H, Minthon L, Lannfelt L, Strid S, Annas P, et al. 2007. Longitudinal stability of CSF biomarkers in Alzheimer's disease. *Neurosci Lett* **419:** 18–22.

Blennow K, Hampel H, Weiner M, Zetterberg H. 2010. Cerebrospinal fluid and plasma biomarkers in Alzheimer disease. *Nat Rev Neurol* **6:** 131–144.

Blom ES, Giedraitis V, Zetterberg H, Fukumoto H, Blennow K, Hyman BT, Irizarry MC, Wahlund LO, Ingelsson M. 2009. Rapid progression from mild cognitive impairment to Alzheimer's disease in subjects with elevated levels of tau in cerebrospinal fluid and the APOE ε4/ε4 genotype. *Dement Geriatr Cogn Disord* **27:** 458–464.

Brys M, Pirraglia E, Rich K, Rolstad S, Mosconi L, Switalski R, Glodzik-Sobanska L, De Santi S, Zinkowski R, Mehta P, et al. 2009a. Prediction and longitudinal study of CSF biomarkers in mild cognitive impairment. *Neurobiol Aging* **30:** 682–690.

Brys M, Glodzik L, Mosconi L, Switalski R, De Santi S, Pirraglia E, Rich K, Kim BC, Mehta P, Zinkowski R, et al. 2009b. Magnetic resonance imaging improves cerebrospinal fluid biomarkers in the early detection of Alzheimer's disease. *J Alzheimer's Dis* **16:** 351–362.

Buerger K, Ewers M, Pirttila T, Zinkowski R, Alafuzoff I, Teipel SJ, DeBernardis J, Kerkman D, McCulloch C, Soininen H, et al. 2006. CSF phosphorylated tau protein correlates with neocortical neurofibrillary pathology in Alzheimer's disease. *Brain* **129:** 3035–3041.

Buerger K, Ernst A, Ewers M, Uspenskaya O, Omerovic M, Morgenthaler NG, Knauer K, Bergmann A, Hampel H. 2009. Blood-based microcirculation markers in Alzheimer's disease-diagnostic value of midregional proatrial natriuretic peptide/C-terminal endothelin-1 precursor fragment ratio. *Biol Psychiat* **65:** 979–984.

Cairns NJ, Ikonomovic MD, Benzinger T, Storandt M, Fagan AM, Shah AR, et al. 2009. Absence of Pittsburgh compound B detection of cerebral amyloid β in a patient with clinical, cognitive, and cerebrospinal fluid markers of Alzheimer disease: A case report. *Arch Neurol* **66:** 1557–1562.

Castano EM, Roher AE, Esh CL, Kokjohn TA, Beach T. 2006. Comparative proteomics of cerebrospinal fluid in neuropathologically-confirmed Alzheimer's disease and non-demented elderly subjects. *Neurol Res* **28:** 155–163.

Choi SR, Golding G, Zhuang Z, Zhang W, Lim N, Hefti F, Benedum TE, Dilbourn MR, Skovronsky D, Kung HF. 2009. Preclinical properties of 18F-AV-45: A PET agent for Aβ plaques in the brain. *J Nucl Med* **50:** 1887–1894.

Clark CM, Xie S, Chittams J, Ewbank D, Peskind E, Galasko D, Morris JC, McKeel DW Jr, Farlow M, Weitlauf SL, et al. 2003. Cerebrospinal fluid tau and β-amyloid: How well do these biomarkers reflect autopsy-confirmed dementia diagnoses? *Arch Neurol* **60:** 1696–1702.

Craig-Schapiro R, Fagan AM, Holtzman DM. 2009. Biomarkers of Alzheimer's disease. *Neurobiol Dis* **35:** 128–140.

Craig-Schapiro R, Perrin RJ, Roe CM, Xiong C, Carter D, Cairns NJ, Mintun MA, Peskind ER, Li F, Galasko DR, et al. 2010. YKL-40: A novel prognostic fluid biomarker for preclinical Alzheimer's disease. *Biol Psychiat* **68**: 903–912.

Cummings JL, Doody R, Clark C. 2007. Disease-modifying therapies for Alzheimer disease: Challenges to early intervention. *Neurology* **69**: 1622–1634.

Das P, Murphy MP, Younkin LH, Younkin SG, Golde TE. 2001. Reduced effectiveness of Aβ1–42 immunization in APP transgenic mice with significant amyloid deposition. *Neurobiol Aging* **22**: 721–727.

Davidsson P, Puchades M, Blennow K. 1999. Identification of synaptic vesicle, pre- and postsynaptic proteins in human cerebrospinal fluid using liquid-phase isoelectric focusing. *Electrophoresis* **20**: 431–437.

Dubois B, Feldman HH, Jacova C, Dekosky ST, Barberger-Gateau P, Cummings J, et al. 2007. Research criteria for the diagnosis of Alzheimer's disease: Revising the NINCDS-ADRDA criteria. *Lancet Neurol* **6**: 734–746.

Engelborghs S, De Vreese K, Van de Casteele T, Vanderstichele H, Van Everbroeck B, Cras P, Martin JJ, Vanmechelen E, De Deyn PP. 2008. Diagnostic performance of a CSF-biomarker panel in autopsy-confirmed dementia. *Neurobiol Aging* **29**: 1143–1159.

Fagan AM, Mintun MA, Mach RH, Lee SY, Dence CS, Shah AR, LaRossa GN, Spinner ML, Klunk WE, Mathis CA, et al. 2006. Inverse relation between in vivo amyloid imaging load and cerebrospinal fluid Aβ42 in humans. *Ann Neurol* **59**: 512–519.

Fagan AM, Roe CM, Xiong C, Mintun MA, Morris JC, Holtzman DM. 2007. Cerebrospinal fluid tau/β-amyloid(42) ratio as a prediction of cognitive decline in nondemented older adults. *Arch Neurol* **64**: 343–349.

Fagan AM, Head D, Shah AR, Marcus D, Mintun M, Morris JC, Holtzman DM. 2009a. Decreased cerebrospinal fluid Aβ(42) correlates with brain atrophy in cognitively normal elderly. *Ann Neurol* **65**: 176–183.

Fagan AM, Mintun MA, Shah AR, Aldea P, Roe CM, Mach RH, et al. 2009b. Cerebrospinal fluid tau and ptau$_{181}$ increase with cortical amyloid deposition in cognitively normal individuals: Implications for future clinical trials of Alzheimer's disease. *EMBO Mol Med* **1**: 371–380.

Fagan AM, Shaw LM, Xiong C, Vanderstichele H, Mintun MA, Trojanowski JQ, Coart E, Morris JC, Holtzman DM. 2011. Comparison of analytical platforms for cerebrospinal fluid measures of {β}-Amyloid 1–42, total tau, and P-tau181 for identifying Alzheimer disease amyloid plaque pathology. *Arch Neurol* **68**: 1137–1144.

Finehout EJ, Franck Z, Choe LH, Relkin N, Lee KH. 2007. Cerebrospinal fluid proteomic biomarkers for Alzheimer's disease. *Ann Neurol* **61**: 120–129.

Fjell AM, Walhovd KB, Fennema-Notestine C, McEvoy LK, Hagler DJ, Holland D, Blennow K, Brewer JB, Dale AM, the Alzheimer's Disease Neuorimaging Initiative. 2010. Brain atrophy in healthy aging is related to CSF levels of Aβ1–42. *Cereb Cortex* **20**: 2069–2079.

Fleisher AS, Raman R, Siemers ER, Becerra L, Clark CM, Dean RA, et al. 2008. Phase 2 safety trial targeting amyloid β production with a γ-secretase inhibitor in Alzheimer disease. *Arch Neurol* **65**: 1031–1038.

Forman MS, Farmer J, Johnson JK, Clark CM, Arnold SE, Coslett HB, Chatterjee A, Hurtig HI, Karlawish JH, Rosen HJ, et al. 2006. Frontotemporal dementia: Clinicopathological correlations. *Ann Neurol* **59**: 952–962.

Forsberg A, Engler H, Almkvist O, Blomquist G, Hagman G, Wall A, Ringheim A, Lángström B, Nordberg A. 2008. PET imaging of amyloid deposition in patients with mild cognitive impairment. *Neurobiol Aging* **29**: 1456–1465.

Friede RL, Samorajski T. 1970. Axon caliber related to neurofilaments and microtubules in sciatic nerve fibers of rats and mice. *Anat Rec* **167**: 379–387.

Frisoni GB, Prestia A, Zanetti O, Galluzzi S, Romano M, Cotelli M, Gennarelli M, Binetti G, Bocchio L, Paghera B, et al. 2009. Markers of Alzheimer's disease in a population attending a memory clinic. *Alzheimer's Dement* **5**: 307–317.

Fukumoto H, Cheung BS, Hyman BT, Irizarry MC. 2002. β-Secretase protein and activity are increased in the neocortex in Alzheimer disease. *Arch Neurol* **59**: 1381–1389.

Fukumoto H, Tokuda T, Kasai T, Ishigami N, Hidaka H, Kondo M, Allsop D, Nakagawa M. 2010. High-molecular-weight {β}-amyloid oligomers are elevated in cerebrospinal fluid of Alzheimer patients. *FASEB J* **24**: 2716–2726.

Galasko D, Chang L, Motter R, Clark CM, Kaye J, Knopman D, Thomas R, Kholodenko D, Schenk D, Lieberburg I, et al. 1998. High cerebrospinal fluid tau and low amyloid β42 levels in the clinical diagnosis of Alzheimer disease and relation to apolipoprotein E genotype. *Arch Neurol* **55**: 937–945.

Ganguli M, Rodriguez E, Mulsant B, Richards S, Pandav R, Bilt JV, Dodge HH, Stoehr GP, Saxton J, Morycz RK, et al. 2004. Detection and management of cognitive impairment in primary care: The Steel Valley Seniors Survey. *J Am Geriatr Soc* **52**: 1668–16675.

Garcia-Alloza M, Subramanian M, Thyssen D, Borrelli LA, Fauq A, Das P, Golde TE, Hyman BT, Bacskai BJ. 2009. Existing plaques and neuritic abnormalities in APP:PS1 mice are not affected by administration of the γ-secretase inhibitor LY-411575. *Mol Neurodegener* **4**: 19.

Georganopoulou DG, Chang L, Nam JM, Thaxton CS, Mufson EJ, Klein WL, Mirkin CA. 2005. Nanoparticle-based detection in cerebral spinal fluid of a soluble pathogenic biomarker for Alzheimer's disease. *Proc Natl Acad Sci* **102**: 2273–2276.

Gilman S, Koller M, Black RS, Jenkins L, Griffith SG, Fox NC, Eisner L, Kirby L, Rovira MB, Forette F, et al. 2005. Clinical effects of Aβ immunization (AN1792) in patients with AD in an interrupted trial. *Neurology* **64**: 1553–1562.

Glenner GG, Wong CW. 1984. Alzheimer's disease: Initial report of the purification and characterization of a novel cerebrovascular amyloid protein. *Biochem Biophys Res Commun* **120**: 885–890.

Gotz J, Chen F, van Dorpe J, Nitsch RM. 2001. Formation of neurofibrillary tangles in P301l tau transgenic mice induced by Aβ 42 fibrils. *Science* **293**: 1491–1495.

Graff-Radford NR, Crook JE, Lucas J, Boeve BF, Knopman DS, Ivnik RJ, Smith GE, Younkin LH, Petersen RC, Younkin SG. 2007. Association of low plasma Aβ42/Aβ40 ratios with increased imminent risk for mild cognitive impairment and Alzheimer disease. *Arch Neurol* **64**: 354–362.

Grimmer T, Riemenschneider M, Förstl H, Henriksen G, Klunk WE, Mathis CA, Shiga T, Wester HJ, Kurz A, Drzezga A. 2009. β Amyloid in Alzheimer's disease: Increased deposition in brain is reflected in reduced concentration in cerebrospinal fluid. *Biol Psychiat* **65**: 927–934.

Grundke-Iqbal I, Iqbal K, Tung YC, Quinlan M, Wisniewski HM, Binder LI. 1986. Abnormal phosphorylation of the microtubule-associated protein tau (tau) in Alzheimer cytoskeletal pathology. *Proc Natl Acad Sci* **83**: 4913–4917.

Gustafson DR, Skoog I, Rosengren L, Zetterberg H, Blennow K. 2007. Cerebrospinal fluid β-amyloid 1–42 concentration may predict cognitive decline in older women. *J Neurol Neurosurg Psychiat* **78**: 461–464.

Hampel H, Buerger K, Zinkowski R, Teipel SJ, Goernitz A, Andreasen N, Sjoegren M, DeBernardis J, Kerkman D, Ishiguro K, et al. 2004. Measurement of phosphorylated tau epitopes in the differential diagnosis of Alzheimer disease: A comparative cerebrospinal fluid study. *Arch Gen Psychiat* **61**: 95–102.

Hampel H, Ewers M, Bürger K, Annas P, Mörtberg A, Bogstedt A, Frölich L, Schröder J, Schönknecht P, Riepe MW, et al. 2009. Lithium trial in Alzheimer's disease: A randomized, single-blind, placebo-controlled, multicenter 10-week study. *J Clin Psychiat* **70**: 922–931.

Hansson O, Zetterberg H, Buchhave P, Londos E, Blennow K, Minthon L. 2006. Association between CSF biomarkers and incipient Alzheimer's disease in patients with mild cognitive impairment: A follow-up study. *Lancet Neurol* **5**: 228–234.

Hansson O, Zetterberg H, Buchhave P, Andreasson U, Londos E, Minthon L, Blennow K. 2007a. Prediction of Alzheimer's disease using the CSF Aβ42/Aβ40 ratio in patients with mild cognitive impairment. *Dement Geriatr Cogn Disord* **23**: 316–320.

Hansson O, Buchhave P, Zetterberg H, Blennow K, Minthon L, Warkentin S. 2007b. Combined rCBF and CSF biomarkers predict progression from mild cognitive impairment to Alzheimer's disease. *Neurobiol Aging* **30**: 165–173.

Hardy J, Selkoe DJ. 2002. The amyloid hypothesis of Alzheimer's disease: Progress and problems on the road to therapeutics. *Science* **297**: 353–356.

Hesse C, Rosengren L, Andreasen N, Davidsson P, Vanderstichele H, Vanmechelen E, Blennow K. 2001. Transient increase in total tau but not phospho-tau in human cerebrospinal fluid after acute stroke. *Neurosci Lett* **297**: 187–190.

Holsinger RM, McLean CA, Collins SJ, Masters CL, Evin G. 2004. Increased β-Secretase activity in cerebrospinal fluid of Alzheimer's disease subjects. *Ann Neurol* **55**: 898–899.

Hu WT, Chen-Plotkin A, Arnold SE, Grossman M, Clark CM, Shaw LM, Pickering E, Kuhn M, Chen Y, McCluskey L, et al. 2010. Novel CSF biomarkers for Alzheimer's disease and mild cognitive impairment. *Acta Neuropathol* **119**: 669–678.

Hye A, Lynham S, Thambisetty M, Causevic M, Campbell J, Byers HL, Hooper C, Rijsdijk F, Tabrizi SJ, Banner S, et al. 2006. Proteome-based plasma biomarkers for Alzheimer's disease. *Brain* **129**: 3042–3050.

Irizarry MC. Biomarkers of Alzheimer disease in plasma. 2004. *NeuroRx* **1**: 226–234.

Jarrett JT, Berger EP, Lansbury PT Jr. 1993. The carboxy terminus of the β amyloid protein is critical for the seeding of amyloid formation: Implications for the pathogenesis of Alzheimer's disease. *Biochemistry* **32**: 4693–4697.

Jellinger KA. 1996. Diagnostic accuracy of Alzheimer's disease: A clinicopathological study. *Acta Neuropathol (Berl)* **91**: 219–220.

Kadir A, Andreasen N, Almkvist O, Wall A, Forsberg A, Engler H, Hagman G, Larksater M, Winblad B, Zetterberg H, et al. 2008. Effect of phenserine treatment on brain functional activity and amyloid in Alzheimer's disease. *Ann Neurol* **63**: 621–631.

Kang J, Lemaire HG, Unterbeck A, Salbaum JM, Masters CL, Grzeschik KH, Multhaup G, Beyreuther K, Müller-Hill B. 1987. The precursor of Alzheimer's disease amyloid A4 protein resembles a cell-surface receptor. *Nature* **325**: 733–736.

Kauwe JS, Cruchaga C, Mayo K, Fenoglio C, Bertelsen S, Nowotny P, Galimberti D, Scarpini E, Morris JC, Fagan AM, et al. 2008. Variation in MAPT is associated with cerebrospinal fluid tau levels in the presence of amyloid-β deposition. *Proc Natl Acad Sci* **105**: 8050–8054.

Kauwe JS, Wang J, Mayo K, Morris JC, Fagan AM, Holtzman DM, Goate AM. 2009. Alzheimer's disease risk variants show association with cerebrospinal fluid amyloid β. *Neurogenetics* **10**: 13–17.

Klyubin I, Betts V, Welzel AT, Blennow K, Zetterberg H, Wallin A, Lemere CA, Cullen WK, Peng Y, Wisniewski T, et al. 2008. Amyloid β protein dimer-containing human CSF disrupts synaptic plasticity: Prevention by systemic passive immunization. *J Neurosci* **28**: 4231–4237.

Knopman DS, DeKosky ST, Cummings JL, Chui H, Corey-Bloom J, Relkin N, Small GW, Miller B, Stevens JC. 2001. Practice parameter: Diagnosis of dementia (an evidence-based review). Report of the Quality Standards Subcommittee of the American Academy of Neurology. *Neurology* **56**: 1143–1153.

Kohnken R, Buerger K, Zinkowski R, Miller C, Kerkman D, DeBernardis J, Shen J, Möller HJ, Davies P, Hampel H. 2000. Detection of tau phosphorylated at threonine 231 in cerebrospinal fluid of Alzheimer's disease patients. *Neurosci Lett* **287**: 187–190.

Koopman K, Le Bastard N, Martin JJ, Nagels G, De Deyn PP, Engelborghs S. 2009. Improved discrimination of autopsy-confirmed Alzheimer's disease (AD) from non-AD dementias using CSF P-tau(181P). *Neurochem Int* **55**: 214–218.

Kotzbauer PT, Trojanowsk JQ, Lee VM. 2001. Lewy body pathology in Alzheimer's disease. *J Mol Neurosci* **17**: 225–232.

Kuo YM, Emmerling MR, Lampert HC, Hempelman SR, Kokjohn TA, Woods AS, Cotter RJ, Roher AE. 1999. High levels of circulating Aβ42 are sequestered by plasma proteins in Alzheimer's disease. *Biochem Biophys Res Commun* **257**: 787–791.

Lannfelt L, Blennow K, Zetterberg H, Batsman S, Ames D, Harrison J, Masters CL, Targum S, Bush AL, Murdoch R, et al. 2008. Safety, efficacy, and biomarker findings of PBT2 in targeting Aβ as a modifying therapy for Alzheimer's disease: A phase IIa, double-blind, randomised, placebo-controlled trial. *Lancet Neurol* **7**: 779–786.

Lanz TA, Hosley JD, Adams WJ, Merchant KM. 2004. Studies of Aβ pharmacodynamics in the brain, cerebrospinal fluid, and plasma in young (plaque-free) Tg2576 mice using the γ-secretase inhibitor N2-[(2S)-2-(3,5-difluorophenyl)-2-hydroxyethanoyl]-N1-[(7S)-5-methyl-6-oxo-6,7-dihydro-5H-dibenzo[b,d]azepin-7-yl]-L-alaninamide (LY-411575). *J Pharmacol Exp Ther* **309:** 49–55.

Laterza OF, Modur VR, Crimmins DL, Olander JV, Landt Y, Lee JM, Ladenson JH. 2006. Identification of novel brain biomarkers. *Clin Chem* **52:** 1713–1721.

Lee JM, Blennow K, Andreasen N, Laterza O, Modur V, Olander J, Gao F, Ohlendorf M, Ladenson JH. 2008. The brain injury biomarker VLP-1 is increased in the cerebrospinal fluid of Alzheimer disease patients. *Clin Chem* **54:** 1617–1623.

Lewczuk P, Esselmann H, Meyer M, Wollscheid V, Neumann M, Otto M, Maler JM, Rüther E, Kornhuber J, Wiltfang J. 2003. The amyloid-β (Aβ) peptide pattern in cerebrospinal fluid in Alzheimer's disease: Evidence of a novel carboxyterminally elongated Aβ peptide. *Rapid Commun Mass Spectrom* **17:** 1291–1296.

Lewczuk P, Kornhuber J, Vanderstichele H, Vanmechelen E, Esselmann H, Bibl M, Wolf S, Otto M, Reulbach U, Kölsch H, et al. 2008. Multiplexed quantification of dementia biomarkers in the CSF of patients with early dementias and MCI: A multicenter study. *Neurobiol Aging* **29:** 812–818.

Lewczuk P, Kamrowski-Kruck H, Peters O, Heuser I, Jessen F, Popp J, Bürger K, Hampel H, Frölich L, Wolf S, et al. 2010. Soluble amyloid precursor proteins in the cerebrospinal fluid as novel potential biomarkers of Alzheimer's disease: A multicenter study. *Mol Psychiat* **15:** 138–145.

Lewis J, Dickson DW, Lin WL, Chisholm L, Corral A, Jones G, Yen SH, Sahara N, Skipper L, Yager D, et al. 2001. Enhanced neurofibrillary degeneration in transgenic mice expressing mutant tau and APP. *Science* **293:** 1487–1491.

Levites Y, Das P, Price RW, Rochette MJ, Kostura LA, McGowan EM, Murphy MP, Golde TE. 2006. Anti-Aβ42- and anti-Aβ40-specific mAbs attenuate amyloid deposition in an Alzheimer disease mouse model. *J Clin Invest* **116:** 193–201.

Li G, Sokal I, Quinn JF, Leverenz JB, Brodey M, Schellenberg GD, et al. 2007. CSF tau/Aβ42 ratio for increased risk of mild cognitive impairment: A follow-up study. *Neurology* **69:** 631–639.

Maddalena A, Papassotiropoulos A, Muller-Tillmanns B, Jung HH, Hegi T, Nitsch RM, Hock C. 2003. Biochemical diagnosis of Alzheimer disease by measuring the cerebrospinal fluid ratio of phosphorylated tau protein to β-amyloid peptide_42. *Arch Neurol* **60:** 1202–1206.

Masters CL, Simms G, Weinman NA, Multhaup G, McDonald BL, Beyreuther K. 1985. Amyloid plaque core protein in Alzheimer disease and Down syndrome. *Proc Natl Acad Sci* **82:** 4245–4249.

Mattsson N, Zetterberg H, Hansson O, Andreasen N, Parnetti L, Jonsson M, Herukka SK, van der Flier WM, Blankenstein MA, Ewers M, et al. 2009. CSF biomarkers and incipient Alzheimer disease in patients with mild cognitive impairment. *JAMA* **302:** 385–393.

Mattsson N, Andreasson U, Persson S, Arai H, Batish SD, Bernardini S, Bocchio-Chiavetto L, Blankenstein MA,

Carrillo MC, Chalbot S. 2011. The Alzheimer's Association external quality control program for cerebrospinal fluid biomarkers. *Alzheimers Dement* **7:** 386–395.

Mawuenyega KG, Sigurdson W, Ovod V, Munsell L, Kasten T, Morris JC, Yarasheski KE, Bateman RJ. 2010. Decreased clearance of CNS β-amyloid in Alzheimer's disease. *Science* **330,** 1774.

Mayeux R, Honig LS, Tang MX, Manly J, Stern Y, Schupf N, Mehta PD. 2003. Plasma Aβ40 and Aβ42 and Alzheimer's disease: Relation to age, mortality, and risk. *Neurology* **61:** 1185–1190.

McKhann G, Drachman D, Folstein M, Katzman R, Price D, Stadlan EM. 1984. Clinical diagnosis of Alzheimer's disease: Report of the NINCDS-ADRDA Work Group under the auspices of Department of Health and Human Services Task Force on Alzheimer's Disease. *Neurology* **34:** 939–944.

McKhann GM, Knopman DS, Chertkow H, Hyman BT, Jack CR Jr, Kawas CH, Klunk WE, Koroshetz WJ, Manly JJ, Mayeux R, et al. 2011. The diagnosis of dementia due to Alzheimer's disease: Recommendations from the National Institute on Aging—Alzheimer's Association workgroups on diagnostic guidelines for Alzheimer's disease. *Alzheimer's Dement* **7,** 263–269.

Mehta PD, Pirttila T, Mehta SP, Sersen EA, Aisen PS, Wisniewski HM. 2000. Plasma and cerebrospinal fluid levels of amyloid β proteins 1–40 and 1–42 in Alzheimer disease. *Arch Neurol* **57:** 100–105.

Montine TJ, Quinn J, Kaye J, Morrow JD. 2007. F(2)-isoprostanes as biomarkers of late-onset Alzheimer's disease. *J Mol Neurosci* **33:** 114–119.

Moonis M, Swearer JM, Dayaw MP, St. George-Hyslop P, Rogaeva E, Kawarai T, Pollen DA. 2005. Familial Alzheimer disease: Decreases in CSF αβ_42 levels precede cognitive decline. *Neurology* **65:** 323–325.

Nyberg S, Jonhagen ME, Cselenyi Z, Halldin C, Julin P, Olsson H, Freund-Levi Y, Andersson J, Varnas K, Svensson S, et al. 2009. Detection of amyloid in Alzheimer's disease with positron emission tomography using [11C]AZD2184. *Eur J Nucl Med Mol Imaging* **36:** 1859–1863.

Okamura N, Arai H, Maruyama M, Higuchi M, Matsui T, Tanji H, Seki T, Hirai H, Chiba H, Itoh M, et al. 2002. Combined analysis of CSF tau levels and [(123)I]Iodoamphetamine SPECT in mild cognitive impairment: Implications for a novel predictor of Alzheimer's disease. *Am J Psychiat* **159:** 474–476.

Olsson A, Hoglund K, Sjogren M, Andreasen N, Minthon L, Lannfelt L, Buerger K, Moller HJ, Hampel H, Davidsson P, et al. 2003. Measurement of α- and β-secretase cleaved amyloid precursor protein in cerebrospinal fluid from Alzheimer patients. *Exp Neurol* **183:** 74–80.

Olsson A, Vanderstichele H, Andreasen N, De Meyer G, Wallin A, Holmberg B, Rosengren L, Vanmechelen E, Blennow K. 2005. Simultaneous measurement of β-amyloid_(1–42), total tau, and phosphorylated tau (Thr181) in cerebrospinal fluid by the xMAP technology. *Clin Chem* **51:** 336–345.

Orgogozo JM, Gilman S, Dartigues JF, Laurent B, Puel M, Kirby LC, Jouanny P, Dubois B, Eisner L, Flitman S, et al. 2003. Subacute meningoencephalitis in a subset of patients with AD after Aβ42 immunization. *Neurology* **61:** 46–54.

Ost M, Nylén K, Csajbok L, Ohrfelt AO, Tullberg M, Wikkelsö C, Nellgárd P, Rosengren L, Blennow K, Nellgárd B. 2006. Initial CSF total tau correlates with 1-year outcome in patients with traumatic brain injury. *Neurology* **67:** 1600–1604.

Otto M, Wiltfang J, Tumani H, Zerr I, Lantsch M, Kornhuber J, Weber T, Kretzschmar HA, Poser S. 1997. Elevated levels of tau-protein in cerebrospinal fluid of patients with Creutzfeldt–Jakob disease. *Neurosci Lett* **225:** 210–212.

Pomara N, Willoughby LM, Sidtis JJ, Mehta PD. 2005. Selective reductions in plasma Aβ 1–42 in healthy elderly subjects during longitudinal follow-up: A preliminary report. *Am J Geriatr Psychiat* **13:** 914–917.

Portelius E, Westman-Brinkmalm A, Zetterberg H, Blennow K. 2006a. Determination of β-amyloid peptide signatures in cerebrospinal fluid using immunoprecipitation–mass spectrometry. *J Proteome Res* **5:** 1010–1016.

Portelius E, Zetterberg H, Andreasson U, Brinkmalm G, Andreasen N, Wallin A, et al. 2006b. An Alzheimer's disease-specific β-amyloid fragment signature in cerebrospinal fluid. *Neurosci Lett* **409:** 215–219.

Portelius E, Hansson SF, Tran AJ, Zetterberg H, Grognet P, Vanmechelen E, Höglund K, Brinkmalm G, Westman-Brickmalm A, Nordhoff E, et al. 2008. Characterization of tau in cerebrospinal fluid using mass spectrometry. *J Proteome Res* **7:** 2114–2120.

Portelius E, Price E, Brinkmalm G, Stiteler M, Olsson M, Persson R, et al. 2009. A novel pathway for amyloid precursor protein processing. *Neurobiol Aging* **32:** 1090–1098.

Portelius E, Andreasson U, Ringman JM, Buerger K, Daborg J, Buchhave P, et al. 2010. Distinct cerebrospinal fluid amyloid β peptide signatures in sporadic and PSEN1 A431E-associated familial Alzheimer's disease. *Mol Neurodegener* **5:** 2.

Price JL, Morris JC. 1999. Tangles and plaques in nondemented aging and "preclinical" Alzheimer's disease. *Ann Neurol* **45:** 358–368.

Raschetti R, Albanese E, Vanacore N, Maggini M. 2007. Cholinesterase inhibitors in mild cognitive impairment: A systematic review of randomised trials. *PLoS Med* **4:** e338.

Ray S, Britschgi M, Herbert C, Takeda-Uchimura Y, Boxer A, Blennow K, Friedman LF, Galasko DR, Jutel M, Karydas A, et al. 2007. Classification and prediction of clinical Alzheimer's diagnosis based on plasma signaling proteins. *Nat Med* **13:** 1359–1362.

Riemenschneider M, Lautenschlager N, Wagenpfeil S, Diehl J, Drzezga A, Kurz A. 2002. Cerebrospinal fluid tau and β-amyloid 42 proteins identify Alzheimer disease in subjects with mild cognitive impairment. *Arch Neurol* **59:** 1729–1734.

Ringman JM, Younkin SG, Pratico D, Seltzer W, Cole GM, Geschwind DH, et al. 2008. Biochemical markers in persons with preclinical familial Alzheimer disease. *Neurology* **71:** 85–92.

Salloway S, Sperling R, Gilman S, Fox NC, Blennow K, Raskind M, Sabbagh M, Honig LS, Doody R, van Dyck CH, et al. 2009. A phase 2 trial of bapineuzumab in mild to moderate Alzheimer's disease. *Neurology* **73:** 2061–2070.

Samgard K, Zetterberg H, Blennow K, Hansson O, Minthon L, Londos E. 2009. Cerebrospinal fluid total tau as a marker of Alzheimer's disease intensity. *Int J Geriatr Psychiat* **25:** 403–410.

Sankaranarayanan S, Holahan MA, Colussi D, Crouthamel MC, Devanarayan V, Ellis J, Espeseth A, Gates AT, Graham SL, Gregro AR, et al. 2009. First demonstration of cerebrospinal fluid and plasma A β lowering with oral administration of a β-site amyloid precursor protein-cleaving enzyme 1 inhibitor in nonhuman primates. *J Pharmacol Exp Ther* **328:** 131–140.

Santos AN, Torkler S, Nowak D, Schlittig C, Goerdes M, Lauber T, Trischmann L, Schaupp M, Penz M, Tiller FW, et al. 2007. Detection of amyloid-β oligomers in human cerebrospinal fluid by flow cytometry and fluorescence resonance energy transfer. *J Alzheimer's Dis* **11:** 117–125.

Schneider JA, Arvanitakis Z, Leurgans SE, Bennett DA. 2009. The neuropathology of probable Alzheimer's disease and mild cognitive impairment. *Ann Neurol* **66:** 200–208.

Schoonenboom NS, Mulder C, Van Kamp GJ, Mehta SP, Scheltens P, Blankenstein MA, Mehta PD. 2005. Amyloid β 38, 40, and 42 species in cerebrospinal fluid: More of the same? *Ann Neurol* **58:** 139–142.

Schoonenboom NS, van der Flier WM, Blankenstein MA, Bouwman FH, Van Kamp GJ, Barkhof F, Scheltens P. 2008. CSF and MRI markers independently contribute to the diagnosis of Alzheimer's disease. *Neurobiol Aging* **29:** 669–675.

Seubert P, Vigo-Pelfrey C, Esch F, Lee M, Dovey H, Davis D, Sinha S, Schlossmacher M, Whaley J, Swindlehurst C, et al. 1992. Isolation and quantification of soluble Alzheimer's β-peptide from biological fluids. *Nature* **359:** 325–327.

Shaw LM, Vanderstichele H, Knapik-Czajka M, Clark CM, Aisen PS, Petersen RC, Blennow K, Soares H, Simon A, Lewczuk P, et al. 2009. Cerebrospinal fluid biomarker signature in Alzheimer's disease neuroimaging initiative subjects. *Ann Neurol* **65:** 403–413.

Siemers ER. 2009. How can we recognize "disease modification" effects? *J Nutr Health Aging* **13:** 341–343.

Sjogren M, Rosengren L, Minthon L, Davidsson P, Blennow K, Wallin A. 2000. Cytoskeleton proteins in CSF distinguish frontotemporal dementia from AD. *Neurology* **54:** 1960–1964.

Sjogren M, Blomberg M, Jonsson M, Wahlund LO, Edman A, Lind K, Rosengren L, Blennow K, Wallin A. 2001a. Neurofilament protein in cerebrospinal fluid: A marker of white matter changes. *J Neurosci Res* **66:** 510–516.

Sjogren M, Davidsson P, Gottfries J, Vanderstichele H, Edman A, Vanmechelen E, Wallin A, Blennow K. 2001b. The cerebrospinal fluid levels of tau, growth-associated protein-43 and soluble amyloid precursor protein correlate in Alzheimer's disease, reflecting a common pathophysiological process. *Dement Geriatr Cogn Disord* **12:** 257–264.

Skoog I, Davidsson P, Aevarsson O, Vanderstichele H, Vanmechelen E, Blennow K. 2003. Cerebrospinal fluid β-amyloid 42 is reduced before the onset of sporadic dementia: A population-based study in 85-year-olds. *Dement Geriatr Cogn Disord* **15:** 169–176.

Snider BJ, Fagan AM, Roe C, Shah AR, Grant EA, Xiong C, Morris JC, Holtzman DM. 2009. Cerebrospinal fluid biomarkers and rate of cognitive decline in very mild dementia of the Alzheimer type. *Arch Neurol* **66:** 638–645.

Snowdon DA. 1997. Aging and Alzheimer's disease: Lessons from the Nun Study. *Gerontologist* **37:** 150–156.

Sperling RA, Aisen PS, Beckett LA, Bennett DA, Craft S, Fagan AM, Iwatsubo T, Jack CR Jr, Kaye J, Montine TJ, et al. 2011. Toward defining the preclinical stages of Alzheimer's disease: Recommendations from the National Institute on Aging—Alzheimer's Association workgroups on diagnostic guidelines for Alzheimer's disease. *Alzheimer's Dement* **7,** 280–292.

Stomrud E, Hansson O, Blennow K, Minthon L, Londos E. 2007. Cerebrospinal fluid biomarkers predict decline in subjective cognitive function over 3 years in healthy elderly. *Dement Geriatr Cogn Disord* **24:** 118–124.

Storandt M, Grant EA, Miller JP, Morris JC. 2006. Longitudinal course and neuropathologic outcomes in original vs revised MCI and in pre-MCI. *Neurology* **67:** 467–473.

Strozyk D, Blennow K, White LR, Launer LJ. 2003. CSF Aβ 42 levels correlate with amyloid-neuropathology in a population-based autopsy study. *Neurology* **60:** 652–656.

Sunderland T, Linker G, Mirza N, Putnam KT, Friedman DL, Kimmel LH, Bergeson J, Manetti GJ, Zimmermann M, Tang B, et al. 2003. Decreased β-amyloid$_{1-42}$ and increased tau levels in cerebrospinal fluid of patients with Alzheimer disease. *JAMA* **289:** 2094–2103.

Tapiola T, Alafuzoff I, Herukka SK, Parkkinen L, Hartikainen P, Soininen H, Pirttilä T. 2009. Cerebrospinal fluid β-amyloid 42 and tau proteins as biomarkers of Alzheimer-type pathologic changes in the brain. *Arch Neurol* **66:** 382–389.

Tarawneh R, D'Angelo G, Macy E, Xiong C, Carter D, Cairns NJ, Fagan AM, Head D, Mintun MA, Ladenson JH, Lee JM, Morris JC, Holtzman DM, et al. 2011. Visin-like protein-1: Diagnostic and prognostic biomarker in Alzheimer disease. *Ann Neurol* **70:** 274–285.

Terry RD, Masliah E, Salmon DP, Butters N, DeTeresa R, Hill R, Hansen LA, Katzman R. 1991. Physical basis of cognitive alterations in Alzheimer's disease: Synapse loss is the major correlate of cognitive impairment. *Ann Neurol* **30:** 572–580.

Tibbling G, Link H, Ohman S. 1977. Principles of albumin and IgG analyses in neurological disorders. I. Establishment of reference values. *Scand J Clin Lab Invest* **37:** 385–390.

Tolboom N, van der Flier WM, Yaqub M, Boellaard R, Verwey NA, Blankenstein MA, Windhorst AD, Scheltens P, Lammertsma AA, van Berckel BN. 2009. Relationship of cerebrospinal fluid markers to ^{11}C-PiB and ^{18}F-FDDNP binding. *J Nucl Med* **50:** 1464–1470.

Vanmechelen E, Vanderstichele H, Davidsson P, Van Kerschaver E, Van Der Perre B, Sjögren M, Andreasen N, Blennow K. 2000. Quantification of tau phosphorylated at threonine 181 in human cerebrospinal fluid: A sandwich ELISA with a synthetic phosphopeptide for standardization. *Neurosci Lett* **285:** 49–52.

van Oijen M, Hofman A, Soares HD, Koudstaal PJ, Breteler MM. 2006. Plasma Aβ(1–40) and Aβ(1–42) and the risk of dementia: A prospective case-cohort study. *Lancet Neurol* **5:** 655–660.

Vellas B. 2009. Editorial: Use of biomarkers in Alzheimer's trials. *J Nutr Health Aging* **13:** 331.

Vemuri P, Wiste HJ, Weigand SD, Shaw LM, Trojanowski JQ, Weiner MW, Knopman DS, Petersen RC, Jack CR Jr, Alzheimer's Disease Neuroimaging Initiative. 2009. MRI and CSF biomarkers in normal, MCI, and AD subjects: Diagnostic discrimination and cognitive correlations. *Neurology* **73:** 287–293.

Visser PJ, Scheltens P, Verhey FR. 2005. Do MCI criteria in drug trials accurately identify subjects with predementia Alzheimer's disease? *J Neurol Neurosurg Psychiat* **76:** 1348–1354.

Visser PJ, Verhey F, Knol DL, Scheltens P, Wahlund LO, Freund-Levi Y, Tsolaki M, Minthon L, Wallin AK, Hampel H, et al. 2009. Prevalence and prognostic value of CSF markers of Alzheimer's disease pathology in patients with subjective cognitive impairment or mild cognitive impairment in the DESCRIPA study: A prospective cohort study. *Lancet Neurol* **8:** 619–627.

Wallin AK, Hansson O, Blennow K, Londos E, Minthon L. 2009. Can CSF biomarkers or pre-treatment progression rate predict response to cholinesterase inhibitor treatment in Alzheimer's disease? *Int J Geriatr Psychiat* **24:** 638–647.

Walsh DM, Selkoe DJ. 2007. A β oligomers—A decade of discovery. *J Neurochem* **101:** 1172–1184.

World Health Organization. 1992. *ICD-10: International statistical classification of diseases*, 10th ed. WHO, Geneva.

Yang LB, Lindholm K, Yan R, Citron M, Xia W, Yang XL, Beach T, Sue L, Wong P, Price D, et al. 2003. Elevated β-secretase expression and enzymatic activity detected in sporadic Alzheimer disease. *Nat Med* **9:** 3–4.

Zetterberg H, Wahlund LO, Blennow K. 2003. Cerebrospinal fluid markers for prediction of Alzheimer's disease. *Neurosci Lett* **352:** 67–69.

Zetterberg H, Andreasen N, Blennow K. 2004. Increased cerebrospinal fluid levels of transforming growth factor-β1 in Alzheimer's disease. *Neurosci Lett* **367:** 194–196.

Zetterberg H, Hietala MA, Jonsson M, Andreasen N, Styrud E, Karlsson I, Edman A, Popa C, Rasulzada A, Wahlund LO, et al. 2006. Neurochemical aftermath of amateur boxing. *Arch Neurol* **63:** 1277–1280.

Zetterberg H, Pedersen M, Lind K, Svensson M, Rolstad S, Eckerström C, Syversen S, Mattsson UB, Ysander C, Mattsson N, et al. 2007. Intra-individual stability of CSF biomarkers for Alzheimer's disease over two years. *J Alzheimer's Dis* **12:** 255–260.

Zetterberg H, Andreasson U, Hansson O, Wu G, Sankaranarayanan S, Andersson ME, Buchhave P, Londos E, Umek RM, Minthon L, et al. 2008. Elevated cerebrospinal fluid BACE1 activity in incipient Alzheimer disease. *Arch Neurol* **65:** 1102–1107.

Zhang Y, Londos E, Minthon L, Wattmo C, Liu H, Aspelin P, Wahlund LO. 2008. Usefulness of computed tomography linear measurements in diagnosing Alzheimer's disease. *Acta Radiol* **49:** 91–97.

Zhong Z, Ewers M, Teipel S, Burger K, Wallin A, Blennow K, He P, McAllister C, Hampel H, Shen Y. 2007. Levels of β-secretase (BACE1) in cerebrospinal fluid as a predictor of risk in mild cognitive impairment. *Arch Gen Psychiat* **64:** 718–726.

Epidemiology of Alzheimer Disease

Richard Mayeux and Yaakov Stern

Gertrude H. Sergievsky Center, Taub Institute for Research on Alzheimer's Disease and the Aging Brain, Columbia University Medical Center, New York, New York 10032

Correspondence: ys11@columbia.edu

The global prevalence of dementia has been estimated to be as high as 24 million, and is predicted to double every 20 years until at least 2040. As the population worldwide continues to age, the number of individuals at risk will also increase, particularly among the very old. Alzheimer disease is the leading cause of dementia beginning with impaired memory. The neuropathological hallmarks of Alzheimer disease include diffuse and neuritic extracellular amyloid plaques in brain that are frequently surrounded by dystrophic neurites and intraneuronal neurofibrillary tangles. The etiology of Alzheimer disease remains unclear, but it is likely to be the result of both genetic and environmental factors. In this review we discuss the prevalence and incidence rates, the established environmental risk factors, and the protective factors, and briefly review genetic variants predisposing to disease.

Alzheimer disease is characterized by progressive cognitive decline usually beginning with impairment in the ability to form recent memories, but inevitably affecting all intellectual functions and leading to complete dependence for basic functions of daily life, and premature death. The pathological manifestations of Alzheimer disease include diffuse and neuritic extracellular amyloid plaques and intracellular neurofibrillary tangles accompanied by reactive microgliosis, dystrophic neurites, and loss of neurons and synapses (see Serrano-Pozo et al. 2011). While these pathological lesions do not fully explain the clinical features of the disease, it has been hypothesized that alterations in the production and processing of amyloid β-protein may be the principal initiating factor. The underlying causes of these multifaceted changes remain unknown, but advancing age, and genetic and nongenetic antecedent factors are thought to play important roles. Alzheimer disease is the most frequent cause of dementia in Western societies. In the US, approximately 5.5 million people are affected, and the prevalence worldwide is estimated to be as high as 24 million. Given that both established and developing nations are rapidly aging, the frequency is expected to double every 20 years until 2040. The magnitude of the impending rise owing to societal aging is considerable and will be a costly public health burden in the years to come.

DEFINITIONS AND CRITERIA

In 1984, representatives from the National Institute of Neurological and Communicative Disorders and Stroke and the Alzheimer Disease and Related Disorders Association (NINCDS-ADRDA) developed a uniform set of criteria to enable clinicians and researchers to maintain consistency in the diagnosis. They included aspects of medical history, clinical examination, neuropsychological testing, and laboratory assessments (McKhann et al. 1984). These criteria have been remarkably reliable and valid for the diagnosis of AD over the past three decades (Galasko et al. 1994; Lim et al. 1999). The criteria were developed with the intent of accurately associating the clinical symptoms with the neuropathological manifestations after death. Levels of certainty were established that were labeled as *definite* for autopsy-confirmed disease, *probable* for the typical clinical syndrome without intervening issues and *possible* for diagnoses complicated by disorders that might contribute to the dementia. The criteria facilitated estimates of the prevalence and incidence rates of clinically diagnosed probable and possible AD.

The NINCDS-ADRDA criteria have very recently been updated (McKhann et al. 2011). With major advances in neuropsychological assessment, brain imaging and the neuropathological, biochemical and genetic understanding of this disease, revisions were considered a necessity. The breadth of the AD phenotype in society is greater than was previously thought. For example, neuropathological changes may precede clinical dementia by a decade or more. The growing use of brain imaging and cerebrospinal fluid biomarkers (see below) may yield both higher specificity and sensitivity in the diagnosis and thus are considered in the updated diagnostic criteria, especially when used for clinical research. It has become increasingly clear that cerebrovascular disease can coexist with AD to a greatly varying extent, further contributing to the cognitive and physical dysfunction.

A set of newly proposed criteria are similar to, but distinct from, those in the 1984 NINCDS-ADRDA criteria, with updates that include the recognition of both amnestic and nonamnestic symptom onset and alterations in numerous other cognitive domains. Further, cerebrovascular disease is now recognized as a contributor to dementia, defined by a history of a stroke temporally related to the onset or worsening of cognitive impairment, the presence of multiple or extensive infarcts, or severe burden of hyperintense white matter lesions by MRI. Accordingly, the presence of substantial cerebrovascular pathology reduces the certainty of a clinical diagnosis of AD to possible. Hallucinations, delusions, Parkinson-like motor manifestations and realted findings can suggest dementia with Lewy bodies or other forms of dementia (see Tarawneh and Holtzman 2011; Weintraub et al. 2011).

In this chapter, we will discuss the prevalence and incidence rates of AD disease in developed and developing countries and summarize the evidence for numerous antecedent risk factors, protective factors and genetic risk factors.

FREQUENCY OF ALZHEIMER DISEASE

In 2005, Alzheimer Disease International commissioned an international group of experts to reach a consensus on dementia prevalence and estimated incidence in 14 World Health Organization regions, based on epidemiological data acquired over recent years. The results suggested that 24.2 million people lived with dementia at that time, with 4.6 million new cases arising every year (Ferri et al. 2005). North America and Western Europe have at age 60 the highest prevalence of dementia (6.4 and 5.4% of the population at age 60), followed by Latin America (4.9%) and China and its developing western-Pacific neighbors (4.0%). The annual incidence rates (per 1000) for these countries were estimated at 10.5 for North America, 8.8 for Western Europe, 9.2 for Latin America and 8.0 for China and its developing western-Pacific neighbors, increasing exponentially with age in all countries, especially through the seventh and eighth decades of life.

The prevalence rates for AD also rise exponentially with age, increasing markedly after 65 years. There is almost a 15-fold increase in the prevalence of dementia, predominately Alzheimer disease, between the ages of 60 and 85 years (Evans et al. 1989). Compared with Africa, Asia and Europe, the prevalence of AD appears to be much higher in the US, which may relate to methods of ascertainment. The prevalence may be higher among African-American and

Cite this article as *Cold Spring Harb Perspect Med* doi: 10.1101/cshperspect.a006239

Hispanic populations living in the US, but lower for Africans in their homelands, for reasons that remain uncertain (Ogunniyi et al. 2000; Hendrie et al. 2001).

In 1998, Brookmeyer et al. estimated the age-specific incidence rates of AD based on studies in Boston, Framingham, Rochester, and Baltimore. These rates doubled every 5 years after the age of 60 and rose from about 0.17% per year at age 65 to 0.71, 1.0, and 2.92% per year, respectively, at 75, 80, and 85 (Brookmeyer et al. 1998). This observation is consistent with the vast majority of studies that have estimated the age-specific incidence of AD by sex and by ethnic group (Fig. 1; Bachman et al. 1993; Letenneur et al. 1994; Brayne et al. 1995; Hebert et al. 1995; Aevarsson and Skoog 1996; Fratiglioni et al. 1997; Andersen et al. 1999; Copeland et al. 1999; Launer et al. 1999; Ganguli et al. 2000; Kawas et al. 2000; Lobo et al. 2000; Chandra et al. 2001; Hendrie et al. 2001; Tang et al. 2001; Di Carlo et al. 2002; Edland et al. 2002; Knopman et al. 2002; Kukull et al. 2002; Fitzpatrick et al. 2004; Lopez-Pousa et al. 2004; Nitrini et al. 2004; Ravaglia et al. 2005a; Jellinger and Attems 2010).

Two factors contribute to the difficulty in establishing accurate incidence rates of AD: (1) determining the age at onset; and (2) defining a disease-free population. Nonetheless, studies illustrate the consistent increase in incidence rates with age from approximately 0.5% per year among individuals aged 65–70 to approximately 6–8% for individuals over age 85. The rapid rise in the frequency of AD with advancing age, combined with the relatively long duration of the illness, accounts in large part for the high prevalence of the disease worldwide. Improvement and standardization of diagnostic methods have provided a means to compare estimates of the frequency of AD across various populations.

ANTECEDENT RISK FACTORS THAT INCREASE THE RISK OF ALZHEIMER DISEASE

A large number of factors has been associated with increased risk of AD, but among those, cerebrovascular disease and it antecedents are the most consistently reported (Table 1). A history of diabetes, hypertension, smoking, obesity, and dyslipidemia have all been found to increase risk. Interestingly cerebrovascular disease, including large cortical infarcts, single strategically placed infarcts, multiple small infarcts, cerebral hemorrhage, cortical changes owing to hypoperfusion, white matter changes and vasculopathies, are all antecedents to dementia in general (Barba et al. 2000; de Koning et al. 2000; Desmond et al. 2000, 2002; Zhu et al. 2000; Henon et al. 2001; Klimkowicz et al. 2002; Honig et al. 2003; Liebetrau et al. 2003; Ivan et al. 2004; Linden et al. 2004; Srikanth et al. 2004; Tang et al. 2004; Zhou et al. 2004; de Koning et al. 2005; Kuller et al. 2005; Gamaldo et al. 2006; Jin et al. 2006; Simons et al. 2006; Srikanth et al. 2006; Yip et al. 2006; Jin et al. 2008; Reitz et al. 2008; Rastas et al. 2010).

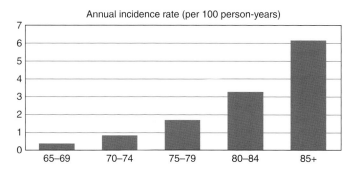

Annual incidence rate (per 100 person-years)

Figure 1. The annual incidence rate (per 100 person-years) for Alzheimer disease. This graph is an estimate of the data collected in 24 published studies.

Table 1. Factors that modify the risk of Alzheimer disease

Antecedent	Direction	Possible mechanisms
Cardiovascular disease	Increased	Parenchymal destruction
		Strategic location
		$\uparrow$ Aβ deposition
Smoking	Increased	Cerebrovascular effects
		Oxidative stress
Hypertension	Increased and decreased	Microvascular disease
Type II diabetes	Increased	Cerebrovascular effect
		Insulin and Aβ compete for clearance
Obesity	Increased	Increased risk of type II diabetes inflammatory
Traumatic head injury	Increased	$\uparrow$Aβ and amyloid precursor protein deposition
Education	Decreased	Provides cognitive reserve
Leisure activity	Decreased	Improves lipid metabolism, mental stimulation
Mediterranean diet	Decreased	Antioxidant, anti-inflammatory
Physical activity	Decreased	Activates brain plasticity, promotes brain vascularization

Cerebrovascular Disease

While it is clear that cerebrovascular disease may present with manifestations resembling dementia, purely vascular dementia is uncommon. More often cerebrovascular disease co-exists with AD, so that evidence of both vascular disease and prototypical AD manifestations is present (Schneider and Bennett 2010). Pendlebury and Rothwell (2009) analyzed data from several hospital- and population-based cohorts (7511 patients) and estimated a frequency of new-onset dementia to be approximately 7% following a first stroke. Interestingly, the twofold increased risk of dementia after incident stroke was independent of the level or the rate of change of prestroke cognitive function, suggesting that prestroke cognitive function is not a major determinant of the effect of stroke on the risk of poststroke dementia (Reitz et al. 2008). The proposed mechanisms by which stroke could lead to cognitive impairment include destruction of brain parenchyma with atrophy (Fein et al. 2000; Jellinger 2002), damage in strategic locations that leads to amnestic syndromes, such as thalamic strokes, an increase in Aβ deposition and the combination of vascular and Alzheimer-type pathology (Blennow et al. 2006). As one possible mechanism for an increase in Aβ, there is evidence from rodent models of ischemia and hypoxia owing to hypoperfusion that a resulting overexpression of

p25 and cdk5 increases levels of BACE1, which in turn increases amyloid precursor protein (APP) processing (Wen et al. 2007, 2008).

White matter hyperintensities are frequently observed by MRI in patients with dementia, but the mechanisms by which white matter changes contribute to cognitive decline are unclear. Moreover because hypertension, diabetes and microvasuclar disease are each associated with these changes, there is no clear process to explain the effect on cognition or their role in Alzheimer disease. Thalamic vascular disease can lead to lower performance on cognitive tasks, particularly those associated with frontal and temporal lobe function, including memory storage and retrieval (Swartz et al. 2008; Wright et al. 2008).

Hypertension

Cross-sectional and longitudinal studies implicate blood pressure as a possible contributor to late-life dementia. Observational studies of the association between elevated blood pressure during middle age and late-life cognitive impairment suggest that mid-life hypertension increases the risk of late-life dementia (Kilander et al. 2000; Launer et al. 2000; Wu et al. 2003; Yamada et al. 2003; Elias et al. 2004; Whitmer et al. 2005b). When hypertension is assessed in later life, the association is somewhat ambiguous, in that both high and abnormally low blood pressure are associated with dementia (Skoog et al. 1996; Knopman et al. 2001; Morris ct al. 2001; Ruitenberg et al. 2001; Tyas et al. 2001; Bohannon et al. 2002; Lindsay et al. 2002; Posner et al. 2002; Elias et al. 2003; Kuller et al. 2003; Piguet et al. 2003; Qiu et al. 2003; Reinprecht et al. 2003; Verghese et al. 2003a; Hebert et al. 2004; Solfrizzi et al. 2004; Tervo et al. 2004; Borenstein et al. 2005; Petitti et al. 2005; Waldstein et al. 2005). With Alzheimer disease onset and progression, blood pressure begins to decrease, possibly related to vessel stiffening, weight loss, and changes in the autonomic regulation of blood flow. Hypertension is a treatable medical disorder, but clinical trials of antihypertensive medications in AD patients have been attempted with inconsistent results (Forette et al. 2002; Lithell et al. 2003; Tzourio et al. 2003; Peters et al. 2010).

Type II Diabetes

The presence of type II diabetes is associated with a approximately twofold increased risk of AD (risk ratios vary between 1.5 and 4.0; Luchsinger et al. 2001; Peila et al. 2002; Farris et al. 2003; Luchsinger et al. 2004a). It has been suggested that diabetes directly affects Aβ accumulation in the brain because hyperinsulinemia, which accompanies type II diabetes, disrupts brain Aβ clearance by competing for the insulin-degrading enzyme (Selkoe 2000; Farris et al. 2003). Receptors for advanced glycation end-products, which also play a role in the pathogenesis of diabetes, are present in cels associated with senile plaques and neurofibrillary tangles have been shown to be one example of a cell surface receptor for Aβ. Excess adipose tissue may also predispose to type II diabetes by producing adipokines critical to metabolism and cytokines important in inflammation. Adiponectin, leptin, resistin, TNF-α and IL-6 are also produced and correlate with insulin resistance and hyperinsulinemia, which in turn may directly or indirectly affect AD risk (Trujillo and Scherer 2005; Yu and Ginsberg 2005). A meta-analysis of longitudinal studies examining type II diabetes and other disorders of glucose or insulin levels found a pooled effect size for diabetes of 1.54 in increasing AD risk (95% confidence interval, CI, 1.33–1.79; $z =$ 5.7; $p < .001$; Profenno et al. 2009).

Reger et al. (2008) showed that the administration of intranasal insulin improved cognitive performance in the early phases of AD and in patients with amnestic mild cognitive impairment, as did a 6-month trial of the PPAR-γ agonist, rosiglitazone (Watson et al. 2005). Another study (Risner et al. 2006) in patients with AD lacking the APOE-ε4 allele showed significant although small improvements in cognitive and functional improvement in response to rosiglitazone, whereas in a study by Sato et al. (2009), treatment with 15–30 mg pioglitazone daily for 6 months led to improvements in cognitive function and regional cerebral blood flow in the parietal lobe.

Body Weight

Several cross-sectional and case–control studies found that low body mass index or being underweight were apparent risk factors for dementia and age-related brain changes such as atrophy (Faxen-Irving et al. 2005). In contrast several prospective studies linked both low and high body weight, weight loss and weight gain to risk of AD (Nourhashemi et al. 2002, 2003; Gustafson et al. 2003; Bagger et al. 2004; Brubacher et al. 2004; Buchman et al. 2005; Goble 2005; Jeong et al. 2005; Kivipelto et al. 2005; Razay and Vreugdenhil 2005; Rosengren et al. 2005; Stewart et al. 2005; Tabet 2005; Whitmer et al. 2005a; Waldstein and Katzel 2006; Arbus et al. 2008; Atti et al. 2008). The strongest effect was in a meta-analysis associating obesity (assessed by high body mass index) and the risk of AD (odds ratio, OR, 1.59 95% CI 1.02–2.5; $z =$ 2.0; $p = .042$) (Profenno et al. 2009). The mechanisms by which body weight alters disease risk are unknown, but may include effects such as insulin resistance or the co-incidence of type II diabetes.

Smoking

Case–control studies initially suggested that smoking lowers the risk of Alzheimer disease, but subsequent prospective studies showed an increased risk or no association (Doll et al. 2000). Smoking may increase the risk of dementia by augmentation of cholinergic metabolism, that is, up-regulating cholinergic nicotinic receptors in the brain (Whitehouse et al. 1988). Cholinergic deficits, characterized by reduced levels of acetylcholine, choline acetyl transferase and/or nicotinic acetyl choline receptors, are invariably found in AD brains. However, nicotine itself increases acetylcholine release, elevates the number of nicotinic receptors, and improves attention and information processing. These actions may be opposed by elevated oxidative stress caused by smoking, and oxidative stress has been implicated as a putative AD mechanism (Rottkamp et al. 2000; Perry et al. 2002) through the generation of free radicals and affecting inflammatory–immune systems, which in turn can activate phagocytes that generate further oxidative damage (Traber et al. 2000).

Traumatic Brain Injury

Compared with those without a history of trauma, individuals having suffered traumatic brain injury have a higher risk of dementia, particularly those who carry the APOE-ε4 allele (Koponen et al. 2004). A meta-analyses demonstrated that the risk of dementia is higher among men (but not women) with a history of traumatic brain injury (Fleminger et al. 2003). Postmortem and experimental studies do support a link: After human brain injury, both Aβ deposition (Hartman et al. 2002; Iwata et al. 2002; Stone et al. 2002) and intraneuronal tau pathology are increased, even in younger patients (Smith et al. 2003). In addition, CSF Aβ levels are elevated and APP is overproduced (Emmerling et al. 2000; Franz et al. 2003).

PROTECTIVE FACTORS THAT REDUCE RISK OF ALZHEIMER DISEASE

Cognitive Reserve

Individuals with intellectually enriched lifestyles, such as those with high educational and/or occupational attainment, have a reduced risk of expressing AD pathology clinically. While several studies reported no association between educational level and risk of AD (Hall et al. 2000; Chandra et al. 2001), a lower risk of dementia in general in subjects with higher education has been reported by several others worldwide (Evans et al. 1993, 1997; Letenneur et al. 1994, 1999; Stern et al. 1994; White et al. 1994; Qiu et al. 2001).

There is also evidence for a role of education in age-related cognitive decline, with several studies of "normal aging" reporting slower cognitive and functional decline in individuals with higher educational attainment (Chodosh et al. 2002). These studies suggest that the same education-related factors that delay the onset of AD-type dementia also allow individuals to cope more effectively with brain changes encountered in normal aging. In an ethnically diverse cohort of nondemented elders in New York City, increased literacy was also associated with slower decline in memory, executive function, and language skills (Manly et al. 2005).

Numerous studies have also explored the relationship between leisure activities and incident dementia. Community activities and gardening were also protective for incident dementia in China (Zhang et al. 1999). Having an extensive social network was protective for the development of dementia (Fratiglioni et al. 2004), and engagement in mental, social, and other productive activities was associated with decreased risk of incident dementia (Wang et al. 2002). Participation in a variety of leisure activities characterized as intellectual (e.g., reading, playing games, going to classes) or social engagements (e.g., visiting friends or relatives) was assessed in another population study of nondemented elderly in New York (Scarmeas et al. 2001). During follow-up, subjects with high leisure activity had 38% less risk of developing dementia. In another prospective study, frequency of participation in common cognitive activities (i.e., reading a newspaper, magazine, or book) was assessed at baseline for 801 elderly Catholic nuns, priests and brothers without dementia (Wilson et al. 2002a). Finally, in another prospective cohort from New York, participation in leisure activities, particularly reading, playing board games or musical instruments, and dancing, was associated with a reduced risk of incident dementia (Verghese et al. 2003b). Increased participation in cognitive activities was also associated with reduced rates of memory decline in this study.

A meta-analysis examined cohort studies of the effects of education, occupation, premorbid IQ and mental activities on dementia risk (Valenzuela and Sachdev 2005). A summary analysis was based on an integrated total of 29,279 individuals from 22 studies. The median follow-up was 7.1 years. The summary odds ratio for incident dementia for individuals with high brain reserve compared with low brain reserve was 0.54 (95% CI 0.49–0.59, $p < 0.0001$), that is, a decreased risk of 46%. Eight out of 33 data sets showed no significant effect, whereas 25 out of 33 demonstrated a significant protective effect. The authors found a significant negative association between incident dementia risk (based on differential education) and the overall dementia rate for each cohort ($r = -0.57$, $p = 0.04$), indicating that in negative studies there was a lower overall risk of incident dementia in the cohort.

In contrast to the studies above, in which greater cognitive reserve was associated with better outcomes, a series of studies of patients with AD suggested that those with higher reserve have poorer outcomes (Table 1). In prospective studies of AD subjects matched for clinical severity at baseline (Geerlings et al. 1999; Stern et al. 1999), patients with greater education or occupational attainment died sooner than those with less attainment. Similarly, higher educational or occupational attainment (Stern et al. 1999; Scarmeas et al. 2006a), increased engagement in leisure activities (Helzner et al. 2007), and greater lifetime cognitive activity (Wilson et al. 2010) have each been associated with more rapid cognitive decline in patients with diagnosed AD. Although at first these findings appear contraintuitive, they are consistent with the cognitive reserve hypothesis. The hypothesis predicts that, at any level of assessed clinical severity, the underlying pathology of Alzheimer disease is more advanced in patients with higher than those with less cognitive reserve. This would result in the clinical disease emerging when pathology was more advanced, as suggested by the incidence studies reviewed above. This disparity in degree of pathology would be present at more advanced clinical stages of the disease as well. At some point the greater degree of pathology in the high-reserve patients would result in more rapid death. Higher educational attainment and greater engagement in leisure activities and lifetime cognitive activities have also been associated with more rapid cognitive decline in patients with Alzheimer disease.

Diet

Dietary fats can increase cholesterol levels, which in turn can increase vascular risk in the brain. This sequence may also increase the risk of AD (Sparks et al. 2000). Intake of saturated fats in the fifth (highest) quintile compared with the first quintile of dietary fats was associated with a doubling of risk of incident Alzheimer disease. Trans-unsaturated fats were associated with a 3-times-higher risk of developing AD, whereas the highest intake of n-6 polyunsaturated fats and monounsaturated fat reduced AD risk (Morris et al. 2003). An increased risk of AD has also been associated with higher intake of total and saturated fat, with no evidence of an association with polyunsaturated fat (Luchsinger et al. 2002).

Omega-3 fatty acids stems are essential dietary components in early brain development. Many studies have found that consumption of fish or omega-3 fatty acids is associated with a reduced risk of AD (Morris et al. 2003; Schaefer et al. 2006; van Gelder et al. 2007). For example, a study in France found that weekly consumption of fish was associated with reduced AD risk, and regular consumption of omega-3 rich oils was associated with increased risk of all causes of dementia (Barberger-Gateau et al. 2007).

Two studies found a lower risk of Alzheimer disease in individuals with a higher dietary intake of vitamin D (Engelhart et al. 2002; Morris et al. 2002). This association was not noted in a third study, perhaps because the level of vitamin D intake was lower (Luchsinger et al. 2003).

Total homocysteine has also been inconsistently associated with AD (Luchsinger et al. 2004b; Seshadri 2006; Reitz et al. 2009). Concentrations of homocysteine are largely determined by certain B vitamins. Based on folate levels measured in serum, there was preliminary evidence from two studies that low folate levels are associated with increased AD risk (Wang et al. 2001; Ravaglia et al. 2005b). Some studies that used estimated dietary intake of folate and B vitamins based on self-reported information reported conflicting results. One reported an association between higher intake of folate and reduced risk of AD (Luchsinger et al. 2007), whereas another did not find a significant reduction in AD risk associated with folate intake (Morris et al. 2006). Neither study found an association between vitamins B6 or B12 and risk of AD.

Inconsistencies in the existing literature regarding some of the above dietary elements and AD risk may be a result of failure to consider possible additive and interactive (antagonistic or synergistic) effects among nutritional components, which may be better captured in a composite dietary pattern such as the Mediterranean diet. The latter is characterized by high intake of vegetables, legumes, fruits, and cereals; high intake of unsaturated fatty acids (mostly in the form of olive oil), but low intake of saturated fatty acids; a moderately high intake of fish; a low-to-moderate intake of dairy products (mostly cheese or yogurt); a low intake of meat and poultry; and regular but moderate amounts of ethanol, primarily in the form of wine and generally during meals (Trichopoulou et al. 2003). In one study (Scarmeas et al. 2006b), higher adherence to the Mediterranean diet was associated with lower risk of AD (hazard ratio, 0.91; 95% CI, 0.83–0.98; $p = 0.015$). Compared with subjects in the lowest Mediterranean diet tertile, subjects in the middle tertile had an AD hazard ratio of 0.85 (95% CI, 0.63–1.16) and those in the highest tertile had a hazard ratio of 0.60 (95% CI, 0.42–0.87) (p for trend = 0.007). In a follow-up analysis, the

Mediterranean diet was also associated with a reduced risk of developing mild cognitive impairment and of progression from mild cognitive impairment to AD (Scarmeas et al. 2009).

Physical Activity

Exercise can enhance learning in both young and aged animals (van Praag et al. 1999), activate brain plasticity mechanisms, remodel neuronal circuitry in the brain (Cotman and Berchtold 2002), promote brain vascularization (Black et al. 1990), and stimulate neurogenesis (van Praag et al. 1999). It may also increase neuronal survival and resistance to brain insults (Carro et al. 2001), increase levels of brain-derived neurotrophic factor, mobilize gene expression profiles that would be predicted to benefit brain plasticity (Cotman and Berchtold 2002), and reduce levels of C-reactive protein and interleukin-6, two inflammatory markers (Ford 2002; Reuben et al. 2003). A Cochrane review (Angevaren et al. 2008) found that eight of 11 random, controlled trials of exercise in older people without known cognitive impairment reported that aerobic exercise interventions were associated with improvements in cognitive function.

Although some studies have failed to detect an association between physical activity and dementia (Wang et al. 2002; Wilson et al. 2002a; Verghese et al. 2003b), others have observed a beneficial role (Podewils et al. 2005; Rovio et al. 2005; Larson et al. 2006; Wang et al. 2006). A study of 1880 community-dwelling elders without dementia living in New York City investigated the combined association of diet and physical activity with Alzheimer risk. A combination of adherence to a strict Mediterranean-type diet and regular physical activity (compared with no or minimal physical activity) was associated with a significant reduction in risk of AD.

Cognitive Enhancement

Several studies have specifically examined the potential effects of cognitive engagement on the risk of AD (Wilson et al. 2002b, 2007;

Verghese et al. 2003b; Akbaraly et al. 2009). The studies used self-report of the frequency of involvement in specific activities that potentially have a cognitive component. In the Three-City cohort study, analyses were carried out on 5698 dementia-free participants aged 65 and over. Stimulating leisure activities were significantly associated with a reduced risk of AD (hazard ratio (HR) = 0.39). This finding was independent of other proxies of cognitive reserve and remained significant after adjusting for vascular risk factors, depressive symptoms and physical functioning.

GENETIC EPIDEMIOLOGY

Rare Variants

Rare mutations in three genes have been firmly implicated in familial early-onset disease: *APP*, *PSEN1*, and *PSEN2* (Table 2; Goate et al. 1991; Levy-Lahad et al. 1995a,b; Rogaev et al. 1995; Sherrington et al. 1995, 1996). These mutations have high penetrance, are mostly inherited in an autosomal dominant pattern and lead with certainty to enhanced relative levels of the Aβ42 peptide, its aggregation and an early onset of disease, typically beginning in the fourth or fifth decade of life. *APP* mutations account for an even smaller fraction (less than 1% of all AD patients). Rare variants such as these are occasionally seen in families of patients with familial Alzheimer disease having later onset (Athan et al. 2001). All *APP* missense mutations influence APP proteolytic processing and/or aggregation, because they are positioned in or near the Aβ-coding exons (16 and 17) of APP (see AD Mutation Database, http://www.molgen.vib-ua.be/ADMutations/). The mutation spectrum also includes microduplication at the *APP* locus on Ch 21. At the time of writing, 182 different AD-related mutations in 401 families have been identified in *PSEN1*, whereas only 14 mutations in 23 families were detected in *PSEN2* (http://www.molgen.vib-ua.be/ADMutations/). The majority of *PSEN* mutations are single-nucleotide substitutions, but small deletions and insertions have also been described. *PSEN* mutations alter the γ-secretase-mediated proteolytic cleavage of *APP*, resulting in an increased $A\beta_{42}/A\beta_{40}$ ratio by an increase in $A\beta_{42}$ and/or a decrease in $A\beta_{40}$, suggesting a partial loss-of-function mechanism rather than a gain-of-function in *PSEN* (see Tanzi 2011 for a detailed review). Although mutations in these three genes represent rare causes of AD, their discovery greatly supported a pivotal role for Aβ in the pathogenesis of AD. According to this amyloid (or Aβ hypothesis), neurodegenerative processes are the consequence of an imbalance between Aβ production and Aβ clearance, suggesting

Table 2. Gene variants associated with Alzheimer disease

Gene	Main alteration	Presumed mechanism
Amyloid precursor protein (*APP*)	Mutation	Autosomal dominant, mostly early onset
Presenilin 1 (*PSEN1*)	Mutation	Autosomal dominant, mostly early onset
Presenilin 2 (*PSEN2*)	Mutation	Autosomal dominant, mostly early onset
Apolipoprotein-E (*APOE*)	Common variant	Familial and sporadic, late onset
Sortilin-related receptor, L(DLR class) A repeats-containing (*SORL1*)	Common variant	Familial and sporadic, late onset
Clusterin (*CLU*)	Common variant	Sporadic, late onset
Phosphatidylinositol binding clathrin assembly protein (*PICALM*)	Common variant	Sporadic, late onset
Complement component (3b/4b) receptor 1 (*CR1*)	Common variant	Sporadic, late onset
Bridging integrator 1 (*BIN1*)	Common variant	Sporadic, late onset

that other genes involved in these pathways might also turn out to be risk factors.

Common Variants

The strongest common genetic variant for typical late-onset AD beginning after age approximately 65 years is apolipoprotein E (*APOE*), a three-allele polymorphism (ε2, ε3, and ε4) where ε3 is considered a neutral allele, ε4 the high-risk allele, and ε2 a protective allele (Table 2). The ε4 allele influences age at onset in a dose-dependent manner (Corder et al. 1993). However, more than half of the patients with late-onset disease do not have the high-risk ε4 allele. The population attributable risk related to APOE-ε4 has been estimated at 20% (Slooter et al. 1998). Genome-wide association (GWA) studies have identified variants in *CLU*, *PICALM*, *CR1*, and *BIN1* as putative susceptibility loci (Harold et al. 2009; Lambert et al. 2009; Seshadri et al. 2010). These genetic variants have been confirmed in other non-Hispanic and Hispanic populations (Carrasquillo et al. 2010; Jun et al. 2010; Lee et al. 2010). The odds ratios for these genes are much lower than for *APOE* (OR = are 3.2 and 14.9 for ε3/ε4 and ε4/ε4, respectively [Farrer et al. 1997]) and range from 1.16 to 1.20 for *CR1*, *CLU*, and *PICALM*.

Familial Late-Onset Alzheimer Disease

Bertram et al. (2008) performed a GWA study in 1376 samples from 410 families with late-onset Alzheimer disease (LOAD) and subsequently replicated their findings. A locus on chromosome 14q31 was strongly associated with LOAD, but the identity of the underlying locus is unknown and may be a modifier of onset age. The results of GWA studies in the NIA-LOAD Family Study, involving 900+ families stratified by APOE genotype, also identified single-nucleotide polymorphisms on chromosome 10p14 in *CUGBP2* with genome wide significance within individuals with one *APOE* ε4 allele, which was replicated in an independent Caribbean Hispanic cohort (Wijsman et al. 2011). The NIA-LOAD Family Study also replicated

the variants in *BIN1* and provided modest confirmation for *CLU*, but not for *CR1* or *PICALM* after *APOE* adjustment (Hollingworth et al. 2011; Naj et al. 2011). The role of these genes in the pathogenesis of Alzheimer's disease remains to be determined, but it is clear that large sample sizes have enabled identification of these putative gene variants.

Finally, variants in *SORL1*, which encodes a protein involved in trafficking of APP, are associated with late-onset AD. Although in line with other recently described genetic links for AD (Lee et al. 2007; Rogaeva et al. 2007), the effect sizes of the *SORL1* associations are modest (Reitz et al. 2011). Variants in the SORL1 homolog, SORCS1, are also modestly associated with AD. Overexpression of either gene leads to a decrease in Aβ levels in cultured cells, whereas inhibition by RNAi increases Aβ. Thus, both genes may play a role in AD pathogenesis.

Although these results of the published GWA studies are informative, the genetic associations need functional validation. GWA studies represent a method of screening the genome, but limitations exist in their ability to detect true associations. The results of such studies might be difficult to replicate if the real effect turns out to be smaller than the effect observed in the initial study. In addition, GWA studies may not detect associations with multiple rare variants at a single site (which are better detected by linkage studies) or with single rare variants (minor allele frequency <5%). Finally, such studies alone cannot prove causality or establish the biological significance of an observed genetic association.

CONCLUSIONS

Our understanding of AD pathogenesis has grown substantially over the past two decades. However, with the large numbers of individuals reaching the age of highest risk, some would say that we have a long way to go toward preventing or limiting the full impact of the disease. Current treatments are palliative at best and newer therapies remain unproven. Knowing who is a risk and why will make prevention and management easier in the future (Aisen et al. 2011; Lee et al. 2011; Schenk et al. 2011).

REFERENCES

Reference is also in this collection.

Aevarsson O, Skoog I. 1996. A population-based study on the incidence of dementia disorders between 85 and 88 years of age. *J Am Geriatr Soc* **44:** 1455–1460.

* Aisen PS, Cummings JL, Schneider LS. 2011. Symptomatic and non-amyloid/Tau-based pharmacologic treatment for Alzheimer disease. *Cold Spring Harb Perspect Med* doi: 10.1101/cshperspect.a006395.

Akbaraly TN, Portet F, Fustinoni S, Dartigues JF, Artero S, Rouaud O, Touchon J, Ritchie K, Berr C. 2009. Leisure activities and the risk of dementia in the elderly: results from the Three-City Study. *Neurology* **73:** 854–861.

Andersen K, Nielsen H, Lolk A, Andersen J, Becker I, Kragh-Sorensen P. 1999. Incidence of very mild to severe dementia and Alzheimer's disease in Denmark: The Odense Study. *Neurology* **52:** 85–90.

Angevaren M, Aufdemkampe G, Verhaar H, Aleman A, Vanhees L. 2008. Physical activity and enhanced fitness to improve cognitive function in older people without known cognitive impairment. *Cochrane Database of Systematic Reviews (Online):* CD005381.

Arbus C, Soto ME, Andrieu S, Nourhashemi F, Camus V, Schmitt L, Vellas B. 2008. The prevalence of clinically significant depressive symptoms in Alzheimer's disease: relationship with other psychological and behavioural symptoms. *Int J Geriatr Psychiat* **23:** 1209–1211.

Athan ES, Williamson J, Ciappa A, Santana V, Romas SN, Lee JH, Rondon H, Lantigua RA, Medrano M, Torres M, et al. 2001. A founder mutation in presenilin 1 causing early-onset Alzheimer disease in unrelated Caribbean Hispanic families. *JAMA* **286:** 2257–2263.

Atti AR, Palmer K, Volpato S, Winblad B, De Ronchi D, Fratiglioni L. 2008. Late-life body mass index and dementia incidence: Nine-year follow-up data from the Kungsholmen Project. *J Am Geriatr Soc* **56:** 111–116.

Bachman DL, Wolf PA, Linn RT, Knoefel JE, Cobb JL, Belanger AJ, White LR, D'Agostino RB. 1993. Incidence of dementia and probable Alzheimer's disease in a general population: The Framingham Study. *Neurology* **43:** 515–519.

Bagger YZ, Tanko LB, Alexandersen P, Qin G, Christiansen C. 2004. The implications of body fat mass and fat distribution for cognitive function in elderly women. *Obesity Res* **12:** 1519–1526.

Barba R, Martinez-Espinosa S, Rodriguez-Garcia E, Pondal M, Vivancos J, Del Ser T. 2000. Poststroke dementia: Clinical features and risk factors. *Stroke* **31:** 1494–1501.

Barberger-Gateau P, Raffaitin C, Letenneur L, Berr C, Tzourio C, Dartigues JF, Alperovitch A. 2007. Dietary patterns and risk of dementia: The Three-City cohort study. *Neurology* **69:** 1921–1930.

Bertram L, Lange C, Mullin K, Parkinson M, Hsiao M, Hogan MF, Schjeide BM, Hooli B, Divito J, Ionita I, et al. 2008. Genome-wide association analysis reveals putative Alzheimer's disease susceptibility loci in addition to APOE. *Am J Hum Genet* **83:** 623–632.

Black JE, Isaacs KR, Anderson BJ, Alcantara AA, Greenough WT. 1990. Learning causes synaptogenesis, whereas motor activity causes angiogenesis, in cerebellar cortex of adult rats. *Proc Natl Acad Sci* **87:** 5568–5572.

Blennow K, de Leon MJ, Zetterberg H. 2006. Alzheimer's disease. *Lancet* **368:** 387–403.

Bohannon AD, Fillenbaum GG, Pieper CF, Hanlon JT, Blazer DG. 2002. Relationship of race/ethnicity and blood pressure to change in cognitive function. *J Am Geriatr Soc* **50:** 424–429.

Borenstein AR, Wu Y, Mortimer JA, Schellenberg GD, McCormick WC, Bowen JD, McCurry S, Larson EB. 2005. Developmental and vascular risk factors for Alzheimer's disease. *Neurobiol Aging* **26:** 325–334.

Brayne C, Gill C, Huppert FA, Barkley C, Gehlhaar E, Girling DM, O'Connor DW, Paykel ES. 1995. Incidence of clinically diagnosed subtypes of dementia in an elderly population. Cambridge Project for Later Life. *Br J Psychiat* **167:** 255–262.

Brookmeyer R, Gray S, Kawas C. 1998. Projections of Alzheimer's disease in the United States and the public health impact of delaying disease onset. *Am J Public Health* **88:** 1337–1342.

Brubacher D, Monsch AU, Stahelin HB. 2004. Weight change and cognitive performance. *Int J Obes Relat Metab Disord* **28:** 1163–1167.

Buchman AS, Wilson RS, Bienias JL, Shah RC, Evans DA, Bennett DA. 2005. Change in body mass index and risk of incident Alzheimer disease. *Neurology* **65:** 892–897.

Carrasquillo MM, Belbin O, Hunter TA, Ma L, Bisceglio GD, Zou F, Crook JE, Pankratz VS, Dickson DW, Graff-Radford NR, et al. 2010. Replication of CLU, CR1, and PICALM associations with Alzheimer disease. *Arch Neurol* **67:** 961–964.

Carro E, Trejo JL, Busiguina S, Torres-Aleman I. 2001. Circulating insulin-like growth factor I mediates the protective effects of physical exercise against brain insults of different etiology and anatomy. *J Neurosci* **21:** 5678–5684.

Chandra V, Pandav R, Dodge HH, Johnston JM, Belle SH, DeKosky ST, Ganguli M. 2001. Incidence of Alzheimer's disease in a rural community in India: The Indo-US study. *Neurology* **57:** 985–989.

Chodosh J, Reuben DB, Albert MS, Seeman TE. 2002. Predicting cognitive impairment in high-functioning community-dwelling older persons: MacArthur Studies of Successful Aging. *J Am Geriat Soc* **50:** 1051–1060.

Copeland JR, McCracken CF, Dewey ME, Wilson KC, Doran M, Gilmore C, Scott A, Larkin BA. 1999. Undifferentiated dementia, Alzheimer's disease and vascular dementia: age- and gender-related incidence in Liverpool. The MRC-ALPHA Study. *Br J Psychiat* **175:** 433–438.

Corder EH, Saunders AM, Strittmatter WJ, Schmechel DE, Gaskell PC, Small GW, Roses AD, Haines JL, Pericak-Vance MA. 1993. Gene dose of apolipoprotein E type 4 allele and the risk of Alzheimer's disease in late onset families. *Science* **261:** 921–923.

Cotman CW. Berchtold NC. 2002. Exercise: A behavioral intervention to enhance brain health and plasticity. *Trends Neurosci* **25:** 295–301.

de Koning I, Dippel DW, van Kooten F, Koudstaal PJ. 2000. A short screening instrument for poststroke dementia: The R-CAMCOG. *Stroke* **31:** 1502–1508.

de Koning I, van Kooten F, Koudstaal PJ, Dippel DW. 2005. Diagnostic value of the Rotterdam-CAMCOG in post-stroke dementia. *J Neurol Neurosurg Psychiat* **76:** 263–265.

Desmond DW, Moroney JT, Paik MC, Sano M, Mohr JP, Aboumatar S, Tseng CL, Chan S, Williams JB, Remien RH, et al. 2000. Frequency and clinical determinants of dementia after ischemic stroke. *Neurology* **54:** 1124–1131.

Desmond DW, Moroney JT, Sano M, Stern Y. 2002. Incidence of dementia after ischemic stroke: Results of a longitudinal study. *Stroke* **33:** 2254–2260.

Di Carlo A, Baldereschi M, Amaducci L, Lepore V, Bracco L, Maggi S, Bonaiuto S, Perissinotto E, Scarlato G, Farchi G, et al. 2002. Incidence of dementia, Alzheimer's disease, and vascular dementia in Italy. The ILSA Study. *J Am Geriatr Soc* **50:** 41–48.

Doll R, Peto R, Boreham J, Sutherland I. 2000. Smoking and dementia in male British doctors: Prospective study. *BMJ* **320:** 1097.

Edland SD, Rocca WA, Petersen RC, Cha RH, Kokmen E. 2002. Dementia and Alzheimer disease incidence rates do not vary by sex in Rochester, Minn. *Arch Neurol* **59:** 1589–1593.

Elias MF, Elias PK, Sullivan LM, Wolf PA, D'Agostino RB. 2003. Lower cognitive function in the presence of obesity and hypertension: The Framingham heart study. *Int J Obes Relat Metab Disord* **27:** 260–268.

Elias PK, Elias MF, Robbins MA, Budge MM. 2004. Blood pressure-related cognitive decline: Does age make a difference? *Hypertension* **44:** 631–636.

Emmerling MR, Morganti-Kossmann MC, Kossmann T, Stahel PF, Watson MD, Evans LM, Mehta PD, Spiegel K, Kuo YM, Roher AE, et al. 2000. Traumatic brain injury elevates the Alzheimer's amyloid peptide Aβ42 in human CSF. A possible role for nerve cell injury. *Ann NY Acad Sci* **903:** 118–122.

Engelhart MJ, Geerlings MI, Ruitenberg A, van Swieten JC, Hofman A, Witteman JC, Breteler MM. 2002. Dietary intake of antioxidants and risk of Alzheimer disease. *JAMA* **287:** 3223–3229.

Evans DA, Funkenstein HH, Albert MS, Scherr PA, Cook NR, Chown MJ, Hebert LE, Hennekens CH, Taylor JO. 1989. Prevalence of Alzheimer's disease in a community population of older persons. Higher than previously reported. *JAMA* **262:** 2551–2556.

Evans DA, Beckett LA, Albert MS, Hebert LE, Scherr PA, Funkenstein HH, Taylor JO. 1993. Level of education and change in cognitive function in a community population of older persons. *Ann Epidemiol* **3:** 71–77.

Evans DA, Hebert LE, Beckett LA, Scherr PA, Albert MS, Chown MJ, Pilgrim DM, Taylor JO. 1997. Education and other measures of socioeconomic status and risk of incident Alzheimer disease in a defined population of older persons. *Arch Neurol* **54:** 1399–1405.

Farrer LA, Cupples LA, Haines JL, Hyman B, Kukull WA, Mayeux R, Myers RH, Pericak-Vance MA, Risch N, van Duijn CM. 1997. Effects of age, sex, and ethnicity on the association between apolipoprotein E genotype and Alzheimer disease. A meta-analysis. APOE and Alzheimer Disease Meta Analysis Consortium. *JAMA* **278:** 1349–1356.

Farris W, Mansourian S, Chang Y, Lindsley L, Eckman EA, Frosch MP, Eckman CB, Tanzi RE, Selkoe DJ, Guenette S. 2003. Insulin-degrading enzyme regulates the levels of insulin, amyloid β-protein, and the β-amyloid precursor protein intracellular domain in vivo. *Proc Natl Acad Sci* **100:** 4162–4167.

Faxen-Irving G, Basun H, Cederholm T. 2005. Nutritional and cognitive relationships and long-term mortality in patients with various dementia disorders. *Age Ageing* **34:** 136–141.

Fein G, Di Sclafani V, Tanabe J, Cardenas V, Weiner MW, Jagust WJ, Reed BR, Norman D, Schuff N, Kusdra L, et al. 2000. Hippocampal and cortical atrophy predict dementia in subcortical ischemic vascular disease. *Neurology* **55:** 1626–1635.

Ferri CP, Prince M, Brayne C, Brodaty H, Fratiglioni L, Ganguli M, Hall K, Hasegawa K, Hendrie H, Huang Y, et al. 2005. Global prevalence of dementia: A Delphi consensus study. *Lancet* **366:** 2112–2117.

Fitzpatrick AL, Kuller LH, Ives DG, Lopez OL, Jagust W, Breitner JC, Jones B, Lyketsos C, Dulberg C. 2004. Incidence and prevalence of dementia in the Cardiovascular Health Study. *J Am Geriatr Soc* **52:** 195–204.

Fleminger S, Oliver DL, Lovestone S, Rabe-Hesketh S, Giora A. 2003. Head injury as a risk factor for Alzheimer's disease: The evidence 10 years on; a partial replication. *J Neurol Neurosurg Psychiat* **74:** 857–862.

Ford ES. 2002. Does exercise reduce inflammation? Physical activity and C-reactive protein among U.S. adults. *Epidemiology* **13:** 561–568.

Forette F, Seux ML, Staessen JA, Thijs L, Babarskiene MR, Babeanu S, Bossini A, Fagard R, Gil-Extremera B, Laks T, et al. 2002. The prevention of dementia with antihypertensive treatment: New evidence from the Systolic Hypertension in Europe (Syst-Eur) study. *Arch Intern Med* **162:** 2046–2052.

Franz G, Beer R, Kampfl A, Engelhardt K, Schmutzhard E, Ulmer H, Deisenhammer F. 2003. Amyloid β 1–42 and tau in cerebrospinal fluid after severe traumatic brain injury. *Neurology* **60:** 1457–1461.

Fratiglioni L, Viitanen M, von Strauss E, Tontodonati V, Herlitz A, Winblad B. 1997. Very old women at highest risk of dementia and Alzheimer's disease: Incidence data from the Kungsholmen Project, Stockholm. *Neurology* **48:** 132–138.

Fratiglioni L, Paillard-Borg S, Winblad B. 2004. An active and socially integrated lifestyle in late life might protect against dementia. *Lancet Neurol* **3:** 343–353.

Galasko D, Hansen LA, Katzman R, Wiederholt W, Masliah E, Terry R, Hill LR, Lessin P, Thal LJ. 1994. Clinical-neuropathological correlations in Alzheimer's disease and related dementias. *Arch Neurol* **51:** 888–895.

Gamaldo A, Moghekar A, Kilada S, Resnick SM, Zonderman AB, O'Brien R. 2006. Effect of a clinical stroke on the risk of dementia in a prospective cohort. *Neurology* 67: 1363–1369.

Ganguli M, Dodge HH, Chen P, Belle S, DeKosky ST. 2000. Ten-year incidence of dementia in a rural elderly US community population: The MoVIES Project. *Neurology* 54: 1109–1116.

Geerlings MI, Deeg DJ, Penninx BW, Schmand B, Jonker C, Bouter LM, van Tilburg W. 1999. Cognitive reserve and mortality in dementia: The role of cognition, functional ability and depression. *Psychol Med* 29: 1219–1226.

Goate A, Chartier-Harlin MC, Mullan M, Brown J, Crawford F, Fidani L, Giuffra L, Haynes A, Irving N, James L, et al. 1991. Segregation of a missense mutation in the amyloid precursor protein gene with familial Alzheimer's disease. *Nature* 349: 704–706.

Goble AJ. 2005. Obesity in middle age and future risk of dementia: Problem is probably greater for women. *BMJ* 331: 454.

Gustafson D, Rothenberg E, Blennow K, Steen B, Skoog I. 2003. An 18-year follow-up of overweight and risk of Alzheimer disease. *Arch Intern Med* 163: 1524–1528.

Hall KS, Gao S, Unverzagt FW, Hendrie HC. 2000. Low education and childhood rural residence: Risk for Alzheimer's disease in African Americans. *Neurology* 54: 95–99.

Harold D, Abraham R, Hollingworth P, Sims R, Gerrish A, Hamshere ML, Pahwa JS, Moskvina V, Dowzell K, Williams A, et al. 2009. Genome-wide association study identifies variants at CLU and PICALM associated with Alzheimer's disease. *Nat Genet* 41: 1088–1093.

Hartman RE, Laurer H, Longhi L, Bales KR, Paul SM, McIntosh TK, Holtzman DM. 2002. Apolipoprotein E4 influences amyloid deposition but not cell loss after traumatic brain injury in a mouse model of Alzheimer's disease. *J Neurosci* 22: 10083–10087.

Hebert LE, Scherr PA, Beckett LA, Albert MS, Pilgrim DM, Chown MJ, Funkenstein HH, Evans DA. 1995. Age-specific incidence of Alzheimer's disease in a community population. *JAMA* 273: 1354–1359.

Hebert LE, Scherr PA, Bennett DA, Bienias JL, Wilson RS, Morris MC, Evans DA. 2004. Blood pressure and late-life cognitive function change: A biracial longitudinal population study. *Neurology* 62: 2021–2024.

Helzner EP, Scarmeas N, Cosentino S, Portet F, Stern Y. 2007. Leisure activity and cognitive decline in incident Alzheimer disease. *Arch Neurol* 64: 1749–1754.

Hendrie HC, Ogunniyi A, Hall KS, Baiyewu O, Unverzagt FW, Gureje O, Gao S, Evans RM, Ogunseyinde AO, Adeyinka AO, et al. 2001. Incidence of dementia and Alzheimer disease in 2 communities: Yoruba residing in Ibadan, Nigeria, and African Americans residing in Indianapolis, Indiana. *JAMA* 285: 739–747.

Henon H, Durieu I, Guerouaou D, Lebert F, Pasquier F, Leys D. 2001. Poststroke dementia: Incidence and relationship to prestroke cognitive decline. *Neurology* 57: 1216–1222.

Hollingworth P, Harold D, Sims R, Gerrish A, Lambert JC, Carrasquillo MM, Abraham R, Hamshere ML, Pahwa JS, Moskvina V, et al. 2011. Common variants at ABCA7, MS4A6A/MS4A4E, EPHA1, CD33 and CD2AP are associated with Alzheimer's disease. *Nat Genet* 43: 429–435.

Honig LS, Tang MX, Albert S, Costa R, Luchsinger J, Manly J, Stern Y, Mayeux R. 2003. Stroke and the risk of Alzheimer disease. *Arch Neurol* 60: 1707–1712.

Ivan CS, Seshadri S, Beiser A, Au R, Kase CS, Kelly-Hayes M, Wolf PA. 2004. Dementia after stroke: The Framingham Study. *Stroke* 35: 1264–1268.

Iwata A, Chen XH, McIntosh TK, Browne KD, Smith DH. 2002. Long-term accumulation of amyloid-β in axons following brain trauma without persistent upregulation of amyloid precursor protein genes. *J Neuropathol Exp Neurol* 61: 1056–1068.

Jellinger KA. 2002. The pathology of ischemic–vascular dementia: An update. *J Neurol Sci* 203–204: 153–157.

Jellinger KA, Attems J. 2010. Prevalence of dementia disorders in the oldest-old: An autopsy study. *Acta Neuropathol* 119: 421–433.

Jeong SK, Nam HS, Son MH, Son EJ, Cho KH. 2005. Interactive effect of obesity indexes on cognition. *Dement Geriatr Cogn Disord* 19: 91–96.

Jin YP, Di Legge S, Ostbye T, Feightner JW, Hachinski V. 2006. The reciprocal risks of stroke and cognitive impairment in an elderly population. *Alzheimer's Dement* 2: 171–178.

Jin YP, Ostbye T, Feightner JW, Di Legge S, Hachinski V. 2008. Joint effect of stroke and APOE 4 on dementia risk: The Canadian Study of Health and Aging. *Neurology* 70: 9–16.

Jun G, Naj AC, Beecham GW, Wang LS, Buros J, Gallins PJ, Buxbaum JD, Ertekin-Taner N, Fallin MD, Friedland R, et al. 2010. Meta-analysis confirms CR1, CLU, and PICALM as Alzheimer disease risk loci and reveals interactions with APOE genotypes. *Arch Neurol* 67: 1473–1484.

Kawas C, Gray S, Brookmeyer R, Fozard J, Zonderman A. 2000. Age-specific incidence rates of Alzheimer's disease: The Baltimore Longitudinal Study of Aging. *Neurology* 54: 2072–2077.

Kilander L, Nyman H, Boberg M, Lithell H. 2000. The association between low diastolic blood pressure in middle age and cognitive function in old age. A population-based study. *Age Ageing* 29: 243–248.

Kivipelto M, Ngandu T, Fratiglioni L, Viitanen M, Kareholt I, Winblad B, Helkala EL, Tuomilehto J, Soininen H, Nissinen A. 2005. Obesity and vascular risk factors at midlife and the risk of dementia and Alzheimer disease. *Arch Neurol* 62: 1556–1560.

Klimkowicz A, Dziedzic T, Slowik A, Szczudlik A. 2002. Incidence of pre- and poststroke dementia: Cracow Stroke Registry. *Dement Geriatr Cogn Disord* 14: 137–140.

Knopman D, Boland LL, Mosley T, Howard G, Liao D, Szklo M, McGovern P, Folsom AR. 2001. Cardiovascular risk factors and cognitive decline in middle-aged adults. *Neurology* 56: 42–48.

Knopman DS, Rocca WA, Cha RH, Edland SD, Kokmen E. 2002. Incidence of vascular dementia in Rochester, Minn, 1985–1989. *Arch Neurol* 59: 1605–1610.

Koponen S, Taiminen T, Kairisto V, Portin R, Isoniemi H, Hinkka S, Tenovuo O. 2004. APOE-ε4 predicts dementia but not other psychiatric disorders after traumatic brain injury. *Neurology* 63: 749–750.

Kukull WA, Higdon R, Bowen JD, McCormick WC, Teri L, Schellenberg GD, van Belle G, Jolley L, Larson EB.

2002. Dementia and Alzheimer disease incidence: A prospective cohort study. *Arch Neurol* **59:** 1737–1746.

Kuller LH, Lopez OL, Newman A, Beauchamp NJ, Burke G, Dulberg C, Fitzpatrick A, Fried L, Haan MN. 2003. Risk factors for dementia in the cardiovascular health cognition study. *Neuroepidemiology* **22:** 13–22.

Kuller LH, Lopez OL, Jagust WJ, Becker JT, DeKosky ST, Lyketsos C, Kawas C, Breitner JC, Fitzpatrick A, Dulberg C. 2005. Determinants of vascular dementia in the Cardiovascular Health Cognition Study. *Neurology* **64:** 1548–1552.

Lambert JC, Heath S, Even G, Campion D, Sleegers K, Hiltunen M, Combarros O, Zelenika D, Bullido MJ, Tavernier B, et al. 2009. Genome-wide association study identifies variants at CLU and CR1 associated with Alzheimer's disease. *Nat Genet* **41:** 1094–1099.

Larson EB, Wang L, Bowen JD, McCormick WC, Teri L, Crane P, Kukull W. 2006. Exercise is associated with reduced risk for incident dementia among persons 65 years of age and older. *Ann Intern Med* **144:** 73–81.

Launer LJ, Andersen K, Dewey ME, Letenneur L, Ott A, Amaducci LA, Brayne C, Copeland JR, Dartigues JF, Kragh-Sorensen P, et al. 1999. Rates and risk factors for dementia and Alzheimer's disease: results from EURODEM pooled analyses. EURODEM Incidence Research Group and Work Groups. European Studies of Dementia. *Neurology* **52:** 78–84.

Launer LJ, Ross GW, Petrovitch H, Masaki K, Foley D, White LR, Havlik RJ. 2000. Midlife blood pressure and dementia: The Honolulu–Asia aging study. *Neurobiol Aging* **21:** 49–55.

Lee JH, Cheng R, Schupf N, Manly J, Lantigua R, Stern Y, Rogaeva E, Wakutani Y, Farrer L, St George-Hyslop P, et al. 2007. The association between genetic variants in SORL1 and Alzheimer disease in an urban, multiethnic, community-based cohort. *Arch Neurol* **64:** 501–506.

Lee JH, Cheng R, Barral S, Reitz C, Medrano M, Lantigua R, Jimenez-Velazquez IZ, Rogaeva E, St George-Hyslop PH, Mayeux R. 2010. Identification of novel loci for Alzheimer disease and replication of CLU, PICALM, and BIN1 in Caribbean Hispanic individuals. *Arch Neurol* **68:** 320–328.

* Lee V, Brunden KR, Hutton M, Trojanowski JQ. 2011. Developing therapeutic approaches to Tau, selected kinases, and related neuronal protein targets. *Cold Spring Harb Perspect Med* doi: 10.1101/cshperspect.a006437.

Letenneur L, Commenges D, Dartigues JF, Barberger-Gateau P. 1994. Incidence of dementia and Alzheimer's disease in elderly community residents of south-western France. *Int J Epidemiol* **23:** 1256–1261.

Letenneur L, Gilleron V, Commenges D, Helmer C, Orgogozo JM, Dartigues JF. 1999. Are sex and educational level independent predictors of dementia and Alzheimer's disease? Incidence data from the PAQUID project. *J Neurol Neurosurg Psychiat* **66:** 177–183.

Levy-Lahad E, Wasco W, Poorkaj P, Romano DM, Oshima J, Pettingell WH, Yu CE, Jondro PD, Schmidt SD, Wang K, et al. 1995a. Candidate gene for the chromosome 1 familial Alzheimer's disease locus. *Science* **269:** 973–977.

Levy-Lahad E, Wijsman EM, Nemens E, Anderson L, Goddard KA, Weber JL, Bird TD, Schellenberg GD. 1995b. A familial Alzheimer's disease locus on chromosome 1. *Science* **269:** 970–973.

Liebetrau M, Steen B, Skoog I. 2003. Stroke in 85-year-olds: Prevalence, incidence, risk factors, and relation to mortality and dementia. *Stroke* **34:** 2617–2622.

Lim A, Tsuang D, Kukull W, Nochlin D, Leverenz J, McCormick W, Bowen J, Teri L, Thompson J, Peskind ER, et al. 1999. Clinico-neuropathological correlation of Alzheimer's disease in a community-based case series. *J Am Geriatr Soc* **47:** 564–569.

Linden T, Skoog I, Fagerberg B, Steen B, Blomstrand C. 2004. Cognitive impairment and dementia 20 months after stroke. *Neuroepidemiology* **23:** 45–52.

Lindsay J, Laurin D, Verreault R, Hebert R, Helliwell B, Hill GB, McDowell I. 2002. Risk factors for Alzheimer's disease: A prospective analysis from the Canadian Study of Health and Aging. *Am J Epidemiol* **156:** 445–453.

Lithell H, Hansson L, Skoog I, Elmfeldt D, Hofman A, Olofsson B, Trenkwalder P, Zanchetti A. 2003. The Study on Cognition and Prognosis in the Elderly (SCOPE): Principal results of a randomized double-blind intervention trial. *J Hypertens* **21:** 875–886.

Lobo A, Launer LJ, Fratiglioni L, Andersen K, Di Carlo A, Breteler MM, Copeland JR, Dartigues JF, Jagger C, Martinez-Lage J, et al. 2000. Prevalence of dementia and major subtypes in Europe: A collaborative study of population-based cohorts. Neurologic Diseases in the Elderly Research Group. *Neurology* **54:** S4–S9.

Lopez-Pousa S, Vilalta-Franch J, Llinas-Regla J, Garre-Olmo J, Roman GC. 2004. Incidence of dementia in a rural community in Spain: The Girona cohort study. *Neuroepidemiology* **23:** 170–177.

Luchsinger JA, Tang MX, Stern Y, Shea S, Mayeux R. 2001. Diabetes mellitus and risk of Alzheimer's disease and dementia with stroke in a multiethnic cohort. *Am J Epidemiol* **154:** 635–641.

Luchsinger JA, Tang MX, Shea S, Mayeux R. 2002. Caloric intake and the risk of Alzheimer disease. *Arch Neurol* **59:** 1258–1263.

Luchsinger JA, Tang MX, Shea S, Mayeux R. 2003. Antioxidant vitamin intake and risk of Alzheimer disease. *Arch Neurol* **60:** 203–208.

Luchsinger JA, Tang MX, Shea S, Mayeux R. 2004a. Hyperinsulinemia and risk of Alzheimer disease. *Neurology* **63:** 1187–1192.

Luchsinger JA, Tang MX, Shea S, Miller J, Green R, Mayeux R. 2004b. Plasma homocysteine levels and risk of Alzheimer disease. *Neurology* **62:** 1972–1976.

Luchsinger JA, Tang MX, Miller J, Green R, Mayeux R. 2007. Relation of higher folate intake to lower risk of Alzheimer disease in the elderly. *Arch Neurol* **64:** 86–92.

Manly JJ, Schupf N, Tang MX, Stern Y. 2005. Cognitive decline and literacy among ethnically diverse elders. *J Geriat Psychiat Neurol* **18:** 213–217.

McKhann G, Drachman D, Folstein M, Katzman R, Price D, Stadlan EM. 1984. Clinical diagnosis of Alzheimer's disease: Report of the NINCDS–ADRDA Work Group under the auspices of Department of Health and Human Services Task Force on Alzheimer's Disease. *Neurology* **34:** 939–944.

McKhann GM, Knopman DS, Chertkow H, Hyman BT, Jack CR Jr, Kawas CH, Klunk WE, Koroshetz WJ, Manly JJ, Mayeux R, et al. 2011. The diagnosis of dementia due to Alzheimer's disease: Recommendations from the National Institute on Aging—Alzheimer's Association workgroups on diagnostic guidelines for Alzheimer's disease. *Alzheimers Dement* **7**: 263–269.

Morris MC, Scherr PA, Hebert LE, Glynn RJ, Bennett DA, Evans DA. 2001. Association of incident Alzheimer disease and blood pressure measured from 13 years before to 2 years after diagnosis in a large community study. *Arch Neurol* **58**: 1640–1646.

Morris MC, Evans DA, Bienias JL, Tangney CC, Bennett DA, Aggarwal N, Wilson RS, Scherr PA. 2002. Dietary intake of antioxidant nutrients and the risk of incident Alzheimer disease in a biracial community study. *JAMA* **287**: 3230–3237.

Morris MC, Evans DA, Bienias JL, Tangney CC, Bennett DA, Aggarwal N, Schneider J, Wilson RS. 2003. Dietary fats and the risk of incident Alzheimer disease. *Arch Neurol* **60**: 194–200.

Morris MC, Evans DA, Schneider JA, Tangney CC, Bienias JL, Aggarwal NT. 2006. Dietary folate and vitamins B-12 and B-6 not associated with incident Alzheimer's disease. *J Alzheimer's Dis* **9**: 435–443.

Naj AC, Jun G, Beecham GW, Wang LS, Vardarajan BN, Buros J, Gallins PJ, Buxbaum JD, Jarvik GP, Crane PK, et al. 2011. Common variants at MS4A4/MS4A6E, CD2AP, CD33 and EPHA1 are associated with late-onset Alzheimer's disease. *Nat Genet* **43**: 436–441.

Nitrini R, Caramelli P, Herrera E Jr, Bahia VS, Caixeta LF, Radanovic M, Anghinah R, Charchat-Fichman H, Porto CS, Carthery MT, et al. 2004. Incidence of dementia in a community-dwelling Brazilian population. *Alzheimer Dis Assoc Disord* **18**: 241–246.

Nourhashemi F, Andrieu S, Gillette-Guyonnet S, Reynish E, Albarede JL, Grandjean H, Vellas B. 2002. Is there a relationship between fat-free soft tissue mass and low cognitive function? Results from a study of 7,105 women. *J Am Geriatr Soc* **50**: 1796–1801.

Nourhashemi F, Deschamps V, Larrieu S, Letenneur L, Dartigues JF, Barberger-Gateau P. 2003. Body mass index and incidence of dementia: The PAQUID study. *Neurology* **60**: 117–119.

Ogunniyi A, Baiyewu O, Gureje O, Hall KS, Unverzagt F, Siu SH, Gao S, Farlow M, Oluwole OS, Komolafe O, et al. 2000. Epidemiology of dementia in Nigeria: Results from the Indianapolis–Ibadan study. *Eur J Neurol* **7**: 485–490.

Peila R, Rodriguez BL, Launer LJ. 2002. Type 2 diabetes, APOE gene, and the risk for dementia and related pathologies: The Honolulu–Asia Aging Study. *Diabetes* **51**: 1256–1262.

Pendlebury ST, Rothwell PM. 2009. Prevalence, incidence, and factors associated with pre-stroke and post-stroke dementia: A systematic review and meta-analysis. *Lancet Neurol* **8**: 1006–1018.

Perry G, Cash AD, Smith MA. 2002. Alzheimer disease and oxidative stress. *J Biomed Biotechnol* **2**: 120–123.

Peters R, Pinto E, Beckett N, Swift C, Potter J, McCormack T, Nunes M, Grimley-Evans J, Fletcher A, Bulpitt C. 2010. Association of depression with subsequent mortality, cardiovascular morbidity and incident dementia in people aged 80 and over and suffering from hypertension. Data from the Hypertension in the Very Elderly Trial (HYVET). *Age Ageing* **39**: 439–445.

Petitti DB, Crooks VC, Buckwalter JG, Chiu V. 2005. Blood pressure levels before dementia. *Arch Neurol* **62**: 112–116.

Piguet O, Grayson DA, Creasey H, Bennett HP, Brooks WS, Waite LM, Broe GA. 2003. Vascular risk factors, cognition and dementia incidence over 6 years in the Sydney Older Persons Study. *Neuroepidemiology* **22**: 165–171.

Podewils LJ, Guallar E, Kuller LH, Fried LP, Lopez OL, Carlson M, Lyketsos CG. 2005. Physical activity, APOE genotype, and dementia risk: Findings from the Cardiovascular Health Cognition Study. *Am J Epidemiol* **161**: 639–651.

Posner HB, Tang MX, Luchsinger J, Lantigua R, Stern Y, Mayeux R. 2002. The relationship of hypertension in the elderly to AD, vascular dementia, and cognitive function. *Neurology* **58**: 1175–1181.

Profenno LA, Porsteinsson AP, Faraone SV. 2009. Meta-analysis of Alzheimer's disease risk with obesity, diabetes, and related disorders. *Biol Psychiat* **67**: 505–512.

Qiu C, Backman L, Winblad B, Aguero-Torres H, Fratiglioni L. 2001. The influence of education on clinically diagnosed dementia incidence and mortality data from the Kungsholmen Project. *Arch Neurol* **58**: 2034–2039.

Qiu C, von Strauss E, Fastbom J, Winblad B, Fratiglioni L. 2003. Low blood pressure and risk of dementia in the Kungsholmen project: A 6-year follow-up study. *Arch Neurol* **60**: 223–228.

Rastas S, Pirttila T, Mattila K, Verkkoniemi A, Juva K, Niinisto L, Lansimies E, Sulkava R. 2010. Vascular risk factors and dementia in the general population aged >85 years: Prospective population-based study. *Neurobiol Aging* **31**: 1–7.

Ravaglia G, Forti P, Maioli F, Martelli M, Servadei L, Brunetti N, Dalmonte E, Bianchin M, Mariani E. 2005a. Incidence and etiology of dementia in a large elderly Italian population. *Neurology* **64**: 1525–1530.

Ravaglia G, Forti P, Maioli F, Martelli M, Servadei L, Brunetti N, Porcellini E, Licastro F. 2005b. Homocysteine and folate as risk factors for dementia and Alzheimer disease. *Am J Clin Nutr* **82**: 636–643.

Razay G, Vreugdenhil A. 2005. Obesity in middle age and future risk of dementia: midlife obesity increases risk of future dementia. *BMJ* **331**.

Reger MA, Watson GS, Green PS, Wilkinson CW, Baker LD, Cholerton B, Fishel MA, Plymate SR, Breitner JC, DeGroodt W, et al. 2008. Intranasal insulin improves cognition and modulates β-amyloid in early AD. *Neurology* **70**: 440–448.

Reinprecht F, Elmstahl S, Janzon L, Andre-Petersson L. 2003. Hypertension and changes of cognitive function in 81-year-old men: a 13-year follow-up of the population study "Men born in 1914," Sweden. *J Hypertens* **21**: 57–66.

Reitz C, Bos MJ, Hofman A, Koudstaal PJ, Breteler MM. 2008. Prestroke cognitive performance, incident stroke, and risk of dementia: The Rotterdam Study. *Stroke* **39**: 36–41.

Reitz C, Tang MX, Miller J, Green R, Luchsinger JA. 2009. Plasma homocysteine and risk of mild cognitive impairment. *Dement Geriatr Cogn Disord* **27:** 11–17.

Reitz C, Cheng R, Rogaeva E, Lee JH, Tokuhiro S, Zou F, Bettens K, Sleegers K, Tan EK, Kimura R, et al. 2011. Meta-analysis of the association between variants in SORL1 and Alzheimer disease. *Arch Neurol* **68:** 99–106.

Reuben DB, Judd-Hamilton L, Harris TB, Seeman TE. 2003. The associations between physical activity and inflammatory markers in high-functioning older persons: MacArthur Studies of Successful Aging. *J Am Geriatr Soc* **51:** 1125–1130.

Risner ME, Saunders AM, Altman JF, Ormandy GC, Craft S, Foley IM, Zvartau-Hind ME, Hosford DA, Roses AD. 2006. Efficacy of rosiglitazone in a genetically defined population with mild-to-moderate Alzheimer's disease. *Pharmacogenom J* **6:** 246–254.

Rogaev EI, Sherrington R, Rogaeva EA, Levesque G, Ikeda M, Liang Y, Chi H, Lin C, Holman K, Tsuda T, et al. 1995. Familial Alzheimer's disease in kindreds with missense mutations in a gene on chromosome 1 related to the Alzheimer's disease type 3 gene. *Nature* **376:** 775–778.

Rogaeva E, Meng Y, Lee JH, Gu Y, Kawarai T, Zou F, Katayama T, Baldwin CT, Cheng R, Hasegawa H, et al. 2007. The neuronal sortilin-related receptor SORL1 is genetically associated with Alzheimer disease. *Nat Genet* **39:** 168–177.

Rosengren A, Skoog I, Gustafson D, Wilhelmsen L. 2005. Body mass index, other cardiovascular risk factors, and hospitalization for dementia. *Arch Intern Med* **165:** 321–326.

Rottkamp CA, Nunomura A, Raina AK, Sayre LM, Perry G, Smith MA. 2000. Oxidative stress, antioxidants, and Alzheimer disease. *Alzheimer Dis Assoc Disord* **14** (Suppl 1)**:** S62–S66.

Rovio S, Kareholt I, Helkala EL, Viitanen M, Winblad B, Tuomilehto J, Soininen H, Nissinen A, Kivipelto M. 2005. Leisure-time physical activity at midlife and the risk of dementia and Alzheimer's disease. *Lancet Neurol* **4:** 705–711.

Ruitenberg A, Skoog I, Ott A, Aevarsson O, Witteman JC, Lernfelt B, van Harskamp F, Hofman A, Breteler MM. 2001. Blood pressure and risk of dementia: results from the Rotterdam study and the Gothenburg H-70 Study. *Dement Geriatr Cogn Disord* **12:** 33–39.

Sato T, Hanyu H, Hirao K, Kanetaka H, Sakurai H, Iwamoto T. 2009. Efficacy of PPAR-γ agonist pioglitazone in mild Alzheimer disease. *Neurobiol Aging* **32:** 1626–1633.

Scarmeas N, Levy G, Tang MX, Manly J, Stern Y. 2001. Influence of leisure activity on the incidence of Alzheimer's disease. *Neurology* **57:** 2236–2242.

Scarmeas N, Albert SM, Manly JJ, Stern Y. 2006a. Education and rates of cognitive decline in incident Alzheimer's disease. *J Neurol Neurosurg Psychiat* **77:** 308–316.

Scarmeas N, Stern Y, Mayeux R, Luchsinger JA. 2006b. Mediterranean diet, Alzheimer disease, and vascular mediation. *Arch Neurol* **63:** 1709–1717.

Scarmeas N, Luchsinger JA, Schupf N, Brickman AM, Cosentino S, Tang MX, Stern Y. 2009. Physical activity, diet, and risk of Alzheimer disease. *JAMA* **302:** 627–637.

Schaefer EJ, Bongard V, Beiser AS, Lamon-Fava S, Robins SJ, Au R, Tucker KL, Kyle DJ, Wilson PW, Wolf PA. 2006. Plasma phosphatidylcholine docosahexaenoic acid content and risk of dementia and Alzheimer disease: The Framingham Heart Study. *Arch Neurol* **63:** 1545–1550.

* Schenk D, Basi GS, Pangalos MN. 2011. Treatment strategies targeting amyloid-protein. *Cold Spring Harb Perspect Med* doi: 10.1101/cshperspect.a006387.

Schneider JA, Bennett DA. 2010. Where vascular meets neurodegenerative disease. *Stroke* **41:** S144–S146.

Selkoe DJ. 2000. The origins of Alzheimer disease: A is for amyloid. *JAMA* **283:** 1615–1617.

* Serrano-Pozo A, Frosch MP, Masliah E, Hyman BT. 2011. Neuropathological alterations in Alzheimer disease. *Cold Spring Harb Perspect Med* doi: 10.1101/cshperspect. a006189.

Seshadri S. 2006. Elevated plasma homocysteine levels: Risk factor or risk marker for the development of dementia and Alzheimer's disease? *J Alzheimer's Dis* **9:** 393–398.

Seshadri S, Fitzpatrick AL, Ikram MA, DeStefano AL, Gudnason V, Boada M, Bis JC, Smith AV, Carassquillo MM, Lambert JC, et al. 2010. Genome-wide analysis of genetic loci associated with Alzheimer disease. *JAMA* **303:** 1832–1840.

Sherrington R, Rogaev EI, Liang Y, Rogaeva EA, Levesque G, Ikeda M, Chi H, Lin C, Li G, Holman K, et al. 1995. Cloning of a gene bearing missense mutations in early-onset familial Alzheimer's disease. *Nature* **375:** 754–760.

Sherrington R, Froelich S, Sorbi S, Campion D, Chi H, Rogaeva EA, Levesque G, Rogaev EI, Lin C, Liang Y, et al. 1996. Alzheimer's disease associated with mutations in presenilin 2 is rare and variably penetrant. *Human Mol Genet* **5:** 985–988.

Simons LA, Simons J, McCallum J, Friedlander Y. 2006. Lifestyle factors and risk of dementia: Dubbo Study of the elderly. *Med J Australia* **184:** 68–70.

Skoog I, Lernfelt B, Landahl S, Palmertz B, Andreasson LA, Nilsson L, Persson G, Oden A, Svanborg A. 1996. 15-Year longitudinal study of blood pressure and dementia. *Lancet* **347:** 1141–1145.

Slooter AJ, Cruts M, Kalmijn S, Hofman A, Breteler MM, Van Broeckhoven C, van Duijn CM. 1998. Risk estimates of dementia by apolipoprotein E genotypes from a population-based incidence study: The Rotterdam Study. *Arch Neurol* **55:** 964–968.

Smith C, Graham DI, Murray LS, Nicoll JA. 2003. Tau immunohistochemistry in acute brain injury. *Neuropathol Appl Neurobiol* **29:** 496–502.

Solfrizzi V, Panza F, Colacicco AM, D'Introno A, Capurso C, Torres F, Grigoletto F, Maggi S, Del Parigi A, Reiman EM, et al. 2004. Vascular risk factors, incidence of MCI, and rates of progression to dementia. *Neurology* **63:** 1882–1891.

Sparks DL, Kuo YM, Roher A, Martin T, Lukas RJ. 2000. Alterations of Alzheimer's disease in the cholesterol-fed rabbit, including vascular inflammation. Preliminary observations. *Ann NY Acad Sci* **903:** 335–344.

Srikanth VK, Anderson JF, Donnan GA, Saling MM, Didus E, Alpitsis R, Dewey HM, Macdonell RA, Thrift AG. 2004. Progressive dementia after first-ever stroke: A community-based follow-up study. *Neurology* **63**: 785–792.

Srikanth VK, Quinn SJ, Donnan GA, Saling MM, Thrift AG. 2006. Long-term cognitive transitions, rates of cognitive change, and predictors of incident dementia in a population-based first-ever stroke cohort. *Stroke* **37**: 2479–2483.

Stern Y, Gurland B, Tatemichi TK, Tang MX, Wilder D, Mayeux R. 1994. Influence of education and occupation on the incidence of Alzheimer's disease. *JAMA* **271**: 1004–1010.

Stern Y, Albert S, Tang MX, Tsai WY. 1999. Rate of memory decline in AD is related to education and occupation: Cognitive reserve? *Neurology* **53**: 1942–1957.

Stewart R, Masaki K, Xue QL, Peila R, Petrovitch H, White LR, Launer LJ. 2005. A 32-year prospective study of change in body weight and incident dementia: The Honolulu-Asia Aging Study. *Arch Neurol* **62**: 55–60.

Stone JR, Okonkwo DO, Singleton RH, Mutlu LK, Helm GA, Povlishock JT. 2002. Caspase-3-mediated cleavage of amyloid precursor protein and formation of amyloid Beta peptide in traumatic axonal injury. *J Neurotrauma* **19**: 601–614.

Swartz RH, Stuss DT, Gao F, Black SE. 2008. Independent cognitive effects of atrophy and diffuse subcortical and thalamico-cortical cerebrovascular disease in dementia. *Stroke* **39**: 822–830.

Tabet N. 2005. Obesity in middle age and future risk of dementia: Dietary fat and sugar may hold the clue. *BMJ* **331**: 454–455.

Tang MX, Cross P, Andrews H, Jacobs DM, Small S, Bell K, Merchant C, Lantigua R, Costa R, Stern Y, et al. 2001. Incidence of AD in African-Americans, Caribbean Hispanics, and Caucasians in northern Manhattan. *Neurology* **56**: 49–56.

Tang WK, Chan SS, Chiu HF, Ungvari GS, Wong KS, Kwok TC, Mok V, Wong KT, Richards PS, Ahuja AT. 2004. Frequency and determinants of poststroke dementia in Chinese. *Stroke* **35**: 930–935.

* Tanzi RE. 2011. The genetics of Alzheimer disease. *Cold Spring Harb Perspect Med* doi: 10.1101/cshperspect.a006296.

* Tarawneh R, Holtzman DM. 2011. The clinical problem of symptomatic Alzheimer disease and mild cognitive impairment. *Cold Spring Harb Perspect Med* doi: 10.1101/cshperspect.a006148.

Tervo S, Kivipelto M, Hanninen T, Vanhanen M, Hallikainen M, Mannermaa A, Soininen H. 2004. Incidence and risk factors for mild cognitive impairment: A population-based three-year follow-up study of cognitively healthy elderly subjects. *Dement Geriatr Cogn Disord* **17**: 196–203.

Traber MG, van dV, Reznick AZ, Cross CE. 2000. Tobacco-related diseases. Is there a role for antioxidant micronutrient supplementation? *Clin Chest Med* **21**: 173.

Trichopoulou A, Costacou T, Bamia C, Trichopoulos D. 2003. Adherence to a Mediterranean diet and survival in a Greek population. *New Engl J Med* **348**: 2599–2608.

Trujillo ME, Scherer PE. 2005. Adiponectin—journey from an adipocyte secretory protein to biomarker of the metabolic syndrome. *J Intern Med* **257**: 167–175.

Tyas SL, Manfreda J, Strain LA, Montgomery PR. 2001. Risk factors for Alzheimer's disease: A population-based, longitudinal study in Manitoba. *Int J Epidemiol* **30**: 590–597.

Tzourio C, Anderson C, Chapman N, Woodward M, Neal B, MacMahon S, Chalmers J. 2003. Effects of blood pressure lowering with perindopril and indapamide therapy on dementia and cognitive decline in patients with cerebrovascular disease. *Arch Intern Med* **163**: 1069–1075.

Valenzuela MJ, Sachdev P. 2005. Brain reserve and dementia: A systematic review. *Psychol Med* **25**: 1–14.

van Gelder BM, Tijhuis M, Kalmijn S, Kromhout D. 2007. Fish consumption, n-3 fatty acids, and subsequent 5-y cognitive decline in elderly men: The Zutphen Elderly Study. *Am J Clin Nutr* **85**: 1142–1147.

van Praag H, Kempermann G, Gage FH. 1999. Running increases cell proliferation and neurogenesis in the adult mouse dentate gyrus. *Nat Neurosci* **2**: 266–270.

Verghese J, Lipton RB, Hall CB, Kuslansky G, Katz MJ. 2003a. Low blood pressure and the risk of dementia in very old individuals. *Neurology* **61**: 1667–1672.

Verghese J, Lipton RB, Katz MJ, Hall CB, Derby CA, Kuslansky G, Ambrose AF, Sliwinski M, Buschke H. 2003b. Leisure activities and the risk of dementia in the elderly. *New Engl J Med* **348**: 2508–2516.

Waldstein SR, Katzel LI. 2006. Interactive relations of central versus total obesity and blood pressure to cognitive function. *Int J Obes* **30**: 201–207.

Waldstein SR, Giggey PP, Thayer JF, Zonderman AB. 2005. Nonlinear relations of blood pressure to cognitive function: The Baltimore Longitudinal Study of Aging. *Hypertension* **45**: 374–379.

Wang HX, Wahlin A, Basun H, Fastbom J, Winblad B, Fratiglioni L. 2001. Vitamin B(12) and folate in relation to the development of Alzheimer's disease. *Neurology* **56**: 1188–1194.

Wang HX, Karp A, Winblad B, Fratiglioni L. 2002. Late-life engagement in social and leisure activities is associated with a decreased risk of dementia: A longitudinal study from the Kungsholmen project. *Am J Epidemiol* **155**: 1081–1087.

Wang L, Larson EB, Bowen JD, van Belle G. 2006. Performance-based physical function and future dementia in older people. *Archiv Intern Med* **166**: 1115–1120.

Watson GS, Cholerton BA, Reger MA, Baker LD, Plymate SR, Asthana S, Fishel MA, Kulstad JJ, Green PS, Cook DG, et al. 2005. Preserved cognition in patients with early Alzheimer disease and amnestic mild cognitive impairment during treatment with rosiglitazone: A preliminary study. *Am J Geriatr Psychiat* **13**: 950–958.

* Weintraub S, Wicklund AH, Salmon DP. 2011. The neuropsychological profile of Alzheimer disease. *Cold Spring Harb Perspect Med* doi: 10.1101/cshperspect.a006171.

Wen Y, Yang SH, Liu R, Perez EJ, Brun-Zinkernagel AM, Koulen P, Simpkins JW. 2007. Cdk5 is involved in NFT-like tauopathy induced by transient cerebral ischemia in female rats. *Biochim Biophys Acta* **1772**: 473–483.

Wen Y, Yu WH, Maloney B, Bailey J, Ma J, Marie I, Maurin T, Wang L, Figueroa H, Herman M, et al. 2008. Transcriptional regulation of β-secretase by p25/cdk5 leads to enhanced amyloidogenic processing. *Neuron* **57**: 680–690.

White L, Katzman R, Losonczy K, Salive M, Wallace R, Berkman L, Taylor J, Fillenbaum G, Havlik R. 1994. Association of education with incidence of cognitive impairment in three established populations for epidemiologic studies of the elderly. *J Clin Epidemiol* **47**: 363–374.

Whitehouse PJ, Martino AM, Wagster MV, Price DL, Mayeux R, Atack JR, Kellar KJ. 1988. Reductions in [^{3}H]nicotinic acetylcholine binding in Alzheimer's disease and Parkinson's disease: An autoradiographic study. *Neurology* **38**: 720–723.

Whitmer RA, Gunderson EP, Barrett-Connor E, Quesenberry CP Jr, Yaffe K. 2005a. Obesity in middle age and future risk of dementia: A 27 year longitudinal population based study. *BMJ* **330**: 1360.

Whitmer RA, Sidney S, Selby J, Johnston SC, Yaffe K. 2005b. Midlife cardiovascular risk factors and risk of dementia in late life. *Neurology* **64**: 277–281.

Wijsman EM, Pankratz ND, Choi Y, Rothstein JH, Faber KM, Cheng R, Lee JH, Bird TD, Bennett DA, Diaz-Arrastia R, et al. 2011. Genome wide association of familial late onset Alzheimer's disease replicates *BIN1* and *CLU*, and nominates *CUGBP2* in interaction with *APOE*. *PLoS Genet* **7**: e1001308.

Wilson RS, Bennett DA, Bienias JL, Aggarwal NT, Mendes De Leon CF, Morris MC, Schneider JA, Evans DA. 2002a. Cognitive activity and incident AD in a population-based sample of older persons. *Neurology* **59**: 1910–1914.

Wilson RS, Mendes De Leon CF, Barnes LL, Schneider JA, Bienias JL, Evans DA, Bennett DA. 2002b. Participation in cognitively stimulating activities and risk of incident Alzheimer disease. *JAMA* **287**: 742–748.

Wilson RS, Scherr PA, Schneider JA, Tang Y, Bennett DA. 2007. Relation of cognitive activity to risk of developing Alzheimer disease. *Neurology* **69**: 1911–1920.

Wilson RS, Barnes LL, Aggarwal NT, Boyle PA, Hebert LE, Mendes de Leon CF, Evans DA. 2010. Cognitive activity and the cognitive morbidity of Alzheimer disease. *Neurology* **75**: 990–996.

Wright CB, Festa JR, Paik MC, Schmiedigen A, Brown TR, Yoshita M, DeCarli C, Sacco R, Stern Y. 2008. White matter hyperintensities and subclinical infarction: Associations with psychomotor speed and cognitive flexibility. *Stroke* **39**: 800–805.

Wu C, Zhou D, Wen C, Zhang L, Como P, Qiao Y. 2003. Relationship between blood pressure and Alzheimer's disease in Linxian County, China. *Life Sci* **72**: 1125–1133.

Yamada M, Kasagi F, Sasaki H, Masunari N, Mimori Y, Suzuki G. 2003. Association between dementia and midlife risk factors: The Radiation Effects Research Foundation Adult Health Study. *J Am Geriatr Soc* **51**: 410–414.

Yamagishi S, Nakamura K, Inoue H, Kikuchi S, Takeuchi M. 2005. Serum or cerebrospinal fluid levels of glyceraldehyde-derived advanced glycation end products (AGEs) may be a promising biomarker for early detection of Alzheimer's disease. *Med Hypoth* **64**: 1205–1207.

Yip AG, Brayne C, Matthews FE. 2006. Risk factors for incident dementia in England and Wales: The Medical Research Council Cognitive Function and Ageing Study. A population-based nested case-control study. *Age Ageing* **35**: 154–160.

Yu YH, Ginsberg HN. 2005. Adipocyte signaling and lipid homeostasis: Sequelae of insulin-resistant adipose tissue. *Circul Res* **96**: 1042–1052.

Zhang X, Li C, Zhang M. 1999. Psychosocial risk factors of Alzheimer's disease. *Zhonghua Yi Xue Za Zhi* **79**: 335–338.

Zhou DH, Wang JY, Li J, Deng J, Gao C, Chen M. 2004. Study on frequency and predictors of dementia after ischemic stroke: The Chongqing stroke study. *J Neurol* **251**: 421–427.

Zhu L, Fratiglioni L, Guo Z, Basun H, Corder EH, Winblad B, Viitanen M. 2000. Incidence of dementia in relation to stroke and the apolipoprotein E ε4 allele in the very old. Findings from a population-based longitudinal study. *Stroke* **31**: 53–60.

Biochemistry and Cell Biology of Tau Protein in Neurofibrillary Degeneration

Eva-Maria Mandelkow and Eckhard Mandelkow

Max-Planck Unit for Structural Molecular Biology, c/o DESY, 22607 Hamburg, Germany; and DZNE, German Center for Neurodegenerative Diseases, and CAESAR Research Center, 53175 Bonn, Germany

Correspondence: mandelkow@mpasmb.desy.de

Tau represents the subunit protein of one of the major hallmarks of Alzheimer disease (AD), the neurofibrillary tangles, and is therefore of major interest as an indicator of disease mechanisms. Many of the unusual properties of Tau can be explained by its nature as a natively unfolded protein. Examples are the large number of structural conformations and biochemical modifications (phosphorylation, proteolysis, glycosylation, and others), the multitude of interaction partners (mainly microtubules, but also other cytoskeletal proteins, kinases, and phosphatases, motor proteins, chaperones, and membrane proteins). The pathological aggregation of Tau is counterintuitive, given its high solubility, but can be rationalized by short hydrophobic motifs forming β structures. The aggregation of Tau is toxic in cell and animal models, but can be reversed by suppressing expression or by aggregation inhibitors. This review summarizes some of the structural, biochemical, and cell biological properties of Tau and Tau fibers. Further aspects of Tau as a diagnostic marker and therapeutic target, its involvement in other Tau-based diseases, and its histopathology are covered by other chapters in this volume.

Curiously, "Tau" the protein and "Tau" the lepton were discovered in the same year, 1975 (Weingarten et al. 1975; Perl et al. 1975). They have fascinated cell biologists and elementary particle physicists since then, yielded one Nobel prize, and produced more than 5000 hits in Pubmed, including more than 100 for the decay of the Higgs boson into Tau pairs. For cell biologists, Tau was one of the first microtubule-associated proteins (MAPs) to be characterized, named by Marc Kirschner when his team was searching for factors that promote the self-assembly of tubulin into microtubules (hence Tau = Tubulin binding protein). This started a line of research centered around the cell biological role of Tau as a stabilizer of microtubules in neurons and other cells, with important roles in cell differentiation and polarization. Early milestones in this research were the biochemical characterization of Tau (Cleveland et al. 1977a,b), its up-regulation, along with tubulin, during neuronal differentiation (Drubin and Kirschner 1986), the demonstration that it was mainly an axonal protein in mature neurons (in contrast to the dendritic MAP2; Binder et al. 1985), and the cloning and isoform characterization of Tau from mouse, cow, and human (Goedert et al. 1989; Himmler 1989; Lee et al. 1988).

A second line of Tau research was triggered by basic neurological research to identify the components of the abnormal protein deposits found in the brains of Alzheimer disease patients. One of them, Aβ, was identified as the core protein of extracellular amyloid plaques by molecular cloning (Kang et al. 1987), and the other, Tau, as the core of intracellular neurofibrillary tangles by antibody reactivity (Brion et al. 1985; Grundke-Iqbal et al. 1986; Kosik et al. 1986; Wood et al. 1986). These discoveries led to concerted efforts by cell biologists and neuroscientists to elucidate the physiological and pathological properties of Tau. Human Tau and its splicing isoforms were identified (Goedert et al. 1988), Tau-specific antibodies against normal and diseased states were developed (Kosik et al. 1988; Wolozin et al. 1986), abnormal posttranslational modifications of Tau were identified (e.g., phosphorylation sites, kinases, phosphatases; Biernat et al. 1992; Hanger et al. 1992; Goedert et al. 1994), and the principles of abnormal aggregation emerged (Wischik et al. 1988; Wille et al. 1992).

Over the years, interest in Tau waxed and waned, depending on new discoveries. After the initial excitement, it took a slump when it became clear that familial Alzheimer disease (AD) was caused by mutations affecting amyloid precursor protein (APP) processing, and therefore Tau pathology appeared secondary to Aβ pathology. Tau research was boosted by the discovery that a number of neurodegenerative diseases displayed Tau deposits independently of Aβ amyloid (e.g., PiD, PSP), including frontotemporal dementias caused by Tau mutations (FTDP17; see Goedert et al. 2011). These observations established a role for Tau in its own right as a disease-causing agent. Why Tau and Aβ enter a special relationship in AD is still a matter of debate, but recent results from transgenic mice suggest that Tau pathology is not simply a downstream consequence of Aβ pathology, but necessary for the appearance of Aβ-induced toxicity (for a review, see Morris et al. 2011).

Regarding therapy, the Tau-based research has led to several approaches (reviewed by Schneider and Mandelkow 2008; Lee et al. 2011). They are directed against hyperphosphorylation (e.g., the search for kinase inhibitors or phosphatase enhancers), aggregation (e.g., aggregation inhibitors), compounds promoting microtubule stability (to compensate for Tau dysfunction), and Tau-based immunotherapy. So far, no treatment has arrived in the clinic.

A number of excellent reviews on the biology and pathology of Tau have appeared over the past few years (Cassimeris and Spittle 2001; Garcia and Cleveland 2001; Terwel et al. 2002; Dehmelt and Halpain 2005; Andreadis 2006; Ballatore et al. 2007; Gotz et al. 2007, 2010; Iqbal and Grundke-Iqbal 2008; Schneider and Mandelkow 2008; Sergeant et al. 2008; Aguzzi and Rajendran 2009; Spires-Jones et al. 2009; Iqbal et al. 2009; Wolfe 2009; Goedert et al. 2010; Morris et al. 2011; Salminen et al. 2011). This brief review will cover a few salient aspects, with an emphasis on Tau structure and interactions.

TAU DOMAINS

Human Tau is encoded on chromosome 17q21 (Neve et al. 1986). The protein occurs mainly in the axons of the CNS and consists largely of six isoforms generated by alternative splicing (Goedert et al. 1989). They differ by the presence or absence of two near-amino-terminal inserts of 29 residues each, encoded by exons 2 and 3, and by one of the repeats (R2, 31 residues) in the carboxy-terminal half. Different names are in use, derived from inserts/repeats, number of residues, or clone names, as summarized in Table 1.

There are additional minor isoforms in the CNS (see review by Andreadis 2006), and a "big Tau" isoform occuring predominantly in the peripheral nervous system (PNS), equivalent to 2N4R plus 242 residues from exon 4a (Couchie et al. 1992; Goedert et al. 1992). The organization of other mammalian Taus (e.g., mouse, rat, cow) is similar, with only a few alterations, mostly in the amino-terminal region, for

Table 1. Isoforms of Tau protein

Clone	Inserts/repeats	Number of amino acids (AA)	MW (kDa)
htau40	2N4R	441	45.9
htau39	2N3R	410	42.6
htau34	1N4R	412	43.0
htau37	1N3R	381	39.7
htau24	0N4R	383	40.0
htau23	0N3R	352	36.7
big Tau	2N4R + exon 4a	695	72.7

example, mouse Tau is 11 residues shorter (ranging from 341 to 430 residues) and has a carboxy-terminal half identical to human Tau (Lee et al. 1988).[1] Tau, together with MAP2 and MAP4, forms a family of proteins with similar domain structure, with up to five repeats of ~31 residues in the carboxy-terminal half and an amino-terminal half of variable size (MAP2, 1858 residues [4R], mostly in neuronal dendrites; MAP4, 1152 residues [4R], ubiquitous in many cell types; Cassimeris and Spittle 2001; Dehmelt and Halpain 2005; Doll et al. 1993).

Domains of Tau (Fig. 1) can be defined on the basis of their microtubule interactions and/or their amino acid character. Chymotryptic cleavage in vitro behind Y197 generates two fragments whose carboxy-terminal part binds to microtubules and promotes their assembly, and hence is termed the "assembly domain" (Steiner et al. 1990). The amino-terminal

---

[1]A note on "repeat" nomenclature. Lee et al. (1988) noticed the repeating character of the Tau sequence and defined as repeats the 18-AA stretches of the motifs VXSK to PGGG because of their high sequence homology. The intervening 13 or 14 residues were less conserved and were termed "interrepeats" (Goode and Feinstein 1994). Later, the comparison of 3R- and 4R-isoforms revealed that the residues encoded by exon 10 correspond exactly to one repeat of 31 residues (VQIINK . . . PGGGS), suggesting this as a natural unit for the definition of a repeat (Himmler et al. 1989). In this paper we adhere to this definition, so that the four repeats of human Tau correspond to the sequences 244–274, 275–305 (exon 10), 306–336, and 337–368. Thus, one repeat in our definition corresponds roughly to one 13-AA interrepeat plus the following 18-AA repeat in the earlier definition.

fragment does not bind to microtubules but projects away from the microtubule surface and hence is termed "projection domain" (Hirokawa et al. 1988). A more detailed analysis, based on nuclear magnetic resonance (NMR) spectroscopy, confirms and refines these features: Pronounced interactions with microtubules (MT) occur beween Tau residues 200 and 400 (Mukrasch et al. 2005; Sillen et al. 2007) and thus cover the repeat domain plus the adjacent flanking domains of ~40 residues each, consistent with binding studies (see below). However, weaker interactions are also distributed elsewhere in the carboxy-terminal half of Tau (Mukrasch et al. 2009).

The overall amino acid composition is unusually hydrophilic, consistent with the unfolded character of the protein. In full-length Tau (2N4R) there are 80 S or T residues, 56 negative (D + E), 58 positive (K + R), and eight aromatic (5 Y, 3 F, and no W). Thus the protein has an overall basic character, but the amino-terminal ~120 residues (including the two inserts) are predominantly acidic, and the carboxy-terminal ~40 residues are roughly neutral. This asymmetry of charges is important for interactions with microtubules and other partners, internal folding, and Tau aggregation. The middle region (AA 150–240) contains numerous prolines, many of them as SP or TP motifs (targets of proline-directed kinases), up to seven PXXP motifs (binding sites of proteins with SH3 domains); hence this region is considered as a "proline-rich domain." Another region (~400) containing several prolines is downstream of the repeat domain. These proline-rich domains have acquired a special importance in the field because they harbor many epitopes of antibodies that become hyperphosphorylated in AD, often at SP or TP motifs, and are therefore diagnostic for the disease state, both in human patients and in animal models.

TAU STRUCTURE

Because of its hydrophilic character, Tau does not adopt the compact folded structure typical of most cytosolic proteins. In fact, evidence from various biophysical methods (circular

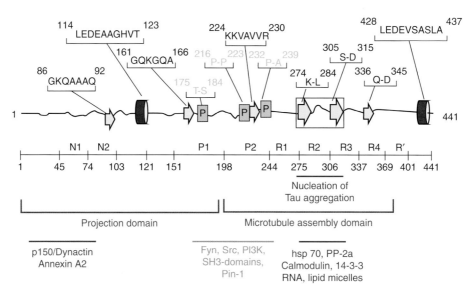

Figure 1. Domains and structural elements in Tau. *Top*: Representation of Tau deduced from NMR (Mukrasch et al. 2009). Most of the chain is unfolded (black lines), with a few short and transient elements of secondary structure (α-helix red, β-strand yellow, poly-proline helix green). The red box indicates the region of the two hexapeptide motifs responsible for Tau aggregation. *Middle*: Domain subdivision (following Gustke et al. 1994). The carboxy-terminal half promotes microtubule assembly, and the amino-terminal half projects out from the microtubule surface. N1, N2 and R2 may be absent owing to alternative splicing. R1–R4 represent the repeat domain; together with the flanking domains, this represents the microtubule interaction domain. *Bottom*: Approximate location of interaction sites with other proteins.

dichroism, NMR and small angle X-ray scattering [SAXS]) show that the entire Tau molecule is "natively unfolded" or "intrinsically disordered" (Schweers et al. 1994; Mukrasch et al. 2009). This means that the polypeptide chain is highly flexible and mobile; there is only a low content of secondary structures (α-helix, β-strand, poly-proline II helix), which are, moreover, transient (Fig. 1, *top*). This corresponds to the observation that Tau can fulfill its physiological function of stabilizing MTs even after harsh treatment (heat, acid), which forms the basis of the biochemical preparation of assembly-competent Tau (Fellous et al. 1977). The loose disordered character of Tau is revealed by its unusually large extent in solution, sweeping out a volume ~27 times that of an equivalent compact molecule (Mylonas et al. 2008). This illustrates that Tau could form transient interactions with a multiplicity of other proteins in the crowded environment of a cell. In spite of the disorder on the local level, Tau

shows a preference for global interactions between domains that can be likened to a "paperclip," where the amino-terminal, carboxy-terminal, and repeat domains approach each other (Jeganathan et al. 2006).

TAU AND MICROTUBULES

Microtubules are protein polymers of the cytoskeleton with diverse cellular tasks, best known for their role in stabilizing cell shape, mitosis, and as tracks for intracellular transport by motor proteins. Microtubules can be prepared from brain extracts by repetitive cycles of assembly and disassembly which can be monitored conveniently by light scattering (Gaskin et al. 1974; Weisenberg 1972). Thereby one copurifies many proteins termed microtubule-associated proteins, including Tau. Tau and other MAPs stabilize microtubules by binding to the MT surface and promote their self-assembly from tubulin subunits, but they are not essential for microtubule structure. Reported dissociation constants range from ∼0.02 to ∼1 µM, depending on isotype, mutations, phosphorylation and other modifications, and method of determination (Cleveland et al. 1977a; Butner and Kirschner 1991; Goode and Feinstein 1994; Gustke et al. 1994; Hong et al. 1998; Makrides et al. 2004; Sillen et al. 2007). Generally, Tau mutations (i.e., those occurring in FTDP17) tend to weaken the binding to microtubules somewhat (Hong et al. 1998; Barghorn et al. 2000); phosphorylation can have small or major inhibitory effects, depending on the type and number of sites (e.g., phosphorylation at sites inside the repeat domain has a larger effect than at sites outside; Biernat et al. 1993). Isoforms with more repeats (e.g., 2N4R) tend to bind more strongly than shorter ones (e.g., 0N3R).

The exact binding site of Tau on MT is not known, despite various attempts by different imaging techniques, and despite the fact that the structure of microtubules is known at high resolution (Fig. 2; Nogales et al. 1999). The uncertainty is largely due to Tau's loose and natively unfolded structure, which obliterates imaging contrast, both for negative staining or cryo-EM and atomic force microscopy (AFM) imaging (Al-Bassam et al. 2002;

Santarella et al. 2004; Schaap et al. 2007). In contrast, other well-folded MT-interacting proteins have been located with high precision, for example, kinesin and doublecortin (Kikkawa et al. 2000; Wendt et al. 2002; Moores et al. 2004; Santarella et al. 2004). The presence of up to four repeats in Tau has led to the idea that Tau repeats and tubulin subunits bind to each other in a commensurate fashion, but this is not supported by other data. For example, Fauquant et al. (2011) recently achieved very tight microtubule binding (K_d ∼ low nanomolar range) for the 117 residue Tau fragment 208–324 (corresponding roughly to domains P2–R3 which stretch across two adjacent αβ-heterodimers of tubulin). This argues that the central part of Tau is aligned along protofilaments, consistent with cryo-electron microscopy data.

In neurons, Tau is strongly substoichiometric compared with tubulin (∼20–40 µM tubulin compared with ∼1 µM Tau or less [Cleveland et al. 1977b; Hiller and Weber 1978]); in vitro binding studies show saturation at Tau:tubulin ratios up to ∼0.5, that is, about one Tau molecule for two tubulin αβ-heterodimers (Gustke et al. 1994; Makrides et al. 2004), and this ratio holds for Tau molecules with different numbers of repeats, consistent with the model

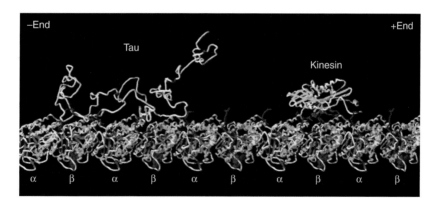

Figure 2. Visualization of Tau and kinesin bound to microtubules. The diagram shows a Tau molecule and a kinesin motor domain bound to a microtubule protofilament (row of αβ-tubulin heterodimers). All molecules are in the same size range (∼350–450 residues), but tubulin and kinesin are compactly folded. Tau is not and therefore occupies a much larger volume, loosely filled with polypeptide chain and highly mobile. Structures modeled after Nogales et al. (1999) (tubulin), Sack et al. (1997) (kinesin), and Hoenger et al. (1998) (docking of kinesin on microtubule). Tau is shown as a random coil; its microtubule-bound conformation is not known. (Figure composed by A. Marx.)

of Knossow and colleagues (Fauquant et al. 2011). The highly acidic carboxy-terminal ~30 residues of tubulin are important for tight binding (Littauer et al. 1986), but they are also natively unfolded and thus structurally invisible. Quick-freeze deep-etching reveals stubs of Tau's projection domain ~18 nm in length, with a low stoichiometry (0.2; Hirokawa et al. 1988). This projection is similar to the length of the repeat domain seen by the glycerol spray technique (Wille et al. 1992), but given that the radius of gyration in solution is only ~6.5 nm, these values probably represent highly extended extremes.

In considering functions of Tau with regard to MTs, it is useful to distinguish direct and indirect interactions. Direct interactions include the binding, stabilization, and promotion of MT assembly that can be modulated by Tau and its phosphorylation (Brandt et al. 2005; Dolan and Johnson 2010). This function requires the MT-binding domain (repeats + flanking domains), but not necessarily the projection domain. A more subtle effect is the protection of microtubule ends against length fluctuations (dynamic instability), that is their ability to shrink and grow in a stochastic manner. Control of the rate of "catastrophe" and "rescue" is important for cellular organization (Hoogenraad and Bradke 2009), and overstabilization by Tau can impair cell viability (Panda et al. 2003; Thies and Mandelkow 2007; this effect is exploited in cancer chemotherapy by using drugs such as taxol; Wilson and Jordan 2004).

Indirect interactions affect other proteins that may or may not interact with MT by themselves, and may require the projection domain of Tau. An example is the spacer function of MAPs, which helps to establish a "clear zone" around microtubules in cells. This spacer function is pronounced for large MAPs (e.g., MAP2), whereas Tau and its cousin MAP2c allow a much closer apposition, suggesting that the long and acidic projection domains of MAP2/MAP4 are responsible for mutual repulsion (Chen et al. 1992; Umeyama et al. 1993). Another indirect function is the inhibition of MT-dependent transport by motor proteins,

which is based on the competition between motors (kinesin, dynein) and MAPs for binding sites on the MT surface (Seitz et al. 2002; Stamer et al. 2002; Dixit et al. 2008). Thirdly, because MTs are distributed throughout cellular space, they provide natural anchoring structures for cell components in general. A classical example is the association of cAMP-dependent kinase (PKA) with the projection domain of MAP2 via the RII-docking subunit (Obar et al. 1990), which is important for phosphorylation of cAMP response element binding protein and neurite outgrowth (Harada et al. 2002). Various other kinases can be found enriched in MAP-microtubule fractions, for example, GSK3β, cdk5, MAP kinase, and others (Mandelkow et al. 1992; Morishima-Kawashima and Kosik 1996). In particular this includes major brain tyrosine kinases (e.g., Fyn, Src, Lck, Abl) that can bind to the PXXP motifs in the proline-rich domain of Tau through their SH3 domain (Fig. 1, *bottom*; Bhaskar et al. 2005; Williamson et al. 2008; Ittner et al. 2010).

STRUCTURE OF TAU FIBERS (PHFs)

Given that Tau is hydrophilic, unstructured, and dynamic, its aggregation into seemingly well-ordered and periodic fibers in AD is counterintuitive. In fact, the solubility of Tau in vitro is ~ millimolar, much higher than its concentration in cells (~ micromolar), which explains in part why it has taken a long time to discover assembly conditions in vitro (Fig. 3; Wille et al. 1992; Crowther et al. 1994; Wilson and Binder 1995). However, two factors contribute to pushing Tau toward aggregation. One is the charge compensation of the basic middle part of Tau by polyanions. In vitro this can be achieved by sulfated glycosaminoglycans (e.g., heparin, heparan sulfate, etc.; Goedert et al. 1996; Perez et al. 1996), which helps to overcome the nucleation barrier. A similar effect can be induced by nucleic acids (Kampers et al. 1996), acidic lipid micelles (e.g., made from arachidonic acid; Wilson and Binder 1997), acidic peptides (Friedhoff et al. 1998) or even carboxylated microbeads (Chirita et al. 2005). In neurons, the inducers of Tau fibrillization are not known,

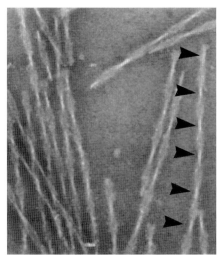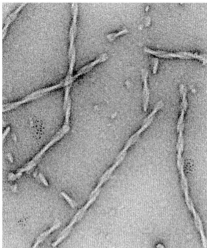

Figure 3. Tau fibers. *Left*: Twisted fibers appearing as "paired helical filaments" isolated from Alzheimer brain tissue, with ∼80 nm periodicity (arrowheads). *Right*: Fibers assembled in vitro from the proaggregant Tau repeat domain (K18ΔK280). Note the similarity of the twisted structures, even though the repeat domain contains only ∼27% of the full-length protein. (Micrographs by E.M. Mandelkow and S. Barghorn.)

but acidic cofactors are likely (intriguingly, Tau can occur in nuclei and near ribosomes, rich in nucleic acids; Papasozomenos and Binder 1987). Of special interest is the case of microtubules that represent an array of acidic proteins, owing to their highly charged carboxy-terminal peptides. Tau binds strongly to the MT surface, but surprisingly does not self-assemble; rather, the MT surface can be overloaded with a coat of Tau molecules in a nonfilamentous form (Ackmann et al. 2000). Since the Tau–Tau interaction site largely overlaps with the Tau–MT interaction site (Mukrasch et al. 2005), it appears that MTs override Tau's capacity for fibrillization, perhaps by stabilizing a nonaggregant conformation. Thus, MTs act effectively as chaperones for Tau to prevent their abnormal aggregation.

The second factor essential for Tau assembly is its propensity for β-structure, encoded in short hexapeptide motifs at the beginning of R2 and R3 (VQIINK and VQIVYK; von Bergen et al. 2000). Disruption of these motifs (e.g., by proline mutations) abrogates Tau's tendency to aggregate, not only in vitro, but also in cell and animal models (Khlistunova et al. 2007; Mocanu et al. 2008; von Bergen et al. 2001). Conversely, strengthening the β-propensity by

mutations (e.g., ΔK280 or P301L) accelerates aggregation in vitro and in animal models. The small size of the β-motifs, embedded in a disordered protein, made it difficult to detect their role, so that the nature of Tau as an "amyloid" protein remained controversial for a long time. However, the β-structure has now been verified by circular dichroism and FTIR (Barghorn et al. 2004), NMR (Mukrasch et al. 2009), electron diffraction (Berriman et al. 2003), X-ray fiber diffraction (Giannetti et al. 2000), and even X-ray crystallography (Sawaya et al. 2007). While the presence of a cross-β structure in the core of PHFs is unambiguous, its arrangement in detail is still unknown. Electron paramagnetic resonance spectroscopy (EPR) studies suggest that the initial ∼20 residues of R2 and R3 are stacked axially in the extended β-structure and in register (Margittai and Langen 2004, 2006). This still leaves various options for the course of the polypeptide chain that are currently being explored by solid-state NMR (A Lange, MPI Göttingen, pers. comm.). These insights will help to define the 3D structure of the core of PHFs, which in turn will allow to design specific inhibitors of aggregation targeting the repeat domain (Pickhardt et al. 2005;

Bulic et al. 2010; Lee et al. 2011). One recent example is the design of a capping peptide blocking the elongation of PHFs (Sievers et al. 2011).

Even if the 3D structure of the repeat domain in the PHF core were known, this would reveal only a minor part (<25%) of the structure of Tau fibers.[2] The remainder, which includes the amino-terminal half and the carboxy-terminal tail, has been remarkably difficult to image by different types of microscopy and has been dubbed the "fuzzy coat" (Crowther and Wischik 1985; Wischik et al. 1988). This coat is still highly mobile even in the aggregated state (Sillen et al. 2005), similar to Tau itself and the projection domain of MT-bound Tau. It can be viewed as a "soft polymer brush" extending from the PHF core, and able to enter multiple interactions with other cellular components (Wegmann et al. 2010).

TAU AND AD

Tau is a major MAP in the brain, but in this regard it is not more or less interesting than other MAPs that have been discovered and classified over the years (MAP1, MAP2, MAP4, etc.; Cassimeris and Spittle 2001; Dehmelt and Halpain 2005). The major interest in Tau stems from its aggregation in AD and other tauopathies. There has been a debate on whether Tau is causal to the disease or just a byproduct of some disease process. For the case of AD the case is still open, and changes in Tau are mostly viewed as a consequence of Aβ pathology (Haass and Selkoe 2007).[3] However, the discovery of mutations in the Tau gene causing frontotemporal dementias has confirmed a causative role of Tau in neurodegeneration (Hutton et al. 1998; Poorkaj et al. 1998; Spillantini et al. 1998), as well as the identification of Tau as one of the risk factors in PSP, PD and others (Hardy and Singleton 2008). Even in the context of AD, the active contribution of Tau was highlighted by animal models, suggesting that Tau is required for the induction of Aβ-induced toxicity (Roberson et al. 2007). In fact, an increased Tau level alone suffices as a risk factor, as demonstrated for the H1c haplotype (Myers et al. 2007). This provides a rationale for the quest for Tau-lowering drugs.

The intense search for disease-related properties of Tau has revealed numerous changes, compared with Tau in nondiseased neurons (Table 2). The problem is to determine which of these changes are causative for disease, whether they are specific, or whether they are simply consequences of an altered state of the cell. We will consider only a few of these mechanisms here. As mentioned above, no mutations in Tau are known that cause bona fide AD. Some changes are common to several tauopathies (e.g., aggregation), others occur not only in disease but also in physiological states. A case in point is phosphorylation: In AD the level is high (eight or more phosphates per Tau molecule, compared with only ~two in normal adult brain; Kopke et al. 1993), but in normal fetal brain it is also high (~four), and likewise it is high in hibernating animals (Hartig et al.

---

[2]A note on "PHF" terminology. The term "paired helical filament" (PHF) was introduced by Kidd (1963) to describe the filaments in AD neurons, long before their composition was known. The term describes the twisting structure with a crossover repeat of ~80 nm and a stain-filled groove running along the center, which appears to divide the fiber into two subfibers ~10 nm wide. Not all fibers have this appearance, some are "straight fibers" (SF), others have variable crossover repeats, but these differences appear to arise from variations in the packing of Tau molecules (Crowther 1991), depending on isoform composition and bound cofactors. There has been an ongoing debate on whether the two subfibers are genuine or merely staining artifacts. An alternative description is that of twisted ribbons, ~22 nm wide and ~10 nm thick (Moreno-Herrero et al. 2004; Pollanen et al. 1997; Wegmann et al. 2010). There is little evidence for the existence of physically separate subfibers; on the contrary, AFM imaging and force application suggest that subunits are stacked axially, not side by side (Wegmann et al. 2010). Thus, the term "Tau fibers" is more appropriate than "PHFs," although the latter is probably too established to fade away.

[3]A note on Tau misfolding. In pathological conditions, Tau is sometimes described as "misfolded," implying that Tau could also be properly folded in normal conditions. However, because Tau is intrinsically disordered, this concept has little explanatory value. In fact, the best folded state of Tau is that in Tau fibers where at least the repeat domain has a well-defined structure, dominated by β-sheet interactions. In this sense, tauopathies are protein aggregation diseases, but not protein misfolding diseases.

Table 2. Changes of Tau protein in tauopathies

Mis-sorting (somatodendritic compartment)
(Hyper-)phosphorylation
Dissociation from microtubules
Aggregation (PHF)
Proteolytic processing
Ubiquitination
Glycation
Glycosylation
Oxidation
Nitration
Acetylation
Amino acid modifications
Altered isoform distribution
Mutations in Tau gene (FTDP17)

2007). Thus hyperphosphorylation is not an absolute indicator of a disease state but rather appears to reflect a state of the cell where the balance of kinases versus phosphatases is tipped in favor of phosphorylation; or conversely a low level of phosphorylation may simply reflect the activity of phosphatases (mainly PP2a) during preparation (Matsuo et al. 1994). The ready response of Tau to such a change is not surprising, considering its disordered structure and numerous potential phosphorylation sites. Other cellular targets should sense the change in biochemical potential in a similar fashion, and in fact this has been demonstrated, for example, for neurofilaments (Ishihara et al. 2001). An overall shift of phosphorylation potential can occur, for example, by a temperature drop during anesthesia or experimental diabetes, which reduces the activity of PP2a and thus mimics an Alzheimer-like phosphorylation state on Tau, reminiscent of the effects of aging (Planel et al. 2007a; Planel et al. 2007b; Veeranna et al. 2009). Conversely, heat stress and oxidative stress activate PP2a and thus generate a low state of Tau phoshorylation, which protects against DNA damage (Davis et al. 1997; Sultan et al. 2011). Therefore, efforts are underway to develop treatments for AD by reducing Tau phosphorylation, either by inhibiting key kinases (e.g., Ahn et al. 2005; Seabrook et al. 2007) or by activating phosphatases such as PP2a (Tanimukai et al. 2005).

The majority of potential P-sites on Tau are found to be phosphorylatable (>45; Hanger et al. 2007), and multiple kinases are able to phosphorylate Tau. A subset of sites have gained prominence because they are recognized by antibodies raised against AD Tau in a phosphorylation-dependent manner and are thus useful as diagnostic reagents. They include PHF1 (pS396 + pS404; Greenberg and Davies 1990), several of the AT series of antibodies (Biernat et al. 1992; Goedert et al. 1994), for example, AT8 (pS202 + pT205), AT180 (pT231 + pS235), AT270 (pT181) and AT100 (pT212 + pS214), and Sternberger monoclonal antibodies of the SMI series (e.g., SMI31, 33, 34; Lichtenberg-Kraag et al. 1992; for a complete list see www.alzforum.org). Most of these sites include SP or TP motifs and are therefore targets of proline-directed kinases (e.g., GSK3β, cdc2, cdk5, MAPK, JNK). Other nonproline directed sites include the KXGS motifs in the repeats whose phosphorylation by MARK or related kinases of the AMPK family (Drewes et al. 1997) strongly decreases the Tau–MT affinity, as recognized by antibody 12E8 (Seubert et al. 1995).

A primary preoccupation of "Tauists" over the years has been the search for functional consequences of the bewildering complexities of phosphorylation. This search has taken two main directions, for consequences regarding microtubule binding and for those affecting Tau aggregation. Owing to differences in experimental procedures and detection methods, it is difficult to summarize the body of data, but there appears to be a consensus that phosphorylation tends to weaken the Tau–microtubule affinity. Some sites are efficient in detaching Tau from MT, notably S262 in R1, phosphorylated by MARK and related kinases (Mandelkow et al. 2004), or S214 in the proline-rich domain, phosphorylated by PKA (Brandt et al. 1994; Illenberger et al. 1998). By contrast, proline-directed sites (SP or TP motifs) are prominently phosphorylated by the proline-directed kinases mentioned above, and although single sites have only a small effect, a combination of them can also considerably weaken the interactions with microtubules

(Hernandez and Avila 2007; Sergeant et al. 2008; Stoothoff and Johnson 2005). For the disease process, the important implication is that Tau is protected against aggregation while bound to MT, but not when it is detached by phosphorylation.

For Tau aggregation the consequences of phosphorylation are even less clear. The fact that Tau phosphorylation precedes aggregation in AD has led to the assumption that phosphorylation drives Tau into aggregation, and certain highly phosphorylated states of Tau may be prone to aggregation (Iqbal et al. 2008). However, in vitro this cannot be confirmed in a general way; on the contrary, phosphorylation at certain sites (e.g., KXGS motifs) protects against aggregation (Schneider et al. 1999). By comparison, polyanionic cofactors are far superior to phosphorylation in stimulating Tau aggregation. In our view it is therefore questionable whether strategies to reduce phosphorylation (e.g., kinase inhibitors) will be effective in preventing Tau aggregation (even though they may be beneficial for other reasons).

Another major modification of Tau in AD is proteolytic cleavage. Tau contains many potential cleavage sites accessible to multiple proteases, yielding breakdown products that could be toxic in various ways. For example, cleavage of the tails by caspases (behind D421 or behind D13; Gamblin et al. 2003; Horowitz et al. 2004; Rissman et al. 2004) perturbs the paperclip folding of Tau (Jeganathan et al. 2006) and makes it more vulnerable to aggregation. Tau can be cleaved by calpain at a number of sites (Canu and Calissano 2003; Park and Ferreira 2005). This generates a metastable fragment A125–R230 that spans several PXXP motifs and therefore has the potential of scavenging SH3-containing proteins including tyrosine kinases (Garg et al. 2011). This Tau fragment of MW = 10.7 kDa or M_r = ∼17 kDa was thought to mediate Aβ toxicity (Park and Ferreira 2005) in neurons, but this remains a matter of debate. A third type of cleavage occurs by PSA (puromycin-sensitive aminopeptidase), discovered by a genomic screen for modifiers of tauopathy in flies (Karsten et al. 2006). This enzyme cleaves substrates into small peptides

and may therefore contribute to the degradation of Tau, independently of the proteasome and/or autophagy (see below). Finally, an inducible cell model of Tau aggregation revealed a complex cleavage pattern whereby a cytosolic protease with thrombin-like characteristics cooperates with a lysosomal protease (cathepsin L) to generate a fragment S258–I360 with a high propensity for aggregation, sufficient to nucleate and coaggregate with endogenous Tau (Wang et al. 2009).

We will mention other biochemical modifications only in passing: Oxidation (which is prominent in aging neurons) affects in the first instance the two cysteines C291 (in R2) and C322 (in R3). They can be cross-linked to form dimers, which greatly enhances the rate of aggregation or as an intra-dimer disulfide bridge, which locks the molecule in a folded conformation (Schweers et al. 1995). Ubiquitination occurs at several lysines (K254, 257, 311, 317, perhaps also 280, 294, 343, 353) that are all in the repeat domain (Morishima-Kawashima et al. 1993). It participates in the protein triage process whereby the chaperone system decides whether to keep the protein for refolding or to send it to the proteasome for degradation (Petrucelli et al. 2004; Shimura et al. 2004b).

O-GlcNac glycosylation is found on many residues, especially in S/T-P motifs, as an alternative for phosphorylation. The reaction protects proteins against aberrant phosphorylation but becomes defective in AD, thus allowing an increase in phosphorylation (Li et al. 2006). Nitration of tyrosine residues occurs via peroxynitrate during oxidative damage (Reynolds et al. 2007). It changes Tau's conformation and reduces MT binding, but also reduces aggregation. Four of the five Tyr residues can be nitrated (Y18, 29, 197, 394); remarkably, the only tyrosine in the repeat domain (Y310) is not affected, possibly because of a protective conformation within R3. Acetylation of lysines affects predominantly K280, impairs MT binding of Tau, promotes aggregation and potentially interferes with ubiquitination and thus degradation of Tau (Cohen et al. 2011; Min et al. 2010). Finally, because Tau and its aggregates are long-lived, they are subject to nonenzymatic modifications. One is glycation by AGEs (advanced glycation end products); this decreases MT binding, promotes aggregation, activates RAGE receptors and thus causes oxidative damage (Ledesma et al. 1994). Other time-dependent changes in Tau include deamidation, isomerization, cross-linking and nonenzymatic cleavage around Asp residues; this is the cause of the "high MW smear" that is typical of Alzheimer Tau preparations run on SDS gels (Watanabe et al. 2004).

The most obvious change of Tau in AD is its aggregation, noticed already by Alois Alzheimer more than 100 years ago. The principles of aggregation are now reasonably well understood from in vitro studies (see above), but it has been difficult to reproduce this in cell and animal models. This is not surprising given the slow growth of aggregates in aging human brains compared with the short lifetimes of cell cultures or transgenic mice. A breakthrough came with the introduction of Tau mutants discovered in FTDP17 (Lewis et al. 2000), because their aggregation was sufficiently fast to be observed in mice. Mouse models of AD and tauopathies have been reviewed extensively in the literature (Gotz and Ittner 2008; Morrissette et al. 2009). Here we focus on some lessons learned from inducible cell and mouse models: An inducible N2a cell model, expressing the Tau repeat domain in a "proaggregant" form (construct K18−ΔK280) that aggregates rapidly because of its high propensity for β structure, develops Tau fibers within 3 days after switching the Tau gene expression on. This is possible, despite the short time window, because endogenous proteases cleave out an even more proaggregant fragment that nucleates Tau fibers and coassembles intact Tau. When switching expression off, aggregates disappear within 4 days. showing that the cell retains the ability to recover. Comparison with an antiaggregant form of the Tau repeat domain (which does not form β structure because of proline mutations in the hexapeptide motifs) reveals that toxicity leading to cell death occurs only with β-structure and aggregation. Toxicity and aggregation can both be prevented by aggregation inhibitors that break

β structure (von Bergen et al. 2001; Khlistunova et al. 2007).

These results can be transferred, cum grano salis, to inducible transgenic mice expressing the same construct of Tau (Mocanu et al. 2008). Only proaggregant Tau_{RD} causes neurofibrillary tangles; these mice have cognitive deficits, correlating with loss of synapses and neurons and impaired LTP. Importantly, cognitive deficits and loss of synapses can be rescued by switching off the expression of the toxic protein (Fig. 5). Nevertheless, aggregates persist in the brain, but change their composition from mixed exogenous + endogenous Tau to endogenous mouse Tau only. The explanation is that proaggregant Tau_{RD} nucleates aggregation, but once the nucleation barrier has been overcome, endogenous Tau coaggregates, and these aggregates persist beyond the switch-off of exogenous Tau because endogenous Tau is still present (Sydow et al. 2011). This observation highlights the dynamic nature of Tau fibers and suggests the possibility of intervention by aggregation inhibitor compounds. Qualitatively similar results were obtained with another inducible mouse expressing Tau with the proaggregant mutation P301L (Santacruz et al. 2005). Here, too, toxicity and memory deficits were related to aggregation, and recovery of memory occurred after switch-off, yet aggregates tended to persist (in this case, the antiaggregant version of the protein was not tested). These results mean that the toxic agent is the continued expression of aggregation-prone Tau. Hyperphosphorylation is a consequence of this, but not the cause. A possible explanation is that exposure of β-strands in cells, ready to interact, represents a toxic burden to the cell and overexerts the cell's chaperone-based defense system, which is designed to "detoxify" such exposed β-strands.

DISTRIBUTION OF TAU

The bulk of Tau is located in the brain, specifically in neurons. It is ubiquitous in immature neurons but becomes axonal during maturation, accompanied by a shift toward higher-molecular-weight isoforms and reduced phosphorylation (Drubin and Kirschner 1986; Kosik et al. 1989). Even after maturation, low levels of Tau are present in other neuronal compartments, for example, the nucleus (Loomis et al. 1990; Sultan et al. 2011) and dendrites (Papasozomenos and Binder 1987), and in other brain cells, notably oligodendrocytes (Goldbaum et al. 2003; LoPresti et al. 1995). Moreover, Tau mRNA can be detected in many cell types (Gu et al. 1996), even in muscle fibers where Tau forms aggregates in inclusion body myositis (Askanas and Engel 2008).

The pathway of neuronal sorting is still incompletely understood; several mechanisms appear to contribute, for example, selective protein transport into axons and selective degradation in dendrites (Hirokawa et al. 1996; Nakata and Hirokawa 2003), selective axonal transport of Tau mRNA (Aronov et al. 2002), and selective up-regulation of translation in axons (Morita and Sobue 2009). Transport of Tau into axons occurs as part of the slow axonal transport component SCa (Mercken et al. 1995), probably as part of a (transient) complex with tubulin

oligomers driven by kinesin, which provides directional bias and yet allows a high rate of diffusion (Baas and Buster 2004; Konzack et al. 2007).

The issue of axonal sorting is important because missorting of Tau into the somatodendritic compartment is recognized as one of the earliest signs of neurodegeneration in AD and in mouse models (Braak et al. 1994; Coleman and Yao 2003). Entry of Tau into dendrites (e.g., triggered by Aβ, glutamate, oxidative stress, etc.) causes a decay of dendritic spines mediated by Ca^{2+} influx through NMDA receptors and thus a decay of neuronal communication (Fig. 4; Mattson 2004; Shankar et al. 2007; Zempel et al. 2010).

Tau is not merely transported as a cargo but can actively interfere with microtubule-dependent traffic because it can compete with motors for binding to microtubules and thereby slow down both anterograde and retrograde transport by kinesin or dynein motors (Stamer et al. 2002; Dixit et al. 2008). Alternatively, Tau could inactivate selected motor complexes, by

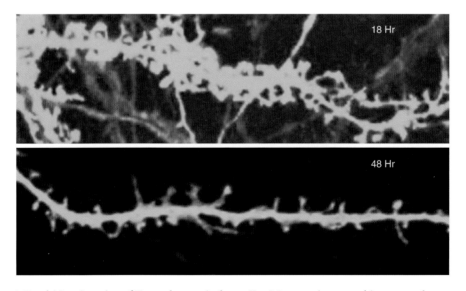

Figure 4. Dendritic missorting of Tau and synaptic decay. *Top*: Mature primary rat hippocampal neuron at 21 DIV with numerous dendritic spines, 18 h after transfection with full-length Tau (2N4R, tagged with CFP, blue). Note that Tau has invaded dendritic shafts and spines. *Bottom*: At 48 h after transfection most spines have shrunk or disappeared. (Adapted from Thies and Mandelkow 2007; reprinted, with permission, from the author.)

direct binding to kinesin (Utton et al. 2005), by sequestering the kinesin-associated protein JIP1 (in case of the K369I mutation; Ittner et al. 2009), or by activating phosphatase PP1 and kinase GSK3β through Tau's amino-terminal 18-residues, leading to the release of cargo vesicles from kinesin light chains (Kanaan et al. 2011). Similarly, the amino-terminal domain of Tau binds to the p150 subunit of dynactin and thereby supports transport by dynein, which can be disrupted by the R5L mutation in Tau (Magnani et al. 2007). These modes of Tau-transport interference could contribute to the movement deficits observed in the first generation of Tau-transgenic mice with pan-neuronal expression of Tau (Lee et al. 2005; Terwel et al. 2002).

Tau is normally a cytosolic protein, but its occurrence outside cells has become important for studying and diagnosing the AD disease process. One reason is that Tau is elevated in the cerebrospinal fluid (CSF) at an early stage of AD and therefore serves as a biomarker (Hampel et al. 2010; Blennow et al. 2011). The origin of CSF-Tau is not clear, but dying and disintegrating neurons could contribute to it. In fact, recent microdialysis experiments suggest that Tau is even higher in the interstitial fluid (Yamada et al. 2011). Another recent development is derived from the earlier observation that Tau pathology spreads in the brain in a well-defined manner, so that its distribution can be correlated with the clinical stages of the disease (Braak stages; Braak and Braak 1991). One hypothesis is that affected neurons release pathological Tau, which is taken up by neighboring cells and thus spreads the pathology in a prion-like fashion (Clavaguera et al. 2009; Frost et al. 2009). Several mechanisms can be envisaged for this release and re-uptake (e.g., via exosomes; Aguzzi and Rajendran 2009). Alternatively, affected neurons could release factors (e.g., cytokines) that then challenge other neurons, either directly or via intermediate cells; an example is the cytosolic accumulation of Tau in neurons encountering activated microglia or exposed to tumor necrosis factor α (Gorlovoy et al. 2009).

TAU BINDING PARTNERS

Since Tau is highly flexible and carries many charges it has the capacity to interact with many partners in the crowded cytosol. This is one of the characteristic features of intrinsically disordered proteins (Dunker et al. 2008). Most of these interactions will be short-lived and difficult to detect. Table 3 presents selected Tau interacting proteins reported in the literature. Various methods to detect these have been employed so that the results are not strictly comparable (e.g., antibody pulldown, FRET,

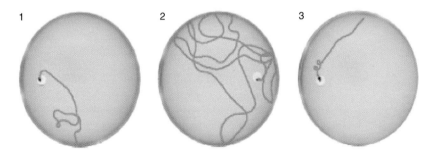

Figure 5. Loss and recovery of memory in regulatable Tau-transgenic mice. The mice express the proaggregant Tau repeat domain (K18ΔK280). Expression is switched OFF in the presence of doxycyclin, and ON without doxycyclin in the drinking water (tet-off system; Gossen and Bujard 2002), and tested in the Morris Water Maze. *Left*: Control mouse learns position of hidden platform quickly, short length of swimming path. *Center*: Mouse after switching the Tau repeat domain ON for 12 months has severe learning deficits, and requires a long time and long path length to find the platform. *Right*: Same mouse as before, after switching Tau expression OFF again for 4 weeks. The memory has returned to control levels (details in Sydow et al. 2011).

Table 3. Binding partners of Tau protein

Binding partner	Binding region of Tau	Remarks	References
Microtubules	Repeat domain + flanking regions		Butner and Kirschner (1991); Gustke et al. (1994)
Actin filaments		MAPs cross-link MT and actin fil.; Tau on actin fil. in growth cone; Tau in stress-induced actin–cofilin rods	Fulga et al. (2007); Griffith and Pollard (1978); Roger et al. (2004); Whiteman et al. (2009)
Neurofilaments		MAPS cross-linking MT-neurofilaments	Aamodt and Williams (1984)
Ribosomes		Colocalization with polysomes	Papasozomenos and Binder (1987)
GSK3b	Amino-terminal; Exon 1–6	In complex with presenilin	Sun et al. (2002); Takashima et al. (1998)
Fyn	Proline-rich domain	Tau binds to SH3 domain, truncated Tau causes accumulation of fyn in cell body	Belkadi and LoPresti (2008); Ittner et al. (2010); Klein et al. (2002); Lee et al. (1998); Reynolds et al. (2008)
Src	Proline-rich domain		Lee et al. (1998); Reynolds et al. (2008)
Lck	Proline-rich domain		Lee et al. (1998); Reynolds et al. (2008)
Pi3K	Proline-rich domain		Reynolds et al. (2008)
JIP1		Competes with kinesin in axonal transport	Ittner et al. (2009)
PP-2a	Repeat domain + AA 221–242	Facilitated binding with Pin1	Lu et al. (1999); Sontag et al. (1999)
Hsp70/Hsc70	Repeat domain		Sarkar et al. (2008); Wang et al. (2009)
Hsp90	VQIVYK motif involved		Dickey et al. (2007); Tortosa et al. (2009)
Hsp27		PHF Tau	Shimura et al. (2004a)
CHIP			Dickey et al. (2007); Shimura et al. (2004b)
BAG-1		Tau-BAG-1 association is Hsc70-dependent	Elliott et al. (2007)
Ubiquitin	Repeat domain	Ubiquitination of PHF Tau	Morishima-Kawashima et al. (1993)
Dynactin	Amino-terminal, Exon1 + 4	Disrupted by R5L mutation	Magnani et al. (2007)
Kinesin LC	Proline-rich domain	Phosphorylation-dependent	Utton et al. (2005)
Pin1	Proline-rich domain, especially pT231– P232 site, also pT212–P213 site		Lu et al. (1999); Smet et al. (2004)
FKBP52		Through heat shock proteins (HSP)	Chambraud et al. (2010)

Continued

Cite this article as *Cold Spring Harb Perspect Med* doi: 10.1101/cshperspect.a006247

Table 3. *Continued*

Binding partner	Binding region of Tau	Remarks	References
FKBP51		Hsp90 cochaperone	Jinwal et al. (2010)
Cdc37		Hsp90 cochaperone (interacts with Tau)	Jinwal et al. (2011)
Calmodulin	Repeat domain, especially R3, AA 318–335	Ca^{2+} dependent	Padilla et al. (1990); Lee and Wolff (1984); Baudier and Cole (1988)
S100b		Ca^{2+}, Zn^{2+}-dependent	Baudier and Cole (1988); Baudier et al. (1987)
α-Synuclein	Repeat domain	Induces fibrillization of Tau	Giasson et al. (2003); Jensen et al. (1999)
14-3-3	Repeat domain, Proline-rich domain, S214, S324, S356	Forms ternary complex with SGK1 and Tau	Chun et al. (2004); Hashiguchi et al. (2000); Sluchanko et al. (2009)
Presenilin	MTBR	Through GSK3	Takashima et al. (1998)
ApoE	MTBR		Strittmatter et al. (1994)
Annexin A2	Involving R406	Linking Tau to plasma membrane	Gauthier-Kemper et al. (2011)
Lipid bilayers	Repeat domain	Anionic lipid vesicles induce aggregation	Chirita et al. (2003); Elbaum-Garfinkle et al. (2010); Wilson and Binder (1997)
Membrane-associated proteins	Amino-terminal projection domain	Interaction with annexin A2, disrupted by R406W mutation. Interaction with Fyn at lipid rafts	Brandt et al. (1995); Gauthier-Kemper et al. (2011); Williamson et al. (2008)
DNA		Tau protects DNA against heat and oxidative stress	Sultan et al. (2011)
mRNA, tRNA, rRNA	Repeat domain	RNAs induce aggregation of Tau Tau on ribosomes, nucleolus	Kampers et al. (1996) Loomis et al. (1990)

colocalization by microscopy, coassembly, yeast 2-hybrid, etc.).

By far the most predominant interaction of Tau is that with microtubules, so that the microtubule network can effectively be imaged by fluorescently labeled Tau, and Tau becomes randomized when MTs break down (curiously, databases of protein–protein interactions tend to ignore this major interaction partner of Tau). However, even with MTs the interaction is short-lived (dwell time ∼4s; Konzack et al. 2007; Samsonov et al. 2004), which explains why Tau can diffuse quite rapidly (diffusion constant $D = \sim 3 \ \mu m^2/s$). This interaction is based on the repeats + flanking domains, but can be interrupted by phosphorylation at key sites (e.g., KXGS motifs in repeats), which leads to the diffuse distribution of Tau in the cytosol and probably contributes to the somatodendritic missorting in degenerating neurons (Zempel et al. 2010). Interactions of Tau with other cytoskeletal elements have been reported as well, notably intermediate filaments (Aamodt and Williams 1984) and microfilaments (F-actin; Griffith and Pollard 1978; Roger et al. 2004). For example, Tau detached from MT by phosphorylation at the KXGS motifs tends to colocalize with actin filaments in growth cones (Biernat et al. 2002; Fulga et al. 2007) or in actin–cofilin rods (Whiteman et al. 2009). These non-MT interactions need not be direct, but could be mediated by other cytoskeleton-associated proteins, consistent with genetic evidence that links modifiers of Tau pathology to the actin network (SUT-1; Kraemer and Schellenberg 2007).

Binding sites of Tau have been reported for several kinases and phosphatases (Reynolds et al. 2008; Sontag et al. 1999). The binding sites lie in or near the MT-binding domain (Fig. 1). Here it is important to distinguish between short-lived interactions that lead to phosphorylation and the longer-lived interactions that characterize the complexes. Unlike MAP2, which has a recognition site for the RII subunit of PKA, Tau does not have a well-characterized binding site for kinase-regulatory proteins. The best-defined kinase interaction sites are the PXXP motifs in the proline-rich domain that can bind to SH3-containing proteins including tyrosine kinases Fyn, Src, or Lck (Reynolds et al. 2008; Williamson et al. 2008). Thus, overexpression of Tau fragments lacking the repeat domain, which stay in the cell body because they cannot be sorted into the axon, also leads to a local accumulation of Fyn (Ittner et al. 2010), and presumably other SH3-domain proteins. A role for Tau–Fyn interactions has been postulated for oligodendrocytes where the complex is transported into cell processes in a MT-dependent manner and is required for myelination (Belkadi and LoPresti 2008; Klein et al. 2002). In neurons, the Tau–Fyn complex becomes enriched in lipid rafts upon exposure to Aβ (Williamson et al. 2008). An analogous cotransport of Tau with Fyn has recently been postulated for neuronal dendrites and spines, enabling Fyn to phosphorylate NMDA receptors and to mediate Aβ-induced excitotoxicity. This way Tau might play a role in the regulation of neuronal network activity (Ittner et al. 2010; Morris et al. 2011).

A number of studies have dealt with the interactions of Tau with the chaperone system. Proteins such as hsp70 and their binding partners (e.g., CHIP) are thought to control the level of soluble Tau and thus help to prevent aggregation in a phosphorylation-dependent manner (Shimura et al. 2004a,b; Dickey et al.

2007; Petrucelli et al. 2004). The binding site has been mapped to the motif VQIVYK, the same as the site responsible for β-structure and aggregation (Sarkar et al. 2008). Since chaperones bind to short peptides with hydrophobic character, this finding suggests that the cell protects itself against aggregation by two types of "chaperones"—microtubules for the bound state, and hsp70 for the unbound state. Independently of this, there is a debate on whether Tau is degraded via the proteasome or the autophagy pathway, which may depend on cell type or phosphorylation state. However, it is noteworthy that the repeat domain possesses two motifs of the consensus type KVERQ, which interact with hsc70 for chaperone-mediated autophagy (Wang et al. 2009). Other interactors of Tau are linked to chaperone components, for example the prolyl isomerase Pin-1 (Liou et al. 2003), FKBP51, FKBP52 (Chambraud et al. 2010; Jinwal et al. 2010). Pin-1 isomerizes the motifs pT212-P and pS231-P in the proline-rich domain from *cis* to *trans* and thus allows the dephosphorylation by PP-2a and recovery of microtubule binding (Smet et al. 2004).

Among the nonprotein interaction partners of Tau, the interactions with the plasma membrane and with nuclear components have been intriguing over the years. The emerging picture is that a small fraction of cellular Tau binds to the membrane through membrane-associated proteins, for example, annexins or proteins of lipid rafts (Williamson et al. 2008; Gauthier-Kemper et al. 2011). Independently of that, Tau can also interact with anionic lipid bilayers and micelles, at least in vitro (Chirita et al. 2003; Elbaum-Garfinkle et al. 2010). The significance in a cellular context is not clear at present, but micelles of arachidonic acid have been suggested as nucleators of Tau aggregation (Wilson and Binder 1997). Likewise, the interaction with nucleic acids was suggested from the observation of nuclear Tau (Loomis et al. 1990); RNAs became interesting as potential nucleators of Tau aggregation (Kampers et al. 1996), but insights into functions came recently with the discovery that Tau can protect DNA against heat and oxidative damage (Sultan et al. 2011).

Given Tau's versatile structure, one can expect that the list of interactors will surely grow; for further details we refer to Table 3. The interaction pathways will hopefully reveal novel insights into approaches that suppress the toxic insults of Tau in the human brain.

ACKNOWLEDGMENTS

We are grateful to Alexander Marx for help with the compilation of material and stimulating discussions.

REFERENCES

*Reference is also in this collection.

Aamodt EJ, Williams RC Jr. 1984. Microtubule-associated proteins connect microtubules and neurofilaments in vitro. *Biochemistry* **23:** 6023–6031.

Ackmann M, Wiech H, Mandelkow E. 2000. Nonsaturable binding indicates clustering of tau on the microtubule surface in a paired helical filament-like conformation. *J Biol Chem* **275:** 30335–30343.

Aguzzi A, Rajendran L. 2009. The transcellular spread of cytosolic amyloids, prions, and prionoids. *Neuron* **64:** 783–790.

Ahn JS, Radhakrishnan ML, Mapelli M, Choi S, Tidor B, Cuny GD, Musacchio A, Yeh LA, Kosik KS. 2005. Defining Cdk5 ligand chemical space with small molecule inhibitors of tau phosphorylation. *Chem Biol* **12:** 811–823.

Al-Bassam J, Ozer RS, Safer D, Halpain S, Milligan RA. 2002. MAP2 and tau bind longitudinally along the outer ridges of microtubule protofilaments. *J Cell Biol* **157:** 1187–1196.

Andreadis A. 2006. Misregulation of tau alternative splicing in neurodegeneration and dementia. *Prog Mol Subcell Biol* **44:** 89–107.

Aronov S, Aranda G, Behar L, Ginzburg I. 2002. Visualization of translated tau protein in the axons of neuronal P19 cells and characterization of tau RNP granules. *J Cell Sci* **115:** 3817–3827.

Askanas V, Engel WK. 2008. Inclusion-body myositis: Muscle-fiber molecular pathology and possible pathogenic significance of its similarity to Alzheimer's and Parkinson's disease brains. *Acta Neuropathol* **116:** 583–595.

Baas PW, Buster DW. 2004. Slow axonal transport and the genesis of neuronal morphology. *J Neurobiol* **58:** 3–17.

Ballatore C, Lee VM, Trojanowski JQ. 2007. Tau-mediated neurodegeneration in Alzheimer's disease and related disorders. *Nat Rev Neurosci* **8:** 663–672.

Barghorn S, Zheng-Fischhofer Q, Ackmann M, Biernat J, von Bergen M, Mandelkow EM, Mandelkow E. 2000. Structure, microtubule interactions, and paired helical filament aggregation by tau mutants of frontotemporal dementias. *Biochemistry* **39:** 11714–11721.

Barghorn S, Davies P, Mandelkow E. 2004. Tau paired helical filaments from Alzheimer's disease brain and assembled in vitro are based on β-structure in the core domain. *Biochemistry* **43:** 1694–1703.

Baudier J, Cole RD. 1988. Interactions between the microtubule-associated tau proteins and S100b regulate tau phosphorylation by the Ca^{2+}/calmodulin-dependent protein kinase II. *J Biol Chem* **263:** 5876–5883.

Baudier J, Mochly-Rosen D, Newton A, Lee SH, Koshland DE Jr, Cole RD. 1987. Comparison of S100b protein with calmodulin: Interactions with melittin and microtubule-associated tau proteins and inhibition of phosphorylation of tau proteins by protein kinase C. *Biochemistry* **26:** 2886–2893.

Belkadi A, LoPresti P. 2008. Truncated Tau with the Fyn-binding domain and without the microtubule-binding domain hinders the myelinating capacity of an oligodendrocyte cell line. *J Neurochem* **107:** 351–360.

Berriman J, Serpell LC, Oberg KA, Fink AL, Goedert M, Crowther RA. 2003. Tau filaments from human brain and from in vitro assembly of recombinant protein show cross-β structure. *Proc Natl Acad Sci* **100:** 9034–9038.

Bhaskar K, Yen SH, Lee G. 2005. Disease-related modifications in tau affect the interaction between Fyn and Tau. *J Biol Chem* **280:** 35119–35125.

Biernat J, Mandelkow EM, Schroter C, Lichtenberg-Kraag B, Steiner B, Berling B, Meyer H, Mercken M, Vandermeeren A, Goedert M, et al. 1992. The switch of tau protein to an Alzheimer-like state includes the phosphorylation of two serine-proline motifs upstream of the microtubule binding region. *EMBO J* **11:** 1593–1597.

Biernat J, Gustke N, Drewes G, Mandelkow EM, Mandelkow E. 1993. Phosphorylation of Ser262 strongly reduces binding of tau to microtubules: Distinction between PHF-like immunoreactivity and microtubule binding. *Neuron* **11:** 153–163.

Biernat J, Wu YZ, Timm T, Zheng-Fischhofer Q, Mandelkow E, Meijer L, Mandelkow EM. 2002. Protein kinase MARK/PAR-1 is required for neurite outgrowth and establishment of neuronal polarity. *Mol Biol Cell* **13:** 4013–4028.

Binder LI, Frankfurter A, Rebhun LI. 1985. The distribution of tau in the mammalian central nervous system. *J Cell Biol* **101:** 1371–1378.

* Blennow K, Zetterberg H, Fagan AM. 2011. Fluid biomarkers in Alzheimer disease. *Cold Spring Harb Perspect Med* doi: 10.1101/cshperspect.a006221.

Braak H, Braak E. 1991. Neuropathological stageing of Alzheimer-related changes. *Acta Neuropathol* **82:** 239–259.

Braak E, Braak H, Mandelkow EM. 1994. A sequence of cytoskeleton changes related to the formation of neurofibrillary tangles and neuropil threads. *Acta Neuropathol* **87:** 554–567.

Brandt R, Lee G, Teplow DB, Shalloway D, Abdel-Ghany M. 1994. Differential effect of phosphorylation and substrate modulation on tau's ability to promote microtubule growth and nucleation. *J Biol Chem* **269:** 11776–11782.

Brandt R, Leger J, Lee G. 1995. Interaction of tau with the neural plasma membrane mediated by tau's amino-terminal projection domain. *J Cell Biol* **131:** 1327–1340.

Brandt R, Hundelt M, Shahani N. 2005. Tau alteration and neuronal degeneration in tauopathies: Mechanisms and models. *Biochim Biophys Acta* **1739:** 331–354.

Brion JP, Couck AM, Passareiro E, Flament-Durand J. 1985. Neurofibrillary tangles of Alzheimer's disease: An immunohistochemical study. *J Submicrosc Cytol* **17:** 89–96.

Bulic B, Pickhardt M, Mandelkow EM, Mandelkow E. 2010. Tau protein and tau aggregation inhibitors. *Neuropharmacology* **59:** 276–289.

Butner KA, Kirschner MW. 1991. Tau protein binds to microtubules through a flexible array of distributed weak sites. *J Cell Biol* **115:** 717–730.

Canu N, Calissano P. 2003. In vitro cultured neurons for molecular studies correlating apoptosis with events related to Alzheimer disease. *Cerebellum* **2:** 270–278.

Cassimeris L, Spittle C. 2001. Regulation of microtubule-associated proteins. *Int Rev Cytol* **210:** 163–226.

Chambraud B, Sardin E, Giustiniani J, Dounane O, Schumacher M, Goedert M, Baulieu EE. 2010. A role for FKBP52 in Tau protein function. *Proc Natl Acad Sci* **107:** 2658–2663.

Chen J, Kanai Y, Cowan NJ, Hirokawa N. 1992. Projection domains of MAP2 and tau determine spacings between microtubules in dendrites and axons. *Nature* **360:** 674–677.

Chirita CN, Necula M, Kuret J. 2003. Anionic micelles and vesicles induce tau fibrillization in vitro. *J Biol Chem* **278:** 25644–25650.

Chirita CN, Congdon EE, Yin H, Kuret J. 2005. Triggers of full-length tau aggregation: A role for partially folded intermediates. *Biochemistry* **44:** 5862–5872.

Chun J, Kwon T, Lee EJ, Kim CH, Han YS, Hong SK, Hyun S, Kang SS. 2004. 14–3–3 Protein mediates phosphorylation of microtubule-associated protein tau by serum- and glucocorticoid-induced protein kinase 1. *Mol Cells* **18:** 360–368.

Clavaguera F, Bolmont T, Crowther RA, Abramowski D, Frank S, Probst A, Fraser G, Stalder AK, Beibel M, Staufenbiel M, et al. 2009. Transmission and spreading of tauopathy in transgenic mouse brain. *Nat Cell Biol* **11:** 909–913.

Cleveland DW, Hwo SY, Kirschner MW. 1977a. Physical and chemical properties of purified tau factor and the role of tau in microtubule assembly. *J Mol Biol* **116:** 227–247.

Cleveland DW, Hwo SY, Kirschner MW. 1977b. Purification of tau, a microtubule-associated protein that induces assembly of microtubules from purified tubulin. *J Mol Biol* **116:** 207–225.

Cohen TJ, Guo JL, Hurtado DE, Kwong LK, Mills IP, Trojanowski JQ, Lee VM. 2011. The acetylation of tau inhibits its function and promotes pathological tau aggregation. *Nat Commun* **2:** 252.

Coleman PD, Yao PJ. 2003. Synaptic slaughter in Alzheimer's disease. *Neurobiol Aging* **24:** 1023–1027.

Couchie D, Mavilia C, Georgieff IS, Liem RK, Shelanski ML, Nunez J. 1992. Primary structure of high molecular weight tau present in the peripheral nervous system. *Proc Natl Acad Sci* **89:** 4378–4381.

Crowther RA. 1991. Straight and paired helical filaments in Alzheimer disease have a common structural unit. *Proc Natl Acad Sci* **88:** 2288–2292.

Crowther RA, Wischik CM. 1985. Image reconstruction of the Alzheimer paired helical filament. *EMBO J* **4:** 3661–3665.

Crowther RA, Olesen OF, Smith MJ, Jakes R, Goedert M. 1994. Assembly of Alzheimer-like filaments from full-length tau protein. *FEBS Lett* **337:** 135–138.

Davis DR, Anderton BH, Brion JP, Reynolds CH, Hanger DP. 1997. Oxidative stress induces dephosphorylation of tau in rat brain primary neuronal cultures. *J Neurochem* **68:** 1590–1597.

Dehmelt L, Halpain S. 2005. The MAP2/Tau family of microtubule-associated proteins. *Genome Biol* **6:** 204.

Dickey CA, Kamal A, Lundgren K, Klosak N, Bailey RM, Dunmore J, Ash P, Shoraka S, Zlatkovic J, Eckman CB, et al. 2007. The high-affinity HSP90–CHIP complex recognizes and selectively degrades phosphorylated tau client proteins. *J Clin Invest* **117:** 648–658.

Dixit R, Ross JL, Goldman YE, Holzbaur EL. 2008. Differential regulation of dynein and kinesin motor proteins by tau. *Science* **319:** 1086–1089.

Dolan PJ, Johnson GV. 2010. The role of tau kinases in Alzheimer's disease. *Curr Opin Drug Discov Devel* **13:** 595–603.

Doll T, Meichsner M, Riederer BM, Honegger P, Matus A. 1993. An isoform of microtubule-associated protein 2 (MAP2) containing four repeats of the tubulin-binding motif. *J Cell Sci* **106:** 633–639.

Drewes G, Ebneth A, Preuss U, Mandelkow EM, Mandelkow E. 1997. MARK, a novel family of protein kinases that phosphorylate microtubule-associated proteins and trigger microtubule disruption. *Cell* **89:** 297–308.

Drubin DG, Kirschner MW. 1986. Tau protein function in living cells. *J Cell Biol* **103:** 2739–2746.

Dunker AK, Silman I, Uversky VN, Sussman JL. 2008. Function and structure of inherently disordered proteins. *Curr Opin Struct Biol* **18:** 756–764.

Elbaum-Garfinkle S, Ramlall T, Rhoades E. 2010. The role of the lipid bilayer in tau aggregation. *Biophys J* **98:** 2722–2730.

Elliott E, Tsvetkov P, Ginzburg I. 2007. BAG-1 associates with Hsc70.Tau complex and regulates the proteasomal degradation of Tau protein. *J Biol Chem* **282:** 37276–37284.

Fauquant C, Redeker V, Landrieu I, Wieruzseski JM, Verdegem D, Laprevote O, Lippens G, Gigant B, Knossow M. 2011. Systematic identification of tubulin interacting fragments of the microtubule-associated protein TAU leads to a highly efficient promoter of microtubule assembly. *J Biol Chem* **286:** 33358–33368.

Fellous A, Francon J, Lennon AM, Nunez J. 1977. Microtubule assembly in vitro. Purification of assembly-promoting factors. *Eur J Biochem* **78:** 167–174.

Friedhoff P, Schneider A, Mandelkow EM, Mandelkow E. 1998. Rapid assembly of Alzheimer-like paired helical filaments from microtubule-associated protein tau monitored by fluorescence in solution. *Biochemistry* **37:** 10223–10230.

Frost B, Jacks RL, Diamond MI. 2009. Propagation of tau misfolding from the outside to the inside of a cell. *J Biol Chem* **284:** 12845–12852.

Fulga TA, Elson-Schwab I, Khurana V, Steinhilb ML, Spires TL, Hyman BT, Feany MB. 2007. Abnormal bundling and accumulation of F-actin mediates tau-induced neuronal degeneration in vivo. *Nat Cell Biol* **9:** 139–148.

Gamblin TC, Chen F, Zambrano A, Abraha A, Lagalwar S, Guillozet AL, Lu M, Fu Y, Garcia-Sierra F, LaPointe N, et al. 2003. Caspase cleavage of tau: Linking amyloid and neurofibrillary tangles in Alzheimer's disease. *Proc Natl Acad Sci* **100:** 10032–10037.

Garcia ML, Cleveland DW. 2001. Going new places using an old MAP: Tau, microtubules and human neurodegenerative disease. *Curr Opin Cell Biol* **13:** 41–48.

Garg S, Timm T, Mandelkow EM, Mandelkow E, Wang Y. 2011. Cleavage of Tau by calpain in Alzheimer's disease: The quest for the toxic 17 kD fragment. *Neurobiol Aging* **32:** 1–14.

Gaskin F, Cantor CR, Shelanski ML. 1974. Turbidimetric studies of the in vitro assembly and disassembly of porcine neurotubules. *J Mol Biol* **89:** 737–755.

Gauthier-Kemper A, Weissmann C, Golovyashkina N, Sebo-Lemke Z, Drewes G, Gerke V, Heinisch JJ, Brandt R. 2011. The frontotemporal dementia mutation R406W blocks tau's interaction with the membrane in an annexin A2-dependent manner. *J Cell Biol* **192:** 647–661.

Giannetti AM, Lindwall G, Chau MF, Radeke MJ, Feinstein SC, Kohlstaedt LA. 2000. Fibers of tau fragments, but not full length tau, exhibit a cross β-structure: Implications for the formation of paired helical filaments. *Protein Sci* **9:** 2427–2435.

Giasson BI, Forman MS, Higuchi M, Golbe LI, Graves CL, Kotzbauer PT, Trojanowski JQ, Lee VM. 2003. Initiation and synergistic fibrillization of tau and α-synuclein. *Science* **300:** 636–640.

Goedert M, Wischik CM, Crowther RA, Walker JE, Klug A. 1988. Cloning and sequencing of the cDNA encoding a core protein of the paired helical filament of Alzheimer disease: Identification as the microtubule-associated protein tau. *Proc Natl Acad Sci* **85:** 4051–4055.

Goedert M, Spillantini MG, Potier MC, Ulrich J, Crowther RA. 1989. Cloning and sequencing of the cDNA encoding an isoform of microtubule-associated protein tau containing four tandem repeats: Differential expression of tau protein mRNAs in human brain. *EMBO J* **8:** 393–399.

Goedert M, Spillantini MG, Crowther RA. 1992. Cloning of a big tau microtubule-associated protein characteristic of the peripheral nervous system. *Proc Natl Acad Sci* **89:** 1983–1987.

Goedert M, Jakes R, Crowther RA, Cohen P, Vanmechelen E, Vandermeeren M, Cras P. 1994. Epitope mapping of monoclonal antibodies to the paired helical filaments of Alzheimer's disease: Identification of phosphorylation sites in tau protein. *Biochem J* **301:** 871–877.

Goedert M, Jakes R, Spillantini MG, Hasegawa M, Smith MJ, Crowther RA. 1996. Assembly of microtubule-associated protein tau into Alzheimer-like filaments induced by sulphated glycosaminoglycans. *Nature* **383:** 550–553.

Goedert M, Clavaguera F, Tolnay M. 2010. The propagation of prion-like protein inclusions in neurodegenerative diseases. *Trends Neurosci* **33:** 317–325.

* Goedert M, Ghetti B, Grazia Spillantini M. 2011. Frontotemporal dementia: Implications for understanding Alzheimer disease. *Cold Spring Harb Perspect Med* doi: 10.1101/cshperspect.a006254.

Goldbaum O, Oppermann M, Handschuh M, Dabir D, Zhang B, Forman MS, Trojanowski JQ, Lee VM, Richter-Landsberg C. 2003. Proteasome inhibition stabilizes tau inclusions in oligodendroglial cells that occur after treatment with okadaic acid. *J Neurosci* **23:** 8872–8880.

Goode BL, Feinstein SC. 1994. Identification of a novel microtubule binding and assembly domain in the developmentally regulated inter-repeat region of tau. *J Cell Biol* **124:** 769–782.

Gorlovoy P, Larionov S, Pham TT, Neumann H. 2009. Accumulation of tau induced in neurites by microglial proinflammatory mediators. *FASEB J* **23:** 2502–2513.

Gossen M, Bujard H. 2002. Studying gene function in eukaryotes by conditional gene inactivation. *Annu Rev Genet* **36:** 153–173.

Gotz J, Ittner LM. 2008. Animal models of Alzheimer's disease and frontotemporal dementia. *Nat Rev Neurosci* **9:** 532–544.

Gotz J, Deters N, Doldissen A, Bokhari L, Ke Y, Wiesner A, Schonrock N, Ittner LM. 2007. A decade of tau transgenic animal models and beyond. *Brain Pathol* **17:** 91–103.

Gotz J, Lim YA, Ke YD, Eckert A, Ittner LM. 2010. Dissecting toxicity of tau and β-amyloid. *Neurodegener Dis* **7:** 10–12.

Greenberg SG, Davies P. 1990. A preparation of Alzheimer paired helical filaments that displays distinct tau proteins by polyacrylamide gel electrophoresis. *Proc Natl Acad Sci* **87:** 5827–5831.

Griffith LM, Pollard TD. 1978. Evidence for actin filament–microtubule interaction mediated by microtubule-associated proteins. *J Cell Biol* **78:** 958–965.

Grundke-Iqbal I, Iqbal K, Tung YC, Quinlan M, Wisniewski HM, Binder LI. 1986. Abnormal phosphorylation of the microtubule-associated protein tau (tau) in Alzheimer cytoskeletal pathology. *Proc Natl Acad Sci* **83:** 4913–4917.

Gu Y, Oyama F, Ihara Y. 1996. Tau is widely expressed in rat tissues. *J Neurochem* **67:** 1235–1244.

Gustke N, Trinczek B, Biernat J, Mandelkow EM, Mandelkow E. 1994. Domains of tau protein and interactions with microtubules. *Biochemistry* **33:** 9511–9522.

Haass C, Selkoe DJ. 2007. Soluble protein oligomers in neurodegeneration: Lessons from the Alzheimer's amyloid β-peptide. *Nat Rev Mol Cell Biol* **8:** 101–112.

Hampel H, Frank R, Broich K, Teipel SJ, Katz RG, Hardy J, Herholz K, Bokde AL, Jessen F, Hoessler YC, et al. 2010. Biomarkers for Alzheimer's disease: Academic, industry and regulatory perspectives. *Nat Rev Drug Discov* **9:** 560–574.

Hanger DP, Hughes K, Woodgett JR, Brion JP, Anderton BH. 1992. Glycogen synthase kinase-3 induces Alzheimer's disease-like phosphorylation of tau: Generation of paired helical filament epitopes and neuronal localisation of the kinase. *Neurosci Lett* **147:** 58–62.

Hanger DP, Byers HL, Wray S, Leung KY, Saxton MJ, Seereeram A, Reynolds CH, Ward MA, Anderton BH. 2007. Novel phosphorylation sites in tau from Alzheimer brain support a role for casein kinase 1 in disease pathogenesis. *J Biol Chem* **282:** 23645–23654.

Harada A, Teng J, Takei Y, Oguchi K, Hirokawa N. 2002. MAP2 is required for dendrite elongation, PKA anchoring in dendrites, and proper PKA signal transduction. *J Cell Biol* **158:** 541–549.

Hardy J, Singleton A. 2008. The HapMap: Charting a course for genetic discovery in neurological diseases. *Arch Neurol* **65:** 319–321.

Hartig W, Stieler J, Boerema AS, Wolf J, Schmidt U, Weissfuss J, Bullmann T, Strijkstra AM, Arendt T. 2007. Hibernation model of tau phosphorylation in hamsters: Selective vulnerability of cholinergic basal forebrain neurons—Implications for Alzheimer's disease. *Eur J Neurosci* **25:** 69–80.

Hashiguchi M, Sobue K, Paudel HK. 2000. 14–3–3ζ is an effector of tau protein phosphorylation. *J Biol Chem* **275:** 25247–25254.

Hernandez F, Avila J. 2007. Tauopathies. *Cell Mol Life Sci* **64:** 2219–2233.

Hiller G, Weber K. 1978. Radioimmunoassay for tubulin: A quantitative comparison of the tubulin content of different established tissue culture cells and tissues. *Cell* **14:** 795–804.

Himmler A. 1989. Structure of the bovine tau gene: Alternatively spliced transcripts generate a protein family. *Mol Cell Biol* **9:** 1389–1396.

Himmler A, Drechsel D, Kirschner MW, Martin DW Jr. 1989. Tau consists of a set of proteins with repeated C-terminal microtubule-binding domains and variable N-terminal domains. *Mol Cell Biol* **9:** 1381–1388.

Hirokawa N, Shiomura Y, Okabe S. 1988. Tau proteins: The molecular structure and mode of binding on microtubules. *J Cell Biol* **107:** 1449–1459.

Hirokawa N, Funakoshi T, Sato-Harada R, Kanai Y. 1996. Selective stabilization of tau in axons and microtubule-associated protein 2C in cell bodies and dendrites contributes to polarized localization of cytoskeletal proteins in mature neurons. *J Cell Biol* **132:** 667–679.

Hoenger A, Sack S, Thormahlen M, Marx A, Muller J, Gross H, Mandelkow E. 1998. Image reconstructions of microtubules decorated with monomeric and dimeric kinesins: Comparison with x-ray structure and implications for motility. *J Cell Biol* **141:** 419–430.

Hong M, Zhukareva V, Vogelsberg-Ragaglia V, Wszolek Z, Reed L, Miller BI, Geschwind DH, Bird TD, McKeel D, Goate A, et al. 1998. Mutation-specific functional impairments in distinct tau isoforms of hereditary FTDP-17. *Science* **282:** 1914–1917.

Hoogenraad CC, Bradke F. 2009. Control of neuronal polarity and plasticity—A renaissance for microtubules?. *Trends Cell Biol* **19:** 669–676.

Horowitz PM, Patterson KR, Guillozet-Bongaarts AL, Reynolds MR, Carroll CA, Weintraub ST, Bennett DA, Cryns VL, Berry RW, Binder LI. 2004. Early N-terminal changes and caspase-6 cleavage of tau in Alzheimer's disease. *J Neurosci* **24:** 7895–7902.

Hutton M, Lendon CL, Rizzu P, Baker M, Froelich S, Houlden H, Pickering-Brown S, Chakraverty S, Isaacs A, Grover A, et al. 1998. Association of missense and 5′-splice-site mutations in tau with the inherited dementia FTDP-17. *Nature* **393:** 702–705.

Illenberger S, Zheng-Fischhofer Q, Preuss U, Stamer K, Baumann K, Trinczek B, Biernat J, Godemann R, Mandelkow EM, Mandelkow E. 1998. The endogenous and cell cycle-dependent phosphorylation of tau protein in living cells: Implications for Alzheimer's disease. *Mol Biol Cell* **9:** 1495–1512.

Iqbal K, Grundke-Iqbal I. 2008. Alzheimer neurofibrillary degeneration: Significance, etiopathogenesis, therapeutics and prevention. *J Cell Mol Med* **12:** 38–55.

Iqbal K, Alonso Adel C, Grundke-Iqbal I. 2008. Cytosolic abnormally hyperphosphorylated tau but not paired helical filaments sequester normal MAPs and inhibit microtubule assembly. *J Alzheimers Dis* **14:** 365–370.

Iqbal K, Liu F, Gong CX, Alonso Adel C, Grundke-Iqbal I. 2009. Mechanisms of tau-induced neurodegeneration. *Acta Neuropathol* **118:** 53–69.

Ishihara T, Higuchi M, Zhang B, Yoshiyama Y, Hong M, Trojanowski JQ, Lee VM. 2001. Attenuated neurodegenerative disease phenotype in tau transgenic mouse lacking neurofilaments. *J Neurosci* **21:** 6026–6035.

Ittner LM, Ke YD, Gotz J. 2009. Phosphorylated Tau interacts with c-Jun N-terminal kinase-interacting protein 1 (JIP1) in Alzheimer disease. *J Biol Chem* **284:** 20909–20916.

Ittner LM, Ke YD, Delerue F, Bi M, Gladbach A, van Eersel J, Wolfing H, Chieng BC, Christie MJ, Napier IA, et al. 2010. Dendritic function of tau mediates amyloid-β toxicity in Alzheimer's disease mouse models. *Cell* **142:** 387–397.

Jeganathan S, von Bergen M, Brutlach H, Steinhoff HJ, Mandelkow E. 2006. Global hairpin folding of tau in solution. *Biochemistry* **45:** 2283–2293.

Jensen PH, Hager H, Nielsen MS, Hojrup P, Gliemann J, Jakes R. 1999. α-Synuclein binds to Tau and stimulates the protein kinase A-catalyzed tau phosphorylation of serine residues 262 and 356. *J Biol Chem* **274:** 25481–25489.

Jinwal UK, Koren J, Borysov SI, Schmid AB, Abisambra JF, Blair LJ, Johnson AG, Jones JR, Shults CL, O'Leary JC, et al. 2010. The Hsp90 cochaperone, FKBP51, increases Tau stability and polymerizes microtubules. *J Neurosci* **30:** 591–599.

Jinwal UK, Trotter JH, Abisambra JF, Koren J, Lawson LY, Vestal GD, O'Leary JC, Johnson AG, Jin Y, Jones JR, et al. 2011. The Hsp90 kinase co-chaperone Cdc37 regulates tau stability and phosphorylation dynamics. *J Biol Chem* **286:** 16976–16983.

Kampers T, Friedhoff P, Biernat J, Mandelkow EM, Mandelkow E. 1996. RNA stimulates aggregation of microtubule-associated protein tau into Alzheimer-like paired helical filaments. *FEBS Lett* **399:** 344–349.

Kanaan NM, Morfini GA, Lapointe NE, Pigino GF, Patterson KR, Song Y, Andreadis A, Fu Y, Brady ST, Binder LI. 2011. Pathogenic forms of Tau inhibit kinesin-dependent axonal transport through a mechanism involving activation of axonal phosphotransferases. *J Neurosci* **31:** 9858–9868.

Kang J, Lemaire HG, Unterbeck A, Salbaum JM, Masters CL, Grzeschik KH, Multhaup G, Beyreuther K, Muller-Hill B. 1987. The precursor of Alzheimer's disease amyloid A4 protein resembles a cell-surface receptor. *Nature* **325:** 733–736.

Karsten SL, Sang TK, Gehman LT, Chatterjee S, Liu J, Lawless GM, Sengupta S, Berry RW, Pomakian J, Oh HS, et al. 2006. A genomic screen for modifiers of tauopathy identifies puromycin-sensitive aminopeptidase as an inhibitor of tau-induced neurodegeneration. *Neuron* **51:** 549–560.

Khlistunova I, Pickhardt M, Biernat J, Wang Y, Mandelkow EM, Mandelkow E. 2007. Inhibition of tau aggregation in cell models of tauopathy. *Curr Alzheimer Res* **4:** 544–546.

Kidd M. 1963. Paired helical filaments in electron microscopy of Alzheimer's disease. *Nature* **197:** 192–193.

Kikkawa M, Okada Y, Hirokawa N. 2000. 15 A resolution model of the monomeric kinesin motor, KIF1A. *Cell* **100:** 241–252.

Klein C, Kramer EM, Cardine AM, Schraven B, Brandt R, Trotter J. 2002. Process outgrowth of oligodendrocytes is promoted by interaction of fyn kinase with the cytoskeletal protein tau. *J Neurosci* **22:** 698–707.

Konzack S, Thies E, Marx A, Mandelkow EM, Mandelkow E. 2007. Swimming against the tide: Mobility of the microtubule-associated protein tau in neurons. *J Neurosci* **27:** 9916–9927.

Kopke E, Tung YC, Shaikh S, Alonso AC, Iqbal K, Grundke-Iqbal I. 1993. Microtubule-associated protein tau. Abnormal phosphorylation of a non-paired helical filament pool in Alzheimer disease. *J Biol Chem* **268:** 24374–24384.

Kosik KS, Joachim CL, Selkoe DJ. 1986. Microtubule-associated protein tau (tau) is a major antigenic component of paired helical filaments in Alzheimer disease. *Proc Natl Acad Sci* **83:** 4044–4048.

Kosik KS, Orecchio LD, Binder L, Trojanowski JQ, Lee VM, Lee G. 1988. Epitopes that span the tau molecule are shared with paired helical filaments. *Neuron* **1:** 817–825.

Kosik KS, Orecchio LD, Bakalis S, Neve RL. 1989. Developmentally regulated expression of specific tau sequences. *Neuron* **2:** 1389–1397.

Kraemer BC, Schellenberg GD. 2007. SUT-1 enables tau-induced neurotoxicity in C. elegans. *Hum Mol Genet* **16:** 1959–1971.

Ledesma MD, Bonay P, Colaco C, Avila J. 1994. Analysis of microtubule-associated protein tau glycation in paired helical filaments. *J Biol Chem* **269:** 21614–21619.

Lee YC, Wolff J. 1984. Calmodulin binds to both microtubule-associated protein 2 and tau proteins. *J Biol Chem* **259:** 1226–1230.

Lee G, Cowan N, Kirschner M. 1988. The primary structure and heterogeneity of tau protein from mouse brain. *Science* **239:** 285–288.

Lee G, Newman ST, Gard DL, Band H, Panchamoorthy G. 1998. Tau interacts with src-family non-receptor tyrosine kinases. *J Cell Sci* **111:** 3167–3177.

Lee VM, Kenyon TK, Trojanowski JQ. 2005. Transgenic animal models of tauopathies. *Biochim Biophys Acta* **1739:** 251–259.

* Lee V, Brunden KR, Hutton M, Trojanowski JQ. 2011. Developing therapeutic approaches to Tau, selected kinases, and related neuronal protein targets. *Cold Spring Harb Perspect Med* doi: 10.1101/cshperspect.a006437.

Lewis J, McGowan E, Rockwood J, Melrose H, Nacharaju P, Van Slegtenhorst M, Gwinn-Hardy K, Paul Murphy M,

Baker M, Yu X, et al. 2000. Neurofibrillary tangles, amyotrophy and progressive motor disturbance in mice expressing mutant (P301L) tau protein. *Nat Genet* **25:** 402–405.

Li X, Lu F, Wang JZ, Gong CX. 2006. Concurrent alterations of O-GlcNAcylation and phosphorylation of tau in mouse brains during fasting. *Eur J Neurosci* **23:** 2078–2086.

Lichtenberg-Kraag B, Mandelkow EM, Biernat J, Steiner B, Schroter C, Gustke N, Meyer HE, Mandelkow E. 1992. Phosphorylation-dependent epitopes of neurofilament antibodies on tau protein and relationship with Alzheimer tau. *Proc Natl Acad Sci* **89:** 5384–5388.

Liou YC, Sun A, Ryo A, Zhou XZ, Yu ZX, Huang HK, Uchida T, Bronson R, Bing G, Li X, et al. 2003. Role of the prolyl isomerase Pin1 in protecting against age-dependent neurodegeneration. *Nature* **424:** 556–561.

Littauer UZ, Giveon D, Thierauf M, Ginzburg I, Ponstingl H. 1986. Common and distinct tubulin binding sites for microtubule-associated proteins. *Proc Natl Acad Sci* **83:** 7162–7166.

Loomis PA, Howard TH, Castleberry RP, Binder LI. 1990. Identification of nuclear tau isoforms in human neuroblastoma cells. *Proc Natl Acad Sci* **87:** 8422–8426.

LoPresti P, Szuchet S, Papasozomenos SC, Zinkowski RP, Binder LI. 1995. Functional implications for the microtubule-associated protein tau: Localization in oligodendrocytes. *Proc Natl Acad Sci* **92:** 10369–10373.

Lu PJ, Wulf G, Zhou XZ, Davies P, Lu KP. 1999. The prolyl isomerase Pin1 restores the function of Alzheimer-associated phosphorylated tau protein. *Nature* **399:** 784–788.

Magnani E, Fan J, Gasparini L, Golding M, Williams M, Schiavo G, Goedert M, Amos LA, Spillantini MG. 2007. Interaction of tau protein with the dynactin complex. *EMBO J* **26:** 4546–4554.

Makrides V, Massie MR, Feinstein SC, Lew J. 2004. Evidence for two distinct binding sites for tau on microtubules. *Proc Natl Acad Sci* **101:** 6746–6751.

Mandelkow EM, Drewes G, Biernat J, Gustke N, Van Lint J, Vandenheede JR, Mandelkow E. 1992. Glycogen synthase kinase-3 and the Alzheimer-like state of microtubule-associated protein tau. *FEBS Lett* **314:** 315–321.

Mandelkow EM, Thies E, Trinczek B, Biernat J, Mandelkow E. 2004. MARK/PAR1 kinase is a regulator of microtubule-dependent transport in axons. *J Cell Biol* **167:** 99–110.

Margittai M, Langen R. 2004. Template-assisted filament growth by parallel stacking of tau. *Proc Natl Acad Sci* **101:** 10278–10283.

Margittai M, Langen R. 2006. Side chain-dependent stacking modulates tau filament structure. *J Biol Chem* **281:** 37820–37827.

Matsuo ES, Shin RW, Billingsley ML, Van deVoorde A, O'Connor M, Trojanowski JQ, Lee VM. 1994. Biopsy-derived adult human brain tau is phosphorylated at many of the same sites as Alzheimer's disease paired helical filament tau. *Neuron* **13:** 989–1002.

Mattson MP. 2004. Pathways towards and away from Alzheimer's disease. *Nature* **430:** 631–639.

Mercken M, Fischer I, Kosik KS, Nixon RA. 1995. Three distinct axonal transport rates for tau, tubulin, and other microtubule-associated proteins: Evidence for dynamic interactions of tau with microtubules in vivo. *J Neurosci* **15:** 8259–8267.

Min SW, Cho SH, Zhou Y, Schroeder S, Haroutunian V, Seeley WW, Huang EJ, Shen Y, Masliah E, Mukherjee C, et al. 2010. Acetylation of tau inhibits its degradation and contributes to tauopathy. *Neuron* **67:** 953–966.

Mocanu MM, Nissen A, Eckermann K, Khlistunova I, Biernat J, Drexler D, Petrova O, Schonig K, Bujard H, Mandelkow E, et al. 2008. The potential for β-structure in the repeat domain of tau protein determines aggregation, synaptic decay, neuronal loss, and coassembly with endogenous Tau in inducible mouse models of tauopathy. *J Neurosci* **28:** 737–748.

Moores CA, Perderiset M, Francis F, Chelly J, Houdusse A, Milligan RA. 2004. Mechanism of microtubule stabilization by doublecortin. *Mol Cell* **14:** 833–839.

Moreno-Herrero F, Perez M, Baro AM, Avila J. 2004. Characterization by atomic force microscopy of Alzheimer paired helical filaments under physiological conditions. *Biophys J* **86:** 517–525.

Morishima-Kawashima M, Hasegawa M, Takio K, Suzuki M, Titani K, Ihara Y. 1993. Ubiquitin is conjugated with amino-terminally processed tau in paired helical filaments. *Neuron* **10:** 1151–1160.

Morishima-Kawashima M, Kosik KS. 1996. The pool of map kinase associated with microtubules is small but constitutively active. *Mol Biol Cell* **7:** 893–905.

Morita T, Sobue K. 2009. Specification of neuronal polarity regulated by local translation of CRMP2 and Tau via the mTOR-p70S6K pathway. *J Biol Chem* **284:** 27734–27745.

Morris M, Maeda S, Vossel K, Mucke L. 2011. The many faces of tau. *Neuron* **70:** 410–426.

Morrissette DA, Parachikova A, Green KN, LaFerla FM. 2009. Relevance of transgenic mouse models to human Alzheimer disease. *J Biol Chem* **284:** 6033–6037.

Mukrasch MD, Biernat J, von Bergen M, Griesinger C, Mandelkow E, Zweckstetter M. 2005. Sites of tau important for aggregation populate {β}-structure and bind to microtubules and polyanions. *J Biol Chem* **280:** 24978–24986.

Mukrasch MD, Bibow S, Korukottu J, Jeganathan S, Biernat J, Griesinger C, Mandelkow E, Zweckstetter M. 2009. Structural polymorphism of 441-residue tau at single residue resolution. *PLoS Biol* **7:** e34.

Myers AJ, Pittman AM, Zhao AS, Rohrer K, Kaleem M, Marlowe L, Lees A, Leung D, McKeith IG, Perry RH, et al. 2007. The MAPT H1c risk haplotype is associated with increased expression of tau and especially of 4 repeat containing transcripts. *Neurobiol Dis* **25:** 561–570.

Mylonas E, Hascher A, Bernado P, Blackledge M, Mandelkow E, Svergun DI. 2008. Domain conformation of tau protein studied by solution small-angle X-ray scattering. *Biochemistry* **47:** 10345–10353.

Nakata T, Hirokawa N. 2003. Microtubules provide directional cues for polarized axonal transport through interaction with kinesin motor head. *J Cell Biol* **162:** 1045–1055.

Neve RL, Harris P, Kosik KS, Kurnit DM, Donlon TA. 1986. Identification of cDNA clones for the human microtubule-associated protein tau and chromosomal localization of the genes for tau and microtubule-associated protein 2. *Brain Res* **387:** 271–280.

Nogales E, Whittaker M, Milligan RA, Downing KH. 1999. High-resolution model of the microtubule. *Cell* **96:** 79–88.

Obar RA, Collins CA, Hammarback JA, Shpetner HS, Vallee RB. 1990. Molecular cloning of the microtubule-associated mechanochemical enzyme dynamin reveals homology with a new family of GTP-binding proteins. *Nature* **347:** 256–261.

Oddo S, Billings L, Kesslak JP, Cribbs DH, LaFerla FM. 2004. Aβ immunotherapy leads to clearance of early, but not late, hyperphosphorylated tau aggregates via the proteasome. *Neuron* **43:** 321–332.

Padilla R, Maccioni RB, Avila J. 1990. Calmodulin binds to a tubulin binding site of the microtubule-associated protein tau. *Mol Cell Biochem* **97:** 35–41.

Panda D, Samuel JC, Massie M, Feinstein SC, Wilson L. 2003. Differential regulation of microtubule dynamics by three- and four-repeat tau: Implications for the onset of neurodegenerative disease. *Proc Natl Acad Sci* **100:** 9548–9553.

Papasozomenos SC, Binder LI. 1987. Phosphorylation determines two distinct species of Tau in the central nervous system. *Cell Motil Cytoskeleton* **8:** 210–226.

Park SY, Ferreira A. 2005. The generation of a 17 kDa neurotoxic fragment: An alternative mechanism by which tau mediates β-amyloid-induced neurodegeneration. *J Neurosci* **25:** 5365–5375.

Perez M, Valpuesta JM, Medina M, Montejo de Garcini E, Avila J. 1996. Polymerization of tau into filaments in the presence of heparin: The minimal sequence required for tau-tau interaction. *J Neurochem* **67:** 1183–1190.

Perl ML, Abrams GS, Boyarski AM, Breidenbach M, Briggs DD, Bulos F, Chinowsky W, Dakin JT, Feldman GJ, Friedberg CE, et al. 1975. Evidence for anomalous lepton production in e$^+$–e$^-$ annihilation. *Phys Rev Lett* **35:** 1489.

Petrucelli L, Dickson D, Kehoe K, Taylor J, Snyder H, Grover A, De Lucia M, McGowan E, Lewis J, Prihar G, et al. 2004. CHIP and Hsp70 regulate tau ubiquitination, degradation and aggregation. *Hum Mol Genet* **13:** 703–714.

Pickhardt M, Gazova Z, von Bergen M, Khlistunova I, Wang Y, Hascher A, Mandelkow EM, Biernat J, Mandelkow E. 2005. Anthraquinones inhibit tau aggregation and dissolve Alzheimer's paired helical filaments in vitro and in cells. *J Biol Chem* **280:** 3628–3635.

Planel E, Richter KE, Nolan CE, Finley JE, Liu L, Wen Y, Krishnamurthy P, Herman M, Wang L, Schachter JB, et al. 2007a. Anesthesia leads to tau hyperphosphorylation through inhibition of phosphatase activity by hypothermia. *J Neurosci* **27:** 3090–3097.

Planel E, Tatebayashi Y, Miyasaka T, Liu L, Wang L, Herman M, Yu WH, Luchsinger JA, Wadzinski B, Duff KE, et al. 2007b. Insulin dysfunction induces in vivo tau hyperphosphorylation through distinct mechanisms. *J Neurosci* **27:** 13635–13648.

Pollanen MS, Markiewicz P, Goh MC. 1997. Paired helical filaments are twisted ribbons composed of two parallel and aligned components: Image reconstruction and modeling of filament structure using atomic force microscopy. *J Neuropathol Exp Neurol* **56:** 79–85.

Poorkaj P, Bird TD, Wijsman E, Nemens E, Garruto RM, Anderson L, Andreadis A, Wiederholt WC, Raskind M, Schellenberg GD. 1998. Tau is a candidate gene for chromosome 17 frontotemporal dementia. *Ann Neurol* **43:** 815–825.

Reynolds MR, Berry RW, Binder LI. 2007. Nitration in neurodegeneration: Deciphering the "Hows" "nYs". *Biochemistry* **46:** 7325–7336.

Reynolds CH, Garwood CJ, Wray S, Price C, Kellie S, Perera T, Zvelebil M, Yang A, Sheppard PW, Varndell IM, et al. 2008. Phosphorylation regulates tau interactions with Src homology 3 domains of phosphatidylinositol 3-kinase, phospholipase Cγ1, Grb2, and Src family kinases. *J Biol Chem* **283:** 18177–18186.

Rissman RA, Poon WW, Blurton-Jones M, Oddo S, Torp R, Vitek MP, LaFerla FM, Rohn TT, Cotman CW. 2004. Caspase-cleavage of tau is an early event in Alzheimer disease tangle pathology. *J Clin Invest* **114:** 121–130.

Roberson ED, Scearce-Levie K, Palop JJ, Yan F, Cheng IH, Wu T, Gerstein H, Yu GQ, Mucke L. 2007. Reducing endogenous tau ameliorates amyloid β-induced deficits in an Alzheimer's disease mouse model. *Science* **316:** 750–754.

Roger B, Al-Bassam J, Dehmelt L, Milligan RA, Halpain S. 2004. MAP2c, but not tau, binds and bundles F-actin via its microtubule binding domain. *Curr Biol* **14:** 363–371.

Sack S, Muller J, Marx A, Thormahlen M, Mandelkow EM, Brady ST, Mandelkow E. 1997. X-ray structure of motor and neck domains from rat brain kinesin. *Biochemistry* **36:** 16155–16165.

Salminen A, Ojala J, Kaarniranta K, Hiltunen M, Soininen H. 2011. Hsp90 regulates tau pathology through co-chaperone complexes in Alzheimer's disease. *Prog Neurobiol* **93:** 99–110.

Samsonov A, Yu JZ, Rasenick M, Popov SV. 2004. Tau interaction with microtubules in vivo. *J Cell Sci* **117:** 6129–6141.

Santacruz K, Lewis J, Spires T, Paulson J, Kotilinek L, Ingelsson M, Guimaraes A, DeTure M, Ramsden M, McGowan E, et al. 2005. Tau suppression in a neurodegenerative mouse model improves memory function. *Science* **309:** 476–481.

Santarella RA, Skiniotis G, Goldie KN, Tittmann P, Gross H, Mandelkow EM, Mandelkow E, Hoenger A. 2004. Surface-decoration of microtubules by human tau. *J Mol Biol* **339:** 539–553.

Sarkar M, Kuret J, Lee G. 2008. Two motifs within the tau microtubule-binding domain mediate its association with the hsc70 molecular chaperone. *J Neurosci Res* **86:** 2763–2773.

Sawaya MR, Sambashivan S, Nelson R, Ivanova MI, Sievers SA, Apostol MI, Thompson MJ, Balbirnie M, Wiltzius JJ, McFarlane HT, et al. 2007. Atomic structures of amyloid cross-β spines reveal varied steric zippers. *Nature* **447:** 453–457.

Schaap IA, Hoffmann B, Carrasco C, Merkel R, Schmidt CF. 2007. Tau protein binding forms a 1 nm thick layer along protofilaments without affecting the radial elasticity of microtubules. *J Struct Biol* **158:** 282–292.

Schneider A, Mandelkow E. 2008. Tau-based treatment strategies in neurodegenerative diseases. *Neurotherapeutics* **5:** 443–457.

Schneider A, Biernat J, von Bergen M, Mandelkow E, Mandelkow EM. 1999. Phosphorylation that detaches tau protein from microtubules (Ser262, Ser214) also protects it against aggregation into Alzheimer paired helical filaments. *Biochemistry* **38:** 3549–3558.

Schweers O, Schonbrunn-Hanebeck E, Marx A, Mandelkow E. 1994. Structural studies of tau protein and Alzheimer paired helical filaments show no evidence for β-structure. *J Biol Chem* **269:** 24290–24297.

Schweers O, Mandelkow EM, Biernat J, Mandelkow E. 1995. Oxidation of cysteine-322 in the repeat domain of microtubule-associated protein tau controls the in vitro assembly of paired helical filaments. *Proc Natl Acad Sci* **92:** 8463–8467.

Scabrook GR, Ray WJ, Shearman M, Hutton M. 2007. Beyond amyloid: The next generation of Alzheimer's disease therapeutics. *Mol Interv* **7:** 261–270.

Seitz A, Kojima H, Oiwa K, Mandelkow EM, Song YH, Mandelkow E. 2002. Single-molecule investigation of the interference between kinesin, tau and MAP2c. *EMBO J* **21:** 4896–4905.

Sergeant N, Bretteville A, Hamdane M, Caillet-Boudin ML, Grognet P, Bombois S, Blum D, Delacourte A, Pasquier F, Vanmechelen E, et al. 2008. Biochemistry of Tau in Alzheimer's disease and related neurological disorders. *Expert Rev Proteomics* **5:** 207–224.

Seubert P, Mawal-Dewan M, Barbour R, Jakes R, Goedert M, Johnson GV, Litersky JM, Schenk D, Lieberburg I, Trojanowski JQ, et al. 1995. Detection of phosphorylated Ser262 in fetal tau, adult tau, and paired helical filament tau. *J Biol Chem* **270:** 18917–18922.

Shankar GM, Bloodgood BL, Townsend M, Walsh DM, Selkoe DJ, Sabatini BL. 2007. Natural oligomers of the Alzheimer amyloid-β protein induce reversible synapse loss by modulating an NMDA-type glutamate receptor-dependent signaling pathway. *J Neurosci* **27:** 2866–2875.

Shimura H, Miura-Shimura Y, Kosik KS. 2004a. Binding of tau to heat shock protein 27 leads to decreased concentration of hyperphosphorylated tau and enhanced cell survival. *J Biol Chem* **279:** 17957–17962.

Shimura H, Schwartz D, Gygi SP, Kosik KS. 2004b. CHIP-Hsc70 complex ubiquitinates phosphorylated tau and enhances cell survival. *J Biol Chem* **279:** 4869–4876.

Sievers SA, Karanicolas J, Chang HW, Zhao A, Jiang L, Zirafi O, Stevens JT, Munch J, Baker D, Eisenberg D. 2011. Structure-based design of non-natural amino-acid inhibitors of amyloid fibril formation. *Nature* **475:** 96–100.

Sillen A, Leroy A, Wieruszeski JM, Loyens A, Beauvillain JC, Buee L, Landrieu I, Lippens G. 2005. Regions of tau implicated in the paired helical fragment core as defined by NMR. *Chembiochem* **6:** 1849–1856.

Sillen A, Barbier P, Landrieu I, Lefebvre S, Wieruszeski JM, Leroy A, Peyrot V, Lippens G. 2007. NMR investigation of the interaction between the neuronal protein tau and the microtubules. *Biochemistry* **46:** 3055–3064.

Sluchanko NN, Seit-Nebi AS, Gusev NB. 2009. Phosphorylation of more than one site is required for tight interaction of human tau protein with 14–3–3ζ. *FEBS Lett* **583:** 2739–2742.

Smet C, Sambo AV, Wieruszeski JM, Leroy A, Landrieu I, Buee L, Lippens G. 2004. The peptidyl prolyl cis/ trans-isomerase Pin1 recognizes the phospho-Thr212– Pro213 site on Tau. *Biochemistry* **43:** 2032–2040.

Sontag E, Nunbhakdi-Craig V, Lee G, Brandt R, Kamibayashi C, Kuret J, White CL 3rd, Mumby MC, Bloom GS. 1999. Molecular interactions among protein phosphatase 2A, tau, and microtubules. Implications for the regulation of tau phosphorylation and the development of tauopathies. *J Biol Chem* **274:** 25490–25498.

Spillantini MG, Murrell JR, Goedert M, Farlow MR, Klug A, Ghetti B. 1998. Mutation in the tau gene in familial multiple system tauopathy with presenile dementia. *Proc Natl Acad Sci* **95:** 7737–7741.

Spires-Jones TL, Stoothoff WH, de Calignon A, Jones PB, Hyman BT. 2009. Tau pathophysiology in neurodegeneration: A tangled issue. *Trends Neurosci* **32:** 150–159.

Stamer K, Vogel R, Thies E, Mandelkow E, Mandelkow EM. 2002. Tau blocks traffic of organelles, neurofilaments, and APP vesicles in neurons and enhances oxidative stress. *J Cell Biol* **156:** 1051–1063.

Steiner B, Mandelkow EM, Biernat J, Gustke N, Meyer HE, Schmidt B, Mieskes G, Soling HD, Drechsel D, Kirschner MW, et al. 1990. Phosphorylation of microtubule-associated protein tau: Identification of the site for Ca2(+)-calmodulin dependent kinase and relationship with tau phosphorylation in Alzheimer tangles. *EMBO J* **9:** 3539–3544.

Stoothoff WH, Johnson GV. 2005. Tau phosphorylation: Physiological and pathological consequences. *Biochim Biophys Acta* **1739:** 280–297.

Strittmatter WJ, Saunders AM, Goedert M, Weisgraber KH, Dong LM, Jakes R, Huang DY, Pericak-Vance M, Schmechel D, Roses AD. 1994. Isoform-specific interactions of apolipoprotein E with microtubule-associated protein tau: Implications for Alzheimer disease. *Proc Natl Acad Sci* **91:** 11183–11186.

Sultan A, Nesslany F, Violet M, Begard S, Loyens A, Talahari S, Mansuroglu Z, Marzin D, Sergeant N, Humez S, et al. 2011. Nuclear tau, a key player in neuronal DNA protection. *J Biol Chem* **286:** 4566–4575.

Sun W, Qureshi HY, Cafferty PW, Sobue K, Agarwal-Mawal A, Neufield KD, Paudel HK. 2002. Glycogen synthase kinase-3β is complexed with tau protein in brain microtubules. *J Biol Chem* **277:** 11933–11940.

Sydow A, Van der Jeugd A, Zheng F, Ahmed T, Balschun D, Petrova O, Drexler D, Zhou L, Rune G, Mandelkow E, et al. 2011. Tau-induced defects in synaptic plasticity, learning, and memory are reversible in transgenic mice after switching off the toxic Tau mutant. *J Neurosci* **31:** 2511–2525.

Takashima A, Murayama M, Murayama O, Kohno T, Honda T, Yasutake K, Nihonmatsu N, Mercken M, Yamaguchi H, Sugihara S, et al. 1998. Presenilin 1 associates with glycogen synthase kinase-3β and its substrate tau. *Proc Natl Acad Sci* **95:** 9637–9641.

Tanimukai H, Grundke-Iqbal I, Iqbal K. 2005. Up-regulation of inhibitors of protein phosphatase-2A in Alzheimer's disease. *Am J Pathol* **166:** 1761–1771.

Terwel D, Dewachter I, Van Leuven F. 2002. Axonal transport, tau protein, and neurodegeneration in Alzheimer's disease. *Neuromolecular Med* **2:** 151–165.

Thies E, Mandelkow EM. 2007. Missorting of tau in neurons causes degeneration of synapses that can be rescued by the kinase MARK2/Par-1. *J Neurosci* **27:** 2896–2907.

Tortosa E, Santa-Maria I, Moreno F, Lim F, Perez M, Avila J. 2009. Binding of Hsp90 to tau promotes a conformational change and aggregation of tau protein. *J Alzheimers Dis* **17:** 319–325.

Umeyama T, Okabe S, Kanai Y, Hirokawa N. 1993. Dynamics of microtubules bundled by microtubule associated protein 2C (MAP2C). *J Cell Biol* **120:** 451–465.

Utton MA, Noble WJ, Hill JE, Anderton BH, Hanger DP. 2005. Molecular motors implicated in the axonal transport of tau and α-synuclein. *J Cell Sci* **118:** 4645–4654.

Veeranna, Yang DS, Lee JH, Vinod KY, Stavrides P, Amin ND, Pant HC, Nixon RA. 2009. Declining phosphatases underlie aging-related hyperphosphorylation of neurofilaments. *Neurobiol Aging* **2010** doi: 10.1016/ j.neurobiolaging.2009.1012.1001.

von Bergen M, Friedhoff P, Biernat J, Heberle J, Mandelkow EM, Mandelkow E. 2000. Assembly of tau protein into Alzheimer paired helical filaments depends on a local sequence motif ((306)VQIVYK(311)) forming β structure. *Proc Natl Acad Sci* **97:** 5129–5134.

von Bergen M, Barghorn S, Li L, Marx A, Biernat J, Mandelkow EM, Mandelkow E. 2001. Mutations of tau protein in frontotemporal dementia promote aggregation of paired helical filaments by enhancing local β-structure. *J Biol Chem* **276:** 48165–48174.

Wang Y, Martinez-Vicente M, Kruger U, Kaushik S, Wong E, Mandelkow EM, Cuervo AM, Mandelkow E. 2009. Tau fragmentation, aggregation and clearance: The dual role of lysosomal processing. *Hum Mol Genet* **18:** 4153–4170.

Watanabe A, Hong WK, Dohmae N, Takio K, Morishima-Kawashima M, Ihara Y. 2004. Molecular aging of tau: Disulfide-independent aggregation and non-enzymatic degradation in vitro and in vivo. *J Neurochem* **90:** 1302–1311.

Wegmann S, Jung YJ, Chinnathambi S, Mandelkow EM, Mandelkow E, Muller DJ. 2010. Human Tau isoforms assemble into ribbon-like fibrils that display polymorphic structure and stability. *J Biol Chem* **285:** 27302–27313.

Weingarten MD, Lockwood AH, Hwo SY, Kirschner MW. 1975. A protein factor essential for microtubule assembly. *Proc Natl Acad Sci* **72:** 1858–1862.

Weisenberg RC. 1972. Microtubule formation in vitro in solutions containing low calcium concentrations. *Science* **177:** 1104–1105.

Wendt TG, Volkmann N, Skiniotis G, Goldie KN, Muller J, Mandelkow E, Hoenger A. 2002. Microscopic evidence for a minus-end-directed power stroke in the kinesin motor ncd. *EMBO J* **21:** 5969–5978.

Whiteman IT, Gervasio OL, Cullen KM, Guillemin GJ, Jeong EV, Witting PK, Antao ST, Minamide LS, Bamburg JR, Goldsbury C. 2009. Activated actin-depolymerizing factor/cofilin sequesters phosphorylated microtubule-associated protein during the assembly of alzheimer-like neuritic cytoskeletal striations. *J Neurosci* **29:** 12994–13005.

Wille H, Drewes G, Biernat J, Mandelkow EM, Mandelkow E. 1992. Alzheimer-like paired helical filaments and antiparallel dimers formed from microtubule-associated protein tau in vitro. *J Cell Biol* **118**: 573–584.

Williamson R, Usardi A, Hanger DP, Anderton BH. 2008. Membrane-bound β-amyloid oligomers are recruited into lipid rafts by a fyn-dependent mechanism. *FASEB J* **22**: 1552–1559.

Wilson DM, Binder LI. 1995. Polymerization of microtubule-associated protein tau under near-physiological conditions. *J Biol Chem* **270**: 24306–24314.

Wilson DM, Binder LI. 1997. Free fatty acids stimulate the polymerization of tau and amyloid β peptides. In vitro evidence for a common effector of pathogenesis in Alzheimer's disease. *Am J Pathol* **150**: 2181–2195.

Wilson L, Jordan MA. 2004. New microtubule/tubulin-targeted anticancer drugs and novel chemotherapeutic strategies. *J Chemother* **16**: 83–85.

Wischik CM, Novak M, Edwards PC, Klug A, Tichelaar W, Crowther RA. 1988. Structural characterization of the core of the paired helical filament of Alzheimer disease. *Proc Natl Acad Sci* **85**: 4884–4888.

Wolfe MS. 2009. Tau mutations in neurodegenerative diseases. *J Biol Chem* **284**: 6021–6025.

Wolozin BL, Pruchnicki A, Dickson DW, Davies P. 1986. A neuronal antigen in the brains of Alzheimer patients. *Science* **232**: 648–650.

Wood JG, Mirra SS, Pollock NJ, Binder LI. 1986. Neurofibrillary tangles of Alzheimer disease share antigenic determinants with the axonal microtubule-associated protein tau (tau). *Proc Natl Acad Sci* **83**: 4040–4043.

Yamada K, Cirrito JR, Stewart FR, Jiang H, Finn MB, Holmes B, Binder LI, Mandelkow EM, Diamond MI, Lee V.M.Y, Holtzman DM. 2011. In vivo microdialysis reveals age-dependent decrease of brain interstitial tau levels in P301S human tau transgenic mice. *J Neurosci* **31**: 13110–13117.

Zempel H, Thies E, Mandelkow E, Mandelkow EM. 2010. Aβ oligomers cause localized Ca(2+) elevation, missorting of endogenous Tau into dendrites, Tau phosphorylation, and destruction of microtubules and spines. *J Neurosci* **30**: 11938–11950.

Frontotemporal Dementia: Implications for Understanding Alzheimer Disease

Michel Goedert[1], Bernardino Ghetti[2], and Maria Grazia Spillantini[3]

[1]MRC Laboratory of Molecular Biology, Cambridge CB2 0QH, United Kingdom

[2]Indiana University School of Medicine, Department of Pathology and Laboratory Medicine, Indianapolis, Indiana 46202

[3]Centre for Brain Repair, Department of Clinical Neurosciences, University of Cambridge, Cambridge CB2 0PY, United Kingdom

Correspondence: mg@mrc-lmb.cam.ac.uk

Frontotemporal dementia (FTD) comprises a group of behavioral, language, and movement disorders. On the basis of the nature of the characteristic protein inclusions, frontotemporal lobar degeneration (FTLD) can be subdivided into the common FTLD-tau and FTLD-TDP as well as the less common FTLD-FUS and FTLD-UPS. Approximately 10% of cases of FTD are inherited in an autosomal-dominant manner. Mutations in seven genes cause FTD, with those in tau *(MAPT)*, chromosome 9 open reading frame 72 (*C9ORF72*), and progranulin (*GRN*) being the most common. Mutations in *MAPT* give rise to FTLD-tau and mutations in *C9ORF72* and *GRN* to FTLD-TDP. The other four genes are transactive response–DNA binding protein-43 (*TARDBP*), fused in sarcoma (*FUS*), valosin-containing protein (*VCP*), and charged multivesicular body protein 2B (*CHMP2B*). Mutations in *TARDBP* and *VCP* give rise to FTLD-TDP, mutations in *FUS* to FTLD-FUS, and mutations in *CHMP2B* to FTLD-UPS. The discovery that mutations in *MAPT* cause neurodegeneration and dementia has important implications for understanding Alzheimer disease.

THE CONCEPT OF FRONTOTEMPORAL DEMENTIA: HISTORICAL OVERVIEW

Frontotemporal dementia (FTD) results from degeneration of the cortex of the frontal and temporal lobes, often in conjunction with the degeneration of subcortical brain regions. This gives rise to a spectrum of behavioral, language, and movement disorders. A link exists between FTD and forms of motor neuron disease (MND). Work on FTD stretches back to the end of the 19th century.

Arnold Pick was Professor of Neuropsychiatry at the German University in Prague from 1886 to 1921. In 1892, he described a 71-year-old man with behavioral disturbances, aphasia, and dementia (Pick 1892). At autopsy, marked atrophy of the left temporal lobe rather than the diffuse atrophy characteristic of senile dementia was present. Although Pick was doubtful of the primacy of these observations, his paper is considered to be the first description of lobar cortical atrophy. At the time, there was much interest in language abnormalities, following the description of motor and sensory aphasias (Broca 1861; Wernicke 1874; see also Freud 1891). A few years later, Déjerine and Sérieux (1897) described a case of sensory aphasia with bilateral temporal atrophy. Pick went on to report four additional cases with temporal lobe atrophy and language disturbances (Pick 1901, 1904). In 1906, he described a patient with disinhibition and mixed apraxia who had severe bilateral frontal and left-sided parietal atrophy, with a more moderate atrophy of the left temporal lobe (Pick 1906). Pick was mainly interested in comparing the clinical picture with the macroscopic appearance of the brain. He made no systematic attempt at identifying histopathological abnormalities. Alzheimer discovered the association of argyrophilic intracytoplasmic inclusions and ballooned neurons with lobar cortical atrophy, in the absence of the plaques and tangles he had described four years earlier (Alzheimer 1907, 1911). This revealed the existence of a second type of intraneuronal inclusion and established that different inclusions can characterize distinct clinical entities.

Richter proposed that lobar cortical atrophies are hereditary diseases (Richter 1918) and Gans, a pupil of Pick, linked his mentor's name to cases of lobar cortical atrophy (Gans 1923). Additional examples of frontal and/or temporal cortical atrophy with or without argyrophilic inclusions were subsequently reported and the clinical condition was called "Pick's disease" (Onari and Spatz 1926; Stertz 1926). Unlike Pick, who believed to have described atypical forms of senile dementia, Onari and Spatz considered Pick's disease to be a distinct entity. One of their patients (Therese Mühlich) had already been described by Alzheimer. Carl Schneider proposed a three-stage model for the clinical course of Pick's disease (Schneider 1927, 1929). In most individuals, the first stage is characterized by disinhibition and impaired judgement, although Schneider recognized that amnestic aphasia is the presenting symptom of temporal lobe atrophy. The second stage is dominated by progressive dementia and focal symptoms, such as apathy in frontal lobe atrophy and sensory aphasia in temporal lobe atrophy. Stereotyped

perseverations of speech, movement, and facial expression also appear. The third stage is characterized by dementia and severe language problems, resulting in a vegetative state with flexion contractures. Schneider concluded that the argyrophilic inclusions and ballooned cells described by Alzheimer were diagnostic of Pick's disease. Similar cases were described in the 1930s, when it became clear that lobar cortical atrophy has a high degree of heritability, irrespective of the presence of argyrophilic inclusions (Grünthal 1930; Verhaart 1930; Von Braunmühl and Leonhard 1934). The link between frontal lobe dementia and MND was also recognized (Meyer 1929; Von Braunmühl 1932). The early work was summarized and discussed by Van Mansvelt (1954) and Lüers and Spatz (1957).

Interest in the focal dementias waned after World War II, before it was rekindled in the 1970s and 1980s. Cases of Pick's disease with argyrophilic inclusions and ballooned neurons (type A) were now distinguished from those with ballooned neurons lacking argyrophilic inclusions (type B) and those lacking both ballooned neurons and argyrophilic inclusions (type C) (Constantinidis 1974). Work by Brun, Gustafson, and Neary showed that some individuals with frontal lobe atrophy lacked a distinctive histopathology (Brun 1987; Gustafson 1987; Neary et al. 1988). Clinically, these patients suffered from a severe personality disorder, which is now known as behavioral-variant FTD (bvFTD). Mesulam described primary progressive aphasia (PPA), with an isolated language deficit as the most prominent presenting feature, in the absence of strokes or tumors (Mesulam 1982, 1987, 2001). PPA has been divided into three syndromes (Gorno-Tempini et al. 2011): (1) Semantic dementia (SD), also known as semantic variant PPA, a fluent aphasia with loss of word meaning (Snowden et al. 1989); (2) progressive nonfluent aphasia (PNFA), also known as nonfluent/ agrammatic variant PPA, a disorder characterized by effortful, nonfluent speech (Grossman et al. 1996); and (3) logopenic progressive aphasia (LPA), also known as logopenic variant PPA, a nonfluent aphasia with deficits in word retrieval and sentence repetition (Gorno-Tempini et al. 2004b).

Symptoms correlate better with specific patterns of brain atrophy than with the underlying neuropathology. Prediction of the neuropathology based on clinical picture remains challenging. FTD is the third most common cause of early-onset dementia (disease onset <65 years), after Alzheimer disease and vascular dementia (Rossor et al. 2010). Approximately 40% of patients with FTD have a family history, but only 10% of cases are inherited in a dominant manner. Links exist with the corticobasal syndrome (CBS), progressive supranuclear palsy (PSP), parkinsonism, and MND.

CLINICAL PRESENTATIONS OF FRONTOTEMPORAL DEMENTIA

Behavioral-Variant Frontotemporal Dementia (bvFTD)

bvFTD comprises more than half of the cases of FTD and is the most heritable form. Presenting features are insidious and include progressive changes in the patient's personality, interpersonal conduct, and emotional modulation (Gustafson 1987; Neary et al. 1988; Piguet et al. 2011a). A variable degree of language impairment is also present. Apathy manifesting as passivity, inertia, reduced motivation, and social withdrawal, associated with a lack of insight, is common. Disinhibition often coexists alongside apathy and manifests itself by impulsivity. Emotional blunting characterized by a lack of empathy is common. Abnormal eating behavior can be extensive, resulting in marked weight gain. Stereotypic and ritualistic behavior is common, as expressed by motor stereotyping, including humming, lip smacking, hand ruffling, and foot tapping. Neglect of self-care and impairment of other activities of daily living are common. Most patients are unable to manage their financial affairs. Memory is relatively spared in the early stages of bvFTD. By neuroimaging, four subtypes have been identified based on relative grey matter loss: frontal-dominant, frontotemporal, temporofrontoparietal, and temporal-dominant (Whitwell et al. 2009a). Combined

frontotemporal and basal ganglion atrophy can also be present, as can atrophy of a number of other subcortical regions. bvFTD and Alzheimer disease lead to divergent network activity patterns, with atrophy in an anterior salience network in bvFTD and a posterior default mode network in Alzheimer disease (Zhou et al. 2010).

Semantic Dementia (SD)

SD is a progressive fluent aphasia, which is characterized by the loss of word meaning (Snowden et al. 1989; Hodges and Patterson 2007). Patients have difficulty in finding words, with anomia being a defining feature. They also complain of memory loss, but this does not in general reflect true amnesia. Although language deficits predominate, behavioral alterations also occur. SD is the least heritable FTD syndrome. A deficit in naming and word comprehension predominates, with the patient's vocabulary being depleted of all but the most common words. However, speech is fluent and the syntax correct. This is often coupled with deficits in person recognition, especially when the right temporal lobe is affected. Although patients are insightful and can be distressed by their condition, lack of empathy and mental inflexibility are common. Restriction of food preferences is present without the overeating characteristic of bvFTD. Compulsive behavior is prominent and centers on visual objects (left temporal lobe predominance) or on letters, words, and symbols (right temporal lobe predominance). By neuroimaging of grey matter, bilateral, often asymmetric, anterior temporal lobe atrophy is most prominent. The hippocampus can also be affected (Mummery et al. 1999). White matter changes are found in the ventral language pathways and the temporal components of the dorsal language pathways (Galantucci et al. 2011).

Progressive Nonfluent Aphasia (PNFA)

PNFA is a disorder of expressive language. Patients lose the ability to speak fluently, with relative preservation of word comprehension and nonlinguistic cognition (Grossman et al.

1996). Several speech changes characterize PNFA. At an early stage, patients speak less than normal and in shorter sentences. They show speech apraxia, with effortful speech and phonological errors. Word finding difficulty is commonly observed, often resulting in muteness. Behavioral features similar to those of bvFTD may occur, but they are usually mild, with apathy being most common. As the disease progresses, extrapyramidal features become widespread and can lead to a change in diagnosis (Gorno-Tempini et al. 2004a). Heritability of PNFA is intermediate between that of bvFTD and SD. Neuroimaging shows a widening of the Sylvian fissure, with atrophy of left posterior frontal and insular regions (Neary et al. 2003; Nestor et al. 2003). In white matter, the most prominent changes are found in the dorsal language pathways (Galantucci et al. 2011).

Logopenic Progressive Aphasia (LPA)

LPA is a progressive nonfluent aphasia, which is characterized by a slow speech rate and word retrieval difficulties (Gorno-Tempini et al. 2004b, 2008). Repetition of phrases is also markedly impaired, in part as a result of limited auditory-verbal short-term memory. Single-word comprehension and semantic association are largely preserved. It differs from the fast output typical of patients with SD and the agrammatism and articulation deficits characteristic of PNFA. However, a language variant of Alzheimer disease overlaps with LPA (Galton et al. 2000; Alladi et al. 2007). It has been suggested that LPA and posterior cortical atrophy are clinical presentations of sporadic, early-onset Alzheimer disease (Migliaccio et al. 2009). This nonmemory phenotype characterizes about one quarter of patients (Van der Flier et al. 2011). Inheritance of the *APOE* ε4 allele appears not to be a risk factor for LPA and posterior cortical atrophy, distinguishing them from the more common amnestic forms of Alzheimer disease (Strittmatter and Roses 1995). Neuroimaging of LPA shows atrophy or hypoperfusion of the left posterior superior and middle temporal regions, and of the inferior parietal region (Gorno-Tempini et al.

2004b). Brain atrophy is located more posteriorly than in SD and PNFA. White matter changes are most marked in the temporoparietal component of the dorsal language pathway (Galantucci et al. 2011).

Frontotemporal Dementia and Corticobasal Syndrome (CBS)

CBS and PSP are atypical parkinsonian disorders. CBS is characterized by extrapyramidal symptoms consisting of progressive asymmetric rigidity and dystonia, and by signs of cortical dysfunction in the form of PNFA, apraxia, cortical sensory loss, alien limb syndrome, myoclonus, and hemineglect. For many years, the emphasis was on the extrapyramidal component, even though similarities with Pick's disease were noticed early on (Rebeiz et al. 1968). More recent work has shown that patients with CBS can have aphasia or a behavioral disorder characteristic of bvFTD (Lippa et al. 1991; Kertesz et al. 1994). Pathologically, CBS is heterogenous, but its most common form is corticobasal degeneration (CBD). Some cases of CBS are dominantly inherited. Neuroimaging shows variable frontoparietal and basal ganglion atrophy (Whitwell et al. 2010).

Frontotemporal Dementia and Progressive Supranuclear Palsy (PSP)

The clinical presentation of PSP includes vertical supranuclear ophtalmoplegia with difficulty looking up, bradykinesia, axial dystonia and rigidity, pseudobulbar palsy and postural instability with backward falls (Steele et al. 1964; Litvan et al. 1996). More than half of the patients develop cognitive impairment. Apathy and emotional blunting, accompanied by mental slowness and reduced verbal fluency, are common. A small percentage of cases of PSP is inherited. By neuroimaging, atrophy in premotor and supplemental motor areas is observed, with sparing of the inferior frontal lobe (Whitwell et al. 2010). Some patients show PNFA with early apraxia of speech (Josephs et al. 2006). Three subtypes of PSP have been described: Richardson's syndrome,

PSP-parkinsonism, and PSP-pure akinesia with gait freezing (Williams and Lees 2009). Cognitive impairment and cortical atrophy are most prominent in Richardson's syndrome, which corresponds to classical PSP.

Frontotemporal Dementia and Parkinsonism Linked to Chromosome 17 (FTDP-17)

In the 1980s and 1990s, dominantly inherited forms of FTD were identified (Ghetti et al. 2011). Extrapyramidal signs resembling CBS and PSP also featured prominently. Amyotrophy was present in some cases. These forms of inherited FTD were given different names according to their predominant clinical and pathological features, including familial Pick's disease, disinhibition-dementia-parkinsonism-amyotrophy complex, familial progressive subcortical gliosis, familial presenile dementia with tangles, autosomal-dominant parkinsonism, dementia with pallido-ponto-nigral degeneration, and multiple system tauopathy with presenile dementia. Despite this heterogeneity, disease was linked to the long arm of chromosome 17 (Wilhelmsen et al. 1994). The syndrome received its name at a consensus conference during which 13 families were presented (Foster et al. 1997). FTDP-17 is divided into a dementia-dominant and a parkinsonism-dominant type. Neuroimaging shows variable frontotemporoparietal and basal ganglion atrophy (Whitwell et al. 2009b).

Frontotemporal Dementia with Motor Neuron Disease (MND)

MND can be associated with cognitive dysfunction (Morita et al. 1987). Mild frontal lobe involvement is found in 30% of cases and in ~3% of cases FTD is present (Shaw 2010). A psychotic phase consisting of vivid delusions is an early sign. Behavioral and cognitive changes tend to predate MND. Bulbar signs are common and electromyography is as in MND. Inherited cases of FTD-MND have been linked to chromosome 9p21 (Vance et al. 2006). Neuroimaging shows posterior frontal lobe atrophy (Whitwell et al. 2006). Based on the presence of isolated upper MND in some cases, further subclassification of FTD-MND has been proposed (Josephs and Dickson 2007).

HISTOPATHOLOGY OF FRONTOTEMPORAL LOBAR DEGENERATION (FTLD)

FTLD-Tau

In 1986, the argyrophilic inclusions of Pick's disease were shown to be immunoreactive for hyperphosphorylated tau (Pollock et al. 1986), a normally soluble microtubule-associated protein that stabilizes microtubules and promotes microtubule assembly. It followed the finding that the intracellular inclusions of Alzheimer disease stain for hyperphosphorylated tau (Brion et al. 1985; Grundke-Iqbal et al. 1986). In adult human brain, six tau isoforms are expressed from a single *MAPT* gene through alternative mRNA splicing (Fig. 1A) (Goedert et al. 1989a,b). Three isoforms have three repeats each and three isoforms have four repeats each. By 1992, the paired helical filament of Alzheimer disease had been shown to be made of the six tau isoforms, each full-length and hyperphosphorylated (Goedert et al. 1988, 1992; Wischik et al. 1988; Lee et al. 1991). Filamentous tau inclusions were subsequently shown to be characteristic of many cases of FTDP-17 (Spillantini et al. 1996, 1998a).

Around 40% of patients with FTD show tau inclusions (Fig. 2). They include most cases of PNFA, ~45% of cases of bvFTD and some cases of SD (Piguet et al. 2011a). Most cases of LPA are characterized by focal Alzheimer disease pathology (Aβ plaques and tau tangles), as are some cases of SD and PNFA (Mesulam et al. 2008; Rabinovici et al. 2008). Focal Alzheimer disease pathology accounts for ~25% of autopsy cases of PPA. A frontal variant of Alzheimer disease has also been described (Johnson et al. 1999). Tau inclusions are characteristic of Pick's disease, PSP, and CBD, which belongs to the CBS spectrum (Goedert and Spillantini 2006). They are not typical of FTD-MND, even though MND can occur in conjunction with FTD and tauopathy (Fu et al. 2010).

M. Goedert et al.

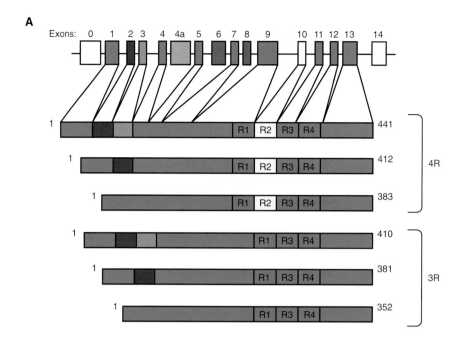

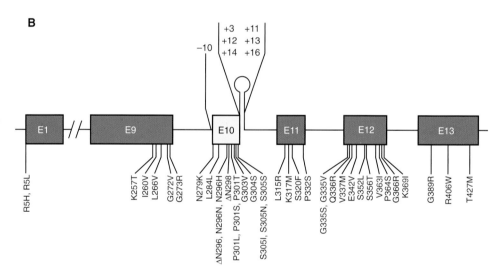

Figure 1. *MAPT* and the six tau isoforms expressed in adult human brain and mutations in *MAPT* in fronto-temporal dementia and parkinsonism linked to chromosome 17. (*A*) *MAPT* consists of 16 exons (E). Alternative mRNA splicing of E2 (red), E3 (green), and E10 (yellow) gives rise to six tau isoforms (352-441 amino acids). The constitutively spliced exons (E1, E4, E5, E7, E9, E11, E12, E13) are indicated in blue. E0, which is part of the promoter, and E14 are noncoding (white). E6 and E8 (violet) are not transcribed in human brain. E4a (orange) is only expressed in the peripheral nervous system. The repeats of tau (R1–R4) are shown, with three isoforms having four repeats each (4R) and three isoforms having three repeats each (3R). Each repeat is 31 or 32 amino acids in length. (*B*) Shown are 39 coding region mutations in E1, E9, E10, E11, E12, and E13 as well as seven intronic mutations flanking E10.

Cite this article as *Cold Spring Harb Perspect Med* doi: 10.1101/cshperspect.a006254

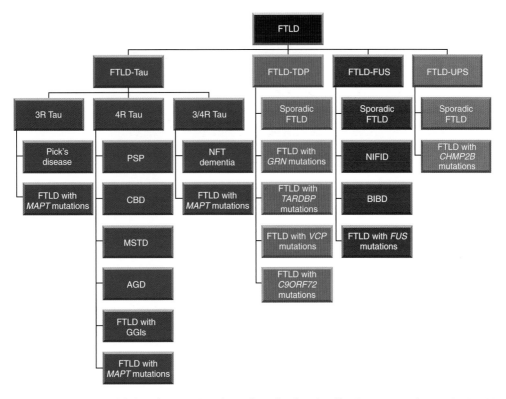

Figure 2. Frontotemporal lobar degeneration (FTLD) molecular classification. Four subtypes (FTLD-Tau, FTLD-TDP, FTLD-FUS, and FTLD-UPS) can be distinguished, based on what is known about the major components that make up the pathological deposits (Tau protein, TDP-43, FUS and unknown protein). FTLD-Tau and FTLD-TDP are more common than FTLD-FUS and FTLD-UPS. Tau deposits are made of either three-repeat (3R), four-repeat (4R) or all six (3/4R) brain isoforms of tau. Together, FTLD-TDP, FTLD-FUS, and FTLD-UPS make up FTLD-U, which is characterized by the presence of tau-negative, ubiquitin-positive inclusions. In some cases of FTLD-U, the ubiquitinated protein is unknown; they are classified as FTLD-UPS, to indicate that the inclusions can currently only be identified by markers of the ubiquitin-proteasome system. Abbreviations: PSP, progressive supranuclear palsy; CBD, corticobasal degeneration; MSTD, multiple system tauopathy with presenile dementia; AGD, argyrophilic grain disease; GGI, globular glial inclusion; NIFID, neuronal intermediate filament inclusion disease; BIBD, basophilic inclusion body disease; UPS, ubiquitin-proteasome system.

The anatomical distribution of pathology rather than its molecular identity determines the nature of the clinical syndromes. In most cases of Alzheimer disease, the locus coeruleus, entorhinal cortex, and hippocampus are the initial targets of neurofibrillary pathology, with the neocortex becoming affected later (Braak and Del Tredici 2011). In Pick's disease, tau inclusions predominate in the cerebral cortex, resulting in FTD (Piguet et al. 2011b). In PSP, patients with Richardson's syndrome have a higher tau burden and a different distribution of inclusions than patients with PSP-parkinsonism (Williams et al. 2007). The subthalamic nucleus, substantia nigra, and globus pallidus are the most affected brain regions. In CBD, apraxia, rigidity, dystonia, and frontal lobe signs reflect the presence of neuronal and glial tau deposits in brainstem, basal ganglia, and cerebral cortex (Feany and Dickson 1995).

The repeats of tau form the core of the filaments whose isoform composition varies between diseases. The assembly of four-repeat tau into filaments is characteristic of PSP,

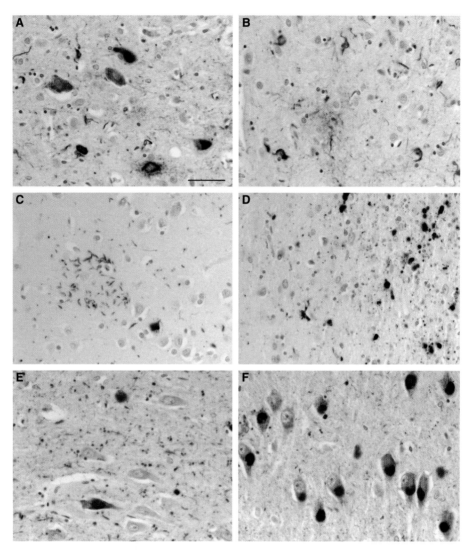

Figure 3. FTLD-Tau. Inclusions in progressive supranuclear palsy (*A,B*), corticobasal degeneration (*C*), white matter tauopathy with globular glial inclusions (*D*), argyrophilic grain disease (*E*), and Pick's disease (*F*). Progressive supranuclear palsy, corticobasal degeneration, white matter tauopathy with globular glial inclusions and argyrophilic grain disease are four-repeat tauopathies with abundant neuronal and glial tau filaments. Pick's disease is a three-repeat tauopathy with abundant neuronal tau filaments. Scale bar, 50 μm.

CBD, and many cases of FTDP-17 (Fig. 3). It is also typical of argyrophilic grain disease and white matter tauopathy with globular glial inclusions, which belong to the FTD spectrum. A combination of neuronal and glial tau pathology is in evidence, with the glial pathology predominating in white matter tauopathy with globular glial inclusions (Kovacs et al. 2008).

In contrast, in Pick's disease and some cases of FTDP-17, three-repeat tau predominates in the neuronal inclusions (Fig. 3), whereas in Alzheimer disease, other diseases with extracellular deposits, Guam Parkinsonism-dementia complex, tangle-only dementia, and some cases of FTDP-17, both three- and four-repeat tau isoforms make up the neurofibrillary lesions.

Distinct sets of tau isoforms in different neuro-degenerative diseases and the presence of morphologically distinct filaments have led to the suggestion that self-propagating conformers of tau may exist (Goedert et al. 2010), akin to the prion strains accounting for the conformational variability of PrP^{Sc} (Colby and Prusiner 2011). In support, experimental evidence for the intercellular transfer of tau aggregates has been adduced (Clavaguera et al. 2009; Frost et al. 2009).

FTLD-TDP

By 2006, most cases of FTLD were known to exhibit either tau-positive or tau-negative inclusions (FTLD-U) (Fig. 2). The latter were first described in patients with MND (Okamoto et al. 1991). Four histological subtypes (A–D)

of FTLD-U can be distinguished (Fig. 4) (Mackenzie et al. 2006, 2011; Sampathu et al. 2006). Type A is associated with bvFTD and PFNA, type B with bvFTD and FTD-MND, type C with SD, and type D with familial inclusion body myopathy with Paget's disease of the bone and frontotemporal dementia (IBMPFD).

In 2006, transactive response-DNA binding protein-43 (TDP-43) was identified as the major component of the inclusions in most cases of FTLD-U (Figs. 2 and 4), MND, and FTLD-MND (Arai et al. 2006; Neumann et al. 2006). Around 50% of patients with FTD have TDP-43 inclusions. They include most cases of SD, ~45% of cases of bvFTD, as well as some cases of PNFA, LPA, FTDP-17, CBS, and PSP (Piguet et al. 2011a). Most cases of FTD-MND belong to the TDP-43 proteinopathy group. In Alzheimer disease, TDP-43 deposits

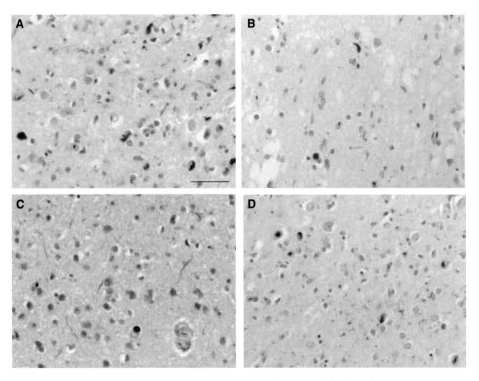

Figure 4. FTLD-TDP: Histological subtypes (A–D). Type A is characterized by abundant TDP-43-immunoreactive compact neuronal cytoplasmic inclusions and short dystrophic neurites, often with neuronal intranuclear inclusions (A); type B by abundant compact and granular cytoplasmic inclusions (B); type C by abundant long dystrophic neurites (C); and type D by abundant lentiform neuronal intranuclear inclusions and many short dystrophic neurites (D). Scale bar, 50 μm.

are found in a minority of cases in conjunction with the characteristic plaques and tangles (Amador-Ortiz et al. 2007).

TDP-43 is a ubiquitously expressed 414 amino acid RNA-binding protein of the heterogenous nuclear ribonucleoprotein (hnRNP) family with two RNA recognition motifs, nuclear localization and export signals, and a carboxy-terminal glycine-rich region. The glycine-rich region is predicted to show a prion domain, based on an algorithm that identifies yeast prion domains (Cushman et al. 2010). TDP-43 binds to noncoding RNAs, introns, and the 3′-untranslated regions of mRNAs, indicating a role in the integration of gene regulation. It functions as a transcriptional repressor and splicing modulator. UV-crosslinking and immunoprecipitation analysis has shown that TDP-43 has thousands of potential targets, with a preference for long clusters of UG-rich intronic sequences (Polymenidou et al. 2011; Tollerey et al. 2011). It binds to ∼30% of the mouse transcriptome. TDP-43 negatively regulates its own mRNA and protein through binding to a long UG-rich region in its 3′-untranslated region (Ayala et al. 2011). It is predominantly nuclear, even though it normally shuttles between nucleus and cytoplasm. In FTD, TDP-43 it is found mainly in the cytoplasm in a hyperphosphorylated, ubiquitinated, and truncated form (Hasegawa et al. 2008).

FTLD-FUS

Most cases of FTLD-U show TDP-43 inclusions. In 2009, inclusions made of fused in sarcoma (FUS) were shown to account for the bulk of TDP-43-negative FTLD-U (Fig. 2) (Neumann et al. 2009a), following the discovery that mutations in *FUS* cause familial forms of ALS (Kwiatkowski et al. 2009; Vance et al. 2009). Less than 10% of cases of FTLD have FUS inclusions. They include atypical cases of FTLD-U, basophilic inclusion body disease, and neuronal intermediate filament inclusion body disease (Munoz et al. 2009; Neumann et al. 2009a,b). Neuroimaging of FTLD-FUS shows atrophy of frontoinsular and cingulate cortex, and of the head of the caudate nucleus (Josephs et al. 2010;

Seelaar et al. 2010). FTD-FUS should be suspected when disease onset is before 40 years of age, in the absence of a family history of FTD, and the presence of caudate atrophy. This is reminiscent of a case from the early literature (Bonfiglio 1938). The existence of cases of PPA with FUS inclusions remains to be demonstrated.

FUS is a widely expressed 526 amino acid protein with an amino-terminal region rich in QGSY residues, a glycine-rich region, an RNA recognition motif, two RGG domains, and a zinc finger motif. Like TDP-43, it is a DNA/RNA-binding protein that is involved in transcriptional and translational regulation, as well as in mRNA splicing and transport. The predicted prion domain of FUS resides in the amino-terminal region (Cushman et al. 2010). In normal brain, FUS is concentrated in the nucleus, with smaller amounts in the cytoplasm. In FTD, the ability of FUS to shuttle to the nucleus is impaired, resulting in its cytoplasmic accumulation. FUS inclusions contain the full-length protein (Neumann et al. 2009a). Staining for TDP-43 and FUS appears to be mutually exclusive, suggestive of distinct subtypes of FTLD-U.

FTLD-UPS

FTLD-TDP and FTLD-FUS account for the majority of cases of FTLD-U. Additional forms remain to be discovered, because inclusions that are negative for TDP-43 and FUS, but positive for components of the ubiquitin-proteasome system (UPS), have been described (Fig. 2) (Holm et al. 2009).

GENETICS OF FRONTOTEMPORAL DEMENTIA

Dominantly inherited FTD is caused by mutations in seven genes. Mutations in *MAPT* (Hutton et al. 1998; Poorkaj et al. 1998; Spillantini et al. 1998b), chromosome 9 open reading frame 72 (*C9ORF72*) (DeJesus-Hernandez et al. 2011; Renton et al. 2011), and progranulin (*GRN*) (Baker et al. 2006; Cruts et al. 2006) are the most common. The other four genes are *TARDBP* (Benajiba et al. 2009; Kovacs et al. 2009), *FUS*

(Ticozzi et al. 2009), valosin-containing protein (*VCP*) (Watts et al. 2004), and charged multivesicular body protein 2B (*CHMP2B*) (Skibinski et al. 2005).

Mutations in *MAPT*

Mutations in *MAPT* account for ∼5% of cases of FTD and are believed to cause disease through a gain of toxic function mechanism. Most mutations are located in exons 9–12 (which encode the repeats) and the adjacent introns (Fig. 1B). It remains to be determined whether the amino acid changes in codon 5 of exon 1 are pathogenic. Mutations fall into two largely nonoverlapping groups: those with a primary effect at the protein level and those influencing the alternative splicing of tau pre-mRNA. Mutations acting at the protein level change or delete single amino acids in tau. This reduces the ability of tau to interact with microtubules, suggesting that this interaction is crucial for preventing the self-assembly of tau (Hasegawa et al. 1998). Some mutations also promote the assembly of tau into filaments (Goedert et al. 1999; Nacharaju et al. 1999). Mutations having their primary effect at the RNA level are intronic or exonic and increase the alternative mRNA splicing of exon 10. This changes the ratio of 3- to 4-repeat isoforms, resulting in the relative overproduction of 4-repeat tau and the formation of filamentous inclusions made of 4-repeat tau.

Cases with *MAPT* mutations show abundant filamentous inclusions made of hyperphosphorylated tau in either nerve cells or in both nerve cells and glial cells. Clinical and neuropathological phenotypes similar or identical to those of Pick's disease, PSP, CBD, and argyrophilic grain disease have been described. A given mutation can lead to different clinical syndromes in an individual family. Thus, mutation P301S in exon 10 of *MAPT* caused bvFTD in a father and CBD in his son (Bugiani et al. 1999), supporting the view that FTD and CBS are part of the same disease spectrum (Kertesz et al. 2000).

Haplotypes H1 and H2 characterize *MAPT* in populations of European descent. They result from a 900 kb inversion/noninversion (H1/H2) polymorphism (Stefansson et al. 2005). Inheritance of the H1 haplotype is a risk factor for PSP and CBD (Williams and Lees 2009). This was confirmed in a genome-wide association study of PSP, which also implicated proteins involved in vesicle traffic, the unfolded protein response and the innate immune system (Höglinger et al. 2011). Heterozygous microdeletions in the chromosomal region, which defines the H1 and H2 haplotypes, give rise to a clinical phenotype consisting of mental retardation, hypotonia, and a characteristic face (Koolen et al. 2006; Sharp et al. 2006; Shaw-Smith et al. 2006). Besides *MAPT*, the deleted region comprises five additional genes [corticotrophin-releasing hormone receptor 1 (*CRHR1*), intramembrane protease 5 (*IMP5*), *NP 689679.1*, *NP 787078.1*, and *KIAA1267*]. Deletions occur on the H2 haplotype through low-copy repeat-mediated nonallelic homologous recombination. An association has also been described between the H1 haplotype and idiopathic Parkinson's disease (Pastor et al. 2000), a disease without tau inclusions. The elevated risk of PSP and CBD conferred by the H1 haplotype appears to promote *MAPT* transcription and incorporation of exon 10, resulting in increased levels of four-repeat tau (Caffrey et al. 2006).

Mutations in *C9ORF72*

The cause of chromosome 9p21-linked FTD-MND has been identified as a hexanucleotide (GGGGCC) expansion in the noncoding region of *C9ORF72*, a gene that encodes a protein of unknown function (DeJesus-Hernandez et al. 2011; Renton et al. 2011). The hexanucleotide expansion leads to the loss of an alternatively spliced transcript and the formation of nuclear RNA foci. The latter may be toxic. The repeat expansion in *C9ORF72* is also a common cause of isolated FTD and MND.

Mutations in *GRN*

Mutations in *GRN* account for ∼5% of cases of FTD and cause disease by a loss of function mechanism. Progranulin is a 593 amino acid glycoprotein consisting of 7.5 tandem repeats of a 12-cysteine granulin motif. Although its function is only incompletely understood, progranulin may be a physiological antagonist of tumor necrosis α signaling (Tang et al. 2011). It has been reported to act on nerve cells by binding to sortilin following release from activated microglial cells (Hu et al. 2010). Mutations in *GRN* include gene deletions, as well as nonsense, frameshift, and splice-site mutations that cause premature termination, creating null alleles with the mutant RNAs being degraded by nonsense-mediated decay (Van Swieten and Heutink 2008). Known mutations result in haploinsufficiency, implying that progranulin is critical for the survival of neurons in adult brain. Reduced levels of plasma progranulin have been used to identify mutation carriers (Ghidoni et al. 2008). Mutations in *GRN* cause diseases belonging to the whole spectrum of FTD, with a predominance of bvFTD and PNFA (Yu et al. 2010). Parietal deficits and CBS have been observed (Spina et al. 2007). This is reflected in frontotemporoparietal cortical atrophy. Cases with *GRN* mutations show type A TDP-43 inclusions (Mackenzie et al. 2006), showing that a reduction in progranulin levels causes the accumulation of TDP-43. Unlike *TARDBP* mutations, mutations in *GRN* do not appear to cause MND. In a genome-wide study of FTLD-TDP, significant association was detected with three single nucleotide polymorphisms in the transmembrane protein 106B locus (*TMEM106B*) (Van Deerlin et al. 2010). It was most significant in patients with *GRN* mutations.

Mutations in *TARDBP*

Mutations in *TARDBP* are mostly associated with inherited forms of MND, consistent with the presence of TDP-43 inclusions in upper and lower motor neurons in patients with the disease (Gitcho et al. 2008; Sreedharan et al. 2008; Yokoseki et al. 2008). *TARDBP* mutations have also been described in two patients with bvFTD and SD who went on to develop MND (Benajiba et al. 2009). Histopathological changes were not documented. One patient

with a K263E change in *TARDBP* developed FTD, supranuclear palsy, and chorea, in the absence of MND. Abundant neuronal and glial TDP-43 deposits were in evidence, especially in brainstem and subcortical nuclei (Kovacs et al. 2009). The mechanisms by which mutations in *TARDBP* cause neurodegeneration are unclear. Pathological assembly is associated with a marked reduction in nuclear TDP-43 staining (Neumann et al. 2006) and the cytoplasmic accumulation of TDP-43 is believed to be an early event (Giordana et al. 2010). A combination of loss of function and gain of toxic function mechanisms may be at play. Wild-type TDP-43 is prone to aggregation and disease-causing mutations increase its aggregation and toxicity (Johnson et al. 2009). Many disease-causing mutations are located in the carboxy-terminal domain of TDP-43.

Mutations in *FUS*

Mutations in *FUS* cause inherited forms of MND (Kwiatkowski et al. 2009; Vance et al. 2009). Patients have FUS inclusions in spinal cord and cerebral cortex. Cases of FTD and/or FTD-MND may also be caused by mutations in *FUS* (Ticozzi et al. 2009), but larger clinico-pathological series must be awaited. Like mutant TDP-43, mutant FUS accumulates in the cytoplasm, where it is found in stress granules (Dormann et al. 2010; Nishimoto et al. 2010). Wild-type FUS is prone to aggregation, but disease-causing mutations do not increase its aggregation or toxicity (Sun et al. 2011). The mutations appear to cause cytoplasmic mislocalization instead. Although several disease-causing mutations are present in its amino-terminal region, most mutations are located in the carboxy-terminus of FUS.

Mutations in *VCP*

Mutations in *VCP* cause IBMPFD through what appears to be a gain of function (Watts et al. 2004), possibly as the result of a dominant negative effect. IBMPFD affects skeletal muscle, bone, and nervous system, with dementia developing in ∼30% of patients. It is characterized by the presence of type D TDP-43 inclusions (Neumann et al. 2007). Some missense mutations in *VCP* cause inherited MND (Johnson et al. 2010) and motor neuron abnormalities are present in many patients with IBMPFD. Furthermore, a missense mutation in *vacuolar protein sorting 54* (*Vps54*), the homolog of *VCP*, causes motor neuron degeneration in the wobbler mouse, a model of MND (Schmitt-John et al. 2005). VCP belongs to the type II AAA$^+$ (ATPases associated with a variety of activities) family and takes part in multiple cellular processes, including protein quality control, nuclear functions, and the regulation of membrane dynamics. It extracts ubiquitinated proteins from complexes, so that they can be degraded by the proteasome. VCP promotes autophagic protein degradation, with disease-causing mutations giving rise to defective autophagosome maturation (Ju and Weihl 2010). Transgenic mice expressing mutant VCP show many characteristics of IBMPFD, including involvement of skeletal muscle, bone and brain, and show increased activation of NF-κB signaling (Custer et al. 2010). In the brain of these mice, TDP-43 is redistributed from the nucleus to the cytoplasm, in the absence of nuclear inclusions. In a *Drosophila* model of IBMPFD, a genetic screen has identified TBPH, the fly ortholog of TDP-43, as one of three RNA-binding proteins that dominantly suppress degeneration (Ritson et al. 2010). In this model, VCP mutations lead to the redistribution of TDP-43 to the cytoplasm.

Mutations in *CHMP2B*

Mutations in *CHMP2B* appear to cause disease through a loss of function (Skibinski et al. 2005). The early signs are those of bvFTD, with extrapyramidal symptoms developing later, resulting in a clinical picture of CBS (Gydesen et al. 2002). In a Danish family with a truncating *CHMP2B* mutation, the intracytoplasmic inclusions are ubiquitin-positive, but negative for TDP-43 and FUS (Holm et al. 2009). CHMP2B is a component of the endosomal-sorting complex required for transport-III (ESCRT-III), which is involved in the

degradation of proteins in the endocytic and autophagic pathways. A disruption of these processes results in the accumulation of autophagosomes, possibly leading to FTD (Lee et al. 2007).

IMPLICATIONS FOR UNDERSTANDING ALZHEIMER DISEASE

For a long time, tau inclusions were believed by many to be epiphenomena of little relevance. Reasons underlying this negative stance were the absence of genetic evidence linking dysfunction of tau to neurodegeneration and the presence of tau pathology in diseases other than Alzheimer disease. Things changed with the identification of mutations in *MAPT* in cases of FTDP-17 with filamentous tau pathology, establishing that dysfunction of tau is sufficient to cause neurodegeneration and dementia (Hutton et al. 1998; Poorkaj et al. 1998; Spillantini et al. 1998b). Thus, a pathway leading from soluble to insoluble, filamentous tau is central to the neurodegenerative process in the human tauopathies. It is therefore important to understand the mechanisms underlying tau aggregation and its downstream consequences for cell function. With the benefit of hindsight, it is clear that Alzheimer's description of silver-positive inclusions in cases with either presenile dementia or lobar cortical atrophy marked the beginning of the tauopathy field.

The crucial importance of FTDP-17T is that it proves that mutations in *MAPT* can lead to neurofibrillary assembly, neurodegeneration and dementia, in the absence of Aβ amyloid deposits. The morphologies of tau filaments observed in the various forms of FTDP-17T vary (Crowther and Goedert 2000). Some mutations, such as V337M and R406W, produce filaments that appear identical to the paired helical and straight filaments of Alzheimer disease (Spillantini et al. 1996; Reed et al. 1997; Hutton et al. 1998; Poorkaj et al. 1998). All six tau isoforms are affected by the mutations and are incorporated into the filaments, which give rise to a pattern of tau bands on SDS-PAGE identical to that seen in Alzheimer disease. Mutation G389R also affects all six tau isoforms and the majority of filaments resemble the straight filaments of Alzheimer disease (Murrell et al. 1999), despite the presence of Pick-like bodies by light microscopy. In contrast, in the case of mutations that increase the splicing of exon 10, the filaments appear as irregularly twisted ribbons, which are made of tau isoforms with four repeats (Spillantini et al. 1997). In the case of mutation P301L in exon 10, which affects only four-repeat tau isoforms, the majority of filaments consists of narrow, irregularly twisted ribbons, with a smaller number of straight filaments (Spillantini et al. 1998c).

Unlike Alzheimer disease and several other neurodegenerative diseases with tau inclusions, most cases of FTD lack extracellular deposits. However, focal Alzheimer disease pathology is diagnostic of a significant proportion of cases of PPA. Crossing mice transgenic for human mutant amyloid precursor protein with mice transgenic for human mutant tau results in increased tau deposition in some brain regions (Lewis et al. 2001). Similarly, in mice transgenic for the Danish mutant form of human BRI2 and mutant tau, the extracellular deposition of Dan-amyloid promotes tau phosphorylation and aggregation (Coomaraswamy et al. 2010). Phosphorylation of tau by GSK3β and AMP-activated protein kinase is a potential mechanism. This is consistent with the coexistence of extracellular amyloid deposits and intraneuronal tau inclusions in Alzheimer disease, familial British and Danish dementias, and in some diseases caused by mutations in the prion protein gene (Ghetti et al. 1994; Vidal et al. 2004; Goedert and Spillantini 2006). It suggests that extracellular amyloid deposits with a certain conformation trigger the intraneuronal assembly of tau into filaments.

Tau is required for Aβ toxicity in experimental models (Roberson et al. 2007). The absence of Aβ toxicity in mice lacking *MAPT* may result from a reduction in excitotoxicity, because of the decreased dendritic localization of the tyrosine kinase Fyn, resulting in hypophosphorylation of the NMDA receptor and a reduced interaction with postsynaptic density protein-95 (Ittner at al. 2010). Haploinsufficiency of p73, a member of the p53 protein family, has been found to be associated with the formation of tau aggregates in nerve cells and to potentiate Aβ toxicity, possibly through the activation of stress-activated protein kinases (Wetzel et al. 2008).

The intraneuronal pathology of Alzheimer disease may originate in a single cell and become self-sustaining, irrespective of upstream factors. Thus, injection of sonicated brain extract from mice with abundant tau inclusions into the cerebral cortex and hippocampus of transgenic mice lacking inclusions induces the assembly of human wild-type tau into filaments and leads to the spreading of pathology from the injection sites to neighboring brain regions (Clavaguera et al. 2009). Injection of brain extract immunodepleted of tau or divided into soluble and insoluble fractions shows that insoluble tau induces aggregation, in the absence of obvious signs of neurodegeneration. Parallel work has shown the transfer of aggregated tau between transfected cells (Frost et al. 2009). It thus appears that the tau species responsible for transmission and toxicity are not identical. An uncoupling of prion infective titre and neurotoxicity has been described (Sandberg et al. 2011).

Although tau inclusions form in many neurodegenerative diseases, their relevance for neurotoxicity remains a subject for debate. Studies using transgenic mice overexpressing human mutant tau in a conditional manner have reported a dissociation between tangle formation and nerve cell death (Santacruz et al. 2005). It appears that soluble hyperphosphorylated tau can contribute to nerve cell dysfunction prior to assembly into filaments. This is reminiscent of *Drosophila* and *Caenorhabditis elegans* lines expressing human wild-type or mutant tau, in which nerve cell loss and a reduced lifespan are observed, in the apparent absence of tau filaments (Wittmann et al. 2001; Kraemer et al. 2003). In genetic modifier screens in *Drosophila*, an increase in kinase activity enhanced tau toxicity, whereas an increase in phosphatase activity was beneficial (Feany et al. 2010). Activation of oxidative defences was also beneficial. In *C. elegans*, loss of *Sut-2* (suppressor of tau pathology-2), eliminated the toxic effects of human mutant tau, possibly via an increase in autophagic clearance (Guthrie et al. 2009).

The main goal behind work on tauopathies is to transform the treatment of common neurodegenerative diseases through an understanding of the underlying molecular pathways. There is an unmet need for mechanism-based therapies of Alzheimer disease. Tau binds to microtubules and boosting this interaction may be beneficial. This may be achieved through a reduction of the hyperphosphorylation of tau (Le Corre et al. 2006). In Alzheimer disease, tau assembles into paired helical and straight filaments. The assembly pathway is being defined and inhibitors of aggregation are being developed (Pickhardt et al. 2005; Taniguchi et al. 2005). Immunotherapy has been shown to clear tau aggregates from transgenic mouse brain and to reduce functional impairment (Asuni et al. 2007). Because aggregation is a concentration-dependent process, a reduction in production and/or increased clearance of tau are also potential targets (Morris et al. 2011).

REFERENCES

Alladi S, Xuereb J, Bak T, Nestor P, Knibb J, Patterson K, Hodges JR. 2007. Focal cortical presentations of Alzheimer's disease. *Brain* 130: 2636–2645.

Alzheimer A. 1907. Über eine eigenartige Erkrankung der Hirnrinde. *Allg Z Psychiat* 64: 146–148.

Alzheimer A. 1911. Über eigenartige Krankheitsfälle des späteren Alters. *Z ges Neurol Psychiat* 4: 356–385.

Amador-Ortiz C, Lin WL, Ahmed Z, Personett D, Davies P, Duara R, Graff-Radford NR, Hutton ML, Dickson DW. 2007. TDP-43 immunoreactivity in hippocampal sclerosis and Alzheimer's disease. *Ann Neurol* 61: 435–445.

Arai T, Hasegawa M, Akiyama H, Ikeda K, Nonaka T, Mori H, Mann D, Tsuchiya K, Yoshida M, Hashizume Y, et al. 2006. TDP-43 is a component of ubiquitin-positive tau-negative inclusions in frontotemporal lobar degeneration and amyotrophic lateral sclerosis. *Biochem Biophys Res Commun* 351: 602–611.

Asuni AA, Boutajangout A, Quartermain D, Sigurdsson EM. 2007. Immunotherapy targeting pathological tau conformers in a transgenic mouse model reduces brain pathology associated with functional improvements. *J Neurosci* 27: 9115–9129.

Ayala YM, De Conti L, Avendano-Vázquez SE, Dhir A, Romano M, D'Ambrogio A, Tollervey J, Ule J, Baralle M, Buratti E, et al. 2011. TDP-43 regulates its mRNA levels through a negative feedback loop. *EMBO J* 30: 277–288.

Baker M, Mackenzie IR, Pickering-Brown SM, Gass J, Rademakers R, Lindholm C, Snowden J, Adamson J, Sadovnick AD, Rollinson S, et al. 2006. Mutations in progranulin cause tau-negative frontotemporal dementia linked to chromosome 17. *Nature* 442: 916–919.

Benajiba L, Le Ber I, Camuzat A, Lacoste M, Thomas-Anterion C, Couratier P, Legallic S, Salachas F, Hannequin D, Decousus M, et al. 2009. *TARDBP* mutations in motoneuron disease with frontotemporal lobar degeneration. *Ann Neurol* 65: 470–474.

Bonfiglio F. 1938. Die umschriebene Atrophie der Basalganglien. *Z Neurol* 160: 306–333.

Braak H, Del Tredici K. 2011. The pathological process underlying Alzheimer's disease in individuals under thirty. *Acta Neuropathol* 121: 171–181.

Brion JP, Passareiro H, Nunez J, Flament-Durand J. 1985. Mise en évidence immunologique de la protéine tau au niveau des lésions de dégénérescence neurofibrillaire de la maladie d'Alzheimer. *Arch Biol* 95: 229–235.

Broca P. 1861. Perte de la parole, ramollissement chronique et destruction partielle du lobe antérieur gauche du cerveau. *Bull Soc Anthropol* 2: 235–238.

Brun A. 1987. Frontal lobe degeneration of non-Alzheimer type. I. Neuropathology. *Arch Gerontol Geriatr* 6: 193–208.

Bugiani O, Murrell JR, Giaccone G, Hasegawa M, Ghigo G, Tabaton M, Morbin M, Primavera A, Carella F, Solaro C, et al. 1999. Frontotemporal dementia and corticobasal degeneration in a family with a P301S mutation in *Tau*. *J Neuropathol Exp Neurol* 58: 667–677.

Caffrey TM, Joachim C, Paracchini S, Esiri MM, Wade-Martins R. 2006. Haplotype-specific expression of exon 10 at the human *MAPT* locus. *Hum Mol Genet* 15: 3529–3537.

Clavaguera F, Bolmont T, Crowther RA, Abramowski D, Frank S, Probst A, Fraser G, Stalder AK, Beibel M, Staufenbiel M, et al. 2009. Transmission and spreading of tauopathy in transgenic mouse brain. *Nat Cell Biol* 11: 909–913.

Colby DW, Prusiner SB. 2011. Prions. *Cold Spring Harb Perspect Biol* 3: a006833.

Constantinidis J, Richard J, Tissot R. 1974. Pick's disease. Histological and clinical correlations. *Eur Neurol* 11: 208–217.

Coomaraswamy J, Kilger E, Wölfing H, Schäfer C, Kaeser SA, Wegenast-Braun BM, Hefendehl JK, Wolburg H, Mazzella M, Ghiso J, et al. 2010. Modeling familial Danish dementia in mice supports the concept of the amyloid hypothesis of Alzheimer's disease. *Proc Natl Acad Sci* 107: 7969–7974.

Crowther RA, Goedert M. 2000. Abnormal tau-containing filaments in neurodegenerative diseases. *J Struct Biol* 130: 271–279.

Cruts M, Gijselinck I, van der Zee J, Engelborghs S, Wils H, Pirici D, Rademakers R, Vandenberghe R, Dermaut B, Martin JJ, et al. 2006. Null mutations in progranulin cause ubiquitin-positive frontotemporal dementia linked to chromosome 17q21. *Nature* 442: 920–924.

Cushman M, Johnson BS, King OD, Gitler AD, Shorter J. 2010. Prion-like disorders: Blurring the divide between transmissibility and infectivity. *J Cell Sci* 123: 1191–1201.

Custer SK, Neumann M, Lu H, Wright AC, Taylor JP. 2010. Transgenic mice expressing mutant forms of VCP/p97 recapitulate the full spectrum of IBMPFD including degeneration in muscle, brain and bone. *Hum Mol Genet* **19**: 1741–1755.

Déjerine J, Sérieux P. 1897. Un cas de surdité verbale pure terminée par aphasie sensorielle, suivi d'autopsie. *CR Acad Sci Paris* **49**: 1074–1077.

DeJesus-Hernandez M, Mackenzie IR, Boeve BF, Boxer AL, Baker M, Rutherford NJ, Nicholson AM, Finch NA, Flynn H, Adamson J, et al. 2011. Expanded GGGGCC hexanucleotide repeat in noncoding region of *C9ORF72* causes chromosome 9p-linked FTD and ALS. *Neuron* doi: 10.1016/j.neuron.2011.09.011.

Dormann D, Rodde R, Edbauer D, Bentmann E, Fischer I, Hruscha A, Than ME, Mackenzie IRA, Capell A, Schmid B, et al. 2010. ALS-associated fused in sarcoma (*FUS*) mutations disrupt transportin-mediated nuclear import. *EMBO J* **29**: 21841–21857.

Feany MB. 2010. New approaches to the pathology and genetics of neurodegeneration. *Am J Pathol* **176**: 2058–2066.

Feany MB, Dickson DW. 1995. Widespread cytoskeletal pathology characterizes corticobasal degeneration. *Am J Pathol* **146**: 1388–1396.

Foster NL, Wilhelmsen K, Sima AA, Jones MZ, D'Amato CJ, Gilman S. 1997. Frontotemporal dementia and parkinsonism linked to chromosome 17: A consensus conference. *Ann Neurol* **41**: 706–715.

Freud S. 1891. *Zur Auffassung der Aphasien.* Franz Deuticke, Leipzig und Wien.

Frost B, Jacks RL, Diamond MI. 2009. Propagation of tau misfolding from the outside to the inside of a cell. *J Biol Chem* **284**: 12845–12852.

Fu YJ, Nishihara Y, Kuroda S, Toyoshima Y, Ishihara T, Shinozaki M, Miyashita A, Piao YS, Tan CF, Tani T, et al. 2010. Sporadic four-repeat tauopathy with frontotemporal lobar degeneration, Parkinsonism, and motor neuron disease: A distinct neuropathological and biochemical disease entity. *Acta Neuropathol* **120**: 21–32.

Galantucci S, Tartaglia MC, Wilson SM, Henry ML, Filippi M, Agosta F, Dronkers NF, Henry RG, Ogar JM, Miller BL, et al. 2011. White matter damage in primary progressive aphasias: A diffusion tensor tractography study. *Brain* **134**: 3011–3029.

Galton CJ, Patterson K, Xuereb JH, Hodges JR. 2000. Atypical and typical presentations of Alzheimer's disease: A clinical, neuropsychological, neuroimaging and pathological study of 13 cases. *Brain* **123**: 484–498.

Gans A. 1923. Betrachtungen über Art und Ausbreitung des krankhaften Prozesses in einem Fall von Pickscher Atrophie des Stirnhirns. *Z Neurol* **80**: 10–28.

Ghetti B, Tagliavini F, Giaccone G, Bugiani O, Frangione B, Farlow MR, Dlouhy SR. 1994. Familial Gerstmann-Sträussler-Scheinker disease with neurofibrillary tangles. *Mol Neurobiol* **8**: 41–48.

Ghetti B, Wszolek ZW, Boeve BF, Spina S, Goedert M. 2011. Frontotemporal dementia and parkinsonism linked to chromosome 17. In *Neurodegeneration: The molecular pathology of dementia and movement disorders*, 2nd ed. (ed. Dickson D, Weller RO), pp. 110–134. Blackwell, Oxford, UK.

Ghidoni R, Benussi L, Glionna M, Franzoni M, Binetti G. 2008. Low plasma progranulin levels predict progranulin mutations in frontotemporal lobar degeneration. *Neurology* **71**: 1235–1239.

Giordana MT, Piccinini M, Grifoni S, De Marco G, Vercellino M, Magistrello M, Pellerino A, Buccinna B, Lupino E, Rinaudo MT. 2010. TDP-43 redistribution is an early event in sporadic amyotrophic lateral sclerosis. *Brain Pathol* **20**: 351–360.

Gitcho MA, Baloh RH, Chakraverty S, Mayo K, Norton JB, Levitch D, Hatanpaa KJ, White CL, Bigio EH, Caselli R, et al. 2008. TDP-43 A315 mutation in familial motor neuron disease. *Ann Neurol* **63**: 535–538.

Goedert M, Spillantini MG. 2006. A century of Alzheimer's disease. *Science* **314**: 777–781.

Goedert M, Wischik CM, Crowther RA, Walker JE, Klug A. 1988. Cloning and sequencing of the cDNA encoding a core protein of the paired helical filament of Alzheimer disease. *Proc Natl Acad Sci* **85**: 4051–4055.

Goedert M, Spillantini MG, Potier MC, Ulrich J, Crowther RA. 1989a. Cloning and sequencing of the cDNA encoding an isoform of microtubule-associated protein tau containing four tandem repeats: Differential expression of tau protein mRNAs in human brain. *EMBO J* **8**: 393–399.

Goedert M, Spillantini MG, Jakes R, Rutherford D, Crowther RA. 1989b. Multiple isoforms of human microtubule-associated protein tau: Sequences and localization in neurofibrillary tangles of Alzheimer's disease. *Neuron* **3**: 519–526.

Goedert M, Spillantini MG, Cairns NJ, Crowther RA. 1992. Tau proteins of Alzheimer paired helical filaments: Abnormal phosphorylation of all six brain isoforms. *Neuron* **8**: 159–168.

Goedert M, Jakes R, Crowther RA. 1999. Effects of frontotemporal dementia FTDP-17 mutations on heparin-induced assembly of tau filaments. *FEBS Lett* **450**: 306–311.

Goedert M, Clavaguera F, Tolnay M. 2010. The propagation of prion-like protein inclusions in neurodegenerative diseases. *Trends Neurosci* **33**: 317–325.

Gorno-Tempini ML, Murray RC, Rankin KP, Weiner MW, Miller BL. 2004a. Clinical, cognitive and anatomical evolution from nonfluent progressive aphasia to corticobasal syndrome: a case report. *Neurocase* **10**: 426–436.

Gorno-Tempini ML, Dronkers NF, Rankin KP, Ogar JM, Phengrasamy L, Rosen HJ, Johnson JK, Weiner MW, Miller BL. 2004b. Cognition and anatomy in three variants of primary progressive aphasia. *Ann Neurol* **55**: 335–346.

Gorno-Tempini ML, Brambati SM, Ginex V, Ogar J, Dronkers NF, Marcone A, Perani D, Garibotto V, Cappa SF, Miller BL. 2008. The logopenic/phonological variant of primary progressive aphasia. *Neurology* **71**: 1227–1234.

Gorno-Tempini ML, Hillis AE, Weintraub S, Kertesz A, Mendez M, Cappa SF, Ogar JM, Rohrer JD, Black S, Boeve BF, et al. 2011. Classification of primary progressive aphasia and its variants. *Neurology* **76**: 1006–1014.

Grossman M, Mickanin J, Onishi K, Hughes E, D'Esposito M, Ding XS, Alavi A, Reivich M. 1996. Progressive nonfluent aphasia: Language, cognitive, and PET mesausres contrasted with probable Alzheimer disease. *J Cogn Neurosci* **8:** 135–154.

Grundke-Iqbal I, Iqbal K, Tung YC, Quinlan M, Wisniewski HM, Binder LI. 1986. Abnormal phosphorylation of the microtubule-associated protein tau in Alzheimer cytoskeletal pathology. *Proc Natl Acad Sci* **83:** 4913–4917.

Grünthal E. 1930. Über ein Brüderpaar mit Pickscher Krankheit. *Z Neurol* **129:** 350–375.

Gustafson L. 1987. Frontal lobe degeneration of non-Alzheimer type. II. Clinical picture and differential diagnosis. *Arch Gerontol Geriatr* **6:** 209–223.

Guthrie CR, Schellenberg GD, Kraemer BC. 2009. SUT-2 potentiates tau-induced neurotoxicity in *Caenorhabditis elegans*. *Hum Mol Genet* **18:** 1825–1838.

Gydesen S, Brown JM, Brun A, Chakrabarti L, Gade A, Johannsen P, Rossor M, Thusgaard T, Grove A, Yancopoulou D, et al. 2002. Chromosome 3 linked frontotemporal dementia (FTD-3). *Neurology* **59:** 1585–1594.

Hasegawa M, Smith MJ, Goedert M. 1998. Tau proteins with FTDP-17 mutations have a reduced ability to promote microtubule assembly. *FEBS Lett* **437:** 207–210.

Hasegawa M, Arai T, Nonaka T, Kametani F, Yoshida M, Hashizume Y, Beach TG, Buratti E, Baralle F, Morita M, et al. 2008. Phosphorylated TDP-43 in frontotemporal lobar degeneration and amyotrophic lateral sclerosis. *Ann Neurol* **64:** 60–70.

Hodges JR, Patterson K. 2007. Semantic dementia: A unique clinicopathological syndrome. *Lancet Neurol* **6:** 1004–1014.

Höglinger GU, Melhem NM, Dickson D, Sleiman PMA, Wang LS, Klei L, Rademakers R, de Silva R, Litvan I, Riley DC, et al. 2011. Common variants affect risk for the tauopathy progressive supranuclear palsy. *Nat Genet* **43:** 699–705.

Holm IE, Isaacs AM, Mackenzie IRA. 2009. Absence of FUS-immunoreactive pathology in frontotemporal dementia linked to chromosome 3 (FTD-3) caused by mutation in the *CHMP2B* gene. *Acta Neuropathol* **118:** 719–720.

Hu F, Padukkavidana T, Vaegter CB, Brady OA, Zheng Y, Mackenzie IR, Feldman HH, Nykjaer A, Strittmatter SM. 2010. Sortilin-mediated endocytosis determines levels of the frontotemporal dementia protein, progranulin. *Neuron* **68:** 654–667.

Hutton M, Lendon CL, Rizzu M, Baker M, Froelich S, Houlden H, Pickering-Brown S, Chakraverty S, Isaacs A, Grover A, et al. 1998. Association of missense and 5′-splice-site mutations in *tau* with the inherited dementia FTDP-17. *Nature* **393:** 702–705.

Ittner LM, Ke YD, Delerue F, Bi M, Gladbach A, Van Eersel J, Wölfing H, Chieng BC, Christie J, Napier IA, et al. 2010. Dendritic function of tau mediates amyloid-β toxicity in Alzheimer's disease mouse models. *Cell* **142:** 387–397.

Johnson JK, Head E, Kim R, Starr A, Cotman CW. 1999. Clinical and pathological evidence for a frontal variant of Alzheimer disease. *Arch Neurol* **56:** 1233–1239.

Johnson BS, Snead D, Lee JJ, McCaffery MM, Shorter J, Gitler AD. 2009. TDP-43 is intrinsically aggregation-prone, and amyotrophic lateral sclerosis-linked mutations accelerate aggregation and toxicity. *J Biol Chem* **284:** 20329–20339.

Johnson JO, Mandrioli J, Benatar M, Abramzon Y, Van Deerlin VM, Trojanowski JQ, Gibbs JR, Brunetti M, Gronka S, Wuu J, et al. 2010. Exome sequencing reveals *VCP* mutations as a cause of familial ALS. *Neuron* **68:** 857–864.

Josephs KA, Dickson DW. 2007. Frontotemporal lobar degeneration with upper motor neuron disease/primary lateral sclerosis. *Neurology* **69:** 1800–1801.

Josephs KA, Duffy JR, Strand EA, Whitwell JL, Layton KF, Parisi JE, Hauser MF, Witte RJ, Boeve BF, Knopman DS, et al. 2006. Clinicopathological and imaging correlates of progressive aphasia and apraxia of speech. *Brain* **129:** 1385–1398.

Josephs KA, Whitwell JL, Parisi JE, Petersen RC, Boeve BF, Jack CR, Dickson DW. 2010. Caudate atrophy on MRI is a characteristic feature of FTLD-FUS. *Eur J Neurol* **17:** 969–975.

Ju JS, Weihl CC. 2010. Inclusion body myopathy, Paget's disease of the bone and frontotemporal dementia: A disorder of autophagy. *Hum Mol Genet* **19:** R38–R45.

Kertesz A, Hudson L, Mackenzie IRA, Munoz DG. 1994. The pathology and nosology of primary progressive aphasia. *Neurology* **44:** 2065–2072.

Kertesz A, Martinez-Lage P, Davidson W, Munoz DG. 2000. The corticobasal degeneration syndrome overlaps progressive aphasia and frontotemporal dementia. *Neurology* **55:** 1368–1375.

Koolen DA, Vissers LELM, Pfundt R, de Leeuw N, Knight SJL, Regan R, Kooy RF, Reyniers E, Romano C, Fichera M, et al. 2006. A new chromosome 17q21.31 microdeletion syndrome associated with a common inversion polymorphism. *Nat Genet* **38:** 999–1001.

Kovacs GG, Majtenyi K, Spina S, Murrell JR, Gelpi E, Höftberger R, Fraser G, Crowther RA, Goedert M, Budka H, et al. 2008. White matter tauopathy with globular glial inclusions: A distinct sporadic frontotemporal lobar degeneration. *J Neuropathol Exp Neurol* **67:** 963–975.

Kovacs GG, Murrell JR, Horvath S, Haraszti L, Majtenyi K, Molnar MJ, Budka H, Ghetti B, Spina S. 2009. *TARDBP* variation associated with frontotemporal dementia, supranuclear gaze palsy, and chorea. *Mov Disord* **24:** 1843–1847.

Kraemer BC, Zhang B, Leverenz JB, Thomas JH, Trojanowski JQ, Schellenberg GD. 2003. Neurodegeneration and defective neurotransmission in a *Caenorhabditis elegans* model of tauopathy. *Proc Natl Acad Sci* **100:** 9980–9985.

Kwiatkowski TJ, Bosco DA, LeClerc AL, Tamrazian E, Vanderburg CR, Russ C, Davis A, Gilchrist J, Kasarskis EJ, Munsat T, et al. 2009. Mutations in the *FUS/TLS* gene on chromosome 16 cause familial amyotrophic lateral sclerosis. *Science* **323:** 1205–1211.

Le Corre S, Klafki HW, Plesnila N, Hübinger G, Obermeier A, Sahagún H, Monse B, Seneci P, Lewis J, Eriksen J, et al. 2006. An inhibitor of tau hyperphosphorylation prevents severe motor impairments in tau transgenic mice. *Proc Natl Acad Sci* **103:** 9673–9678.

Lee VMY, Balin BJ, Otvos L, Trojanowski JQ. 1991. A68—a major subunit of paired helical filaments and derivatized forms of normal tau. *Science* **251:** 675–678.

Lee JA, Beigneux A, Tariq Ahmad S, Young SG, Gao FB. 2007. ESCRT-III dysfunction causes autophagosome accumulation and neurodegeneration. *Curr Biol* **17:** 1561–1567.

Lewis J, Dickson DW, Lin WL, Chisholm L, Corral A, Jones G, Yen SH, Sahara N, Skipper L, Yager D, et al. 2001. Enhanced neurofibrillary degeneration in transgenic mice expressing mutant tau and APP. *Science* **293:** 1487–1491.

Lippa CF, Cohen R, Smith TW, Drachman DA. 1991. Primary progressive aphasia with focal neuronal achromasia. *Neurology* **41:** 882–886.

Litvan I, Agid Y, Calne D, Campbell G, Dubois B, Duvoisin RC, Goetz CG, Golbe LI, Grafman J, Growdon JH, et al. 1996. Clinical research criteria for the diagnosis of progressive supranuclear palsy (Steele-Richardson-Olszewski syndrome). *Neurology* **47:** 1–9.

Lüers T, Spatz H. 1957. Picksche Krankheit. In *Handbuch der speziellen Anatomie und Histologie* (ed. Henke F, Lubarsch O), Vol. 13, pp. 614–715. Springer, Berlin.

Mackenzie IRA, Baborie A, Pickering-Brown S, Du Plessis D, Jaros E, Perry RH, Neary D, Snowden JS, Mann DMA. 2006. Heterogeneity of ubiquitin pathology in frontotemporal lobar degeneration. Classification and relation to clinical phenotype. *Acta Neuropathol* **112:** 539–549.

Mackenzie IRA, Neumann M, Baborie A, Sampathu DM, Du Plessis D, Jaros E, Perry RH, Trojanowski JQ, Mann DMA, Lee VMY. 2011. A harmonized classification system for FTLD-TDP pathology. *Acta Neuropathol* **122:** 111–113.

Mesulam MM. 1982. Slowly progressive aphasia without generalized dementia. *Ann Neurol* **11:** 592–598.

Mesulam MM. 1987. Primary progressive aphasia—differentiation from Alzheimer's disease. *Ann Neurol* **22:** 533–534.

Mesulam MM. 2001. Primary progressive aphasia. *Ann Neurol* **49:** 425–432.

Mesulam MM, Wicklund A, Johnson N, Rogalski E, Léger GC, Rademaker A, Weintraub S, Bigio EH. 2008. Alzheimer and frontotemporal pathology in subsets of primary progressive aphasia. *Ann Neurol* **63:** 709–719.

Meyer A. 1929. Über eine der amyotrophischen Lateralsklerose nahestehende Erkrankung mit psychischen Störungen. *Z Neurol* **121:** 107–128.

Migliaccio R, Agosta F, Rascovsky K, Karydas A, Bonasera S, Rabinovici GD, Miller BL, Gorno-Tempini ML. 2009. Clinical syndromes associated with posterior atrophy. *Neurology* **73:** 1571–1578.

Morita K, Kaiya H, Ikeda T, Namba M. 1987. Presenile dementia combined with amyotrophy: A review of 34 Japanese cases. *Arch Gerontol Geriatr* **6:** 263–277.

Morris M, Maeda S, Vossel K, Mucke L. 2011. The many faces of tau. *Neuron* **70:** 410–426.

Mummery CJ, Patterson K, Wise RJS, Vandenberghe R, Price CJ, Hodges JR. 1999. Disrupted temporal lobe connections in semantic dementia. *Brain* **122:** 61–73.

Munoz DG, Neumann M, Kusaka H, Yokota O, Ishihara K, Terada S, Kuroda S, Mackenzie IR. 2009. FUS pathology in basophilic inclusion body disease. *Acta Neuropathol* **118:** 617–627.

Murrell JR, Spillantini MG, Zolo P, Guazzelli M, Smith MJ, Hasegawa M, Redi F, Crowther RA, Pietrini P, Ghetti B, et al. 1999. Tau gene mutation G389R causes a tauopathy with abundant Pick body-like inclusions and axonal deposits. *J Neuropathol Exp Neurol* **58:** 1207–1226.

Nacharaju P, Lewis J, Easson C, Yen S, Hackett J, Hutton M, Yen SH. 1999. Accelerated filament formation from tau protein with specific FTDP-17 mutations. *FEBS Lett* **447:** 195–199.

Neary D, Snowden JS, Northen B, Goulding P. 1988. Dementia of frontal type. *J Neurol Neurosurg Psychiatry* **51:** 353–361.

Neary D, Snowden JS, Gustafson L, Passant U, Stuss D, Black S, Freedman M, Kertesz A, Robert PH, Albert M, et al. 2003. Progressive non-fluent aphasia is associated with hypometabolism centred on the left anterior insula. *Brain* **126:** 2406–2418.

Nestor PJ, Graham NL, Fryer TD, Williams GB, Patterson K, Hodges JR. 2003. Progressive non-fluent aphasia is associated with hypometabolism centred on the left anterior insula. *Brain* **126:** 2406–2418.

Neumann M, Sampathu DM, Kwong LK, Truax AC, Micsenyi MC, Chou TT, Bruce J, Schuck T, Grossman M, Clark CM, et al. 2006. Ubiquitinated TDP-43 in frontotemporal lobar degeneration and amyotrophic lateral sclerosis. *Science* **314:** 130–133.

Neumann M, Mackenzie IR, Cairns NJ, Boyer PJ, Markesbery WR, Smith CD, Taylor JP, Kretzschmar HA, Kimonis VE, Forman MS. 2007. TDP-43 in the ubiquitin pathology of frontotemporal dementia with *VCP* gene mutations. *J Neuropathol Exp Neurol* **66:** 152–157.

Neumann M, Rademakers R, Roeber S, Baker M, Kretzschmar HA, Mackenzie IRA. 2009a. A new subtype of frontotemporal lobar degeneration with FUS pathology. *Brain* **132:** 2922–2931.

Neumann A, Roeber S, Kretzschmar HA, Rademakers R, Baker M, Mackenzie IRA. 2009b. Abundant FUS-immunoreactive pathology in neuronal intermediate filament inclusion disease. *Acta Neuropathol* **118:** 605–616.

Nishimoto Y. Ito D, Yagi T, Nihei Y, Tsunoda Y, Suzuki N. 2010. Characterization of alternative isoforms and inclusion body of the TAR DNA-binding protein-43. *J Biol Chem* **285:** 608–619.

Okamoto K, Hirai S, Yamazaki T, Sun X, Nakazato Y. 1991. New ubiquitin-positive intraneuronal inclusions in the extra-motor cortices in patients with amyotrophic lateral sclerosis. *Neurosci Lett* **129:** 233–236.

Onari K, Spatz H. 1926. Anatomische Beiträge zur Lehre von der Pickschen umschriebenen Grosshirnrinden-Atrophie ("Picksche Krankheit"). *Z Neurol* **101:** 470–511.

Pastor P, Ezquerra M, Munoz E, Marti MJ, Blesa R, Tolosa E, Oliva R. 2000. Significant association between the tau gene A0/A0 genotype and Parkinson's disease. *Ann Neurol* **47:** 242–245.

Pick A. 1892. Ueber die Beziehungen der senilen Hirnatrophie zur Aphasie. *Prager med Wschr* **17:** 165–167.

Pick A. 1901. Senile Hirnatrophie als Grundlage von Herderscheinungen. *Wiener klin Wschr* **14:** 403–404.

Pick A. 1904. Zur Symptomatologie der linksseitigen Schläfenlappenatrophie. *Mschr Psychiat Neurol* **16:** 378–388.

Pick A. 1906. Über einen weiteren Symptomcomplex im Rahmen der Dementia senilis, bedingt durch umschriebene stärkere Hirnatrophie (gemischte Apraxie). *Mschr Psychiat Neurol* **19:** 97–108.

Pickhardt M, Gazova Z, von Bergen M, Khlistunova I, Wang Y, Hascher A, Mandelkow EM, Biernat J, Mandelkow E. 2005. Anthraquinones inhibit tau aggregation and dissolve Alzheimer paired helical filaments in vitro and in cells. *J Biol Chem* **280:** 3628–3635.

Piguet O, Hornberger M, Mioshi E, Hodges JR. 2011a. Behavioural-variant frontotemporal dementia: Diagnosis, clinical staging, and management. *Lancet Neurol* **10:** 162–172.

Piguet O, Halliday GW, Reid WGJ, Casey B, Carman R, Huang Y, Xuereb JH, Hodges JR, Kril JJ. 2011b. Clinical phenotypes in autopsy-confirmed Pick disease. *Neurology* **76:** 253–259.

Pollock NJ, Mirra SS, Binder LI, Hansen LA, Wood JG. 1986. Filamentous aggregates in Pick's disease, progressive supranuclear palsy, and Alzheimer's disease share antigenic determinants with microtubule-associated protein, tau. *Lancet* **328:** 1211.

Polymenidou M, Lagier-Tourenne C, Hutt KR, Huelga SC, Moran J, Liang TY, Ling SC, Sun E, Wancewicz E, Mazur C, et al. 2011. Long pre-mRNA depletion and RNA missplicing contribute to neuronal vulnerability from loss of TDP-43. *Nat Neurosci* **14:** 459–468.

Poorkaj P, Bird TD, Wijsman E, Nemens E, Garruto RM, Anderson L, Andreadis A, Wiederholt WC, Raskind M, Schellenberg GD. 1998. Tau is a candidate gene for chromosome 17 frontotemporal dementia. *Ann Neurol* **43:** 815–825.

Rabinovici GD, Jagust WJ, Furst AJ, Ogar JM, Racine CA, Mormino EC, O'Neil JP, Lal RA, Dronkers NF, Miller BL, et al. 2008. Aβ amyloid and glucose metabolism in three variants of primary progressive aphasia. *Ann Neurol* **64:** 388–401.

Rebeiz JJ, Kolodny EM, Richardson EP. 1968. Corticodentonigral degeneration with neuronal achromasia. *Arch Neurol* **18:** 20–33.

Reed LA, Grabowski TJ, Schmidt ML, Morris JC, Goate A, Solodkin A, Van Hoesen GW, Schelper RL, Talbot CJ, Wragg MA, et al. 1997. Autosomal dominant dementia with widespread neurofibrillary tangles. *Ann Neurol* **42:** 564–572.

Renton AE, Majounie E, Waite A, Simón-Sanchez J, Rollinson S, Gibbs JR, Schymick JC, Laaksovirta H, Van Swieten JC, Myllykangas L, et al. 2011. A hexanucleotide repeat expansion in *C9ORF72* is the cause of chromosome 9p21-linked ALS-FTD. *Neuron* doi: 10.1016/j.neuron.2011.09.010.

Richter H. 1918. Eine besondere Art von Stirnhirnschwund mit Verblödung. *Z Neurol* **38:** 127–159.

Ritson GP, Custer SK, Freibaum BD, Guinto JB, Geffel D, Moore J, Tang W, Winton MJ, Neumann M, Trojanowski JQ, et al. 2010. TDP-43 mediates degeneration in a novel *Drosophila* model of disease caused by mutations in VCP/p97. *J Neurosci* **30:** 7729–7739.

Roberson ED, Scearce-Levie K, Palop JJ, Yan F, Cheng IH, Wu T, Gerstein H, Yu GQ, Mucke L. 2007. Reducing endogenous tau ameliorates amyloid β-induced deficits in an Alzheimer's disease mouse model. *Science* **316:** 750–754.

Rossor MN, Fox NC, Mummery CM, Schott JM, Warren JD. 2010. The diagnosis of young-onset dementia. *Lancet Neurol* **9,** 793–806.

Sampathu DM, Neumann M, Kwong LK, Chou TT, Micsenyi M, Truax A, Bruce J, Grossman M, Trojanowski JQ, Lee VMY. 2006. Pathological heterogeneity of frontotemporal lobar degeneration with ubiquitin-positive inclusions delineated by ubiquitin immunohistochemistry and novel monoclonal antibodies. *Am J Pathol* **169:** 1343–1352.

Sandberg MK, Al-Doujaily H, Sharps B, Clarke AR, Collinge J. 2011. Prion propagation and toxicity *in vivo* occur in two distinct mechanistic phases. *Nature* **470:** 540–542.

Santacruz K, Lewis J, Spires T, Paulson J, KKotilinek L, Ingelsson M, Guimares A, DeTure M, Ramsden M, McGowan E, et al. 2005. Tau suppression in a neurodegenerative mouse model improves memory function. *Science* **309:** 476–481.

Schmitt-John T, Drepper C, Mussmann A, Hahn P, Kuhlmann M, Thiel C, Hafner M, Lengeling A, Heimann P, Jones JM, et al. 2005. Mutation of *Vps54* causes motor neuron disease and defective spermiogenesis in the wobbler mouse. *Nat Genet* **37:** 1213–1215.

Schneider C. 1927. Über Picksche Krankheit. *Mschr Psychiat Neurol* **65:** 230–275.

Schneider C. 1929. Weitere Beiträge zur Lehre von der Pickschen Krankheit. *Z Neurol* **120:** 340–384.

Seelaar H, Klijnsma KY, de Koning I, Van der Lugt A, Chiu WZ, Azmani A, Rozemuller AJM, Van Swieten JC. 2010. Frequency of ubiquitin and FUS-positive, TDP-43-negative frontotemporal lobar degeneration. *J Neurol* **257:** 747–753.

Sharp AJ, Hansen S, Selzer RR, Cheng Z, Regan R, Hurst JA, Stewart H, Price SM, Blair E, Hennekam RC, et al. 2006. Discovery of previously unidentified genomic disorders from the duplication architecture of the human genome. *Nat Genet* **38:** 1038–1042.

Shaw CE. 2010. Capturing VCP: Another molecular piece in the ALS jigsaw puzzle. *Neuron* **68:** 812–814.

Shaw-Smith C, Pittman AM, Willatt L, Martin H, Rickman L, Gribble S, Curley R, Cumming S, Dunn C, Kalaitzopoulos D, et al. 2006. Microdeletion encompassing *MAPT* at chromosome 17q21.3 is associated with developmental delay and learning disability. *Nat Genet* **38:** 1032–1037.

Skibinski G, Parkinson NJ, Brown JM, Charkrabarti L, Lloyd SL, Hummerich H, Nielsen JE, Hodges JR, Spillantini MG, Thusgaard T, et al. 2005. Mutations in the endosomal ESCRTIII-complex subunit CHMP2B in frontotemporal dementia. *Nat Genet* **37:** 806–808.

Snowden JS, Goulding PJ, Neary D. 1989. Semantic dementia: A form of circumscribed atrophy. *Behav Neurol* **2:** 167–182.

Spillantini MG, Crowther RA, Goedert M. 1996. Comparison of the neurofibrillary pathology in Alzheimer's disease and familial presenile dementia with tangles. *Acta Neuropathol* **92:** 42–48.

Spillantini MG, Goedert M, Crowther RA, Murrell JR, Farlow MR, Ghetti B. 1997. Familial multiple system tauopathy with presenile dementia: A disease with abundant neuronal and glial tau filaments. *Proc Natl Acad Sci* **94:** 4113–4118.

Spillantini MG, Bird TD, Ghetti B. 1998a. Frontotemporal dementia and parkinsonism linked to chromosome 17: A new group of tauopathies. *Brain Pathol* **8:** 387–402.

Spillantini MG, Murrell JR, Goedert M, Farlow MR, Klug A, Ghetti B. 1998b. Mutation in the tau gene in familial multiple system tauopathy with presenile dementia. *Proc Natl Acad Sci* **95:** 7737–7741.

Spillantini MG, Crowther RA, Kamphorst W, Heutink P, Van Swieten JC. 1998c. Tau pathology in two Dutch families with mutations in the microtubule-binding region of tau. *Am J Pathol* **153:** 1359–1363.

Spina S, Murrell JR, Huey ED, Wassermann EM, Pietrini P, Grafman J, Ghetti B. 2007. Corticobasal syndrome associated with the A90D *progranulin* mutation. *J Neuropathol Exp Neurol* **66:** 892–900.

Sreedharan J, Blair IP, Tripathi VB, Hu X, Vance C, Rogelj B, Ackerley S, Durnall JC, Williams KL, Buratti E, et al. 2008. TDP-43 mutations in familial and sporadic amyotrophic lateral sclerosis. *Science* **319:** 1668–1672.

Stefansson H, Helgason A, Thorleifsson G, Steinthorsdottir V, Masson G, Barnard J, Baker A, Jonasdottir A, Ingason A, Gudnadottir VG, et al. 2005. A common inversion under selection in Europeans. *Nat Genet* **37:** 129–137.

Steele JC, Richardson JC, Olszewski J. 1964. Progressive supranuclear palsy. *Arch Neurol* **10:** 333–359.

Stertz G. 1926. Über die Picksche Atrophie. *Z Neurol* **101:** 729–749.

Strittmatter WJ, Roses AD. 1995. Apolipoprotein E and Alzheimer disease. *Proc Natl Acad Sci* **92:** 4725–4727.

Sun Z, Diaz Z, Fang X, Hart MP, Chesi A, Shorter J, Gitler AD. 2011. Molecular determinants and genetic modifiers of aggregation and toxicity for the ALS disease protein FUS/TLS. *PLoS Biol* **9:** e1000614.

Tang W, Lu Y, Tian QY, Zhang Y, Guo FJ, Liu GY, Syed NM, Lai Y, Lin EA, Kong L, et al. 2011. The growth factor progranulin binds to TNF receptors and is therapeutic against inflammatory arthritis in mice. *Science* **332:** 478–484.

Taniguchi S, Suzuki N, Masuda M, Hisanaga SI, Iwatsubo T, Goedert M, Hasegawa M. 2005. Inhibition of heparin-induced tau filament formation by phenothiazines, polyphenols and porphyrins. *J Biol Chem* **280:** 7614–7623.

Ticozzi N, Silani V, LeClerc AL, Keagle P, Gellera C, Ratti A, Taroni F, Kwiatkowski TJ, McKenna-Yasek DN, Sapp PC, et al. 2009. Analysis of *FUS* gene mutation in familial amyotrophic lateral sclerosis within an Italian cohort. *Neurology* **73:** 1180–1185.

Tollervey JR, Curk T, Rogelj B, Riese M, Cereda M, Kayikci M, König J, Hortobágyi T, Nishimura AL, Zupunski V, et al. 2011. Characterizing the RNA targets and position-dependent splicing regulation by TDP-43. *Nat Neurosci* **14:** 452–458.

Vance C, Al-Chalabi A, Ruddy D, Smith BN, Hu X, Sreedharan J, Siddique T, Schelhaas HJ, Kusters B, Troost D, et al. 2006. Familial amyotrophic lateral sclerosis with frontotemporal dementia is linked to a locus on chromosome 9p13.2–21.3. *Brain* **129:** 868–876.

Vance C, Rogelj B, Hortobágyi T, De Vos KJ, Nihimura AL, Sreedharan J, Hu X, Smith B, Ruddy D, Wright P, et al. 2009. Mutations in FUS, an RNA processing protein, cause familial amyotrophic sclerosis type 6. *Science* **323:** 1208–1211.

Van Deerlin VM, Sleiman PMA, Martinez-Lage M, Chen-Plotkin A, Wang LS, Graff-Radford NR, Dickson DW, Rademakers R, Boeve BF, Grossman M, et al. 2010. Common variants at 7p21 are associated with frontotemporal lobar degeneration with TDP-43 inclusions. *Nat Genet* **42:** 234–239.

Van der Flier WM, Pijnenburg YAL, Fox NC, Scheltens P. 2011. Early-onset versus late-onset Alzheimer's disease: The case of the missing *APOE* ε4 allele. *Lancet Neurol* **10:** 280–288.

Van Mansvelt J. 1954. *Pick's disease*. MJvd Loeff, Enschede.

Van Swieten JC, Heutink P. 2008. Mutations in progranulin (*GRN*) within the spectrum of clinical and pathological phenotypes of frontotemporal dementia. *Lancet Neurol* **7:** 965–974.

Verhaart WJC. 1930. Over de ziekte van Pick. *Nederl Tijdschr Geneesk* **74:** 5586–5598.

Vidal R, Delisle MB, Ghetti B. 2004. Neurodegeneration caused by proteins with an aberrant carboxyl-terminus. *J Neuropathol Exp Neurol* **63:** 787–800.

Von Braunmühl A. 1932. Picksche Krankheit und amyotrophische Lateralsklerose. *Allg Z Psychiat* **96:** 364–366.

Von Braunmühl A, Leonhard K. 1934. Über ein Schwesternpaar mit Pickscher Krankheit. *Z Neurol* **150:** 209–241.

Watts GDJ, Wymer J, Kovach MJ, Mehta SG, Mumm S, Darvish D, Pestronk A, Whyte MP, Kimonis VE. 2004. Inclusion body myopathy associated with Paget disease of bone and frontotemporal dementia is caused by mutant valosin-containing protein. *Nat Genet* **36:** 377–381.

Wernicke C. 1874. *Der aphasische Symptomencomplex: Eine psychologische Studie auf anatomischer Basis.* Max Cohn & Weigert, Breslau.

Wetzel MK, Naska S, Laliberte CL, Rymar VV, Fujitani M, Biernaskie JA, Cole CJ, Lerch JP, Spring S, Wang SH, et al. 2008. p73 regulates neurodegeneration and phospho-tau accumulation in aging and Alzheimer's disease. *Neuron* **59:** 708–721.

Whitwell JL, Jack CR, Senjem ML, Josephs KA. 2006. Patterns of atrophy in pathologically confirmed FTLD with and without motor neuron degeneration. *Neurology* **66:** 102–104.

Whitwell JL, Przybelski SA, Weigand SD, Ivnik RJ, Vemuri P, Gunter JL, Senjem ML, Shiung MM, Boeve BF, Knopman DS, et al. 2009a. Distinct anatomical subtypes of the behavioural variant of frontotemporal dementia: A cluster analysis study. *Brain* **132:** 2932–2946.

Whitwell JL, Jack CR, Boeve BF, Senjem ML, Baker M, Rademakers R, Ivnik RJ, Knopman DS, Wszolek ZK, Petersen RC, et al. 2009b. Voxel-based morphometry patterns of atrophy in FTLD with mutations in *MAPT* or *PGRN*. *Neurology* **72:** 813–820.

Whitwell JL, Avula R, Senjem ML, Kantarci K, Weigand SD, Samikoglu A, Edmonson HA, Vemuri P, Knopman DS, Boeve BF, et al. 2010a. Gray and white matter water diffusion in the syndromic variants of frontotemporal dementia. *Neurology* **74:** 1279–1287.

Whitwell JL, Jack CR, Boeve BF, Parisi JE, Ahlskog JE, Drubach DA, Senjem ML, Knopman DS, Petersen RC, Dickson DW, et al. 2010b. Imaging correlates of pathology in corticobasal syndrome. *Neurology* **75:** 1879–1887.

Cite this article as *Cold Spring Harb Perspect Med* doi: 10.1101/cshperspect.a006254

Wilhelmsen KC, Lynch T, Pavlou E, Higgins M, Nygaard TG. 1994. Localization of disinhibition-dementia-parkinsonism-amyotrophy complex to 17q21–22. *Am J Hum Genet* **55:** 1159–1164.

Williams DR, Lees AJ. 2009. Progressive supranuclear palsy: Clinicopathological concepts and diagnostic challenges. *Lancet Neurol* **8:** 270–279.

Williams DR, Holton JL, Strand C, Pittman A, de Silva R, Lees AJ, Revesz T. 2007. Pathological tau burden and distribution distinguishes progressive supranuclear palsy-parkinsonism from Richardson's syndrome. *Brain* **130:** 1566–1576.

Wischik CM, Novak M, Thogersen HC, Edwards PC, Runswick MJ, Jakes R, Walker JE, Milstein C, Roth M, Klug A. 1988. Isolation of a fragment of tau derived from the core of the paired helical filament of Alzheimer disease. *Proc Natl Acad Sci* **85:** 4506–4510.

Wittmann CW, Wszolek ZF, Shulman JM, Salvaterra PM, Lewis J, Hutton M, Feany MB. 2001. Tauopathy in *Drosophila*: Neurodegeneration without neurofibrillary tangles. *Science* **293:** 711–714.

Yokoseki A, Shiga A, Tan CF, Tagawa A, Kaneko H, Koyama A, Eguchi H, Tsujino A, Ikeuchi T, Kakita A, et al. 2008. *TDP-43* mutation in familial amyotrophic lateral sclerosis. *Ann Neurol* **63:** 538–542.

Yu CE, Bird TD, Bekris LM, Montine TJ, Leverenz JB, Steinbart E, Galloway NM, Feldman H, Woltjer R, Miller CA, et al. 2010. The spectrum of mutations in progranulin. *Arch Neurol* **67:** 161–170.

Zhou J, Greicius MD, Gennatas ED, Growdon ME, Jang JY, Rabinovici GD, Kramer JH, Weiner M, Miller BL, Seeley WW. 2010. Divergent network connectivity changes in behavioural variant frontotemporal dementia and Alzheimer's disease. *Brain* **133:** 1352–1367.

Biochemistry of Amyloid β-Protein and Amyloid Deposits in Alzheimer Disease

Colin L. Masters[1] and Dennis J. Selkoe[2]

[1]The Mental Health Research Institute, The University of Melbourne, Parkville 3010, Australia

[2]Center for Neurologic Diseases, Harvard Medical School and Brigham and Women's Hospital, Boston, Massachusetts 02115

Correspondence: c.masters@unimelb.edu.au

Progressive cerebral deposition of the amyloid β-protein (Aβ) in brain regions serving memory and cognition is an invariant and defining feature of Alzheimer disease. A highly similar but less robust process accompanies brain aging in many nondemented humans, lower primates, and some other mammals. The discovery of Aβ as the subunit of the amyloid fibrils in meningocerebral blood vessels and parenchymal plaques has led to innumerable studies of its biochemistry and potential cytotoxic properties. Here we will review the discovery of Aβ, numerous aspects of its complex biochemistry, and current attempts to understand how a range of Aβ assemblies, including soluble oligomers and insoluble fibrils, may precipitate and promote neuronal and glial alterations that underlie the development of dementia. Although the role of Aβ as a key molecular factor in the etiology of Alzheimer disease remains controversial, clinical trials of amyloid-lowering agents, reviewed elsewhere in this book, are poised to resolve the question of its pathogenic primacy.

THE LASTING IMPACT OF THE DISCOVERY OF AMYLOID β-PROTEIN ON THE ELUCIDATION OF ALZHEIMER DISEASE

With the benefit of hindsight, it is now clear that the isolation and partial sequencing of the meningovascular amyloid β-protein (Aβ) by George Glenner and Caine Wong in 1984 provided a turning point for modern research on the fundamental mechanism of Alzheimer disease (AD). Ever since Alzheimer peered through the microscope at the brain of his first patient and wrote prophetically "scattered through the entire cortex ... one found miliary foci that were caused by the deposition of a peculiar substance ...," neuropathologists had sought the nature of the amyloid material found in the senile plaque. By the early 1980s, as compositional analyses of the neurofibrillary tangle were beginning (see Mandelkow and Mandelkow 2011), a few investigators turned their attention to the identity of the amyloid protein in vascular and plaque deposits. In this chapter, we will review how our biochemical understanding of the amyloid deposits emerged and has advanced, and we will describe many features of the peptides that comprise this hallmark lesion of AD and certain molecules associated with them. The trafficking and proteolytic processing of amyloid precursor protein (APP), including the generation of

Cite this article as *Cold Spring Harb Perspect Med* doi: 10.1101/cshperspect.a006262

Aβ, and the proteolytic degradation of the peptide are covered in other chapters (see Haass et al. 2011; Saido and Leissring 2011, respectively) and will not be discussed here.

BIOCHEMISTRY OF Aβ IN MENINGOVASCULAR AMYLOID DEPOSITS AND AMYLOID PLAQUE CORES

Because George Glenner's earlier research on the circulating precursors of nonneural amyloid deposits (e.g., AL amyloid) convinced him that the amyloid in AD might well be derived from a serum precursor, he focused his attention on the amyloid in meningeal vessel walls. By stripping the meninges from postmortem AD brains, Glenner and Wong enriched for amyloid-bearing microvessels and discarded the cerebral tissue with its potentially "contaminating" amyloid plaques and neurofibrillary tangles (Glenner and Wong 1984b). They used the chaotropic salt guanidine hydrochloride (at 6M) to solubilize and then chromatographically enrich the amyloid subunit, which ran as a 4.2 kDa band on SDS-PAGE. HPLC purification of the protein and amino-terminal sequencing to residue 24 revealed a unique sequence (their report of a glutamine rather than glutamate at position 11 was corrected in their subsequent sequencing of Down's syndrome meningovascular Aβ). In this initial report, Glenner and Wong suggested that this novel peptide might turn out to be derived from a serum precursor and that it could "provide a diagnostic test for Alzheimer's disease and a means to understand its pathogenesis." Whereas the first of these three predictions turned out not to be true, the second and third clearly did.

Shortly after this paper appeared, Glenner and Wong published a highly similar study (Glenner and Wong 1984a) which showed that the meningovascular amyloid subunit in Down's syndrome brains was the same "β-protein," as they had dubbed it. Glenner called attention to this evidence of a key biochemical relationship between Down's syndrome and AD, a concept he had touted as early as 1979 in a prescient article in *Medical Hypotheses* (Glenner 1979). He stressed that Down's

syndrome may be a "predictable model" for AD and further suggested that "the genetic defect in Alzheimer's disease is localized on chromosome 21." Glenner reasoned that, because trisomy 21 led to Alzheimer-type Aβ accumulation in vessels and plaques, familial AD itself might well involve a defect in the precursor of the β-protein on this chromosome. This prediction turned out to be true in part; the first gene implicated in a familial form of AD was indeed the β-amyloid precursor protein. What Glenner apparently did not recognize—or at least state at the time—was the heterogeneity of familial forms of AD as well as the notion that many cases may not be genetically determined. Nevertheless, these two brief papers in *Biochemical and Biophysical Research Communications*, although not viewed as potentially seminal in the months after their publication, turned out to provide both the factual and conceptual underpinnings for all subsequent research on β-amyloidosis in AD.

During the years 1983–1985, efforts independent of those of Glenner were made in several laboratories to isolate and sequence the amyloid in senile plaque cores (Fig. 1) from AD brains. These efforts began before the identification of the vascular Aβ peptide by Glenner and Wong, but they were greatly facilitated by it. In 1983, Allsop, Landon, and Kidd reported a method for isolating intact neuritic plaque cores from postmortem AD brain and found them to be insoluble in various denaturants (Allsop et al. 1983). They published an amino acid composition which did not resemble any previously described amyloid protein. The authors described a variety of contaminants in their final preparations, including bacteria, leading to concerns about the accuracy of this composition, although subsequent methods produced core preparations of greater purity but generally similar composition, signifying the relative insensitivity of the amino acid composition of partially purified proteins as a biochemical comparator.

In the laboratories of Masters and Beyreuther, Roher, Selkoe, and Frangione, distinct but partially related methods for purifying

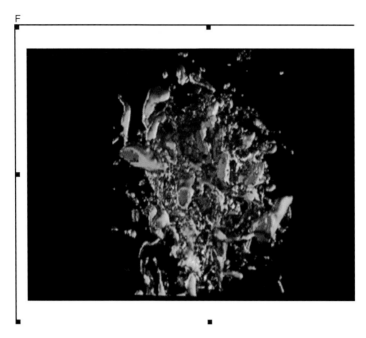

Figure 1. Three-dimensional reconstructed image by confocal microscopy of a neuritic (senile) plaque in the cortex of a patient dying with Alzheimer disease. Red labeling is by an antibody to amyloid β-protein which reveals the extracellular amyloid; green labeling is with an antibody against p-Tau which reveals intimately associated dystrophic neurites. Note that this plaque core is not a solid mass of amyloid but is fragmented and porous and contains abnormal cell processes intercalated within it. (Image courtesy of Dr. Eliezer Masliah, University of California, San Diego, CA.)

and solubilizing amyloid plaque cores from postmortem AD brain were developed. Masters and colleagues first reported the protein subunit of amyloid plaque cores, using a method which used nonionic detergent extraction of brain, pepsin digestion, and sucrose density gradient fractionation (Masters et al. 1985). The resultant cores were found to be approximately 90% pure by microscopy and were partially soluble in high concentrations (10%) of SDS and BME and fully soluble in approximately 70% formic acid. By both HPLC and SDS/urea PAGE, the formic acid-solubilized core protein ran not only at ~4.3 kDa but also at ~8, 12, and 16 kDa, demonstrating the ready association of the monomer into SDS-stable oligomers. Masters and Beyreuther pointed out that the molecular mass, amino acid composition and amino-terminal sequence of the protein they isolated from cores were essentially identical to those described for vascular Aβ

by Glenner, although their analyses showed considerable amino-terminal "raggedness" in the plaque-derived protein. They concluded that the shared 4 kDa subunit indicated a common origin for the plaque and vascular amyloids in AD. Again, Aβ peptides isolated from AD and Down's syndrome plaques were indistinguishable. The amino-terminal heterogeneity reported by Masters and Beyreuther was striking, in that only 12% of the sequenced protein began at Asp1, with 64% starting at Phe4 and the remainder at downstream residues, perhaps deriving in part from their use of pepsin digestion during plaque purification. In Masters' report, Glenner's 24-residue sequence was extended to residue 28, although the identities of two of those additional four residues were later revised.

Plaque core purifications and analyses performed at that time in three other laboratories provided largely consistent findings.

The various methods employed took advantage of the insolubility of the amyloid cores in detergents such as SDS and their relative resistance to quantitative digestion by proteases. In the studies of Roher et al. (1986) and Gorevic et al. (1986), as in that of Masters et al. (1985), peptidases were used to diminish contaminants, but this approach raised the possibility of partial digestion of Aβ itself and the creation of some of the observed amino-terminal heterogeneity. In the study of Selkoe et al. (1986) the use of extensive SDS extraction of the cores, then sucrose gradient centrifugation, and then a two-step fluorescence-activated particle sorting (FACS) led to SDS-insoluble plaque cores that were >90–95% pure by electron microscopy, enabling an estimate (via amino acid analysis) of the protein content of a single plaque core: 60–130 pg. However, the attempts of Selkoe and colleagues to sequence this purified plaque amyloid after its solubilization in formic acid or saturated guanidine thiocyanate showed a blocked amino terminus. In subsequent years, biochemical and immunocytochemical studies from several laboratories made clear that the amino termini of plaque Aβ peptides are heterogeneous and include derivatized and amino-terminally blocked species, e.g., pyroglutamate at residue 3. It is likely that the degree of amino-terminal heterogeneity and the precise termini obtained in various biochemical analyses of plaque cores depends in considerable part on the biochemical nature and harshness of the extraction protocol. It has been shown that particular purification reagents can chemically alter Aβ structure, for example, the oxidation of Met35 in the presence of formic acid. Other types of amino acid modifications of plaque Aβ, such as racemization and isomerization of its aspartates (e.g., D-aspartate and L- and D-isoaspartates) or formylation of serines during formic acid solubilization, have been reported. The former changes may occur during the prolonged aging of the deposited amyloid proteins in vivo, whereas the latter is an artifact of an in vitro method of solubilization.

One amino-terminal modification that has received particular attention is the proteolytic removal of residues 1 and 2 (Asp and Ala) and the subsequent cyclizing of residue 3 (Glu) to a pyroglutamate (designated N-3pE). First described in biochemical extracts of AD cortex (Mori et al. 1992), this truncated species was found to be detectable immunohistochemically in many diffuse (i.e., mostly nonfibrillar) plaques in AD and DS cortex (Saido et al. 1995). This truncation increases the aggregation kinetics of Aβ (D'Arrigo et al. 2009; Sanders et al. 2009; Wirths et al. 2010) and also obviates the amino-terminal binding of those therapeutic antibodies which target Asp1 of Aβ (Gardberg et al. 2009). Recent work has shown that glutaminyl cyclase, an enzyme in brain and other tissues which cyclizes exposed glutamates, can do so with high efficiency at Glu3 (Seifert et al. 2009) after removal of the first two residues by aminopeptidases (Schlenzig et al. 2009; Sevalle et al. 2009). The amount of AβpE3 in the brains of APP transgenic mice can increase with time, suggesting that the deposits begin with full-length $Aβ_{1-x}$, some of which is first truncated by local aminopeptidase activity and then modified by glutaminyl cyclase (Wirths et al. 2010). Other changes in the amino terminus, including pathogenic mutations at residues 6 and 7 (Ono et al. 2010), may have major effects on oligomerization.

Taken together, the early biochemical analyses of the amyloid fibrils in meningeal vessels and cerebral plaque cores established that the subunit in both cases was a highly hydrophobic ~4 kDa protein with a unique sequence that had a strong tendency to self-aggregate into stable dimers, trimers, and tetramers, higher oligomers and, ultimately, typical 8 nm amyloid fibrils. One interesting sidelight of these studies was the observation that the Aβ derived from plaque cores was generally more insoluble than that from vascular deposits. For example, 6 M guanidine hydrochloride could effectively solubilize the latter but not the former, whereas the stronger chaotropic salt, guanidine thiocyanate, at saturated (6.8 M) concentrations, could solubilize the cores (Selkoe et al. 1986). The use of concentrated formic acid by Masters and coworkers provided a reagent that appeared to bring even the most insoluble amyloid fibers in AD brains into solution, and it has subsequently been widely used for this purpose. That it can do so indicates that, in general, cerebral Aβ proteins which assemble into amyloid fibrils undergo little or no covalent cross-linking.

Although the identity of the protein subunit of Alzheimer amyloid was thus well established by 1986, the carboxy-terminal sequence beyond residue 28 and the molecular origin of this small peptide remained unclear. As detailed in Haass et al. (2011), it was the power of molecular biological approaches that enabled the elucidation of its full length and how it actually arose from proteolysis of a large precursor polypeptide (Kang et al. 1987).

In the almost 30 years since the biochemical characterization of AD amyloid deposits commenced, we have come to realize that the complexity of this relatively short peptide is determined in part by the microenvironment in which it is generated and resides. Although small amounts can be produced in the endoplasmic reticulum and other vesicular organelles in the secretory pathway, much of the peptide appears to arise from APP that has trafficked to the cell surface and is then sequentially processed by β- and γ-secretase (both are aspartyl proteases) in the mildly acidic environment of recycling endosomes (Selkoe 1994; Kaether et al. 2006; Cirrito et al. 2008; and see Haass et al. 2011). As mentioned above, the peptide isolated from fibrillar amyloid plaques shows substantial heterogeneity at both its amino and carboxyl termini. Its biochemical properties vary significantly depending on its terminal residues, particularly at the hydrophobic carboxyl terminus. Although the field has focused until recently on two peptide lengths, the most abundantly produced species (Aβ1–40) and the far less abundant but more aggregation prone Aβ1–42, this is a simplification, as the variability of carboxy-terminal lengths created by γ-secretase extends at least from $A\beta_{36}$ to $A\beta_{43}$ (Kang et al. 1987). This heterogeneity arises secondary to the initial ε-cleavage of APP by the presenilin/γ-secretase complex at the membrane/cytoplasmic interface, namely at Leu49-Val50 (Weidemann et al. 2002), followed by processive intramembrane processing

by this protease in an amino-terminal direction (i.e., first ε, then ζ and then γ cleavages) (Qi-Takahara et al. 2005; Takami et al. 2009; and see Haass et al. 2011).

AMYLOID FIBRILS OF Aβ: STUDIES OF THEIR STRUCTURE AND PROPERTIES

The pathognomonic lesions of AD are the fibrillar extracellular deposits of Aβ in parenchymal plaques and vascular amyloid and the intraneuronal neurofibrillary tangles, which also have the tinctorial properties of amyloid (Serrano-Pozo et al. 2011). How Aβ, including its buffer-soluble oligomeric forms, may induce the formation of intracellular tangles of the tau protein is discussed elsewhere (Mandelkow and Mandelkow 2011; Mucke and Selkoe 2011). Here we will review the pathway which converts the Aβ region from its largely α-helical conformation when APP is embedded in the lipid membrane to its gradual aggregation into large polymers (filaments) rich in cross-β sheet structure in the extracellular space of the brain. The conversion of α-helix or random coil stretches within normally soluble proteins into principally β-sheet rich assemblies is a common theme in several neurodegenerative diseases. Drawing on the analogous prion theory, it is also possible for a β-sheet conformer to induce or "seed" an α-helical conformer (or some other metastable intermediate) to adopt β-sheet structure (Eisele et al. 2009, 2010). What structural relationship such intermediates in fibrilogenesis have to the soluble, diffusible oligomers of Aβ detected in AD brain remains uncertain. Despite more than 50 years of structural analysis, the atomic resolution of classical amyloid fibrils remains incomplete. Although many techniques have been applied (including solid-state nuclear magnetic resonance and cryo-electron microscopy), the basic noncrystalline subunit in the Aβ fibril has prevented progress (Caspar 2009; Kajava et al. 2010). Moreover, most of the data available on the structure of Aβ and its fibrils come from studies of synthetic Aβ peptides, and it remains unclear whether these accurately model the natural Aβ assemblies found in AD brain.

Theoretical Computational and Molecular Dynamic Models of the Aβ Amyloid Fibril

Although the monomeric subunit of fibrils is thought to consist of two β-strands connected by a turn, the ambiguous nature of the amino and carboxyl termini have precluded development of a detailed model (Olofsson et al. 2009b; Paparcone and Buehler 2009; Ramos et al. 2009). The convoluted carboxy-terminal folding seen in a constrained oligomeric structure (Streltsov et al. 2011) provides a caveat that the simple, U-shape β-turn may be an oversimplification. Some variability in this turn region has now been identified using molecular dynamic (MD) simulations of dimers compared to trimers/pentamers (Horn and Sticht 2010) and a triangular subunit forming a threefold hexamer (Zheng et al. 2010). Constraining the β-turn by linking Asp23 to Lys28 also results in a system with increased fibrillogenic propensity (Reddy et al. 2009a). Placing the β-turn on a constraining physical interface also affects assembly (Fu et al. 2009), and this could have implications for Aβ assembly when some of the peptide is bound to cell membranes, as is likely in the brain. Assembly at low or neutral pH may have an effect on the registration of the subunits within the fibril (Negureanu and Baumketner 2009). Interpeptide hydrogen bonds may play a major role in fibril growth, based on MD modeling (Reddy et al. 2009b; Takeda and Klimov 2009b, 2010). Oxidation of Met35 and assembly in quiescent versus agitated conditions have also been modeled and found to have effects on the hydrophobic surfaces exposed on the fibrils (Wu et al. 2010a).

Structural Studies of Synthetic Aβ Fibrils

Low-resolution (8 Å) cryo-electron microscopy of synthetic Aβ$_{40}$ and Aβ$_{42}$ reveals similar protofilament structures, with approximately 2.5 peptides per cross-β repeat per protofilament (Schmidt et al. 2009). The lack of an integral number per repeat suggests that the assembly may have undefinable amino termini within a tetrameric structure (Caspar 2009). Other low-resolution (10 Å) cryo-EM reconstructions have suggested that the carboxyl terminus forms the inside wall of a hollow core (Zhang et al. 2009d). Two-dimensional infrared spectroscopy discloses intramolecular water molecules around residues 17/34 and 18/36 in a conformation with a presumptive β-turn at 23/28. Substitutions around Glu22 and Asp23, either artificial or mimicking the pathogenic "Arctic" or "Iowa" FAD mutations, produce major effects on rates of aggregation (Perálvarez-Marín et al. 2009; Tycko et al. 2009), perhaps through a mechanism that involves off-registry side chain interactions (Takeda and Klimov 2009c).

DIFFUSIBLE OLIGOMERS OF Aβ

If one considers the trajectory of biochemical studies of Aβ, it is clear that the field has moved over the last dozen years from an initial emphasis on the fibrillar state found in amyloid plaques and meningocerebral vessels to a range of smaller, oligomeric Aβ assemblies that are relatively soluble and diffusible and thus more able to exert a toxic effect on the neuronal plasma membrane, including synapses. A rich and confusing vocabulary has developed to describe the oligomers of Aβ as they assemble along pathways which may or may not lead to the classical 8 nm amyloid fibrils found in plaques and blood vessels (Table 1). The methods of analysis often determine nomenclature: biochemical characterization of synthetic or natural (cellular and brain) Aβ peptides using SDS-PAGE or size exclusion chromatography has led to descriptions of assemblies containing a few (e.g., 2–20) monomers, usually designated soluble oligomers; other methods, particularly those using morphological or biophysical approaches on synthetic Aβ such as electron microscopy or atomic force microscopy, may describe linear protofilaments (often ∼4 nm in diameter) or spherical/globular particles, each of which has been interpreted as a precursor of amyloid fibrils. It is important to emphasize here that many of the synthetic Aβ assembly forms reported in the literature have been made in vitro using supraphysiological concentrations of a single-length peptide (e.g., Aβ1–40), and

Table 1. Aβ assemblies described in the literature

A rich vocabulary that depends on the source of the peptide, the method of analysis, and the laboratory involved

Aβ oligomers of natural or synthetic origin, as visualized chromatographically and/or on denaturing protein gels: monomers (A_4), dimers (A_8), trimers, tetramers (A_{16}), pentamers, hexamers, dodecamer/12-mer (Aβ*56), lower/higher order oligomers [(Aβ)$_n$]

Other synthetic oligomeric Aβ assemblies: amyloid-β-derived diffusible ligands (ADDLs); Aβ micelles, annular (pore-like) structures, (pre-)globulomers (globular oligomers), growth-arrested colloid particles, metastable aggregates, nanopore-like structures, neuroparticles, paranuclei/nucleating seeds, on/off pathway intermediate states, spherical aggregates, etc.

Synthetic Aβ fibrillar assemblies: protofibrils, prefibrils, fibrillar oligomers, nanofibrils

the occurrence of closely similar or identical species in AD brain tissue may not have been explicitly confirmed structurally (immuno-chemical cross-reaction would not be sufficient confirmation). One caveat in this regard is that natural Aβ oligomers isolated from AD brain tissue or APP-expressing cell cultures are far more potent in electrophysiological or cytotoxicity assays than are synthetic assembly mixtures such as ADDLs ("Aβ-derived diffusible ligands") (Lambert et al. 1998) or protofibrils (Harper et al. 1997; Walsh et al. 1997), which require high nanomolar concentrations to induce biological effects, suggesting that they contain many "off-pathway" (unnatural) assembly forms that do not interact with neuronal membranes the way natural oligomers do. Indeed, some such synthetic "oligomers" have not been proven to be truly soluble in aqueous buffers (i.e., not pelletable at 100,000 g in an ultracentrifuge), which is the case for natural oligomers (see, for further reviews of the complexity of Aβ assembly forms, Haass and Selkoe 2007; Walsh and Selkoe 2007; Di Carlo 2010; Sakono and Zako 2010).

Synthetic Aβ as a Substrate for Oligomer Formation

Ever since the sequence of Aβ became known, the easiest approach to study assembly has been to aggregate synthetic peptides at supra-physiological concentrations in vitro (Castano et al. 1986; Gorevic et al. 1986; Kirschner et al. 1987). Classical biochemical analyses of the synthetic aggregates have been supplemented with

newer biophysical methods such as scanning tunneling microscopy (Liu et al. 2009a; Ma et al. 2009), atomic force microscopy (Wu et al. 2010b), quartz crystal microbalance (Ogi et al. 2009), hydrogen exchange mass spectrometry (Zhang et al. 2009a), electron capture dissociation Fourier-transform ion cyclotron resonance mass spectroscopy (Sargaeva et al. 2009), single-molecule spectroscopy (Ding et al. 2009), fluorescence photobleaching and quenching (Reinke et al. 2009; Edwin et al. 2010), click peptide technique (Taniguchi et al. 2009), and ion mobility coupled with mass spectrometry (Bernstein et al. 2009). The experimental conditions for assembling synthetic Aβ monomers into oligomers vary enormously with regard to the roles of temperature, salts, detergents, lipids, metal ions, fatty acids, and other molecules (Sahoo et al. 2009; Yu et al. 2009; Ahmed et al. 2010; Ladiwala et al. 2010; Ryan et al. 2010), and each such condition provides constraints on the techniques the can be used to study the synthetic peptide. Stabilization of synthetic dimers by cross-linking oxidized tyrosine-10 residues (Ono et al. 2009) or introduced cysteine residues (O'Nuallain et al. 2010) also provides a way to study this smallest oligomer and its role in the dynamic equilibrium of Aβ assembly.

Amino acid substitutions and modifications can readily be introduced into synthetic peptides. However, to what degree these synthetic changes adequately model the in vivo situation is often disregarded by investigators. For example, the familial intra-Aβ mutations that occur in dominant fashion at position 22 or

23 (E22G, E22Q, E22K, and D23N) result in the accrual in vivo of a mixture of mutant and wild-type peptides of heterogeneous lengths, but this is often not modeled in vitro (Masuda et al. 2009; Murray et al. 2009b; Brorsson et al. 2010). Nevertheless, synthetic Aβ studies of this critical region do provide some information on the effects of these mutations on the β-turn at 25/26 versus 22/23 and consequent effects on oligomerization and toxicity in vitro.

Molecular Dynamic Approaches to Understanding Synthetic Aβ Oligomers

Although some progress in obtaining atomic resolution of the amino terminus and carboxyl terminus of synthetic Aβ has been made, the overall structure(s) of the oligomer(s) at different assembly points remains elusive. A plethora of MD simulations and theoretical modeling has emerged. Starting at the amino terminus, Takeda and Klimov (2009a) find that amino-terminal truncation has an effect on oligomer (dimer) formation. The metal-binding region of Aβ around residues 6–14 has not yet been adequately addressed by MD studies (see below), and there are conflicting results on models obtained for the loop and β-strands associated with the residue 16–35 region (Chebaro et al. 2009; Miller et al. 2009; Murray et al. 2009a; Hamley et al. 2010; Wei et al. 2010). The oxidation state of Met35 has long been of interest (Haeffner et al. 2010); this residue in the hydrophobic carboxyl terminus may play a role in oligomerization driven by hydrophobic interactions (Zhao et al. 2009). Although it has long been suspected that the highly hydrophobic carboxyl terminus of Aβ42 is a principal determinant of aggregation, its biophysical role in oligomerization has only recently begun to be addressed using synthetic peptides (Murray et al. 2009a; Li et al. 2010). The structure of the carboxyl terminus may involve novel meta-stable conformations (β-hairpin at 35–37), but these remain to be confirmed by crystallo-graphic methods (Wu et al. 2009). Higher order oligomers (pentameric/hexameric assemblies) have been studied by MD and show different effects between the central hydrophobic and carboxy-terminal regions when $A\beta_{40}$ and $A\beta_{42}$ are compared (Urbanc et al. 2010). Synthetic oligomers are also being used in attempts to discover small molecules which are able to target these specific assemblies (Davis and Berkowitz 2009a; Davis et al. 2009; Feng et al. 2009; Liu et al. 2009a; Nerelius et al. 2009; Pitt et al. 2009; Riviere et al. 2009; Smith et al. 2009; Sun et al. 2009; Yamin et al. 2009; Hawkes et al. 2010; Ladiwala et al. 2010).

Recombinant Aβ Oligomers

Aβ oligomers obtained using recombinant techniques appear to be as challenging to work with as their synthetic counterparts (Picone et al. 2009; Walsh et al. 2009; Streltsov et al. 2011). Nevertheless, recombinant constructs have provided a way to conformationally constrain oligomerized Aβ assemblies and are beginning to provide novel insights into lower-order oligomers (e.g., dimers and tetramers) at atomic resolution (see Fig. 2; Streltsov et al. 2011). Recombinant $A\beta_{42}$ with its strong fibrillogenic propensity, is coming under study (Zhang et al. 2009c; Finder et al. 2010). As a bacterially derived product, it is difficult to fully exclude impurities and adventitious factors that might interact with and co-purify with the recombinant peptide. Although purified synthetic Aβ peptides can also contain impurities (e.g., racemized or truncated peptides), the faster aggregating and more potent toxic properties of the recombinant material raise the question of the presence of pro-aggregating seeds and are worthy of further investigation (Finder et al. 2010).

Tissue- and Cell-Derived Natural Oligomers

The ultimate goal of studying the biochemistry of Aβ is to understand its nature and biological properties as it accumulates in the human brain. Early studies detected SDS-stable low-n oligomers on western blots of AD brain extracts (e.g., Masters et al. 1985; Roher et al. 1993), although their biological activities were not studied at that juncture. The major advance of generating mouse lines transgenic for human

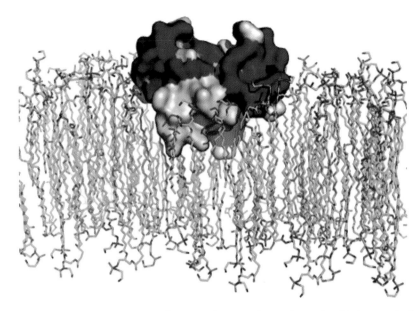

Figure 2. Model of potential interactions of $A\beta_{18-41}$ dimer with membrane lipid bilayers. The hydrophobic dimer–dimer interface of the $A\beta_{18-41}$ tetramer is intercalated into the membrane surface through non-electrostatic interactions, whereas hydrophilic aspects (blue) with metal-binding sites (black) are on the membrane surface. (From Streltsov et al. 2011; reprinted, with permission, from the author.)

APP (Games et al. 1995; Hsiao et al. 1996) has provided dynamic information about which species accrue most quickly (principally Aβ ending at residue 42) and how they aggregate and deposit over time (e.g., Hamaguchi et al. 2009; Philipson et al. 2009; Tomiyama et al. 2010; and see LaFerla and Duff 2011). The in situ association of Aβ oligomers with lipid membranes (Liu et al. 2010b), including post-synaptic densities (Koffie et al. 2009), in APP transgenic mouse brains helps us understand how these potentially toxic Aβ species are compartmentalized. However, only a small number of studies characterizing soluble oligomers per se in transgenic mouse brains has been published (Kawarabayashi et al. 2001; Lesne et al. 2006; Shankar et al. 2009; Pham et al. 2010).

Turning now to studies of human brain tissue, soluble (aqueously extractable and non-pelletable) forms of Aβ in postmortem AD cortex, which include monomers and various oligomers, have become recognized as stronger quantitative correlates of degree of cognitive impairment shortly before death than are amyloid plaques (see Fig. 3; McLean et al. 1999; Tomic et al. 2009; Woltjer et al. 2009; McDonald et al. 2010). Soluble Aβ oligomers extracted from the cortex of typical AD subjects have been shown to potently inhibit long-term potentiation (LTP), enhance long-term depression (LTD), and reduce dendritic spine density in slices of normal rodent hippocampus (Shankar et al. 2008). The extracts of soluble oligomers also disrupted the memory of a learned behavior after intracerebroventricular injection in normal rats. These effects could be principally attributed to dimers, the major SDS-stable oligomer detected on western blots of AD cortex. Importantly, insoluble amyloid plaque cores from the same brains did not impair LTP unless they were first solubilized to release Aβ dimers and other oligomers, suggesting that plaque cores per se have low bioactivity but sequester Aβ dimers that can be synapto-toxic if released (Shankar et al. 2008). There is also evidence that soluble Aβ oligomers isolated from AD cortex can induce hyperphosphorylation of tau protein at AD-relevant epitopes, followed by progressive collapse of the

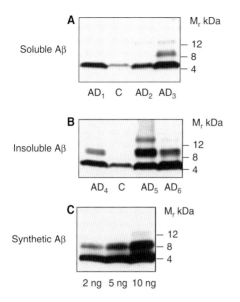

Figure 3. Representative western blots showing Aβ in frontal cortex of selected Alzheimer disease (AD) and control subjects. (*A*) Soluble Aβ in 175,000 g supernatants after a single extraction in phosphate-buffered saline. (*B*) Insoluble Aβ extracted from the 175,000 g pellets. (*C*) To enable quantification and between-gel comparisons, synthetic Aβ$_{40}$ standard curves were run on each gel. The markers designate monomeric (4 kDa), dimeric (8 kDa), and trimeric (12 kDa) forms of Aβ. (From McLean et al. 1999; reprinted, with permission, from the author.)

microtubule cytoskeleton and neuritic dystrophy (Jin et al. 2011).

Although these results suggest a synaptotoxic role for dimers, there are other soluble oligomers detectable in AD brain, including a ~56 kDa putative dodecamer (Lesne et al. 2009). A similar species has been detected in the brains of some APP transgenic mice and its level is shown to correlate with the occurrence of behavioral deficits; isolation of this species from mouse brain and subsequent icv injection into wild-type rats induced decreased spatial memory performance (Lesne et al. 2006; LaFerla and Duff 2011). In vivo, it is likely that there exists an array of low- and medium-sized oligomers, at least some of which appear to be in equilibrium with fibrils in plaques. The latter notion is supported by the occurrence of a halo

of dystrophic neurites immediately around fibrillar plaques, with the neuritic dystrophy diminishing as one moves farther from the plaque; this halo zone is also immunoreactive with certain antibodies that selectively detect small oligomers of Aβ (Meyer-Luehmann et al. 2008; Koffie et al. 2009).

Using immunoaffinity techniques, Noguchi et al. (2009) have isolated 10–15 nm spherical Aβ assemblies (mass >100 kDa) from AD cortex. How these relate to the lower order SDS-stable oligomers discussed above remains to be determined. Other post-translationally modified Aβ species, such as partial aspartate isomerization (Tomidokoro et al. 2010) and carboxy-terminal heterogeneity that includes longer Aβ$_{43}$ peptides (Welander et al. 2009), are being uncovered by isolating Aβ directly from postmortem human brain. In addition, direct analysis of human brain Aβ fibrils may disclose structural differences not predictable from similar analyses of synthetic fibrils (Paravastu et al. 2009).

Neuronally generated Aβ monomers and perhaps various oligomers are presumed to equilibrate within the interstitial fluid of the brain and to turn over in relation to the rates of Aβ production, clearance, and aggregation into amyloid fibrils. From the interstitial compartment or brain parenchyma, soluble Aβ monomers and oligomers may enter into the CSF compartment (Englund et al. 2009; Fukumoto et al. 2010) and even the peripheral blood circulation (Roher et al. 2009; Xia et al. 2009). Although much more work is required to establish the existence of blood-borne Aβ oligomers and confirm their cerebral origin, there is preliminary evidence that blood dimer levels may correlate with clinical features of AD (Villemagne et al. 2010; see also Blennow et al. 2011). Interestingly, such blood-borne dimers are associated with blood cellular membranes (mainly white cells and platelets) and may increase as the natural history of AD advances (Villemagne et al. 2010). In contrast, levels of Aβ42 monomers in both the CSF and plasma are generally considered to fall as AD progresses (Lui et al. 2010a; Blennow et al. 2011).

THE INTERACTIONS OF Aβ WITH OTHER MOLECULES: SERENDIPITOUS BYSTANDERS AND/OR INTIMATE PARTNERS IN PATHOGENESIS?

Early compositional analyses performed on isolated amyloid plaque cores suggested that Aβ, although clearly the major component, was not the sole protein constituent. Moreover, nonproteinaceous components were also identified to varying degrees in enriched—albeit not fully purified—plaque core preparations. It has been difficult to determine on a biochemical basis alone which of these additional constituents are important and integral components of the amyloid plaques and which might become adventitiously associated with Aβ during plaque purification from homogenized brain tissue. When a non-Aβ component of plaques is identified and antibodies are raised to it, these can be used to attempt to label amyloid plaques in situ at both the light and electron microscopic levels. Positive results suggest that a particular protein is indeed associated with the amyloid deposits, although not an integral component of the amyloid fibrils because, like other tissue amyloids, the fibrils should be composed solely of the specific subunit protein. Indeed, the ability to reconstitute amyloid fibrils with an ultrastructure closely resembling the fibrils seen in situ from synthetic Aβ peptides alone has strongly suggested that the sole component of the amyloid filaments in vivo is Aβ. A careful proteomic analysis of amyloid plaque cores isolated from postmortem AD cortex by laser capture microdissection concluded that the only protein constituent detectable by mass spectrometry in the isolated cores was Aβ (Soderberg et al. 2006), supporting the conclusion that the plaque amyloid fibrils are composed of just this protein type. It should be noted, however, that the fibrils may consist in part of heteropolymers of slightly different Aβ peptides, rather than just homopolymers of a single peptide length (e.g., Aβ1–42).

Nevertheless, a variety of other molecules has been found to be loosely or more tightly associated with amyloid deposits during their isolation and can sometimes be shown immunocytochemically in diffuse and/or compacted plaques in situ. Because the morphology of senile plaques indicates the presence of several distinct cellular elements that are intimately apposed, including dystrophic axons and dendrites (Fig. 1) and the processes of activated microglia and reactive astrocytes, any of these as well as local microvessels could potentially be sources of various non-Aβ constituents of the plaques. In short, mature amyloid (neuritic) plaques are heterogeneous mixtures of proteinaceous and nonproteinaceous constituents, and the temporal sequence of accrual of these elements onto the presumed initial Aβ polymer has been difficult to determine.

A recently completed interactome of APP disclosed more than 200 different entities which interact with different domains of APP (128 validated, 74 putative), including a significant proportion interacting with the Aβ region (Perreau et al. 2010). One of the earliest to be identified was the enzyme acetylcholinesterase (AChE; Friede 1965), perhaps paradoxical because of its subsequent role as a therapeutic target for AD and surprising in that the mechanistic basis for the co-location of AChE with the amyloid plaques remains uncertain (De Ferrari et al. 2001). Most of the identified molecular interactors of Aβ in the brain remain equally mysterious and often raise the question of bystander versus functionally significant partner.

Metal Ions

Because of their ubiquitous presence in human tissues, the bioavailable metal ions, Cu, Zn, and Fe, have been obvious choices for investigation of amyloid association. For decades, uncertainty has reigned over the quantitative elemental analysis of whole brain homogenates—and of isolated plaques or tangles—in AD compared to normal aged controls and other neurodegenerative diseases. At the level of grey matter homogenates, there is no agreement that any particular metal ion is specifically elevated or lowered in AD brain. Most techniques have detected elevations in Cu, Zn, or Fe in AD amyloid plaques, either in situ or after their purification (see, for example, Rajendran et al. 2009), but such analytical approaches have never been entirely convincing. The observations that both APP and Aβ have sequences consistent with metal-binding motifs and metallo-complexing activities add a new dimension to this line of enquiry (Faller 2009; Duce et al. 2010). Measuring the affinities of metal–protein interactions is challenging (Xiao and Wedd 2010) but, as technologies have improved, the general rule has emerged that the metal affinities increase as the proteins move toward their sites of final subcellular compartmentalization and utilization. Thus, certain other proteins act as chaperones to take the metal ions into compartments where their higher affinity end-user proteins reside. The synapse has proven to be a subcellular site where ions such as Zn^{2+} and Cu^{2+} are used to modulate the activities of key excitatory NMDA/AMPA receptors. It is in the vicinity of this cellular compartment that Aβ may interact with these divalent cations in a fashion that can alter the peptide's conformation. This metal-based mechanism, as well as the overall level of local excitatory neurotransmission (Cirrito et al. 2005), could help provide an explanation for the topographic selectivity of Aβ aggregation and extracellular deposition in the AD brain, as there is an intriguing overlap between those areas of the brain rich in glutamatergic terminals, free vesicular zinc, and Aβ amyloid plaques in certain APP transgenic mice (Stoltenberg et al. 2007).

With an emerging understanding of the pathways leading to soluble oligomer or insoluble fibril production, therapeutic strategies loosely termed as "anti-Aβ aggregation" need to be refocused on the specific steps being targeted (Rodriguez-Rodriguez et al. 2009; Yadav and Sonker 2009; Dickens and Franz 2010), particularly with regard to the concept of "therapeutic chelation" of metal ions. The concept of therapeutic chelation needs to be qualified by the relative affinities each metal ion has for its target protein. Thus, metal "chaperone" is a preferred concept when discussing the reversible interactions divalent cations can have with Aβ, regardless of which oligomeric or fibrillar assembly is being considered.

Aβ and Copper

The average K_D of Cu^{2+} for Aβ is about 10^{-10} M (i.e., low nanomolar) for both soluble and fibrillar forms of the synthetic peptide in vitro (Rózga et al. 2010; Xiao and Wedd 2010). This means that other metallo-chaperone proteins with higher (i.e., high picomolar or greater) affinities will prevent Cu^{2+} binding to Aβ. This criterion would include human serum albumin (Perrone et al. 2009), suggesting that Aβ in locations (e.g., CSF or blood) remote from parenchymal brain compartments such as neurites and synapses should be unmetallated. Furthermore, therapeutic compounds designed to act as metal-ion chaperones with low picomolar affinities would be expected to compete with Aβ for Cu^{2+} binding only within the brain parenchyma.

Aβ may have more than one Cu^{2+}-binding site (Behbehani and Mirzaie 2009; Jun et al. 2009; Sarell et al. 2009). Depending on the stoichiometry, Cu^{2+}–Aβ interactions can cause synthetic Aβ to aggregate in vitro principally via an oligomer-forming pathway or a fibrillogenic pathway (Brzyska et al. 2009; Moore et al. 2009; Olofsson et al. 2009a; Tõugu et al. 2009; Haeffner et al. 2010). That is, at subequimolar Cu^{2+}:Aβ ratios, amyloid fibrils form; at supra-equimolar ratios, stable oligomers form first, then dityrosine cross-linkages occur (Smith et al. 2007). The principal Cu^{2+}-binding site is coordinated within the first 16 residues and involves His6, His13, and His14, together with the first two residues (Asp1, Ala2) (Dorlet et al. 2009; Drew et al. 2009a,b; Hureau et al. 2009a,b). This coordination environment is pleiotropic (Drew et al. 2009b), adding to the complexity of the analysis (Drochioiu et al. 2009; Hureau et al. 2009a). As was predicted when the Aβ sequence became known, the protonation of the histidine residues, dependent on pH, should have a major effect in the Aβ folding pathway: metallation and folding of Aβ in the endosome/lysosome pathway will probably be quite different from that in the extracellular or peri-synaptic compartments.

Cu^{2+} as a redox-active entity can also induce oxidative modification to Aβ, particularly at Tyr10 with consequent dityrosine covalent cross-links (Drew et al. 2009a,b; Moore et al. 2009; Jiang et al. 2010). Other residues, such as Met35, may participate (Barman et al. 2009; Butterfield et al. 2010), but this is not proven (da Silva et al. 2009). Whether the metal-modified Aβ is capable of pro- or anti-oxidant activity is also uncertain (Baruch-Suchodolsky and Fischer 2009), but it is an important question that needs to be resolved in terms of understanding the toxicity of Aβ oligomers. Reducing intracellular Cu^{2+} bioavailability has an inhibitory effect on Aβ oligomer formation (Crouch et al. 2009a).

Aβ and Zinc

In contrast to Cu^{2+}, Zn^{2+} is redox inactive and therefore cannot be directly involved in any oxidative processes involving Aβ. In common with Cu^{2+}, Zn^{2+} has pleotropic binding sites on Aβ (Damante et al. 2009; Talmard et al. 2009; Miller et al. 2010) which can serve to drive synthetic Aβ aggregation in vitro. The Zn^{2+}-induced formation of cytotoxic Aβ oligomers in proximity to excitatory glutamatergic synapses is believed to be a mechanism contributing to synaptic degeneration in AD (Deshpande et al. 2009). Zn–Aβ complexes also become more resistant to proteolytic degradation in in vitro experiments (Crouch et al. 2009b), potentially allowing metal-bound Aβ fibrils to accumulate in the extracellular space.

Aβ and Iron

Studies of Fe^{3+}/Fe^{2+} complexes with Aβ indicate a potential pro-aggregating role for this abundant metal (Jiang et al. 2009a; Uranga et al. 2010), especially if evidence that Aβ has significantly higher affinity for Fe^{2+} than does transferrin (Jiang et al. 2009a) is confirmed.

Aβ INTERACTIONS WITH CELL MEMBRANES, LIPOPROTEINS, AND MEMBRANE-ASSOCIATED PROTEINS

The proteolytic release of Aβ from APP is believed to occur principally in an endosomal/lysosomal compartment or from the surface of the plasma membrane (see Haass et al. 2011). Given the amphiphilic nature of Aβ, it is not surprising that many potential interactions can occur once it is a free peptide. These interactions can be driven by phase/interface effects, electrostatic (charge) interactions dependent on the pH of the microenvironment, and hydrophobic interactions if the hydrophobic carboxy-terminal region is able to re-associate with the lipid bilayer. These types of bonding apply also to Aβ interactions with the lipoprotein particles formed with ApoE, ApoA, and ApoJ, as well as with other membrane-associated macromolecular complexes in the vicinity of synapses such as NMDA, AMPA, insulin, and nicotinic ACh receptors. All of these complex protein interactions are dependent in part on the conformation and state of assembly of Aβ itself. When sequential fractions of postmortem AD brain homogenates are analyzed, the major pool of Aβ lies in the detergent-insoluble (e.g., formic acid- or guanidine-extractable) fraction, presumably representing rather insoluble amyloid plaques, but a considerable amount is apparently loosely associated with cellular membranes (e.g., the sodium carbonate-extractable fraction). The diffusible, aqueously extractable fraction (e.g., buffered saline extract) is generally less than 1–2% of the total recoverable brain Aβ. It is the membrane-associated pool of brain Aβ which can be recovered in sodium carbonate or Triton that we will focus on now (see Relini et al. 2009 for a recent review).

Phase/Interface Effects

Most in vitro studies of the α-helix to β-sheet conversion and aggregation of Aβ peptides are conducted at concentrations 3–4 orders of magnitude greater than those found in vivo. Moreover, the special microenvironment in which Aβ aggregation is believed to occur in vivo is not always taken into account, e.g., the relatively high concentrations of metal ions in and around synapses. The interface between the interstitial fluid phase and the surface of the plasma membrane is likely to be a critical factor in influencing the aggregation pathway of Aβ. A number of in vitro studies find this, showing interface clustering of Aβ (Chi et al. 2010) that slows the lag phase of fibril formation (Hellstrand et al. 2010) by providing an environment for a hydrophobic layer adjacent to the membrane interface (Jiang et al. 2009b). Physical movement/agitation at the water–membrane interface may also promote fibrillogenesis (Morinaga et al. 2010; Wu et al. 2010a). The nature of this interface may therefore strongly affect the Aβ folding pathway (Kayed et al. 2009). In contrast to the hydrophilic ectodomains of various proteins proposed to function as Aβ receptors, membrane lipid surfaces seem a more biophysically plausible receptor for the highly hydrophobic Aβ oligomers.

Electrostatic/Charge Effects

The role of negatively charged phospholipid head groups, sphingolipids, sialic acid, etc. in affecting the binding and oligomerization of Aβ is being increasingly examined (Kayed et al. 2009; Salay et al. 2009; Kotarek and Moss 2010; Sureshbabu et al. 2010). Smaller (1–2 nm diameter) synthetic Aβ oligomers have a greater tendency to bind such charged species than do those of larger (4–5 nm) size (Cizas et al. 2010). Local membrane charge may also alter the β-turn of synthetic Aβ peptides (Grimaldi et al. 2010). Exposed phosphatidylserine has been proposed as a mediator of Aβ–membrane surface interactions (Simakova and Arispe 2007). MD modeling (Davis and Berkowitz 2009a,b) suggests the induction of subtle changes in conformation around the β-turn of Aβ fold on its membrane binding, and in vitro studies show the effect of pH and the protonation of His13 and/or His14 when the amphiphilic domain Aβ$_{11-22}$ is used for membrane binding studies (Ravault et al. 2009). Using L- and D-handed enantiomers of Aβ$_{42}$, Ciccotosto et al. (2011) have reported that synthetic Aβ binds directly to cell membranes in vivo through phosphatidylserine and that this interaction is stereospecific. The toxicity of Aβ oligomers may therefore be related in part to some aspect of its specific electrostatic interactions with phosphatidylserine. Gangliosides

provide another charged interactor for Aβ on the cell surface (Nakazawa et al. 2009; Peters et al. 2009; Utsumi et al. 2009; Yagi-Utsumi et al. 2010), with potential effects on the folding pattern of the peptide (Mao et al. 2010; Ogawa et al. 2011).

Hydrophobic Interactions of Aβ

After the release of the Aβ monomer from its partially transmembrane location, a portion of resultant Aβ assemblies may bind and re-insert into the hydrophobic lipid bilayer. There has been a longstanding controversy in the field as to whether this re-insertion event leads to the formation of a complete transmembrane pore or whether membrane association and partial insertion can disrupt the bilayer to such an extent that its structural integrity is compromised. MD simulations and in vitro artificial lipid membrane models of this insertional event are plentiful (Friedman et al. 2009; Lemkul and Bevan 2009; Miyashita et al. 2009; Qiu et al. 2009; Song et al. 2009; Yang et al. 2009a,b; Morita et al. 2010; Schauerte et al. 2010; Wang et al. 2010), but rigorous evidence for a hydrophobic membrane-traversing interaction in vivo is lacking. Using photobleaching Förster resonance energy transfer, there was a loss of signal from the hydrophobic carboxyl terminus of Aβ as it interacts with the plasma membrane of PC12 cells, which may indicate its sequestration within the lipid bilayer (Bateman and Chakrabartty 2009). Addition of synthetic Aβ$_{42}$ oligomers to N2a and HT22 neuronal cell lines led to significant cellular stiffening/rigidity (Lulevich et al. 2010). Peripheral membrane association of Aβ$_{42}$ (but not Aβ$_{40}$) oligomers with lysosmes has also been suggested as evidence of in vivo membrane insertion (Liu et al. 2010b). Clearly, more evidence is required to prove actual transmembrane insertion of the peptide in vivo.

Aβ Interaction with Lipoproteins

Electrostatic or hydrophobic interactions of Aβ with the various lipoprotein particles (ApoE, ApoA, ApoJ) are discussed elsewhere in this volume (Holtzman et al. 2011). We note in vivo evidence of direct ApoE–Aβ and ApoA1–Aβ interactions (Bales et al. 2009; Paula-Lima et al. 2009), and that ApoE found in the brain is more heavily sialylated than that in the peripheral circulation (Kawasaki et al. 2009), potentially facilitating electrostatic interactions with Aβ (see above).

Aβ Interactions with Selected Membrane Polypeptides (e.g., NMDA and ACh Receptors)

Growing evidence suggests the occurrence of at least functional—if not physical—interactions of Aβ oligomers with NMDA or α7-nicotinic ACh receptors or the cellular prion protein (Hu et al. 2009; Lauren et al. 2009; Li et al. 2009; Liu et al. 2009b; Zhang et al. 2009b). However, much of this evidence comes from studies showing that antagonists or downstream regulators of these and other cell-surface receptors (e.g., AMPA and insulin receptors) can mitigate or fully prevent the effects of soluble Aβ oligomers on synaptic form and function (see, e.g., Shankar et al. 2007; Li et al. 2009). Such studies only indicate that the expression and normal function of the receptor in question is necessary for some of the downstream effects of Aβ on neurons to occur, not that these cell-surface polypeptides are the direct receptors for Aβ in vivo. Instead, the binding of extracellular Aβ oligomers—via their exposed hydrophobic residues—to certain lipids in the plasma membrane could alter the biophysical properties of the bilayer and secondarily and somewhat nonspecifically perturb the structures (and thus the functions) of a variety of membrane-anchored neuronal receptor proteins. Moreover, as mentioned above, the high concentrations of Zn^{2+} and Cu^{2+} found in and around NMDAR-containing post-synaptic elements may be involved in the actions of Aβ oligomers at the membrane.

Other Aβ Interactions

Over the past 30 years, many other proteins have been described as being associated with Aβ extracellular deposits, using a variety of immunohistochemical or biochemical approaches. Among these, two broad categories of proteins stand out: extracellular matrix factors and inflammatory/stress response factors. The latter include members of the complement cascade, cytokines, immunoglobulins, acute phase proteins, components of the inflammosome, etc. The serine protease inhibitor, α1-antichymotrypsin, is an acute phase protein that may be tightly associated with amyloid plaque cores (Abraham et al. 1988). Biochemical isolation approaches have also yielded co-purifying proteins of unknown pathogenic significance, e.g., a fragment (residues 60–95) of the neuronal protein, α-synuclein, namely, its NAC peptide (i.e., "non-amyloid component" of plaques). The fact that some cortical neurons in AD accumulate aggregates of α-synuclein (Lewy bodies and neurites) provides a possible explanation for the co-purification of this protein fragment from homogenized AD cortex. Many other polypeptides of unknown mechanistic importance in the disease pathogenesis could be cited here. The fact that some amyloid-associated proteins differ in their primary sequences and amounts between human and mouse brain could help explain why APP transgenic mice deposit plaques of human Aβ but not always with the same local associations and consequences (e.g., without significant neuronal loss).

CONCLUSIONS

Even the wealth of details and accompanying references that we have discussed above cannot do the subject of Aβ biochemistry justice. Since Glenner and Wong's seminal paper in 1984, innumerable studies of this small, hydrophobic, and potentially lethal protein have been published. Indeed, several important aspects of its biology, including its mechanisms of formation (Haass et al. 2011) and clearance (Saido and Leissring 2011) and its measurement by brain imaging (Johnson et al. 2011) and in biological fluids (Blennow et al. 2011), are covered extensively in other parts of this volume. The genetics of dominantly inherited AD and the pathobiology of the apolipoprotein ε4 allele in AD have combined to give Aβ an apparent initiating role in at least some forms of the AD syndrome. Because these familial forms are largely indistinguishable from "sporadic" late-onset AD, parsimony suggests that an imbalance between Aβ production and clearance—an Aβ dyshomeostasis—is a driving force for many or all cases of AD as we define this eponymic syndrome. And yet, precisely why Aβ accumulates and what upstream events can lead to this accumulation remains unknown for the majority of cases of the disease. Perhaps only through the results of clinical trials of agents that must be working solely on Aβ (e.g., highly specific anti-Aβ antibodies) can we adequately test the theory that Aβ accumulation is a central pathogenic event in AD. For the sake of our patients and their families, one can only hope that the answer to this provocative question lies not too far in the future.

REFERENCES

*Reference is also in this collection.

Abraham CR, Selkoe DJ, Potter H. 1988. Immunochemical identification of the serine protease inhibitor, α_1-antichymotrypsin in the brain amyloid deposits of Alzheimer's disease. Cell 52: 487–501.

Ahmed M, Davis J, Aucoin D, Sato T, Ahuja S, Aimoto S, Elliott JI, Van Nostrand WE, Smith SO. 2010. Structural conversion of neurotoxic amyloid-β_{1-42} oligomers to fibrils. Nat Struct Mol Biol 17: 561–567.

Allsop D, Landon M, Kidd M. 1983. The isolation and amino acid composition of senile plaque core protein. Brain Res 259: 348–352.

Bales KR, Liu F, Wu S, Lin SZ, Koger D, DeLong C, Hansen JC, Sullivan PM, Paul SM. 2009. Human APOE isoform-dependent effects on brain β-amyloid levels in PDAPP transgenic mice. J Neurosci 29: 6771–6779.

Barman A, Taves W, Prabhakar R. 2009. Insights into the mechanism of methionine oxidation catalyzed by metal (Cu^{2+}, Zn^{2+}, and Fe^{3+})-amyloid beta (Aβ) peptide complexes: A computational study. J Comput Chem 30: 1405–1413.

Baruch-Suchodolsky R, Fischer B. 2009. Aβ$_{40}$, either soluble or aggregated, is a remarkably potent antioxidant in cell-free oxidative systems. Biochemistry 48: 4354–4370.

Bateman DA, Chakrabartty A. 2009. Two distinct conformations of Aβ aggregates on the surface of living PC12 cells. Biophys J 96: 4260–4267.

Behbehani GR, Mirzaie M. 2009. A high performance method for thermodynamic study on the binding of copper ion and glycine with Alzheimer's amyloid β peptide. J Therm Anal Calorim 96: 631–635.

Bernstein SL, Dupuis NF, Lazo ND, Wyttenbach T, Condron MM, Bitan G, Teplow DB, Shea J-E, Ruotolo BT, Robinson CV, et al. 2009. Amyloid-β protein oligomerization and the importance of tetramers and dodecamers in the aetiology of Alzheimer's disease. Nat Chem 1: 326–331.

*Blennow K, Zetterberg H, Fagan AM. 2011. Fluid biomarkers in Alzheimer disease. Cold Spring Harb Perspect Med doi: 10.1101/cshperspect.a006221.

Brorsson AC, Bolognesi B, Tartaglia GG, Shammas SL, Favrin G, Watson I, Lomas DA, Chiti F, Vendruscolo M, Dobson CM, et al. 2010. Intrinsic determinants of neurotoxic aggregate formation by the amyloid β peptide. Biophys J 98: 1677–1684.

Brzyska M, Trzesniewska K, Wieckowska A, Szczepankiewicz A, Elbaum D. 2009. Electrochemical and conformational consequences of copper (Cu-I and Cu-II) binding to β-amyloid(1–40). Chembiochem 10: 1045–1055.

Butterfield DA, Galvan V, Lange MB, Tang H, Sowell RA, Spilman P, Fombonne J, Gorostiza O, Zhang J, Sultana R, et al. 2010. In vivo oxidative stress in brain of Alzheimer disease transgenic mice: Requirement for methionine 35 in amyloid β-peptide of APP. Free Radic Biol Med 48: 136–144.

Caspar DL. 2009. Inconvenient facts about pathological amyloid fibrils. Proc Natl Acad Sci 106: 20555–20556.

Castano EM, Ghiso J, Prelli F, Gorevic PD, Migheli A, Frangione B. 1986. In vitro formation of amyloid fibrils from two synthetic peptides of different lengths homologous to Alzheimer's disease β-protein. Biochem Biophys Res Commun 141: 782–789.

Chebaro Y, Mousseau N, Derreumaux P. 2009. Structures and thermodynamics of Alzheimer's amyloid-β Aβ(16–35) monomer and dimer by replica exchange molecular dynamics simulations: Implication for full-length Aβ fibrillation. J Phys Chem B 113: 7668–7675.

Chi EY, Frey SL, Winans A, Lam KLH, Kjaer K, Majewski J, Lee KYC. 2010. Amyloid-β fibrillogenesis seeded by interface-induced peptide misfolding and self-assembly. Biophys J 98: 2299–2308.

Ciccotosto GD, Tew DJ, Drew SC, Smith DG, Johanssen T, Lal V, Lau TL, Perez K, Curtain CC, Wade JD, et al. 2011. Stereospecific interactions are necessary for Alzheimer disease amyloid-β toxicity. Neurobiol Aging 32: 235–248.

Cirrito JR, Yamada KA, Finn MB, Sloviter RS, Bales KR, May PC, Schoepp DD, Paul SM, Mennerick S, Holtzman DM. 2005. Synaptic activity regulates interstitial fluid amyloid-β levels in vivo. Neuron 48: 913–922.

Cirrito JR, Kang JE, Lee J, Stewart FR, Verges DK, Silverio LM, Bu G, Mennerick S, Holtzman DM. 2008. Endocytosis is required for synaptic activity-dependent release of amyloid-beta in vivo. Neuron 58: 42–51.

Cizas P, Budvytyte R, Morkuniene R, Moldovan R, Broccio M, Losche M, Niaura G, Valincius G, Borutaite V. 2010. Size-dependent neurotoxicity of β-amyloid oligomers. Arch Biochem Biophy 496: 84–92.

Crouch PJ, Hung LW, Adlard PA, Cortes M, Lal V, Filiz G, Perez KA, Nurjono M, Caragounis A, Du T, et al. 2009a. Increasing Cu bioavailability inhibits Aβ oligomers and tau phosphorylation. *Proc Natl Acad Sci* **106:** 381–386.

Crouch PJ, Tew DJ, Du T, Nguyen DN, Caragounis A, Filiz G, Blake RE, Trounce IA, Soon CPW, Laughton K, et al. 2009b. Restored degradation of the Alzheimer's amyloid-β peptide by targeting amyloid formation. *J Neurochem* **108:** 1198–1207.

D'Arrigo C, Tabaton M, Perico A. 2009. N-terminal truncated pyroglutamyl β amyloid peptide Aβpy3–42 shows a faster aggregation kinetics than the full-length Aβ1–42. *Biopolymers* **91:** 861–873.

da Silva GFZ, Lykourinou VAngerhofer A, L-J Ming. 2009. Methionine does not reduce Cu(II)-β-amyloid!—Rectification of the roles of methionine-35 and reducing agents in metal-centered oxidation chemistry of Cu(II)-β-amyloid. *Biochim Biophy Acta* **1792:** 49–55.

Damante CA, Osz K, Nagy Z, Pappalardo G, Grasso G, Impellizzeri G, Rizzarelli E, Sovago I. 2009. Metal loading capacity of Aβ N-terminus: a combined potentiometric and spectroscopic study of zinc(II) complexes with Aβ(1–16), its short or mutated peptide fragments and its polyethylene glycol-ylated analogue. *Inorg Chem* **48:** 10405–10415.

Davis CH, Berkowitz ML. 2009a. Interaction between amyloid-β (1–42) peptide and phospholipid bilayers: A molecular dynamics study. *Biophys J* **96:** 785–797.

Davis CH, Berkowitz ML. 2009b. Structure of the amyloid-β (1–42) monomer absorbed to model phospholipid bilayers: A molecular dynamics study. *J Phys Chem B* **113:** 14480–14486.

Davis TJ, Soto-Ortega DD, Kotarek JA, Gonzalez-Velasquez FJ, Sivakumar K, Wu LY, Wang Q, Moss MA. 2009. Comparative study of inhibition at multiple stages of amyloid-β self-assembly provides mechanistic insight. *Mol Pharmacol* **76:** 405–413.

De Ferrari GV, Canales MA, Shin I, Weiner LM, Silman I, Inestrosa NC. 2001. A structural motif of acetylcholinesterase that promotes amyloid β-peptide fibril formation. *Biochemistry* **40:** 10447–10457.

Deshpande A, Kawai H, Metherate R, Glabe CG, Busciglio J. 2009. A role for synaptic zinc in activity-dependent Aβ oligomer formation and accumulation at excitatory synapses. *J Neurosci* **29:** 4004–4015.

Di Carlo M. 2010. Beta amyloid peptide: From different aggregation forms to the activation of different biochemical pathways. *Eur Biophys J Biophys Lett* **39:** 877–888.

Dickens MG, Franz KJ. 2010. A prochelator activated by hydrogen peroxide prevents metal-induced amyloid β aggregation. *Chembiochem* **11:** 59–62.

Ding H, Wong PT, Lee EL, Gafni A, Steel DG. 2009. Determination of the oligomer size of amyloidogenic protein β-amyloid(1–40) by single-molecule spectroscopy. *Biophys J* **97:** 912–921.

Dorlet P, Gambarelli S, Faller P, Hureau C. 2009. Pulse EPR spectroscopy reveals the coordination sphere of copper(II) ions in the 1–16 amyloid-β peptide: A key role of the first two N-terminus residues. *Angew Chem Int Ed Engl* **48:** 9273–9276.

Drew SC, Masters CL, Barnham KJ. 2009a. Alanine-2 carbonyl is an oxygen ligand in Cu^{2+} coordination of Alzheimer's disease amyloid-β peptide—relevance to N-

terminally truncated forms. *J Am Chem Soc* **131:** 8760–8761.

Drew SC, Noble CJ, Masters CL, Hanson GR, Barnham KJ. 2009b. Pleomorphic copper coordination by Alzheimer's disease amyloid-β peptide. *J Am Chem Soc* **131:** 1195–1207.

Drochioiu G, Manea M, Dragusanu M, Murariu M, Dragan ES, Petre BA, Mezo G, Przybylski M. 2009. Interaction of β-amyloid (1–40) peptide with pairs of metal ions: An electrospray ion trap mass spectrometric model study. *Biophys Chem* **144:** 9–20.

Duce JA, Tsatsanis A, Cater MA, James SA, Robb E, Wikhe K, Leong SL, Perez K, Johanssen T, Greenough MA, et al. 2010. Iron-export ferroxidase activity of β-amyloid precursor protein is inhibited by zinc in Alzheimer's disease. *Cell* **142:** 857–867.

Edwin NJ, Hammer RP, McCarley RL, Russo PS. 2010. Reversibility of β-amyloid self-assembly: Effects of pH and added salts assessed by fluorescence photobleaching recovery. *Biomacromolecules* **11:** 341–347.

Eisele YS, Bolmont T, Heikenwalder M, Langer F, Jacobson LH, Yan ZX, Roth K, Aguzzi A, Staufenbiel M, Walker LC, et al. 2009. Induction of cerebral β-amyloidosis: Intracerebral versus systemic Aβ inoculation. *Proc Natl Acad Sci* **106:** 12926–12931.

Eisele YS, Obermüller U, Heilbronner G, Baumann F, Kaeser SA, Wolburg H, Walker LC, Staufenbiel M, Heikenwalder M, Jucker M. 2010. Peripherally applied Aβ-containing inoculates induce cerebral β-amyloidosis. *Science* **330:** 980–982.

Englund H, Degerman Gunnarsson M, Brundin RM, Hedlund M, Kilander L, Lannfelt L, Pettersson FE. 2009. Oligomerization partially explains the lowering of Aβ42 in Alzheimer's disease cerebrospinal fluid. *Neurodegener Dis* **6:** 139–147.

Faller P. 2009. Copper and zinc binding to amyloid-β: Coordination, dynamics, aggregation, reactivity and metal-ion transfer. *Chembiochem* **10:** 2837–2845.

Feng Y, Wang XP, Yang SG, Wang YJ, Zhang X, Du XT, Sun XX, Zhao M, Huang L, Liu RT. 2009. Resveratrol inhibits beta-amyloid oligomeric cytotoxicity but does not prevent oligomer formation. *Neurotoxicology* **30:** 986–995.

Finder VH, Vodopivec I, Nitsch RM, Glockshuber R. 2010. The recombinant amyloid-β peptide Aβ1-42 aggregates faster and is more neurotoxic than synthetic Aβ1-42. *J Mol Biol* **396:** 9–18.

Friede RL. 1965. Enzyme histochemical studies of senile plaques. *J Neuropathol Exp Neurol* **24:** 477–491.

Friedman R, Pellarin R, Caflisch A. 2009. Amyloid aggregation on lipid bilayers and its impact on membrane permeability. *J Mol Biol* **387:** 407–415.

Fu ZM, Luo Y, Derreumaux P, Wei GH. 2009. Induced β-barrel formation of the Alzheimer's Aβ 25–35 oligomers on carbon nanotube surfaces: Implication for amyloid fibril inhibition. *Biophys J* **97:** 1795–1803.

Fukumoto H, Tokuda T, Kasai T, Ishigami N, Hidaka H, Kondo M, Allsop D, Nakagawa M. 2010. High-molecular-weight β-amyloid oligomers are elevated in cerebrospinal fluid of Alzheimer patients. *FASEB J* **24:** 2716–2726.

Games D, Adams D, Alessandrini R, Barbour R, Berthelette P, Blackwell C, Carr T, Clemens J, Donaldson T, Gillespie F, et al. 1995. Alzheimer-type neuropathology in transgenic mice overexpressing V717F β-amyloid precursor protein. *Nature* **373:** 523–527.

Gardberg A, Dice L, Pridgen K, Ko J, Patterson P, Ou S, Wetzel R, Dealwis C. 2009. Structures of Aβ-related peptide-monoclonal antibody complexes. *Biochemistry* **48:** 5210–5217.

Glenner GG. 1979. Congophilic microangiopathy in the pathogenesis of Alzheimer's syndrome (presenile dementia). *Med Hypotheses* **5:** 1231–1236.

Glenner GG, Wong CW. 1984a. Alzheimer's disease and Down's syndrome: Sharing of a unique cerebrovascular amyloid fibril protein. *Biochem Biophys Res Commun* **122:** 1131–1135.

Glenner GG, Wong CW. 1984b. Alzheimer's disease: Initial report of the purification and characterization of a novel cerebrovascular amyloid protein. *Biochem Biophys Res Commun* **120:** 885–890.

Gorevic P, Goni F, Pons-Estel B, Alvarez F, Peress R, Frangione B. 1986. Isolation and partial characterization of neurofibrillary tangles and amyloid plaque cores in Alzheimer's disease: Immunohistological studies. *J Neuropathol Exp Neurol* **45:** 647–664.

Grimaldi M, Scrima M, Esposito C, Vitiello G, Ramunno A, Limongelli V, D'Errico G, Novellino E, D'Ursi AM. 2010. Membrane charge dependent states of the β-amyloid fragment Aβ (16–35) with differently charged micelle aggregates. *Biochim Biophys Acta* **1798:** 660–671.

Haass C, Selkoe DJ. 2007. Soluble protein oligomers in neurodegeneration: Lessons from the Alzheimer's amyloid β-peptide. *Nat Rev Mol Cell Biol* **8:** 101–112.

* Haass C, Kaether C, Sisodia S, Thinakaran G. 2011. Trafficking and proteolytic processing of APP. *Cold Spring Harb Perspect Med* doi: 10.1101/cshperspect.a006270.

Haeffner F, Barnham KJ, Bush AI, Brinck T. 2010. Generation of soluble oligomeric β-amyloid species via copper catalyzed oxidation with implications for Alzheimer's disease: A DFT study. *J Mol Model* **16:** 1103–1108.

Hamaguchi T, Ono K, Murase A, Yamada M. 2009. Phenolic compounds prevent Alzheimer's pathology through different effects on the amyloid-β aggregation pathway. *Am J Pathol* **175:** 2557–2565.

Hamley IW, Nutt DR, Brown GD, Miravet JF, Escuder B, Rodriguez-Llansola F. 2010. Influence of the solvent on the self-assembly of a modified amyloid beta peptide fragment. II. NMR and computer simulation investigation. *J Phys Chem B* **114:** 940–951.

Harper JD, Wong SS, Lieber CM., Lansbury PT Jr. 1997. Observation of metastable Aβ amyloid protofibrils by atomic force microscopy. *Chem Biol* **4:** 119–125.

Hawkes CA, Deng LH, Shaw JE, Nitz M, McLaurin J. 2010. Small molecule β-amyloid inhibitors that stabilize protofibrillar structures in vitro improve cognition and pathology in a mouse model of Alzheimer's disease. *Eur J Neurosci* **31:** 203–213.

Hellstrand E, Sparr E, Linse S. 2010. Retardation of Aβ fibril formation by phospholipid vesicles depends on membrane phase behavior. *Biophys J* **98:** 2206–2214.

* Holtzman D, Herz J, Bu Guojun. 2011. Apolipoprotein E and apolipoprotein E receptors: Normal biology and roles in Alzheimer disease. *Cold Spring Harb Perspect Med* doi: 10.1101/cshperspect.a006312.

Horn AH, Sticht H. 2010. Amyloid-β42 oligomer structures from fibrils: A systematic molecular dynamics study. *J Phys Chem B* **114:** 2219–2226.

Hsiao K, Chapman P, Nilsen S, Ekman C, Harigaya Y, Younkin S, Yang F, Cole G. 1996. Correlative memory deficits, Aβ elevation, and amyloid plaques in transgenic mice. *Science* **274:** 99–102.

Hu NW, Klyubin I, Anwy R, Rowan MJ. 2009. GluN2B subunit-containing NMDA receptor antagonists prevent Aβ-mediated synaptic plasticity disruption in vivo. *Proc Natl Acad Sci* **106:** 20504–20509.

Hureau C, Balland V, Coppel Y, Solari PL, Fonda E, Faller P. 2009a. Importance of dynamical processes in the coordination chemistry and redox conversion of copper amyloid-β complexes. *J Biol Inorg Chem* **14:** 995–1000.

Hureau C, Coppel Y, Dorlet P, Solari PL, Sayen S, Guillon E, Sabater L, Faller P. 2009b. Deprotonation of the Asp1-Ala2 peptide bond induces modification of the dynamic copper(II) environment in the amyloid-β peptide near physiological pH. *Angew Chem Int Ed Engl* **48:** 9522–9525.

Jiang D, Li X, Williams R, Patel S, Men L, Wang Y, Zhou F. 2009a. Ternary complexes of iron, amyloid-β, and nitrilotriacetic acid: Binding affinities, redox properties, and relevance to iron-induced oxidative stress in Alzheimer's disease. *Biochemistry* **48:** 7939–7947.

Jiang DL, Dinh KL, Ruthenburg TC, Zhang Y, Su L, Land DP, Zhou FM. 2009b. A kinetic model for β-amyloid adsorption at the air/solution interface and its implication to the β-amyloid aggregation process. *J Phys Chem B* **113:** 3160–3168.

Jiang DL, Li XJ, Liu L, Yagnik GB, Zhou FM. 2010. Reaction rates and mechanism of the ascorbic acid oxidation by molecular oxygen facilitated by Cu(II)-containing amyloid-β complexes and aggregates. *J Phys Chem B* **114:** 4896–4903.

Jin M, Shepardson N, Yang T, Walsh D, Selkoe D. 2011. Soluble amyloid β-protein dimers isolated from Alzheimer cortex directly induce Tau hyperphosphorylation and neuritic degeneration. *Proc Natl Acad Sci* **108:** 5819–5824.

* Johnson KA, Fox NC, Sperling RA, Klunk WE. 2011. Brain imaging in Alzheimer disease. *Cold Spring Harb Perspect Med* doi: 10.1101/cshperspect.a006213.

Jun S, Gillespie JR, Shin BK, Saxena S. 2009. The second Cu(II)-binding site in a proton-rich environment interferes with the aggregation of amyloid-β(1–40) into amyloid fibrils. *Biochemistry* **48:** 10724–10732.

Kaether C, Schmitt S, Willem M, Haass C. 2006. Amyloid precursor protein and Notch intracellular domains are generated after transport of their precursors to the cell surface. *Traffic* **7:** 408–415.

Kajava AV, Baxa U, Steven AC. 2010. β arcades: Recurring motifs in naturally occurring and disease-related amyloid fibrils. *FASEB J* **24:** 1311–1319.

Kang J, Lemaire H-G, Unterbeck A, Salbaum JM, Masters CL, Grzeschik K-H, Multhaup G, Beyreuther K, Muller-Hill B. 1987. The precursor of Alzheimer's disease amyloid A4 protein resembles a cell-surface receptor. *Nature* **325**: 733–736.

Kawarabayashi T, Younkin LH, Saido TC, Shoji M, Ashe KH, Younkin SG. 2001. Age-dependent changes in brain, CSF, and plasma amyloid β protein in the Tg2576 transgenic mouse model of Alzheimer's disease. *J Neurosci* **21**: 372–381.

Kawasaki K, Ogiwara N, Sugano M, Okumura N, Yamauchi K. 2009. Sialic acid moiety of apolipoprotein E and its impact on the formation of lipoprotein particles in human cerebrospinal fluid. *Clin Chim Acta* **402**: 61–66.

Kayed R, Pensalfini A, Margol L, Sokolov Y, Sarsoza F, Head E, Hall J, Glabe C. 2009. Annular protofibrils are a structurally and functionally distinct type of amyloid oligomer. *J Biol Chem* **284**: 4230–4237.

Kirschner DA, Inouye H, Duffy LK, Sinclair A, Lind M, Selkoe DJ. 1987. Synthetic peptide homologous to β protein from Alzheimer disease forms amyloid-like fibrils in vitro. *Proc Natl Acad Sci* **84**: 6953–6957.

Koffie RM, Meyer-Luehmann M, Hashimoto T, Adams KW, Mielke ML, Garcia-Alloza M, Micheva KD, Smith SJ, Kim ML, Lee VM, et al. 2009. Oligomeric amyloid β associates with postsynaptic densities and correlates with excitatory synapse loss near senile plaques. *Proc Natl Acad Sci* **106**: 4012–4017.

Kotarek JA, Moss MA. 2010. Impact of phospholipid bilayer saturation on amyloid-β protein aggregation intermediate growth: A quartz crystal microbalance analysis. *Anal Biochem* **399**: 30–38.

Ladiwala AR, Lin JC, Bale SS, Marcelino-Cruz AM, Bhattacharya A, Dordick JS, Tessier PM. 2010. Resveratrol selectively remodels soluble oligomers and fibrils of amyloid Aβ into off-pathway conformers. *J Biol Chem* **285**: 24228–24237.

* LaFerla F, Duff K. 2011. Animal models of Alzheimer disease. *Cold Spring Harb Perspect Med* doi: 10.1101/cshperspect.a006320.

Lambert MP, Barlow AK, Chromy BA, Edwards C, Freed R, Iosatos M, Morgan TE, Rozovsky I, Trommer B, Viola KL, et al. 1998. Diffusible, nonfribrillar ligands derived from $A\beta_{1-42}$ are potent central nervous system neurotoxins. *Proc Natl Acad Sci* **95**: 6448–6453.

Laurén J, Gimbel DA, Nygaard HB, Gilbert JW, Strittmatter SM. 2009. Cellular prion protein mediates impairment of synaptic plasticity by amyloid-β oligomers. *Nature* **457**: 1128–1132.

Lemkul JA Bevan DR. 2009. Perturbation of membranes by the amyloid β-peptide—a molecular dynamics study. *FEBS J* **276**: 3060–3075.

Lesné S, Koh MT, Kotilinek L, Kayed R, Glabe CG, Yang A, Gallagher M, Ashe KH. 2006. A specific amyloid-β protein assembly in the brain impairs memory. *Nature* **440**: 352–357.

Lesné S, Sherman MA, Handoka MA, Schneider JA, Bennett DA, Ashe KH. 2009. Distinct brain Aβ oligomers are associated with different stages of Alzheimer's disease. *Soc Neurosci* (Abstr 62720).

Li S, Hong S, Shepardson NE, Walsh DM, Shankar GM, Selkoe D. 2009. Soluble oligomers of amyloid β protein facilitate hippocampal long-term depression by disrupting neuronal glutamate uptake. *Neuron* **62**: 788–801.

Li H, Monien BH, Fradinger EA, Urbanc B, Bitan G. 2010. Biophysical characterization of Aβ42 C-terminal fragments: Inhibitors of Aβ42 neurotoxicity. *Biochemistry* **49**: 1259–1267.

Liu L, Zhang L, Mao X, Niu L, Yang Y, Wang C. 2009a. Chaperon-mediated single molecular approach toward modulating Aβ peptide aggregation. *Nano Lett* **9**: 4066–4072.

Liu Q, Huang Y, Xue FQ, Simard A, DeChon J, Li G, Zhang JL, Lucero L, Wang M, Sierks M, et al. 2009b. A novel nicotinic acetylcholine receptor subtype in basal gorebrain cholinergic neurons with high sensitivity to amyloid peptides. *J Neurosci* **29**: 918–929.

Lui JK, Laws SM, Li QX, Villemagne VL, Ames D, Brown B, Bush AI, De Ruyck K, Dromey J, Ellis KA, et al. 2010a. Plasma amyloid-β as a biomarker in Alzheimer's disease: The AIBL study of aging. *J Alzheimers Dis* **20**: 1233–1242.

Liu RQ, Zhou QH, Ji SR, Zhou Q, Feng D, Wu Y, Sui SF. 2010b. Membrane localization of β-amyloid 1–42 in lysosomes: A possible mechanism for lysosome labilization. *J Biol Chem* **285**: 19986–19996.

Lulevich V, Zimmer CC, Hong HS, Jin LW, Liu GY. 2010. Single-cell mechanics provides a sensitive and quantitative means for probing amyloid-β peptide and neuronal cell interactions. *Proc Natl Acad Sci* **107**: 13872–13877.

Ma XJ, Liu L, Mao XB, Niu L, Deng K, Wu WH, Li YM, Yang YL, Wang C. 2009. Amyloid β (1–42) folding multiplicity and single-molecule binding behavior studied with STM. *J Mol Biol* **388**: 894–901.

* Mandelkow E-M, Mandelkow E. 2011. Biochemistry and cell biology of Tau protein in neurofibrillary degeneration. *Cold Spring Harb Perspect Med* doi: 10.1101/cshperspect.a006247.

Mao YL, Shang ZG, Imai Y, Hoshino T, Tero R, Tanaka M, Yamamoto N, Yanagisawa K, Urisu T. 2010. Surface-induced phase separation of a sphingomyelin/cholesterol/ganglioside GM1-planar bilayer on mica surfaces and microdomain molecular conformation that accelerates Aβ oligomerization. *Biochim Biophys Acta* **1798**: 1090–1099.

Masters CL, Simms G, Weinman NA, Multhaup G, McDonald BL, Beyreuther K. 1985. Amyloid plaque core protein in Alzheimer disease and Down syndrome. *Proc Natl Acad Sci* **82**: 4245–4249.

Masuda Y, Uemura S, Ohashi R, Nakanishi A, Takegoshi K, Shimizu T, Shirasawa T, Irie K. 2009. Identification of physiological and toxic conformations in Aβ 42 aggregates. *Chembiochem* **10**: 287–295.

McDonald JM, Savva GM, Brayne C, Welzel AT, Forster G, Shankar GM, Selkoe DJ, Ince PG, Walsh DM, Medical Research Council Cognitive Function and Aging Study. 2010. The presence of sodium dodecyl sulphate-stable Aβ dimers is strongly associated with Alzheimer-type dementia. *Brain* **133**: 1328–1341.

McLean CA, Cherny RA, Fraser FW, Fuller SJ, Smith MJ, Beyreuther K, Bush AI, Masters CL. 1999. Soluble pool of Aβ amyloid as a determinant of severity of neurodegeneration in Alzheimer's disease. *Ann Neurol* **46**: 860–866.

Meyer-Luehmann M, Spires-Jones TL, Prada C, Garcia-Alloza M, de Calignon A, Rozkalne A, Koenigsknecht-Talboo J, Holtzman DM, Bacskai BJ, Hyman BT. 2008.

Rapid appearance and local toxicity of amyloid-β plaques in a mouse model of Alzheimer's disease. *Nature* **451:** 720–724.

Miller Y, Ma BY, Nussinov R. 2009. Polymorphism of Alzheimer's Aβ(17–42) (p3) oligomers: The importance of the turn location and its conformation. *Biophys J* **97:** 1168–1177.

Miller Y, Ma B, Nussinov R. 2010. Zinc ions promote Alzheimer Aβ aggregation via population shift of polymorphic states. *Proc Natl Acad Sci* **107:** 9490–9495.

Miyashita N, Straub JE, Thirumalai D. 2009. Structures of β-amyloid peptide 1–40, 1–42, and 1–55—the 672–726 fragment of APP-in a membrane environment with implications for interactions with gamma-secretase. *J Am Chem Soc* **131:** 17843–17852.

Moore BD, Rangachari V, Tay WM, Milkovic NM, Rosenberry TL. 2009. Biophysical analyses of synthetic amyloid-β(1–42) aggregates before and after covalent cross-linking. Implications for deducing the structure of endogenous amyloid-β oligomers. *Biochemistry* **48:** 11796–11806.

Mori H, Takio K, Ogawara M, Selkoe DJ. 1992. Mass spectrometry of purified amyloid β protein in Alzheimer's disease. *J Biol Chem* **267:** 17082–17086.

Morinaga A, Hasegawa K, Nomura R, Ookoshi T, Ozawa D, Goto Y, Yamada M, Naiki H. 2010. Critical role of interfaces and agitation on the nucleation of Aβ amyloid fibrils at low concentrations of Aβ monomers. *Biochim Biophy Acta* **1804:** 986–995.

Morita M, Vestergaard M, Hamada T, Takagi M. 2010. Real-time observation of model membrane dynamics induced by Alzheimer's amyloid beta. *Biophys Chem* **147:** 81–86.

* Mucke L, Selkoe D. 2011. Neurotoxicity of amyloid β-protein: Synaptic and network dysfunction. *Cold Spring Harb Perspect Med* doi: 10.1101/cshperspect.a006338.

Murray MM, Bernstein SL, Nyugen V, Condron MM, Teplow DB, Bowers MT. 2009a. Amyloid β protein: Aβ40 inhibits Aβ42 oligomerization. *J Am Chem Soc* **131:** 6316–6317.

Murray MM, Krone MG, Bernstein SL, Baumketner A, Condron MM, Lazo ND, Teplow DB, Wyttenbach T, Shea JE, Bowers MT. 2009b. Amyloid β-protein: Experiment and theory on the 21–30 fragment. *J Phys Chem B* **113:** 6041–6046.

Nakazawa Y, Suzuki Y, Williamson MP, Saito H, Asakura T. 2009. The interaction of amyloid Aβ(1–40) with lipid bilayers and ganglioside as studied by ^{31}P solid-state NMR. *Chem Phys Lipids* **158:** 54–60.

Negureanu L, Baumketner A. 2009. Microscopic factors that control β-sheet registry in amyloid fibrils formed by fragment 11–25 of amyloid β peptide: Insights from computer simulations. *J Mol Biol* **389:** 921–937.

Nerelius C, Sandegren A, Sargsyan H, Raunak R, Leijonmarck H, Chatterjee U, Fisahn A, Imarisio S, Lomas DA, Crowther DC, et al. 2009. α-Helix targeting reduces amyloid-β peptide toxicity. *Proc Natl Acad Sci* **106:** 9191–9196.

Noguchi A, Matsumura S, Dezawa M, Tada M, Yanazawa M, Ito A, Akioka M, Kikuchi S, Sato M, Ideno S, et al. 2009. Isolation and characterization of patient-derived, toxic, high mass amyloid β-protein (Aβ) assembly

from Alzheimer disease brains. *J Biol Chem* **284:** 32895–32905.

O'Nuallain B, Freir DB, Nicoll AJ, Risse E, Ferguson N, Herron CE, Collinge J, Walsh DM. 2010. Amyloid β-protein dimers rapidly form stable synaptotoxic protofibrils. *J Neurosci* **30:** 14411–14419.

Ogawa M, Tsukuda M, Yamaguchi T, Ikeda K, Okada T, Yano Y, Hoshino M, Matsuzaki K. 2011. Ganglioside-mediated aggregation of amyloid β-proteins (Aβ): Comparison between Aβ-(1–42) and Aβ-(1–40). *J Neurochem* **116:** 851–857.

Ogi H, Hatanaka K, Fukunishi Y, Nagai H, Hirao M, Nishiyama M. 2009. Aggregation behavior of amyloid β$_{1-42}$ peptide studied using 55 MHz wireless-electrodeless quartz crystal microbalance—article no. 07GF01. *Jpn J Appl Phys* **48:** doi: 10.1143/JJAP.48.07GF01.

Olofsson A, Lindhagen-Persson M, Vestling M, Sauer-Eriksson AE, Öhman A. 2009a. Quenched hydrogen/deuterium exchange NMR characterization of amyloid-β peptide aggregates formed in the presence of Cu^{2+} or Zn^{2+}. *FEBS J* **276:** 4051–4060.

Olofsson A, Sauer-Eriksson AE, Öhman A. 2009b. Amyloid fibril dynamics revealed by combined hydrogen/deuterium exchange and nuclear magnetic resonance. *Anal Biochem* **385:** 374–376.

Ono K, Condron MM, Teplow DB. 2009. Structure-neurotoxicity relationships of amyloid β-protein oligomers. *Proc Natl Acad Sci* **106:** 14745–14750.

Ono K, Condron MM, Teplow DB. 2010. Effects of the English (H6R) and Tottori (D7N) familial Alzheimer disease mutations on amyloid β-protein assembly and toxicity. *J Biol Chem* **285:** 23186–23197.

Paparcone R, Buehler MJ. 2009. Microscale structural model of Alzheimer Aβ(1–40) amyloid fibril—article no. 243904. *Appl Phys Lett* **94:** 43904–43904.

Paravastu AK, Qahwash I, Leapman RD, Meredith SC, Tycko R. 2009. Seeded growth of β-amyloid fibrils from Alzheimer's brain-derived fibrils produces a distinct fibril structure. *Proc Natl Acad Sci* **106:** 7443–7448.

Paula-Lima AC, Tricerri MA, Brito-Moreira J, Bomfim TR, Oliveira FF, Magdesian MH, Grinberg LT, Panizzutti R, Ferreira ST. 2009. Human apolipoprotein A-I binds amyloid-β and prevents A β-induced neurotoxicity. *Int J Biochem Cell Biol* **41:** 1361–1370.

Perálvarez-Marín A, Mateos L, Zhang C, Singh S, Cedazo-Minguez A, Visa N, Morozova-Roche L, Graslund A, Barth A. 2009. Influence of residue 22 on the folding, aggregation profile, and toxicity of the Alzheimer's amyloid β peptide. *Biophys J* **97:** 277–285.

Perreau VM, Orchard S, Adlard PA, Bellingham SA, Cappai R, Ciccotosto GD, Cowie TF, Crouch PJ, Duce JA, Evin G, et al. 2010. A domain level interaction network of amyloid precursor protein and Aβ of Alzheimer's disease. *Proteomics* **10:** 2377–2395.

Perrone L, Mothes E, Vignes M, Mockel A, Figueroa C, Miquel MC, Maddelein ML, Faller P. 2009. Copper transfer from Cu-Aβ to human serum albumin inhibits aggregation, radical production and reduces Aβ toxicity. *Chembiochem* **11:** 110–118.

Peters I, Igbavboa U, Schütt T, Haidari S, Hartig U, Rosello X, Bottner S, Copanaki E, Deller T, Kogel D, et al. 2009. The interaction of beta-amyloid protein with cellular membranes stimulates its own production. *Biochim Biophys Acta* **1788:** 964–972.

Pham E, Crews L, Ubhi K, Hansen L, Adame A, Cartier A, Salmon D, Galasko D, Michael S, Savas JN, et al. 2010. Progressive accumulation of amyloid-β oligomers in Alzheimer's disease and in amyloid precursor protein transgenic mice is accompanied by selective alterations in synaptic scaffold proteins. *FEBS J* **277:** 3051–3067.

Philipson O, Hammarström P, Nilsson KPR, Portelius E, Olofsson T, Ingelsson M, Hyman BT, Blennow K, Lannfelt L, Kalimo H, et al. 2009. A highly insoluble state of Aβ similar to that of Alzheimer's disease brain is found in Arctic APP transgenic mice. *Neurobiol Aging* **30:** 1393–1405.

Picone P, Carrotta R, Montana G, Nobile MR, Biagio PLS, Di Carlo M. 2009. Aβ oligomers and fibrillar aggregates induce different apoptotic pathways in LAN5 neuroblastoma cell cultures. *Biophys J* **96:** 4200–4211.

Pitt J, Roth W, Lacor P, Smith AB, Blankenship M, Velasco P, De Felice F, Breslin P, Klein WL. 2009. Alzheimer's-associated Aβ oligomers show altered structure, immunoreactivity and synaptotoxicity with low doses of oleocanthal. *Toxicol Appl Pharmacol* **240:** 189–197.

Qi-Takahara Y, Morishima-Kawashima M, Tanimura Y, Dolios G, Hirotani N, Horikoshi Y, Kametani F, Maeda M, Saido TC, Wang R, et al. 2005. Longer forms of amyloid β protein: Implications for the mechanism of intramembrane cleavage by γ-secretase. *J Neurosci* **25:** 436–445.

Qiu L, Lewis A, Como J, Vaughn MW, Huang J, Somerharju P, Virtanen J, Cheng KH. 2009. Cholesterol modulates the interaction of β-amyloid peptide with lipid bilayers. *Biophys J* **96:** 4299–4307.

Rajendran R, Minqin R, Ynsa MD, Casadesus G, Smith MA, Perry G, Halliwell B, Watt F. 2009. A novel approach to the identification and quantitative elemental analysis of amyloid deposits—insights into the pathology of Alzheimer's disease. *Biochem Biophys Res Commun* **382:** 91–95.

Ramos I, Fabris D, Qi W, Fernandez EJ, Good TA. 2009. Kinetic study of β-amyloid residue accessibility using reductive alkylation and mass spectrometry. *Biotechnol Bioeng* **104:** 181–192.

Ravault S, Flore C, Saurel O, Milon A, Brasseur R, Lins L. 2009. Study of the specific lipid binding properties of Aβ 11–22 fragment at endosomal pH. *Langmuir* **25:** 10948–10953.

Reddy G, Straub JE, Thirumalai D. 2009a. Influence of preformed Asp23-Lys28 salt bridge on the conformational fluctuations of monomers and dimers of Aβ peptides with implications for rates of fibril formation. *J Phys Chem B* **113:** 1162–1172.

Reddy G, Straubb JE, Thirumalai D. 2009b. Dynamics of locking of peptides onto growing amyloid fibrils. *Proc Natl Acad Sci* **106:** 11948–11953.

Reinke AA, Seh HY, Gestwicki JE. 2009. A chemical screening approach reveals that indole fluorescence is quenched by pre-fibrillar but not fibrillar amyloid-β. *Bioorg Med Chem Lett* **19:** 4952–4957.

Relini A, Cavalleri O, Rolandi R, Gliozzi A. 2009. The two-fold aspect of the interplay of amyloidogenic proteins with lipid membranes. *Chem Phys Lipids* **158:** 1–9.

Riviere C, Delaunay JC, Immel F, Cullin C, Monti JP. 2009. The polyphenol piceid destabilizes preformed amyloid fibrils and oligomers in vitro: Hypothesis on possible molecular mechanisms. *Neurochem Res* **34:** 1120–1128.

Rodríguez-Rodríguez C, Sánchez de Groot N, Rimola A, Alvarez-Larena A, Lloveras V, Vidal-Gancedo J, Ventura S, Vendrell J, Sodupe M, González-Duarte P. 2009. Design, selection, and characterization of thioflavin-based intercalation compounds with metal chelating properties for application in Alzheimer's disease. *J Am Chem Soc* **131:** 1436–1451.

Roher A, Wolfe D, Palutke M, KuKuruga D. 1986. Purification, ultrastructure, and chemical analyses of Alzheimer disease amyloid plaque core protein. *Proc Natl Acad Sci* **83:** 2662–2666.

Roher AE, Lowenson JD, Clarke S, Wolkow C, Wang R, Cotter RJ, Reardon I, Zürcher-Neely HA, Heinrikson RL, Ball MJ, et al. 1993. Structural alterations in the peptide backbone of β-amyloid core protein may account for its deposition and stability in Alzheimer's disease. *J Biol Chem* **268:** 3072–3083.

Roher AE, Esh CL, Kokjohn TA, Castano EM, Van Vickle GD, Kalback WM, Patton RL, Luehrs DC, Daugs ID, Kuo YM, et al. 2009. Amyloid beta peptides in human plasma and tissues and their significance for Alzheimer's disease. *Alzheimers Dement* **5:** 18–29.

Ryan DA, Narrow WC, Federoff HJ, Bowers WJ. 2010. An improved method for generating consistent soluble amyloid-beta oligomer preparations for in vitro neurotoxicity studies. *J Neurosci Methods* **190:** 171–179.

Rózga M, Kłoniecki M, Dadlez M, Bal W. 2010. A direct determination of the dissociation constant for the Cu(II) complex of amyloid β1–40 peptide. *Chem Res Toxicol* **23:** 336–340.

Sahoo B, Nag S, Sengupta P, Maiti S. 2009. On the stability of the soluble amyloid aggregates. *Biophys J* **97:** 1454–1460.

* Saido T, Leissring MA. 2011. Proteolytic degradation of amyloid β-protein. *Cold Spring Harb Perspect Med* doi: 10.1101/cshperspect.a006379.

Saido TC, Iwatsubo T, Mann DMA, Shimada H, Ihara Y, Kawashima S. 1995. Dominant and differential deposition of distinct β-amyloid peptide species, $Aβ_{N3(p3)}$, in senile plaques. *Neuron* **14:** 457–466.

Sakono M, Zako T. 2010. Amyloid oligomers: Formation and toxicity of Aβ oligomers. *FEBS J* **277:** 1348–1358.

Salay LC, Qi W, Keshet B, Tamm LK, Fernandez EJ. 2009. Membrane interactions of a self-assembling model peptide that mimics the self-association, structure and toxicity of Aβ(1–40). *Biochim Biophys Acta* **1788:** 1714–1721.

Sanders HM, Lust R, Teller JK. 2009. Amyloid-beta peptide Aβ p3–42 affects early aggregation of full-length Aβ 1–42. *Peptides* **30:** 849–854.

Sarell CJ, Syme CD, Rigby SEJ, Viles JH. 2009. Copper(II) binding to amyloid-β fibrils of Alzheimer's disease reveals a picomolar affinity: Stoichiometry and coordination geometry are independent of Aβ oligomeric form. *Biochemistry* **48:** 4388–4402.

Sargaeva NP, Lin C, O'Connor PB. 2009. Identification of aspartic and isoaspartic acid residues in amyloid β peptides, including Aβ1−42, using electron-ion reactions. *Anal Chem* **81**: 9778−9786.

Schauerte JA, Wong PT, Wisser KC, Ding H, Steel DG, Gafni A. 2010. Simultaneous single-molecule fluorescence and conductivity studies reveal distinct classes of Aβ species on lipid bilayers. *Biochemistry* **49**: 3031−3039.

Schlenzig D, Manhart S, Cinar Y, Kleinschmidt M, Hause G, Willbold D, Funke SA, Schilling S, Demuth HU. 2009. Pyroglutamate formation influences solubility and amyloidogenicity of amyloid peptides. *Biochemistry* **48**: 7072−7078.

Schmidt M, Sachse C, Richter W, Xu C, Fändrich M, Grigorieff N. 2009. Comparison of Alzheimer Aβ(1−40) and Aβ(1−42) amyloid fibrils reveals similar protofilament structures. *Proc Natl Acad Sci* **106**: 19813−19818.

Seifert F, Schulz K, Koch B, Manhart S, Demuth HU, Schilling S. 2009. Glutaminyl cyclases display significant catalytic proficiency for glutamyl substrates. *Biochemistry* **48**: 11831−11833.

Selkoe DJ. 1994. Cell biology of the amyloid β-protein precursor and the mechanism of Alzheimer's disease. *Ann Rev Cell Biol* **10**: 373−403.

Selkoe DJ, Abraham CR, Podlisny MB, Duffy LK. 1986. Isolation of low-molecular-weight proteins from amyloid plaque fibers in Alzheimer's disease. *J Neurochem* **146**: 1820−1834.

* Serrano-Pozo A, Frosch MP, Masliah E, Hyman BT. 2011. Neuropathological alterations in Alzheimer disease. *Cold Spring Harb Perspect Med* doi: 10.1101/cshperspect.a006189.

Sevalle J, Amoyel A, Robert P, Fournié-Zaluski MC, Roques B, Checler F. 2009. Aminopeptidase A contributes to the N-terminal truncation of amyloid β-peptide. *J Neurochem* **109**: 248−256.

Shankar GM, Bloodgood BL, Townsend M, Walsh DM, Selkoe DJ, Sabatini BL. 2007. Natural oligomers of the Alzheimer amyloid-β protein induce reversible synapse loss by modulating an NMDA-type glutamate receptor-dependent signaling pathway. *J Neurosci* **27**: 2866−2875.

Shankar GM, Li S, Mehta TH, Garcia-Munoz A, Shepardson NE, Smith I, Brett FM, Farrell MA, Rowan MJ, Lemere CA, et al. 2008. Amyloid-β protein dimers isolated directly from Alzheimer's brains impair synaptic plasticity and memory. *Nat Med* **14**: 837−842.

Shankar GM, Leissring MA, Adame A, Sun X, Spooner E, Masliah E, Selkoe DJ, Lemere CA, Walsh DM. 2009. Biochemical and immunohistochemical analysis of an Alzheimer's disease mouse model reveals the presence of multiple cerebral Aβ assembly forms throughout life. *Neurobiol Dis* **36**: 293−302.

Simakova O, Arispe NJ. 2007. The cell-selective neurotoxicity of the Alzheimer's Aβ peptide is determined by surface phosphatidylserine and cytosolic ATP levels. Membrane binding is required for Aβ toxicity. *J Neurosci* **27**: 13719−13729.

Smith DP, Ciccotosto GD, Tew DJ, Fodero-Tavoletti MT, Johanssen T, Masters CL, Barnham KJ, Cappai R. 2007. Concentration dependent Cu2+ induced aggregation and dityrosine formation of the Alzheimer's disease amyloid-β peptide. *Biochemistry* **46**: 2881−2891.

Smith NW, Annunziata O, Dzyuba SV. 2009. Amphotericin B interactions with soluble oligomers of amyloid Aβ 1−42 peptide. *Bioorg Med Chem* **17**: 2366−2370.

Söderberg L, Bogdanovic N, Axelsson B, Winblad B, Näslund J, Tjernberg LO. 2006. Analysis of single Alzheimer solid plaque cores by laser capture microscopy and nano-electrospray/tandem mass spectrometry. *Biochemistry* **45**: 9849−9856.

Song HP, Ritz S, Knoll W, Sinner EK. 2009. Conformation and topology of amyloid β-protein adsorbed on a tethered artificial membrane probed by surface plasmon field-enhanced fluorescence spectroscopy. *J Struct Biol* **168**: 117−124.

Stoltenberg M, Bush AI, Bach G, Smidt K, Larsen A, Rungby J, Lund S, Doering P, Danscher G. 2007. Amyloid plaques arise from zinc-enriched cortical layers in APP/PS1 transgenic mice and are paradoxically enlarged with dietary zinc deficiency. *Neuroscience* **150**: 357−369.

Streltsov VA, Varghese JN, Masters CL, Nuttall SD. 2011. Crystal structure of the amyloid-β p3 fragment provides a model for oligomer formation in Alzheimer's disease. *J Neurosci* **31**: 1419−1426.

Sun X, Wu WH, Liu Q, Chen MS, Yu YP, Ma Y, Zhao YF, Li YM. 2009. Hybrid peptides attenuate cytotoxicity of β-amyloid by inhibiting its oligomerization: Implication from solvent effects. *Peptides* **30**: 1282−1287.

Sureshbabu N, Kirubagaran R, Thangarajah H, Malar EJP, Jayakumar R. 2010. Lipid-induced conformational transition of amyloid β peptide fragments. *J Mol Neurosci* **41**: 368−382.

Takami M, Nagashima Y, Sano Y, Ishihara S, Morishima-Kawashima M, Funamoto S, Ihara Y. 2009. γ-Secretase: Successive tripeptide and tetrapeptide release from the transmembrane domain of β-carboxyl terminal fragment. *J Neurosci* **29**: 13042−13052.

Takeda T, Klimov DK. 2009a. Probing the effect of amino-terminal truncation for Aβ(1−40) peptides. *J Phys Chem B* **113**: 6692−6702.

Takeda T, Klimov DK. 2009b. Replica exchange simulations of the thermodynamics of Aβ fibril growth. *Biophys J* **96**: 442−452.

Takeda T, Klimov DK. 2009c. Side chain interactions can impede amyloid fibril growth: Replica exchange simulations of Aβ peptide mutant. *J Phys Chem B* **113**: 11848−11857.

Takeda T, Klimov DK. 2010. Computational backbone mutagenesis of Aβ peptides: Probing the role of backbone hydrogen bonds in aggregation. *J Phys Chem B* **114**: 4755−4762.

Talmard C, Yona RL, Faller P. 2009. Mechanism of zinc(II)-promoted amyloid formation: Zinc(II) binding facilitates the transition from the partially α-helical conformer to aggregates of amyloid-β protein(1−28). *J Biol Inorg Chem* **14**: 449−455.

Taniguchi A, Sohma Y, Hirayama Y, Mukai H, Kimura T, Hayashi Y, Matsuzaki K, Kiso Y. 2009. "Click peptide": pH-triggered in situ production and aggregation of monomer Aβ 1−42. *Chembiochem* **10**: 710−715.

Tomic JL, Pensalfini A, Head E, Glabe CG. 2009. Soluble fibrillar oligomer levels are elevated in Alzheimer's disease brain and correlate with cognitive dysfunction. *Neurobiol Dis* **35**: 352−358.

Tomidokoro Y, Rostagno A, Neubert TA, Lu Y, Rebeck GW, Frangione B, Greenberg SM, Ghiso J. 2010. Iowa variant of familial Alzheimer's disease. Accumulation of post-translationally modified Aβ D23N in parenchymal and cerebrovascular amyloid deposits. *Am J Pathol* **176:** 1841–1854.

Tomiyama T, Matsuyama S, Iso H, Umeda T, Takuma H, Ohnishi K, Ishibashi K, Teraoka R, Sakama N, Yamashita T, et al. 2010. A mouse model of amyloid β oligomers: Their contribution to synaptic alteration, abnormal tau phosphorylation, glial activation, and neuronal loss in vivo. *J Neurosci* **30:** 4845–4856.

Tõugu V, Karafin A, Zovo K, Chung RS, Howells C, West AK, Palumaa P. 2009. Zn(II)- and Cu(II)-induced non-fibrillar aggregates of amyloid-β (1–42) peptide are transformed to amyloid fibrils, both spontaneously and under the influence of metal chelators. *J Neurochem* **110:** 1784–1795.

Tycko R, Sciarretta KL, Orgel J, Meredith SC. 2009. Evidence for novel β-sheet structures in Iowa mutant β-amyloid fibrils. *Biochemistry* **48:** 6072–6084.

Uranga RM, Giusto NM, Salvador GA. 2010. Effect of transition metals in synaptic damage induced by amyloid beta peptide. *Neuroscience* **170:** 381–389..

Urbanc B, Betnel M, Cruz L, Bitan G, Teplow DB. 2010. Elucidation of amyloid β-protein oligomerization mechanisms: Discrete molecular dynamics study. *J Am Chem Soc* **132:** 4266–4280.

Utsumi M, Yamaguchi Y, Sasakawa H, Yamamoto N, Yanagisawa K, Kato K. 2009. Up-and-down topological mode of amyloid β-peptide lying on hydrophilic/hydrophobic interface of ganglioside clusters. *Glycoconj J* **26:** 999–1006.

Villemagne VL, Perez KA, Pike KE, Kok WM, Rowe CC, White AR, Bourgeat P, Salvado O, Bedo J, Hutton CA, et al. 2010. Blood-borne amyloid-β dimer correlates with clinical markers of Alzheimer's disease. *J Neurosci* **30:** 6315–6322.

Walsh DM, Selkoe DJ. 2007. Aβ oligomers—a decade of discovery. *J Neurochem* **101:** 1172–1184.

Walsh DM, Lomakin A, Benedek GB, Maggio JE, Condron MM, Teplow DB. 1997. Amyloid β-protein fibrillogenesis: Detection of a protofibrillar intermediate. *J Biol Chem* **272:** 22364–22374.

Walsh DM, Thulin E, Minogue AM, Gustavsson N, Pang E, Teplow DB, Linse S. 2009. A facile method for expression and purification of the Alzheimer's disease-associated amyloid β-peptide. *FEBS J* **276:** 1266–1281.

Wang QM, Zhao C, Zhao J, Wang JD, Yang JC, Yu X, Zhen J. 2010. Comparative molecular dynamics study of Aβ adsorption on the self-assembled monolayers. *Langmuir* **26:** 3308–3316.

Wei GH, Jewett AI, Shea JE. 2010. Structural diversity of dimers of the Alzheimer amyloid-β(25–35) peptide and polymorphism of the resulting fibrils. *Phys Chem Chem Phys* **12:** 3622–3629.

Weidemann A, Eggert S, Reinhard FB, Vogel M, Paliga K, Baier G, Masters CL, Beyreuther K, Evin G. 2002. A novel ε-cleavage within the transmembrane domain of the Alzheimer amyloid precursor protein demonstrates homology with Notch processing. *Biochemistry* **41:** 2825–2835.

Welander H, Frånberg J, Graff C, Sundström E, Winblad B, Tjernberg LO. 2009. Aβ 43 is more frequent than Aβ 40 in amyloid plaque cores from Alzheimer disease brains. *J Neurochem* **110:** 697–706.

Wirths O, Bethge T, Marcello A, Harmeier A, Jawhar S, Lucassen PJ, Multhaup G, Brody DL, Esparza T, Ingelsson M, et al. 2010. Pyroglutamate Abeta pathology in APP/PS1KI mice, sporadic and familial Alzheimer's disease cases. *J Neural Transm* **117:** 85–96.

Woltjer RL, Sonnen JA, Sokal I, Rung LG, Yang W, Kjerulf JD, Klingert D, Johnson C, Rhew I, Tsuang D, et al. 2009. Quantitation and mapping of cerebral detergent-insoluble proteins in the elderly. *Brain Pathol* **19:** 365–374.

Wu C, Murray MM, Bernstein SL, Condron MM, Bitan G, Shea JE, Bowers MT. 2009. The structure of Aβ 42 C-terminal fragments probed by a combined experimental and theoretical study. *J Mol Biol* **387:** 492–501.

Wu C, Bowers MT, Shea JE. 2010a. Molecular structures of quiescently grown and brain-derived polymorphic fibrils of the Alzheimer amyloid Aβ₉₋₄₀ peptide: A comparison to agitated fibrils. *PLoS Comput Biol* **6:** e1000693. doi: 10.1372/journal/pcbi.1000693.

Wu JW, Breydo L, Isas JM, Lee J, Kuznetsov YG, Langen R, Glabe C. 2010b. Fibrillar oligomers nucleate the oligomerization of monomeric amyloid β but do not seed fibril formation. *J Biol Chem* **285:** 6071–6079.

Xia WM, Yang T, Shankar G, Smith IM, Shen Y, Walsh DM, Selkoe DJ. 2009. A specific enzyme-linked immunosorbent assay for measuring β-amyloid protein oligomers in human plasma and brain tissue of patients with Alzheimer disease. *Arch Neurol* **66:** 190–199.

Xiao Z, Wedd AG. 2010. The challenges of determining metal-protein affinities. *Nat Prod Rep* **27:** 768–789.

Yadav A, Sonker M. 2009. Perspectives in designing anti-aggregation agents as Alzheimer disease drugs. *Euro J Med Chem* **44:** 3866–3873.

Yagi-Utsumi M, Kameda T, Yamaguchi Y, Kato K. 2010. NMR characterization of the interactions between lyso-GM1 aqueous micelles and amyloid-β. *FEBS Lett* **584:** 831–836.

Yamin G, Ruchala P, Teplow DB. 2009. A peptide hairpin inhibitor of amyloid β-protein oligomerization and fibrillogenesis. *Biochemistry* **48:** 11329–11331.

Yang C, Li JY, Li Y, Zhu XL. 2009a. The effect of solvents on the conformations of Amyloid β-peptide (1–42) studied by molecular dynamics simulation. *J Mol Struct: THEOCHEM* **895:** 1–8.

Yang C, Zhu XL, Li JY, Chen K. 2009b. Molecular dynamics simulation study on conformational behavior of Aβ(1–40) and Aβ(1–42) in water and methanol. *J Mol Struct: THEOCHEM* **907:** 51–56.

Yu LP, Edalji R, Harlan JE, Holzman TF, Lopez AP, Labkovsky B, Hillen H, Barghorn S, Ebert U, Richardson PL, et al. 2009. Structural characterization of a soluble amyloid β-peptide oligomer. *Biochemistry* **48:** 1870–1877.

Zhang A, Qi W, Good TA, Fernandez EJ. 2009a. Structural differences between Aβ(1–40) intermediate oligomers and fibrils elucidated by proteolytic fragmentation and hydrogen/deuterium exchange. *Biophys J* **96:** 1091–1104.

Zhang JF, Hou L, Gao XP, Guo F, Jing W, Qi JS, Qiao JT. 2009b. Amyloid β-protein differentially affects NMDA receptor- and GABA$_A$ receptor-mediated currents in rat hippocampal CA1 neurons. *Prog Natl Sci* **19:** 963–972.

Zhang L, Yu HX, Song CC, Lin XF, Chen B, Tan C, Cao GX, Wang ZW. 2009c. Expression, purification, and characterization of recombinant human β-amyloid42 peptide in Escherichia coli. *Protein Expres Purif* **64:** 55–62.

Zhang R, Hu XY, Khant H, Ludtke SJ, Chiu W, Schmid MF, Frieden C, Lee JM. 2009d. Interprotofilament interactions between Alzheimer's Aβ$_{1-42}$ peptides in amyloid fibrils revealed by cryoEM. *Proc Natl Acad Sci* **106:** 4653–4658.

Zhao JH, Liu HL, Liu YF, Lin HY, Fang HW, Ho Y, Tsai WB. 2009. Molecular dynamics simulations to investigate the aggregation behaviors of the Aβ(17–42) oligomers. *J Biomol Struct Dyn* **26:** 481–490.

Zheng J, Yu X, Wang J, Yang JC, Wang Q. 2010. Molecular modeling of two distinct triangular oligomers in amyloid β-protein. *J Phys Chem B* **114:** 463–470.

Trafficking and Proteolytic Processing of APP

Christian Haass[1], Christoph Kaether[2], Gopal Thinakaran[3], and Sangram Sisodia[3]

[1]DZNE—German Center for Neurodegenerative Diseases, 80336 Munich, Germany; and Adolf Butenandt-Institute, Biochemistry, Ludwig-Maximilians University, 80336 Munich, Germany

[2]Leibniz Institut für Altersforschung, D-07745 Jena, Germany

[3]Department of Neurobiology, University of Chicago, Chicago, Illinois 60637

Correspondence: christian.haass@dzne.lmu.de; ssisodia@bsd.uchicago.edu

Accumulations of insoluble deposits of amyloid β-peptide are major pathological hallmarks of Alzheimer disease. Amyloid β-peptide is derived by sequential proteolytic processing from a large type I trans-membrane protein, the β-amyloid precursor protein. The proteolytic enzymes involved in its processing are named secretases. β- and γ-secretase liberate by sequential cleavage the neurotoxic amyloid β-peptide, whereas α-secretase prevents its generation by cleaving within the middle of the amyloid domain. In this chapter we describe the cell biological and biochemical characteristics of the three secretase activities involved in the proteolytic processing of the precursor protein. In addition we outline how the precursor protein maturates and traffics through the secretory pathway to reach the subcellular locations where the individual secretases are preferentially active. Furthermore, we illuminate how neuronal activity and mutations which cause familial Alzheimer disease affect amyloid β-peptide generation and therefore disease onset and progression.

PROTEOLYTIC PROCESSING OF APP

APP Processing: The Amyloidogenic and Anti-Amyloidogenic Pathways

The 37–43 amino acid amyloid β-peptide (Aβ) is generated by proteolytic processing from its precursor, the β-amyloid precursor protein (APP) in a physiologically normal pathway (Haass et al. 1992, 1993a; Seubert et al. 1992; Shoji et al. 1992; Busciglio et al. 1993; Haass and Selkoe 1993). APP is a type-I oriented membrane protein with its amino terminus within the lumen/extracellular space and its carboxyl terminus within the cytosol (Kang et al. 1987; Dyrks et al. 1988). Although APP

is initially targeted into the secretory pathway (see below), it is proteolytically processed at several different subcellular sites (Weidemann et al. 1989). Three protease activities called α-, β-, and γ-secretase are involved in specific processing steps (Haass 2004). The name "secretases" refers to the secretion of the proteolytically cleaved substrates. All three protease activities have been identified and are described below.

We discriminate two principal processing pathways: the amyloidogenic pathway, which leads to Aβ generation; and the anti-myloidogenic pathway, which prevents Aβ generation (Fig. 1). Aβ is produced in the amyloidogenic

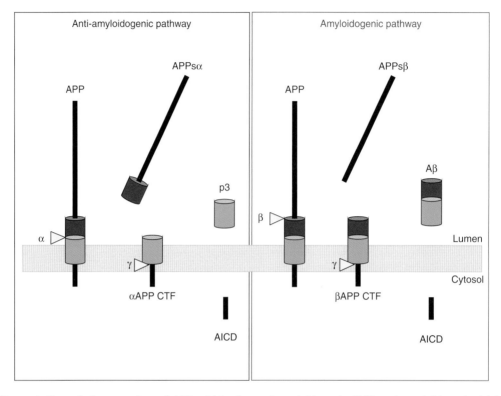

Figure 1. Proteolytic processing of APP within the anti-amyloidogenic (*left*) and amyloidogenic (*right*) pathways.

pathway by the consecutive action of β- and γ-secretase (Haass 2004). The β-secretase activity initiates Aβ generation by shedding a large part of the ectodomain of APP (APPsβ) and generating an APP carboxy-terminal fragment (βCTF or C99), which is then cleaved by γ-secretase. The latter cleavage occurs within the hydrophobic environment of biological membranes. Consecutive shedding and intramembrane proteolysis is now summarized under the term "regulated intramembrane proteolysis" (Brown et al. 2000; Rawson 2002; Lichtenthaler et al. 2011), a cellular process, which is frequently involved in important signaling pathways (Selkoe and Kopan 2003; see DeStrooper et al. 2011). On γ-secretase cleavage, Aβ is liberated and then found in extracellular fluids such as plasma or cerebrospinal fluid (Seubert et al. 1992). In the anti-amyloidogenic pathway, APP is cleaved approximately in the middle of the Aβ region by the α-secretase activity (Esch et al. 1990; Sisodia et al. 1990). This processing step generates a truncated APP CTF (αCTF or C83), which lacks the amino-terminal portion of the Aβ domain. The subsequent intramembrane cut by γ-secretase liberates a truncated Aβ peptide called p3 (Haass et al. 1993b), which apparently is pathologically irrelevant. γ-Secretase not only liberates Aβ (from C99) and p3 (from C83) but also generates the APP intracellular domain (AICD) (Gu et al. 2001; Sastre et al. 2001; Weidemann et al. 2002), which is released into the cytosol and which may have a function in nuclear signaling (Cao and Sudhof 2001; von Rotz et al. 2004). The amyloidogenic and the anti-amyloidogenic processing pathways compete with each other at least in some subcellular loci, since enhancing α-secretase activity in animal models of Alzheimer disease (AD) or in cultured cells can significantly lower Aβ generation and even amyloid plaque formation (Nitsch et al. 1992; Postina et al. 2004).

Familial Alzheimer Disease–Associated Mutations within the APP Gene Affect Aβ Generation and Aggregation

A number of familial Alzheimer disease (FAD)-associated mutations have been found within and around the Aβ domain (Chartier-Harlin et al. 1991; Selkoe 2001; discussed in detail in Schenk et al. 2011). These mutations accelerate disease progression via diverse mechanisms. The Swedish mutation at the amino terminus of the Aβ region (Mullan et al. 1992) results in a significant increase of total Aβ production (such as Aβ40 and Aβ42) by providing a better substrate for the β-secretase activity (Citron et al. 1992; Cai et al. 1993). Mutations located just beyond the carboxyl terminus of Aβ (such as the so-called Austrian, Iranian, French, German, London, and Florida mutations) cause the increased production of longer Aβ species (Aβ42), which aggregate more rapidly and are believed to be the major neurotoxic Aβ species (Suzuki et al. 1994). Mutations in the mid region, such as the Arctic (Nilsberth et al. 2001) and Dutch mutations (Levy et al. 1990), affect the primary sequence of Aβ and apparently change the structure of Aβ, resulting in its enhanced aggregation propensity. Some of these intra-Aβ mutations can lead to mixed amyloid pathologies: marked cerebral angiopathy and marked amyloid plaque formation. For the Flemish mutation, an unexpected pathological mechanism was described recently. This mutation is located in an apparent substrate inhibitory domain that negatively regulates γ-secretase activity by binding to an unknown allosteric site within the complex. The Flemish mutation can reduce the activity of this inhibitory domain and consequently increase Aβ generation (Tian et al. 2010).

The Amyloidogenic Proteases: β- and γ-Secretase

β-Secretase

β-Secretase mediates the initial and rate-limiting processing step during Aβ generation (Vassar 2004). Expression cloning or biochemical purification led to the identification of a unique β-secretase enzyme (Sinha et al. 1999; Vassar et al. 1999; Yan et al. 1999; Hussain et al. 2000; Lin et al. 2000). Although many different names were originally used to describe this activity, such as memapsin, aspartyl protease 2, or BACE1 (β-site APP cleaving enzyme-1), BACE1 is now the generally accepted term for the enzyme harboring β-secretase activity. BACE1 is a membrane-bound aspartyl protease with its active site in the lumen/extracellular space and with structural similarities to the pepsin family (Hong et al. 2000). Besides BACE1, a homologous protease called BACE2 was identified (Vassar 2004). However, BACE2 is not involved in amyloidogenesis and may rather exert an anti-amyloidogenic activity in non-neuronal cells somewhat similar to α-secretase (Bennett et al. 2000a; Farzan et al. 2000; Fluhrer et al. 2002; Basi et al. 2003). BACE1 is the sole β-secretase, because its knockout completely blocks Aβ generation (Cai et al. 2001; Roberds et al. 2001; Luo et al. 2003). The protease is ubiquitously expressed, with highest levels in brain and pancreas; the physiological relevance of high pancreatic expression is currently not understood. Because APP is also expressed at very high levels in the brain, the concomitant high levels of BACE1 and APP make the brain the primary tissue for high Aβ generation and help explain why AD is a brain disease even though APP is expressed ubiquitously.

BACE1 is an important therapeutic target (Citron 2004), because its inhibition not only reduces Aβ levels but also prevents the accumulation of βCTFs, which contain the entire Aβ domain and serve as the final substrate for Aβ production (see Fig. 1). This is an important issue, because accumulation of such CTFs may cause additional, poorly understood toxic effects. Progress has been made toward the generation of BACE1 inhibitors, and clinical studies are on the way (Citron 2004; Schenk et al. 2011). However, one must be aware that such an approach also inhibits the physiological function of BACE1. So far, only very few physiological substrates have been validated whose cleavage by BACE1 is associated with a clear biological function. BACE1 knockout mice are viable and fertile and do not show any major behavioral, morphological, or developmental deficits (Cai et al. 2001; Roberds et al. 2001; Luo et al. 2003). However, subtle behavioral phenotypes such as some memory impairment and changes in spontaneous activity (Harrison et al. 2003; Dominguez et al. 2005) indicate that a loss of function of BACE1 can have detrimental consequences. Very high postnatal expression levels of BACE1 (Willem et al. 2006) revealed a function of BACE1 in myelination, a process which occurs after birth. Indeed all available BACE1 knockout mice show a significant hypomyelination phenotype in the peripheral nervous system (Fig. 2A; Hu et al. 2006; Willem et al. 2006). Whether myelination within the CNS is also under the control of BACE1, as described by Hu et al. (2006), is currently under debate. Schwann cell-mediated myelination in the peripheral nervous system is regulated via the Neuregulin-1 (NRG1) signaling pathway (Birchmeier and Nave 2008). Interestingly, proteolytic processing of NRG1 (Fig. 2B) is believed to facilitate its signaling activity. Indeed, in the BACE1 knockout animals, uncleaved NRG1

accumulates. Thus, NRG1 is a physiological substrate for BACE1, and at least one of the physiological functions of BACE1 concerns myelination. BACE1 has also been shown to be involved in the regulation of voltage-dependent sodium channels (Kim et al. 2007). Moreover, other substrates such as Type II α-2,6-sialyltransferase, platelet selectin glyco-protein ligand-1, APP-like proteins, Aβ itself, and the interleukin-like receptor type II have also been shown to be processed by BACE1 (summarized in Willem et al. 2009). However, the physiological consequences of these cleavages are unclear, and one should keep in mind that most substrates were identified on overexpression of BACE1 and/or the substrate, which is likely to generate conditions allowing artificial substrate/protease interactions.

γ-Secretase

The Aβ-liberating cleavage of APP is mediated by γ-secretase and occurs within the transmembrane domain (TMD). γ-Secretase structure and function is discussed in DeStrooper et al. (2011). Here, we will briefly introduce

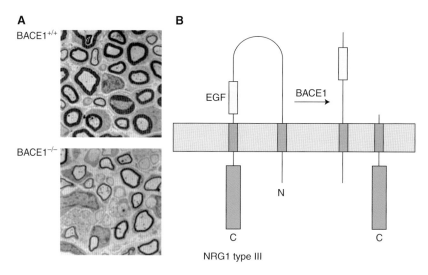

Figure 2. Biological function of BACE1 in myelination. (*A*) A BACE1 knockout in mice results in a hypomyelination phenotype within the peripheral nervous system. Cross-sections through the sciatic nerve of wild-type mice and BACE knockout mice are shown. (*B*) Proteolytic processing of NRG1 type III. NRG1 type III is cleaved by BACE1. This processing step leads to the exposure of EGF-containing domain and facilitates signaling via ErbB4 in Schwann cells.

γ-secretase and then focus on the cellular assembly of γ-secretase and its subcellular sites of activity.

γ-Secretase is a protease complex consisting of four subunits (reviewed in Steiner et al. 2008). Presenilin (PS) 1 or PS2 contain the two critical aspartyl residues within TMDs 6 and 7, which are part of the catalytic domain of the aspartyl protease activity of γ-secretase (Wolfe et al. 1999). Additional complex components are nicastrin (NCT), anterior pharynx defective (APH)-1a or APH-1b, and the PS enhancer (PEN)-2 (Yu et al. 2000; Francis et al. 2002). These four components are necessary and sufficient for full γ-secretase activity (Edbauer et al. 2003). Little is known about the biological function of NCT, APH-1, and PEN-2. NCT is probably required as a size-selecting substrate receptor (Shah et al. 2005; Dries et al. 2009), although recent findings may challenge such a function (Chavez-Gutier-rez et al. 2008; Martin et al. 2009). PEN-2 apparently facilitates PS endoproteolysis into its active heterodimeric state and stabilizes PS within the γ-secretase complex (Hasegawa et al. 2004; Prokop et al. 2004). No specific function has so far been assigned to APH-1, although it may act as a scaffold for the initial binding of NCT and assembly of the complex (LaVoie et al. 2003).

The intramembrane processing of APP by γ-secretase is not restricted to a single site. Rather, it appears that γ-secretase substrates are cleaved several times within their TMDs. Cleavages at the so-called ε-, ζ-, and γ-sites that are separated by approximately three amino acids are postulated (Fig. 3; Sastre et al. 2001; Weidemann et al. 2002; Qi-Takahara et al. 2005; Takami et al. 2009). To make things even more complicated, the final γ-cleavage is also not precise and can occur under physiological conditions at least between amino acids 37 and 43 of the Aβ domain. This difference is of greatest relevance for the understanding of AD pathology, because the longer Aβ42 species is more aggregation prone and believed to be the toxic building block of Aβ oligomers, which affect memory and cell survival (Haass and Selkoe 2007). How can these multiple cleavages be explained? Although it is not yet finally proven, it is likely that this phenomenon is due to a stepwise cleavage mechanism performed by one and the same γ-secretase. Moreover, stepwise endoproteolysis may be a general phenomenon of intramembrane proteolysis mediated by all γ-secretase-like proteases (Fluhrer et al. 2006, 2008, 2009). Apparently, once APP (or another substrate) is bound to the active site of the γ-secretase complex, intramembrane proteolysis begins with the ε-cleavage after amino acids

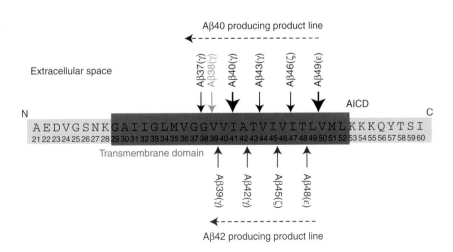

Figure 3. Sequential processing of APP by γ-secretase.

49 or 48. This is then followed by cleavage after amino acids 46 or 45 (ζ-cleavage) and terminates with the cleavage at the γ-site mostly at amino acids 42 or 40 (but also after amino acids 37, 38, 39, and 43; Fig. 3). Two product lines are discussed (Fig. 3): one leading predominantly to Aβ42 generation (starting with the ε-cleavage after amino acid 48 and followed by cleavages after amino acids 45 and 42); and the other leading predominantly to Aβ40 (starting with the ε-cleavage after amino acid 49 and followed by cleavages after amino acids 46 and 43). As discussed in Schenk et al. (2011), these cleavages may be therapeutically modulated to selectively prevent Aβ42 generation.

The Anti-Amyloidogenic α-Secretase

As mentioned above, the anti-amyloidogenic processing of APP occurs within the Aβ domain between residues Lys16 and Leu17 (Esch et al. 1990; Sisodia et al. 1990; Wang et al. 1991) and results in the secretion of the large APP amino-terminal domain and the generation of α-CTF (C83). This cleavage is performed by a set of proteases termed α-secretases. Shortly after the identification of the α-secretase cleavage site, it was noted that in cultured cells this cleavage predominantly occurs at the cell surface, suggesting that α-secretases are plasma membrane (PM)-bound proteases (Sisodia 1992). Activation of protein kinase C by phorbol esters stimulates α-secretase processing and secretion of the APP ectodomain (Buxbaum et al. 1990). This protein kinase C-dependent APP processing was dubbed "regulated α-secretase cleavage" of APP. Several zinc metalloproteinases that are members of the "a disintegrin and metalloprotease" family such as ADAM9, ADAM10, TACE/ADAM17 and ADAM19 can function as α-secretase (Allinson et al. 2003). Targeted disruption of individual genes that encode ADAM10, TACE/ADAM17, or ADAM19 has no effect on constitutive α-secretase processing of APP, indicating that α-secretase activity is shared by a set of ADAM proteases (Buxbaum et al. 1998b; Merlos-Suarez et al. 1998; Hartmann et al. 2002; Weskamp et al. 2002). However, recent evidence suggests that, at least in neurons, the principal constitutive α-secretase activity is exerted by ADAM10 (Kuhn et al. 2010). Besides APP, Notch receptors and ligands, tumor necrosis factor α, cadherins and IL-6 receptor, EGF receptor ligands, and several other type I transmembrane proteins are cleaved by α-secretases to release their extracellular domain. Consequently, the process of ectodomain shedding mediated by α-secretases appears to be largely sequence independent. At a minimum, α-secretase cleavage of APP is determined by an α-helical conformation and the distance (12–13 residues) of the hydrolyzed bond from the membrane (Sisodia 1992).

Amyloidogenic processing appears to be the favored pathway of APP metabolism in neurons, largely because of the greater abundance of BACE1, whereas anti-amyloidogenic pathway is predominant in all other cell types. Overexpression of ADAM10 and other putative α-secretases in cultured cells as well as in transgenic mice increases the secretion of the APP ectodomain ending at the α-secretase site. Interestingly, neuronal overexpression of ADAM10 in transgenic mice reduces BACE1 processing of APP and amyloid deposition (Postina et al. 2004). This finding is of physiological relevance because ADAM10 is expressed throughout the cortex and hippocampus in the adult central nervous system, and APP, BACE1, and ADAM10 are co-expressed in human cortical neurons (Marcinkiewicz et al. 2000). Other putative α-secretases such as ADAM9, TACE/ADAM17 and ADAM19 are also expressed in the adult brain. Thus, up-regulation of α-secretase activity to promote anti-amyloidogenic processing of APP is potentially of therapeutic value (Postina et al. 2004).

Commitment of APP to amyloidogenic and anti-amyloidogenic pathways can be differentially modulated by the activation of cell-surface receptors such as the serotonin/5-hydroxytryptamine (5-HT$_4$) receptor, metabotropic glutamate receptors, muscarinic acetylcholine receptors, and platelet-derived growth factor receptor (Allinson et al. 2003). Signaling downstream from these receptors regulates APPsα and Aβ secretion by engaging intermediates including protein kinase C, protein kinase A, phosphatidylinositol-3-kinase, mitogen-activated protein kinase kinase, extracellular signal-regulated kinase, Src tyrosine kinase, small GTPase Rac, inositol 1,4,5-trisphosphate, cAMP, and cytosolic calcium (reviewed in Gandy et al. 1994; Allinson et al. 2003). Lowering cholesterol levels in cultured cells stimulates α-secretase cleavage of APP through mechanisms involving impaired APP endocytosis and increased steady-state levels of ADAM10 (Kojro et al. 2001). The effect of cholesterol depletion is not specific to APP cleavage, because the shedding of the human interleukin-6 receptor by ADAM10 and TACE/ADAM17 is also stimulated under these conditions (Matthews et al. 2003).

CELLULAR TRAFFICKING OF APP

Biosynthesis and Trafficking through the Secretory Pathway

The pathways of APP trafficking in a nonpolarized mammalian cell are depicted in Figure 4. During its transit from the ER to the PM, nascent APP is posttranslationally modified by N- and O-linked glycosylation, ectodomain and cytoplasmic phosphorylation, and tyrosine sulphation. Only a small fraction of nascent APP molecules reach the PM (estimated at ∼10% based on APP overexpression in cultured cells), whereas the majority of APP at steady-state localizes to the Golgi apparatus and trans-Golgi network (TGN). APP which is not shed from the cell surface is internalized within minutes of arrival at the cell surface because of the presence of its "YENPTY" internalization motif near the carboxyl terminus of APP (residues 682–687 of APP695 isoform) (Lai et al. 1995; Marquez-Sterling et al. 1997). Following endocytosis, APP is delivered to endosomes, and a fraction of endocytosed molecules is recycled to the cell surface. Measurable amounts of internalized APP also undergo degradation in lysosomes (Haass et al. 1992).

Endocytic APP Sorting and Aβ Production

Although attempts to characterize the role of endocytic APP trafficking by expression of dominant-negative dynamin mutants resulted in discrepant findings (Chyung et al. 2003; Ehehalt et al. 2003; Carey et al. 2005), mutations

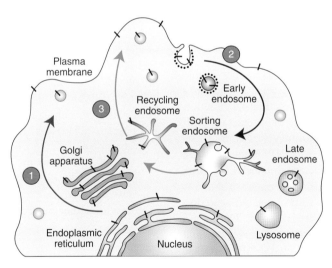

Figure 4. Intracellular trafficking of APP. Nascent APP molecules (black bars) mature through the constitutive secretory pathway (1). Once APP reaches the cell surface, it is rapidly internalized (2) and subsequently trafficked through endocytic and recycling organelles to the TGN or the cell surface (3). A small fraction is also degraded in the lysosome. Nonamyloidogenic processing mainly occurs at the cell surface where α-secretases are present. Amyloidogenic processing involves transit through the endocytic organelles where APP encounters β- and γ-secretases.

within the APP cytosolic YENPTY motif selectively inhibit APP internalization and decrease Aβ generation (Perez et al. 1999). This motif and the flanking region serve as the binding site for many cytosolic adaptors that have phosphotyrosine-binding domains, including Fe65, Fe65L1, Fe65L2, Mint 1 (also called X11α), Mint 2, Mint 3, Dab1, sorting nexin 17, and c-Jun amino-terminal kinase-interacting protein family members. Overexpression of Mint 1, Mint 2, or Fe65 causes reduction in Aβ generation and less deposition in the brains of APP transgenic mice, strongly suggesting a physiological role for these adaptors in regulating amyloidogenic processing of APP in the nervous system (Miller et al. 2006). In addition to binding APP, Mint proteins can directly bind ADP-ribosylation factors, raising the intriguing possibility that Mints may regulate vesicular trafficking of APP by serving as coat proteins (Hill et al. 2003). A conformational change introduced by phosphorylation at Thr-668 (14 amino acids proximal to the YENPTY motif) interferes with Fe65 binding to APP and facilitates BACE1 and γ-secretase cleavage of APP in cultured cells (Ando et al. 2001; Lee et al. 2003). However, analysis of Thr-668-Ala knock-in mice indicates that the phosphorylation status of Thr-668 does not affect physiological processing of APP into Aβ peptides in vivo (Sano et al. 2006). In addition to its potential role in APP endocytosis, Fe65 stabilizes the highly labile AICD, which may serve as a regulatory step in modulating the physiological function of AICD. Fe65 is capable of interacting with APP and LRP (a multifunctional endocytosis receptor containing two NPXY motifs) via distinct protein interaction domains (Trommsdorff et al. 1998). Lack of LRP expression causes reduced APP internalization and Aβ secretion (Ulery et al. 2000; Pietrzik et al. 2002; Cam et al. 2005), leading to the conclusion that endocytosis of LRP is coupled to APP internalization and processing, and Fe65 acts as a functional linker between APP and LRP in modulating endocytic APP trafficking (Pietrzik et al. 2004). In addition, Ran-binding protein 9 promotes APP interaction with APP and facilitates APP internalization in a Fe65-independent manner (Lakshmana et al. 2009). Finally, the type I transmembrane protein sorLA/LR11 (a member of the VPS10p-domain receptor family), which functionally interacts with cytosolic adaptors GGA and PACS-1, regulates Aβ production by acting as a Golgi/TGN retention factor for APP (Andersen et al. 2005; Offe et al. 2006; Schmidt et al. 2007). Aβ levels are reduced on overexpression of sorLA/LR11 in cultured cells and increased in the brains of sorLA/LR11 knockout mice (Andersen et al. 2005; Offe et al. 2006). sorLA/LR11 is also genetically associated with AD and its steady-state levels are markedly reduced in the brains of patients with AD, further implicating this sorting molecule in the physiological regulation of APP metabolism (Andersen et al. 2005; Offe et al. 2006; Rogaeva et al. 2007).

Polarized Trafficking of APP in Non-Neuronal Cells

Obviously, neurons are of pivotal interest for the analysis of APP trafficking and processing. Because of the polarized nature of neurons, a strong interest emerged in understanding how APP is targeted to selected destinations and where during its cellular transport APP is processed into its cleavage products by the three secretase activities described above. Cellular model systems have been developed that allow analysis of polarized sorting in relatively simple peripheral cells. Madin–Darby canine kidney (MDCK) cells are a suitable cell system, as they form polarized monolayers with defined apical and basolateral surfaces on culturing in Transwell chambers. This widely used tool in cell biology not only allows the separate collection of apically and basolaterally secreted proteins but also the detection of membrane-bound proteins on either surface, for example, via biotinylation.

Polarized Trafficking of APP via Two Independent Sorting Mechanisms

Using MDCK cells, it has been shown that a number of cleavage products of APP including soluble APP (α-secretase generated APP; αAPPs), Aβ, and p3 are selectively targeted to the basolateral compartment (Haass et al. 1994; De Strooper et al. 1995a). In addition, surface APP also accumulates on the basolateral surface, and APPsα shed from surface APP accumulates in the basolateral media (Fig. 5). These findings suggested that APP contains a sorting signal that selectively targets it to the basolateral side of polarized cells. Deletion of the last 42 amino acids of the cytoplasmic domain of APP (aa 654–695 according to the numbering of APP695) causes a random (default) transport of the resultant APP-ΔC to both surfaces (Fig. 5C). Moreover, Tyr 653 was identified as a critical amino acid required for efficient basolateral APP sorting (Haass et al. 1995a). Interestingly, this signal acts independently of a re-internalization signal between aa 684–687 (see above). Surprisingly, when a Tyr653-mutant APP was expressed, the bulk of αAPPs was still sorted efficiently to the basolateral compartment, although the membrane-bound holoprotein was transported equally to both surfaces (De Strooper et al. 1995a; Haass et al. 1995a). This result indicates two independent sorting mechanisms, one for membrane-bound APP and one for soluble APPsα (Fig. 5A–C). Whereas the first sorting pathway is dependent on a cytoplasmic sorting signal similar to other polarized sorted proteins, the soluble ectodomain of APP apparently contains an independent basolateral sorting signal (De Strooper et al. 1995b; Haass et al. 1995a). Indeed, when APPsα was expressed as a recombinant protein, it was still rather efficiently sorted to the basolateral compartment (Haass et al. 1995a). Evidence exists that alternative splicing of APP can affect polarized secretion of soluble APP (Hartmann et al. 1996). APP variants lacking the exon 15 encoded domain are sorted equally into both compartments. It is assumed that the 3D structure by itself, not a linear sequence motif, determines polarized sorting of secreted APPsα. Cellular fractionation studies show that a large amount of APPsα is already generated by α-secretase within the Golgi compartment long before it reaches the cell surface of MDCK cells (Haass et al. 1995a). Based on previous findings it was assumed that sorting of soluble proteins occurs within a pH-sensitive compartment (De Strooper et al. 1995a; Haass et al. 1995a). Indeed NH$_4$Cl treatment randomizes polarized secretion of αAPPs. Thus, two distinct pathways mediate polarized sorting of APP in MDCK cells (Fig. 5A–C).

Polarized Sorting of Secretases

The above findings have major implications for the polarized trafficking of all three secretase activities. As described in the first publication on polarized secretion of Aβ, only small amounts of authentic Aβ beginning with Asp1 of the Aβ sequence are observed in the basolateral media (Haass et al. 1994). This is consistent with the finding that BACE1, which cleaves at Asp1, is predominantly targeted to the apical surface of MDCK, a process which markedly limits Aβ generation in polarized cells (Capell et al. 2002). Indeed, when APP is mis-sorted to the apical surface, it is almost exclusively processed by BACE-1. This also indicates that little α-secretase activity is present in the apical sorting pathway, because apparently there is almost no competition for BACE-1 cleavage of APP on the apical side. Indeed ADAM-10, the major α-secretase activity (see above), is targeted basolaterally (Wild-Bode et al. 2006); here, it competes efficiently with the rather small amount of BACE1 present within the basolateral pathway. ADAM-10, like many other members of the ADAM family, contains two cytoplasmic Src homology 3 (SH3)-binding domains. Sequential deletion revealed critical Pro residues within the juxtamembrane SH3-binding domain. This trafficking signal was required to target ADAM-10 to adherens junctions and to support its function in cell migration and E-cadherin processing (Wild-Bode et al. 2006). Therapeutic strategies aimed at increasing α-secretase-mediated anti-amyloidogenic processing of APP have to take this important physiological function—and numerous other functions which depend on α-secretase-mediated shedding—into consideration.

In contrast to BACE1 and ADAM-10, γ-secretase activity is found on both surfaces (Capell et al. 2002), a finding, which is consistent with the observation that Aβ and p3 can be found

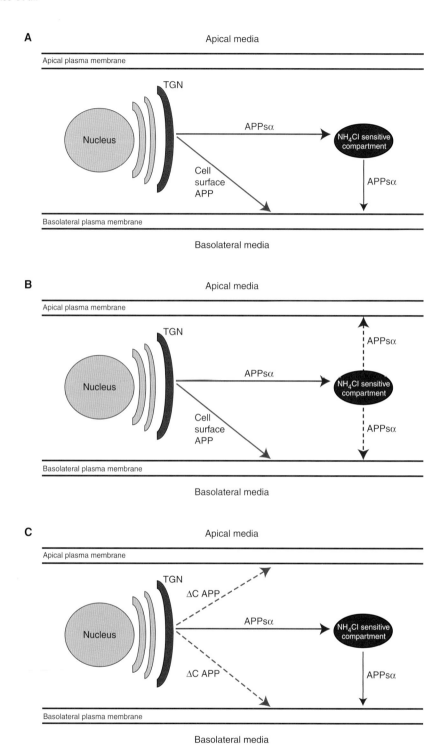

Figure 5. Polarized sorting of APP in MDCK cells. (*A*) Two independent basolateral sorting pathways for αAPPs via a NH$_4$Cl-sensitive compartment (blue) and full-length APP (red). (*B*) Inhibition of vesicular acidification by NH$_4$Cl leads to random secretion of αAPPs whereas full-length APP is still sorted to the basolateral membrane. (*C*) APP lacking a cytoplasmic signal for basolateral sorting (ΔC APP) undergoes random surface transport.

in both compartments, dependent on the APP variant expressed (i.e., with or without a baso-lateral sorting sequence) (Haass et al. 1995a). Thus the two competing proteases, ADAM-10 and BACE1, are sorted differentially to the baso-lateral or apical surface, whereas γ-secretase is found on both sides (Fig. 6).

As described above, several familial autoso-mal dominant mutations were linked to APP. One of these mutations, the so-called Swedish mutation (Mullan et al. 1992) occurs imme-diately adjacent to the BACE1 cleavage site (Met-Asp). This mutation strongly facilitates BACE-1-mediated processing of APP and there-fore results in enhanced Aβ generation (Citron et al. 1992; Cai et al. 1993). In parallel, a sig-nificantly enhanced amount of the shorter var-iant of sAPP (APPsβ) is secreted (Haass et al. 1995). Interestingly, when Swedish mutant APP was expressed in MDCK cells, APPsβ was found to be secreted apically, while the endoge-nous APPs (mainly consisting of APPsα) and membrane-bound holoAPP still underwent basolateral sorting (Lo et al. 1994; De Strooper et al. 1995a). Based on the findings described above, this observation may reflect the Swe-

dish mutation-induced processing of the small amounts of APP targeted to the apical surface by the predominantly apically targeted BACE1.

Trafficking of APP in Neurons

Although MDCK cells have yielded important insights into the polarized trafficking and proc-essing of APP, these findings had to be con-firmed in neurons, which are presumably the primary source of Aβ production in vivo. Neu-rons are highly polarized into soma, axons, and dendrites, all of which perform different func-tions and therefore are equipped with distinct sets of proteins and lipids that regulate pro-tein trafficking. To complicate matters fur-ther, axons and dendrites are subdivided into separate compartments, e.g., dendritic shafts, dendritic spines, axonal shaft, axonal presynap-tic endings, and others. An elaborate system of tracks (microtubules), trucks (kinesin and dynein motor proteins), and address labels (specific sorting signals) ensures proper deliv-ery of proteins to their respective destina-tions. Disturbances in this system could affect APP processing and have been linked to AD

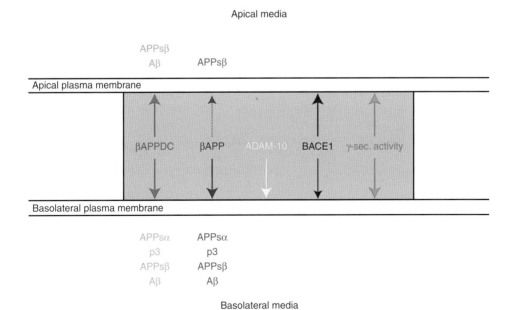

Figure 6. Polarized sorting APP, its processing products, and its secretases.

pathogenesis (De Vos et al. 2008; Morfini et al. 2009). It is therefore essential to understand in detail the trafficking and processing of APP in neurons.

The transport from ER to Golgi and TGN described earlier is thought to be similar in nonpolarized cells and in the neuronal soma. But after leaving the TGN in neurons, APP is transported to axons and dendrites in post-Golgi transport vesicles (reviewed in Kins et al. 2006). APP delivery to the axon makes use of the fast axonal transport system (Koo et al. 1990; Sisodia et al. 1993), with kinesin-1 as the microtubule motor protein (reviewed in Kins et al. 2006). As visualized by GFP-tagged fusion proteins, APP is transported in vesicular and often elongated tubular structures which move with special characteristics along the axon (Kaether et al. 2000; Stamer et al. 2002; Goldsbury et al. 2006; Szodorai et al. 2009). Whereas most other proteins are axonally transported in vesicles that display a saltatory movement, often changing directions, the APP tubules continuously move unidirectionally, with an average speed of 4.5 μm/s, reaching maximal speeds up to 10 μm/s (Kaether et al. 2000). This is among the fastest transport velocities measured in cultured neurons. Significant retrograde transport with slightly slower kinetics was also observed (Kaether et al. 2000; Stamer et al. 2002). Little is known about the fate of the axonal transport carrier vesicles. Where do they fuse with the axonal PM? What are their fusion kinetics? Where do the retrograde carriers go? A small fraction of the axonal APP has been suggested to undergo transcytotic transport to dendrites, but the significance and kinetics of this process need to be determined (Simons et al. 1995; Yamazaki et al. 1995). Likewise a detailed study of dendritic transport kinetics of APP is lacking.

What are the sorting signals mediating axonal and/or dendritic transport? An axonal sorting signal was mapped to a juxtamembrane domain which includes the Aβ-domain (Tienari et al. 1996); however, a recent report showed that APP is transported into axons and dendrites without apparent sorting signals (Back et al. 2007). Along this line, APP lacking the cytoplasmic domain (ΔC) (where the basolateral sorting signal is located; see above) is transported along neurites with characteristics indistinguishable from wild-type APP (Fig. 7a; Back et al. 2007; Szodorai et al. 2009). Therefore, the basolateral sorting signal in the carboxy-terminal region of APP documented in MDCK studies seems to have no function for polarized sorting in neurons. What emerges at this point is that the sorting of APP in neurons is fundamentally different from that of other polarized cells, and much more work has to be done to fully understand polarized trafficking of APP in neurons.

SUBCELLULAR SITES OF APP PROCESSING

Subcellular Sites of α-Secretase-Mediated APP Processing

As described above, α-secretase-mediated shedding occurs predominantly on the cell surface. However, substantial cleavage by α-secretase has also been reported to occur within TGN, for example in MDCK cells (see above).

Subcellular Sites of β-Secretase-Mediated APP Processing

As described above, BACE1 is a type-1 membrane protein that is co-translationally translocated into the ER as an immature pro-enzyme. During maturation, BACE1 undergoes a number of post/co-translational modifications, including N-glycosylation, disulfide bridge formation, and palmitoylation (Bennett et al. 2000b; Capell et al. 2000; Huse et al. 2000; Benjannet et al. 2001). The propeptide of immature BACE1 is removed by Furin and related proteases during maturation (Capell et al. 2000; Creemers et al. 2001). Surprisingly, the propeptide seems not to significantly affect BACE1 proteolytic function (Creemers et al. 2001). BACE1 reaches the PM and becomes enriched in lipid rafts (Riddell et al. 2001; Cordy et al. 2003). Rafts are discussed as potential sites for efficient Aβ generation, as APP and BACE1 apparently come into immediate contact within this compartment (Ehehalt et al. 2003; Abad-

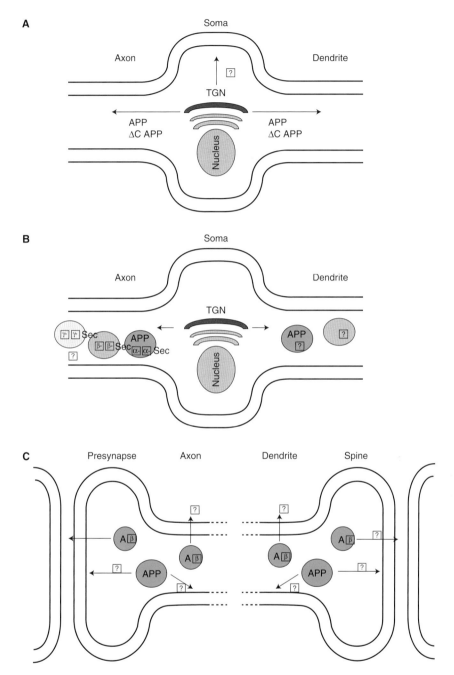

Figure 7. Neuronal APP transport and processing. (*A*) Post-Golgi sorting of APP. APP as well as APPΔC is transported by fast axonal transport along the axon and by as yet uncharacterized transport into dendrites. Transport to and fusion with the plasma membrane in the neuronal soma is likely, but has not been characterized. (*B*) Transport and sorting of APP and secretases. APP and α-secretase are transported in axonal carriers that do not contain β- or γ-secretase. Whether β- and γ-secretase are transported together is not known. Colocalization of APP and secretases in dendritic transport vesicles has not been studied. (*C*) Release of Aβ occurs at presynaptic sites, but whether it is also released from axon shafts is unknown. Aβ is released from dendrites, but the exact location has not been determined. Where APP fuses with the axonal and dendritic plasma membrane and where processing by secretases occurs remains elusive.

Rodriguez et al. 2004). This would be consistent with the finding that BACE1 undergoes palmitoylation. However, inhibition of palmitoylation and raft localization still permits relatively normal Aβ production (Vetrivel et al. 2009). Thus, the role of rafts in Aβ generation is still under debate. On reaching the PM, BACE1 undergoes internalization. Internalization and targeting to endosomes is dependent on a di-leucine motif located within the short cyto-plasmic domain of BACE1 (Huse et al. 2000; Pastorino et al. 2002). From endosomes, BACE1 can recycle to the TGN (Walter et al. 2001). A single phosphorylation at serine 498 within the carboxy-terminal domain of BACE1 is sufficient for its transport from endosomes to the trans-Golgi. Recycling requires the Golgi-localized, gamma-ear containing ADP (GGA) ribosylation-binding factor (He et al. 2005; Wahle et al. 2005, 2006), and two such GGA proteins are involved in BACE1 trafficking, GGA1 and GGA2. GGA1 is involved in endoso-mal retrieval of BACE1 and its recycling to the PM, whereas GGA2 targets BACE1 to lysosomes for its final degradation.

As an aspartyl protease, BACE1 has an acidic pH optimum (around pH 4.5) (Vassar et al. 1999), which is consistent with a major β-secretase activity within endosomes. Indeed, βCTFs accumulate in this compartment on inhibition of endosomal/lysosomal protein degradation (Golde et al. 1992; Haass et al. 1992). Selective processing of APP by BACE1 within endosomes has been used to design and generate highly effective BACE1 inhibitors. To ensure their accumulation within endo-somes, a membrane-anchored BACE1 transi-tion-state inhibitor was linked to a sterol moiety. Because of its selective accumulation within endosomes, the membrane-bound in-hibitor reduced BACE1 activity much more effi-ciently than a nonmembrane anchored version (Rajendran et al. 2008). However, BACE1 activ-ity is not exclusively restricted to endosomes. For example, Swedish mutant APP which, because of its missense mutation at the Met-Asp cleavage site is more efficiently processed by BACE1, can already be cleaved within late Golgi compartments (see above).

Subcellular Sites of γ-Secretase-Mediated APP Processing

Early studies on APP processing indicated that γ-secretase cleaves APP to generate Aβ at or near the PM. However, initial characterization of PS subcellular localization—before it was clear that it is not only implicated in γ-secretase processing but is its catalytic subunit—sug-gested that PS is mainly localized to the ER. This apparent contradiction was coined the spa-tial paradox by Annaert and De Strooper (1999). Although still not resolved completely, the work of many labs now indicates that mature, proteolytically active PS/γ-secretase is principally localized not in ER, Golgi, or post-Golgi transport vesicles but rather at the PM and in the endosomal/lysosomal system, in-cluding phagosomes and autophagosomes (reviewed in Pasternak et al. 2004; Kaether et al. 2006a; Nixon 2007; Dries and Yu 2008). The γ-secretase subunits found in the ER/early secretory pathway most likely represent unas-sembled or partially assembled subcomplexes, but not the active enzyme. The evidence sup-porting such a model is manifold and, because of space constraints, only key arguments will be highlighted: (1) APP/C99/C83 are not cleaved by γ-secretase in the ER (Cupers et al. 2001; Maltese et al. 2001; Grimm et al. 2003; Kaether et al. 2006b); (2) by immuno-electron micro-scopy, PS1 is not detected in Golgi or TGN but in ER and PM (Rechards et al. 2003); whereas the ER pool most likely reflects un-assembled PS1, the PM pool has assembled, active complex; (3) only the mature, glycosy-lated NCT, not immature unglycosylated NCT, is present in the fully assembled, active γ-secre-tase complex (Edbauer et al. 2002; Kaether et al. 2002), and therefore γ-secretase-associated NCT must have passed the Golgi; (4) γ-secretase has been shown by various methods, including cell surface biotinylation, binding of biotiny-lated inhibitors specific for the active complex, and microscopic techniques, to be present at the PM (Kaether et al. 2002; Tarassishin et al. 2004; Chyung et al. 2005). It has been shown that the ε-cleavage of APP differs in endosomes and PM (Fukumori et al. 2006), suggesting that γ-secretase has different properties depending on its subcellular localization, maybe because of differences in pH or lipid composition. One can speculate that changing the ratio of γ-secretase present in the different subcellular compartments might have an impact on AD pathology. Taken together, γ-secretase cleaves APP on the surface and in endosomes/lysosomes, but the relative contribution of the two remains to be determined and may vary among cell types.

Where in neurons do secretases process APP? Given the complex morphology of neurons, it is not surprising that even less is known about the precise subcellular site of γ-secretase processing in neurons (axonal or somal or dendritic endosomes/lysosomes? dendritic or axonal autophagosomes? other organelles?) than in non-neuronal cells (Fig. 7B). A major secretion site of Aβ seems to be distal axons/synapses (Lazarov et al. 2002; Sheng et al. 2002), but recently it was reported that Aβ can be secreted from axons and dendrites and can elicit local effects on neighboring neurons (Fig. 7C; Wei et al. 2010). A detailed analysis aimed at determining the ratio of axonally versus dendritically secreted Aβ, using for example cultured neurons in compartmentalized chambers, has not been performed. It has been suggested that APP is transported in axonal vesicles which harbor β- and γ-secretase and that consequently Aβ is produced in these vesicles (Kamal et al. 2001). This view has been challenged, and several experiments indicate that APP is not processed in axonal transport vesicles, with the exception of limited processing by α-secretase. Ligation experiments in sciatic nerve indicated that APP, but not PS as component of the γ-secretase, accumulated at the ligation site, indicating completely different transport kinetics of these proteins (Lazarov et al. 2005). In addition, using video microscopy, it was shown that APP and β-secretase are not transported in the same vesicles (Goldsbury et al. 2006). Also, by analyzing immuno-isolated APP-carrying transport vesicles, only α- but not the other secretases were found to colocalize in these vesicles (Szodorai et al. 2009). γ-secretase is present in synapses/distal axons (Beher et al. 1999; Ri-

baut-Barassin et al. 2003; Inoue et al. 2009; Frykman et al. 2010); therefore Aβ could be produced there, but the precise subcellular site(s) of APP processing by β- and γ-secretase in neurons remains to be determined.

Degradation of APP

It should be noted that alternative, secretase-independent processing of APP exists. Early studies showed that the half-life of APP is very short and that not all APP is secreted as APPs, suggesting secretase-independent processing pathways (Weidemann et al. 1989). Later it was shown that APP is degraded in lysosomes to amyloidogenic and nonamyloidogenic fragments (Golde et al. 1992; Haass et al. 1992). In addition, APP was shown to be a caspase substrate (Weidemann et al. 1999; Lu et al. 2003), but the impact of this processing on Aβ generation and/or AD pathology is probably minor (Harris et al. 2010).

Activity-Dependent APP Processing

Emerging evidence from a variety of human studies has suggested that Aβ levels and metabolism might be regulated by neuronal activity. In this regard, some patients with temporal lobe epilepsy, who experience elevated neuronal activity, develop Aβ-containing plaques as early as 30 years of age (Mackenzie and Miller 1994; Gouras et al. 1997). Moreover, regions of the brain that develop the highest levels of Aβ plaques, including the frontal and parietal lobes and posterior cingulate cortex, exhibit the highest baseline metabolic activity in the so-called "default network" (Gusnard et al. 2001; Raichle et al. 2001; Buckner et al. 2005). This high metabolic activity is a reflection of elevated neuronal and synaptic activity. Parallel studies in animal models and cell culture have linked APP transport, neuronal activity, and Aβ metabolism. APP is axonally transported from the entorhinal cortex to the hippocampal formation via the perforant pathway (Buxbaum et al. 1998a), and lesions of this pathway in transgenic mice overexpressing FAD-linked mutant APP and PS1 transgenes results in substantially less Aβ deposition within the hippocampus (Lazarov et al. 2002). Early studies showed that electrical depolarization increases the release of soluble APP-α in rat hippocampal brain slices (Nitsch et al. 1993), and it appears that these effects are mediated by activation of muscarinic M1 acetylcholine receptors which leads to parallel decreases in Aβ levels (Beach et al. 2001; Hock et al. 2003). On the other hand, specific stimulation of NMDA receptors up-regulates APP, inhibits α-secretase activity, and promotes Aβ production (Lesne et al. 2005).

To determine the effects of neuronal activity on Aβ secretion, Kamenetz et al. (2003) prepared hippocampal slices from transgenic mice overexpressing APP harboring the FAD-linked Swedish mutation (APP$_{SWE}$) and maintained these preparations in the presence of pharmacological agents that either decrease neuronal activity [tetrodotoxin (TTX), high magnesium, or flunitrazepam than in non-neuronal cells (Fig. 7B). A major secretion site of Aβ seems to be distal axons/synapses a GABA-A receptor potentiator)] or increase it (picrotoxin [a GABA-A channel blocker]). Agents that decreased or increased activity resulted in significant reductions or elevations, respectively, in levels of Aβ (both Aβ40 and Aβ42) detected in the slice medium, indicating that the secretion of Aβ from neuronal cells that overexpress APP can be controlled by neuronal activity. Western blot analyses revealed that increasing neuronal activity significantly enhanced the levels of β-CTF, the penultimate precursor of Aβ peptides, and elevated levels of secreted APPsβ, findings which suggested that the level of BACE cleavage can be controlled by neuronal activity. To address whether APP or its products can control synaptic function, wild-type rat hippocampal slice neurons were transduced with viruses expressing APP or APP mutants, and synaptic responses were evoked onto side-by-side pairs of simultaneously recorded postsynaptic neurons where only one neuron expresses the exogenous protein. Excitatory AMPA and NMDA responses onto neurons expressing recombinant APP were significantly depressed, whereas inhibitory (GABA) currents were unaffected. Neurons expressing APP showed

a significant decrease in the frequency of miniature EPSCs, with no change in their amplitude nor in paired-pulse facilitation, suggesting that the depressive effects of APP overexpression are due to a decrease in the number of functional synapses. Indeed, expression of an APP variant harboring an experimental mutation (APP$_{MV}$) just before Aβ Asp1 that blocks β-secretase cleavage produced no significant depression of transmission. Furthermore, transduced slices treated with a highly potent and selective γ-secretase inhibitor (L-685,458) failed to show synaptic depression onto nearby control cells. These results indicate that γ-secretase processing of APP is required for the depressive effects of APP and that this phenotype is independent of the formation of the large ectodomain of APP following either α or β cleavage events. The results indicate that processing of APP into Aβ is dependent on neuronal activity and that formation of Aβ results in synaptic depression. Treatment of transduced slices with NBQX (an AMPA receptor antagonist) or D,L-AP5, an agent that blocks NMDA-Rs, prevented the synaptic depression caused by APP overexpression. Finally, Kamenetz et al. (2003) tested whether Aβ produced from overexpressing neurons can affect neighboring neurons in a cell nonautonomous manner. Here, synaptic function in two uninfected cells, one from a region containing many infected cells and another from a region with no infected cells, was examined. Uninfected neurons surrounded by APP$_{SWE}$-infected neurons had significantly depressed transmission when compared to distant control neurons, suggesting that uninfected neurons in infected regions were responding to the local high concentrations of Aβ. These results are consistent with the notion that high Aβ levels may disrupt synaptic function and, more importantly, that Aβ may also have a normal negative feedback function: increased neuronal activity produces more Aβ; the enhanced Aβ production depresses synaptic function; the depressed synaptic function will decrease neuronal activity.

How do high levels of released Aβ mediate synaptic depression? To address this issue, Hsieh and colleagues (2006) examined the effects of increased Aβ levels on the structure of dendritic spines of CA1 pyramidal dendrites in organotypic slices that acutely overexpress APP. In this setting, spine density in APP-expressing cells was decreased compared to cells expressing the APP(MV) variant that undergoes much less processing by β-secretase. Similar to earlier studies showing that application of synthetic Aβ reduces the levels of surface NMDA and GluR1 receptors in dissociated cultured hippocampal neurons (Almeida et al. 2005; Snyder et al. 2005), Hsieh et al. (2006) confirmed that Aβ generated in situ also leads to decreases in surface and synaptic AMPA receptors on both spines and dendrites. Using an AMPA-R subunit tagged on its amino terminus with a pH-sensitive GFP variant, Hsieh revealed that APP overexpression led to a significant decrease of spine and dendritic surface AMPA receptors compared to cells expressing the APP(MV) variant.

Although these studies made clear that APP overexpression and resultant Aβ secretion can lead to synaptic dysfunction, the subcellular sites from which Aβ acts remained uncertain. To examine this issue, Wei and colleagues (2010) isolated the sites of increased Aβ production by selectively expressing APP in pre- or postsynaptic neurons. Using two-photon laser-scanning imaging to monitor the synaptic deficits caused by such dendritic or axonal Aβ, Wei and colleagues found that either dendritic or axonal Aβ overproduction was sufficient to cause local spine loss and compromise synaptic plasticity in the nearby dendrites of neurons that did not overexpress APP. The Aβ-mediated synaptic dysfunction could be pharmacologically ameliorated by blockade of either neural activity, NMDA receptors, or nicotinic acetylcholine receptors.

Extending these latter studies to an in vivo setting, Cirrito et al. (2005) asked whether synaptic activity influences the levels of Aβ in brain interstitial fluid (ISF). A microdialysis probe with concurrent hippocampal electrophysiological recording was used to assess whether there are dynamic changes in ISF Aβ levels in conjunction with differing levels of neuronal activity in awake, behaving mice. Here, a recording electrode was attached to a microdialysis probe to monitor electroencephalographic (EEG) activity (extracellular field potentials) and simultaneously collect ISF Aβ in the hippocampus of Tg2576 mice at 3–5 months of age. Neuronal and synaptic activity within the hippocampus was enhanced by electrically stimulating the perforant pathway, the major afferent projection from the entorhinal cortex to the hippocampus, conditions that created transient epileptiform discharges within the hippocampus noted on hippocampal EEGs. During these electrical seizures, ISF Aβ levels increased, showing a direct relationship between increased neuronal activity and increases in ISF Aβ in vivo. To determine if endogenous neural activity of the perforant pathway modulates ISF Aβ levels within the hippocampus, a selective metabotropic glutamate receptor 2/3 agonist, LY354740, was infused into the hippocampus via reverse microdialysis, and ISF Aβ levels were monitored. This treatment caused a decrease in ISF Aβ within the hippocampus, consistent with the hypothesis that modulation of endogenous neuronal activity in this pathway can alter hippocampal Aβ production. Indeed, strong depression of local activity using the sodium channel blocker TTX revealed that a decline in EEG amplitude was paralleled by a concomitant decrease in Aβ levels. Taken together with the studies of Kamenetz and colleagues, these studies by Cirrito et al. establish that neuronal or synaptic activity can directly influence Aβ levels.

The question remained as to the mechanism by which increased synaptic activity elevates Aβ secretion. One possibility is that the half-life of extracellular Aβ is extended; alternatively, this effect may involve increased APP processing. Using a γ-secretase inhibitor in TTX or vehicle-treated mice, Cirrito et al. (2005) showed that Aβ half-life was unaltered by the depression of neuronal activity. Additionally, expression of the Aβ-degrading enzyme neprilysin was unchanged in TTX-treated mice.

In further attempts to delineate the mechanism(s) responsible for activity-dependent elevations of ISF Aβ, Cirritto and colleagues (2008) hypothesized that Aβ released into the brain ISF following synaptic transmission requires an intermediate event involving APP endocytosis, analogous to that shown by Koo and Squazzo (1994) in cultured immortalized mammalian cells. To assess the influence of endocytosis on ISF Aβ levels under normal conditions, a myristylated, cell-permeable peptide (dynamin-DN) which inhibits clathrin-mediated endocytosis was infused into hippocampus by reverse microdialysis. As an in vivo control, the dynamin-DN reduced biotinylated transferrin uptake into cells within the dentate gyrus. Importantly, ISF Aβ levels were significantly decreased. Because inhibition of synaptic activity (Cirrito et al. 2005) and inhibition of endocytosis (Cirrito et al. 2008) each reduce ISF Aβ levels, there remained the question of the extent as to which (or both) contributes to ISF Aβ levels. Cirritto et al (2008) co-administered TTX and dynamin-DN. Administration of dynamin-DN first led to a decrease in ISF Aβ levels by 70%, but if the microdialysis perfusion buffer was then switched to contain dynamin-DN and TTX, no additional change in ISF Aβ levels were observed. These findings suggested that all of the ISF Aβ that is produced by synaptic activity requires endocytosis. On the other hand, if animals were pretreated with TTX followed by dynamin-DN, ISF Aβ levels were further reduced when endocytosis was inhibited, a finding that strongly suggested that a "releasable" stored pool of ISF Aβ that is generated via endocytosis is distinct from an Aβ pool that is acutely released by synaptic activity.

Although these studies using hippocampal slices and in vivo microdialysis provide compelling support for activity-dependent Aβ production, most such studies have been performed in acute settings. Studies by Tampellini and colleagues (2010) chronically reduced synaptic activity in vivo via unilateral ablation of whiskers or chronic diazepam treatment. For the whisker ablation experiments, bulbs were unilaterally removed in 2- to 3-month-old Tg19959 mice that express the FAD-linked Swedish (KM-NL) and London (V717F) APP mutations and develop plaques by age 3 months. At 6 months, cytochrome oxidase (COX) staining was reduced in the deafferented versus the synaptically active (control) barrel cortices, indicating that the lesion reduced synaptic activity. The barrel cortices with reduced activity showed a striking decrease in both the number of Aβ plaques and the area covered by plaques compared to the control side. Parallel studies in which the transgenic mice were chronically treated with diazepam for 1 month beginning at age 3 months also led to reduced plaque burden in cortex and hippocampus.

Despite evidence from these elegant in vitro, ex vivo and in vivo studies for an important role for synaptic activity in modulating Aβ production and subsequent synaptotoxicity, there remain gaps in our understanding of the underlying neurobiology. For example, does synaptic activity alter the trafficking of APP and/or the secretases to axonal and/or dendritic compartments? How does synaptic activity elevate the steady-state levels of βCTF, the precursor of Aβ? What are the pre- and postsynaptic receptor(s) involved in binding Aβ and/or its oligomeric forms (see Mucke and Selkoe 2011)? What are the signaling mechanisms by which activated postsynaptic Aβ receptor(s) lead to removal of AMPA and NMDA receptors and how do these changes alter structural plasticity? Finally, is there selectivity in specific neuronal circuits that underlies selectivity vulnerability of certain neuronal populations early in the disease process (i.e., preclinically)?

CONCLUSIONS

APP is the central protein involved in AD pathology as it serves as the precursor for Aβ generation. Intensive analysis of the cell biology of this protein and its proteolytic processing led not only to a detailed understanding of Aβ generation but also allowed the generation of therapeutically relevant secretase inhibitors. Moreover, understanding the biology of secretases allowed major progress in other fields of cell biological research. For example, research on secretases paved the road toward the understanding of RIP and the signaling pathways triggered by this process.

REFERENCES

*Reference is also in this collection.

Abad-Rodriguez J, Ledesma MD, Craessaerts K, Perga S, Medina M, Delacourte A, Dingwall C, De Strooper B, Dotti CG. 2004. Neuronal membrane cholesterol loss enhances amyloid peptide generation. *J Cell Biol* **167:** 953–960.

Allinson TM, Parkin ET, Turner AJ, Hooper NM. 2003. ADAMs family members as amyloid precursor protein α-secretases. *J Neurosci Res* **74:** 342–352.

Almeida CG, Tampellini D, Takahashi RH, Greengard P, Lin MT, Snyder EM, Gouras GK. 2005. Beta-amyloid accumulation in APP mutant neurons reduces PSD-95 and GluR1 in synapses. *Neurobiol Dis* **20:** 187–198.

Andersen OM, Reiche J, Schmidt V, Gotthardt M, Spoelgen R, Behlke J, von Arnim CA, Breiderhoff T, Jansen P, Wu X, et al. 2005. Neuronal sorting protein-related receptor sorLA/LR11 regulates processing of the amyloid precursor protein. *Proc Natl Acad Sci* **102:** 13461–13466.

Ando K, Iijima KI, Elliott JI, Kirino Y, Suzuki T. 2001. Phosphorylation-dependent regulation of the interaction of amyloid precursor protein with Fe65 affects the production of beta-amyloid. *J Biol Chem* **276:** 40353–40361.

Annaert W, De Strooper B. 1999. Presenilins: Molecular switches between proteolysis and signal transduction. *Trends Neurosci* **22:** 439–443.

Back S, Haas P, Tschape JA, Gruebl T, Kirsch J, Muller U, Beyreuther K, Kins S. 2007. Beta-amyloid precursor protein can be transported independent of any sorting signal to the axonal and dendritic compartment. *J Neurosci Res* **85:** 2580–2590.

Basi G, Frigon N, Barbour R, Doan T, Gordon G, McConlogue L, Sinha S, Zeller M. 2003. Antagonistic effects of beta-site amyloid precursor protein-cleaving enzymes 1 and 2 on beta-amyloid peptide production in cells. *J Biol Chem* **278:** 31512–31520.

Beach TG, Kuo YM, Schwab C, Walker DG, Roher AE. 2001. Reduction of cortical amyloid beta levels in guinea pig brain after systemic administration of physostigmine. *Neurosci Lett* **310:** 21–24.

Beher D, Elle C, Underwood J, Davis JB, Ward R, Karran E, Masters CL, Beyreuther K, Multhaup G. 1999. Proteolytic fragments of Alzheimer's disease-associated presenilin 1 are present in synaptic organelles and growth cone membranes of rat brain. *J Neurochem* **72:** 1564–1573.

Benjannet S, Elagoz A, Wickham L, Mamarbachi M, Munzer JS, Basak A, Lazure C, Cromlish JA, Sisodia S, Checler F, et al. 2001. Post-translational processing of beta-secretase (beta-amyloid-converting enzyme) and its ectodomain shedding. The pro- and transmembrane/cytosolic domains affect its cellular activity and amyloid-beta production. *J Biol Chem* **276:** 10879–10887.

Bennett BD, Babu-Khan S, Loeloff R, Louis JC, Curran E, Citron M, Vassar R. 2000a. Expression analysis of BACE2 in brain and peripheral tissues. *J Biol Chem* **275:** 20647–20651.

Bennett BD, Denis P, Haniu M, Teplow DB, Kahn S, Louis JC, Citron M, Vassar R. 2000b. A furin-like convertase mediates propeptide cleavage of BACE, the Alzheimer's beta-secretase. *J Biol Chem* **275:** 37712–37717.

Birchmeier C, Nave KA. 2008. Neuregulin-1, a key axonal signal that drives Schwann cell growth and differentiation. *Glia* **56:** 1491–1497.

Brown MS, Ye J, Rawson RB, Goldstein JL. 2000. Regulated intramembrane proteolysis: A control mechanism conserved from bacteria to humans. *Cell* **100:** 391–398.

Buckner RL, Snyder AZ, Shannon BJ, LaRossa G, Sachs R, Fotenos AF, Sheline YI, Klunk WE, Mathis CA, Morris JC, et al. 2005. Molecular, structural, and functional characterization of Alzheimer's disease: Evidence for a relationship between default activity, amyloid, and memory. *J Neurosci* **25:** 7709–7717.

Busciglio J Gabuzda DH, Matsudaira P, Yankner BA. 1993. Generation of beta-amyloid in the secretory pathway in neuronal and nonneuronal cells. *Proc Natl Acad Sci* **90:** 2092–2096.

Buxbaum JD, Gandy SE, Cicchetti P, Ehrlich ME, Czernik AJ, Fracasso RP, Ramabhadran TV, Unterbeck AJ, Greengard P. 1990. Processing of Alzheimer beta/A4 amyloid precursor protein: Modulation by agents that regulate protein phosphorylation. *Proc Natl Acad Sci* **87:** 6003–6006.

Buxbaum JD, Thinakaran G, Koliatsos V, O'Callahan J, Slunt HH, Price DL, Sisodia SS. 1998a. Alzheimer amyloid protein precursor in the rat hippocampus: Transport and processing through the perforant path. *J Neurosci* **18:** 9629–9637.

Buxbaum JD, Liu KN, Luo Y, Slack JL, Stocking KL, Peschon JJ, Johnson RS, Castner BJ, Cerretti DP, Black RA. 1998b. Evidence that tumor necrosis factor alpha converting enzyme is involved in regulated alpha-secretase cleavage of the Alzheimer amyloid protein precursor. *J Biol Chem* **273:** 27765–27767.

Cai XD, Golde TE, Younkin SG. 1993. Release of excess amyloid beta protein from a mutant amyloid beta protein precursor. *Science* **259:** 514–516.

Cai H, Wang Y, McCarthy D, Wen H, Borchelt DR, Price DL, Wong PC. 2001. BACE1 is the major beta-secretase for generation of Abeta peptides by neurons. *Nat Neurosci* **4:** 233–234.

Cam JA, Zerbinatti CV, Li Y, Bu G. 2005. Rapid endocytosis of the LDL receptor-related protein modulates cell surface distribution and processing of the beta amyloid precursors protein. *J Biol Chem* **280:** 15464–15470.

Cao X, Sudhof TC. 2001. A transcriptionally [correction of transcriptively] active complex of APP with Fe65 and histone acetyltransferase Tip60. *Science* **293:** 115–120.

Capell A, Steiner H, Willem M, Kaiser H, Meyer C, Walter J, Lammich S, Multhaup G, Haass C. 2000. Maturation and pro-peptide cleavage of beta-secretase. *J Biol Chem* **275:** 30849–30854.

Capell A, Meyn L, Fluhrer R, Teplow DB, Walter J, Haass C. 2002. Apical sorting of beta-secretase limits amyloid beta-peptide production. *J Biol Chem* **277:** 5637–5643.

Carey RM, Balcz BA, Lopez-Coviella I, Slack BE. 2005. Inhibition of dynamin-dependent endocytosis increases shedding of the amyloid precursor protein ectodomain and reduces generation of amyloid beta protein. *BMC Cell Biol* **6:** 30.

Chartier-Harlin MC, Crawford F, Houlden H, Warren A, Hughes D, Fidani L, Goate A, Rossor M, Roques P, Hardy J, et al. 1991. Early-onset Alzheimer's disease caused by mutations at codon 717 of the beta-amyloid precursor protein gene. *Nature* **353**: 844–846.

Chavez-Gutierrez L, Tolia A, Maes E, Li T, Wong PC, de Strooper B. 2008. Glu(332) in the Nicastrin ectodomain is essential for gamma-secretase complex maturation but not for its activity. *J Biol Chem* **283**: 20096–20105.

Chyung JH, Selkoe DJ. 2003. Inhibition of receptor-mediated endocytosis demonstrates generation of amyloid beta-protein at the cell surface. *J Biol Chem* **278**: 51035–51043.

Chyung JH, Raper DM, Selkoe DJ. 2005. Gamma-secretase exists on the plasma membrane as an intact complex that accepts substrates and effects intramembrane cleavage. *J Biol Chem* **280**: 4383–4392.

Cirrito JR, Yamada KA, Finn MB, Sloviter RS, Bales KR, May PC, Schoepp DD, Paul SM, Mennerick S, Holtzman DM. 2005. Synaptic activity regulates interstitial fluid amyloid-beta levels in vivo. *Neuron* **48**: 913–922.

Cirrito JR, Kang JE, Lee J, Stewart FR, Verges DK, Silverio LM, Bu G, Mennerick S, Holtzman DM. 2008. Endocytosis is required for synaptic activity-dependent release of amyloid-beta in vivo. *Neuron* **58**: 42–51.

Citron M. 2004. Beta-secretase inhibition for the treatment of Alzheimer's disease—promise and challenge. *Trends Pharmacol Sci* **25**: 92–97.

Citron M, Oltersdorf T, Haass C, McConlogue L, Hung AY, Seubert P, Vigo-Pelfrey C, Lieberburg I, Selkoe DJ. 1992. Mutation of the beta-amyloid precursor protein in familial Alzheimer's disease increases beta-protein production. *Nature* **360**: 672–674.

Cordy JM, Hussain I, Dingwall C, Hooper NM, Turner AJ. 2003. Exclusively targeting beta-secretase to lipid rafts by GPI-anchor addition up-regulates beta-site processing of the amyloid precursor protein. *Proc Natl Acad Sci* **100**: 11735–11740.

Creemers JW, Ines Dominguez D, Plets E, Serneels L, Taylor NA, Multhaup G, Craessaerts K, Annaert W, De Strooper B. 2001. Processing of beta-secretase by furin and other members of the proprotein convertase family. *J Biol Chem* **276**: 4211–4217.

Cupers P, Bentahir M, Craessaerts K, Orlans I, Vanderstichele H, Saftig P, De Strooper B, Annaert W. 2001. The discrepancy between presenilin subcellular localization and gamma-secretase processing of amyloid precursor protein. *J Cell Biol* **154**: 731–740.

De Strooper B, Craessaerts K, Dewachter I, Moechars D, Greenberg B, Van Leuven F, Van den Berghe H. 1995a. Basolateral secretion of amyloid precursor protein in Madin–Darby canine kidney cells is disturbed by alterations of intracellular pH and by introducing a mutation associated with familial Alzheimer's disease. *J Biol Chem* **270**: 4058–4065.

De Strooper B, Craessaerts K, Van Leuven F, Van Den Berghe H. 1995b. Exchanging the extracellular domain of amyloid precursor protein for horseradish peroxidase does not interfere with alpha-secretase cleavage of the beta-amyloid region, but randomizes secretion in Madin–Darby canine kidney cells. *J Biol Chem* **270**: 30310–30314.

* De Strooper B, Iwatsubo T, Wolfe MS. 2011. Presenilins and γ-secretase: Structure, function, and role in Alzheimer

disease. *Cold Spring Harb Perspect Med* doi: 10.1101/cshperspect.a006304.

De Vos KJ, Grierson AJ, Ackerley S, Miller CC. 2008. Role of axonal transport in neurodegenerative diseases. *Annu Rev Neurosci* **31**: 151–173.

Dominguez D, Tournoy J, Hartmann D, Huth T, Cryns K, Deforce S, Serneels L, Camacho IE, Marjaux E, Craessaerts K, et al. 2005. Phenotypic and biochemical analyses of BACE1- and BACE2-deficient mice. *J Biol Chem* **280**: 30797–30806.

Dries DR, Yu G. 2008. Assembly, maturation, and trafficking of the gamma-secretase complex in Alzheimer's disease. *Curr Alzheimer Res* **5**: 132–146.

Dries DR, Shah S, Han YH, Yu C, Yu S, Shearman MS, Yu G. 2009. GLU333 of nicastrin directly participates in gamma-secretase activity. *J Biol Chem* **284**: 29714–29724.

Dyrks T, Weidemann A, Multhaup G, Salbaum JM, Lemaire HG, Kang J, Muller-Hill B, Masters CL, Beyreuther K. 1988. Identification, transmembrane orientation and biogenesis of the amyloid A4 precursor of Alzheimer's disease. *EMBO J* **7**: 949–957.

Edbauer D, Winkler E, Haass C, Steiner H. 2002. Presenilin and nicastrin regulate each other and determine amyloid beta-peptide production via complex formation. *Proc Natl Acad Sci* **99**: 8666–8671.

Edbauer D, Winkler E, Regula JT, Pesold B, Steiner H, Haass C. 2003. Reconstitution of gamma-secretase activity. *Nat Cell Biol* **5**: 486–488.

Ehehalt R, Keller P, Haass C, Thiele C, Simons K. 2003. Amyloidogenic processing of the Alzheimer beta-amyloid precursor protein depends on lipid rafts. *J Cell Biol* **160**: 113–123.

Esch FS, Keim PS, Beattie EC, Blacher RW, Culwell AR, Oltersdorf T, McClure D, Ward PJ. 1990. Cleavage of amyloid beta peptide during constitutive processing of its precursor. *Science* **248**: 1122–1124.

Farzan M, Schnitzler CE, Vasilieva N, Leung D, Choe H. 2000. BACE2, a beta-secretase homolog, cleaves at the beta site and within the amyloid-beta region of the amyloid-beta precursor protein. *Proc Natl Acad Sci* **97**: 9712–9717.

Fluhrer R, Capell A, Westmeyer G, Willem M, Hartung B, Condron MM, Teplow DB, Haass C, Walter J. 2002. A non-amyloidogenic function of BACE-2 in the secretory pathway. *J Neurochem* **81**: 1011–1020.

Fluhrer R, Grammer G, Israel L, Condron MM, Haffner C, Friedmann E, Bohland C, Imhof A, Martoglio B, Teplow DB, et al. 2006. A gamma-secretase-like intramembrane cleavage of TNFalpha by the GxGD aspartyl protease SPPL2b. *Nat Cell Biol* **8**: 894–896.

Fluhrer R, Fukumori A, Martin L, Grammer G, Haug-Kroper M, Klier B, Winkler E, Kremmer E, Condron MM, Teplow DB, et al. 2008. Intramembrane proteolysis of GXGD-type aspartyl proteases is slowed by a familial Alzheimer disease-like mutation. *J Biol Chem* **283**: 30121–30128.

Fluhrer R, Steiner H, Haass C. 2009. Intramembrane proteolysis by signal peptide peptidases: A comparative discussion of GXGD-type aspartyl proteases. *J Biol Chem* **284**: 13975–13979.

Francis R, McGrath G, Zhang J, Ruddy DA, Sym M, Apfeld J, Nicoll M, Maxwell M, Hai B, Ellis MC, et al. 2002. aph-1 and pen-2 are required for Notch pathway signaling, gamma-secretase cleavage of betaAPP, and presenilin protein accumulation. *Dev Cell* **3:** 85–97.

Frykman S, Hur JY, Franberg J, Aoki M, Winblad B, Nahalkova J, Behbahani H, Tjernberg LO. 2010. Synaptic and endosomal localization of active gamma-secretase in rat brain. *PloS One* **5:** e8948.

Fukumori A, Okochi M, Tagami S, Jiang J, Itoh N, Nakayama T, Yanagida K, Ishizuka-Katsura Y, Morihara T, Kamino K, et al. 2006. Presenilin-dependent gamma-secretase on plasma membrane and endosomes is functionally distinct. *Biochemistry* **45:** 4907–4914.

Gandy S, Greengard P. 1994. Regulated cleavage of the Alzheimer amyloid precursor protein: Molecular and cellular basis. *Biochimie* **76:** 300–303.

Golde TE, Estus S, Younkin LH, Selkoe DJ, Younkin SG. 1992. Processing of the amyloid protein precursor to potentially amyloidogenic derivatives. *Science* **255:** 728–730.

Goldsbury C, Mocanu MM, Thies E, Kaether C, Haass C, Keller P, Biernat J, Mandelkow E, Mandelkow EM. 2006. Inhibition of APP trafficking by tau protein does not increase the generation of amyloid-beta peptides. *Traffic* **7:** 873–888.

Gouras GK, Relkin NR, Sweeney D, Munoz DG, Mackenzie IR, Gandy S. 1997. Increased apolipoprotein E epsilon 4 in epilepsy with senile plaques. *Ann Neurol* **41:** 402–404.

Grimm HS, Beher D, Lichtenthaler SF, Shearman MS, Beyreuther K, Hartmann T. 2003. Gamma-secretase cleavage site specificity differs for intracellular and secretory amyloid beta. *J Biol Chem* **278:** 13077–13085.

Gu Y, Misonou H, Sato T, Dohmae N, Takio K, Ihara Y. 2001. Distinct intramembrane cleavage of the beta-amyloid precursor protein family resembling gamma-secretase-like cleavage of Notch. *J Biol Chem* **276:** 35235–35238.

Gusnard DA, Raichle ME, Raichle ME. 2001. Searching for a baseline: Functional imaging and the resting human brain. *Nat Rev Neurosci* **2:** 685–694.

Haass C. 2004. Take five—BACE and the gamma-secretase quartet conduct Alzheimer's amyloid beta-peptide generation. *EMBO J* **23:** 483–488.

Haass C, Selkoe DJ. 1993. Cellular processing of beta-amyloid precursor protein and the genesis of amyloid beta-peptide. *Cell* **75:** 1039–1042.

Haass C, Selkoe DJ. 2007. Soluble protein oligomers in neurodegeneration: Lessons from the Alzheimer's amyloid beta-peptide. *Nat Rev Mol Cell Biol* **8:** 101–112.

Haass C, Koo EH, Mellon A, Hung AY, Selkoe DJ. 1992a. Targeting of cell-surface beta-amyloid precursor protein to lysosomes: Alternative processing into amyloid-bearing fragments. *Nature* **357:** 500–503.

Haass C, Scholssmacher M, Hung AY, Vigo-Pelfrey C, Mellon A, Ostaszewski B, Liederburg I, Koo F, Schenk D, Teplow D, et al. 1992b. Amyloid β-peptide is produced by cultured cells during normal metabolism. *Nature* **359:** 322–325.

Haass C, Hung AY, Schlossmacher MG, Oltersdorf T, Teplow DB, Selkoe DJ. 1993a. Normal cellular processing of the beta-amyloid precursor protein results in the secretion of the amyloid beta peptide and related molecules. *Ann NY Acad Sci* **695:** 109–116.

Haass C, Hung AY, Schlossmacher MG, Teplow DB, Selkoe DJ. 1993b. Beta-amyloid peptide and a 3-kDa fragment are derived by distinct cellular mechanisms. *J Biol Chem* **268:** 3021–3024.

Haass C, Koo EH, Teplow DB, Selkoe DJ. 1994. Polarized secretion of beta-amyloid precursor protein and amyloid beta-peptide in MDCK cells. *Proc Natl Acad Sci* **91:** 1564–1568.

Haass C, Koo EH, Capell A, Teplow DB, Selkoe DJ. 1995a. Polarized sorting of beta-amyloid precursor protein and its proteolytic products in MDCK cells is regulated by two independent signals. *J Cell Biol* **128:** 537–547.

Haass C, Lemere CA, Capell A, Citron M, Seubert P, Schenk D, Lannfelt L, Selkoe DJ. 1995b. The Swedish mutation causes early-onset Alzheimer's disease by beta-secretase cleavage within the secretory pathway. *Nat Med* **1:** 1291–1296.

Harris JA, Devidze N, Halabisky B, Lo I, Thwin MT, Yu GQ, Bredesen DE, Masliah E, Mucke L. 2010. Many neuronal and behavioral impairments in transgenic mouse models of Alzheimer's disease are independent of caspase cleavage of the amyloid precursor protein. *J Neurosci* **30:** 372–381.

Harrison SM, Harper AJ, Hawkins J, Duddy G, Grau E, Pugh PL, Winter PH, Shilliam CS, Hughes ZA, Dawson LA, et al. 2003. BACE1 (beta-secretase) transgenic and knockout mice: Identification of neurochemical deficits and behavioral changes. *Mol Cell Neurosci* **24:** 646–655.

Hartmann T, Bergsdorf C, Sandbrink R, Tienari PJ, Multhaup G, Ida N, Bieger S, Dyrks T, Weidemann A, Masters CL, et al. 1996. Alzheimer's disease betaA4 protein release and amyloid precursor protein sorting are regulated by alternative splicing. *J Biol Chem* **271:** 13208–13214.

Hasegawa H, Sanjo N, Chen F, Gu YJ, Shier C, Petit A, Kawarai T, Katayama T, Schmidt SD, Mathews PM, et al. 2004. Both the sequence and length of the C terminus of PEN-2 are critical for intermolecular interactions and function of presenilin complexes. *J Biol Chem* **279:** 46455–46463.

Hartmann D, de Strooper B, Serneels L, Craessaerts K, Herreman A, Annaert W, Umans L, Lubke T, Lena Illert A, von Figura K, et al. 2002. The disintegrin/metalloprotease ADAM 10 is essential for Notch signalling but not for alpha-secretase activity in fibroblasts. *Hum Mol Genet* **11:** 2615–2624.

He X, Li F, Chang WP, Tang J. 2005. GGA proteins mediate the recycling pathway of memapsin 2 (BACE). *J Biol Chem* **280:** 11696–11703.

Hill K, Li Y, Bennett M, McKay M, Zhu X, Shern J, Torre E, Lah JJ, Levey AI, Kahn RA. 2003. Munc18 interacting proteins: ADP-ribosylation factor-dependent coat proteins that regulate the traffic of beta-Alzheimer's precursor protein. *J Biol Chem* **278:** 36032–36040.

Hock C, Maddalena A, Raschig A, Muller-Spahn F, Eschweiler G, Hager K, Heuser I, Hampel H, Muller-Thomsen T, Oertel W, et al. 2003. Treatment with the selective muscarinic m1 agonist talsaclidine decreases cerebrospinal fluid levels of A beta 42 in patients with Alzheimer's disease. *Amyloid* **10:** 1–6.

Hong L, Koelsch G, Lin X, Wu S, Terzyan S, Ghosh AK, Zhang XC, Tang J. 2000. Structure of the protease domain of memapsin 2 (beta-secretase) complexed with inhibitor. *Science* **290:** 150–153.

Hsieh H, Boehm J, Sato C, Iwatsubo T, Tomita T, Sisodia S, Malinow R. 2006. AMPA-R removal underlies Aβ-induced synaptic depression and dendritic spine loss. *Neuron* **52:** 831–843.

Hu X, Hicks CW, He W, Wong P, Macklin WB, Trapp BD, Yan R. 2006. Bace1 modulates myelination in the central and peripheral nervous system. *Nat Neurosci* **9:** 1520–1525.

Huse JT, Pijak DS, Leslie GJ, Lee VM, Doms RW. 2000. Maturation and endosomal targeting of beta-site amyloid precursor protein-cleaving enzyme. The Alzheimer's disease beta-secretase. *J Biol Chem* **275:** 33729–33737.

Hussain I, Powell DJ, Howlett DR, Chapman GA, Gilmour L, Murdock PR, Tew DG, Meek TD, Chapman C, Schneider K, et al. 2000. ASP1 (BACE2) cleaves the amyloid precursor protein at the beta-secretase site. *Mol Cell Neurosci* **16:** 609–619.

Inoue E, Deguchi-Tawarada M, Togawa A, Matsui C, Arita K, Katahira-Tayama S, Sato T, Yamauchi E, Oda Y, Takai Y. 2009. Synaptic activity prompts gamma-secretase-mediated cleavage of EphA4 and dendritic spine formation. *J Cell Biol* **185:** 551–564.

Kaether C, Skehel P, Dotti CG. 2000. Axonal membrane proteins are transported in distinct carriers: A two-color video microscopy study in cultured hippocampal neurons. *Mol Biol Cell* **11:** 1213–1224.

Kaether C, Lammich S, Edbauer D, Ertl M, Rietdorf J, Capell A, Steiner H, Haass C. 2002. Presenilin-1 affects trafficking and processing of betaAPP and is targeted in a complex with nicastrin to the plasma membrane. *J Cell Biol* **158:** 551–561.

Kaether C, Haass C, Steiner H. 2006a. Assembly, trafficking and function of gamma-secretase. *Neurodegener Dis* **3:** 275–283.

Kaether C, Schmitt S, Willem M, Haass C. 2006b. Amyloid precursor protein and notch intracellular domains are generated after transport of their precursors to the cell surface. *Traffic* **7:** 408–415.

Kamal A, Almenar-Queralt A, LeBlanc JF, Roberts EA, Goldstein LS. 2001. Kinesin-mediated axonal transport of a membrane compartment containing beta-secretase and presenilin-1 requires APP. *Nature* **414:** 643–648.

Kamenetz F, Tomita T, Seabrook G, Borchelt D, Iwatsubo T, Sisodia SS, Malinow R. 2003. APP processing and synaptic function. *Neuron* **37:** 925–937.

Kang J, Lemaire HG, Unterbeck A, Salbaum JM, Masters CL, Grzeschik KH, Multhaup G, Beyreuther K, Muller-Hill B. 1987. The precursor of Alzheimer's disease amyloid A4 protein resembles a cell-surface receptor. *Nature* **325:** 733–736.

Kim DY, Carey BW, Wang H, Ingano LA, Binshtok AM, Wertz MH, Pettingell WH, He P, Lee VM, Woolf CJ, et al. 2007. BACE1 regulates voltage-gated sodium channels and neuronal activity. *Nat Cell Biol* **9:** 755–764.

Kins S, Lauther N, Szodorai A, Beyreuther K. 2006. Subcellular trafficking of the amyloid precursor protein gene family and its pathogenic role in Alzheimer's disease. *Neurodegener Dis* **3:** 218–226.

Kojro E, Gimpl G, Lammich S, Marz W, Fahrenholz F. 2001. Low cholesterol stimulates the nonamyloidogenic pathway by its effect on the alpha-secretase ADAM 10. *Proc Natl Acad Sci* **98:** 5815–5820.

Koo EH, Squazzo SL. 1994. Evidence that production and release of amyloid beta-protein involves the endocytic pathway. *J Biol Chem* **269:** 17386–17389.

Koo EH, Sisodia SS, Archer DR, Martin LJ, Weidemann A, Beyreuther K, Fischer P, Masters CL, Price DL. 1990. Precursor of amyloid protein in Alzheimer disease undergoes fast anterograde axonal transport. *Proc Natl Acad Sci* **87:** 1561–1565.

Kuhn PH, Wang H, Dislich B, Colombo A, Zeitschel U, Ellwart JW, Kremmer E, Rossner S, Lichtenthaler SF. 2010. ADAM10 is the physiologically relevant, constitutive alpha-secretase of the amyloid precursor protein in primary neurons. *EMBO J* **29:** 3020–3032.

Lai A, Sisodia SS, Trowbridge IS. 1995. Characterization of sorting signals in the beta-amyloid precursor protein cytoplasmic domain. *J Biol Chem* **270:** 3565–3573.

Lakshmana MK, Yoon IS, Chen E, Bianchi E, Koo EH, Kang DE. 2009. Novel role of RanBP9 in BACE1 processing of amyloid precursor protein and amyloid beta peptide generation. *J Biol Chem* **284:** 11863–11872.

LaVoie MJ, Fraering PC, Ostaszewski BL, Ye W, Kimberly WT, Wolfe MS, Selkoe DJ. 2003. Assembly of the gamma-secretase complex involves early formation of an intermediate subcomplex of Aph-1 and nicastrin. *J Biol Chem* **278:** 37213–37222.

Lazarov O, Lee M, Peterson DA, Sisodia SS. 2002. Evidence that synaptically released beta-amyloid accumulates as extracellular deposits in the hippocampus of transgenic mice. *J Neurosci* **22:** 9785–9793.

Lazarov O, Morfini GA, Lee EB, Farah MH, Szodorai A, DeBoer SR, Koliatsos VE, Kins S, Lee VM, Wong PC, et al. 2005. Axonal transport, amyloid precursor protein, kinesin-1, and the processing apparatus: Revisited. *J Neurosci* **25:** 2386–2395.

Lee MS, Kao SC, Lemere CA, Xia W, Tseng HC, Zhou Y, Neve R, Ahlijanian MK, Tsai LH. 2003. APP processing is regulated by cytoplasmic phosphorylation. *J Cell Biol* **163:** 83–95.

Lesne S, Ali C, Gabriel C, Croci N, MacKenzie ET, Glabe CG, Plotkine M, Marchand-Verrecchia C, Vivien D, Buisson A. 2005. NMDA receptor activation inhibits alpha-secretase and promotes neuronal amyloid-beta production. *J Neurosci* **25:** 9367–9377.

Levy E, Carman MD, Fernandez-Madrid IJ, Power MD, Lieberburg I, van Duinen SG, Bots GT, Luyendijk W, Frangione B. 1990. Mutation of the Alzheimer's disease amyloid gene in hereditary cerebral hemorrhage, Dutch type. *Science* **248:** 1124–1126.

Lichtenthaler SF, Haass C, Steiner H. 2011. Regulated intramembrane proteolysis—lessons from amyloid precursor protein processing. *J Neurochem* **117:** 779–796.

Lin X, Koelsch G, Wu S, Downs D, Dashti A, Tang J. 2000. Human aspartic protease memapsin 2 cleaves the beta-secretase site of beta-amyloid precursor protein. *Proc Natl Acad Sci* **97:** 1456–1460.

Lo AC, Haass C, Wagner SL, Teplow DB, Sisodia SS. 1994. Metabolism of the "Swedish" amyloid precursor protein variant in Madin–Darby canine kidney cells. *J Biol Chem* **269:** 30966–30973.

Lu DC, Soriano S, Bredesen DE, Koo EH. 2003. Caspase cleavage of the amyloid precursor protein modulates amyloid beta-protein toxicity. *J Neurochem* **87:** 733–741.

Luo Y, Bolon B, Damore MA, Fitzpatrick D, Liu H, Zhang J, Yan Q, Vassar R, Citron M. 2003. BACE1 (beta-secretase) knockout mice do not acquire compensatory gene expression changes or develop neural lesions over time. *Neurobiol Dis* **14:** 81–88.

Mackenzie IR. Miller LA. 1994. Senile plaques in temporal lobe epilepsy. *Acta Neuropathol* **87:** 504–510.

Maltese WA, Wilson S, Tan Y, Suomensaari S, Sinha S, Barbour R, McConlogue L. 2001. Retention of the Alzheimer's amyloid precursor fragment C99 in the endoplasmic reticulum prevents formation of amyloid beta-peptide. *J Biol Chem* **276:** 20267–20279.

Marcinkiewicz M, Seidah NG. 2000. Coordinated expression of beta-amyloid precursor protein and the putative beta-secretase BACE and alpha-secretase ADAM10 in mouse and human brain. *J Neurochem* **75:** 2133–2143.

Marquez-Sterling NR, Lo ACY, Sisodia SS, Koo EH. 1997. Trafficking of cell-surface beta-amyloid precursor protein: Evidence that a sorting intermediate participates in synaptic vesicle recycling. *J Neurosci* **17:** 140–151.

Martin L, Fluhrer R, Haass C. 2009. Substrate requirements for SPPL2b-dependent regulated intramembrane proteolysis. *J Biol Chem* **284:** 5662–5670.

Matthews V, Schuster B, Schutze S, Bussmeyer I, Ludwig A, Hundhausen C, Sadowski T, Saftig P, Hartmann D, Kallen KJ, et al. 2003. Cellular cholesterol depletion triggers shedding of the human interleukin-6 receptor by ADAM10 and ADAM17 (TACE). *J Biol Chem* **278:** 38829–38839.

Merlos-Suarez A, Fernandez-Larrea J, Reddy P, Baselga J, Arribas J. 1998. Pro-tumor necrosis factor-alpha processing activity is tightly controlled by a component that does not affect notch processing. *J Biol Chem* **273:** 24955–24962.

Miller CC, McLoughlin DM, Lau KF, Tennant ME, Rogelj B. 2006. The X11 proteins, Abeta production and Alzheimer's disease. *Trends Neurosci* **29:** 280–285.

Morfini GA, Burns M, Binder LI, Kanaan NM, LaPointe N, Bosco DA, Brown RH Jr, Brown H, Tiwari A, Hayward L, et al. 2009. Axonal transport defects in neurodegenerative diseases. *J Neurosci* **29:** 12776–12786.

* Mucke L. Selkoe DJ. 2011. Neurotoxicity of amyloid β-protein: Synaptic and network dysfunction. *Cold Harbor Perspect Med* doi: 10.1101/cshperspect.a006338.

Mullan M, Crawford F, Axelman K, Houlden H, Lilius L, Winblad B, Lannfelt L. 1992. A pathogenic mutation for probable Alzheimer's disease in the APP gene at the N-terminus of beta-amyloid. *Nat Genet* **1:** 345–347.

Nilsberth C, Westlind-Danielsson A, Eckman CB, Condron MM, Axelman K, Forsell C, Stenh C, Luthman J, Teplow DB, Younkin SG, et al. 2001. The "Arctic" APP mutation (E693G) causes Alzheimer's disease by enhanced A-beta protofibril formation. *Nat Neurosci* **4:** 887–893.

Nitsch RM, Slack BE, Wurtman RJ, Growdon JH. 1992. Release of Alzheimer amyloid precursor derivatives stimulated by activation of muscarinic acetylcholine receptors. *Science* **258:** 304–307.

Nitsch RM, Farber SA, Growdon JH, Wurtman RJ. 1993. Release of amyloid beta-protein precursor derivatives by electrical depolarization of rat hippocampal slices. *Proc Natl Acad Sci* **90:** 5191–5193.

Nixon RA. 2007. Autophagy, amyloidogenesis and Alzheimer disease. *J Cell Sci* **120:** 4081–4091.

Offe K, Dodson SE, Shoemaker JT, Fritz JJ, Gearing M, Levey AI, Lah JJ. 2006. The lipoprotein receptor LR11 regulates amyloid beta production and amyloid precursor protein traffic in endosomal compartments. *J Neurosci* **26:** 1596–1603.

Pasternak SH, Callahan JW, Mahuran DJ. 2004. The role of the endosomal/lysosomal system in amyloid-beta production and the pathophysiology of Alzheimer's disease: Reexamining the spatial paradox from a lysosomal perspective. *J Alzheimers Dis* **6:** 53–65.

Pastorino L, Ikin AF, Nairn AC, Pursnani A, Buxbaum JD. 2002. The carboxyl-terminus of BACE contains a sorting signal that regulates BACE trafficking but not the formation of total A(beta). *Mol Cell Neurosci* **19:** 175–185.

Perez RG, Soriano S, Hayes JD, Ostaszewski B, Xia W, Selkoe DJ, Chen X, Stokin GB, Koo EH. 1999. Mutagenesis identifies new signals for beta-amyloid precursor protein endocytosis, turnover, and the generation of secreted fragments, including Abeta42. *J Biol Chem* **274:** 18851–18856.

Pietrzik CU, Busse T, Merriam DE, Weggen S, Koo EH. 2002. The cytoplasmic domain of the LDL receptor-related protein regulates multiple steps in APP processing. *EMBO J* **21:** 5691–5700.

Pietrzik CU, Yoon IS, Jaeger S, Busse T, Weggen S, Koo EH. 2004. FE65 constitutes the functional link between the low-density lipoprotein receptor-related protein and the amyloid precursor protein. *J Neurosci* **24:** 4259–4265.

Postina R, Schroeder A, Dewachter I, Bohl J, Schmitt U, Kojro E, Prinzen C, Endres K, Hiemke C, Blessing M, et al. 2004. A disintegrin-metalloproteinase prevents amyloid plaque formation and hippocampal defects in an Alzheimer disease mouse model. *J Clin Invest* **113:** 1456–1464.

Prokop S, Shirotani K, Edbauer D, Haass C, Steiner H. 2004. Requirement of PEN-2 for stabilization of the presenilin N-/C-terminal fragment heterodimer within the gamma-secretase complex. *J Biol Chem* **279:** 23255–23261.

Qi-Takahara Y, Morishima-Kawashima M, Tanimura Y, Dolios G, Hirotani N, Horikoshi Y, Kametani F, Maeda M, Saido TC, Wang R, et al. 2005. Longer forms of amyloid beta protein: Implications for the mechanism of intramembrane cleavage by gamma-secretase. *J Neurosci* **25:** 436–445.

Raichle ME, MacLeod AM, Snyder AZ, Powers WJ, Gusnard DA, Shulman GL. 2001. A default mode of brain function. *Proc Natl Acad Sci* **98:** 676–682.

Rajendran L, Schneider A, Schlechtingen G, Weidlich S, Ries J, Braxmeier T, Schwille P, Schulz JB, Schroeder C, Simons M, et al. 2008. Efficient inhibition of the Alzheimer's disease beta-secretase by membrane targeting. *Science* **320:** 520–523.

Rawson RB. 2002. Regulated intramembrane proteolysis: From the endoplasmic reticulum to the nucleus. *Essays Biochem* **38:** 155–168.

Rechards M, Xia W, Oorschot VM, Selkoe DJ, Klumperman J. 2003. Presenilin-1 exists in both pre- and post-Golgi compartments and recycles via COPI-coated membranes. *Traffic* **4:** 553–565.

Ribaut-Barassin C, Dupont JL, Haeberle AM, Bombarde G, Huber G, Moussaoui S, Mariani J, Bailly Y. 2003. Alzheimer's disease proteins in cerebellar and hippocampal synapses during postnatal development and aging of the rat. *Neuroscience* **120:** 405–423.

Riddell DR, Christie G, Hussain I, Dingwall C. 2001. Compartmentalization of beta-secretase (Asp2) into low-buoyant density, noncaveolar lipid rafts. *Curr Biol* **11:** 1288–1293.

Roberds SL, Anderson J, Basi G, Bienkowski MJ, Branstetter DG, Chen KS, Freedman SB, Frigon NL, Games D, Hu K, et al. 2001. BACE knockout mice are healthy despite lacking the primary beta-secretase activity in brain: Implications for Alzheimer's disease therapeutics. *Hum Mol Genet* **10:** 1317–1324.

Rogaeva E, Meng Y, Lee JH, Gu Y, Kawarai T, Zou F, Katayama T, Baldwin CT, Cheng R, Hasegawa H, et al. 2007. The neuronal sortilin-related receptor SORL1 is genetically associated with Alzheimer disease. *Nature Genet* **39:** 168 177.

Sano Y, Nakaya T, Pedrini S, Takeda S, Iijima-Ando K, Iijima K, Mathews PM, Itohara S, Gandy S, Suzuki T. 2006. Physiological mouse brain Abeta levels are not related to the phosphorylation state of threonine-668 of Alzheimer's APP. *PLoS One* **1:** e51.

Sastre M, Steiner H, Fuchs K, Capell A, Multhaup G, Condron MM, Teplow DB, Haass C. 2001. Presenilin-dependent gamma-secretase processing of beta-amyloid precursor protein at a site corresponding to the S3 cleavage of Notch. *EMBO Rep* **2:** 835–841.

* Schenk D, Basi GS, Pangalos MN. 2011. Treatment strategies targeting amyloid beta-protein. *Cold Spring Harb Perspect Med* doi: 10.1101/cshperspect.a006387.

Schmidt V, Sporbert A, Rohe M, Reimer T, Rehm A, Andersen OM, Willnow TE. 2007. SorLA/LR11 regulates processing of amyloid precursor protein via interaction with adaptors GGA and PACS-1. *J Biol Chem* **282:** 32956–32964.

Selkoe DJ. 2001. Alzheimer's disease: Genes, proteins, and therapy. *Physiol Rev* **81:** 741–766.

Selkoe D, Kopan R. 2003. Notch and presenilin: Regulated intramembrane proteolysis links development and degeneration. *Annu Rev Neurosci* **26:** 565–597.

Seubert P, Vigo-Pelfrey C, Esch F, Lee M, Dovey H, Davis D, Sinha S, Schlossmacher M, Whaley J, Swindlehurst C, et al. 1992. Isolation and quantification of soluble Alzheimer's beta-peptide from biological fluids. *Nature* **359:** 325–327.

Shah S, Lee SF, Tabuchi K, Hao YH, Yu C, LaPlant Q, Ball H, Dann CE 3rd, Sudhof T, Yu G. 2005. Nicastrin functions as a gamma-secretase-substrate receptor. *Cell* **122:** 435–447.

Sheng JG, Price DL, Koliatsos VE. 2002. Disruption of corticocortical connections ameliorates amyloid burden in terminal fields in a transgenic model of Abeta amyloidosis. *J Neurosci* **22:** 9794–9799.

Shoji M, Golde TE, Ghiso J, Cheung TT, Estus S, Shaffer LM, Cai XD, McKay DM, Tintner R, Frangione B, et al. 1992. Production of the Alzheimer amyloid beta protein by normal proteolytic processing. *Science* **258:** 126–129.

Simons M, Ikonen E, Tienari PJ, Cid AA, Monning U, Beyreuther K, Dotti CG. 1995. Intracellular routing of human amyloid protein precursor: Axonal delivery followed by transport to the dendrites. *J Neurosci Res* **41:** 121–128.

Sinha S, Anderson JP, Barbour R, Basi GS, Caccavello R, Davis D, Doan M, Dovey HF, Frigon N, Hong J, et al. 1999. Purification and cloning of amyloid precursor protein beta-secretase from human brain. *Nature* **402:** 537–540.

Sisodia SS. 1992. Beta-amyloid precursor protein cleavage by a membrane-bound protease. *Proc Natl Acad Sci* **89:** 6075–6079.

Sisodia SS, Koo EH, Beyreuther K, Unterbeck A, Price DL. 1990. Evidence that β-amyloid protein in Alzheimer's disease is not derived by normal processing. *Science* **248:** 492–495.

Sisodia SS, Koo EH, Hoffman PN, Perry G, Price DL. 1993. Identification and transport of full-length amyloid precursor proteins in rat peripheral nervous system. *J Neurosci* **13:** 3136–3142.

Snyder EM, Nong Y, Almeida CG, Paul S, Moran T, Choi EY, Nairn AC, Salter MW, Lombroso PJ, Gouras GK, Greengard P. 2005. Regulation of NMDA receptor trafficking by amyloid-beta. *Nat Neurosci* **8:** 1051–1058.

Stamer K, Vogel R, Thies E, Mandelkow E, Mandelkow EM. 2002. Tau blocks traffic of organelles, neurofilaments, and APP vesicles in neurons and enhances oxidative stress. *J Cell Biol* **156:** 1051–1063.

Steiner H, Fluhrer R, Haass C. 2008. Intramembrane proteolysis by gamma-secretase. *J Biol Chem* **283:** 29627–29631.

Suzuki N, Cheung TT, Cai XD, Odaka A, Otvos L Jr, Eckman C, Golde TE, Younkin SG. 1994. An increased percentage of long amyloid beta protein secreted by familial amyloid beta protein precursor (beta APP717) mutants. *Science* **264:** 1336–1340.

Szodorai A, Kuan YH, Hunzelmann S, Engel U, Sakane A, Sasaki T, Takai Y, Kirsch J, Muller U, Beyreuther K, et al. 2009. APP anterograde transport requires Rab3A GTPase activity for assembly of the transport vesicle. *J Neurosci* **29:** 14534–14544.

Takami M, Nagashima Y, Sano Y, Ishihara S, Morishima-Kawashima M, Funamoto S, Ihara Y. 2009. Gamma-secretase: Successive tripeptide and tetrapeptide release from the transmembrane domain of beta-carboxyl terminal fragment. *J Neurosci* **29:** 13042–13052.

Tampellini D, Capetillo-Zarate E, Dumont M, Huang Z, Yu F Lin MT, Gouras GK. 2010. Effects of synaptic modulation on beta-amyloid, synaptophysin, and memory performance in Alzheimer's disease transgenic mice. *J Neurosci* **30:** 14299–14304.

Tarassishin L, Yin YI, Bassit B, Li YM. 2004. Processing of Notch and amyloid precursor protein by gamma-secretase is spatially distinct. *Proc Natl Acad Sci* **101:** 17050–17055.

Tian Y, Bassit B, Chau D, Li YM. 2010. An APP inhibitory domain containing the Flemish mutation residue modulates gamma-secretase activity for Abeta production. *Nat Struct Mol Biol* **17:** 151–158.

Tienari PJ, De SB, Ikonen E, Simons M, Weidemann A, Czech C, Hartmann T, Ida N, Multhaup G, Masters CL, et al. 1996. The beta-amyloid domain is essential for axonal sorting of amyloid precursor protein. *Embo J* **15:** 5218–5229.

Trommsdorff M, Borg JP, Margolis B, Herz J. 1998. Interaction of cytosolic adaptor proteins with neuronal apolipoprotein E receptors and the amyloid precursor protein. *J Biol Chem* **273:** 33556–33560.

Ulery PG, Beers J, Mikhailenko I, Tanzi RE, Rebeck GW, Hyman BT, Strickland DK. 2000. Modulation of beta-amyloid precursor protein processing by the low density lipoprotein receptor-related protein (LRP). Evidence that LRP contributes to the pathogenesis of Alzheimer's disease. *J Biol Chem* **275:** 7410–7415.

Vassar R. 2004. BACE1: The beta-secretase enzyme in Alzheimer's disease. *J Mol Neurosci* **23:** 105–114.

Vassar R, Bennett BD, Babu-Khan S, Kahn S, Mendiaz EA, Denis P, Teplow DB, Ross S, Amarante P, Loeloff R, et al. 1999. Beta-secretase cleavage of Alzheimer's amyloid precursor protein by the transmembrane aspartic protease BACE. *Science* **286:** 735–741.

Vetrivel KS, Meckler X, Chen Y, Nguyen PD, Seidah NG, Vassar R, Wong PC, Fukata M, Kounnas MZ, Thinakaran G. 2009. Alzheimer disease Abeta production in the absence of S-palmitoylation-dependent targeting of BACE1 to lipid rafts. *J Biol Chem* **284:** 3793–3803.

von Rotz RC, Kohli BM, Bosset J, Meier M, Suzuki T, Nitsch RM, Konietzko U. 2004. The APP intracellular domain forms nuclear multiprotein complexes and regulates the transcription of its own precursor. *J Cell Sci* **117:** 4435–4448.

Wahle T, Prager K, Raffler N, Haass C, Famulok M, Walter J. 2005. GGA proteins regulate retrograde transport of BACE1 from endosomes to the trans-Golgi network. *Mol Cell Neurosci* **29:** 453–461.

Wahle T, Thal DR, Sastre M, Rentmeister A, Bogdanovic N, Famulok M, Heneka MT, Walter J. 2006. GGA1 is expressed in the human brain and affects the generation of amyloid beta-peptide. *J Neurosci* **26:** 12838–12846.

Walter J, Fluhrer R, Hartung B, Willem M, Kaether C, Capell A, Lammich S, Multhaup G, Haass C. 2001. Phosphorylation regulates intracellular trafficking of beta-secretase. *J Biol Chem* **276:** 14634–14641.

Wang R, Meschia JF, Cotter RJ, Sisodia SS. 1991. Secretion of the β/A4 amyloid precursor protein. Identification of a cleavage site in cultured mammalian cells. *J Biol Chem* **266:** 16960–16964.

Wei W, Nguyen LN, Kessels HW, Hagiwara H, Sisodia S, Malinow R. 2010. Amyloid beta from axons and dendrites reduces local spine number and plasticity. *Nat Neurosci* **13:** 190–196.

Weidemann A, Konig G, Bunke D, Fischer P, Salbaum JM, Masters CL, Beyreuther K. 1989. Identification, biogenesis, and localization of precursors of Alzheimer's disease A4 amyloid protein. *Cell* **57:** 115–126.

Weidemann A, Paliga K, U, D., Reinhard FB, Schuckert O, Evin G, Masters CL. 1999. Proteolytic processing of the Alzheimer's disease amyloid precursor protein within its cytoplasmic domain by caspase-like proteases. *J Biol Chem* **274:** 5823–5829.

Weidemann A, Eggert S, Reinhard FB, Vogel M, Paliga K, Baier G, Masters CL, Beyreuther K, Evin G. 2002. A novel epsilon-cleavage within the transmembrane domain of the Alzheimer amyloid precursor protein demonstrates homology with Notch processing. *Biochemistry* **41:** 2825–2835.

Weskamp G, Cai H, Brodie TA, Higashyama S, Manova K, Ludwig T, Blobel CP. 2002. Mice lacking the metalloprotease-disintegrin MDC9 (ADAM9) have no evident major abnormalities during development or adult life. *Mol Cell Biol* **22:** 1537–1544.

Wild-Bode C, Fellerer K, Kugler J, Haass C, Capell A. 2006. A basolateral sorting signal directs ADAM10 to adherens junctions and is required for its function in cell migration. *J Biol Chem* **281:** 23824–23829.

Willem M, Garratt AN, Novak B, Citron M, Kaufmann S, Rittger A, DeStrooper B, Saftig P, Birchmeier C, Haass C. 2006. Control of peripheral nerve myelination by the beta-secretase BACE1. *Science* **314:** 664–666.

Willem M, Lammich S, Haass C. 2009. Function, regulation and therapeutic properties of beta-secretase (BACE1). *Semin Cell Dev Biol* **20:** 175–182.

Wolfe MS, Xia W, Ostaszewski BL, Diehl TS, Kimberly WT, Selkoe DJ. 1999. Two transmembrane aspartates in presenilin-1 required for presenilin endoproteolysis and gamma-secretase activity. *Nature* **398:** 513–517.

Yamazaki T, Selkoe DJ, Koo EH. 1995. Trafficking of cell surface beta-amyloid precursor protein: Retrograde and transcytotic transport in cultured neurons. *J Cell Biol* **129:** 431–442.

Yan R, Bienkowski MJ, Shuck ME, Miao H, Tory MC, Pauley AM, Brashier JR, Stratman NC, Mathews WR, Buhl AE, et al. 1999. Membrane-anchored aspartyl protease with Alzheimer's disease beta-secretase activity. *Nature* **402:** 533–537.

Yu G, Nishimura M, Arawaka S, Levitan D, Zhang L, Tandon A, Song YQ, Rogaeva E, Chen F, Kawarai T, et al. 2000. Nicastrin modulates presenilin-mediated notch/glp-1 signal transduction and betaAPP processing. *Nature* **407:** 48–54.

Physiological Functions of APP Family Proteins

Ulrike C. Müller[1] and Hui Zheng[2]

[1]Institute for Pharmacy and Molecular Biotechnology, University of Heidelberg, D-69120 Heidelberg, Germany

[2]Huffington Center on Aging and Departments of Molecular & Human Genetics, Molecular & Cellular Biology and Neuroscience, Baylor College of Medicine, Houston, Texas 77030

Correspondence: u.mueller@urz.uni-hd.de; huiz@bcm.edu

Biochemical and genetic evidence establishes a central role of the amyloid precursor protein (APP) in Alzheimer disease (AD) pathogenesis. Biochemically, deposition of the β-amyloid (Aβ) peptides produced from proteolytic processing of APP forms the defining pathological hallmark of AD; genetically, both point mutations and duplications of wild-type APP are linked to a subset of early onset of familial AD (FAD) and cerebral amyloid angiopathy. As such, the biological functions of APP and its processing products have been the subject of intense investigation, and the past 20+ years of research have met with both excitement and challenges. This article will review the current understanding of the physiological functions of APP in the context of APP family members.

Synaptic dysfunction, cognitive decline, and plaque deposition of the β-amyloid peptide Aβ, derived from the β-amyloid precursor protein APP, are hallmark features of Alzheimer disease (AD). Since the molecular cloning of APP, more than 20 years ago (Goldgaber et al. 1987; Kang et al. 1987; Tanzi et al. 1987), a large body of biochemical and genetic evidence has accumulated that identified Aβ as a central trigger for AD pathogenesis. Despite this, the physiological role of APP and the question of whether a loss of its functions contributes to AD are still unclear. The secretases involved in APP processing and Aβ generation have been cloned (see De Strooper et al. 2011; Haass et al. 2011) and have since become major therapeutic targets. Understanding the physiological function of APP is also of immediate relevance for AD pathogenesis. As Aβ is generated as part of normal APP processing (Haass et al. 1992), deregulation of Aβ production (either during pathogenesis or as a consequence of secretase inhibitors) is expected to simultaneously affect other APP processing products and may thus compromise physiologically important signaling pathways. Two major obstacles complicate the analysis of functions of APP in vivo: (1) APP is subject to complex proteolytical processing that generates several polypeptides each of which likely performs specific functions, and (2) APP is part of a gene family with partially overlapping functions.

CELL BIOLOGY AND EXPRESSION

APP Processing

APP is an integral type I transmembrane protein with a single transmembrane domain, a large extracellular ectodomain, and a short cytoplasmic tail (Fig. 1). Processing is initiated either by cleavage of APP by α-secretase within the Aβ region, or by cleavage by β-secretase (BACE) at the amino terminus of Aβ, leading to the secretion of large soluble ectodomains, termed APPsα and APPsβ, respectively. Subsequent processing of the carboxy-terminal fragments (CTFβ or CTFα) by γ-secretase results in the production of Aβ, p3, and the APP intracellular domain (AICD). More recently, a novel amino-terminal fragment (N-APP$_{286}$) derived from APPsβ was identified as a ligand for death receptor 6 (DR6), a member of the TNFR gene family (Nikolaev et al. 2009). Whereas in fibroblasts and nonneuronal cell lines (e.g., HEK293 cells) α-secretase processing is the dominant pathway, primary neuronal cultures express high levels of BACE and thus generate considerable amounts of APPsβ and Aβ (Simons et al. 1996; Kuhn

et al. 2010). In adult mouse brain, secreted total APPs constitutes at least 50% of all APP isoforms and in vivo studies using cycloheximide injections revealed a half-life of 4–5 h for both APPsα and APPsβ, whereas APP-FL is turned over much more rapidly (half-life of ca. 1 h) (Morales-Corraliza et al. 2009).

APP Gene Family and Structure

APP is a member of an evolutionary conserved gene family including APL-1 in *Caenorhabditis elegans* (Daigle and Li 1993), APPL in *Drosophila* (Rosen et al. 1989; Luo et al. 1990), appa and appb in zebrafish (Musa et al. 2001), and in mammals besides APP the two amyloid precursor-like proteins, APLP1 and APLP2 (Wasco et al. 1992, 1993; Slunt et al. 1994). APP family proteins share conserved regions within the ectodomain, in particular the E1 and E2 domains and the intracellular tail that shows the largest sequence identity (Fig. 1). Interestingly, the extracellular juxtamembrane regions are highly divergent with the Aβ sequence being unique for APP. The E1 domain can be further subdivided into a heparin-binding/growth

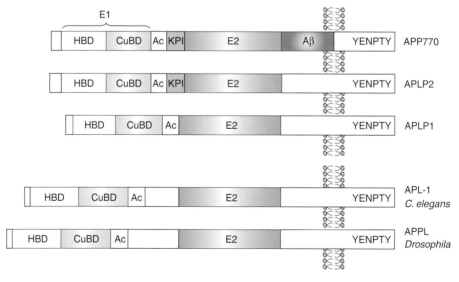

Figure 1. Schematic overview of domain structure of APP family proteins. All APP family members share conserved E1 and E2 extracellular domains, an acidic domain (Ac) and the YENPTY motif in the carboxyl terminus. Note that Aβ is unique for APP. HBD, Heparin binding domain; CuBD, Copper binding domain; KPI, Kunitz-type protease inhibitor domain.

factor-like domain and a metal (copper and zinc) binding domain. The E1 domain is followed by an acidic region and a Kunitz-type protease inhibitor (KPI) domain (that is subject to alternative splicing in both APP and APLP2). The E2 region contains a second heparin binding domain and a RERMS motif implicated in trophic functions (Ninomiya et al. 1993; Roch et al. 1994). APP family proteins are posttranslationally modified including N- and O-glycosylation, sialylation, and CS GAG modification of the ectodomain and are phosphorylated at multiple sites within the intracellular carboxy-terminal domain (reviewed in Suzuki and Nakaya 2008; Jacobsen and Iverfeldt 2009). Crystal structures of several subdomains (reviewed in Reinhard et al. 2005; Gralle and Ferreira 2007), including the recently determined complete E1 structure (Dahms et al. 2010) and AICD bound to the adaptor protein Fe65 are available (Radzimanowski et al. 2010). Membrane bound APP/APLP holoproteins resemble cell surface receptors and have been shown to bind to extracellular matrix components (see below), but also interact with cell surface proteins including Alcadein (Araki et al. 2003), F-spondin (Ho and Südhof 2004), Reelin (Hoe et al. 2009b), LRP1 (Pietrzik et al. 2004), sorL1/LR11 (Schmidt et al. 2007), Nogo-66 receptor (Park et al. 2006), Notch2 (Chen et al. 2006), and Netrin (Lourenco et al. 2009). Although several of these interactions regulate APP processing, the physiological relevance of these interactions is poorly understood. Interaction screens have led to the identification of multiple intracellular binding partners (reviewed in Jacobsen and Iverfeldt 2009). Notably, the YENPTY motif that is conserved from *C. elegans* to mammalian APP/APLPs, confers clathrin mediated endocytosis, modulates Aβ generation (Perez et al. 1999; Ring et al. 2007), and binds several kinases, as well as adaptor proteins including mDab1, JIP, Shc, Grb2, Numb, X11/mint family, and Fe65 family proteins. Although in vitro studies have shown that these interactions may not only modulate APP processing but may also mediate cell signaling, the in vivo relevance is only starting to be revealed.

Although APLP1 and APLP2 lack the Aβ region they are similarly processed. Both APLPs undergo ectodoamin shedding and soluble APLPs have been detected in conditioned medium of transfected cell lines or human cerebrospinal fluid (Slunt et al. 1994; Webster et al. 1995; Paliga et al. 1997). Likewise, p3/Aβ-like fragments (Eggert et al. 2004; Minogue et al. 2009), as well as APLP1 and APLP2 intracellular fragments (termed ALIDs) are generated in a γ-secretase dependent manner (Scheinfeld et al. 2002; Walsh et al. 2003). Whereas there has been robust evidence indicating that APLP2 is processed by α- and β-secretase (Eggert et al. 2004; Pastorino et al. 2004; Endres et al. 2005), APLP1 shedding appeared to be independent of BACE activity as it was not affected by BACE inhibitors (Eggert et al. 2004; Minogue et al. 2009). A recent study using BACE-KO and overexpressing mice showed, however, that BACE deficiency substantially reduces brain APLP1s levels and that ICDs of APP family members are released in the absence of BACE (Frigerio et al. 2010).

Expression, Subcellular Localization, and Axonal Transport

APP and APLP2 are expressed ubiquitously, with particularly high expression in neurons, in largely overlapping patterns during embryonic development and in adult tissue (Slunt et al. 1994; Lorent et al. 1995; Thinakaran et al. 1995). In contrast, APLP1 is found primarily in the nervous system (Lorent et al. 1995). Regarding their subcellular localization, APP/APLPs are found both in somata and dendrites as well as in axons (Yamazaki et al. 1995; Back et al. 2007; Hoe et al. 2009a). APP/APLP expression is up-regulated during neuronal maturation and differentiation, undergoes rapid anterograde transport, and is targeted in vesicles distinct from synaptophysin transport vesicles to synaptic sites (Koo et al. 1990; Sisodia et al. 1993; Kaether et al. 2000; Szodorai et al. 2009). The initial hypothesis that APP anchors these vesicles via its carboxyl terminus to kinesin (Kamal et al. 2001), has been broadly questioned (Tienari et al. 1996; Lazarov et al. 2005;

Back et al. 2007). Using time-lapse microscopy, Szodorai recently showed unaltered velocity of APPΔCT-GFP transport and a requirement for Rab3A GTPase activity for vesicle assembly (Szodorai et al. 2009).

IN VITRO AND EX VIVO STUDIES OF APP

Cell and Synaptic Adhesion

Investigations of conserved domains support an adhesion property for all members of the APP family. The extracellular sequence of APP has been found to interact with various extracellular matrix components, such as heparin (Clarris et al. 1997; Mok et al. 1997), collagen type I (Beher et al. 1996), and laminin (Kibbey et al. 1993), indicating a role of APP in cell-matrix adhesion. Structural and functional studies also implicate a role of the APP extracellular domains in facilitating cell–cell adhesion through transcellular interactions. Of interest, X-ray analysis revealed that the E2 domain of APP could form antiparallel dimers (Wang and Ha 2004). Both Dahms et al. (2010) and Gralle et al. (2006) reported that heparin binding to the extracellular E1 or E2 domain induces APP/APP dimerization. Cell culture studies revealed that APP family members form homo- or heterotypic *cis*-dimers, mainly via the E1 domain and the GxxxG motif in the transmembrane domain (Kaden et al. 2008), and that *cis*-dimerization modulates γ-secretase cleavage (Richter et al. 2010). *Trans*-dimerization of APP family members can promote cell–cell adhesion (Soba et al. 2005). Using a primary neuron/HEK293 mixed culture assay, Wang et al. (2009) reported that transcellular APP/APP interaction induces presynaptic specializations in cocultured neurons. These studies identify APP proteins as a novel class of synaptic adhesion molecules (SAM) with shared biochemical properties as neurexins (NX)/neuroligins (NL), SynCAMs, and leucine-rich repeat transmembrane neuronal proteins (LRRTM) (Scheiffele et al. 2000; Biederer et al. 2002; Graf et al. 2004; Sara et al. 2005; Fogel et al. 2007; Linhoff et al. 2009). Like NX/NL and SynCAM-mediated synaptic adhesion in which extracellular sequences engage transsynaptic interactions and the intracellular domains recruit pre- or postsynaptic complexes (reviewed in Dalva et al. 2007), both the extracellular and intracellular domains of APP are required to mediate the synaptogenic activity. Consistent with Soba et al. (2005), the E1 domain plays a more active role in synaptic adhesion. Interestingly, the highly conserved GYENPTY sequence of the APP intracellular domain could form a tripartite complex with Munc 18 interacting protein (Mint/X11) and calcium/calmodulin-dependent serine protein kinase (CASK) similar to that of neurexin and SynCAM (Hata et al. 1996; Biederer and Südhof 2000; Biederer et al. 2002), and the SynCAM carboxy-terminal sequence could functionally replace the corresponding APP domain in the coculture assay (Wang et al. 2009), suggesting that the Mint/CASK complexes may be the common mediators for the different classes of synaptic adhesion proteins. Thus, the precise role of APP-mediated synaptic adhesion in central synapses, whether it involves interaction with other SAMs, and the relationship between APP-mediated synaptogenesis and synaptic dysfunction occurring in AD are interesting questions that warrant further investigation.

Besides a direct role of APP/APP interaction in cell and synaptic adhesion, APP has been shown to colocalize with integrins on the surface of axons and at the sites of adhesion (Storey et al. 1996; Yamazaki et al. 1997; Young-Pearse et al. 2008). It has also been reported to interact with other cell adhesion molecules including NCAM (Ashley et al. 2005), NgCAM (Osterfield et al. 2008), and TAG 1 (Ma et al. 2008). As such, APP may play a modulatory role through interacting with these cell adhesion molecules.

Neural and Synapto-Trophic Functions

A large body of evidence supports a trophic function of APP in neurons and synapses. Consistent with its expression pattern, deletion or reduction of APP is associated with impaired neuronal viability in vitro and reduced synaptic activity in vivo (Allinquant et al. 1995; Perez et al. 1997; Hérard et al. 2006). Hippocampal neurons deficient for APP (or APLPs) show initially reduced neurite outgrowth, whereas, after prolonged culture axons are elongated and neurite branching is reduced (Perez et al. 1997; Young-Pearse et al. 2008). However, it should be noted that studies using neuronal cultures derived from various APP/APLP1/APLP2 knockout combinations or obtained by differentiation of embryonic stem cells lacking APP family members failed to detect a requirement of APP proteins in either neuronal differentiation or survival (Heber et al. 2000; Bergmans et al. 2010).

The trophic activity of APP can be mediated by the full-length protein and likely involves the APP adhesion properties discussed above. In particular, binding of APP to extracellular proteoglycans has been suggested to play a role in inducing neurite outgrowth, and a peptide homologous to the APP heparin-binding domain blocked this effect (Small et al. 1994, 1999). Qiu et al. found that when APP-transfected CHO cells were used as a substrate for the growth of primary rat hippocampal neurons, increased surface APP expression stimulated short-term neuronal adhesion and longer-term neurite outgrowth (Qiu et al. 1995). Nevertheless, ample literature points to a potent role of the α-secretase processed soluble fragment (APPsα) in the growth promoting and neurotrophic activities. One of the earliest indications came from the observation that secreted APPs, through the "RERMS" motif in the E2 domain, promoted fibroblast proliferation (Saitoh et al. 1989; Ninomiya et al. 1993a; Jin et al. 1994). Moderate overexpression of APP in transgenic mice, infusion of APPsα or the RERMS pentapeptide into the ventricle, or an indirect increase of APPsα levels because of overexpression of α-secretase, has been shown to increase synaptic density (Mucke et al. 1994; Roch et al. 1994; Meziane et al. 1998; Bell et al. 2008). Moreover, gain- or loss-of-function studies with either intraventricular APPsα infusion, down-regulation by antibody infusion or pharmacological inhibition of α-secretase coherently showed a function for APPsα in spatial memory and for LTP (Turner et al. 2003; Taylor et al. 2008).

Caille et al. provided evidence that APPsα and APLP2s act as cofactors for epidermal growth factor (EGF) to stimulate the proliferation of neurosphere cultures in vitro and neural stem cells in the subventricular zone of adult rodent brain in vivo (Caille et al. 2004). Gakhar-Koppole et al. (2008) and Rohe et al. (2008) also reported that APPs stimulated neurogenesis and neurite outgrowth, but suggested that it is mediated through enhanced ERK phosphorylation and may be dependent on membrane-bound APP. Han et al. (2005) offered yet a different mechanism that the growth promoting property is mediated by the ability of APPsα to down-regulate CDK5 and inhibit τ hyperphosphorylation. Of direct physiological relevance, growth and neuronal phenotypes reported in *APP* deficient mice were shown to be fully restored by expressing only APPsα (Ring et al. 2007), and the lethality of the *C. elegans apl-1* null mutant can be rescued by expressing only the APL-1 extracellular domain (Hornsten et al. 2007; Wiese et al. 2010).

Axon Pruning and Degeneration

APPsα has shown synaptotrophic and neuroprotective functions, whereas APPsβ was reported to be much less active or may even be toxic (reviewed in Turner et al. 2003). Recently, employing organotypic slice cultures, Copanaki et al. showed that APPsα (and not APPsβ) antagonizes dendritic degeneration and neuron death triggered by proteasomal stress (Copanaki et al. 2010). The most striking difference came from the study of Nikolaev et al. (2009), which reported that soluble APPsβ, but not APPsα, undergoes further cleavage to produce an amino-terminal ~35 kDa APP derivative (N-APP), which in turn binds to the death receptor DR6 and mediates axon pruning and degeneration under trophic withdrawal conditions. The investigators attempted to link this pathway to both axonal pruning during normal development and axon- and neurodegeneration in AD. The APPsβ isoform specific cleavage and the differential, or opposite activities between APPsα and APPsβ, are intriguing as there is only 17 amino acids differences between the two isoforms.

Intracellular Signaling

Besides the γ-secretase cleavage that yields Aβ40 and Aβ42, PS-dependent proteolysis also occurs at the ε-site of the membrane-intracellular boundary to generate AICD (Sastre et al. 2001; Weidemann et al. 2002; Zhao et al. 2005). This cleavage is highly reminiscent of the PS-mediated release of the Notch intracellular domain (NICD) obligatory for Notch signaling (reviewed in Selkoe and Kopan 2003). Accordingly, AICD has been shown to translocate to the nucleus (Cupers et al. 2001; Gao and Pimplikar 2001; Kimberly et al. 2001). AICD is labile but can be stabilized by Fe65 (Kimberly et al. 2001). Using a heterologous reporter system, AICD was shown to form a transcriptionally active complex with Fe65 and the chromatin-remodeling factor Tip60 (Cao and Südhof 2001; Gao and Pimplikar 2001). However, subsequent analyses painted a more complex picture: (1) Follow-up studies by Cao et al. provided a modified model, whereby Fe65 is first recruited to the membrane-anchored APP where it is activated through an unknown mechanism. γ-secretase cleavage then releases Fe65 together with AICD, thereby allowing Fe65 to enter the nucleus and to interact with Tip60 (Cao and Südhof 2004); (2) Hass and Yankner revealed that PS-dependent AICD production is not required for the APP signaling activity as it proceeds normally in PS null cells and on PS inhibitor treatment (Hass and Yankner 2005). Instead, the investigators provided an alternative pathway involving Tip60 phosphorylation; (3) a later report documented that the proposed signaling activity is, in fact, executed by Fe65 independently of APP (Yang et al. 2006). Last, the link of Fe65 to chromatin remodeling instead of transcription suggests that APP may not act on specific genes, but rather modulates the overall transcriptional state of a cell (Giliberto et al. 2008).

Regardless of the molecular mechanisms, a *trans*-activating role of the APP/Fe65/Tip60 complex has been consistently documented, at least in overexpression systems using artificial reporter constructs. Accordingly, effort has been taken to identify the downstream targets, which reportedly include KAI (Baek et al. 2002), GSK3β (Kim et al. 2003; Ryan and Pimplikar 2005), neprilysin (Pardossi-Piquard et al. 2005), EGFR (Zhang et al. 2007), p53 (Checler et al. 2007), LRP (Liu et al. 2007), APP itself (von Rotz et al. 2004), and genes involved in calcium regulation (Leissring et al. 2002) and cytoskeletal dynamics (Müller et al. 2007). However, the validity of these proposed targets have been either questioned or disputed (Hebert et al. 2006; Yang et al. 2006; Chen and Selkoe 2007; Repetto et al. 2007; Giliberto et al. 2008; Tamboli et al. 2008; Waldron et al. 2008; Aydin et al. 2011). Overall, as attractive as the APP/AICD signaling model is, and regardless of the intense effort devoted to this topic in the past 10 years, neither the molecular pathways nor the downstream targets have been unambiguously established.

Apoptosis

Interestingly, AICD has been shown to be further cleaved by caspases at amino acid 664 of APP (695 numbering) to release two smaller fragments, Jcasp and C31; the latter contains the last 31 amino acids of APP and has been proposed to mediate cytoxicity in a full-length APP dependent manner (Bertrand et al. 2001; Lu et al. 2003; Park et al. 2009). In support of a functional role of this pathway, neuronal cultures generated from AICD transgenic mice are found to be more susceptible to toxic stimuli (Giliberto et al. 2008), and impaired synaptic plasticity and learning and memory seen in APP transgenic models were corrected in a mouse line in which the caspase site was mutated despite the presence of abundant amyloid pathology (Galvan et al. 2006). However, a more recent publication challenged these findings (Harris et al. 2010), and the physiological significance of this cleavage event thus requires further investigation.

IN VIVO LOSS-OF-FUNCTION STUDIES OF APP FAMILY PROTEINS

C. elegans and Drosophila

Drosophila deficient for the single APPL gene are viable, show a defect in fast phototaxis (Luo et al. 1992), and reduced synaptic bouton numbers at the neuromuscular junction NMJ. This activity involves a complex between APPL, the cell adhesion molecule fasciclin and *Drosophila* Mint/X11 (Torroja et al. 1999; Ashley et al. 2005). Knockout of the *C. elegans* ortholog APL-1, which is expressed in multiple tissue including neurons and muscle, disrupts molting and morphogenesis and results in laval lethality. Interestingly, this lethality could be rescued by neuronal expression of only the extracellular domain of APL-1, suggesting a key physiological role for this APPsα related fragment (Hornsten et al. 2007).

APP/APLP Single Knockout Mice

Three APP mouse mutants, one carrying a hypomorphic mutation of APP (APPΔ) (Müller et al. 1994) and two with complete deficiencies of APP (Zheng et al. 1995; Li et al. 1996) have been generated and revealed comparable phenotypes (Anliker and Müller 2006). APP-KO mice are viable and fertile, showing reduced body weight (about 15%–20% smaller) and brain weight (about 10% less) that was associated with reduced size of forebrain commissures and agenesis of the corpus callosum, consistent with a role of APP for neurite outgrowth and/or axonal pathfinding (Zheng et al. 1995; Magara et al. 1999). APP-KO mice also showed increased brain levels of copper (White et al. 1999), cholesterol and sphingolipid (Grimm et al. 2005). In addition, APP-KO animals showed hypersensitivity to kainate-induced seizures (Steinbach et al. 1998), suggesting a role of APP for neuronal excitation/inhibition balance. Behavioral studies revealed reduced locomotor and exploratory activity, altered circadian activity (Müller et al. 1994; Zheng et al. 1995; Ring et al. 2007), and a deficit in grip strength (Zheng et al. 1995; Ring et al. 2007), indicating compromised neuronal or muscular function (see also NMJ phenotype of double knockouts below). In the Morris water maze, APP-KO mice show impairments, both in learning and spatial memory, that are associated with a defect in long-term potentiation (LTP) (Dawson et al. 1999; Phinney et al. 1999; Seabrook et al. 1999; Ring et al. 2007). However, these impairments are not caused by a gross loss of neurons or synapses, as stereological quantification revealed normal neuron and synaptic bouton counts in the hippocampus of aged APP null mice (Phinney et al. 1999). Surprisingly, a recent study showed that APP deficiency leads to an increase in spine density in apical dendrites of cortical (layers 3 and 5) neurons (Bittner et al. 2009). The same group had previously reported an increase in synapse density in low-density cultures of self-innervating (autaptic) hippocampal neurons (Priller et al. 2006), but normal synaptic density in adult APP-KO mice (Priller et al. 2006). Thus, adaptive mechanisms (e.g., activity-dependent synaptic elimination) likely counteract early developmental changes. It remains to be seen whether alterations in spine density are also present in other brain areas of APP family KOs, which signaling pathways are involved, and how this may relate to functional changes.

Although basal glutamatergic synaptic transmission and paired pulse facilitation was unaffected in hippocampal slice recordings of APP-KO mice, a deficit in paired pulse depression of GABAergic IPSCs may contribute to the LTP defect of APP-KO mice (Seabrook et al. 1999). This may involve, as hypothesized (Seabrook et al. 1999), a reduction in feedback suppression mediated by presynaptic $GABA_B$ autoreceptors (but see below Yang et al. 2009). Although the molecular mechanisms of these alterations remain to be determined, these studies indicate that defects in Ca^{2+}-handling, synaptic plasticity and/or neuronal network properties, rather than gross structural changes, cause functional impairments of APP knockout mice. Indeed, recently it was shown that APP is involved in the regulation of L-type Ca channel LTCCs level (Yang et al. 2009). APP-KO mice showed increased levels of $Ca_V1.2$ channels in the striatum that lead to alterations in GABAergic short term plasticity in striatal and hippocampal neurons, such as reduced GABAergic paired pulse inhibition and increased GABAergic posttetanic potentiation (Yang et al. 2009). Moreover, there is recent evidence from overexpression and APP knockdown studies in hippocampal neurons indicating an Aβ independent role of APP for the regulation of Ca^{2+}-oscillations (Santos et al. 2009).

Combined Knockouts of APP Family Members

To test whether APLPs may functionally compensate for APP deficiency, mice lacking individual or all possible combinations of APP family proteins have been generated (reviewed in Anliker and Müller 2006; Zheng and Koo 2006). APLP1-KO mice revealed a somatic growth deficit as the only abnormality (Heber et al. 2000a), whereas, to date, no abnormalities have been found for APLP2-KO mice (von Koch et al. 1997). It should be kept in mind, however, that APLP deficient mice have not been examined in comparable detail as APP-KOs. In contrast to the subtle phenotypes of single mutants, double knockout mice (DKO) carrying APLP2/APLP1 and APLP2/APP-deficiencies proved lethal shortly after birth (von Koch et al. 1997; Heber et al. 2000). Surprisingly, APLP1/APP-deficient mice turned out to be viable, fertile, and without any additional abnormalities (Heber et al. 2000). These data indicated redundancy between APLP2 and both other family members, and corroborate a key physiological role for APLP2. None of the lethal double mutants, however, displayed obvious histopathological abnormalities (examined at the light microscopic level) in the brain. So far, the postnatal lethality of the APP/APLP2-DKO precluded the analysis of APP/APLP2 mediated functions in the postnatal and adult nervous system. However, organotypic hippocampal slice cultures can be studied in case of early postnatal lethality. Of note, using this technique, APP/APLP2-DKO mutants revealed defects in basal glutamatergic synaptic transmission that were absent in single mutants (Schrenk-Siemens et al. 2008). Thus, a more complete picture of APP/APLP function in the CNS will await the generation of brain specific conditional mutants.

In the peripheral nervous system, APP and APLP2 play a redundant and essential role for neuromuscular synapse formation and function, as diaphragm preparations from newborn APP/APLP2-DKO mice show excessive nerve growth, a widened endplate pattern, reduced apposition of pre- and postsynaptic components, and severely impaired (spontaneous and evoked) neurotransmission (Wang et al. 2005). Moreover, submandibular ganglia of APP/APLP2-DKO mice showed a reduction in active zone size, synaptic vesicle density, and number of docked vesicles (Yang et al. 2005) pointing to primarily presynaptic defects (but see conditional mutants). Thus, impaired function of the NMJ likely causes early postnatal lethality of combined mutants and defects in grip strength in APP single KOs. Indeed, subsequent analysis of neuromuscular transmission of APP-KO mice showed reduced paired pulse facilitation that was associated with an increase in asynchronous presynaptic transmitter release mediated by N- and L-type Ca^{2+} channels (Yang et al. 2007).

Triple KO mice lacking all three APP family members die shortly after birth. Unlike the DKO mutants, which did not display histological alterations in the brain, 80% of all triple knockouts showed cranial abnormalities (Herms et al. 2004). The majority of animals showed focal dysplasia resembling human type II lissencephaly and a partial loss of cortical Cajal-Retzius cells (Herms et al. 2004). Within affected areas, neuronal cells from the cortical plate migrated beyond their normal positions and protruded into the marginal zone and the subarachnoid space, indicating a critical role for APP family members in neuronal adhesion and/or positioning (Herms et al. 2004). Interestingly, a very similar phenotype was detected in mice lacking the APP interactors Fe65 and Fe65L1 (Guénette et al. 2006). These data suggest that APP family proteins may mediate some of their function(s) via an APP/Fe65 signaling complex. A role of APP family members in neuronal positioning/migration is further supported by acute in utero knockdown of APP (Young-Pearse et al. 2007) in rats using shRNA electroporation. In summary, these data corroborate an essential role of the APP gene family for normal brain development.

APP CONDITIONAL KNOCKOUT

Germline deletion of APP and APLP2 in mice results in a general impairment in pre- and post-synaptic patterning and a specific defect in pre-synaptic targeting of CHT (Wang et al. 2005, 2007). Conditional alleles of APP and APLP2 have been generated (Wang et al. 2009; Mallm et al. 2010). Consistent with the synaptic adhesion property of APP, deletion of APP (on a global APLP2-KO background) in either presynaptic motor neurons or in postsynaptic muscle was shown to lead to similar neuromuscular synapse defects (Wang et al. 2009). Interestingly, postsynaptic APP expression is required to mediate presynaptic CHT targeting and synaptic transmission, suggesting that transsynaptic APP/APP interaction is necessary in recruiting the presynaptic APP/CHT complex and cholinergic synaptic function. Whether APP modulates other synaptic processes through similar recruitment of synaptic proteins is an interesting question requiring further investigation.

In Vivo Defined Genetic Modifications of APP Proteins

The above knockout animals provide important information concerning the physiological functions of APP proteins, which may be executed either as a full-length protein or as various processing products. The creation of knockin alleles expressing defined proteolytic fragments of APP offers a powerful system to delineate the APP functional domains in vivo. In this regard, knockin mice that express α- or β-secretase processed soluble APP (APPsα or APPsβ) or membrane anchored APP containing mutations of the highly conserved carboxy-terminal sequences have been generated. These alleles are summarized in Figure 2 and will be discussed in this section.

APPsα and APPsβ Knockin

Ring et al. (2007) created a strain of APPsα knockin mice by introducing a stop codon immediately after the α-secretase cleavage site. Interestingly, all of the phenotypes reported in APP deficient mice including body and brain weight deficits, grip strength deficits, alterations in locomotor activity, and impaired spatial learning and LTP have been shown to be fully restored by expressing only APPsα (Ring et al. 2007). Consistently, Taylor et al. (2008) showed a requirement for APPsα for in vivo LTP employing infusion of α-secretase inhibitor or recombinant APPsα, respectively. This crucial function of APPsα for synaptic plasticity and cognition is also of relevance for AD, as reduced CSF levels of APPsα and α-secretase ADAM10 are prominent features of sporadic AD cases (Lannfelt et al. 1995; Sennvik et al. 2000; Colciaghi et al. 2002; Tyler et al. 2002).

Li et al. (2010a) generated an APPsβ knockin allele that allows investigation of the stability and possible cleavage of APPsβ in the absence of APPsα. Contrary to Nikolaev (2009), the APPsβ protein was shown to be highly stable in vivo and does not undergo further cleavage under regular cell culture conditions in vitro. Crossing the APPsβ allele to APLP2 null background revealed that APPsβ failed to rescue the nerve sprouting phenotype of the APP/APLP2 null neuromuscular junction or early postnatal lethality (Li et al. 2010a). These data support the view that APPsβ exists as a stable protein and that the neuromuscular synapse defects present in APP/APLP2 null mice is not caused by the lack of APPsβ and, by extension, a defective APPsβ/DR6 pathway. However, when crossing the APPsα knockin allele (Ring et al. 2007) to an APLP2 null background, most of the combined mutants survived into adulthood (Weyer et al. 2011). These data suggest a distinct functional role of secreted APPsα sufficient to partially rescue the lethality of APP/APLP2-DKO mice, and revealed a synergistic role of both APP and APLP2 for hippocampal function and synaptic plasticity (Weyer et al. 2011).

Deletion or Mutation of the APP Intracellular Domain

Two APP carboxy-terminal deletion knockin mice have been reported. One deletes the last 15 amino acids of the APP sequence (APPΔCT15) (Ring et al. 2007); the other replaces mouse Aβ

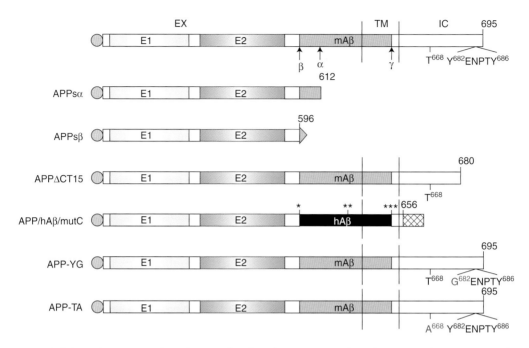

Figure 2. Schematic representation of APP and its knock-in constructs (not drawn to scale). EX, TM, and IC stand for extracellular, transmembrane, and intracellular region, respectively. E1 and E2 domains are marked in yellow and orange, respectively. mAβ and hAβ represent mouse and human Aβ, respectively. β, α, and γ indicate the cleavage sites by β-, α-, and γ-secretase, respectively. * represents signal peptide. ** symbolizes the FLAG tag. Residue T[668], and YENPTY motif are labeled to illustrate the corresponding point mutations in APP-YG knock-in and APP-TA knock-in mice. *, Swedish mutation (K595M596-N595L596); **, Arctic mutation (E618-G618); ***, London mutation (V642-I618), which are introduced in the APP/hAβ/mutC knock-in allele. All residues are numbered according to APP695 numbering.

with the human Aβ sequence containing the Swedish, Arctic, and London FAD mutations and simultaneously deletes the last 39 residues of the APP sequence (APP/hAβ/mutC) (Li et al. 2010b). Crossing the APP/hAβ/mutC allele to APLP2 null background resulted in similar neuromuscular synapse defects and early postnatal lethality as in mice doubly deficient in APP and APLP2, supporting a functional role of the APP carboxy-terminal domain in these development activities. Nevertheless, Aβ production and amyloid pathology could proceed without the carboxy-terminal sequences (Li et al. 2010b). An essential role of the APP carboxy-terminal domain, specifically the YENPTY motif, in development was shown by the creation of APP knockin mice in which the Tyr[682] residue of the Y[682]ENPTY sequence was changed to Gly (APP[YG]). Crossing the

homozygous knockin mice on APLP2-KO background showed that the APP[YG/YG]/APLP2[−/−] mice show neuromuscular synapse deficits and early lethality similar to APP/APLP2 double KO mice (Barbagallo et al. 2011a). In sharp contrast, similar analysis of the knockin mice with mutation of the highly conserved Thr[668] residue (APP[TA]) showed that this site is dispensable for the APP-mediated development function (Barbagallo et al. 2011b).

CONCLUDING REMARKS

Because of the central role of APP in AD pathogenesis, a great deal of effort has been devoted to understanding the biological functions of APP since its cloning in 1988. In vitro and in vivo studies have shown important activities of APP in various neuronal and synaptic processes, which can be executed either as a full-length protein or as one of the processing products. However, the underlying mechanisms remain largely undefined and often controversial. Key questions regarding whether APP is a receptor or a ligand or both, whether APP is by itself a signaling molecule or rather plays a secondary role in gene regulation, how APP function is coordinated between its full-length form and the proteolytic cleavage products and by its many intracellular binding partners awaits further investigation. The creation of the comprehensive panel of APP mouse strains including global inactivation, tissue-specific knockout and defined genetic modifications, combined with modern biological tools such as powerful large-scale experimentation and exciting neuroimaging technology, place us in an excellent position to address these questions.

ACKNOWLEDGMENTS

We thank Edith Gibson for editorial support and Hongmei Li for graphic assistance. The investigators' work cited in this review was supported by grants from NIH (AG032051 and AG033467 to H.Z.), the American Health and Assistance Foundation (A2008-052 to H.Z.), the Deutsche Forschungsgemeinschaft (MU 1457/5-1 and MU 1457/8-1 to U.C.M.), and NGFNplus (01GS08128 to U.C.M.).

REFERENCES

*Reference is also in this collection.

Allinquant B, Hantraye P, Mailleux P, Moya K, Bouillot C, Prochiantz A. 1995. Downregulation of amyloid precursor protein inhibits neurite outgrowth in vitro. *J Cell Biol* **128:** 919–927.

Anliker B, Müller U. 2006. The functions of mammalian amyloid precursor protein and related amyloid precursor-like proteins. *Neurodegener Dis* **3:** 239–246.

Araki Y, Tomita S, Yamaguchi H, Miyagi N, Sumioka A, Kirino Y, Suzuki T. 2003. Novel cadherin-related membrane proteins, Alcadeins, enhance the X11-like protein-mediated stabilization of amyloid β-protein precursor metabolism. *J Biol Chem* **278:** 49448–49458.

Ashley J, Packard M, Ataman B, Budnik V. 2005. Fasciclin II signals new synapse formation through amyloid precursor protein and the scaffolding protein dX11/Mint. *J Neurosci* **25:** 5943–5955.

Aydin D, Filippov MA, Tschäpe JA, Gretz N, Prinz M, Eils R, Brors B, Müller UC. 2011. Comparative transcriptome profiling of amyloid precursor protein family members in the adult cortex. *BMC Genomics* **12:** 160.

Back S, Haas P, Tschape JA, Gruebl T, Kirsch J, Müller U, Beyreuther K, Kins S. 2007. β-amyloid precursor protein can be transported independent of any sorting signal to the axonal and dendritic compartment. *J Neurosci Res* **85:** 2580–2590.

Baek SH, Ohgi KA, Rose DW, Koo EH, Glass CK, Rosenfeld MG. 2002. Exchange of N-CoR corepressor and Tip60 coactivator complexes links gene expression by NF-κB and β-amyloid precursor protein. *Cell* **110:** 55–67.

Barbagallo APM, Wang Z, Zheng H, D'Adamio L. 2011a. A single tyrosine residue in the amyloid precursor protein intracellular domain is essential for developmental function. *J Biol Chem* (in press) (JBC/2011/219837).

Barbagallo APM, Wang Z, Zheng H, D'Adamio L. 2011b. The intracellular threonine of amyloid precursor protein that is essential for docking of Pin1 is dispensable for developmental function. *PLoS ONE* (in press).

Beher D, Hesse L, Masters CL, Multhaup G. 1996. Regulation of amyloid protein precursor (APP) binding to collagen and mapping of the binding sites on APP and collagen type I. *J Biol Chem* **271:** 1613–1620.

Bell KF, Zheng L, Fahrenholz F, Cuello AC. 2008. ADAM-10 over-expression increases cortical synaptogenesis. *Neurobiol Aging* **29:** 554–565.

Bergmans BA, Shariati SA, Habets RL, Verstreken P, Schoonjans L, Müller U, Dotti CG, De Strooper B. 2010. Neurons generated from APP/APLP1/APLP2 triple knockout embryonic stem cells behave normally in vitro and in vivo: Lack of evidence for a cell autonomous role of the amyloid precursor protein in neuronal differentiation. *Stem Cells* **28:** 399–406.

Bertrand E, Brouillet E, Caille I, Bouillot C, Cole GM, Prochiantz A, Allinquant B. 2001. A short cytoplasmic domain of the amyloid precursor protein induces apoptosis in vitro and in vivo. *Mol Cell Neurosci* **18:** 503–511.

Biederer T, Südhof TC. 2000. Mints as adaptors. Direct binding to neurexins and recruitment of munc18. *J Biol Chem* **275:** 39803–39806.

Biederer T, Sara Y, Mozhayeva M, Atasoy D, Liu X, Kavalali ET, Südhof TC. 2002. SynCAM, a synaptic adhesion molecule that drives synapse assembly. *Science* **297:** 1525–1531.

Bittner T, Fuhrmann M, Burgold S, Jung CK, Volbracht C, Steiner H, Mitteregger G, Kretzschmar HA, Haass C, Herms J. 2009. γ-Secretase inhibition reduces spine density in vivo via an amyloid precursor protein-dependent pathway. *J Neurosci* **29:** 10405–10409.

Caille I, Allinquant B, Dupont E, Bouillot C, Langer A, Müller U, Prochiantz A. 2004. Soluble form of amyloid precursor protein regulates proliferation of progenitors in the adult subventricular zone. *Development* **131:** 2173–2181. Epub 2004 Apr 8.

Cao X, Südhof TC. 2001. A transcriptionally [correction of transcriptively] active complex of APP with Fe65 and histone acetyltransferase Tip60. *Science* **293:** 115–120.

Cao X, Südhof TC. 2004. Dissection of amyloid-β precursor protein-dependent transcriptional transactivation. *J Biol Chem* **279:** 24601–24611. Epub 22004 Mar 24.

Checler F, Sunyach C, Pardossi-Piquard R, Sevalle J, Vincent B, Kawarai T, Girardot N, St George-Hyslop P, da Costa CA. 2007. The γ/ε-secretase-derived APP intracellular domain fragments regulate 53. *Curr Alzheimer Res* **4**: 423–426.

Chen AC, Selkoe DJ. 2007. Response to: Pardossi-Piquard et al., "Presenilin-dependent transcriptional control of the Aβ-degrading enzyme neprilysin by intracellular domains of βAPP and APLP." *Neuron* **46**, 541–554. *Neuron* **53**: 479–483.

Chen F, Hasegawa H, Schmitt-Ulms G, Kawarai T, Bohm C, Katayama T, Gu Y, Sanjo N, Glista M, Rogaeva E, et al. 2006. TMP21 is a presenilin complex component that modulates γ-secretase but not ε-secretase activity. *Nature* **440**: 1208–1212.

Clarris HJ, Cappai R, Heffernan D, Beyreuther K, Masters CL, Small DH. 1997. Identification of heparin-binding domains in the amyloid precursor protein of Alzheimer's disease by deletion mutagenesis and peptide mapping. *J Neurochem* **68**: 1164–1172.

Colciaghi F, Borroni B, Pastorino L, Marcello E, Zimmermann M, Cattabeni F, Padovani A, Di Luca M. 2002. [α]-Secretase ADAM10 as well as [α]APPs is reduced in platelets and CSF of Alzheimer disease patients. *Mol Med* **8**: 67–74.

Copanaki E, Chang S, Vlachos A, Tschape JA, Müller UC, Kogel D, Deller T. 2010. εAPPα antagonizes dendritic degeneration and neuron death triggered by proteasomal stress. *Mol Cell Neurosci* **44**: 386–393.

Cupers P, Orlans I, Craessaerts K, Annaert W, De Strooper B. 2001. The amyloid precursor protein (APP)-cytoplasmic fragment generated by γ-secretase is rapidly degraded but distributes partially in a nuclear fraction of neurones in culture. *J Neurochem* **78**: 1168–1178.

Dahms SO, Hoefgen S, Roeser D, Schlott B, Guhrs KH, Than ME. 2010. Structure and biochemical analysis of the heparin-induced E1 dimer of the amyloid precursor protein. *Proc Natl Acad Sci* **107**: 5381–5386.

Daigle I, Li C. 1993. apl-1, a *Caenorhabditis elegans* gene encoding a protein related to the human β-amyloid protein precursor. *Proc Natl Acad Sci* **90**: 12045–12049.

Dalva MB, McClelland AC, Kayser MS. 2007. Cell adhesion molecules: Signalling functions at the synapse. *Nat Rev Neurosci* **8**: 206–220. Epub 2007 Feb 14.

Dawson GR, Seabrook GR, Zheng H, Smith DW, Graham S, O'Dowd G, Bowery BJ, Boyce S, Trumbauer ME, Chen HY, et al. 1999. Age-related cognitive deficits, impaired long-term potentiation and reduction in synaptic marker density in mice lacking the β-amyloid precursor protein. *Neuroscience* **90**: 1–13.

* De Strooper B, Iwatsubo T, Wolfe MS. 2011. Presenilins and γ-secretase: Structure, function and role in Alzheimer disease. *Cold Spring Harb Perspect Med* doi: 10.1101/cshperspect.a006304.

Eggert S, Paliga K, Soba P, Evin G, Masters CL, Weidemann A, Beyreuther K. 2004. The proteolytic processing of the amyloid precursor protein gene family members APLP-1 and APLP-2 involves α-, β-, γ-, and ε-like cleavages: Modulation of APLP-1 processing by n-glycosylation. *J Biol Chem* **279**: 18146–18156.

Endres K, Postina R, Schroeder A, Mueller U, Fahrenholz F. 2005. Shedding of the amyloid precursor protein-like protein APLP2 by disintegrin-metalloproteinases. *FEBS J* **272**: 5808–5820.

Fogel AI, Akins MR, Krupp AJ, Stagi M, Stein V, Biederer T. 2007. SynCAMs organize synapses through heterophilic adhesion. *J Neurosci* **27**: 12516–12530.

Frigerio CS, Fadeeva JV, Minogue AM, Citron M, Van Leuven F, Staufenbiel M, Paganetti P, Selkoe DJ, Walsh DM. 2010. β-Secretase cleavage is not required for generation of the intracellular C-terminal domain of the amyloid precursor family of proteins. *FEBS J* **277**: 1503–1518.

Gakhar-Koppole N, Hundeshagen P, Mandl C, Weyer SW, Allinquant B, Müller U, Ciccolini F. 2008. Activity requires soluble amyloid precursor protein α to promote neurite outgrowth in neural stem cell-derived neurons via activation of the MAPK pathway. *Eur J Neurosci* **28**: 871–882.

Galvan V, Gorostiza OF, Banwait S, Ataie M, Logvinova AV, Sitaraman S, Carlson E, Sagi SA, Chevallier N, Jin K, et al. 2006. Reversal of Alzheimer's-like pathology and behavior in human APP transgenic mice by mutation of Asp664. *Proc Natl Acad Sci* **103**: 7130–7135.

Gao Y, Pimplikar SW. 2001. The γ-secretase-cleaved C-terminal fragment of amyloid precursor protein mediates signaling to the nucleus. *Proc Natl Acad Sci* **98**: 14979–14984.

Giliberto L, Zhou D, Weldon R, Tamagno E, De Luca P, Tabaton M, D'Adamio L. 2008. Evidence that the amyloid β precursor protein-intracellular domain lowers the stress threshold of neurons and has a "regulated" transcriptional role. *Mol Neurodegener* **3**: 12.

Goldgaber D, Lerman MI, McBride OW, Saffiotti U, Gajdusek DC. 1987. Characterization and chromosomal localization of a cDNA encoding brain amyloid of Alzheimer's disease. *Science* **235**: 877–880.

Graf ER, Zhang X, Jin SX, Linhoff MW, Craig AM. 2004. Neurexins induce differentiation of GABA and glutamate postsynaptic specializations via neuroligins. *Cell* **119**: 1013–1026.

Gralle M, Ferreira ST. 2007. Structure and functions of the human amyloid precursor protein: The whole is more than the sum of its parts. *Prog Neurobiol* **82**: 11–32.

Gralle M, Oliveira CL, Guerreiro LH, McKinstry WJ, Galatis D, Masters CL, Cappai R, Parker MW, Ramos CH, Torriani I, et al. 2006. Solution conformation and heparin-induced dimerization of the full-length extracellular domain of the human amyloid precursor protein. *J Mol Biol* **357**: 493–508.

Grimm MO, Grimm HS, Patzold AJ, Zinser EG, Halonen R, Duering M, Tschape JA, De Strooper B, Müller U, Shen J, et al. 2005. Regulation of cholesterol and sphingomyelin metabolism by amyloid-β and presenilin. *Nat Cell Biol* **7**: 1118–1123.

Guénette S, Chang Y, Hiesberger T, Richardson JA, Eckman CB, Eckman EA, Hammer RE, Herz J. 2006. Essential roles for the FE65 amyloid precursor protein-interacting proteins in brain development *EMBO J* **25**: 420–431.

Haass C, Schlossmacher MG, Hung AY, Vigo-Pelfrey C, Mellon A, Ostaszewski BL, Lieberburg I, Koo EH, Schenk D, Teplow DB, et al. 1992. Amyloid β-peptide is produced by cultured cells during normal metabolism. *Nature* **359**: 322–325.

Han P, Dou F, Li F, Zhang X, Zhang YW, Zheng H, Lipton SA, Xu H, Liao FF. 2005. Suppression of cyclin-dependent kinase 5 activation by amyloid precursor protein: A novel excitoprotective mechanism involving modulation of τ phosphorylation. *J Neurosci* **25:** 11542–11552.

Harris J, Devidze N, Halabisky B, Lo I, Thwin MT, Yu GQ, Bredesen DE, Masliah E, Mucke L. 2010. Many neuronal and behavioral impairments in transgenic mouse models of Alzheimer's disease are independent of caspase cleavage of the amyloid precursor protein. *J Neurosci* **30:** 372–381.

Hass MR, Yankner BA. 2005. A {γ}-secretase-independent mechanism of signal transduction by the amyloid precursor protein. *J Biol Chem* **280:** 36895–36904.

* Haass C. 2011. Trafficking and proteolytic processing of APP. *Cold Spring Harb Perspect Med* doi: 10.1101/cshperspect.a006270.

Hata Y, Butz S, Südhof TC. 1996. CASK: A novel dlg/PSD95 homolog with an N-terminal calmodulin-dependent protein kinase domain identified by interaction with neurexins. *J Neurosci* **16:** 2488–2494.

Heber S, Herms J, Gajic V, Hainfellner J, Aguzzi A, Rulicke T, von Kretzschmar H, von Koch C, Sisodia S, Tremml P, et al. 2000. Mice with combined gene knock-outs reveal essential and partially redundant functions of amyloid precursor protein family members. *J Neurosci* **20:** 7951–7963.

Hebert SS, Serneels L, Tolia A, Craessaerts K, Derks C, Filippov MA, Müller U, De Strooper B. 2006. Regulated intramembrane proteolysis of amyloid precursor protein and regulation of expression of putative target genes. *EMBO Rep* **7:** 739–745.

Hérard AS, Besret L, Dubois A, Dauguet J, Delzescaux T, Hantraye P, Bonvento G, Moya KL. 2006. siRNA targeted against amyloid precursor protein impairs synaptic activity in vivo. *Neurobiol Aging* **27:** 1740–1750.

Herms J, Anliker B, Heber S, Ring S, Fuhrmann M, Kretzschmar H, Sisodia S, Müller U. 2004. Cortical dysplasia resembling human type 2 lissencephaly in mice lacking all three APP family members. *Embo J* **23:** 4106–4115.

Ho A, Südhof TC. 2004. Binding of F-spondin to amyloid-β precursor protein: A candidate amyloid-β precursor protein ligand that modulates amyloid-β precursor protein cleavage. *Proc Natl Acad Sci* **101:** 2548–2553.

Hoe HS, Fu Z, Makarova A, Lee JY, Lu C, Feng L, Pajoohesh-Ganji A, Matsuoka Y, Hyman BT, Ehlers MD, et al. 2009a. The effects of amyloid precursor protein on postsynaptic composition and activity. *J Biol Chem* **284:** 8495–8506.

Hoe HS, Lee KJ, Carney RS, Lee J, Markova A, Lee JY, Howell BW, Hyman BT, Pak DT, Bu G, et al. 2009b. Interaction of reelin with amyloid precursor protein promotes neurite outgrowth. *J Neurosci* **29:** 7459–7473.

Hornsten A, Lieberthal J, Fadia S, Malins R, Ha L, Xu X, Daigle I, Markowitz M, O'Connor G, Plasterk R, et al. 2007. APL-1, a *Caenorhabditis elegans* protein related to the human β-amyloid precursor protein, is essential for viability. *Proc Natl Acad Sci* **104:** 1971–1976.

Jacobsen KT, Iverfeldt K. 2009. Amyloid precursor protein and its homologues: A family of proteolysis-dependent receptors. *Cell Mol Life Sci* **66:** 2299–2318.

Jin LW, Ninomiya H, Roch JM, Schubert D, Masliah E, Otero DA, Saitoh T. 1994. Peptides containing the RERMS sequence of amyloid β/A4 protein precursor bind cell surface and promote neurite extension. *J Neurosci* **14:** 5461–5470.

Kaden D, Munter LM, Joshi M, Treiber C, Weise C, Bethge T, Voigt P, Schaefer M, Beyermann M, Reif B, et al. 2008. Homophilic interactions of the amyloid precursor protein (APP) ectodomain are regulated by the loop region and affect β-secretase cleavage of APP. *J Biol Chem* **283:** 7271–7279.

Kaether C, Skehel P, Dotti CG. 2000. Axonal membrane proteins are transported in distinct carriers: A two-color video microscopy study in cultured hippocampal neurons. *Mol Biol Cell* **11:** 1213–1224.

Kamal A, Almenar-Queralt A, LeBlanc JF, Roberts EA, Goldstein LS. 2001. Kinesin-mediated axonal transport of a membrane compartment containing β-secretase and presenilin-1 requires APP. *Nature* **414:** 643–648.

Kang J, Lemaire HG, Unterbeck A, Salbaum JM, Masters CL, Grzeschik KH, Multhaup G, Beyreuther K, Müller-Hill B. 1987. The precursor of Alzheimer's disease amyloid A4 protein resembles a cell-surface receptor. *Nature* **325:** 733–736.

Kibbey MC, Jucker M, Weeks BS, Neve RL, Van Nostrand WE, Kleinman HK. 1993. β-Amyloid precursor protein binds to the neurite-promoting IKVAV site of laminin. *Proc Natl Acad Sci* **90:** 10150–10153.

Kim HS, Kim EM, Lee JP, Park CH, Kim S, Seo JH, Chang KA, Yu E, Jeong SJ, Chong YH, et al. 2003. C-terminal fragments of amyloid precursor protein exert neurotoxicity by inducing glycogen synthase kinase-3β expression. *FASEB J* **17:** 1951–1953.

Kimberly WT, Zheng JB, Guenette SY, Selkoe DJ. 2001. The intracellular domain of the β-amyloid precursor protein is stabilized by Fe65 and translocates to the nucleus in a notch-like manner. *J Biol Chem* **276:** 40288–40292.

Koo EH, Sisodia SS, Archer DR, Martin LJ, Weidemann A, Beyreuther K, Fischer P, Masters CL, Price DL. 1990. Precursor of amyloid protein in Alzheimer disease undergoes fast anterograde axonal transport. *Proc Natl Acad Sci* **87:** 1561–1565.

Kuhn PH, Wang H, Dislich B, Colombo A, Zeitschel U, Ellwart JW, Kremmer E, Rossner S, Lichtenthaler SF. 2010. ADAM10 is the physiologically relevant, constitutive α-secretase of the amyloid precursor protein in primary neurons. *EMBO J* **29:** 3020–3032.

Lannfelt L, Basun H, Vigo-Pelfrey C, Wahlund LO, Winblad B, Lieberburg I, Schenk D. 1995. Amyloid β-peptide in cerebrospinal fluid in individuals with the Swedish Alzheimer amyloid precursor protein mutation. *Neurosci Lett* **199:** 203–206.

Lazarov O, Morfini GA, Lee EB, Farah MH, Szodorai A, DeBoer SR, Koliatsos VE, Kins S, Lee VM, Wong PC, et al. 2005. Axonal transport, amyloid precursor protein, kinesin-1, and the processing apparatus: Revisited. *J Neurosci* **25:** 2386–2395.

Leissring MA, Murphy MP, Mead TR, Akbari Y, Sugarman MC, Jannatipour M, Anliker B, Müller U, Saftig P, De Strooper B, et al. 2002. A physiologic signaling role for the γ-secretase-derived intracellular fragment of APP. *Proc Natl Acad Sci* **99:** 4697–4702.

Li ZW, Stark G, Gotz J, Rulicke T, Gschwind M, Huber G, Müller U, Weissmann C. 1996. Generation of mice with a 200-kb amyloid precursor protein gene deletion by Cre recombinase-mediated site-specific recombination in embryonic stem cells. *Proc Natl Acad Sci* **93:** 6158–6162.

Li H, Wang B, Wang Z, Guo Q, Tabuchi K, Hammer RE, Südhof TC, Wang R, Zheng H. 2010a. Soluble APP regulates transthyretin and Klotho gene expression without rescuing the essential function of APP. *Proc Natl Acad Sci* **107:** 17362–17367.

Li H, Wang Z, Wang B, Guo Q, Dolios G, Tabuchi K, Hammer RE, Südhof TC, Wang R, Zheng H. 2010b. Genetic dissection of the amyloid precursor protein in developmental function and amyloid pathogenesis. *J Biol Chem* **285:** 30598–30605.

Linhoff MW, Lauren J, Cassidy RM, Dobie FA, Takahashi H, Nygaard HB, Airaksinen MS, Strittmatter SM, Craig AM. 2009. An unbiased expression screen for synaptogenic proteins identifies the LRRTM protein family as synaptic organizers. *Neuron* **61:** 734–749.

Liu Q, Zerbinatti CV, Zhang J, Hoe HS, Wang B, Cole SL, Herz J, Muglia L, Bu G. 2007. Amyloid precursor protein regulates brain apolipoprotein E and cholesterol metabolism through lipoprotein receptor LRP1. *Neuron* **56:** 66–78.

Lorent K, Overbergh L, Moechars D, De Strooper B, Van Leuven F, Van den Berghe H. 1995. Expression in mouse embryos and in adult mouse brain of three members of the amyloid precursor protein family, of the α-2-macroglobulin receptor/low density lipoprotein receptor-related protein and of its ligands apolipoprotein E, lipoprotein lipase, α-2-macroglobulin and the 40,000 molecular weight receptor-associated protein. *Neuroscience* **65:** 1009–1025.

Lourenco FC, Galvan V, Fombonne J, Corset V, Llambi F, Müller U, Bredesen DE, Mehlen P. 2009. Netrin-1 interacts with amyloid precursor protein and regulates amyloid-β production. *Cell Death Differ* **16:** 655–663.

Lu DC, Soriano S, Bredesen DE, Koo EH. 2003. Caspase cleavage of the amyloid precursor protein modulates amyloid β-protein toxicity. *J Neurochem* **87:** 733–741.

Luo LQ, Martin-Morris LE, White K. 1990. Identification, secretion, and neural expression of APPL, a *Drosophila* protein similar to human amyloid protein precursor. *J Neurosci* **10:** 3849–3861.

Luo L, Tully T, White K. 1992. Human amyloid precursor protein ameliorates behavioral deficit of flies deleted for Appl gene. *Neuron* **9:** 595–605.

Ma QH, Futagawa T, Yang WL, Jiang XD, Zeng L, Takeda Y, Xu RX, Bagnard D, Schachner M, Furley AJ, et al. 2008. A TAG1-APP signalling pathway through Fe65 negatively modulates neurogenesis [see comment]. *Nat Cell Biol* **10:** 283–294.

Magara F, Müller U, Li ZW, Lipp HP, Weissmann C, Stagljar M, Wolfer DP. 1999. Genetic background changes the pattern of forebrain commissure defects in transgenic mice underexpressing the β-amyloid-precursor protein. *Proc Natl Acad Sci* **96:** 4656–4661.

Mallm JP, Tschape JA, Hick M, Filippov MA, Müller UC. 2010. Generation of conditional null alleles for APP and APLP2. *Genesis* **48:** 200–206.

Meziane H, Dodart JC, Mathis C, Little S, Clemens J, Paul SM, Ungerer A. 1998. Memory-enhancing effects of secreted forms of the β-amyloid precursor protein in normal and amnestic mice. *Proc Natl Acad Sci* **95:** 12683–12688.

Minogue AM, Stubbs AK, Frigerio CS, Boland B, Fadeeva JV, Tang J, Selkoe DJ, Walsh DM. 2009. γ-secretase processing of APLP1 leads to the production of a p3-like peptide that does not aggregate and is not toxic to neurons. *Brain Res* **1262:** 89–99.

Mok SS, Sberna G, Heffernan D, Cappai R, Galatis D, Clarris HJ, Sawyer WH, Beyreuther K, Masters CL, Small DH. 1997. Expression and analysis of heparin-binding regions of the amyloid precursor protein of Alzheimer's disease. *FEBS Lett* **415:** 303–307.

Morales-Corraliza J, Mazzella MJ, Berger JD, Diaz NS, Choi JH, Levy E, Matsuoka Y, Planel E, Mathews PM. 2009. In vivo turnover of τ and APP metabolites in the brains of wild-type and Tg2576 mice: Greater stability of sAPP in the β-amyloid depositing mice. *PLoS One* **4:** e7134.

Mucke L, Masliah E, Johnson WB, Ruppe MD, Alford M, Rockenstein EM, Forss-Petter S, Pietropaolo M, Mallory M, Abraham CR. 1994. Synaptotrophic effects of human amyloid β protein precursors in the cortex of transgenic mice. *Brain Res* **666:** 151–167.

Müller U, Cristina N, Li ZW, Wolfer DP, Lipp HP, Rulicke T, Brandner S, Aguzzi A, Weissmann C. 1994. Behavioral and anatomical deficits in mice homozygous for a modified β-amyloid precursor protein gene. *Cell* **79:** 755–765.

Müller T, Concannon CG, Ward MW, Walsh CM, Tirniceriu AL, Tribl F, Kogel D, Prehn JH, Egensperger R. 2007. Modulation of gene expression and cytoskeletal dynamics by the amyloid precursor protein intracellular domain (AICD). *Mol Biol Cell* **18:** 201–210.

Munter LM, Voigt P, Harmeier A, Kaden D, Gottschalk KE, Weise C, Pipkorn R, Schaefer M, Langosch D, Multhaup G. 2007. GxxxG motifs within the amyloid precursor protein transmembrane sequence are critical for the etiology of Aβ42. *EMBO J* **26:** 1702–1712.

Musa A, Lehrach H, Russo VA. 2001. Distinct expression patterns of two zebrafish homologues of the human APP gene during embryonic development. *Dev Genes Evol* **211:** 563–567.

Nikolaev A, McLaughlin T, O'Leary DDM, Tessier-Lavigne M. 2009. APP binds DR6 to trigger axon pruning and neuron death via distinct caspases. *Nature* **457:** 981–990.

Ninomiya H, Roch JM, Sundsmo MP, Otero DA, Saitoh T. 1993. Amino acid sequence RERMS represents the active domain of amyloid β/A4 protein precursor that promotes fibroblast growth. *J Cell Biol* **121:** 879–886.

Osterfield M, Egelund R, Young LM, Flanagan JG. 2008. Interaction of amyloid precursor protein with contactins and NgCAM in the retinotectal system. *Development* **135:** 1189–1199.

Paliga K, Peraus G, Kreger S, Durrwang U, Hesse L, Multhaup G, Masters CL, Beyreuther K, Weidemann A. 1997. Human amyloid precursor-like protein 1–cDNA cloning, ectopic expression in COS-7 cells and identification of soluble forms in the cerebrospinal fluid. *Eur J Biochem* **250:** 354–363.

Pardossi-Piquard R, Petit A, Kawarai T, Sunyach C, Alves da Costa C, Vincent B, Ring S, D'Adamio L, Shen J, Müller

U, et al. 2005. Presenilin-dependent transcriptional control of the Aβ-degrading enzyme neprilysin by intracellular domains of βAPP and APLP. *Neuron* **46**: 541–554.

Park JH, Gimbel DA, GrandPre T, Lee JK, Kim JE, Li W, Lee DH, Strittmatter SM. 2006. Alzheimer precursor protein interaction with the Nogo-66 receptor reduces amyloid-β plaque deposition. *J Neurosci* **26**: 1386–1395.

Park SA, Shaked GM, Bredesen DE, Koo EH. 2009. Mechanism of cytotoxicity mediated by the C31 fragment of the amyloid precursor protein. *Biochem Biophys Res Commun* **388**: 450–455.

Pastorino L, Ikin AF, Lamprianou S, Vacaresse N, Revelli JP, Platt K, Paganetti P, Mathews PM, Harroch S, Buxbaum JD. 2004. BACE (β-secretase) modulates the processing of APLP2 in vivo. *Mol Cell Neurosci* **25**: 642–649.

Perez RG, Zheng H, Van der Ploeg LH, Koo EH. 1997. The β-amyloid precursor protein of Alzheimer's disease enhances neuron viability and modulates neuronal polarity. *J Neurosci* **17**: 9407–9414.

Perez RG, Soriano S, Hayes JD, Ostaszewski B, Xia W, Selkoe DJ, Chen X, Stokin GB, Koo EH. 1999. Mutagenesis identifies new signals for β-amyloid precursor protein endocytosis, turnover, and the generation of secreted fragments, including Aβ42. *J Biol Chem* **274**: 18851–18856.

Phinney AL, Calhoun ME, Wolfer DP, Lipp HP, Zheng H, Jucker M. 1999. No hippocampal neuron or synaptic bouton loss in learning-impaired aged β-amyloid precursor protein-null mice. *Neuroscience* **90**: 1207–1216.

Pietrzik CU, Yoon IS, Jaeger S, Busse T, Weggen S, Koo EH. 2004. FE65 constitutes the functional link between the low-density lipoprotein receptor-related protein and the amyloid precursor protein. *J Neurosci* **24**: 4259–4265.

Priller C, Bauer T, Mitteregger G, Krebs B, Kretzschmar HA, Herms J. 2006. Synapse formation and function is modulated by the amyloid precursor protein. *J Neurosci* **26**: 7212–7221.

Qiu WQ, Ferreira A, Miller C, Koo EH, Selkoe DJ. 1995. Cell-surface β-amyloid precursor protein stimulates neurite outgrowth of hippocampal neurons in an isoform-dependent manner. *J Neurosci* **15**: 2157–2167.

Radzimanowski J, Simon B, Sattler M, Beyreuther K, Sinning I, Wild K. 2010. Structure of the intracellular domain of the amyloid precursor protein in complex with Fe65-PTB2. *EMBO Rep* **9**: 1136–1140.

Reinhard C, Hebert SS, De Strooper B. 2005. The amyloid-β precursor protein: Integrating structure with biological function. *EMBO J* **24**: 3996–4006.

Repetto E, Yoon IS, Zheng H, Kang DE. 2007. Presenilin 1 regulates epidermal growth factor receptor turnover and signaling in the endosomal-lysosomal pathway. *J Biol Chem* **282**: 31504–31516.

Richter L, Munter LM, Ness J, Hildebrand PW, Dasari M, Unterreitmeier S, Bulic B, Beyermann M, Gust R, Reif B, et al. 2010. Amyloid β 42 peptide (Aβ42)-lowering compounds directly bind to Aβ and interfere with amyloid precursor protein (APP) transmembrane dimerization. *Proc Natl Acad Sci* **107**: 14597–14602.

Ring S, Weyer SW, Kilian SB, Waldron E, Pietrzik CU, Filippov MA, Herms J, Buchholz C, Eckman CB, Korte M, et al. 2007. The secreted β-amyloid precursor protein ectodomain APPs α is sufficient to rescue the anatomical,

behavioral, and electrophysiological abnormalities of APP-deficient mice. *J Neurosci* **27**: 7817–7826.

Roch JM, Masliah E, Roch-Levecq AC, Sundsmo MP, Otero DA, Veinbergs I, Saitoh T. 1994. Increase of synaptic density and memory retention by a peptide representing the trophic domain of the amyloid β/A4 protein precursor. *Proc Natl Acad Sci* **91**: 7450–7454.

Rohe M, Carlo AS, Breyhan H, Sporbert A, Militz D, Schmidt V, Wozny C, Harmeier A, Erdmann B, Bales KR, et al. 2008. Sortilin-related receptor with A-type repeats (SORLA) affects the amyloid precursor protein-dependent stimulation of ERK signaling and adult neurogenesis. *J Biol Chem* **283**: 14826–14834.

Rosen DR, Martin-Morris L, Luo LQ, White K. 1989. A *Drosophila* gene encoding a protein resembling the human β-amyloid protein precursor. *Proc Natl Acad Sci* **86**: 2478–2482.

Ryan KA, Pimplikar SW. 2005. Activation of GSK-3 and phosphorylation of CRMP2 in transgenic mice expressing APP intracellular domain. *J Cell Biol* **171**: 327–335. Epub 2005 Oct 17.

Saitoh T, Sundsmo M, Roch JM, Kimura N, Cole G, Schubert D, Oltersdorf T, Schenk DB. 1989. Secreted form of amyloid β protein precursor is involved in the growth regulation of fibroblasts. *Cell* **58**: 615–622.

Santos SF, Pierrot N, Morel N, Gailly P, Sindic C, Octave JN. 2009. Expression of human amyloid precursor protein in rat cortical neurons inhibits calcium oscillations. *J Neurosci* **29**: 4708–4718.

Sara Y, Biederer T, Atasoy D, Chubykin A, Mozhayeva MG, Südhof TC, Kavalali ET. 2005. Selective capability of SynCAM and neuroligin for functional synapse assembly. *J Neurosci* **25**: 260–270.

Sastre M, Steiner H, Fuchs K, Capell A, Multhaup G, Condron MM, Teplow DB, Haass C. 2001. Presenilin-dependent γ-secretase processing of β-amyloid precursor protein at a site corresponding to the S3 cleavage of Notch. *EMBO Rep* **2**: 835–841.

Scheiffele P, Fan J, Choih J, Fetter R, Serafini T. 2000. Neuroligin expressed in nonneuronal cells triggers presynaptic development in contacting axons. *Cell* **101**: 657–669.

Scheinfeld MH, Ghersi E, Laky K, Fowlkes BJ, D'Adamio L. 2002. Processing of β-amyloid precursor-like protein-1 and -2 by γ-secretase regulates transcription. *J Biol Chem* **277**: 44195–44201.

Schmidt V, Sporbert A, Rohe M, Reimer T, Rehm A, Andersen OM, Willnow TE. 2007. SorLA/LR11 regulates processing of amyloid precursor protein via interaction with adaptors GGA and PACS-1. *J Biol Chem* **282**: 32956–32964.

Schrenk-Siemens K, Perez-Alcala S, Richter J, Lacroix E, Rahuel J, Korte M, Müller U, Barde YA, Bibel M. 2008. Embryonic stem cell-derived neurons as a cellular system to study gene function: Lack of amyloid precursor proteins APP and APLP2 leads to defective synaptic transmission. *Stem Cells* **26**: 2153–2163.

Seabrook GR, Smith DW, Bowery BJ, Easter A, Reynolds T, Fitzjohn SM, Morton RA, Zheng H, Dawson GR, Sirinathsinghji DJ, et al. 1999. Mechanisms contributing to the deficits in hippocampal synaptic plasticity in mice lacking amyloid precursor protein. *Neuropharmacology* **38**: 349–359.

Selkoe D, Kopan R. 2003. Notch and Presenilin: Regulated intramembrane proteolysis links development and degeneration. *Annu Rev Neurosci* **26:** 565–597.

Sennvik K, Fastbom J, Blomberg M, Wahlund LO, Winblad B, Benedikz E. 2000. Levels of α- and β-secretase cleaved amyloid precursor protein in the cerebrospinal fluid of Alzheimer's disease patients. *Neurosci Lett* **278:** 169–172.

Simons M, de Strooper B, Multhaup G, Tienari PJ, Dotti CG, Beyreuther K. 1996. Amyloidogenic processing of the human amyloid precursor protein in primary cultures of rat hippocampal neurons. *J Neurosci* **16:** 899–908.

Sisodia SS, Koo EH, Hoffman PN, Perry G, Price DL. 1993. Identification and transport of full-length amyloid precursor proteins in rat peripheral nervous system. *J Neurosci* **13:** 3136–3142.

Slunt HH, Thinakaran G, Von Koch C, Lo AC, Tanzi RE, Sisodia SS. 1994. Expression of a ubiquitous, cross-reactive homologue of the mouse β-amyloid precursor protein (APP). *J Biol Chem* **269:** 2637–2644.

Small DH, Nurcombe V, Reed G, Clarris H, Moir R, Beyreuther K, Masters CL. 1994. A heparin-binding domain in the amyloid protein precursor of Alzheimer's disease is involved in the regulation of neurite outgrowth. *J Neurosci* **14:** 2117–2127.

Small DH, Clarris HL, Williamson TG, Reed G, Key B, Mok SS, Beyreuther K, Masters CL, Nurcombe V. 1999. Neurite-outgrowth regulating functions of the amyloid protein precursor of Alzheimer's disease. *J Alzheimers Dis* **1:** 275–285.

Soba P, Eggert S, Wagner K, Zentgraf H, Siehl K, Kreger S, Lower A, Langer A, Merdes G, Paro R, et al. 2005. Homo- and heterodimerization of APP family members promotes intercellular adhesion. *EMBO J* **24:** 3624–3634. Epub 2005 Sep 29.

Steinbach JP, Müller U, Leist M, Li ZW, Nicotera P, Aguzzi A. 1998. Hypersensitivity to seizures in β-amyloid precursor protein deficient mice. *Cell Death Differ* **5:** 858–866.

Storey E, Spurck T, Pickett-Heaps J, Beyreuther K, Masters CL. 1996. The amyloid precursor protein of Alzheimer's disease is found on the surface of static but not activity motile portions of neurites. *Brain Res* **735:** 59–66.

Suzuki T, Nakaya T. 2008. Regulation of amyloid β-protein precursor by phosphorylation and protein interactions. *J Biol Chem* **283:** 29633–29637.

Szodorai A, Kuan YH, Hunzelmann S, Engel U, Sakane A, Sasaki T, Takai Y, Kirsch J, Müller U, Beyreuther K, et al. 2009. APP anterograde transport requires Rab3A GTPase activity for assembly of the transport vesicle. *J Neurosci* **29:** 14534–14544.

Tamboli IY, Prager K, Thal DR, Thelen KM, Dewachter I, Pietrzik CU, St George-Hyslop P, Sisodia SS, De Strooper B, Heneka MT, et al. 2008. Loss of γ-secretase function impairs endocytosis of lipoprotein particles and membrane cholesterol homeostasis. *J Neurosci* **28:** 12097–12106.

Tanzi RE, Gusella JF, Watkins PC, Bruns GA, St George-Hyslop P, Van Keuren ML, Patterson D, Pagan S, Kurnit DM, Neve RL. 1987. Amyloid β protein gene: cDNA, mRNA distribution, and genetic linkage near the Alzheimer locus. *Science* **235:** 880–884.

Taylor CJ, Ireland DR, Ballagh I, Bourne K, Marechal NM, Turner PR, Bilkey DK, Tate WP, Abraham WC. 2008. Endogenous secreted amyloid precursor protein-α regulates hippocampal NMDA receptor function, long-term potentiation and spatial memory. *Neurobiol Dis* **31:** 250–260.

Thinakaran G, Kitt CA, Roskams AJ, Slunt HH, Masliah E, von Koch C, Ginsberg SD, Ronnett GV, Reed RR, Price DL, et al. 1995. Distribution of an APP homolog, APLP2, in the mouse olfactory system: A potential role for APLP2 in axogenesis. *J Neurosci* **15:** 6314–6326.

Tienari PJ, De Strooper B, Ikonen E, Simons M, Weidemann A, Czech C, Hartmann T, Ida N, Multhaup G, Masters CL, et al. 1996. The β-amyloid domain is essential for axonal sorting of amyloid precursor protein. *EMBO J* **15:** 5218–5229.

Torroja L, Packard M, Gorczyca M, White K, Budnik V. 1999. The *Drosophila* β-amyloid precursor protein homolog promotes synapse differentiation at the neuromuscular junction. *J Neurosci* **19:** 7793–7803.

Turner PR, O'Connor K, Tate WP, Abraham WC. 2003. Roles of amyloid precursor protein and its fragments in regulating neural activity, plasticity and memory. *Prog Neurobiol* **70:** 1–32.

Tyler SJ, Dawbarn D, Wilcock GK, Allen SJ. 2002. α- and β-secretase: Profound changes in Alzheimer's disease. *Biochem Biophys Res Commun* **299:** 373–376.

von Koch CS, Zheng H, Chen H, Trumbauer M, Thinakaran G, van der Ploeg LH, Price DL, Sisodia SS. 1997. Generation of APLP2 KO mice and early postnatal lethality in APLP2/APP double KO mice. *Neurobiol Aging* **18:** 661–669.

von Rotz RC, Kohli BM, Bosset J, Meier M, Suzuki T, Nitsch RM, Konietzko U. 2004. The APP intracellular domain forms nuclear multiprotein complexes and regulates the transcription of its own precursor. *J Cell Sci* **117:** 4435–4448.

Waldron E, Isbert S, Kern A, Jaeger S, Martin AM, Hebert SS, Behl C, Weggen S, De Strooper B, Pietrzik CU. 2008. Increased AICD generation does not result in increased nuclear translocation or activation of target gene transcription. *Exp Cell Res* **314:** 2419–2433.

Walsh DM, Fadeeva JV, LaVoie MJ, Paliga K, Eggert S, Kimberly WT, Wasco W, Selkoe DJ. 2003. γ-Secretase cleavage and binding to FE65 regulate the nuclear translocation of the intracellular C-terminal domain (ICD) of the APP family of proteins. *Biochemistry* **42:** 6664–6673.

Wang Y, Ha Y. 2004. The X-ray structure of an antiparallel dimer of the human amyloid precursor protein E2 domain. *Mol Cell* **15:** 343–353.

Wang P, Yang G, Mosier DR, Chang P, Zaidi T, Gong YD, Zhao NM, Dominguez B, Lee KF, Gan WB, et al. 2005. Defective neuromuscular synapses in mice lacking amyloid precursor protein (APP) and APP-Like protein 2. *J Neurosci* **25:** 1219–1225.

Wang B, Yang L, Wang Z, Zheng H. 2007. Amyloid precursor protein mediates presynaptic localization and activity of the high-affinity choline transporter. *Proc Natl Acad Sci* **104:** 14140–14145.

Wang Z, Wang B, Yang L, Guo Q, Aithmitti N, Songyang Z, Zheng H. 2009. Presynaptic and postsynaptic interaction of the amyloid precursor protein promotes peripheral and central synaptogenesis. *J Neurosci* **29:** 10788–10801.

Wasco W, Bupp K, Magendantz M, Gusella JF, Tanzi RE, Solomon F. 1992. Identification of a mouse brain cDNA that encodes a protein related to the Alzheimer disease-associated amyloid β protein precursor. *Proc Natl Acad Sci* **89:** 10758–10762.

Wasco W, Gurubhagavatula S, Paradis MD, Romano DM, Sisodia SS, Hyman BT, Neve RL, Tanzi RE. 1993. Isolation and characterization of APLP2 encoding a homologue of the Alzheimer's associated amyloid β protein precursor. *Nat Genet* **5:** 95–100.

Webster MT, Groome N, Francis PT, Pearce BR, Sherriff FE, Thinakaran G, Felsenstein KM, Wasco W, Tanzi RE, Bowen DM. 1995. A novel protein, amyloid precursor-like protein 2, is present in human brain, cerebrospinal fluid and conditioned media. *Biochem J* **310** (Pt 1): 95–99.

Weidemann A, Eggert S, Reinhard FB, Vogel M, Paliga K, Baier G, Masters CL, Beyreuther K, Evin G. 2002. A novel ε-cleavage within the transmembrane domain of the Alzheimer amyloid precursor protein demonstrates homology with Notch processing. *Biochemistry* **41:** 2825–2835.

Weyer SA, Klevanski M, Delekate A, Voikar V, Aydin D, Hick M, Filippov MA, Drost N, Schaller KL, Saar M, et al. 2011. APP and APLP2 are essential at PNS and CNS synapses for transmission, spatial learning and LTP. *EMBO J* **30:** 2266–2280.

White AR, Reyes R, Mercer JF, Camakaris J, Zheng H, Bush AI, Multhaup G, Beyreuther K, Masters CL, Cappai R. 1999. Copper levels are increased in the cerebral cortex and liver of APP and APLP2 knockout mice. *Brain Res* **842:** 439–444.

Wiese M, Antebi A, Zheng H. 2010. Intracellular trafficking and synaptic function of APL-1 in *Caenorhabditis elegans*. *PLoS ONE* **5:** e12790.

Yamazaki T, Selkoe DJ, Koo EH. 1995. Trafficking of cell surface β-amyloid precursor protein: Retrograde and transcytotic transport in cultured neurons. *J Cell Biol* **129:** 431–442.

Yamazaki T, Koo EH, Selkoe DJ. 1997. Cell surface amyloid β-protein precursor colocalizes with β 1 integrins at substrate contact sites in neural cells. *J Neurosci* **17:** 1004–1010.

Yang G, Gong YD, Gong K, Jiang WL, Kwon E, Wang P, Zheng H, Zhang XF, Gan WB, Zhao NM. 2005. Reduced synaptic vesicle density and active zone size in mice lacking amyloid precursor protein (APP) and APP-like protein 2. *Neurosci Lett* **384:** 66–71.

Yang Z, Cool BH, Martin GM, Hu Q. 2006. A dominant role for FE65 (APBB1) in nuclear signaling. *J Biol Chem* **281:** 4207–4214.

Yang L, Wang B, Long C, Wu G, Zheng H. 2007. Increased asynchronous release and aberrant calcium channel activation in amyloid precursor protein deficient neuromuscular synapses. *Neuroscience* **149:** 768–778.

Yang L, Wang Z, Wang B, Justice NJ, Zheng H. 2009. Amyloid precursor protein regulates Cav1.2 L-type calcium channel levels and function to influence GABAergic short-term plasticity. *J Neurosci* **29:** 15660–15668.

Young-Pearse TL, Bai J, Chang R, Zheng JB, LoTurco JJ, Selkoe DJ. 2007. A critical function for β-amyloid precursor protein in neuronal migration revealed by in utero RNA interference. *J Neurosci* **27:** 14459–14469.

Young-Pearse TL, Chen AC, Chang R, Marquez C, Selkoe DJ. 2008. Secreted APP regulates the function of full-length APP in neurite outgrowth through interaction with integrin β1. *Neural Dev* **3:** 15.

Zhang YW, Wang R, Liu Q, Zhang H, Liao FF, Xu H. 2007. Presenilin/γ-secretase-dependent processing of β-amyloid precursor protein regulates EGF receptor expression. *Proc Natl Acad Sci* **104:** 10613–10618.

Zhao G, Cui MZ, Mao G, Dong Y, Tan J, Sun L, Xu X. 2005. {γ}-Cleavage is dependent on {ζ}-cleavage during the proteolytic processing of amyloid precursor protein within its transmembrane domain. *J Biol Chem* **280:** 37689–37697.

Zheng H, Koo EH. 2006. The amyloid precursor protein: Beyond amyloid. *Mol Neurodegener* **1:** 5.

Zheng H, Jiang M, Trumbauer ME, Sirinathsinghji DJ, Hopkins R, Smith DW, Heavens RP, Dawson GR, Boyce S, Conner MW, et al. 1995. β-Amyloid precursor protein-deficient mice show reactive gliosis and decreased locomotor activity. *Cell* **81:** 525–531.

The Genetics of Alzheimer Disease

Rudolph E. Tanzi

Genetics and Aging Research Unit, Department of Neurology, MassGeneral Institute for Neurodegenerative Disease, Massachusetts General Hospital, Harvard Medical School, Boston, Massachusetts 02129

Correspondence: tanzi@helix.mgh.harvard.edu

Family history is the second strongest risk factor for Alzheimer disease (AD) following advanced age. Twin and family studies indicate that genetic factors are estimated to play a role in at least 80% of AD cases. The inheritance of AD exhibits a dichotomous pattern. On one hand, rare mutations in *APP*, *PSEN1*, and *PSEN2* virtually guarantee early-onset (<60 years) familial AD, which represents ~5% of AD. On the other hand, common gene polymorphisms, such as the ε4 and ε2 variants of the *APOE* gene, can influence susceptibility for ~50% of the common late-onset AD. These four genes account for 30%–50% of the inheritability of AD. Genome-wide association studies have recently led to the identification of 11 additional AD candidate genes. This paper reviews the past, present, and future attempts to elucidate the complex and heterogeneous genetic underpinnings of AD.

GENETICS OF EARLY-ONSET FAMILIAL ALZHEIMER DISEASE

Following advanced age, family history is the second greatest risk factor for Alzheimer disease (AD). AD is considered to be a genetically dichotomous disease presenting in two forms: early-onset familial cases usually characterized by Mendelian inheritance (EO-FAD), and late-onset (≥60 years), with no consistent mode of transmission (LOAD; Bertram and Tanzi 2005; Tanzi and Bertram 2005). Familial clustering of AD cases is more obvious for the early-onset form that strikes under the age of 60 years. However, it is estimated that up to 80% of AD involves the inheritance of genetic factors, based on twin and family studies (Gatz et al. 2006). So-called "sporadic" AD is strongly influenced by genetic variants combined with life exposure factors. EO-FAD is most often caused by rare, fully penetrant mutations in three different genes.

In 1987, we as well as others isolated the amyloid β (A4) protein precursor (*APP*; Goldgaber et al. 1987; Kang et al. 1987; Tanzi et al. 1987a, 1988) and mapped it to chromosome 21. The cloning of APP was carried out based on the hypothesis that it would be an AD gene. Glenner and Wong (1984) first put forward the prediction that the gene responsible for the production β-amyloid, which makes up senile plaques and cerebral blood vessel deposits of amyloid, would be on chromosome 21 and carry mutations causing AD. In that same seminal study, they were able to analyze cerebral β-amyloid deposits to derive the partial amino acid sequence of the amyloid β protein (Aβ). Glenner also proposed that AD is a cerebral amyloidosis, in which cerebral β-amyloid drives all subsequent pathology (see Fig. 1). This central thesis was later reinterpreted and reported as the "amyloid cascade hypothesis" of AD (Hardy and Higgins 1992; Hardy and Selkoe 2002; Tanzi and Bertram 2005).

In the same issue of *Science* reporting the isolation of APP (Goldgaber et al. 1987; Tanzi et al. 1987a), we simultaneously reported genetic linkage of EO-FAD to genetic markers on chromosome 21 in the vicinity of APP (St George-Hyslop et al. 1987). Interestingly, we would later show that the four large EO-FAD families used in that study were not genetically linked to *APP* (Tanzi et al. 1987b); they were ultimately demonstrated to carry *PSEN1* mutations (Sherrington et al. 1995). The concurrent genetic linkage of these four EO-FAD families to both *PSEN1* and markers on the proximal portion of chromosome 21 remains to be resolved.

These studies prompted other groups, including that of John Hardy, to test and confirm the genetic linkage of other independent EO-FAD families to our markers on chromosome 21. In 1991, the first EO-FAD mutation was found in *APP* by resequencing these independent EO-FAD families that were tightly linked to chromosome 21 (Goate et al. 1991). However, prior to the Goate et al. (1991) paper, Frangione and colleagues had already reported the first pathogenic mutation in APP (Levy et al. 1990). Their sequencing of exons 16 and 17 of *APP*, encoding the Aβ portion, uncovered a pathogenic mutation in APP responsible for Dutch hereditary cerebral hemorrhage with amyloidosis. Goate et al. (1991), then resequenced the same two *APP* exons to reveal the first EO-FAD mutation (London mutation; V717I) in *APP*.

By 1992, it was clear that mutations in *APP* accounted for only a tiny proportion of EO-FAD. In fact, none of the 50 EO-FAD families that we resequenced in our laboratory between

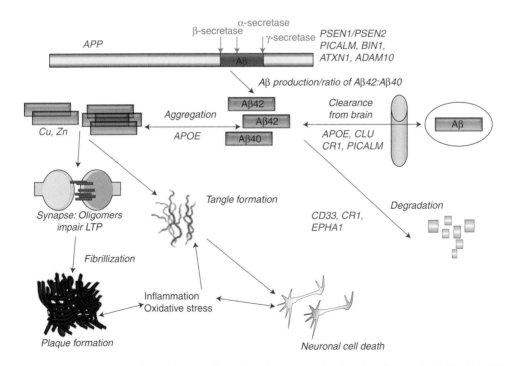

Figure 1. Potential roles of select Alzheimer disease (AD) genes in Aβ-related pathogenesis of AD. (Modified from Bertram and Tanzi 2008; reprinted with permission from the author.)

1987 and 1988 revealed *APP* mutations. In 1995, several EO-FAD mutations were found in presenilin 1 (*PSEN1*; Sherrington et al. 1995) on chromosome 14. This was reported in a study led by Peter St. George-Hyslop and a large host of collaborators, including our laboratory. Shortly thereafter, we first reported a homolog of *PSEN1* called presenilin (*PSEN2*; Levy-Lahad et al. 1995) on chromosome 1 and showed that it harbors the N141I mutation in Volga-German EO-FAD families. This was confirmed by Rogaev et al. (1995) shortly afterward.

To date, 24 mutations (plus duplications) have been reported for *APP*, 185 for *PSEN1*, and 13 for *PSEN2* (Table 1; Alzheimer Disease and Frontotemporal Dementia Mutation Database; http://www.molgen.ua.ac.be/ADMutations). All but one of these mutations (*PSEN2*-N141I) is inherited with EO-FAD in a fully penetrant, autosomal-dominant manner. Another mutation in *APP* is transmitted in a recessive manner.

All but a handful of the more than 200 EO-FAD mutations in *APP*, *PSEN1* and *PSEN2* lead to a common molecular phenotype: an increase in the ratio of $A\beta_{42}$:$A\beta_{40}$ (Scheuner et al. 1996; Tanzi and Bertram 2005). One mutation (Swedish) in APP increases all species of $A\beta$ and several others, resulting in amino acid substitution within the $A\beta$ domain and leading to increased aggregation of $A\beta$. However, most EO-FAD mutations increase the ratio of $A\beta_{42}$:$A\beta_{40}$ (Table 2). The relative increase in $A\beta_{42}$ promotes the aggregation of the peptide into oligomers and ultimately amyloid fibrils (Jarrett et al. 1993).

Three years after their discovery in 1995, the presenilins were shown to be necessary for the generation of $A\beta$ from APP (De Strooper et al. 1998). One year later, Wolfe et al. (1999) showed that the presenilins act as aspartyl proteases that carry out γ-secretase cleavage of APP to produce $A\beta$. γ-Secretase can generate a variety of $A\beta$ species ranging in size from 37 to 46 amino acids. Whether EO-FAD mutations appear in APP near the γ-secretase cleavage site or in the presenilins, the vast majority of them serve to increase the ratio of $A\beta_{42}$:$A\beta_{40}$. γ-Secretase modulators are aimed at reversing this ratio and represent very promising compounds for treating and preventing AD based on what has been garnered from studies addressing the molecular mechanism of EOFAD mutations (Table 1) in *APP*, *PSEN1* and *PSEN1* (Kounnas et al. 2010).

ADDITIONAL EO-FAD CANDIDATE GENES

Beyond *APP*, *PSEN1*, and *PSEN2* attempts to identify additional EO-FAD genes have led to potentially pathogenic mutations in three other genes. A missense mutation (R406W) in the tau gene (*MAPT*) on chromosome 17q was reported to be tightly linked to AD in a Belgian family (Rademakers et al. 2003; Ostojic et al. 2004). However, before, this mutation can be validated to cause AD, autopsy confirmation will be necessary to rule out a diagnosis of frontotemporal lobe dementia (FTDP-17). EO-FAD in a family from the Netherlands was also linked to chromosome 7q36 (Rademakers et al. 2005) near the PAX transcription activation domain interacting protein gene (*PAXIP1*). Finally, the gene for PEN2 on chromosome 19, encoding the γ-secretase component, pen-2, was reported to harbor a missense mutation, D90N, in an AD family (Frigerio et al. 2005). To date, no functional consequences have been demonstrated for this mutation. Clearly, all three

Table 1. Early-onset familial Alzheimer disease genes and their pathogenic effects

Gene	Protein	Chromosome	Mutations	Molecular phenotype
APP	Amyloid β (A4) protein precursor	21q21	24 (duplication)	Increased $A\beta_{42}/A\beta_{40}$ ratio Increased $A\beta$ production Increased $A\beta$ aggregation
PSEN1	Presenilin 1	14q24	185	Increased $A\beta_{42}/A\beta_{40}$ ratio
PSEN2	Presenilin 2	1q31	14	Increased $A\beta_{42}/A\beta_{40}$ ratio

Table 2. Results of select genome-wide association studies of late-onset Alzheimer disease

Genome-wide association studies	Study design	Population	Major genes identified
Reiman et al. 2007	Case–control	US	*APOE, GAB2*
Bertram 2008	Family-based	US	*APOE, ATXN1, CD33, GWA_14q31*
Lambert et al. 2009	Case–control	US, Europe	*APOE, CLU, CR1*
Harold et al. 2009	Case–control	US, Europe	*APOE, CLU, PICALM*
Seshadri et al. 2010	Case–control	US, Europe	*APOE, BIN1*
Naj et al. 2011	Case–control	US, Europe	*MS4A6A/MS4A4E, EPHA1, CD33, CD2AP*
Hollingworth et al. 2011	Case–control	US, Europe	*ABCA7, MS4A6A/MS4A4E, EPHA1, CD33, CD2AP*

of these additional EO-FAD candidate genes will require further confirmation.

GENETICS OF LATE-ONSET AD: *APOE*

Late-onset Alzheimer is the most common form of the disease and is defined by onset age >65 years. Whereas EO-FAD is characterized by classic Mendelian inheritance usually in an autosomal-dominant manner, for LOAD, we observe a genetically complex pattern of inheritance in which genetic risk factors work together with environmental factors and life exposure events to determine lifetime risk for AD. Consequently, it is much more difficult to reliably identify novel LOAD loci, especially because efforts at replication are often plagued by a mixture of replications and refutations.

Thus far, the only gene variant considered to be an *established* LOAD risk factor is the ε4 allele of the apolipoprotein E gene (*APOE*; Strittmatter et al. 1993) on chromosome 19q13. The road to the identification of *APOE* as an AD gene began with genetic linkage of LOAD to chromosome 19 in the vicinity of *APOE* followed by the finding that apoE binds Aβ in cerebrospinal fluid leading. Thus, *APOE* represented a viable AD candidate gene based on both functional data *and* genomic position. The three major alleles of *APOE* correspond to combinations of amino acids at residues 112 and 158 (ε2: Cys_{112}/Cys_{158}; ε3: Cys_{112}/Arg_{158}; ε4: Arg_{112}/Arg_{158}). The ε4-allele of *APOE* increases AD risk by approximately fourfold when inherited in one copy and by greater than 10-fold for two doses of the allele. In contrast, the ε2 allele

of *APOE* exerts "protective" effects (Corder et al. 1994).

Whereas the EO-FAD mutations are sufficient, but not necessary, to cause AD, the *APOE* ε4 allele is neither necessary nor sufficient to cause AD. Instead, it operates as a genetic risk factor for AD that decreases the age of onset in a dose-dependent manner. Functionally, APOE normally plays a role in lipid metabolism and transport. However, in AD, it is believed to play a role in the clearance of Aβ from brain.

Roses et al. (2010) has proposed that other genes in the genomic neighborhood of *APOE* may actually confer risk for AD, for example, a polymorphic poly-T variant in the *TOMM40* gene encoding the translocase of outer mitochondrial membrane 40 homolog. This gene is in complete linkage disequilibrium with *APOE* as it maps only ∼2000 base pairs away. "Long" poly-T repeats have been reported to be associated with earlier onset regardless of *APOE* genotype. Whereas it is theoretically possible that both *APOE* and *TOMM40* contribute to AD risk and just happen to reside next to each other in the genome, "Occam's razor" and simple reason would dictate that only one of these genes is responsible for AD risk in this region of chromosome 19. Because functional studies have shown that *APOE* genotype influences cerebral Aβ clearance, *APOE* would appear to be the more likely candidate versus *TOMM40*.

It should also be noted that several other genes in linkage disequilibrium with *APOE*, in addition to *TOMM40*, also exhibit significant association with AD including *BCAM*, *PVRL2*, and *APOC1*. However, in our own family-based association studies of AD, the strength of association of *APOE* with AD is 15 orders of magnitude higher than that observed for any of these other genes in this region, including *TOMM40* (unpublished data). This adds further support to the notion that *APOE* is the sole AD genetic risk factor in this region of linkage disequilibrium on chromosome 19.

GENETICS OF LATE-ONSET AD: ALZGENE

Since the original report of *APOE* as a genetic risk factor for LOAD, hundreds of genes have been tested for association with AD and reported in the literature. With the rapidly growing number of AD genetic studies published every month, it has become increasingly difficult to follow and interpret the published data. To address this problem, Lars Bertram, colleagues, and I started the online database, AlzGene.org, which provides a routinely updated online database and meta-analyses for the growing list of AD candidate genes ("AlzGene"; URL: www.alzgene.org; Bertram 2007; Bertram and Tanzi 2008).

Meta-analysis results on AlzGene reveal more than three dozen loci that show nominally significant association with risk for AD and 10 with nominal *p*-values $< 10^{-5}$. The 10 genes with the strongest signals for association with AD include *APOE* and nine others, all of which came from genome-wide association studies (GWASs). The GWAS hits are discussed in a separate section below.

Many genes with weak but significant meta-analysis signals have in common that they did not derive from GWASs. These include, for example, *SORL1* (sortilin-related receptor), which is a sorting receptor that regulates the intracellular trafficking of a variety of proteins, including APP (Andersen et al. 2005; Rogaeva et al. 2007). Another is *ACE* (angiotensin converting enzyme 1; Kehoe et al. 1999), a zinc metalloprotease involved in controlling blood pressure, which may increase the risk for AD. ACE is also able to degrade Aβ in vitro (Hu et al. 2001; Hemming et al. 2005). A third

example is *IL8* (interleukin 8), a cytokine mediating inflammatory responses (Mines et al. 2007). A final example is *LDLR* (low-density lipoprotein receptor), which serves as a receptor for APOE and removes low-density lipoproteins (LDL and VLDL) from circulation (Kim et al. 2009).

GENETICS OF LATE-ONSET AD: GENOME-WIDE ASSOCIATION STUDIES

Over the past several years, the most common strategy for finding novel AD gene candidates has been the genome-wide association study. In a GWAS, as many as one million genetic markers (single nucleotide polymorphisms, SNPs) are tested for genetic association with disease risk and/or phenotypic endophenotypes such as age-of-onset, biomarkers, imaging results, and neuropathological endpoints. More than a dozen GWASs have been reported for AD (reviewed in Bertram et al. 2009, 2010; Table 2). The first genome-wide significant finding was reported for *GAB2* (GRB2-associated binding protein 2) by (Reiman et al. 2007); however, it required post hoc stratification by APOE to reach significance. This association was followed up with a series of replications and refutations. GAB2 has been proposed to influence tau phosphorylation (Reiman et al. 2007) and to modulate Aβ production by binding growth factor receptor-bound protein 2 (GRB2), which binds APP and the presenilins (Nizzari et al. 2007).

In 2008, we reported the first genes to directly exhibit genome-wide significant association with AD without the need for stratification on APOE. We employed a family-based GWAS approach (Bertram et al. 2008) and discovered three novel AD genes candidates including *ATXN1* (ataxin 1), *CD33* (siglec 3), and an uncharacterized locus on chromosome 14 (GWA_14q31.2). *ATXN1* can harbor an expanded polyglutamine repeat that causes spinocerebellar ataxia type 1. With regard to AD, we later showed that *ATXN1* affects Aβ levels by modulating β-secretase levels and cleavage of APP (Zhang et al. 2010). This finding was confirmed in vivo in ATXN1 knockout mice, which also suffer cognitive impairment after 6 mo of age (unpublished data). *CD33* is a member of the family of sialic acid–binding, immunoglobulin-like lectins. These molecules promote cell–cell interactions that regulate the innate immune system (Crocker et al. 2007), including inflammation. Interestingly, the innate immune system has recently gained increased attention in AD, with our discovery that Aβ may act as an antimicrobial peptide in the brain's innate immune system (Soscia et al. 2010). *CD33* also resides in the top ten meta-analysis hits on AlzGene.org.

In 2009, two large case–control GWASs (Harold et al. 2009; Lambert et al. 2009) reported three novel AD genes: *CLU* (clusterin; apolipoprotein J), *CR1* (complement component (3b/4b) receptor 1), and *PICALM* (phosphatidylinositol binding clathrin assembly protein). These three loci have been widely replicated in independent follow-up studies and are listed in the top 10 of AlzGene.org meta-analysis hits. Like *APOE*, two of these genes (*CLU* on chromosome 8 and *CR1* on chromosome 1) map in previously implicated LOAD genetic linkage peaks (Butler et al. 2009). Despite the strong statistical support for these three candidates, the effects of these genes on risk for AD are exceedingly small with allelic odds ratios (ORs) of ~1.15 for all three genes, that is, increasing or decreasing risk by ~1.15×. In contrast, the OR for APOE ε4 is ~4 or 15 for one or two alleles, respectively.

At the functional level, clusterin (CLU) has been reported to be involved in transport of Aβ from plasma to brain and Aβ fibrillization (DeMattos et al. 2004; Nuutinen et al. 2009). PICALM is involved in clathrin-mediated endocytosis (Tebar et al. 1999), which is necessary for APP to be processed by γ-secretase into Aβ (Koo and Squazzo 1994). CR1 is the receptor for complement C3b, a key inflammatory molecule that is activated as part of the brain's innate immune system in AD (Khera et al. 2009), and may be able to protect against Aβ-induced neurotoxicity (Rogers et al. 2006).

In 2010, the results of another large case–control GWAS were reported, suggesting the existence of additional AD genetic risk factors (Seshadri et al. 2010). Among them was the gene *BIN1* (bridging integrator 1), which had previously been reported to be associated with AD with subgenome-wide significance (Lambert et al. 2009). *BIN1* is also a top 10 meta-analysis hit on AlzGene and has a tiny effect on AD risk with an allelic OR of ~1.15. *BIN1* (amphiphysin II) is highly expressed in the central nervous system and plays a role in receptor-mediated endocytosis (Pant et al. 2009), which could theoretically affect APP processing and Aβ production or Aβ clearance from brain.

In 2011, two more large case–control GWASs were reported, leading to four more Alzheimer gene candidates: *CD2AP, MS4A6A/ MS4A4E, EPHA1*, and *ABCA7* (Hollingworth et al. 2011; Naj et al. 2011). These studies also identified an additional SNP in *CD33* that influenced risk for AD. Whereas we had previously reported a *CD33* SNP that increased risk for AD with genome-wide significant association (Bertram et al. 2008) using family-based GWASs, these two case–control GWASs reported an SNP roughly 1400 base pairs away that conferred protection against AD. Collectively, our 2008 study along with this 2011 study shows that *CD33* is now the only gene besides *APOE* that exhibits genome-wide significance for association with AD in both case–control and family-based GWASs. Additionally, both genes harbor SNPs that can confer either risk or protection for AD.

When one considers the three EO-FAD genes (*APP, PSEN1*, and *PSEN2*), the LOAD gene (*APOE*), and the 11 genes (*CD33, GWA_14q31.2, ATXN1, CLU, PICALM, CR1, BIN1, ABCA7, MS4A6E/MS4A4E, CD2AP,* and *EPHA1*) exhibiting genome-wide significance for association with LOAD, we now have 15 established AD genes (Table 2). However, we only know the pathogenic gene variants/ mutations for the original four. With regard to function, roles for these genes in AD pathogenesis can be divided into three basic categories: production, degradation, and clearance of Aβ, lipid metabolism, innate immunity, and cellular signaling (Table 3 and Fig. 1).

Table 3. Predicted pathogenic mechanisms of late-onset Alzheimer disease genes from GWASs

Gene	Protein	Location	Risk change (%)	Proposed molecular phenotype
APOE	Apolipoprotein E	19q13	~400%–1500%	Clearance of Aβ; lipid metabolism
CD33	CD33 (Siglec 3)	19q13.3	~10%	Innate immunity; degradation of Aβ
CLU	Clusterin	8p21.1	~10%	Clearance of Aβ; innate immunity
CR1	Complement component (3b/4b) receptor 1	1q32	~15%	Clearance of Aβ; innate immunity
PICALM	Phosphatidylinositol binding clathrin assembly molecule	11q14	~15%	Production and clearance of Aβ; cellular signaling
BIN1	Bridging integrator 1	2q14	~15%	Production and clearance of Aβ; cellular signaling
ABCA7	ATP-binding cassette subfamily A member 7	19p13.3	~20%	Lipid metabolism; cellular signaling
CD2AP	CD2-associated protein	6p12.3	~10%	Cellular signaling
EPHA1	EPH receptor A1	7q34	~10%	Cellular signaling; innate immunity
MS4A6A/MS4A4E	Membrane-spanning 4-domains, subfamily A, members 6A and 4E	11q12.1	~10%	Cellular signaling
ATXN1	Ataxin 1	6p22.3	NA	Production of Aβ

GENETICS OF LATE-ONSET AD: MISSING HERITABILITY AND *ADAM10*

The GWAS approach involves genotyping common ancestral polymorphisms that usually occur in >5% of the general population. The risk effects exerted by the GWAS-derived genes discussed above are tiny, that is they confer only an ~0.10- to 0.15-fold increase or decrease in AD risk in carriers versus noncarriers of the associated alleles, as compared with a four- to 15-fold increase in AD risk owing to the inheritance of *APOE* ε4. A substantial proportion of the genetic variance of LOAD remains unexplained by the currently known susceptibility genes.

The "missing heritability" of complex and heterogeneous disease has been coined the "dark matter" of GWASs because we know it exists but cannot yet observe it (Manolio et al. 2009). The "dark matter" may be explained by common variants that are not included on existing microarrays, copy number variants including genomic insertion/deletions and rearrangements, and rare sequence variants. With regard to rare variants conferring large effects on risk for LOAD, we recently reported two rare LOAD mutations in the *ADAM10* gene that caused AD at an average age of 70 years in seven of 1000 LOAD families tested (Kim et al. 2009).

ADAM10 encodes the major α-secretase in the brain. This enzyme cleaves within the Aβ domain of APP to preclude the formation of β-amyloid. The two novel *ADAM10* LOAD mutations, Q170H and R181G, are located in the prodomain region, and dramatically impair the ability of ADAM10 to carry out α-secretase cleavage of APP both in vitro (Kim et al. 2008) and in vivo (unpublished observation). Thus, the two LOAD-associated mutations in *ADAM10* would appear to be strong candidates for the first rare, highly penetrant pathogenic mutations to be genetically associated with late-onset AD (Kim et al. 2009). This study then becomes the first (and to date, only) to challenge the rare mutation–rare disease (EO-FAD)/common variant–common disease (LOAD) paradigm that postulates that LOAD is only associated with common variants, (e.g., *APOE* ε4).

The two LOAD mutations in *ADAM10* also argue that, in addition to GWASs, resequencing, for example, using novel high-throughput ("next-generation") technologies and whole-genome or exome sequencing, will be necessary to search for additional rare variants causing LOAD. Along these lines, large-scale resequencing has been employed to create a comprehensive array of all rare mutations in the human genome, known as the "1000 Genomes project" (http://www.1000genomes.org/). This database will aid immensely in determining whether rare mutations found in disease cases are novel and pathogenic. Ultimately, the validation of bona fide pathogenic mutations will require comprehensive functional studies in in vitro systems, in vivo animal models, and clinical samples.

SUMMARY

Our understanding of the etiology and pathogenesis of AD can be arguably be divided into two eras: before and after the identification of the AD genes. The past three decades of genetic research in AD have revolutionized our understanding of the causes of AD and accelerated the discovery and development of novel therapeutics aimed at the treatment and prevention of AD (Tanzi and Bertram 2005). The modern era of AD research guided by genetics began in the 1980s and 1990s with genetic linkage studies and positional cloning efforts that led to the identification of the three EO-FAD genes: *APP*, *PSEN1*, and *PSEN2*. The late-onset AD gene *APOE* was discovered using a similar strategy, but was ultimately validated by genetic association studies. Genetic association studies remain the most common method for identifying novel LOAD genes and are most often employed in the form of large-scale GWASs that screen the entire human genome for novel disease loci. Recently, our family-based and others' case–control GWASs (reviewed in Bertram et al. 2009,

2010) led to the elucidation of novel susceptibility variants, all of which confer only small effects on risk. Moreover, up to 50% the heritability of AD remains unexplained by the known genes and AD candidate loci that have been derived from GWASs.

Our initial understanding of the etiology of AD began with the identification of rare causal mutations in the three EO-FAD genes. More recently, we discovered two rare pathogenic mutations in *ADAM10* that impair ADAM10 enzyme activity and lead to AD by 70 years old with high penetrance (Kim et al. 2009). Based on the roughly 200 EO-FAD gene mutations and two ADAM10 LOAD mutations, it will be important to search for additional rare sequence variants in other genes that predispose to AD. Ultimately, the insights into the etiology and pathogenesis of AD garnered from genetic studies of AD will continue to enhance our understanding of the pathological mechanisms leading to AD. Moreover, these findings will aid in the development of novel therapeutic strategies for preventing, stopping and even reversing AD.

REFERENCES

Andersen OM, Reiche J, Schmidt V, Gotthardt M, Spoelgen R, Behlke J, von Arnim CAF, Breiderhoff T, Jansen P, Wu X, et al. 2005. Neuronal sorting protein-related receptor sorLA/LR11 regulates processing of the amyloid precursor protein. *Proc Natl Acad Sci* **102:** 13461–13466.

Bertram L, Tanzi RE. 2005. The genetic epidemiology of neurodegenerative disease. *J Clin Invest* **115:** 1449–1457.

Bertram L, Tanzi RE. 2008. Thirty years of Alzheimer's disease genetics: Systematic meta-analyses herald a new era. *Nat Rev Neurosci* **9:** 768–778.

Bertram L, Tanzi RE. 2009. Genome-wide association studies in Alzheimer's disease. *Hum Mol Genet* **18:** R137–145.

Bertram L, McQueen MB, Mullin K, Blacker D, Tanzi RE. 2007. Systematic meta-analyses of Alzheimer disease genetic association studies: The AlzGene database. *Nat Genet* **39:** 17–23.

Bertram L, Lange C, Mullin K, Parkinson M, Hsiao M, Hogan MF, Schjeide BMM, Hooli B, Divito J, Ionita I, et al. 2008. Genome-wide association analysis reveals putative Alzheimer's disease susceptibility loci in addition to APOE. *Am J Hum Genet* **83:** 623–632.

Bertram L, Lill CM, Tanzi RE. 2010. The genetics of Alzheimer disease: Back to the future. *Neuron* **68:** 270–281.

Butler AW, Ng MYM, Hamshere ML, Forabosco P, Wroe R, Al-Chalabi A, Lewis CM, Powell JF. 2009. Meta-analysis of linkage studies for Alzheimer's disease—A web resource. *Neurobiol Aging* **30:** 1037–1047.

Corder EH, Saunders AM, Risch NJ, Strittmatter WJ, Schmechel DE, Gaskell PC Jr, Rimmler JB, Locke PA, Conneally PM, Schmader KE, et al. 1994. Protective effect of apolipoprotein E type 2 allele for late onset Alzheimer disease. *Nat Genet* **7**, 180–184.

Crocker PR, Paulson JC, Varki A. 2007. Siglecs and their roles in the immune system. *Nat Rev Immunol* **7:** 255–266.

DeMattos RB, Cirrito JR, Parsadanian M, May PC, O'Dell MA, Taylor JW, Harmony JA, Aronow BJ, Bales KR, Paul SM, et al. 2004. ApoE and clusterin cooperatively suppress Aβ levels and deposition: Evidence that ApoE regulates extracellular Aβ metabolism in vivo. *Neuron* **41**, 193–202.

De Strooper B, Saftig P, Craessaerts K, Vanderstichele H, Guhde G, Annaert W, Von Figura K, Van Leuven F 1998. Deficiency of presenilin-1 inhibits the normal cleavage of amyloid precursor protein. *Nature* **391**, 387–390.

Frigerio C, Piscopo P, Calabrese E, Crestini A, Malvezzi Campeggi L, Civita di Fava R, Fogliarino S, Albani D, Marcon G, Cherchi R, et al. 2005. PEN-2 gene mutation in a familial Alzheimer's disease case. *J Neurol* **252:** 1033–1036.

Gatz M, Reynolds CA, Fratiglioni L, Johansson B, Mortimer JA, Berg S, Fiske A, Pedersen NL. 2006. Role of genes and environments for explaining Alzheimer disease. *Arch Gen Psychiatry* **63**, 168–174.

Glenner GG, Wong CW. 1984. Alzheimer's disease and Down's syndrome: Sharing of a unique cerebrovascular amyloid fibril protein. *Biochem Biophys Res Commun* **122**, 1131–1135.

Goate A, Chartier-Harlin MC, Mullan M, Brown J, Crawford F, Fidani L, Giuffra L, Haynes A, Irving N, James L, et al. 1991. Segregation of a missense mutation in the amyloid precursor protein gene with familial Alzheimer's disease. *Nature* **349:** 704–706.

Goldgaber D, Lerman MI, McBride OW, Saffiotti U, Gajdusek DC. 1987. Characterization and chromosomal localization of a cDNA encoding brain amyloid of Alzheimer's disease. *Science* **235**, 877–880.

Hardy JA, Higgins GA. 1992. Alzheimer's disease: The amyloid cascade hypothesis. *Science* **256**, 184–185.

Hardy J, Selkoe DJ. 2002. The amyloid hypothesis of Alzheimer's disease: Progress and problems on the road to therapeutics. *Science* **297**, 353–356.

Harold D, Abraham R, Hollingworth P, Sims R, Gerrish A, Hamshere ML, Pahwa JS, Moskvina V, Dowzell K, Williams A, et al. 2009. Genome-wide association study identifies variants at CLU and PICALM associated with Alzheimer's disease. *Nat Genet* **41:** 1088–1093.

Hemming ML, Selkoe DJ. 2005. Amyloid β-protein is degraded by cellular angiotensin-converting enzyme (ACE) and elevated by an ACE inhibitor. *J Biol Chem* **280:** 37644–37650.

Hollingworth P, Harold D, Sims R, Gerrish A, Lambert JC, Carrasquillo MM, Abraham R, Hamshere ML, Pahwa JS, Moskvina V, et al. 2011. Common variants at ABCA7, MS4A6A/MS4A4E, EPHA1, CD33 and CD2AP are associated with Alzheimer's disease. *Nat Genet* **43:** 429–435.

Hu J, Igarashi A, Kamata M, Nakagawa H. 2001. Angiotensin-converting enzyme degrades Alzheimer amyloid β-peptide (Aβ); retards Aβ aggregation, deposition, fibril formation; and inhibits cytotoxicity. *J Biol Chem* **276:** 47863–47868.

Jarrett JT, Berger EP, Lansbury PT Jr 1993. The carboxy terminus of the β amyloid protein is critical for the seeding of amyloid formation: Implications for the pathogenesis of Alzheimer's disease. *Biochemistry* **32**, 4693–4697.

Kang J, Lemaire HG, Unterbeck A, Salbaum JM, Masters CL, Grzeschik KH, Multhaup G, Beyreuther K, Muller-Hill B. 1987. The precursor of Alzheimer's disease amyloid A4 protein resembles a cell-surface receptor. *Nature* **325**, 733–736.

Kehoe PG, Russ C, McIlory S, Williams H, Holmans P, Holmes C, Liolitsa D, Vahidassr D, Powell J, McGleenon B, et al. 1999. Variation in DCP1, encoding ACE, is associated with susceptibility to Alzheimer disease. *Nat Genet* **21:** 71–72.

Khera R, Das N. 2009. Complement receptor 1: Disease associations and therapeutic implications. *Mol Immunol* **46:** 761–772.

Kim J, Castellano JM, Jiang H, Basak JM, Parsadanian M, Pham V, Mason SM, Paul SM, Holtzman DM. 2009. Overexpression of low-density lipoprotein receptor in the brain markedly inhibits amyloid deposition and increases extracellular Aβ clearance. *Neuron* **64:** 632–644.

Koo EH, Squazzo SL. 1994. Evidence that production and release of amyloid β-protein involves the endocytic pathway. *J Biol Chem* **269:** 17386–17389.

Kounnas MZ, Danks AM, Cheng S, Tyree C, Ackerman E, Zhang X, Ahn K, Nguyen P, Comer P, Mao L, et al. 2010. Modulation of γ-secretase reduces β-amyloid deposition in a transgenic mouse model of Alzheimer's disease. *Neuron* **67:** 769–780.

Lambert J, Heath S, Even G, Campion D, Sleegers K, Hiltunen M, Combarros O, Zelenika D, Bullido MJ, Tavernier B, et al. 2009. Genome-wide association study identifies variants at CLU and CR1 associated with Alzheimer's disease. *Nat Genet* **41:** 1094–1099.

Levy E, Carman MD, Fernandez-Madrid IJ, Power MD, Lieberburg I, van Duinen SG, Bots GT, Luyendijk W, Frangione B. 1990. Mutation of the Alzheimer's disease amyloid gene in hereditary cerebral hemorrhage, Dutch type. *Science* **248**, 1124–1126.

Levy-Lahad E, Wasco W, Poorkaj P, Romano DM, Oshima J, Pettingell WH, Yu CE, Jondro PD, Schmidt SD, Wang K. 1995. Candidate gene for the chromosome 1 familial Alzheimer's disease locus. *Science* **269:** 973–977.

Manolio TA, Collins FS, Cox NJ, Goldstein DB, Hindorff LA, Hunter DJ, McCarthy MI, Ramos EM, Cardon LR, Chakravarti A, et al. 2009. Finding the missing heritability of complex diseases. *Nature* **461:** 747–753.

Mines M, Ding Y, Fan G. 2007. The many roles of chemokine receptors in neurodegenerative disorders: Emerging new therapeutical strategies. *Curr Med Chem* **14:** 2456–2470.

Naj AC, Jun G, Beecham GW, Wang LS, Vardarajan BN, Buros J, Gallins PJ, Buxbaum JD, Jarvik GP, Crane PK, et al. 2011. Common variants at MS4A4/MS4A6E,

CD2AP, CD33 and EPHA1 are associated with late-onset Alzheimer's disease. *Nat Genet* **43:** 436–441.

Nizzari M, Venezia V, Repetto E, Caorsi V, Magrassi R, Gagliani MC, Carlo P, Florio T, Schettini G, Tacchetti C, et al. 2007. Amyloid precursor protein and Presenilin1 interact with the adaptor GRB2 and modulate ERK 1,2 signaling. *J Biol Chem* **282:** 13833–13844.

Nuutinen T, Suuronen T, Kauppinen A, Salminen A. 2009. Clusterin: A forgotten player in Alzheimer's disease. *Brain Res Rev* **61:** 89–104.

Ostojic J, Elfgren C, Passant U, Nilsson K, Gustafson L, Lannfelt L, Froelich Fabre S. 2004. The tau R406W mutation causes progressive presenile dementia with bitemporal atrophy. *Dement Geriatr Cogn Disord* **17:** 298–301.

Pant S, Sharma M, Patel K, Caplan S, Carr CM, Grant BD. 2009. AMPH-1/Amphiphysin/Bin1 functions with RME-1/Ehd1 in endocytic recycling. *Nat Cell Biol* **11:** 1399–1410.

Rademakers R, Dermaut B, Peeters K, Cruts M, Heutink P, Goate A, Van Broeckhoven C. 2003. Tau (MAPT) mutation Arg406Trp presenting clinically with Alzheimer disease does not share a common founder in Western Europe. *Hum Mutat* **22:** 409–411.

Rademakers R, Cruts M, Sleegers K, Dermaut B, Theuns J, Aulchenko Y, Weckx S, De Pooter T, Van den Broeck M, Corsmit E, et al. 2005. Linkage and association studies identify a novel locus for Alzheimer disease at 7q36 in a Dutch population-based sample. *Am J Hum Genet* **77:** 643–652.

Reiman EM, Webster JA, Myers AJ, Hardy J, Dunckley T, Zismann VL, Joshipura KD, Pearson JV, Hu-Lince D, Huentelman MJ, et al. 2007. Papassotiropoulos A, Stephan DA. GAB2 alleles modify Alzheimer's risk in APOE ε4 carriers. *Neuron* **54:** 713–720.

Rogaev EI, Sherrington R, Rogaeva EA, Levesque G, Ikeda M, Liang Y, Chi H, Lin C, Holman K, Tsuda T. 1995. Familial Alzheimer's disease in kindreds with missense mutations in a gene on chromosome 1 related to the Alzheimer's disease type 3 gene. *Nature* **376:** 775–778.

Rogaeva E, Meng Y, Lee JH, Gu Y, Kawarai T, Zou F, Katayama T, Baldwin CT, Cheng R, Hasegawa H, et al. 2007. The neuronal sortilin-related receptor SORL1 is genetically associated with Alzheimer disease. *Nat Genet* **39:** 168–177.

Rogers J, Li R, Mastroeni D, Grover A, Leonard B, Ahern G, Cao P, Kolody H, Vedders L, Kolb WP, et al. 2006. Peripheral clearance of amyloid β peptide by complement C3-dependent adherence to erythrocytes. *Neurobiol Aging* **27:** 1733–1739.

Roses AD, Lutz MW, Amrine-Madsen H, Saunders AM, Crenshaw DG, Sundseth SS, Huentelman MJ, Welsh-Bohmer KA, Reiman EM. 2010. A TOMM40 variable-length polymorphism predicts the age of late-onset Alzheimer's disease. *Pharmacogenom J* **10,** 375–384.

Scheuner D, Eckman C, Jensen M, Song X, Citron M, Suzuki N, Bird TD, Hardy J, Hutton M, Kukull W, et al. 1996. Secreted amyloid β-protein similar to that in the senile plaques of Alzheimer's disease is increased in vivo by the presenilin 1 and 2 and APP mutations linked to familial Alzheimer's disease. *Nat Med* **2:** 864–870.

Seshadri S, Fitzpatrick AL, Ikram MA, DeStefano AL, Gudnason V, Boada M, Bis JC, Smith AV, Carassquillo MM, Lambert JC, et al. 2010. Genome-wide analysis of genetic loci associated with Alzheimer disease. *JAMA* **303:** 1832–1840.

Sherrington R, Rogaev EI, Liang Y, Rogaeva EA, Levesque G, Ikeda M, Chi H, Lin C, Li G, Holman K, et al. 1995. Cloning of a gene bearing missense mutations in early-onset familial Alzheimer's disease. *Nature* **375:** 754–760.

Soscia SJ, Kirby JE, Washicosky KJ, Tucker SM, Ingelsson M, Hyman B, Burton MA, Goldstein LE, Duong S, Tanzi RE, et al. 2010. The Alzheimer's disease-associated amyloid β-protein is an antimicrobial peptide. *PLoS ONE* **5:** e9505.

St. George-Hyslop PH, Tanzi RE, Polinsky RJ, Haines JL, Nee L, Watkins PC, Myers R, Feldman R, Pollen D, Drachman D, et al. 1987. The genetic defect causing familial Alzheimer's disease maps on Chromosome 21. *Science* **235:** 885–890.

Strittmatter WJ, Saunders AM, Schmechel D, Pericak-Vance M, Enghild J, Salvesen GS, Roses AD. 1993. Apolipoprotein E: High-avidity binding to β-amyloid and increased frequency of type 4 allele in late-onset familial Alzheimer disease. *Proc Natl Acad Sci* **90:** 1977–1981.

Tanzi RE, Bertram L. 2005. Twenty years of the Alzheimer's disease amyloid hypothesis: A genetic perspective. *Cell* **120:** 545–555.

Tanzi RE, Gusella JF, Watkins PC, Bruns GA, St George-Hyslop P, Van Keuren ML, Patterson D, Pagan S, Kurnit DM, Neve RL. 1987a. Amyloid β protein gene: cDNA, mRNA distribution, and genetic linkage near the Alzheimer locus. *Science* **235:** 880–884.

Tanzi RE, St. George-Hyslop PH, Haines JL, Polinsky RJ, Nee L, Foncin J-F, Neve RL, McClatchey AI, Conneally PM, Gusella JF. 1987b. The genetic defect in familial Alzheimer's disease is not tightly linked to the amyloid β protein gene. *Nature* **329:** 156–157.

Tanzi RE, McClatchey AI, Lamperti ED, V-Komaroff L, Gusella JF, Neve R. 1988. Protease inhibitor domain encoded by an amyloid protein precursor mRNA associated with Alzheimer's disease. *Nature* **331:** 528–530.

Tebar F, Bohlander SK, Sorkin A. 1999. Clathrin assembly lymphoid myeloid leukemia (CALM) protein: Localization in endocytic-coated pits, interactions with clathrin, and the impact of overexpression on clathrin-mediated traffic. *Mol Biol Cell* **10:** 2687–2702.

Wolfe MS, Xia W, Ostaszewski BL, Diehl TS, Kimberly WT, Selkoe DJ. 1999. Two transmembrane aspartates in presenilin-1 required for presenilin endoproteolysis and γ-secretase activity. *Nature* **398,** 513–517.

Zhang C, Browne A, Child D, Divito JR, Stevenson JA, Tanzi RE. 2010. Loss of function of ATXN1 increases amyloid β-protein levels by potentiating β-secretase processing of β-amyloid precursor protein. *J Biol Chem* **285:** 8515–8526.

Presenilins and γ-Secretase: Structure, Function, and Role in Alzheimer Disease

Bart De Strooper[1,2], Takeshi Iwatsubo[3], and Michael S. Wolfe[4]

[1]Center for Human Genetics, Leuven Institute for Neurodegenerative Diseases, KULeuven, 3000 Leuven, Belgium

[2]Department for Molecular and Developmental Genetics, VIB, 3000 Leuven, Belgium

[3]Department of Neuropathology, Graduate School of Medicine, University of Tokyo, Tokyo 113-0033, Japan

[4]Center for Neurologic Diseases, Brigham and Women's Hospital and Harvard Medical School, Boston, Massachusetts 02115

Correspondence: mwolfe@rics.bwh.harvard.edu

Presenilins were first discovered as sites of missense mutations responsible for early-onset Alzheimer disease (AD). The encoded multipass membrane proteins were subsequently found to be the catalytic components of γ-secretases, membrane-embedded aspartyl protease complexes responsible for generating the carboxyl terminus of the amyloid β-protein (Aβ) from the amyloid protein precursor (APP). The protease complex also cleaves a variety of other type I integral membrane proteins, most notably the Notch receptor, signaling from which is involved in many cell differentiation events. Although γ-secretase is a top target for developing disease-modifying AD therapeutics, interference with Notch signaling should be avoided. Compounds that alter Aβ production by γ-secretase without affecting Notch proteolysis and signaling have been identified and are currently at various stages in the drug development pipeline.

As described in Haas et al. (2011), the amyloid protein precursor (APP) undergoes successive proteolysis by β- and γ-secretases to produce the amyloid β-protein (Aβ) that characteristically deposits in the brain in Alzheimer disease (AD). Both of these proteases are top targets for AD drug discovery, although each presents challenges for developing safe and effective therapeutics. γ-Secretase is a large complex of four different integral membrane proteins, with presenilin as the catalytic component comprising an unusual membrane-embedded aspartyl protease. Herein, we describe the discovery of the γ-secretase components,

the biological functions of γ-secretase, as well as other roles of presenilin outside the protease complex, what is known so far about the structure of the complex, the role of γ-secretase in disease (especially in AD), and the current status and direction of γ-secretase inhibitors and modulators as candidate AD therapeutics.

THE IDENTIFICATION OF THE PRESENILINS AND THE OTHER γ-SECRETASE SUBUNITS

The name "γ-secretase" was used for the first time in 1993 to describe the proteolytic activity that cleaves APP in the transmembrane domain

(TMD) (Haass and Selkoe 1993). It took about 10 years to identify all of the components of the molecular machine responsible for this cleavage (De Strooper 2003). The first step forward was in 1995 when two lines of genetic investigation merged unexpectedly into the identification of the presenilins. Analysis of families with inherited forms of AD were found to contain mutations in the until then unknown genes *presenilin 1* (*PSEN1*; see Fig. 1 for protein sequence, topology, and sites of mutations) on chromosome 14q24.3 (Alzheimer's Disease Collaborative Group 1995; Sherrington et al. 1995) and *presenilin 2* (*PSEN2*) on chromosome 1q42.2 (Levy-Lahad et al. 1995; Rogaev et al. 1995). A second line of genetic investigation, in the worm *Caenorhabditis elegans*, inde-

pendently identified a presenilin gene as a suppressor of *lin-12* gain-of-function mutants (Levitan and Greenwald 1995). *lin-12* is the worm ortholog of *Notch*, a gene critical for cell signaling during development. Thus, presenilin was important in the pathogenesis of AD and at the same time for development by regulating Notch signaling. However, the link between these two functions remained unclear, and it was proposed that presenilins could act as a channel, a receptor, or a transporter protein or even affect tau phosphorylation and dysfunction.

The first clue to the role of presenilins in APP processing came from observations that AD-causing mutations in *PSEN1* and *PSEN2* (more than 150 different mutations in these

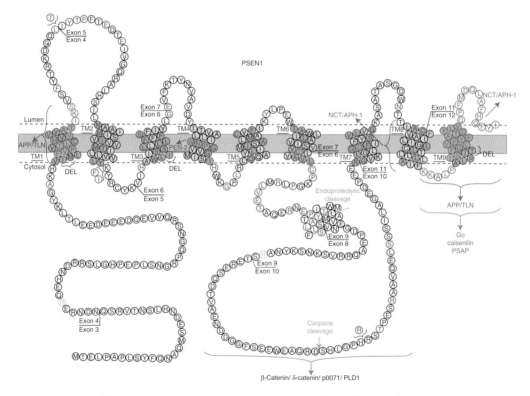

Figure 1. Amino acid sequence, topology, and mutations in *presenilin 1*. Single amino acid residues that have been found to be substituted by mutations causing familial AD are indicated in red. Exon/intron boundaries, the different transmembrane domains (TM1-TM9), residues (blue) involved in the interaction with amyloid precursor protein (APP), telencephalin (TLN), PEN-2, Nicastrin (NCT), and APH-1 are indicated with brackets. (This figure was adapted from Dillen and Annaert 2006; reprinted, with permission, from Elsevier ©2006. It is based on a figure published on the Alzforum website http://www.alzforum.org/res/com/mut/pre/diagram1.asp.)

genes have been identified) affect the generation of Aβ peptides, changing the relative amount of Aβ42 peptide (Aβ containing 42 amino acid residues) versus the shorter Aβ40 (the more abundantly generated peptide, containing 40 amino acid residues; see Haas et al. 2011). This was shown in fibroblasts derived from patients (Scheuner et al. 1996), by overexpressing the mutant presenilins in cell lines (Borchelt et al. 1996; Citron et al. 1997), and by experiments in living mice, either overexpressing the mutant presenilin in brain using various promoters (Borchelt et al. 1996, 1997; Duff et al. 1996; Citron et al. 1997) or by knocking in mutations in the endogenous mouse presenilin gene (Siman et al. 2000; Flood et al. 2002).

The function of presenilin in the γ-secretase proteolytic activity became apparent when neurons were derived from *PSEN1* knockout mice and used to show that PSEN1 was critically involved in the generation of all Aβ peptides (De Strooper et al. 1998). This experiment established presenilin as an important AD drug target (Haass and Selkoe 1998). The central role of presenilin in the γ-secretase processing of Notch was established a year later in mouse and *Drosophila* (De Strooper et al. 1999; Struhl and Greenwald 1999). Furthermore, because a γ-secretase inhibitor was shown to block not only APP processing but also Notch cleavage (De Strooper et al. 1999), it was suggested that a presenilin-dependent protease was responsible for both cleavages, and that blocking this enzyme would cause major side effects in patients. Notch is indeed not only involved in embryogenesis and development but also in differentiation of immune cells, the goblet cells in the intestine, and others (van Es et al. 2005).

At the same time, other studies suggested that presenilin was actually the catalytic subunit of γ-secretase. Site-directed mutagenesis of two aspartyl residues embedded in the TMDs VI and VII of PSEN1 resulted in a dominant-negative effect on γ-secretase activity, suggesting that presenilin was a protease, specifically of the aspartyl type (Wolfe et al. 1999b). These mutations did not affect the expression or the incorporation of presenilin into the γ-secretase

complex (Nyabi et al. 2003), and are in a conserved region of the presenilin proteins (Steiner et al. 2000). They are found in a family of related intramembrane-cleaving proteases, the signal peptide peptidases (SPP) (Ponting et al. 2002; Weihofen et al. 2002). Finally, transition-state analog (i.e., active site-directed) γ-secretase inhibitors were shown to directly bind to the presenilin subunit of the γ-secretase complex (Esler et al. 2000; Li, Xu et al. 2000), providing convincing evidence that presenilin is indeed a protease.

In mammals, two homologous proteins exist, i.e., PSEN1 and PSEN2. They are both synthesized as precursor proteins of 50 kDa with nine TMDs (Laudon et al. 2005; Spasic et al. 2006), and are cleaved into a 30 kDa amino-terminal fragment (NTF) and a 20 kDa carboxy-terminal fragment (CTF) during maturation (Thinakaran et al. 1996), probably by autocatalysis (Wolfe et al. 1999b,c; Fukumori et al. 2010).

Together with other proteases, presenilins represent a novel class of intramembrane-cleaving proteases or *i*-clips (Wolfe et al. 1999c; Wolfe and Kopan 2004). However, the presenilins are different from other *i*-clips, in the sense that they need three other protein subunits to achieve optimal activity. Early reports already suggested that it is not possible to overexpress presenilin in a functionally active way, as additional proteins ("limiting factors") are needed for presenilin to mature into stable NTF plus CTF heterodimers (Baumann et al. 1997; Thinakaran et al. 1997). The first "limiting" factor was coisolated in an immuno-chemical purification protocol using antibodies against presenilin. The resultant 130 kDa type I integral membrane protein was baptized Nicastrin (Yu et al. 2000). The genes for Nicastrin and for the two other proteins of the γ-secretase complex were also identified independently in screens for modifiers of Notch homologs *glp-1* and *lin-12* in *C. elegans*. Aph-1 (for "anterior pharynx-defective phenotype") is a 30 kDa protein with 7 TMDs (Goutte et al. 2000; Levitan et al. 2001; Goutte et al. 2002), and Pen-2 (for "presenilin enhancer") is a 12 kDa hairpinlike, two-transmembrane protein (Francis et al. 2002). A series of reconstitution and knockdown experiments established that the four proteins (Fig. 2) are necessary and sufficient for γ-secretase processing (Edbauer et al. 2003; Kimberly et al. 2003; Takasugi et al. 2003). Both genetic screens (Francis et al. 2002) and recent purifications of the γ-secretase complex (Teranishi et al. 2009; Wakabayashi et al. 2009; Winkler et al. 2009) were not able to identify additional proteins stably associated with the complex, suggesting strongly that the core of the complex has been identified. Additional proteins might, however, be involved in the regulation of the activity or subcellular localization of the complex (Chen et al. 2006; Wakabayashi et al. 2009; He et al. 2010).

The stoichiometry of the γ-secretase complex is likely 1:1:1:1, based on molecular mass estimates in blue native electrophoresis (Kimberly et al. 2003), quantitative western blot analysis (Sato et al. 2007), and electron microscopy (EM) studies of the purified complex (Osenkowski et al. 2009). Thus, as there are two different *PSEN* genes and two different *Aph1* genes (Aph1a and Aph1b) encoded in the human genome, it follows that at least four different γ-secretase complexes exist (De Strooper 2003). The situation is actually even more complicated, as alternatively spliced forms for the presenilins and for Aph-1a have been reported (Alzheimer's Disease Collaborative Group 1995; Gu et al. 2003). The biological significance of this heterogeneity is only now being explored.

THE BIOLOGICAL FUNCTIONS OF PRESENILIN

As discussed, the main function of the presenilins is to provide the catalytic subunits to the different γ-secretases (De Strooper et al. 1998, 1999; Wolfe et al. 1999b; Esler et al. 2000; Li et al. 2000). Over the years, other presenilin functions have been proposed—in protein trafficking and turnover, in calcium homeostasis, in regulation of β-catenin signaling, and others—sometimes within and sometimes outside of the γ-secretase complex. These putatively "nonproteolytic" functions can be shown using presenilins in which the catalytic aspartyl residues (Wolfe et al. 1999b) are replaced by other amino acid residues and showing that a particular function is not dependent on these aspartyl residues. This criterion has been met in several

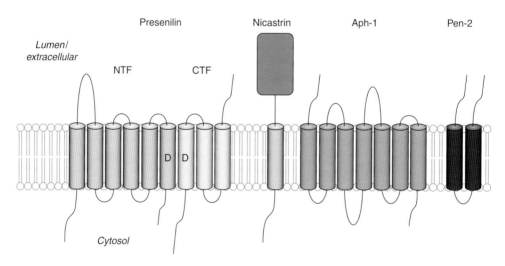

Figure 2. Subunits of the γ-secretase complex and their membrane topologies. Presenilin is proteolytically processed into two fragments during maturation of the complex, an amino-terminal fragment (NTF) and a carboxy-terminal fragment (CTF). The two transmembrane catalytic aspartic acid residues, one in the NTF and one in the CTF, are indicated by D. Other subunits are Nicastrin, APH-1, and PEN-2.

instances, e.g., for the calcium leak function of presenilin in the endoplasmic reticulum (Tu et al. 2006; Nelson et al. 2007), for the growth alterations caused by deficiencies in cytoskeleton function in a presenilin-deficient variant of the moss *Physcomitrella patens* (Khandelwal et al. 2007), or in the turnover of the membrane protein telencephalin (Esselens et al. 2004).

To focus first on the proteolytic functions of γ-secretase (Fig. 3), the crucial and conserved role of presenilin in Notch signaling (Levitan and Greenwald 1995; De Strooper et al. 1999; Struhl and Greenwald 1999) has been repeatedly shown. In all species, severe developmental defects are associated with altered expression of Notch target genes such as the "hairy and enhancer of split" (HES) family. By using conditionally targeted alleles or partial knockouts of presenilin or else γ-secretase inhibitors, it is

possible to evaluate the role of presenilin in Notch signaling in adulthood. Deficiencies in T- and B-cell differentiation (Doerfler et al. 2001; Hadland et al. 2001; Qyang et al. 2004; Tournoy et al. 2004; Wong et al. 2004), bloody diarrhea as a consequence of hampered intestinal goblet cell differentiation (Searfoss et al. 2003; Wong et al. 2004; van Es et al. 2005), and skin and hair defects (Xia et al. 2001; Tournoy et al. 2004), have been observed. Conditional knockout of presenilins in the forebrain (using an *αCaMKII* promoter to drive Cre expression) leads to progressive neurodegeneration, which has been proposed as an argument that loss of presenilin function could contribute to the pathogenesis of sporadic AD independently of affecting $A\beta_{42}$ generation (discussed in Shen and Kelleher 2007). However, the predictable absence of Aβ deposition in these

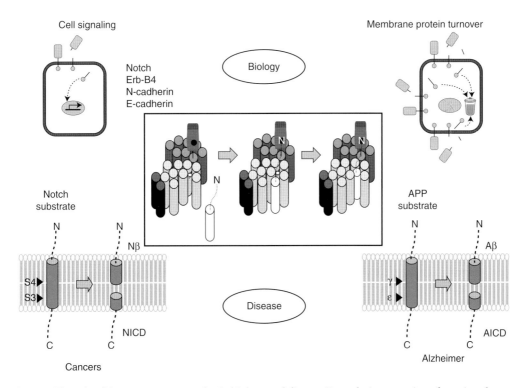

Figure 3. The role of the γ-secretase complex in biology and disease. Proteolytic processing of certain substrates (e.g., Notch, ErbB4, N-cadherin, E-cadherin) leads to cell signaling. Alternatively, processing of substrates by γ-secretase is simply a means of clearing protein stubs from the membrane. Excessive signaling from the Notch receptor leads to certain forms of cancer, and formation of the amyloid β-protein from its precursor APP by γ-secretase is involved in the pathogenesis of Alzheimer disease.

knockout mice means that they do not constitute a model of AD.

It is clear that Notch phenotypes are predominant in presenilin-deficient animals, and interference with the Notch signaling pathway is the greatest concern when developing γ-secretase inhibitors to treat AD patients. However, over the years, more than 60 other proteins have been proposed as substrates for the γ-secretases (for an overview, see Hemming et al. 2008, Wakabayashi and De Strooper 2008, and McCarthy et al. 2009). Interestingly, the phenotypes of the mice in which individual subunits of γ-secretase (i.e., PSEN1 or PSEN2 and Aph1a or Aph1b/c) have been knocked out are quite divergent, suggesting some specificity in the substrates cleaved by the different γ-secretase complexes in vivo. The Aph1b/c containing γ-secretase complexes can, for instance, be completely removed from the mouse genome without causing any Notch defects, whereas similar inactivation of the Aph1a-complexes leads to severe embryonic phenotypes (Ma et al. 2005; Serneels et al. 2005, 2009). Interestingly, Aph1b/c knockout mice display subtle behavioral phenotypes characterized by disturbed prepulse inhibition, increased amphetamine sensitivity, and alterations in an operational memory task (Dejaegere et al. 2008). Accumulation of neuregulin CTFs in brain extracts of these mice suggested that neuregulin is a substrate of Aph1b/c-γ-secretase. Similar phenotypes have been seen in neuregulin-deficient mice (Stefansson et al. 2002) and interestingly, also in BACE-1 knockout mice (Savonenko et al. 2008), in agreement with the fact that BACE-1 is the principal sheddase of neuregulin (Willem et al. 2006).

The biochemical evidence that the APP and its close relatives, amyloid precursor-like protein (APLP)-1 and -2 are substrates of γ-secretase in vivo is also beyond discussion (De Strooper et al. 1998; Naruse et al. 1998; Scheinfeld et al. 2002; Eggert et al. 2004; Yanagida et al. 2009). As described in Müller and Zheng (2011), APP-deficient animals have yielded little direct information with regard to the specific molecular pathways for which APP is required, and it therefore remains unclear to what extent

γ-secretase processing of APP (apart from generating the infamous Aβ peptide) has biological consequences. γ-Secretase inactivation causes accumulation of APP carboxy-terminal fragments (APP-CTF) to levels which are two- to threefold higher than what is observed in wild-type cells, and Aβ peptide is no longer produced. It is possible that the main role of γ-secretase processing of the APP membrane-bound fragments is to clear these hydrophobic remnants (Kopan and Ilagan 2004), although some evidence suggests that the released APP intracellular domain might be involved in signaling processes (critically discussed in Reinhard et al. 2005). Importantly, also in the context of the development of γ-secretase inhibitors for the clinic, it seems that additional clearance mechanisms can compensate for the loss of γ-secretase processing by removing APP CTFs via alternative pathways. Other substrates that have been well studied are the N- and E-cadherins. Presenilin-1 forms complexes with these proteins and the α- and β-catenins at the cell surface (Georgakopoulos et al. 1999). γ-Secretase proteolysis of E-cadherin results in the release of the associated β- (and α-) catenins and disassembly of the adherens junction (Marambaud et al. 2002). N-cadherin cleavage by γ-secretase is stimulated by NMDA agonists. The cleavage gives rise to an intracellular N-cadherin fragment that binds to CBP (the cyclic AMP response element binding protein [CREB] binding protein) (Marambaud et al. 2003).

Presenilins have also been implicated in the cellular trafficking of proteins. Given the many substrates of presenilin, it is not unexpected that interference with proteolysis will lead to abnormal accumulation of protein fragments in the cell. However, a number of cell-surface proteins that are apparently not substrates of γ-secretase, including intercellular adhesion molecule 5 (ICAM5) or telencephalin (Esselens et al. 2004), epidermal growth factor receptor (EGFR) (Repetto et al. 2007), and β1-integrins (Zou et al. 2008), are also mislocalized in presenilin-deficient cells. Defective transport between endosomes and lysosomes or other deficits in late endosomal or other degradative organelles have been proposed to explain the abnormal accumulation of these proteins in presenilin knockout cells (Esselens et al. 2004; Wilson et al. 2004; Repetto et al. 2007; Lee et al. 2010).

The role of presenilin in Ca^{2+} homeostasis is even more controversial. There is consensus that clinical mutations in presenilin disturb the Ca^{2+} pool at the level of the ER (Bezprozvanny and Mattson 2008). The mechanisms, however, are debated and include higher expression of the Ryanodine receptor (RyR) (Chan et al. 2000; Hayrapetyan et al. 2008), stimulation of inositol-3-phosphate (IP3)-induced ER Ca^{2+} release (Leissring et al. 1999; Kasri et al. 2006; Cheung et al. 2008), or stimulation of sarco(endo)plasmic reticulum Ca^{2+}-ATPase (SERCA) pumps (Green et al. 2008). Presenilins might act as Ca^{2+} leak channels themselves (Tu et al. 2006). This leakage function is only observed with full-length presenilin-1 (i.e., before it becomes incorporated into the γ-secretase complex), and again, presenilin-containing aspartate mutations are able to maintain this function.

STRUCTURE-FUNCTION RELATIONSHIP OF γ-SECRETASE

The first step in understanding the structure of a membrane protein complex such as γ-secretase is to determine the membrane topology of the individual components. Presenilin 1 (PSEN1) and PSEN2 are integral membrane proteins that span membranes multiple times: Initially, the amino and carboxyl termini of PSEN1 and PSEN2 were predicted to be oriented to the cytoplasmic side (Doan et al. 1996), but a later N-linked glycosylation scanning approach revealed that PSEN spans the membrane nine times, with amino and carboxyl termini being oriented to the cytoplasmic and luminal sides, respectively (Laudon et al. 2005). Nicastrin is a type I single-span membrane protein with a large extracellular domain, the latter being heavily glycosylated and tightly folded on maturation (Shirotani et al. 2003). Aph-1 is apparently a 7-TMD protein with its amino and carboxyl termini located on the luminal and cytoplasmic sides, respectively (Fortna et al. 2004). Pen-2 spans the membrane twice, with

both the amino and carboxyl termini being found on the luminal side (Crystal et al. 2003).

Another fundamental issue toward elucidating the structure of the γ-secretase complex is determining its protein–protein contacts. Which components are bound to each other, and what are the binding domains? Nicastrin and Aph-1 form an initial subcomplex in the endoplasmic reticulum (LaVoie et al. 2003), and multiple TMDs of Aph-1 are involved in the binding to Nicastrin (Pardossi-Piquard et al. 2009; Chiang et al. 2010). The Nicastrin/Aph-1 subcomplex then interacts with the PSEN and Pen-2 subcomplex (Fraering et al. 2004a). Site-directed mutagenesis combined with coimmunoprecipitation studies showed that the carboxy-terminal domain of PSEN interacts with the TMD of Nicastrin (Capell et al. 2003; Kaether et al. 2004). Aph-1 also directly interacts with the carboxy-terminal region of PSEN (Steiner et al. 2008). Binding of Pen-2 to PSEN occurs independently of the Nct/Aph-1 interaction (Fraering et al. 2004a). It has also been shown that PSEN1 interacts with Pen-2 through its fourth TMD (Kim and Sisodia 2005; Watanabe et al. 2005).

Because of the unique features of γ-secretase as a membrane-embedded protein complex harboring at least 19 membrane-spanning regions and executing intramembrane hydrolysis of substrate proteins, there is great interest in its precise structure. However, crystallization of the purified γ-secretase complex has not been achieved yet. Hence, a couple of indirect approaches have been conducted to begin to predict the structure of the complex. EM and single-particle image analysis on human γ-secretase complexes purified from mammalian cells revealed a cylindrical interior chamber of ~20–40 Å length, consistent with a proteolytic site occluded from the hydrophobic environment of the lipid bilayer. Lectin tagging of the Nicastrin ectodomain enabled proper orientation of the globular, ~120 Å-long complex within the membrane (Lazarov et al. 2006). Further analysis of the structure of γ-secretase complex by cryoelectron microscopy and single-particle image reconstruction at 12 Å resolution revealed several domains on the extracellular side, three low-density cavities, and a surface groove in the transmembrane region of the complex (Osenkowski et al. 2009). Human γ-secretase complexes reconstituted in Sf9 cells have also been purified and analyzed by EM and 3D reconstruction (Ogura et al. 2006). The resultant three-dimensional structure of γ-secretase at 48 Å resolution occupied a volume of 560 × 320 × 240 Å, which resembled a flattened heart comprised of two oppositely faced, dimpled domains; a low-density space containing multiple pores resided between the domains, which may house the catalytic site. The differences in the predicted shape and size of the complex between the two studies may reflect monomeric versus dimeric or oligomeric states and may stem from the distinct conditions for reconstitution, detergent extraction and purification, as well as the limitation of the resolution of the method for revealing the internal structure of γ-secretase at the atomic level.

The most intriguing aspect in the structure-function relationship of γ-secretase is how it executes the proteolytic cleavage of the membrane-spanning segment of substrate proteins within the hydrophobic lipid bilayer. To examine the water accessibility of the regions flanking the catalytic aspartate residues in the sixth and seventh TMDs of PSEN1, the substituted cysteine accessibility method (SCAM) was applied. This involves the use of disulfide-forming reagents to probe accessibility of specific amino acids that have been changed to cysteines. Via SCAM, TMD6 and TMD7 were found to be partly facing a hydrophilic environment (i.e., in a catalytic pore structure) that enables the intramembrane proteolysis (Fig. 4A) (Sato et al. 2006; Tolia et al. 2006). Residues at the luminal portion of TMD6 are predicted to form a subsite for substrate or inhibitor binding on the α-helix facing a hydrophilic milieu, whereas those around the GxGD catalytic motif within TMD7 are highly water accessible, suggesting formation of a hydrophilic cavity within the membrane region. The SCAM data also suggested that the two catalytic aspartates are closely opposed to each other. Subsequently, the structures of TMD 8, 9, and the carboxyl

terminus of PSEN1, which are located carboxy terminally to the catalytic domain and include the conserved PAL motif and the hydrophobic carboxy-terminal tip, both of which are implicated in the formation of the γ-secretase complex and its catalytic activity, were analyzed by SCAM (Fig. 4B) (Sato et al. 2008; Tolia et al. 2008). The amino acid residues around the proline-alanine-leucine (PAL) motif and the luminal side of TMD9 were highly water accessible and located in proximity to the catalytic center. The region starting from the luminal end of TMD9 toward the carboxyl terminus formed an amphipathic α-helix-like structure that extended along the interface between the membrane and the extracellular milieu. Competition analysis using γ-secretase inhibitors showed the involvement of TMD9 in the initial binding of substrates, as well as in the subsequent catalytic process as a subsite. Recently, TMD1 of PS1 also was shown to be involved in the hydrophilic catalytic pore, serving as a part of subsite for γ-secretase cleavage, together with TMD 6, 7, and 9 (Takagi et al. 2010).

Recently, the structure of the CTF of human PS1 was analyzed by nuclear magnetic resonance studies in SDS micelles (Sobhanifar et al. 2010). The structure revealed a topology where the membrane was likely traversed three times in accordance with the nine TMD model of PS1, but containing unique structural features adapted to accommodate intramembrane catalysis, including a putative half-membrane-spanning helix amino-terminally harboring the second catalytic aspartate (residue 385), a severely kinked helical structure toward the carboxyl terminus, as well as a soluble helix in the unstructured amino-terminal loop of the CTF. These predicted structures were in good accordance with those obtained by SCAM analysis.

PRESENILINS AND DISEASE

As mentioned earlier, presenilin mutations were first identified in connection with familial AD, and subsequent work established that presenilin is the catalytic component of the γ-secretase complex that produces Aβ. This and other

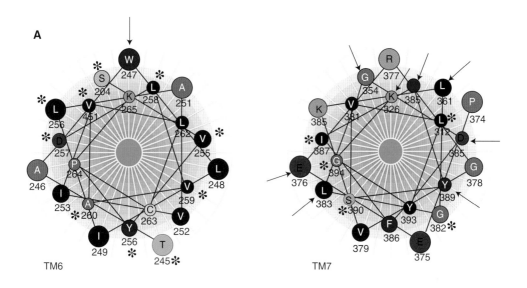

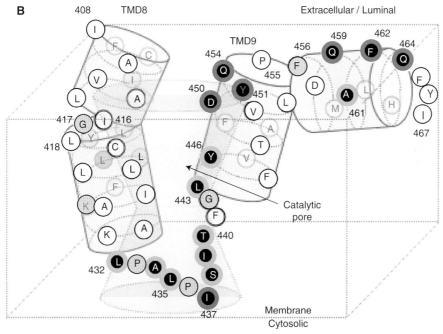

Figure 4. Predicted structure in and around the putative catalytic pore of PS1 based on the results of SCAM analysis. (*A*) Helical wheel model of TMD6 and 7 viewed from the amino terminus. The arrows and asterisks indicate amino acids reactive and nonreactive to biotin-HPDP, respectively, by the SCAM analysis (Tolia et al. 2006). Note that most of the accessible residues cluster on one side, although this domain does not seem to be a classically amphipathic helix. (*B*) Hypothetical structure around TMD8, 9, and the extreme carboxyl terminus of PS1 in relation to the catalytic pore. Residues labeled by 2-aminoethyl methanethiosulfonate (MTSEA)-biotin by the SCAM analysis (that are accessible to hydrophilic environment; Sato et al. 2008) are shown by a white letter in a black circle.

evidence strongly implicate Aβ, particularly Aβ42, in the pathogenesis of monogenic, dominant familial AD cases (i.e., those with missense mutations in *APP*, *PSEN1*, or *PSEN2* genes). AD-associated mutations in the presenilins alter the ratio of Aβ42/Aβ40, a critical factor in the tendency of Aβ to aggregate into neurotoxic species, whether the deleterious aggregates are fibrillar plaques or (according to current thinking) soluble oligomers (reviewed in Mucke 2011). Thus, these missense mutations alter the biochemical character of the γ-secretase complex and its interaction with the APP substrate to skew the transmembrane cleavage toward longer, more aggregation-prone forms of Aβ.

Interestingly, most of the AD-associated mutations in presenilin also cause a reduction in overall proteolytic activity (Song et al. 1999; Moehlmann et al. 2002; Schroeter et al. 2003; Bentahir et al. 2006), raising the question of whether a partial loss of presenilin function causes familial AD. Indeed, conditional knockout of *PSEN1* and *PSEN2* in the mouse brain results in neurodegeneration and memory deficits reminiscent of AD, albeit with no Aβ production (Saura et al. 2004; Wines-Samuelson et al. 2010). However, all of the mutations in the presenilins associated with AD (over 160 such mutations have been identified) are dominant, one mutant allele being sufficient to cause the carrier to develop AD in midlife. Furthermore, none of these AD-associated mutations result in truncation or loss of the presenilin protein, and the mutant protein assembles with other γ-secretase components into full complexes that are proteolytically active (and thus compatible with entirely normal development). Complete loss-of-function mutations in *PSEN1*, *Pen-2*, and *Nicastrin* in humans cause familial forms of a severe skin disorder, not neurodegeneration or AD (Wang et al. 2010). Although many of the AD-mutant forms of PSEN1 lead to some reduction in proteolytic function, some mutants display only subtle reductions, if any at all (Kulic et al. 2000). Moreover, no familial AD mutations have been found in any other γ-secretase substrate besides APP, strongly suggesting that it is alteration of APP

proteolysis by the mutant presenilins that is the key to the pathogenesis of AD. Together, these observations suggest that an altered Aβ42/Aβ40 ratio is the critical factor by which presenilin mutations cause familial AD. Such mutations may or may not be accompanied by a reduction of proteolytic activity, but a complete loss of activity is not observed with any of these mutations. The phenotypes observed in the conditional knockout mice may reflect an essential role of presenilins in neuronal health or function (e.g., neurotransmitter release; Zhang et al. 2009) that is only revealed on complete removal of these proteins, and deficient Notch signaling is certainly to be considered as a contributing factor in AD pathogenesis (Costa et al. 2003, 2005; Ge et al. 2004; Presente et al. 2004; Wang et al. 2004). Nevertheless, reduced function in certain signaling pathways may be a secondary contributing factor in the early-onset AD cases associated with presenilin mutations, although they cause no other known medical consequences.

Aside from onset in middle age and dominant genetic inheritance, the relatively rare familial AD cases mostly display essentially the same progression of symptoms and the same plaque and tangle pathology as late-onset sporadic AD. Thus, the clear involvement of Aβ in familial AD also implicates this peptide in the pathogenesis of the much more common sporadic form of the disease. As the presenilin-containing γ-secretase complex carries out the proteolysis that determines the carboxyl terminus of Aβ and the critical Aβ42/Aβ40 ratio, the protease complex is likewise implicated in the pathogenic pathway of sporadic AD. That being said, there is little evidence that the structure and properties of presenilin/γ-secretase are different in sporadic AD patients versus non-AD controls, or that sporadic AD involves specific changes in the Aβ42/Aβ40 ratio that are produced by γ-secretase. Nevertheless, it remains possible that local cellular changes alter APP proteolysis by γ-secretase to produce longer forms of Aβ. For instance, environmental factors such as diet may influence membrane composition to elicit such changes. Whether or not such speculations are ultimately borne out, all Aβ is produced via the γ-secretase complex, which makes the protease critical to the disease process. Without γ-secretase-mediated production of Aβ, the disease process should not occur.

In addition to its role in Aβ generation and AD, presenilin/γ-secretase is an essential component of the Notch signaling pathway, as noted earlier. As Notch signaling often keeps precursor cells in a dividing, less specialized state, overactivation of this pathway can cause cancer. Indeed, mutations in Notch are implicated in various forms of cancer (Shih Ie and Wang 2007). These mutations result in a Notch protein that can signal even in the absence of its cognate protein ligand (such as Delta and Jagged). For instance, a chromosomal translocation that results in a truncated, constitutively active form of Notch1 is found in rare cases of human T-cell acute lymphoblastic leukemia (T-ALL) (Ellisen et al. 1991; Grabher et al. 2006), whereas activating point mutations in Notch1 have been found in 50% of all T-ALL (Weng et al. 2004). Elevation of Notch3 expression is implicated in subsets of non-small-cell lung cancer (Dang et al. 2000) and ovarian cancer (Park et al. 2006), and activation of Notch signaling is also implicated in breast cancer (Hu et al. 2006). For this reason, γ-secretase is considered a potential anticancer target, i.e., blocking the overactivated Notch signaling pathway by preventing the release of the Notch intracellular domain, a transcriptional activator (e.g., Tammam et al. 2009). However, some cancer-causing Notch mutations bypass γ-secretase altogether, producing a truncated form of the receptor comprised of only the intracellular domain (i.e., not membrane localized) (Pear and Aster 2004). Thus, knowledge of the specific Notch mutations in individual patients would be critical in deciding whether to use a γ-secretase inhibitor to treat cancers. In contrast, in the skin, Notch acts as a tumor suppressor, and γ-secretase inhibition can cause skin cancer by interfering with Notch signaling (Demehri et al. 2009) (see below). This further complicates the use of such inhibitors to treat other types of cancer that involve Notch overactivation.

γ-SECRETASE AS A DRUG TARGET

Because the presenilin-containing γ-secretase complex plays an essential role in producing the Aβ peptide, considerable efforts have gone into the discovery and development of small-molecule inhibitors as potential therapeutics for AD. Early inhibitors were useful chemical tools for characterizing γ-secretase as an aspartyl protease (Wolfe et al. 1999a; Shearman et al. 2000), for labeling presenilin to provide evidence that the active site resides at the interface between PS1 NTF and CTF (Esler et al. 2000; Li et al. 2000), for purification of the protease complex (Esler et al. 2002; Beher et al. 2003; Fraering et al. 2004b), and for addressing its mechanism of action (Esler et al. 2002; Kornilova et al. 2005). Most of these compounds, however, were peptidomimetics with poor drug-like qualities. The development of inhibitors with better in vivo activity led to the demonstration of Aβ lowering in the brains of transgenic mice overexpressing AD-associated human APP mutants (Dovey et al. 2001; Lanz et al. 2004). However, treatment over an extended period (e.g., 2 wk) resulted in gastrointestinal toxicity and immunosuppression, owing to interference with the Notch signaling pathway (Searfoss et al. 2003; Wong et al. 2004).

Other evidence shows that, in contrast to its role in cell proliferation in many other cell types, Notch signaling acts as a tumor suppressor in epithelia (Nicolas et al. 2003; Proweller et al. 2006; Demehri et al. 2009), and that reduction of γ-secretase components can result in skin cancers (Xia et al. 2001; Li et al. 2007). Indeed, it has become clear that compounds targeting γ-secretase for the potential treatment of AD should alter Aβ production without significantly lowering the normal, physiologically regulated release of the Notch intracellular domain. The γ-secretase inhibitor that had advanced the furthest in clinical trials, LY450139 (semagacestat; Fig. 5) from Eli Lilly (Fleisher et al. 2008), displayed very little, if any, selectivity for APP compared to Notch, raising concern that doses that effectively lower brain Aβ production would cause systemic toxicity owing to inhibition of Notch signaling. Indeed, a phase 3 trial

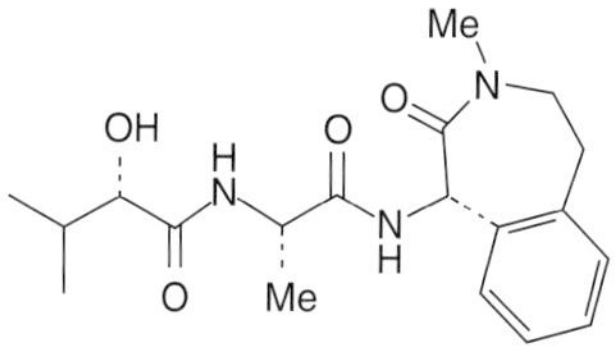

LY-450139

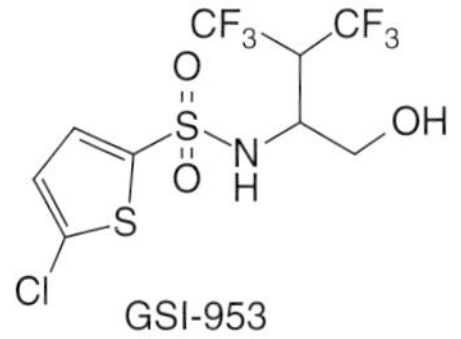

GSI-953

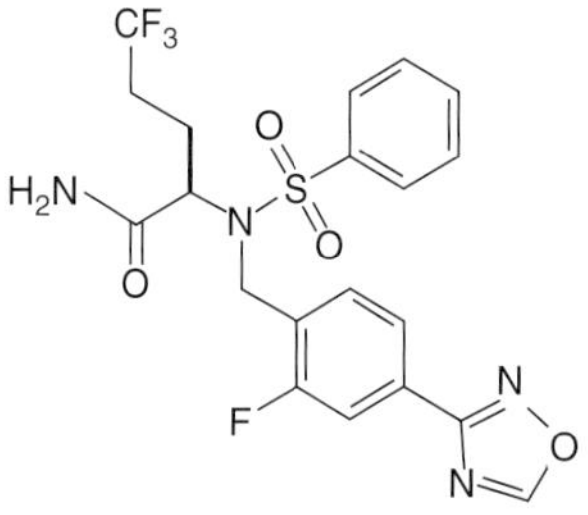

BMS-708, 163

Figure 5. γ-Secretase inhibitors recently or currently in clinical trials for the treatment of Alzheimer disease. LY450139 shows little selectivity for APP with respect to the Notch receptor, whereas GSI-953 and BMS-708,163 are clearly selective.

of this compound was halted owing to increased incidences of skin cancer, GI side effects, and some worsening of cognitive function.

Two general classes of compounds targeting γ-secretase have been found to alter Aβ production with varying degrees of selectivity with respect to Notch. The first are so-called γ-secretase modulators, which do not inhibit Aβ production, but instead shift production away from the more aggregation-prone Aβ42 and increase formation of a more soluble 38-residue form (Aβ38). These γ-secretase modulators are exemplified by a subset of nonsteroidal antiinflammatory drugs (NSAIDs) (such as ibuprofen and sulindac sulfide) that were the first compounds discovered to alter the γ-secretase processing of APP in this therapeutically important manner (Weggen et al. 2001). Only certain NSAIDs display this

property, and in a manner that does not depend on inhibition of cyclooxygenase (the target of NSAIDs that mediates their antiinflammatory activity). The first compound in this class to enter into clinical trials, R-flurbiprofen (tarenflurbil, Flurizan), is a single enantiomer of a clinically approved racemic NSAID (Eriksen et al. 2003; Galasko et al. 2007; Kukar et al. 2007). Unlike its mirror image, R-flurbiprofen does not inhibit cyclooxygenase, but it nevertheless retains the ability to lower Aβ42. This drug candidate, however, eventually failed owing to lack of efficacy (Green et al. 2009), a result that was not surprising given the very poor potency and brain penetration of this agent. Other compounds with similar properties, but that are much more potent, are in various stages of development. How these compounds elicit their effects is unclear. Some evidence suggests that the compounds selectively target the APP substrate (Kukar et al. 2008), whereas other studies suggest a direct interaction with the protease complex, even in the absence of substrate (Beher et al. 2004). The former mode of interaction (substrate targeting) would be unusual, while the latter mode (allosteric inhibition) is more common.

The second class of therapeutically promising molecules is the so-called "Notch-sparing" γ-secretase inhibitors. These compounds are capable of decreasing the proteolysis of APP by γ-secretase (and thereby decreasing the production of all forms of Aβ) while allowing the enzyme to continue processing the Notch receptor. Early compounds reported with this property were weak inhibitors identified by screening kinase inhibitors: The screen was based on the finding that the γ-secretase complex contains an ATP-binding site that affects the processing of APP but not that of Notch (Fraering et al. 2005). As kinase inhibitors typically interact with ATP-binding sites, the thought was that some kinase inhibitors might interact with an ATP-binding site on γ-secretase. The abl kinase inhibitor imatinib (Gleevec) was the first reported Notch-sparing γ-secretase inhibitor, doing so in an abl kinase-independent manner (Netzer et al. 2003). Recent affinity isolation of the imatinib target apparently responsible for the Aβ-lowering effects identified γ-secretase activating protein (GSAP), a novel 16 kDa protein that can interact stably with the γ-secretase complex (He et al. 2010).

Since the identification of these initial, weak agents, a number of much more potent Notch-sparing inhibitors have been reported, with several that are currently in early- to mid-stage clinical trials (Kreft et al. 2009). These include BMS-708,163 (Fig. 5) from Bristol-Myers-Squibb (BMS) (Gillman et al. 2010), PF-3,084,014 from Pfizer (Lanz et al. 2010), and GSI-953 (begacestat; Fig. 5) from Wyeth (now part of Pfizer) (Mayer et al. 2008). The Wyeth compound displays nanomolar potency but only 14-fold selectivity for APP over Notch, which may not be sufficient to avoid peripheral Notch-related toxicities. The BMS and Pfizer compounds are both highly potent (nanomolar to subnanomolar) and selective (~200- to 300-fold); however, it is still unclear whether this selectivity will be sufficient if the compounds do not have high brain penetration.

Avoiding interference with γ-secretase proteolysis of Notch could provide compounds that will have other toxicities that had been masked by the Notch-deficient phenotypes. As mentioned earlier, γ-secretase cleaves many type I membrane proteins after ectodomain release by cell surface sheddases (Beel and Sanders 2008). In some cases, proteolysis of the substrate results in a signaling event or other specific cellular function, for example, the γ-secretase proteolysis of N-cadherin (Marambaud et al. 2003) mentioned earlier. Also, neuregulin-1-triggered γ-secretase cleavage of ErbB4 inhibits astrocyte differentiation by interacting with repressors of astrocyte gene expression (Sardi et al. 2006). It is presently unclear whether interference with these cellular functions will result in toxicity in vivo. In other cases, however, proteolysis of a substrate by γ-secretase may not serve a specific cellular function but may simply be a means of clearing the membrane of protein stubs left behind after ectodomain shedding (Kopan and Ilagan 2004). Although this might appear to be an essential housekeeping function, no general

mechanism-based cell toxicity has been observed from γ-secretase inhibitors, perhaps owing to redundant function by other membrane-embedded proteases. Another important issue is selectivity with respect to the family of presenilin homologs exemplified by signal peptide peptidase (Golde et al. 2009). Such "off-target" interactions could also result in toxicity in vivo.

CONCLUDING REMARKS

Since the discovery of PSEN mutations associated with early-onset AD in 1995, our understanding of the nature of the γ-secretase complex and the normal and pathological functions of presenilins has come far. Challenges for the future include elucidating the detailed structure of this 19-TMD complex and translating our understanding into practical therapeutics for AD. The hope is that a second edition of this collection will describe major advances on these and other research fronts, and perhaps even some success in the clinic.

ACKNOWLEDGMENTS

B.D. is Arthur Bax and Anna Vanluffelen chair for Alzheimer disease research, and is supported by a Methusalem grant from the K.U. Leuven and the Flemisch government, by the Fund for Scientific Research Flanders (FWO-V), the Foundation for Alzheimer Research (SAO/FRMA), and the Interuniversity Attraction Pole Program (IAP P6/43) of the Belgian Federal Science Policy Office. T.I. is Professor of Neuropathology and supported by the Ministry of Education, Culture, Sports, Science, and Technology, and by Core Research for Evolutional Science and Technology of Japan. M.S.W. is Professor of Neurology and is supported by grants from the National Institutes of Health, the Alzheimer's Association, and the American Health Assistance Foundation.

REFERENCES

*Reference is also in this collection.

Alzheimer's Disease Collaborative Group. 1995. The structure of the presenilin 1 (S182) gene and identification of six novel mutations in early onset AD families. *Nat Genet* **11:** 219–222.

Baumann K, Paganetti PA, Sturchler-Pierrat C, Wong C, Hartmann H, Cescato R, Frey P, Yankner BA, Sommer B, Staufenbiel M. 1997. Distinct processing of endogenous and overexpressed recombinant presenilin 1. *Neurobiol Aging* **18:** 181–189.

Beel AJ, Sanders CR. 2008. Substrate specificity of γ-secretase and other intramembrane proteases. *Cell Mol Life Sci* **65:** 1311–1334.

Beher D, Fricker M, Nadin A, Clarke EE, Wrigley JD, Li YM, Culvenor JG, Masters CL, Harrison T, Shearman MS. 2003. In vitro characterization of the presenilin-dependent γ-secretase complex using a novel affinity ligand. *Biochemistry* **427:** 8133–8142.

Beher D, Clarke EE, Wrigley JD, Martin AC, Nadin A, Churcher I, Shearman MS. 2004. Selected non-steroidal anti-inflammatory drugs and their derivatives target γ-secretase at a novel site. Evidence for an allosteric mechanism. *J Biol Chem* **279:** 43419–43426.

Bentahir M, Nyabi O, Verhamme J, Tolia A, Horre K, Wiltfang J, Esselmann H, De Strooper B. 2006. Presenilin clinical mutations can affect γ-secretase activity by different mechanisms. *J Neurochem* **96:** 732–742.

Bezprozvanny I, Mattson MP. 2008. Neuronal calcium mishandling and the pathogenesis of Alzheimer's disease. *Trends Neurosci* **31:** 454–463.

Borchelt DR, Thinakaran G, Eckman CB, Lee MK, Davenport F, Ratovitsky T, Prada CM, Kim G, Seekins S, Yager D, et al. 1996. Familial Alzheimer's disease-linked presenilin 1 variants elevate Aβ1–42/1–40 ratio in vitro and in vivo. *Neuron* **17:** 1005–1013.

Borchelt DR, Ratovitski T, van Lare J, Lee MK, Gonzales V, Jenkins NA, Copeland NG, Price DL, Sisodia SS. 1997. Accelerated amyloid deposition in the brains of transgenic mice coexpressing mutant presenilin 1 and amyloid precursor proteins. *Neuron* **19:** 939–945.

Capell A, Kaether C, Edbauer D, Shirotani K, Merkl S, Steiner H, Haass C. 2003. Nicastrin interacts with γ-secretase complex components via the N-terminal part of its transmembrane domain. *J Biol Chem* **278:** 52519–52523.

Chan SL, Mayne M, Holden CP, Geiger JD, Mattson MP. 2000. Presenilin-1 mutations increase levels of ryanodine receptors and calcium release in PC12 cells and cortical neurons. *J Biol Chem* **275:** 18195–18200.

Chen F, Hasegawa H, Schmitt-Ulms G, Kawarai T, Bohm C, Katayama T, Gu Y, Sanjo N, Glista M, Rogaeva E, et al. 2006. TMP21 is a presenilin complex component that modulates γ-secretase but not ε-secretase activity. *Nature* **440:** 1208–1212.

Cheung KH, Shineman D, Muller M, Cardenas C, Mei L, Yang J, Tomita T, Iwatsubo T, Lee VM, Foskett JK. 2008. Mechanism of Ca^{2+} disruption in Alzheimer's disease by presenilin regulation of InsP3 receptor channel gating. *Neuron* **58:** 871–883.

Chiang PM, Fortna RR, Price DL, Li T, Wong PC. 2010. Specific domains in anterior pharynx-defective 1 determine its intramembrane interactions with nicastrin and presenilin. *Neurobiol Aging* doi: 10.1016/j.neurobiolaging.2009.12.028.

Citron M, Westaway D, Xia W, Carlson G, Diehl T, Levesque G, Johnson-Wood K, Lee M, Seubert P, Davis A, et al. 1997. Mutant presenilins of Alzheimer's disease increase production of 42-residue amyloid β-protein in both transfected cells and transgenic mice. *Nat Med* **3:** 67–72.

Costa RM, Honjo T, Silva AJ. 2003. Learning and memory deficits in Notch mutant mice. *Curr Biol* **13:** 1348–1354.

Costa RM, Drew C, Silva AJ. 2005. Notch to remember. *Trends Neurosci* **28:** 429–435.

Crystal AS, Morais VA, Pierson TC, Pijak DS, Carlin D, Lee VM, Doms RW. 2003. Membrane topology of γ-secretase component PEN-2. *J Biol Chem* **278:** 20117–20123.

Dang TP, Gazdar AF, Virmani AK, Sepetavec T, Hande KR, Minna JD, Roberts JR, Carbone DP. 2000. Chromosome 19 translocation, overexpression of Notch3, and human lung cancer. *J Natl Cancer Inst* **92:** 1355–1357.

Dejaegere T, Serneels L, Schafer MK, Van Biervliet J, Horre K, Depboylu C, Alvarez-Fischer D, Herreman A, Willem M, Haass C, et al. 2008. Deficiency of Aph1B/C-γ-secretase disturbs Nrg1 cleavage and sensorimotor gating that can be reversed with antipsychotic treatment. *Proc Natl Acad Sci* **105:** 9775–9780.

Demehri S, Turkoz A, Kopan R. 2009. Epidermal Notch1 loss promotes skin tumorigenesis by impacting the stromal microenvironment. *Cancer Cell* **16:** 55–66.

De Strooper B. 2003. Aph-1, Pen-2, and nicastrin with presenilin generate an active γ-secretase complex. *Neuron* **38:** 9–12.

De Strooper B, Saftig P, Craessaerts K, Vanderstichele H, Guhde G, Annaert W, Von Figura K, Van Leuven F. 1998. Deficiency of presenilin-1 inhibits the normal cleavage of amyloid precursor protein. *Nature* **391:** 387–390.

De Strooper B, Annaert W, Cupers P, Saftig P, Craessaerts K, Mumm JS, Schroeter EH, Schrijvers V, Wolfe MS, Ray WJ, et al. 1999. A presenilin-1-dependent γ-secretase-like protease mediates release of Notch intracellular domain. *Nature* **398:** 518–522.

Doan A, Thinakaran G, Borchelt DR, Slunt HH, Ratovitsky T, Podlisny M, Selkoe DJ, Seeger M, Gand SE, Price DL, et al. 1996. Protein topology of presenilin 1. *Neuron* **17:** 1023–1030.

Doerfler P, Shearman MS, Perlmutter RM. 2001. Presenilin-dependent γ-secretase activity modulates thymocyte development. *Proc Natl Acad Sci* **98:** 9312–9317.

Dovey HF, John V, Anderson JP, Chen LZ, de Saint Andrieu P, Fang LY, Freedman SB, Folmer B, Goldbach E, Holztynska EJ, et al. 2001. Functional γ-secretase inhibitors reduce β-amyloid peptide levels in brain. *J Neurochem* **76:** 173–181.

Duff K, Eckman C, Zehr C, Yu X, Prada CM, Perez-tur J, Hutton M, Buee L, Harigaya Y, Yager D, et al. 1996. Increased amyloid-β42(43) in brains of mice expressing mutant presenilin 1. *Nature* **383:** 710–713.

Edbauer D, Winkler E, Regula JT, Pesold B, Steiner H, Haass C. 2003. Reconstitution of γ-secretase activity. *Nat Cell Biol* **5:** 486–488.

Eggert S, Paliga K, Soba P, Evin G, Masters CL, Weidemann A, Beyreuther K. 2004. The proteolytic processing of the amyloid precursor protein gene family members APLP-1 and APLP-2 involves α-, β-, γ-, and ε-like cleavages: Modulation of APLP-1 processing by *n*-glycosylation. *J Biol Chem* **279:** 18146–18156.

Ellisen LW, Bird J, West DC, Soreng AL, Reynolds TC, Smith SD, Sklar J. 1991. TAN-1, the human homolog of the *Drosophila* notch gene, is broken by chromosomal translocations in T lymphoblastic neoplasms. *Cell* **66**: 649–661.

Eriksen JL, Sagi SA, Smith TE, Weggen S, Das P, McLendon DC, Ozols VV, Jessing KW, Zavitz KH, Koo EH, et al. 2003. NSAIDs and enantiomers of flurbiprofen target γ-secretase and lower Aβ 42 in vivo. *J Clin Invest* **112**: 440–449.

Esler WP, Kimberly WT, Ostaszewski BL, Diehl TS, Moore CL, Tsai J-Y, Rahmati T, Xia W, Selkoe DJ, Wolfe MS. 2000. Transition-state analogue inhibitors of γ-secretase bind directly to presenilin-1. *Nature Cell Biol* **2**: 428–434.

Esler WP, Kimberly WT, Ostaszewski BL, Ye W, Diehl TS, Selkoe DJ, Wolfe MS. 2002. Activity-dependent isolation of the presenilin/γ-secretase complex reveals nicastrin and a γ substrate. *Proc Natl Acad Sci* **99**: 2720–2725.

Esselens C, Oorschot V, Baert V, Raemaekers T, Spittaels K, Serneels L, Zheng H, Saftig P, De Strooper B, Klumperman J, et al. 2004. Presenilin 1 mediates the turnover of telencephalin in hippocampal neurons via an autophagic degradative pathway. *J Cell Biol* **166**: 1041–1054.

Fleisher AS, Raman R, Siemers ER, Becerra L, Clark CM, Dean RA, Farlow MR, Galvin JE, Peskind ER, Quinn JF, et al. 2008. Phase 2 safety trial targeting amyloid β production with a γ-secretase inhibitor in Alzheimer disease. *Arch Neurol* **65**: 1031–1038.

Flood DG, Reaume AG, Dorfman KS, Lin YG, Lang DM, Trusko SP, Savage MJ, Annaert WG, De Strooper B, Siman R, et al. 2002. FAD mutant PS-1 gene-targeted mice: Increased Aβ42 and Aβ deposition without APP overproduction. *Neurobiol Aging* **23**: 335–348.

Fortna RR, Crystal AS, Morais VA, Pijak DS, Lee VM, Doms RW. 2004. Membrane topology and nicastrin-enhanced endoproteolysis of APH-1, a component of the γ-secretase complex. *J Biol Chem* **279**: 3685–3693.

Fraering PC, LaVoie MJ, Ye W, Ostaszewski BL, Kimberly WT, Selkoe DJ, Wolfe MS. 2004a. Detergent-dependent dissociation of active γ-secretase reveals an interaction between Pen-2 and PS1-NTF and offers a model for subunit organization within the complex. *Biochemistry* **43**: 323–333.

Fraering PC, Ye W, Strub JM, Dolios G, LaVoie MJ, Ostaszewski BL, Van Dorsselaer A, Wang R, Selkoe DJ, Wolfe MS. 2004b. Purification and characterization of the human γ-Secretase complex. *Biochemistry* **43**: 9774–9789.

Fraering PC, Ye W, Lavoie MJ, Ostaszewski BL, Selkoe DJ, Wolfe MS. 2005. γ-Secretase substrate selectivity can be modulated directly via interaction with a nucleotide binding site. *J Biol Chem* **280**: 41987–41996.

Francis R, McGrath G, Zhang J, Ruddy DA, Sym M, Apfeld J, Nicoll M, Maxwell M, Hai B, Ellis MC, et al. 2002. aph-1 and pen-2 are required for Notch pathway signaling, γ-secretase cleavage of βAPP, and presenilin protein accumulation. *Dev Cell* **3**: 85–97.

Fukumori A, Fluhrer R, Steiner H, Haass C. 2010. Three-amino acid spacing of presenilin endoproteolysis suggests a general stepwise cleavage of γ-secretase-mediated intramembrane proteolysis. *J Neurosci* **30**: 7853–7862.

Galasko DR, Graff-Radford N, May S, Hendrix S, Cottrell BA, Sagi SA, Mather G, Laughlin M, Zavitz KH, Swabb

E, et al. 2007. Safety, tolerability, pharmacokinetics, and Aβ levels after short-term administration of R-flurbiprofen in healthy elderly individuals. *Alzheimer Dis Assoc Disord* **21**: 292–299.

Ge X, Hannan F, Xie Z, Feng C, Tully T, Zhou H, Xie Z, Zhong Y. 2004. Notch signaling in *Drosophila* long-term memory formation. *Proc Natl Acad Sci* **101**: 10172–10176.

Georgakopoulos A, Marambaud P, Efthimiopoulos S, Shioi J, Cui W, Li HC, Schutte M, Gordon R, Holstein GR, Martinelli G, et al. 1999. Presenilin-1 forms complexes with the cadherin/catenin cell-cell adhesion system and is recruited to intercellular and synaptic contacts. *Mol Cell* **4**: 893–902.

Gillman KW, Starrett JE, Parker MF, Xie K, Bronson JJ, Marcin LR, McElhone KE, Bergstrom CP, Mate RA, Williams R, et al. 2010. Discovery and evaluation of BMS-708163, a potent, selective and orally bioavailable γ-secretase inhibitor. *ACS Med Chem Lett* **1**: 120–124.

Golde TE, Wolfe MS, Greenbaum DC. 2009. Signal peptide peptidases: A family of intramembrane-cleaving proteases that cleave type 2 transmembrane proteins. *Semin Cell Dev Biol* **20**: 225–230.

Goutte C, Hepler W, Mickey KM, Priess JR. 2000. aph-2 encodes a novel extracellular protein required for GLP-1-mediated signaling. *Development* **127**: 2481–2492.

Goutte C, Tsunozaki M, Hale VA, Priess JR. 2002. APH-1 is a multipass membrane protein essential for the Notch signaling pathway in *Caenorhabditis elegans* embryos. *Proc Natl Acad Sci* **99**: 775–779.

Grabher C, von Boehmer H, Look AT. 2006. Notch 1 activation in the molecular pathogenesis of T-cell acute lymphoblastic leukaemia. *Nat Rev Cancer* **6**: 347–359.

Green KN, Demuro A, Akbari Y, Hitt BD, Smith IF, Parker I, LaFerla FM. 2008. SERCA pump activity is physiologically regulated by presenilin and regulates amyloid-β production. *J Cell Biol* **181**: 1107–1116.

Green RC, Schneider LS, Amato DA, Beelen AP, Wilcock G, Swabb EA, Zavitz ZH. 2009. Effect of tarenflurbil on cognitive decline and activities of daily living in patients with mild Alzheimer disease: A randomized controlled trial. *JAMA* **302**: 2557–2564.

Gu Y, Chen F, Sanjo N, Kawarai T, Hasegawa H, Duthie M, Li W, Ruan X, Luthra A, Mount HT, et al. 2003. APH-1 interacts with mature and immature forms of presenilins and nicastrin and may play a role in maturation of presenilin.nicastrin complexes. *J Biol Chem* **278**: 7374–7380.

Haass C, Selkoe DJ. 1993. Cellular processing of β-amyloid precursor protein and the genesis of amyloid β-peptide. *Cell* **75**: 1039–1042.

Haass C, Selkoe DJ. 1998. Alzheimer's disease. A technical KO of amyloid-β peptide. *Nature* **391**: 339–340.

* Haass C, Kaether C, Sisodia S, Thinakaran G. 2011. Trafficking and proteolytic processing of APP. *Cold Spring Harb Perspect Med* doi: 10.1101/cshperspect.a006270.

Hadland BK, Manley NR, Su D, Longmore GD, Moore CL, Wolfe MS, Schroeter EH, Kopan R. 2001. γ-secretase inhibitors repress thymocyte development. *Proc Natl Acad Sci* **98**: 7487–7491.

Hayrapetyan V, Rybalchenko V, Rybalchenko N, Koulen P. 2008. The N-terminus of presenilin-2 increases single channel activity of brain ryanodine receptors through direct protein-protein interaction. *Cell Calcium* **44:** 507–518.

He G, Luo W, Li P, Remmers C, Netzer WJ, Hendrick J, Bettayeb K, Flajolet M, Gorelick F, Wennogle LP, et al. 2010. γ-secretase activating protein is a therapeutic target for Alzheimer's disease. *Nature* **467:** 95–98.

Hemming ML, Elias JE, Gygi SP, Selkoe DJ. 2008. Proteomic profiling of γ-secretase substrates and mapping of substrate requirements. *PLoS Biol* **6:** e257.

Hu C, Dievart A, Lupien M, Calvo E, Tremblay G, Jolicoeur P. 2006. Overexpression of activated murine Notch1 and Notch3 in transgenic mice blocks mammary gland development and induces mammary tumors. *Am J Pathol* **168:** 973–990.

Kaether C, Capell A, Edbauer D, Winkler E, Novak B, Steiner H, Haass C. 2004. The presenilin C-terminus is required for ER-retention, nicastrin-binding and γ-secretase activity. *Embo J* **23:** 4738–4748.

Kasri NN, Kocks SL, Verbert L, Hebert SS, Callewaert G, Parys JB, Missiaen L, De Smedt H. 2006. Up-regulation of inositol 1,4,5-trisphosphate receptor type 1 is responsible for a decreased endoplasmic-reticulum Ca^{2+} content in presenilin double knock-out cells. *Cell Calcium* **40:** 41–51.

Khandelwal A, Chandu D, Roe CM, Kopan R, Quatrano RS. 2007. Moonlighting activity of presenilin in plants is independent of γ-secretase and evolutionarily conserved. *Proc Natl Acad Sci* **104:** 13337–13342.

Kim SH, Sisodia SS. 2005. Evidence that the "NF" motif in transmembrane domain 4 of presenilin 1 is critical for binding with PEN-2. *J Biol Chem* **280:** 41953–41966.

Kimberly WT, LaVoie MJ, Ostaszewski BL, Ye W, Wolfe MS, Selkoe DJ. 2003. γ-Secretase is a membrane protein complex comprised of presenilin, nicastrin, aph-1, and pen-2. *Proc Natl Acad Sci* **100:** 6382–6387.

Kopan R, Ilagan MX. 2004. γ-Secretase: Proteasome of the membrane? *Nat Rev Mol Cell Biol* **5:** 499–504.

Kornilova AY, Bihel F, Das C, Wolfe MS. 2005. The initial substrate binding site of γ-secretase is located on presenilin near the active site. *Proc Natl Acad Sci* **102:** 3230–3235.

Kreft AF, Martone R, Porte A. 2009. Recent advances in the identification of γ-secretase inhibitors to clinically test the Aβ oligomer hypothesis of Alzheimer's disease. *J Med Chem* **52:** 6169–6188.

Kukar T, Prescott S, Eriksen JL, Holloway V, Murphy MP, Koo EH, Golde TE, Nicolle MM. 2007. Chronic administration of R-flurbiprofen attenuates learning impairments in transgenic amyloid precursor protein mice. *BMC Neurosci* **8:** 54.

Kukar TL, Ladd TB, Bann MA, Fraering PC, Narlawar R, Maharvi GM, Healy B, Chapman R, Welzel AT, Price RW, et al. 2008. Substrate-targeting γ-secretase modulators. *Nature* **453:** 925–929.

Kulic L, Walter J, Multhaup G, Teplow DB, Baumeister R, Romig H, Capell A, Steiner H, Haass C. 2000. Separation of presenilin function in amyloid β-peptide generation and endoproteolysis of Notch. *Proc Natl Acad Sci* **97:** 5913–5918.

Lanz TA, Hosley JD, Adams WJ, Merchant KM. 2004. Studies of Aβ pharmacodynamics in the brain, cerebrospinal fluid, and plasma in young (plaque-free) Tg2576 mice using the γ-secretase inhibitor N2-[(2S)-2-(3,5-difluorophenyl)-2-hydroxyethanoyl]-N1-[(7S)-5-methyl-6-oxo-6,7-di hydro-5H-dibenzo[b,d]azepin-7-yl]-L-alaninamide (LY-411575). *J Pharmacol Exp Ther* **309:** 49–55.

Lanz TA, Wood KM, Richter KE, Nolan CE, Becker SL, Pozdnyakov N, Martin BA, Du P, Oborski CE, Wood DE, et al. 2010. Pharmacodynamics and pharmacokinetics of the γ-secretase inhibitor, PF-3084014. *J Pharmacol Exp Ther* **334:** 269–277.

Laudon H, Hansson EM, Melen K, Bergman A, Farmery MR, Winblad B, Lendahl U, von Heijne G, Naslund J. 2005. A nine-transmembrane domain topology for presenilin 1. *J Biol Chem* **280:** 35352–35360.

LaVoie MJ, Fraering PC, Ostaszewski BL, Ye W, Kimberly WT, Wolfe MS, Selkoe DJ. 2003. Assembly of the γ-secretase complex involves early formation of an intermediate subcomplex of Aph-1 and nicastrin. *J Biol Chem* **278:** 37213–37222.

Lazarov VK, Fraering PC, Ye W, Wolfe MS, Selkoe DJ, Li H. 2006. Electron microscopic structure of purified, active γ-secretase reveals an aqueous intramembrane chamber and two pores. *Proc Natl Acad Sci* **103:** 6889–6894.

Lee JH, Yu WH, Kumar A, Lee S, Mohan PS, Peterhoff CM, Wolfe DM, Martinez-Vicente M, Massey AC, Sovak G, et al. 2010. Lysosomal proteolysis and autophagy require presenilin 1 and are disrupted by Alzheimer-related PS1 mutations. *Cell* **141:** 1146–1158.

Leissring MA, Paul BA, Parker I, Cotman CW, LaFerla FM. 1999. Alzheimer's presenilin-1 mutation potentiates inositol 1,4,5-trisphosphate-mediated calcium signaling in Xenopus oocytes. *J Neurochem* **72:** 1061–1068.

Levitan D, Greenwald I. 1995. Facilitation of lin-12-mediated signalling by sel-12, a *Caenorhabditis elegans* S182 Alzheimer's disease gene. *Nature* **377:** 351–354.

Levitan D, Yu G, St George Hyslop P, Goutte C. 2001. APH-2/nicastrin functions in LIN-12/Notch signaling in the *Caenorhabditis elegans* somatic gonad. *Dev Biol* **240:** 654–661.

Levy-Lahad E, Wasco W, Poorkaj P, Romano DM, Oshima J, Pettingell WH, Yu CE, Jondro PS, Schmidt SD, Wang K, et al. 1995. Candidate gene for the chromosome 1 familial Alzheimer's disease locus. *Science* **269:** 973–977.

Li YM, Xu M, Lai MT, Huang Q, Castro JL, DiMuzio-Mower J, Harrison T, Lellis C, Nadin A, Neduvelil JG, et al. 2000. Photoactivated γ-secretase inhibitors directed to the active site covalently label presenilin 1. *Nature* **405:** 689–694.

Li T, Wen H, Brayton C, Das P, Smithson LA, Fauq A, Fan X, Crain BJ, Price DL, Golde TE, et al. 2007. Epidermal growth factor receptor and notch pathways participate in the tumor suppressor function of γ-secretase. *J Biol Chem* **282:** 32264–32273.

Ma G, Li T, Price DL, Wong PC. 2005. APH-1a is the principal mammalian APH-1 isoform present in γ-secretase complexes during embryonic development. *J Neurosci* **25:** 192–198.

Marambaud P, Shioi J, Serban G, Georgakopoulos A, Sarner S, Nagy V, Baki L, Wen P, Efthimiopoulos S, Shao Z, et al.

2002. A presenilin-1/γ-secretase cleavage releases the E-cadherin intracellular domain and regulates disassembly of adherens junctions. *Embo J* **21**: 1948–1956.

Marambaud P, Wen PG, Dutt A, Shioi J, Takashima A, Siman R, Robakis NK. 2003. A CBP binding transcriptional repressor produced by the PS1/ε-cleavage of N-cadherin is inhibited by PS1 FAD mutations. *Cell* **114**: 635–645.

Mayer SC, Kreft AF, Harrison B, Abou-Gharbia M, Antane M, Aschmies S, Atchison K, Chlenov M, Cole DC, Comery T, et al. 2008. Discovery of begacestat, a Notch-1-sparing γ-secretase inhibitor for the treatment of Alzheimer's disease. *J Med Chem* **51**: 7348–7351.

McCarthy JV, Twomey C, Wujek P. 2009. Presenilin-dependent regulated intramembrane proteolysis and γ-secretase activity. *Cell Mol Life Sci* **66**: 1534–1555.

Moehlmann T, Winkler E, Xia X, Edbauer D, Murrell J, Capell A, Kaether C, Zheng H, Ghetti B, Haass C, et al. 2002. Presenilin-1 mutations of leucine 166 equally affect the generation of the Notch and APP intracellular domains independent of their effect on Aβ 42 production. *Proc Natl Acad Sci* **99**: 8025–8030.

* Mucke L. 2011. Neurotoxicity of amyloid β-protein: Synaptic and network dysfunction. *Cold Spring Harb Perspect Med* doi: 10.1101/cshperspect.a006338.

* Müller UC, Zheng H. 2011. Physiological functions of APP family proteins. *Cold Spring Harb Perspect Med* doi: 10.1101/cshperspect.a006288.

Naruse S, Thinakaran G, Luo JJ, Kusiak JW, Tomita T, Iwatsubo T, Qian X, Ginty DD, Price DL, Borchelt DR, et al. 1998. Effects of PS1 deficiency on membrane protein trafficking in neurons. *Neuron* **21**: 1213–1221.

Nelson O, Tu H, Lei T, Bentahir M, de Strooper B, Bezprozvanny I. 2007. Familial Alzheimer disease-linked mutations specifically disrupt Ca²⁺ leak function of presenilin 1. *J Clin Invest* **117**: 1230–1239.

Netzer WJ, Dou F, Cai D, Veach D, Jean S, Li Y, Bornmann WG, Clarkson B, Xu H, Greengard P. 2003. Gleevec inhibits β-amyloid production but not Notch cleavage. *Proc Natl Acad Sci* **100**: 12444–12449.

Nicolas M, Wolfer A, Raj K, Kummer JA, Mill P, van Noort M, Hui CC, Clevers H, Dotto GP, Radtke F. 2003. Notch1 functions as a tumor suppressor in mouse skin. *Nat Genet* **33**: 416–441.

Nyabi O, Bentahir M, Horre K, Herreman A, Gottardi-Littell N, Van Broeckhoven C, Merchiers P, Spittaels K, Annaert W, De Strooper B. 2003. Presenilins mutated at Asp-257 or Asp-385 restore Pen-2 expression and Nicastrin glycosylation but remain catalytically inactive in the absence of wild type Presenilin. *J Biol Chem* **278**: 43430–43436.

Ogura T, Mio K, Hayashi I, Miyashita H, Fukuda R, Kopan R, Kodama T, Hamakubo T, Iwatsubo T, Tomita T, et al. 2006. Three-dimensional structure of the γ-secretase complex. *Biochem Biophys Res Commun* **343**: 525–534.

Osenkowski P, Li H, Ye W, Li D, Aeschbach L, Fraering PC, Wolfe MS, Selkoe DJ, Li H. 2009. Cryoelectron microscopy structure of purified γ-secretase at 12 Å resolution. *J Mol Biol* **385**: 642–652.

Pardossi-Piquard R, Yang SP, Kanemoto S, Gu Y, Chen F, Bohm C, Sevalle J, Li T, Wong PC, Checler F, et al. 2009. APH1 polar transmembrane residues regulate the assembly and activity of presenilin complexes. *J Biol Chem* **284**: 16298–16307.

Park JT, Li M, Nakayama K, Mao TL, Davidson B, Zhang Z, Kurman RJ, Eberhart CG, Shih Ie M, Wang TL. 2006. Notch3 gene amplification in ovarian cancer. *Cancer Res* **66**: 6312–6318.

Pear WS, Aster JC. 2004. T cell acute lymphoblastic leukemia/lymphoma: A human cancer commonly associated with aberrant NOTCH1 signaling. *Curr Opin Hematol* **11**: 426–433.

Ponting CP, Hutton M, Nyborg A, Baker M, Jansen K, Golde TE. 2002. Identification of a novel family of presenilin homologues. *Hum Mol Genet* **11**: 1037–1044.

Presente A, Boyles RS, Serway CN, de Belle JS, Andres AJ. 2004. Notch is required for long-term memory in *Drosophila*. *Proc Natl Acad Sci* **101**: 1764–1768.

Proweller A, Tu L, Lepore JJ, Cheng L, Lu MM, Seykora J, Millar SE, Pear WS, Parmacek MS. 2006. Impaired notch signaling promotes de novo squamous cell carcinoma formation. *Cancer Res* **66**: 7438–7444.

Qyang Y, Chambers SM, Wang P, Xia X, Chen X, Goodell MA, Zheng H. 2004. Myeloproliferative disease in mice with reduced presenilin gene dosage: Effect of γ-secretase blockage. *Biochemistry* **43**: 5352–5359.

Reinhard C, Hebert SS, De Strooper B. 2005. The amyloid-β precursor protein: Integrating structure with biological function. *EMBO J* **24**: 3996–4006.

Repetto E, Yoon IS, Zheng H, Kang DE. 2007. Presenilin 1 regulates epidermal growth factor receptor turnover and signaling in the endosomal-lysosomal pathway. *J Biol Chem* **282**: 31504–31516.

Rogaev EI, Sherrington R, Rogaeva EA, Levesque G, Ikeda M, Liang Y, Chi H, Lin C, Holman K, Tsuda T, et al. 1995. Familial Alzheimer's disease in kindreds with missense mutations in a gene on chromosome 1 related to the Alzheimer's disease type 3 gene. *Nature* **376**: 775–778.

Sardi SP, Murtie J, Koirala S, Patten BA, Corfas G. 2006. Presenilin-dependent ErbB4 nuclear signaling regulates the timing of astrogenesis in the developing brain. *Cell* **127**: 185–197.

Sato C, Morohashi Y, Tomita T, Iwatsubo T. 2006. Structure of the catalytic pore of γ-secretase probed by the accessibility of substituted cysteines. *J Neurosci* **26**: 12081–12088.

Sato T, Diehl TS, Narayanan S, Funamoto S, Ihara Y, De Strooper B, Steiner H, Haass C, Wolfe MS. 2007. Active γ-secretase complexes contain only one of each component. *J Biol Chem* **282**: 33985–33993.

Sato C, Takagi S, Tomita T, Iwatsubo T. 2008. The C-terminal PAL motif and transmembrane domain 9 of presenilin 1 are involved in the formation of the catalytic pore of the γ-secretase. *J Neurosci* **28**: 6264–6271.

Saura CA, Choi SY, Beglopoulos V, Malkani S, Zhang D, Shankaranarayana Rao BS, Chattarji SRS, Kelleher RJ III, Kandel ER, Duff K, et al. 2004. Loss of presenilin function causes impairments of memory and synaptic plasticity followed by age-dependent neurodegeneration. *Neuron* **42**: 23–36.

Savonenko AV, Melnikova T, Laird FM, Stewart KA, Price DL, Wong PC. 2008. Alteration of BACE1-dependent NRG1/ErbB4 signaling and schizophrenia-like phenotypes in BACE1-null mice. *Proc Natl Acad Sci* **105**: 5585–5590.

Scheinfeld MH, Ghersi E, Laky K, Fowlkes BJ, D'Adamio L. 2002. Processing of β-amyloid precursor-like protein-1 and -2 by γ-secretase regulates transcription. *J Biol Chem* **277**: 44195–44201.

Scheuner D, Eckman C, Jensen M, Song X, Citron M, Suzuki N, Bird TD, Hardy J, Hutton M, Kukull W, et al. 1996. Secreted amyloid β-protein similar to that in the senile plaques of Alzheimer's disease is increased in vivo by the presenilin 1 and 2 and APP mutations linked to familial Alzheimer's disease. *Nat Med* **2**: 864–870.

Schroeter EH, Ilagan MX, Brunkan AL, Hecimovic S, Li YM, Xu M, Lewis HD, Saxena MT, De Strooper D, Coonrod A, et al. 2003. A presenilin dimer at the core of the γ-secretase enzyme: Insights from parallel analysis of Notch 1 and APP proteolysis. *Proc Natl Acad Sci* **100**: 13075–13080.

Searfoss GH, Jordan WH, Calligaro DO, Galbreath EJ, Schirtzinger LM, Berridge BR, Gao H, Higgins MA, May PC, Ryan TP. 2003. Adipsin: A biomarker of gastrointestinal toxicity mediated by a functional γsecretase inhibitor. *J Biol Chem* **278**: 46107–46116.

Serneels L, Dejaegere T, Craessaerts K, Horre K, Jorissen E, Tousseyn T, Hebert S, Coolen M, Martens G, Zwijsen A, et al. 2005. Differential contribution of the three Aph1 genes to γ-secretase activity in vivo. *Proc Natl Acad Sci* **102**: 1719–1724.

Serneels L, Van Biervliet J, Craessaerts K, Dejaegere T, Horre K, Van Houtvin T, Esselmann H, Paul S, Schafer MK, Berezovska O, et al. 2009. γ-Secretase heterogeneity in the Aph1 subunit: Relevance for Alzheimer's disease. *Science* **324**: 639–642.

Shearman MS, Beher D, Clarke EE, Lewis HD, Harrison T, Hunt P, Nadin A, Smith AL, Stevenson G, Castro JL. 2000. L-685,458, an aspartyl protease transition state mimic, is a potent inhibitor of amyloid β-protein precursor γ-secretase activity. *Biochemistry* **39**: 8698–8704.

Shen J, Kelleher RJ III. 2007. The presenilin hypothesis of Alzheimer's disease: Evidence for a loss-of-function pathogenic mechanism. *Proc Natl Acad Sci* **104**: 403–409.

Sherrington R, Rogaev EI, Liang Y, Rogaeva EA, Levesque G, Ikeda M, Chi H, Lin C, Li G, Holman K, et al. 1995. Cloning of a gene bearing missense mutations in early-onset familial Alzheimer's disease. *Nature* **375**: 754–760.

Shih Ie M, Wang TL. 2007. Notch signaling, γ-secretase inhibitors, and cancer therapy. *Cancer Res* **67**: 1879–1882.

Shirotani K, Edbauer D, Capell A, Schmitz J, Steiner H, Haass C. 2003. γ-Secretase activity is associated with a conformational change of nicastrin. *J Biol Chem* **278**: 16474–16477.

Siman R, Reaume AG, Savage MJ, Trusko S, Lin YG, Scott RW, Flood DG. 2000. Presenilin-1 P264L knock-in mutation: Differential effects on Aβ production, amyloid deposition, and neuronal vulnerability. *J Neurosci* **20**: 8717–8726.

Sobhanifar S, Schneider B, Lohr F, Gottstein F, Ikeya T, Mlynarczyk K, Pulawski W, Ghoshdastider U, Kolinski M, Filipek S, et al. 2010. Structural investigation of the C-terminal catalytic fragment of presenilin 1. *Proc Natl Acad Sci* **107**: 9644–9649.

Song W, Nadeau P, Yuan M, Yang X, Shen J, Yankner BA. 1999. Proteolytic release and nuclear translocation of Notch-1 are induced by presenilin-1 and impaired by pathogenic presenilin-1 mutations. *Proc Natl Acad Sci* **96**: 6959–6963.

Spasic D, Tolia A, Dillen K, Baert V, De Strooper B, Vrijens S, Annaert W. 2006. Presenilin-1 maintains a nine-trans-membrane topology throughout the secretory pathway. *J Biol Chem* **281**: 26569–26577.

Stefansson H, Sigurdsson E, Steinthorsdottir V, Bjornsdottir S, Sigmundsson T, Ghosh S, Brynjolfsson J, Gunnarsdottir S, Ivarsson O, Chou TT, et al. 2002. Neuregulin 1 and susceptibility to schizophrenia. *Am J Hum Genet* **71**: 877–892.

Steiner H, Kostka M, Romig H, Basset G, Pesold B, Hardy JA, Capell A, Meyn L, Grim MG, Baumeister R, et al. 2000. Glycine 384 is required for presenilin-1 function and is conserved in bacterial polytopic aspartyl proteases. *Nature Cell Biol* **2**: 848–851.

Steiner H, Winkler E, Haass C. 2008. Chemical crosslinking provides a model of the γ-secretase complex subunit architecture and evidence for close proximity of the C-terminal fragment of presenilin with APH-1. *J Biol Chem* **283**: 34677–34686.

Struhl G, Greenwald I. 1999. Presenilin is required for activity and nuclear access of Notch in *Drosophila*. *Nature* **398**: 522–525.

Takagi S, Tominaga A, Sato C, Tomita T, Iwatsubo T. 2010. Participation of transmembrane domain 1 of presenilin 1 in the catalytic pore structure of the γ-secretase. *J Neurosci* **30**: 15943–15950.

Takasugi N, Tomita T, Hayashi I, Tsuruoka M, Niimura M, Takahashi Y, Thinakaran G, Iwatsubo T. 2003. The role of presenilin cofactors in the γ-secretase complex. *Nature* **422**: 438–441.

Tammam J, Ware C, Efferson C, O'Neil J, Rao S, Qu X, Gorenstein J, Angagaw M, Kim H, Kenific C, et al. 2009. Down-regulation of the Notch pathway mediated by a γ-secretase inhibitor induces anti-tumour effects in mouse models of T-cell leukaemia. *Br J Pharmacol* **158**: 1183–1195.

Teranishi Y, Hur JY, Welander H, Franberg J, Aoki M, Winblad B, Frykman S, Tjernberg LO. 2009. Affinity pulldown of γ-secretase and associated proteins from human and rat brain. *J Cell Mol Med* **14**: 2675–2686.

Thinakaran G, Borchelt DR, Lee MK, Slunt HH, Spitzer L, Kim G, Ratovitsky T, Davenport F, Nordstedt C, Seeger M, et al. 1996. Endoproteolysis of presenilin 1 and accumulation of processed derivatives in vivo. *Neuron* **17**: 181–190.

Thinakaran G, Harris CL, Ratovitski T, Davenport F, Slunt HH, Price DL, Borchelt DR, Sisodia SS. 1997. Evidence that levels of presenilins (PS1 and PS2) are coordinately regulated by competition for limiting cellular factors. *J Biol Chem* **272**: 28415–28422.

Tolia A, Chavez-Gutierrez L, De Strooper B. 2006. Contribution of presenilin transmembrane domains 6 and 7 to a water-containing cavity in the γ-secretase complex. *J Biol Chem* **281**: 27633–27642.

Tolia A, Horre K, De Strooper B. 2008. Transmembrane domain 9 of presenilin determines the dynamic conformation of the catalytic site of γ-secretase. *J Biol Chem* **283:** 19793–19803.

Tournoy J, Bossuyt X, Snellinx A, Regent M, Garmyn M, Serneels L, Saftig P, Craessaerts K, De Strooper B, Hartmann D. 2004. Partial loss of presenilins causes seborrheic keratosis and autoimmune disease in mice. *Hum Mol Genet* **13:** 1321–1331.

Tu H, Nelson O, Bezprozvanny A, Wang Z, Lee SF, Hao YH, Serneels L, De Strooper B, Yu G, Bezprozvanny I. 2006. Presenilins form ER Ca^{2+} leak channels, a function disrupted by familial Alzheimer's disease-linked mutations. *Cell* **126:** 981–993.

van Es JH, van Gijn ME, Riccio O, van den Born M, Vooijs M, Begthel H, Cozijnsen M, Robine S, Winton DJ, Radtke F, et al. 2005. Notch/γ-secretase inhibition turns proliferative cells in intestinal crypts and adenomas into goblet cells. *Nature* **435:** 959–963.

Wakabayashi T, De Strooper B. 2008. Presenilins: Members of the γ-secretase quartets, but part-time soloists too. *Physiology (Bethesda)* **23:** 194–204.

Wakabayashi T, Craessaerts K, Bammens L, Bentahir M, Borgions F, Herdewijn P, Staes A, Timmerman E, Vandekerckhove J, Rubinstein E, et al. 2009. Analysis of the γ-secretase interactome and validation of its association with tetraspanin-enriched microdomains. *Nat Cell Biol* **11:** 1340–1346.

Wang Y, Chan SL, Miele L, Yao PJ, Mackes J, Ingram DK, Mattson MP, Furukawa K. 2004. Involvement of Notch signaling in hippocampal synaptic plasticity. *Proc Natl Acad Sci* **101:** 9458–9462.

Wang B, Yang W, Wen W, Sun J, Su B, Liu B, Ma D, Lv D, Wen Y, Qu T, et al. 2010. γ-Secretase gene mutations in familial acne inversa. *Science* **330:** 1065.

Watanabe N, Tomita T, Sato C, Kitamura T, Morohashi Y, Iwatsubo T. 2005. Pen-2 is incorporated into the γ-secretase complex through binding to transmembrane domain 4 of presenilin 1. *J Biol Chem* **280:** 41967–41975.

Weggen S, Eriksen JL, Das P, Sagi SA, Wang R, Pietrzik CU, Findlay KA, Smith TE, Murphy MP, Bulter T, et al. 2001. A subset of NSAIDs lower amyloidogenic Aβ42 independently of cyclooxygenase activity. *Nature* **414:** 212–216.

Weihofen A, Binns K, Lemberg MK, Ashman K, Martoglio B. 2002. Identification of signal peptide peptidase, a presenilin-type aspartic protease. *Science* **296:** 2215–2218.

Weng AP, Ferrando AA, Lee W, Morris JPT, Silverman LB, Sanchez-Irizarry C, Blacklow SC, Look AT, Aster JC. 2004. Activating mutations of NOTCH1 in human T cell acute lymphoblastic leukemia. *Science* **306:** 269–271.

Willem M, Garratt AN, Novak B, Citron M, Kaufmann S, Rittger A, DeStrooper B, Saftig P, Birchmeier C, Haass C. 2006. Control of peripheral nerve myelination by the β-secretase BACE1. *Science* **314:** 664–666.

Wilson CA, Murphy DD, Giasson BI, Zhang B, Trojanowski JQ, Lee VM. 2004. Degradative organelles containing mislocalized α- and β-synuclein proliferate in presenilin-1 null neurons. *J Cell Biol* **165:** 335–346.

Wines-Samuelson M, Schulte EC, Smith MJ, Aoki C, Liu X, Kelleher RJ III, Shen J. 2010. Characterization of age-dependent and progressive cortical neuronal degeneration in presenilin conditional mutant mice. *PLoS One* **5:** e10195.

Winkler E, Hobson S, Fukumori A, Dumpelfeld B, Luebbers T, Baumann K, Haass C, Hopf C, Steiner H. 2009. Purification, pharmacological modulation, and biochemical characterization of interactors of endogenous human γ-secretase. *Biochemistry* **48:** 1183–1197.

Wolfe MS, Kopan R. 2004. Intramembrane proteolysis: Theme and variations. *Science* **305:** 1119–1123.

Wolfe MS, Xia W, Moore CL, Leatherwood DD, Ostaszewski B, Donkor IO, Selkoe DJ. 1999a. Peptidomimetic probes and molecular modeling suggest Alzheimer's γ-secretases are intramembrane-cleaving aspartyl proteases. *Biochemistry* **38:** 4720–4727.

Wolfe MS, Xia W, Ostaszewski BL, Diehl TS, Kimberly WT, Selkoe DJ. 1999b. Two transmembrane aspartates in presenilin-1 required for presenilin endoproteolysis and γ-secretase activity. *Nature* **398:** 513–517.

Wolfe MS, De Los Angeles J, Miller DD, Xia W, Selkoe DJ. 1999c. Are presenilins intramembrane-cleaving proteases? Implications for the molecular mechanism of Alzheimer's disease. *Biochemistry* **38:** 11223–11230.

Wong GT, Manfra D, Poulet FM, Zhang Q, Josien H, Bara T, Engstrom L, Pinzon-Ortiz M, Fine JS, Lee HJ, et al. 2004. Chronic treatment with the γ-secretase inhibitor LY-411,575 inhibits β-amyloid peptide production and alters lymphopoiesis and intestinal cell differentiation. *J Biol Chem* **279:** 12876–12882.

Xia X, Qian S, Soriano S, Wu Y, Fletcher AM, Wang XJ, Koo EH, Wu X, Zheng H. 2001. Loss of presenilin 1 is associated with enhanced β-catenin signaling and skin tumorigenesis. *Proc Natl Acad Sci* **98:** 10863–10868.

Yanagida K, Okochi M, Tagami S, Nakayama T, Kodama TS, Nishitomi K, Jiang J, Mori K, Tatsumi S, Arai T, et al. 2009. The 28-amino acid form of an APLP1-derived Aβ-like peptide is a surrogate marker for Aβ42 production in the central nervous system. *EMBO Mol Med* **1:** 223–235.

Yu G, Nishimura M, Arawaka S, Levitan D, Zhang L, Tandon A, Song YQ, Rogaeva E, Chen F, Kawarai T, et al. 2000. Nicastrin modulates presenilin-mediated notch/glp-1 signal transduction and βAPP processing. *Nature* **407:** 48–54.

Zhang C, Wu B, Beglopoulos V, Wines-Samuelson M, Zhang D, Dragatsis I, Sudhof TC, Shen J. 2009. Presenilins are essential for regulating neurotransmitter release. *Nature* **460:** 632–636.

Zou K, Hosono T, Nakamura T, Shiraishi H, Maeda T, Komano H, Yanagisawa K, Michikawa M. 2008. Novel role of presenilins in maturation and transport of integrin β1. *Biochemistry* **47:** 3370–3378.

Apolipoprotein E and Apolipoprotein E Receptors: Normal Biology and Roles in Alzheimer Disease

David M. Holtzman[1], Joachim Herz[2], and Guojun Bu[3]

[1]Department of Neurology, Alzheimer's Disease Research Center, Hope Center for Neurological Disorders, Washington University School of Medicine, St. Louis, Missouri 63110

[2]Departments of Molecular Genetics, Neuroscience, and Neurology and Neurotherapeutics, University of Texas, Southwestern, Dallas, Texas 75390-9046

[3]Department of Neuroscience, Mayo Clinic, Jacksonville, Florida 32224

Correspondence: holtzman@neuro.wustl.edu

Apolipoprotein E (*APOE*) genotype is the major genetic risk factor for Alzheimer disease (AD); the ε4 allele increases risk and the ε2 allele is protective. In the central nervous system (CNS), apoE is produced by glial cells, is present in high-density-like lipoproteins, interacts with several receptors that are members of the low-density lipoprotein receptor (LDLR) family, and is a protein that binds to the amyloid-β (Aβ) peptide. There are a variety of mechanisms by which apoE isoform may influence risk for AD. There is substantial evidence that differential effects of apoE isoform on AD risk are influenced by the ability of apoE to affect Aβ aggregation and clearance in the brain. Other mechanisms are also likely to play a role in the ability of apoE to influence CNS function as well as AD, including effects on synaptic plasticity, cell signaling, lipid transport and metabolism, and neuroinflammation. ApoE receptors, including LDLRs, Apoer2, very low-density lipoprotein receptors (VLDLRs), and lipoprotein receptor-related protein 1 (LRP1) appear to influence both the CNS effects of apoE as well as Aβ metabolism and toxicity. Therapeutic strategies based on apoE and apoE receptors may include influencing apoE/Aβ interactions, apoE structure, apoE lipidation, LDLR receptor family member function, and signaling. Understanding the normal and disease-related biology connecting apoE, apoE receptors, and AD is likely to provide novel insights into AD pathogenesis and treatment.

Alzheimer disease (AD), specifically the late-onset form of AD (LOAD), is the most common cause of dementia in individuals older than 60 years of age. Although mutations in the genes *PS1*, *PS2*, and *APP* cause less common forms of early-onset, autosomal dominant familial AD (FAD), these cases represent <1% of AD. In addition to the genes that cause FAD, LOAD also has a strong genetic component. Although several susceptibility genes for AD have been reported, by far the strongest genetic risk factor for LOAD is apolipoprotein

E (*APOE*) genotype, with the ε4 allele being an AD risk factor and the ε2 allele being protective relative to the prevalent ε3 allele (Corder et al. 1993; Strittmatter et al. 1993a). Strong evidence suggests a major mechanism by which apoE influences AD and cerebral amyloid angiopathy (CAA) is via its effects on Aβ metabolism (Kim et al. 2009a; Castellano et al. 2011). Current understanding of apoE biology in the CNS and how apoE/Aβ interactions are relevant to AD will be reviewed in the first section. There are several apoE receptors that are members of the LDLR family (Fig. 1). Some of these receptors, such as LDLR and LRP1, influence apoE levels (Fryer et al. 2005a; Liu et al. 2007). Others, such as Apoer2 and VLDLR, although apoE receptors, are also receptors for other ligands such as the neuromodulatory signaling protein

Reelin, which plays an important role in neuro-development and synaptic function. These receptors are involved in neural signaling and tau phosphorylation, and there is evidence that apoE can counteract some of the neurotoxicity caused by Aβ. Apoer2 and VLDLR will be reviewed in the second section. LDLR and LRP1 are important receptors for apoE in the brain that regulate CNS apoE levels. Although LDLR has no known ligand other than apoE in the CNS, LRP is somewhat unique in that it has multiple ligands, binds to both APP and Aβ, and influences APP and Aβ metabolism. LDLR and LRP1 will be reviewed in the third section. Although there are currently no apoE-based therapies for AD, given the effects of apoE and apoE receptors on both Aβ and CNS development and function, a variety of

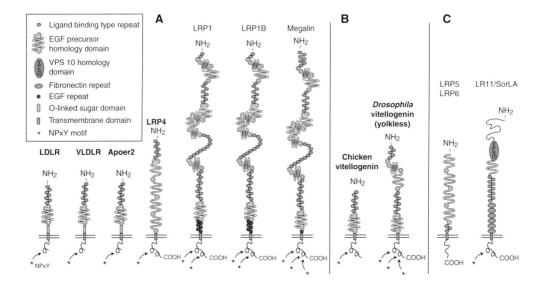

Figure 1. The low-density lipoprotein (LDL) receptor gene family. (*A*) The core LDL receptor gene family as it exists in mammalian species. These family members are characterized by one or more ligand-binding domains, epidermal growth factor (EGF), homology domains consisting of EGF repeats and YWTD propeller (β-propeller) domains involved in pH-dependent release of ligands in the endosomes, a single transmembrane domain and a cytoplasmic tail containing at least one NPxY motif. The latter represents both the endocytosis signal as well as a binding site for adaptor proteins linking the receptor to intracellular signaling pathways. Furthermore, LDLR, VLDLR, and Apoer2 carry an O-linked sugar domain. (*B*) Equivalent receptors that are structurally and functionally distinct family members in nonmammalian species. (*C*) A subgroup of functionally important, but more distantly related family members that share some, but not all, of the structural requirements of the "core members." In addition, they could also contain domains, e.g., vacuolar protein sorting (VPS) domains, which are not present in the core family. (From Dieckmann et al. 2010; reprinted, with permission, from Walter de Gruyter GmbH © 2010.)

apoE/apoE receptor-based approaches will be discussed.

ApoE: POTENTIAL ROLE IN AD

Neurobiology of ApoE

The human apoE protein is a 299 amino acid glycoprotein that is expressed by several cell types, but with highest expression in the liver and in the CNS (Mahley 1988). In the brain, apoE is expressed predominantly by astrocytes but also by microglia (Fig. 2) (Pitas et al. 1987; Grehan et al. 2001). Under certain conditions, such as after excitotoxic injury, some neurons appear to be able to synthesize apoE (Xu et al. 1999; Xu et al. 2006). Under physiological conditions, apoE is present in lipoprotein particles (Fig. 2). Although it is present in lipoproteins of different size classes in plasma, in the CNS, it is the most abundantly produced apoprotein and is secreted by glial cells in nascent high-density lipoprotein (HDL)-like particles (Pitas et al. 1987; DeMattos et al. 2001) that are discoidal in shape and contain phospholipids and cholesterol. ApoE is also present in cerebrospinal fluid (CSF) at a concentration of ~5 μg/ml, in spherical particles that are similar to glial-secreted HDL, except that they also contain a cholesteryl ester core (LaDu et al. 1998). Although apoE-containing lipoproteins may play a role in reverse cholesterol transport as well as in cholesterol and lipid delivery, their role in CNS lipid and cholesterol homeostasis is not yet clearly defined. As in the periphery, apoE functions as a ligand in receptor-mediated endocytosis of lipoprotein particles in the CNS. In vitro studies have shown that cholesterol released from apoE-containing lipoprotein particles is used to support synaptogenesis (Mauch et al. 2001) and the maintenance of synaptic connections (Pfrieger 2003). Although there is some in vitro (Nathan et al. 1994; Holtzman et al. 1995) and in vivo (Masliah et al. 1995; Poirier 2003) data suggesting that apoE can play a role in neuronal sprouting after injury, whether apoE plays a major role in supporting synaptogenesis and maintenance of synaptic connections in vivo in the uninjured brain has not

yet been proven. For example, several studies have shown that the brain of apoE knockout mice, for the most part, appears normal in the absence of injury (Anderson et al. 1998; Fagan et al. 1998). Moreover, no overt cognitive defects have been reported in humans with genetic ApoE deficiency. In addition to apoE, several other apolipoliproteins are present in the CNS, the most abundant being apoAI and apoJ, also called clusterin. ApoE in the CNS is derived from the CNS; the same appears to be true for clusterin. In contrast, apoAI in CNS is derived from the periphery (Sorci-Thomas et al. 1988). Whether apoAI and clusterin play a role in CNS lipid metabolism, or in normal brain function, is not clear. Genetic deficiency of either protein in humans or mice does not result in an obvious CNS phenotype (Schaefer et al. 1982; McLaughlin et al. 2000). Interestingly, single-nucleotide polymorphisms in clusterin have been shown to be a risk factor for AD (Harold et al. 2009; Lambert et al. 2009). The mechanism for this is unclear, although animal model data have shown that clusterin strongly influences Aβ aggregation and toxicity in vivo (DeMattos et al. 2002; DeMattos et al. 2004).

Genetic, Clinical, and Biomarker Observations on Relationship of ApoE and AD

The human apoE gene contains several single-nucleotide polymorphisms (SNPs) distributed across the gene (Nickerson et al. 2000). The most common three SNPs lead to changes in the coding sequence and result in the three common isoforms of apoE: apoE2 (cys112, cys158), apoE3 (cys112, arg158), and apoE4 (arg112, arg158). Although the three common isoforms differ by only one or two amino acids at residues 112 or 158, these differences alter apoE structure and function (Mahley et al. 2006). In regard to the connection between apoE and AD, apoE was found to colocalize with amyloid plaques in the early 1990s (Namba et al. 1991; Wisniewski and Frangione 1992). After that, the ε4 allele of the *APOE* gene was discovered to be a strong genetic risk factor for AD (Corder et al. 1993; Strittmatter

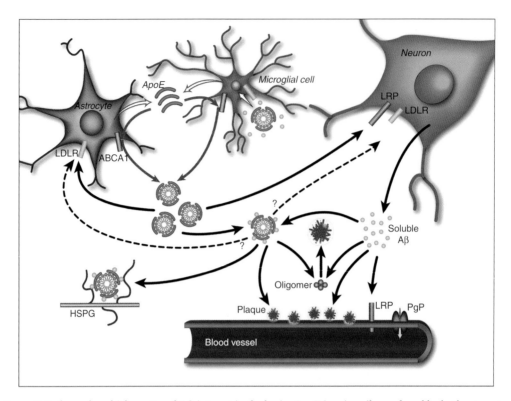

Figure 2. Pathways by which apoE and Aβ interact in the brain. ApoE is primarily produced by both astrocytes and microglia and is subsequently lipidated by ABCA1 to form lipoprotein particles. In the extracellular space, lipidated apoE binds to soluble Aβ in an isoform-dependent pattern (E2 > E3 > E4) and influences the formation of parenchymal amyloid plaques and transport of Aβ within the CNS. ApoE is endocytosed into various cell types within the brain by different members of the LDL receptor family, including LDLR and LRP1. ApoE may also facilitate the cellular uptake of Aβ through the endocytosis of a complex of apoE-containing lipoprotein particles bound to Aβ in a manner that likely depends on the isoforms and its level of lipidation. Furthermore, apoE has been shown to directly enhance both the degradation of Aβ within microglial cells and the ability of astrocytes to clear diffuse Aβ deposits (Koistinaho et al. 2004; Jiang et al. 2008). Aβ associated with apoE-containing lipoprotein particles may also be retained within the CNS through their binding to heparin sulfate proteoglycan (HSPG) moieties present in the extracellular space (Mahley and Rall 2000). At the blood–brain barrier (BBB), soluble Aβ is predominantly transported from the interstitial fluid into the bloodstream via LRP1 and P-glycoprotein (Cirrito et al. 2005; Zlokovic 2008). ApoE has been shown to slow the transport of Aβ across the BBB in an isoform-dependent manner (E4 > E3 > E2) (Bell et al. 2007; Ito et al. 2007; Deane et al. 2008). In addition, apoE can influence the pathogenesis of CAA in an amyloid protein precursor (APP)-transgenic mouse model, with apoE4 increasing the amount of vascular plaques in comparison to apoE3 (Fryer et al. 2005b). (From Kim et al. 2009; reprinted, with permission, from Elsevier © 2009.)

et al. 1993a). Since then, numerous studies have confirmed that the ε4 allele is the strongest genetic risk factor for both AD and CAA, or a combination of both disorders (Schmechel et al. 1993; Greenberg et al. 1995; Bertram et al. 2007). As compared to individuals with no ε4 alleles, the increased risk for AD is approximately threefold in people with one ε4 allele and ∼ 12-fold in those with two ε4 alleles. The odds ratio for ε4 versus ε3 alleles by meta-analysis of multiple studies is 3.68 as of June 2011 (www.alzgene.org). Importantly, the ε2 allele of apoE is associated with a lower risk for AD (Corder et al. 1994; Farrer et al. 1997) with an odds ratio of ε2 versus ε3 of 0.62 as of June 2011 (www.alzgene.org).

Evidence of a Key Role for ApoE on Aβ Metabolism in AD Pathogenesis

In vitro and in vivo data including data in humans and animal models suggests that the physical interaction of apoE with Aβ plays an important role in AD and CAA pathogenesis (Fig. 1). It was first proposed that apoE was an Aβ-binding protein in the brain that induces a pathological β-sheet conformational change in Aβ (Wisniewski and Frangione 1992). Pathological studies showed a positive correlation between plaque density and ε4 allele dose in AD patients at autopsy (Rebeck et al. 1993; Schmechel et al. 1993). Although some studies reported conflicting findings (Benjamin et al. 1995; Heinonen et al. 1995), a large autopsy study strongly suggested that ε4 dosage is associated with increased neuritic plaques in AD (Tiraboschi et al. 2004). If the effect of apoE4 is to accelerate the average onset of Aβ deposition in the brain, an expectation would be that middle-aged individuals at risk to develop AD in the future who are still cogntively normal would have larger amounts of Aβ deposition in the brain. This has now been shown to be the case as evidenced by amyloid-imaging studies with Pittsburgh compound B as well as CSF studies using CSF Aβ42 in which a decrease has been shown to indicate brain amyloid deposition. Cognitively normal apoE4-positive middle-aged and elderly individuals are much more likely to have brain amyloid (Reiman et al. 2009; Morris et al. 2010) and low CSF Aβ42 (Sunderland et al. 2004; Morris et al. 2010) than apoE4-negative individuals. Further, apoE2-positive individuals rarely develop fibrillar Aβ as defined by a positive amyloid-imaging scan (Morris et al. 2010).

Whereas human data supports the idea that apoE isoforms result in differential susceptibilty to Aβ aggregation in the brain, animal studies utilizing genetically modified mice that develop Aβ deposition and express human apoE isoforms show more directly that human apoE isoforms have a strong effect on the time of onset of Aβ aggregation as well as the amount, location, and conformation of Aβ in the brain. Early studies with APP-transgenic (Tg) mice that develop Aβ deposition in the brain (PDAPP and Tg2576 models) showed that when these mice were crossed with apoE$^{-/-}$ mice, there was less Aβ deposition and a virtual abolishment of true amyloid plaques, plaque-associated neuritic dystrophy, CAA, and CAA-associated microhemorrhage in the absence of apoE (Bales et al. 1997; Bales et al. 1999; Holtzman et al. 2000b; Fryer et al. 2003). In addition, the anatomical pattern of Aβ deposition differs in the absence of apoE (Holtzman et al. 2000a; Irizarry et al. 2000). The expression of human apoE isoforms in either PDAPP or Tg2576 Tg mice resulted in a marked delay in the deposition of Aβ and formation of neuritic plaques, compared with APP Tg mice expressing no apoE or mouse apoE (Fagan et al. 2002; Fryer et al. 2005b). Importantly, expression of human apoE isoforms in APP Tg mice results in an isoform-specific effect on the amount of Aβ accumulation as well as true amyloid deposits (E4 > E3 > E2) (Holtzman et al. 2000a; Fagan et al. 2002; Fryer et al. 2005b). In addition to the isoform-specific effects of human apoE on parenchymal Aβ pathology, crossing human apoE knockin mice to Tg2576 mice resulted in a relative shift of Aβ deposition from the brain parenchyma to arterioles in the form of CAA in apoE4 expressing mice relative to apoE3 or mouse apoE (Fryer et al. 2005b). A similar effect of apoE4 predisposing to CAA is seen in humans. These data strongly suggest that understanding the in vivo mechanisms underlying the apoE isoform-mediated difference in Aβ accumulation is critical for relating these findings to the pathogenesis of AD.

The underlying mechanism underlying how apoE influences Aβ aggregation and accumulation in the brain is on its way to being elucidated. In vitro and in vivo studies suggest that apoE may influence Aβ seeding and fibrillogenesis, as well as soluble Aβ clearance. Lipid-free and lipidated (physiological) forms of apoE can interact with Aβ in vitro (Strittmatter et al. 1993b; LaDu et al. 1994; Sanan et al. 1994; Aleshkov et al. 1997; Yang et al. 1997; Tokuda et al. 2000). Most studies show that the efficiency of complex formation between lipidated apoE and Aβ follows the order of apoE2 > apoE3 >> apoE4. The effect of apoE isoforms on Aβ aggregation has also been investigated extensively in vitro. Some studies show apoE causing greater fibrillization (E4 > E3 > E2) (Ma et al. 1994; Wisniewski et al. 1994; Castano et al. 1995), whereas others show that apoE inhibits fibrillization (Evans et al. 1994; Wood et al. 1996). Conflicting results between in vitro studies may be owing to the differences in apoE and Aβ preparations or other factors. Altering the lipidation state of apoE in the brain is associated with strong effects on Aβ fibrillization in vivo. ATP-binding cassette A1 (ABCA1) normally lipidates apoE in the brain. When APP Tg mice are crossed onto an $Abca1^{-/-}$ background, this decreases apoE lipidation and increases amyloid deposition (Hirsch-Reinshagen et al. 2005; Koldamova et al. 2005a; Wahrle et al. 2005), whereas increasing ABCA1 increases apoE lipidation and decreases amyloid deposition (Wahrle et al. 2008).

In addition to the effects of apoE on fibrillogenesis, there is evidence that apoE alters both the transport and clearance of soluble Aβ in the brain (Fig. 1). A recent study shows that apoE isoforms do not differentially influence Aβ production in vivo; however, apoE isoforms differentially affect Aβ clearance before Aβ deposition with E4 resulting in clearance that is slower than E3 and E2 (Castellano et al. 2011). These results suggest the difference in Aβ accumulation between apoE isoforms is likely because of isoform-specific differences in Aβ clearance. ApoE seems to play an important role in the clearance of Aβ through several possible mechanisms. ApoE-containing lipoprotein particles may sequester Aβ and modulate the cellular uptake of an apoE-Aβ complex by receptor-mediated endocytosis. Alternatively, apoE may modulate Aβ removal from the brain to the systemic circulation by transport across the blood–brain barrier. Data from in vitro studies support the idea that apoE facilitates the binding and internalization of soluble Aβ by cells or its clearance via enzymes such as neprilysn (Beffert et al. 1998; Yang et al. 1999; Cole and Ard 2000; Koistinaho et al. 2004; Jiang et al. 2008). Although in vitro studies suggest

that apoE enhances cellular Aβ uptake and degradation (Kim et al. 2009a), there is in vivo evidence that apoE retards Aβ clearance from the brain (DeMattos et al. 2004; Bell et al. 2007; Deane et al. 2008), possibly via an effect at the blood–brain barrier (BBB) (Fig. 1) (Zlokovic 2008). More work is clearly needed to determine the exact role that apoE has in modifying brain Aβ clearance, the role of the BBB in the process, and whether isoform-specific effects exist.

Several key questions remain to be further addressed regarding the effect of apoE on Aβ. Whether it is better to increase or decrease human apoE levels (regardless of isoform) to reduce Aβ levels is still unanswered. Analyzing whether, and to what extent, altering human apoE level affects Aβ pathology will help determine whether targeting apoE levels may be a viable therapeutic option for influencing Aβ levels and toxicity, and ultimately treating AD.

ApoE RECEPTORS AND SYNAPTIC PLASTICITY

The strong association of ApoE4 with late-onset AD raised the possibility that ApoE is mediating its powerful effect on the average age of disease onset at least in part through the receptors to which it binds. These ApoE receptors include the core, as well as potentially several more distantly related members of the LDLR gene family (Fig. 1). LRP1 has been repeatedly, albeit weakly, associated with AD risk (Beffert et al. 1999; Vazquez-Higuera et al. 2009), and a coding polymorphism in the distantly related Wnt coreceptor LRP6 has also been implicated (De Ferrari et al. 2007). None of the other family members have so far been convincingly associated with AD by human genetic data. The absence of genetic association, however, does not preclude important roles for these multifunctional receptors in the molecular mechanisms that underlie the disease process. The very nature of their essential functions during the development of the embryo in general (Herz et al. 1992; Johnson et al. 2005; Dietrich et al. 2010; Karner et al. 2010), and the brain, in particular (Willnow et al. 1996; Trommsdorff et al. 1999; May et al. 2004; Boycott et al. 2005; Boycott et al. 2009), may occlude their participation in AD pathogenesis, which would manifest itself much later in life.

Mechanisms by which ApoE receptors may contribute to AD development and progression may include roles in the control of inflammation (Lillis et al. 2008; Zurhove et al. 2008), cholesterol metabolism (reviewed in Herz et al. 2009), neurogenesis (Gajera et al. 2010), or the generation and trafficking of APP and Aβ (reviewed in the third section). Other potential mechanisms by which ApoE receptors may promote neuronal survival (Beffert et al. 2006b) during aging involve signaling pathways that control microtubule and actin dynamics (Beffert et al. 2002; Assadi et al. 2003; Brich et al. 2003; Ohkubo et al. 2003; Chai et al. 2009; Forster et al. 2010; Rust et al. 2010), dendritogenesis (Niu et al. 2004), spine formation (Niu et al. 2008), glutamate receptor function and synaptic plasticity (Zhuo et al. 2000; Weeber et al. 2002; Beffert et al. 2005; Chen et al. 2005; D'Arcangelo 2005; Sinagra et al. 2005; Groc et al. 2007; Durakoglugil et al. 2009; Korwek et al. 2009; Chen et al. 2010), as well as learning and memory (reviewed in Herz and Beffert 2000; Herz and Chen 2006; Bu 2009; Herz 2009). In this section we will mainly focus on the role of the ApoE receptors Apoer2 and Vldlr and their ligand Reelin in these processes.

Molecular Basis of Signal Transduction by Neuronal ApoE Receptors

ApoE receptors contain only short cytoplasmic tails, which lack functional enzymatic domains through which many cell-surface receptors transmit extracellular signals into the cell. However, they harbor a variety of short conserved sequence stretches, such as the tetra-amino acid NPxY motif, which serve as docking sites for a wide array of cytoplasmic adaptor and scaffolding proteins (Trommsdorff et al. 1998; Gotthardt et al. 2000; Beffert et al. 2005; Hoe et al. 2006a; Hoe et al. 2006b). The receptors can also interact as coreceptors through their extracellular domains with other types of signaling

proteins and modules, and thereby modulate their intrinsic activity (Boucher et al. 2002; Loukinova et al. 2002; Huang et al. 2003; Lillis et al. 2008; Zurhove et al. 2008), including that of the N-methyl-D-aspartate (NMDA) receptor (May et al. 2004; Beffert et al. 2005; Hoe et al. 2006b).

Apoer2 and Vldlr are a notable exception, inasmuch as they do not need to associate with another protein with intrinsic signal transduction activity to elicit an intracellular signal. Both receptors bind the large homo-oligomeric signaling protein Reelin with high affinity (D'Arcangelo et al. 1999; Hiesberger et al. 1999), resulting in their clustering at the plasma membrane (Strasser et al. 2004). The simultaneous interaction of the adapter protein Disabled 1 (Dab1) with NPxY motifs in their intracellular domains (ICDs) (Trommsdorff et al. 1998; Stolt et al. 2005) results in the progressive recruitment and transphosphorylation of Src family tyrosine kinases (SFKs) (Howell et al. 1997; Arnaud et al. 2003; Bock and Herz 2003). This in turn initiates a kinase casade inside the neuron, starting with the activation of phosphoinositide-3-kinase (PI3K), which subsequently activates protein kinase B (also known as Akt), and ending with the inhibition of glycogen synthase 3β (GSK3β) (Beffert et al. 2002), one of the primary kinases that phosphorylate the microtubule stabilizing protein tau on the same sites that are typically abnormally phosphorylated in the neurofibrillary tangles in the AD-afflicted brain.

Reelin signaling is essential for normal brain development by regulating a pathway that controls the migration and positioning of the neuronal cell bodies in their appropriate cortical layers of the neocortex and the cerebellum (Tissir and Goffinet 2003), as well as neuronal connectivity (Del Rio et al. 1997). Activation of SFKs is the "master switch" that is required for the initiation of all subsequent downstream signaling events, which are not limited to the control of GSK3β activity but also involve the regulation of Lis1-dependent nuclear translocation (Shu et al. 2004), n-cofilin-mediated actin reorganization (Chai et al. 2009; Frotscher 2010), and tyrosine phosphorylation of NMDA receptor subunits (Beffert et al. 2005; Chen et al. 2005).

Regulation of Tau Phosphorylation

Genetic disruption of any component of this Reelin-Apoer2/Vldlr-Dab1 signaling pathway in the mouse, i.e., loss-of-function mutations in the ligand, the receptors, or the adaptor protein, results in reduced phosphorylation of GSK3β on an inhibitory serine residue, which leads to disinhibition of the enzyme and hyperphosphorylation of tau (Hiesberger et al. 1999; Beffert et al. 2002; Brich et al. 2003; Ohkubo et al. 2003). High levels of tau phosphorylation disrupt neuronal vesicle transport by compromising microtubule stability (Mudher et al. 2004), and consequently lead to variable degrees of neuronal dysfunction and premature death of signaling defective mutant mice (Sheldon et al. 1997; Trommsdorff et al. 1999; Brich et al. 2003). Intriguingly, genetic deficiency of tau prevents APP/Aβ-induced cognitive defects as well as excitotoxicity in mice (Roberson et al. 2007), indicating that the presence of abnormally phosphorylated tau, rather than its functional loss, is the likely reason for the severe motor defects that cause the premature death in the Reelin pathway mutants. This is further supported by a series of recent studies that showed a broad effect of mislocalized, phosphorylated tau on the spinodendritic targeting of Fyn (Ittner et al. 2010) and of the scaffolding protein JIP1 (Ittner et al. 2010), as well as on the disruption of glutamate receptor trafficking and recycling (Hoover et al. 2010). Intriguingly, the tau-induced synaptic defects are prevented or reversed by reducing the tau levels (Roberson et al. 2011; Sydow et al. 2011).

Loss of LRP1 also results in increased GSK3β activity, at least in fibroblasts and adipocytes, as a result of a loss of autocrine Wnt5a expression (Terrand et al. 2009). Conditional LRP1 knockout mice, lacking LRP1 expression exclusively in postmitotic neurons, also display severe locomotor abnormalities (May et al. 2004), raising the possibility that these dysfunctions could also be caused in part by defective regulation of tau phosphorylation, although

this has not been explored at the time of this writing.

Tau hyperphosphorylation in Reelin signaling defective animals on a mixed strain background is highly variable (Hiesberger et al. 1999) and strongly dependent on the background strains. This observation was exploited in an unbiased approach to map genetic modifiers of ApoE receptor/Dab1-dependent tau phosphorylation in the mouse (Brich et al. 2003). Surprisingly, the strongest modifier mapped to a narrow genomic region centered around APP on mouse chromosome 16, in addition to a suggestive quantitative trait in the vicinity of Presenilin 1 on chromosome 12. Together these findings add further support to a model in which ApoE receptors functionally interact with APP, Aβ, and tau to control the molecular mechanisms that underlie the pathogenesis of AD.

Regulation of Dendritic Spines, Glutamatergic Neurotransmission, and Synaptic Plasticity

Numerous independent studies and observations point toward a role for Reelin and ApoE receptors in the formation of neuronal connections (Del Rio et al. 1997; Borrell et al. 2007) and the generation of dendritic complexity (Trommsdorff et al. 1999; Costa et al. 2001; Niu et al. 2004; Matsuki et al. 2008; Hoe et al. 2009). The latter may, however, not be entirely dependent on Apoer2 and Vldlr (Chameau et al. 2009) and may also involve interactions with APP (Hoe et al. 2009). Reelin signaling also regulates dendritic spine morphology (Costa et al. 2001; Niu et al. 2008; Pujadas et al. 2010), which likely involves regulation of actin dynamics and the participation of n-cofilin (Chai et al. 2009; Rust et al. 2010). It activates LIM kinase (LIMK), which inhibits the actin-depolymerizing activity of n-cofilin. The dynamic remodeling of synaptic connections requires constant reorganization of actin filaments (Dillon and Goda 2005). Consequently, postnatal disruption of n-cofilin in mice leads to increased synapse density and enlargement of axospinous synapses (Rust et al.

2010) with defects in long-term potentiation (LTP) and long-term depression (LTD). Although synaptic AMPA receptor mobility is not affected, diffusion of extrasynaptic AMPA receptors is reduced owing to F-actin stabilization, preventing efficient egress of AMPA receptors from the synaptic into the extrasynaptic domain, and thus LTD, in the n-cofilin mutants. Similarly, Reelin has been shown to regulate surface mobility and synaptic residency of NMDA receptor NR2B subunits (Groc et al. 2007). It is thus required for NMDA receptor maturation (Sinagra et al. 2005) and for the maintenance of normal NR2A/B ratios (Campo et al. 2009).

These findings explain the profound effect of Reelin on glutamatergic neurotransmission and synaptic plasticity ex corpore (Weeber et al. 2002; Beffert et al. 2005; Beffert et al. 2006b; Qiu et al. 2006; Campo ct al. 2009) and in vivo (Pujadas et al. 2010) (E Weeber, pers. comm.). Reelin potently increases LTP, which requires the presence of both receptors, Apoer2 and Vldlr (Weeber et al. 2002). This increase of synaptic plasticity is mediated by the effect Reelin has on NMDA and AMPA receptor trafficking and conductance, which determine the synaptic acitivity of these glutamate receptors (Qiu et al. 2006). It further requires the presence of a 59 amino acid insert encoded by an alternatively spliced exon in the cytoplasmic domain of Apoer2 (Beffert et al. 2005). Only when the insert is present can Apoer2 functionally couple with NMDA receptors and induce tyrosine phosphorylation of NR2 subunits in response to Reelin. Increased tyrosine phosphorylation of the NMDA receptor increases ion gating and reduces its endocytosis, thereby increasing NMDA receptor activity overall (Salter and Kalia 2004; Snyder et al. 2005). Intriguingly, differential splicing of this exon is regulated in a circadian, activity-driven manner (Beffert et al. 2005), suggesting that periodic variation of NMDA receptor activity by Reelin is physiologically significant for synapse function, learning, and memory (Beffert et al. 2002; Weeber et al. 2002; Beffert et al. 2005; D'Arcangelo 2005; Beffert et al. 2006b; Pujadas et al. 2010).

ApoE Receptors as Antagonists of Aβ-Induced Synaptic Suppression

Aβ$_{1-42}$ oligomers are strong inducers of synaptic suppression, and several mechanisms have been proposed to explain this effect (Lambert et al. 1998; Walsh et al. 2002; Lacor et al. 2004; Snyder et al. 2005; Lesne et al. 2006; Townsend et al. 2006; Haass and Selkoe 2007; Shankar et al. 2007; Berman et al. 2008; Puzzo et al. 2008; Shankar et al. 2008; Nygaard and Strittmatter 2009; Gimbel et al. 2010; Palop and Mucke 2010; Renner et al. 2010; Ronicke et al. 2010) (see Mucke and Selkoe 2011). Synaptic suppression by the oligomers correlates with reduced NMDA receptor activity (Snyder et al. 2005; Shankar et al. 2007), which is caused by NMDA receptor dephosphorylation and accelerated endocytosis (Snyder et al. 2005). Snyder, Greengard, and colleagues (Snyder et al. 2005) proposed that this is mediated by the Aβ-mediated activation of phosphatases (STEP and calcineurin). The concomitant reduction of NMDA receptor activity induces dendritic spine loss and, intriguingly, this requires calcineurin, as well as the active, i.e., Ser3-unphosphorylated form of n-cofilin (Shankar et al. 2007). A dominant negative form of n-cofilin, in which Ser3 is replaced with a phosphomimetic amino acid (Ser3Asp), prevents oligomer-induced spine loss (Shankar et al. 2007).

Reelin induces the phosphorylation of n-cofilin at the inhibitory Ser3 residue, thereby promoting spine stability (Chai et al. 2009; Frotscher 2010). Moreover, Reelin signaling activates SFKs (Chen et al. 2005), which would directly oppose the activity of the phosphatases on the NMDA receptor (Snyder et al. 2005). This hypothesis was tested by measuring the effect of different Aβ preparations, including Aβ-containing extracts from human AD brain, on hippocampal synaptic plasticity, NMDA receptor tyrosine phosphorylation, and activity in response to Reelin (Durakoglugil et al. 2009). At low to intermediate, but not at unphysiologically high ($>$400 nM) Aβ concentrations, activation of Reelin signaling can completely prevent the synaptic suppression induced by the oligomers, suggesting that Reelin is a physiological mediator of neuroprotection. Importantly, ApoE4 strongly interferes with these synapse-enhancing functions of Reelin by sequestering ApoE receptors in intracellular compartments (Chen et al. 2010) (Fig. 3), thus providing a novel mechanism by which accelerated spine loss, increased tau phosphorylation (Kocherhans et al. 2010), loss of network homeostasis (Palop et al. 2007; Palop and Mucke 2010), and earlier disease onset through loss of neuroprotective compensatory bandwidth (Korwek et al. 2009) can be readily explained. This mechanism is also consistent with the finding that ApoE4 reduces spine density and dendritic complexity in cortical neurons in vivo (Dumanis et al. 2009). Moreover, Reelin expression levels are reduced in the brains of AD patients and in the entorhinal

cortex of APP overexpressing mice (Chin et al. 2007), suggesting that Aβ can reduce Reelin expression in a subset of entorhinal pyramidal neurons, thereby adding further support to a role of diminished Reelin signaling in AD progression (Herz and Chen 2006).

ApoE Receptors Protect against Neurodegeneration

Recent evidence shows that ApoE receptors, specifically Apoer2 and LRP1, directly protect against the loss of neurons and dendrites in vivo (Beffert et al. 2006b). Apoer2 was found to protect against the loss of corticospinal neurons during the normal aging process (Beffert et al. 2006b). This protection requires the presence of the alternatively spliced cytoplasmic

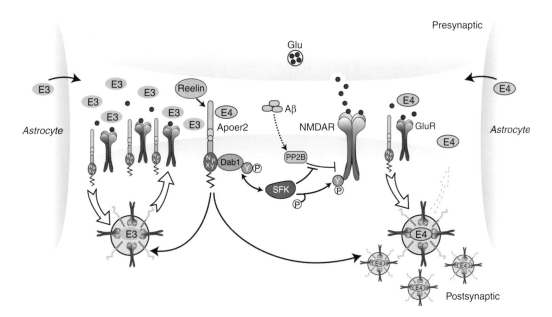

Figure 3. ApoE isoforms differentially impair ApoE receptor and glutamate receptor recycling at the synapse. Apoer2 induces *N*-methyl-D-aspartate receptor (NMDAR) tyrosine phosphorylation by activating Src family tyrosine kinases (SFKs) in response to Reelin in the postsynaptic neuron. Astrocyte-derived ApoE3 (green ovals) or ApoE4 (gray ovals) bind to Apoer2 and are constitutively but slowly internalized. Apoer2 undergoes accelerated endocytosis in response to Reelin signaling. ApoE4 sequesters Apoer2 in intracellular compartments along with glutamate receptors (NMDAR and GluR), thereby reducing the ability of the postsynaptic neuron to recycle these proteins with normal kinetics, whereas ApoE2 or ApoE3 efficiently recycle back to the cell surface and thus deplete surface Apoer2 and glutamate receptor levels to a lesser extent (illustrated on the left for ApoE3). Aβ oligomers interfere with NMDAR tyrosine phosphorylation by activating tyrosine phosphatases (Snyder et al. 2005). (Modified from Chen et al. 2010; reprinted, with permission, from the National Academy of Sciences © 2010.)

insert, which functionally couples Apoer2 to NMDA receptors, presumably through a PSD95-mediated interaction (Beffert et al. 2005; Hoe et al. 2006b), but also serves to recruit a c-jun amino-terminal kinase (JNK) signaling complex to the cytoplasmic tail of Apoer2 (Gott-hardt et al. 2000; Stockinger et al. 2000). Intri-guingly, JNK3 knockout mice and Apoer2 mutants lacking the alternatively spliced insert are resistant to lesion-induced neuronal death, suggesting that JNK recruitment to the Apoer2 cytoplasmic domain can promote both, neuro-nal loss or survival, depending on context (Bef-fert et al. 2006b).

Apoer2 also protects against neurodegener-ation through another, mechanistically distinct mechanism, which involves its role in the uptake of essential selenoproteins into the brain (Burk et al. 2007). Loss of Apoer2 sensitizes the animals to low dietary selenium levels resulting in death from rapid and severe neurodegenera-tion. Selenoprotein 1 (Sepp1)-deficient animals show a pronounced LTP defect owing to sele-nium deficiency in the CNS when fed a sele-nium-reduced diet (Peters et al. 2006). However, the synaptic defects of Apoer2 knockin mutants (Beffert et al. 2005; Beffert et al. 2006a; Beffert et al. 2006b) are not caused by selenium deple-tion, but by the loss of NMDA and AMPA recep-tor regulation (Masiulis et al. 2009). LRP2 also mediates transport of this essential micronu-trient (Chiu-Ugalde et al. 2010).

Neuroprotection by Apoer2 is further likely to involve its potent ability to mediate phos-phorylation of cyclic AMP response element binding protein (CREB), a neuroprotective transcription factor that is also involved in long-term memory formation. Ca^{2+} influx through synaptic NMDA receptors stimulates CREB phosphorylation and promotes neuronal sur-vival, whereas excitotoxic stimulation of extra-synaptic NMDA receptors shuts off CREB phosphorylation and promotes neuronal death (Hardingham et al. 2002). Reelin signaling strongly promotes CREB phosphorylation in cultured primary cortical neurons and this requires NMDA receptor activity (Chen et al. 2005). However, this is almost completely pre-vented by ApoE4 (Chen et al. 2010), suggesting

another potential mechanism by which this apolipoprotein may contribute to the pre-mature onset of neurodegeneration in ApoE4 carriers.

LRP1: EFFECTS ON APP, Aβ, AND ApoE METABOLISM

Regulation of APP Trafficking and Processing by LRP1 and Other ApoE Receptors

The β-secretase BACE1 is abundantly present and active in acidic endosomes (Cole and Vassar 2007). Consequently, increased APP endocyto-sis and distribution in endosomes lead to increased amyloidogenic processing and Aβ production. Conversely, if APP is retained at the cell surface, it has a greater availability for the cell-surface-localized α-secretase and is cleaved to sAPPα and a minimally toxic pep-tide p3 (see Haass et al. 2011 for details). There-fore, APP-interacting proteins or cellular conditions that alter APP trafficking and/or distribution are expected to impact APP proc-essing to Aβ. Indeed, several apoE receptors interact with APP and modulate its trafficking and processing. LRP1 interacts with APP extrac-ellularly by binding to the Kunitz-type protease inhibitor (KPI) domain that is present in the longer forms of APP (APP751 and APP770) (Kounnas et al. 1995). Further studies showed that LRP1 also interacts with the neuronal isoform of APP lacking the KPI domain (APP695). Two different phosphotyrosine-binding (PTB) domains within the adaptor protein FE65 bind to the NPxY motifs within APP and LRP1, thus bridging an interaction between these two membrane proteins intracell-ularly (Trommsdorff et al. 1998; Kinoshita et al. 2001; Pietrzik et al. 2004). Because of the rapid endocytosis rate of LRP1 compared with that of APP (Cam et al. 2005), the consequence of APP and LRP1 interaction is accelerated APP endo-cytic trafficking and processing to Aβ (Ulery et al. 2000; Zerbinatti et al. 2004; Cam et al. 2005; Zerbinatti et al. 2006). The in vivo role of LRP1 in APP trafficking and processing requires further investigation.

Several other apoE receptors also interact with APP and regulate its trafficking and processing to Aβ. LRP1B, which shares high sequence homology with LRP1 but has a significantly slower rate of endocytosis retains APP at the cell surface and reduces its processing to Aβ (Cam et al. 2004). Apoer2 either decreases or increases Aβ production depending on the experimental conditions. In the presence of F-spondin, a common ligand that bridges APP and Apoer2 extracellular interaction, the slow endocytosis rate of Apoer2 inhibits APP endocytic trafficking and reduces Aβ production (Hoe et al. 2005). However, in the absence of common ligands, Apoer2 increases the distribution of APP into lipid rafts and APP processing to Aβ (Fuentealba et al. 2007). A third apoE receptor that modulates APP trafficking and processing to Aβ is sorLA/LR11 whose expression is significantly reduced in AD brains (Scherzer et al. 2004). Cell biological studies show that sorLA in neurons shifts APP distribution to the Golgi compartment and decreases its processing to Aβ (Andersen et al. 2005). Importantly, a deletion of the *Sorla* gene in mice increases concentration of Aβ in the brain (Andersen et al. 2005). Supporting a role for sorLA in AD pathogenesis, a genetic study showed that inherited variants in the *SORL1* gene (which encodes sorLA) are associated with LOAD (Rogaeva et al. 2007). Collectively, these studies show that apoE receptors are intimately associated with APP in neurons and regulate APP trafficking and processing.

LRP1 and LDLR in Cellular and Brain Aβ Metabolism

Impaired Aβ clearance is likely a major pathogenic event for LOAD. There are two major pathways by which Aβ is cleared from the brain: (1) receptor-mediated clearance by cells in brain parenchyma (microglia, astrocytes, neurons), along the interstitial fluid (ISF) drainage pathway or through the BBB and (2) through endopeptidase-mediated proteolytic degradation (see Saido and Leissring 2011 for details on proteolytic degradation of Aβ). Receptor-mediated clearance of Aβ in the brain is at least partially mediated by the apoE receptors LRP1, LDLR, and VLDLR, which are widely expressed in neurons, astrocytes, and microglia of brain parenchyma, as well as in endothelial cells, astrocytes, and smooth muscle cells at the BBB and cerebral arteries.

The best-characterized Aβ clearance receptor in the brain is LRP1, which along with several of its ligands are present in amyloid plaques (Rebeck et al. 1995). The important function of LRP1 in brain Aβ clearance was shown in amyloid mouse model with decreased LRP1 expression owing to a deletion of their chaperone RAP (Van Uden et al. 2002). Recombinant RAP and LRP1 antibody also reduce Aβ efflux from mouse brain (Shibata et al. 2000). In humans, a decreased LRP1 expression in the brain capillaries in AD brains may contribute to impaired Aβ clearance (Deane et al. 2004), whereas circulating soluble LRP1 (sLRP) might provide peripheral "sink" activity for Aβ clearance through the BBB (Sagare et al. 2007).

LRP1 binds Aβ directly (Deane et al. 2004) or indirectly via its ligands, which include α2-macroglobulin (Narita et al. 1997), RAP (Kanekiyo and Bu 2009), and apoE (Bu 2009; Kim et al. 2009a). ApoE is the best-characterized Aβ chaperone. Because apoE immunoreactivity is commonly found in amyloid plaques (Namba et al. 1991; Wisniewski and Frangione 1992), it is likely that apoE interacts with Aβ directly in the human brain. The region of apoE that is responsible for Aβ binding is in the carboxy-terminal domain overlapping with the lipid-binding region (Strittmatter et al. 1993b; Tamamizu-Kato et al. 2008), suggesting that the lipophilic Aβ peptide associates with apoE in a process that is analogous to lipid binding. Indeed, Aβ binding to apoE compromises its lipid-binding function (Tamamizu-Kato et al. 2008). Furthermore, Aβ peptides modulate the binding of apoE isoforms differently to apoE receptors (Beffert et al. 1998; Hone et al. 2005). These results show that Aβ peptides can interfere with the normal function of apoE under in vitro conditions. It is unclear if in vivo this is the case. A fraction of apoE3/lipoprotein binds to Aβ with higher affinity than apoE4/lipoprotein (LaDu et al. 1994). However, whether Aβ binding to apoE/lipoprotein leads to enhanced or reduced Aβ clearance, has not yet been clarifed (Kim et al. 2009a). If Aβ is cleared more efficiently through apoE/lipoprotein-independent pathway, one would expect that Aβ binding to apoE/lipoprotein will impede its clearance. On the other hand, if apoE/lipoprotein/Aβ complexes enter cells via apoE receptor (e.g., LRP1 and LDLR) pathways more efficiently than Aβ alone, apoE/lipoprotein likely promotes Aβ clearance. The in vivo role of apoE/lipoprotein in Aβ clearance is likely influenced by apoE lipidation state, receptor expression, and local Aβ concentration (Bu 2009; Kim et al. 2009a). Interestingly, a recent study shows that Aβ binding to apoE4 redirects its clearance from LRP1 to VLDLR, which internalizes Aβ-apoE4 complexes at the BBB more slowly than LRP1 (Deane et al. 2008). In contrast, Aβ-apoE2 and Aβ-apoE3 complexes are cleared at the BBB via both VLDLR and LRP1 at a substantially faster rate than Aβ-apoE4 complexes.

LDLR is another receptor that is implicated in brain Aβ clearance, although the effects of LDLR loss-of-function on Aβ clearance are still being worked out. One study showed that LDLR deficiency was associated with increased amyloid deposition in Tg2576 APP-transgenic mice (Cao et al. 2006). In contrast, another study using PDAPP-transgenic mice did not find a significant effect of *Ldlr* deletion on Aβ level or deposition although there was a trend for increased Aβ in the absence of LDLR (Fryer et al. 2005a). Using a gain-of-function approach, a more recent study showed that overexpression of the LDLR in the brain of transgenic mice enhanced Aβ clearance and decreased Aβ deposition (Kim et al. 2009b). It is not clear whether the effect of LDLR overexpression on Aβ clearance is because of the reduced level of apoE in the LDLR transgenic mice, or a direct effect on Aβ, or both. Nonetheless, these findings indicate that increasing LDLR expression may represent a novel therapeutic strategy to treat AD.

The receptor-mediated clearance is, in principle, an efficient way of reducing brain Aβ because most Aβ that is internalized by apoE

receptors is delivered to lysosomes for degradation (see Fig. 4) or transcytosed into the plasma via BBB. However, it is possible that receptor-mediated clearance of Aβ into neurons can lead to intraneuronal accumulation of Aβ (Fig. 3), which under certain conditions may be toxic (Billings et al. 2005). A portion of Aβ that is internalized by neurons, in particular oligomeric Aβ42, accumulates in multivesicular bodies (MVBs)/late endosomes and lysosomes, and contributes to lysosomal dysfunction and neuronal toxicity. In contrast, receptor-mediated internalization of Aβ by astrocytes (Koistinaho et al. 2004) and microglia (Mandrekar et al. 2009) is likely to represent a more functional pathway to clear and eventually degrade Aβ.

Evidence that LRP1 and LDLR Are Key Metabolic Receptors for ApoE/Lipoprotein in the Brain

Although several LDLR family members are expressed in the brain, accumulating evidence indicates that the LDLR and LRP1 are the two primary metabolic receptors for apoE/lipoprotein. Deletion of the *Ldlr* gene in mice increases apoE levels in brain parenchyma and CSF (Fryer et al. 2005a), suggesting impaired metabolism of apoE. In contrast, overexpression of the LDLR in the brain decreases apoE levels, reflecting an increased metabolism of apoE (Kim et al. 2009b). Similarly, conditional deletion of the *Lrp1* gene in mouse forebrain neurons increases apoE levels (Liu et al. 2007) and overexpression of a functional LRP1 minireceptor in mouse brain decreases brain apoE levels (Zerbinatti et al. 2006). Although both LDLR and LRP1 play roles in brain apoE/lipoprotein metabolism, there are important differences between them. First, whereas LRP1 is highly expressed in neurons and to a lesser degree in glia, LDLR is more prominently expressed in glia than neurons (Rebeck et al. 1993; Rapp et al. 2006). Second, deletion of the *Lrp1* gene in mouse forebrain neurons reduces brain cholesterol levels (Liu et al. 2007), whereas cholesterol levels in *Ldlr* knockout mice are unchanged (Fryer et al. 2005a). Third, apoE/lipoprotein

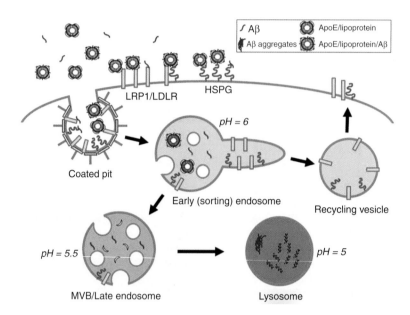

Figure 4. Schematic model of LRP1/LDLR-mediated cellular transport of apoE/lipoprotein and Aβ. Three cell-surface receptors, LRP1, LDLR, and HSPG, are capable of binding to apoE/lipoprotein, Aβ, and apoE/lipoprotein/Aβ complexes. On clathrin-mediated endocytosis, ligands are mostly dissociated from the receptors within the early/sorting endosomes owing to lower pH. Whereas receptors are typically recycled back to the cell surface, ligands are delivered to multivesicular bodies (MVBs)/late endosomes and eventually to lysosomes for degradation. Lipid components are transported out of the lysosomes for storage or reutilization. Depending on the concentrations and cellular conditions, some Aβ molecules might aggregate within the lysosomes as intracellular Aβ, which could eventually serve to seed amyloid plaques (Hu et al. 2009).

particles secreted by astrocytes have higher affinity for LDLR than LRP1 (Fryer et al. 2005a), whereas recombinant apoE (Narita et al. 2002), apoE-enriched lipoprotein particles (Kowal et al. 1990), and CSF-isolated HDL particles (Fagan et al. 1996) bind more avidly to LRP1. The receptor-binding specificity of apoE is likely influenced by its conformation and lipidation state. It is possible that apoE/lipoprotein particles secreted by astrocytes recruit additional apoE molecules, perhaps bound to heparan sulfate proteoglycan (HSPG), before being transported to the CSF or binding to LRP1 at the neuronal cell surface.

There is some evidence that apoE isoforms may differ in their function in regard to cholesterol transport and efflux (Michikawa et al. 2000; Gong et al. 2002; Rapp et al. 2006), although not all studies show this (Hirsch-Reinshagen et al. 2004). Thus the roles of apoE isoforms in brain cholesterol metabolism require

further investigation. The structural differences among apoE isoforms that determine their lipid- and receptor-binding specificities in the brain environment could account for their differences in modulating brain cholesterol metabolism. It is important to note that there are likely LRP1-mediated cholesterol transport mechanisms in the brain that are independent of apoE because LRP1 deficiency in the brain, but not apoE deficiency, leads to decreased brain cholesterol levels. Other LRP1 ligands such as lipoprotein lipase might also play a role. Alternatively, LRP1 may serve as a cholesterol sensor that influences cholesterol synthesis and/or intracellular transport.

In addition to cholesterol, apoE also mediates the transport of other brain lipids, some of which are not produced in astrocytes. For example, sulfatide, an oligodendrocyte-synthesized lipid that is crucial for neuronal spine and myelin sheath integrity, is actively transported

Cite this article as *Cold Spring Harb Perspect Med* doi: 10.1101/cshperspect.a006312

by an apoE- and LRP1-dependent mechanism (Han 2007). It is possible that apoE/lipoprotein particles are modified by myelin-associated lipids before being transported into neurons. Interestingly, sulfatide is a potential biomarker for AD diagnosis as its levels are decreased in AD brains (Han 2007). Whether LRP1/LDLR-mediated apoE/cholesterol transport is impaired in AD brains and how this in turn contributes to AD pathogenesis is currently not clear. However, because of the important role of apoE/cholesterol in injury repair, the cholesterol transport pathway should be considered when apoE/LRP1/LDLR pathways are explored as therapeutic targets for AD.

SUMMARY

APOE genotype is the strongest genetic risk factor for AD, and understanding the mechanism underlying this relationship has the potential to lead to new therapeutic approaches. A major reason that appears to underlie this relationship is the fact that apoE isoforms result in differential onset of Aβ accumulation in the brain with the onset E4 earlier than E3, which is earlier than E2. There is direct in vivo evidence that differences in Aβ clearance is one factor that accounts for this (Castellano et al. 2011), although effects of apoE on Aβ aggregation independent of clearance may also be important. From a therapeutic standpoint, pathways that stimulate Aβ clearance via apoE-dependent mechanisms are one possible approach to decrease Aβ accumulation and its toxic effects. Targeting the liver X receptor (LXR) pathway (Koldamova et al. 2005b), apoE lipidation state via ABCA1, as well as LDLR, LRP1, and other apoE receptors are potential ways to stimulate apoE-dependent Aβ clearance. In terms of apoE-dependent Aβ aggregation, interrupting the apoE-Aβ interaction may also have therapeutic potential (Sadowski et al. 2006). In addition to effects on the apoE/Aβ pathway, apoE receptors such as Apoer2 and Vldlr play important roles in synaptic plasticity, tau phosphorylation, and neuroprotection. Determining ways to activate these receptors may be

another strategy to delay or halt the progressive neurodegenerative process that occurs in AD.

REFERENCES

*Reference is also in this collection.

Aleshkov S, Abraham CR, Zannis VI. 1997. Interaction of nascent apoE2, apoE3, and apoE4 isoforms expressed in mammalian cells with amyloid peptide β(1-40). Relevance to Alzheimer's disease. *Biochemistry* **36:** 10571–10580.

Andersen OM, Reiche J, Schmidt V, Gotthardt M, Spoelgen R, Behlke J, von Arnim CA, Breiderhoff T, Jansen P, Wu X, et al. 2005. Neuronal sorting protein-related receptor sorLA/LR11 regulates processing of the amyloid precursor protein. In *Proc Natl Acad Sci* **102:** 13461–13466.

Anderson R, Barnes JC, Bliss TV, Cain DP, Cambon K, Davies HA, Errington ML, Fellows LA, Gray RA, Hoh T, et al. 1998. Behavioural, physiological and morphological analysis of a line of apolipoprotein E knockout mouse. *Neuroscience* **85:** 93–110.

Arnaud L, Ballif BA, Forster E, Cooper JA. 2003. Fyn tyrosine kinase is a critical regulator of disabled-1 during brain development. *Curr Biol* **13:** 9–17.

Assadi AH, Zhang G, Beffert U, McNeil RS, Renfro AL, Niu S, Quattrocchi CC, Antalffy BA, Sheldon M, Armstrong DD, et al. 2003. Interaction of reelin signaling and Lis1 in brain development. *Nat Genet* **35:** 270–276.

Bales KR, Verina T, Dodel RC, Du Y, Altstiel L, Bender M, Hyslop P, Johnstone EM, Little SP, Cummins DJ, et al. 1997. Lack of apolipoprotein E dramatically reduces amyloid β-peptide deposition. *Nat Genet* **17:** 263–264.

Bales KR, Verina T, Cummins DJ, Du Y, Dodel JC, Saura J, Fishman CE, DeLong CA, Piccardo P, Petegnief V, et al. 1999. Apolipoprotein E is essential for amyloid deposition in the APPV717F transgenic mouse model of Alzheimer's disease. *Proc Natl Acad Sci* **96:** 15233–15238.

Beffert U, Arguin C, Poirier J. 1999. The polymorphism in exon 3 of the low density lipoprotein receptor-related protein gene is weakly associated with Alzheimer's disease. *Neurosci Lett* **259:** 29–32.

Beffert U, Aumont N, Dea D, Lussier-Cacan S, Davignon J, Poirier J. 1998. β-amyloid peptides increase the binding and internalization of apolipoprotein E to hippocampal neurons. *J Neurochem* **70:** 1458–1466.

Beffert U, Morfini G, Bock HH, Reyna H, Brady ST, Herz J. 2002. Reelin-mediated signaling locally regulates protein kinase B/Akt and glycogen synthase kinase 3β. *J Biol Chem* **277:** 49958–49964.

Beffert U, Weeber EJ, Durudas A, Qiu S, Masiulis I, Sweatt JD, Li WP, Adelmann G, Frotscher M, Hammer RE, et al. 2005. Modulation of synaptic plasticity and memory by Reelin involves differential splicing of the lipoprotein receptor Apoer2. *Neuron* **47:** 567–579.

Beffert U, Durudas A, Weeber EJ, Stolt PC, Giehl KM, Sweatt JD, Hammer RE, Herz J. 2006a. Functional dissection of Reelin signaling by site-directed disruption of Disabled-1 adaptor binding to apolipoprotein E receptor 2: Distinct roles in development and synaptic plasticity. *J Neurosci* **26:** 2041–2052.

Beffert U, Nematollah Farsian F, Masiulis I, Hammer RE, Yoon SO, Giehl KM, Herz J. 2006b. ApoE receptor 2 controls neuronal survival in the adult brain. *Curr Biol* **16:** 2446–2452.

Bell RD, Sagare AP, Friedman AE, Bedi GS, Holtzman DM, Deane R, Zlokovic BV. 2007. Transport pathways for clearance of human Alzheimer's amyloid β-peptide and apolipoproteins E and J in the mouse central nervous system. *J Cereb Blood Flow Metab* **27:** 909–918.

Benjamin R, Leake A, Ince PG, Perry RH, McKeith IG, Edwardson JA, Morris CM. 1995. Effects of apolipoprotein E genotype on cortical neuropathology in senile dementia of the Lewy body and Alzheimer's disease. *Neurodegeneration* **4:** 443–448.

Berman DE, Dall'Armi C, Voronov SV, McIntire LB, Zhang H, Moore AZ, Staniszewski A, Arancio O, Kim TW, Di Paolo G. 2008. Oligomeric amyloid-β peptide disrupts phosphatidylinositol-4,5-bisphosphate metabolism. *Nat Neurosci* **11:** 547–554.

Bertram L, McQueen MB, Mullin K, Blacker D, Tanzi RE. 2007. Systematic meta-analyses of Alzheimer disease genetic association studies: The AlzGene database. *Nat Genet* **39:** 17–23.

Billings LM, Oddo S, Green KN, McGaugh JL, Laferla FM. 2005. Intraneuronal Aβ causes the onset of early Alzheimer's disease-related cognitive deficits in transgenic mice. *Neuron* **45:** 675–688.

Bock HH, Herz J. 2003. Reelin activates SRC family tyrosine kinases in neurons. *Curr Biol* **13:** 18–26.

Borrell V, Pujadas L, Simo S, Dura D, Sole M, Cooper JA, Del Rio JA, Soriano E. 2007. Reelin and mDab1 regulate the development of hippocampal connections. *Mol Cell Neurosci* **36:** 158–173.

Boucher P, Liu P, Gotthardt M, Hiesberger T, Anderson RG, Herz J. 2002. Platelet-derived growth factor mediates tyrosine phosphorylation of the cytoplasmic domain of the low density lipoprotein receptor-related protein in caveolae. *J Biol Chem* **277:** 15507–15513.

Boycott KM, Flavelle S, Bureau A, Glass HC, Fujiwara TM, Wirrell E, Davey K, Chudley AE, Scott JN, McLeod DR, et al. 2005. Homozygous deletion of the very low density lipoprotein receptor gene causes autosomal recessive cerebellar hypoplasia with cerebral gyral simplification. *Am J Human Genet* **77:** 477–483.

Boycott KM, Bonnemann C, Herz J, Neuert S, Beaulieu C, Scott JN, Venkatasubramanian A, Parboosingh JS. 2009. Mutations in VLDLR as a cause for autosomal recessive cerebellar ataxia with mental retardation (dysequilibrium syndrome). *J Child Neurol* **24:** 1310–1315.

Brich J, Shie FS, Howell BW, Li R, Tus K, Wakeland EK, Jin LW, Mumby M, Churchill G, Herz J, et al. 2003. Genetic modulation of tau phosphorylation in the mouse. *J Neurosci* **23:** 187–192.

Bu G. 2009. Apolipoprotein E and its receptors in Alzheimer's disease: Pathways, pathogenesis and therapy. *Nat Rev Neurosci* **10:** 333–344.

Burk RF, Hill KE, Olson GE, Weeber EJ, Motley AK, Winfrey VP, Austin LM. 2007. Deletion of apolipoprotein E receptor-2 in mice lowers brain selenium and causes severe neurological dysfunction and death when a low-selenium diet is fed. *J Neurosci* **27:** 6207–6211.

Cam JA, Zerbinatti CV, Knisely JM, Hecimovic S, Li Y, Bu G. 2004. The low density lipoprotein receptor-related protein 1B retains β-amyloid precursor protein at the cell surface and reduces amyloid-β peptide production. *J Biol Chem* **279:** 29639–29646.

Cam JA, Zerbinatti CV, Li Y, Bu G. 2005. Rapid endocytosis of the low density lipoprotein receptor-related protein modulates cell surface distribution and processing of the β-amyloid precursor protein. *J Biol Chem* **280:** 15464–15470.

Campo CG, Sinagra M, Verrier D, Manzoni OJ, Chavis P. 2009. Reelin secreted by GABAergic neurons regulates glutamate receptor homeostasis. *PLoS One* **4:** e5505. doi: 10.1371/journal.pone.0005505.

Cao D, Fukuchi K, Wan H, Kim H, Li L. 2006. Lack of LDL receptor aggravates learning deficits and amyloid deposits in Alzheimer transgenic mice. *Neurobiol Aging* **27:** 1632–1643.

Castano EM, Prelli F, Wisniewski T, Golabek A, Kumar RA, Soto C, Frangione B. 1995. Fibrillogenesis in Alzheimer's disease of amyloid β peptides and apolipoprotein E. *Biochem J* **306:** 599–604.

Castellano JM, Kim J, Stewart FR, DeMattos RB, Patterson BW, Fagan AM, Morris JC, Mawuenyega KG, Paul SM, Bateman RJ, et al. 2011. Human apoE isoforms differentially regulate brain amyloid-β peptide clearance. *Sci Transl Med* **3:** 89ra57.

Chai X, Forster E, Zhao S, Bock HH, Frotscher M. 2009. Reelin acts as a stop signal for radially migrating neurons by inducing phosphorylation of n-cofilin at the leading edge. *Commun Integr Biol* **2:** 375–377.

Chameau P, Inta D, Vitalis T, Monyer H, Wadman WJ, van Hooft JA. 2009. The N-terminal region of reelin regulates postnatal dendritic maturation of cortical pyramidal neurons. *Proc Natl Acad Sci* **106:** 7227–7232.

Chen Y, Beffert U, Ertunc M, Tang TS, Kavalali ET, Bezprozvanny I, Herz J. 2005. Reelin modulates NMDA receptor activity in cortical neurons. *J Neurosci* **25:** 8209–8216.

Chen Y, Durakoglugil MS, Xian X, Herz J. 2010. ApoE4 reduces glutamate receptor function and synaptic plasticity by selectively impairing ApoE receptor recycling. *Proc Natl Acad Sci* **107:** 12011–12016.

Chin J, Massaro CM, Palop JJ, Thwin MT, Yu GQ, Bien-Ly N, Bender A, Mucke L. 2007. Reelin depletion in the entorhinal cortex of human amyloid precursor protein transgenic mice and humans with Alzheimer's disease. *J Neurosci* **27:** 2727–2733.

Chiu-Ugalde J, Theilig F, Behrends T, Drebes J, Sieland C, Subbarayal P, Kohrle J, Hammes A, Schomburg L, Schweizer U. 2010. Mutation of megalin leads to urinary loss of selenoprotein P and selenium deficiency in serum, liver, kidneys and brain. *Biochem J* **431:** 103–111.

Cirrito JR, Deane R, Fagan AM, Spinner ML, Parsadanian M, Finn MB, Jiang H, Prior JL, Sagare A, Bales KR, et al. 2005. P-glycoprotein deficiency at the blood-brain barrier increases amyloid-β deposition in an Alzheimer disease mouse model. *J Clin Invest* **115:** 3285–3290.

Cole GM, Ard MD. 2000. Influence of lipoproteins on microglial degradation of Alzheimer's amyloid β-protein. *Microsc Res Tech* **50:** 316–324.

Cole SL, Vassar R. 2007. The Alzheimer's disease β-secretase enzyme, BACE1. *Mol Neurodegener* **2:** 22.

Corder EH, Saunders AM, Strittmatter WJ, Schmechel DE, Gaskell PC, Small GW, Roses AD, Haines JL, Pericak-Vance MA. 1993. Gene dose of apolipoprotein E type 4 allele and the risk of Alzheimer's disease in late onset families. *Science* **261:** 921–923.

Corder EH, Saunders AM, Risch NJ, Strittmatter WJ, Schmechel DE, Gaskell PC Jr, Rimmler JB, Locke PA, Conneally PM, Schmader KE, et al. 1994. Protective effect of apolipoprotein E type 2 allele for late onset Alzheimer disease. *Nat Genet* **7:** 180–184.

Costa E, Davis J, Grayson DR, Guidotti A, Pappas GD, Pesold C. 2001. Dendritic spine hypoplasticity and downregulation of reelin and GABAergic tone in schizophrenia vulnerability. *Neurobiol Dis* **8:** 723–742.

D'Arcangelo G. 2005. Apoer2: A reelin receptor to remember. *Neuron* **47:** 471–473.

D'Arcangelo G, Homayouni R, Keshvara L, Rice DS, Sheldon M, Curran T. 1999. Reelin is a ligand for lipoprotein receptors. *Neuron* **24:** 471–479.

Deane R, Wu Z, Sagare A, Davis J, Du Yan S, Hamm K, Xu F, Parisi M, LaRue B, Hu HW, et al. 2004. LRP/amyloid β-peptide interaction mediates differential brain efflux of Aβ isoforms. *Neuron* **43:** 333–344.

Deane R, Sagare A, Hamm K, Parisi M, Lane S, Finn MB, Holtzman DM, Zlokovic BV. 2008. apoE isoform-specific disruption of amyloid β peptide clearance from mouse brain. *J Clin Invest* **118:** 4002–4013.

De Ferrari GV, Papassotiropoulos A, Biechele T, Wavrant De-Vrieze F, Avila ME, Major MB, Myers A, Saez K, Henriquez JP, Zhao A, et al. 2007. Common genetic variation within the low-density lipoprotein receptor-related protein 6 and late-onset Alzheimer's disease. *Proc Natl Acad Sci* **104:** 9434–9439.

Del Rio JA, Heimrich B, Borrell V, Forster E, Drakew A, Alcantara S, Nakajima K, Miyata T, Ogawa M, Mikoshiba K, et al. 1997. A role for Cajal-Retzius cells and reelin in the development of hippocampal connections. *Nature* **385:** 70–74.

DeMattos RB, Brendza RP, Heuser JE, Kierson M, Cirrito JR, Fryer JD, Sullivan PM, Fagan AM, Han X, Holtzman DM. 2001. Purification and characterization of astrocyte-secreted apolipoprotein E and J-containing lipoproteins from wild-type and human apoE transgenic mice. *Neurochem Int* **39:** 415–425.

DeMattos RB, O'dell MA, Parsadanian M, Taylor JW, Harmony JAK, Bales KR, Paul SM, Aronow BJ, Holtzman DM. 2002. Clusterin promotes amyloid plaque formation and is critical for neuritic toxicity in a mouse model of Alzheimer's disease. *Proc Natl Acad Sci* **10:** 10843–10848.

DeMattos RB, Cirrito JR, Parsadanian M, May PC, O'Dell MA, Taylor JM, Harmony JAK, Aronow BJ, Bales KR, Paul SM, et al. 2004. ApoE and clusterin cooperatively suppress Ab levels and deposition: Evidence that apoE regulates extracellular Ab metabolism in vivo. *Neuron* **41:** 193–202.

Dieckmann M, Dietrich MF, Herz J. 2010. Lipoprotein receptors—An evolutionarily ancient multifunctional receptor family. *Biol Chem* **391:** 1341–1363.

Dietrich MF, van der Weyden L, Prosser HM, Bradley A, Herz J, Adams DJ. 2010. Ectodomains of the LDL receptor-related proteins LRP1b and LRP4 have anchorage independent functions in vivo. *PLoS One* **5:** e9960. doi: 10.1371/journal.pone.0009960.

Dillon C, Goda Y. 2005. The actin cytoskeleton: Integrating form and function at the synapse. *Annu Rev Neurosci* **28:** 25–55.

Dumanis SB, Tesoriero JA, Babus LW, Nguyen MT, Trotter JH, Ladu MJ, Weeber EJ, Turner RS, Xu B, Rebeck GW, et al. 2009. ApoE4 decreases spine density and dendritic complexity in cortical neurons in vivo. *J Neurosci* **29:** 15317–15322.

Durakoglugil MS, Chen Y, White CL, Kavalali ET, Herz J. 2009. Reelin signaling antagonizes β-amyloid at the synapse. *Proc Natl Acad Sci* **106:** 15938–15943.

Evans KC, Berger EP, Cho C-G, Weisgraber KH, Lansbury PT. 1994. Apolipoprotein E is a kinetic but not a thermodynamic inhibitor of amyloid formation: Implications for the pathogenesis and treatment of Alzheimer's disease. *Proc Natl Acad Sci* **92:** 763–767.

Fagan AM, Bu G, Sun Y, Daugherty A, Holtzman DM. 1996. Apolipoprotein E-containing high density lipoprotein promotes neurite outgrowth and is a ligand for the low density lipoprotein receptor-related protein. *J Biol Chem* **271:** 30121–30125.

Fagan AM, Murphy BA, Patel SN, Kilbridge JF, Mobley WC, Bu G, Holtzman DM. 1998. Evidence for normal aging of the septo-hippocampal cholinergic system in apoE$^{-/-}$ mice but impaired clearance of axonal degeneration products following injury. *Exp Neurol* **151:** 314–325.

Fagan AM, Watson M, Parsadanian M, Bales KR, Paul SM, Holtzman DM. 2002. Human and murine apoE markedly influence Aβ metabolism both prior and subsequent to plaque formation in a mouse model of Alzheimer's disease. *Neurobiol Dis* **9:** 305–318.

Farrer LA, Cupples LA, Haines JL, Hyman B, Kukull WA, Mayeux R, Myers RH, Pericak-Vance MA, Risch N, van Duijn CM. 1997. Effects of age, sex, and ethnicity on the association between apolipoprotein E genotype and Alzheimer disease. A meta-analysis. APOE and Alzheimer Disease Meta Analysis Consortium. *JAMA* **278:** 1349–1356.

Forster E, Bock HH, Herz J, Chai X, Frotscher M, Zhao S. 2010. Emerging topics in Reelin function. *Eur J Neurosci* **31:** 1511–1518.

Frotscher M. 2010. Role for Reelin in stabilizing cortical architecture. *Trends Neurosci* **33:** 407–414.

Fryer JD, Taylor JW, DeMattos RB, Bales KR, Paul SM, Parsadanian M, Holtzman DM. 2003. Apolipoprotein E markedly facilitates age-dependent cerebral amyloid angiopathy and spontaneous hemorrhage in APP transgenic mice. *J Neurosci* **23:** 7889–7896.

Fryer JD, Demattos RB, McCormick LM, O'Dell M A, Spinner ML, Bales KR, Paul SM, Sullivan PM, Parsadanian M, Bu G, et al. 2005a. The low density lipoprotein receptor regulates the level of central nervous system human and murine apolipoprotein E but does not modify amyloid plaque pathology in PDAPP mice. *J Biol Chem* **280:** 25754–25759.

Fryer JD, Simmons K, Parsadanian M, Bales KR, Paul SM, Sullivan PM, Holtzman DM. 2005b. ApoE4 alters the amyloid-β 40:42 ratio and promotes the formation of cerebral amyloid angiopathy in an APP transgenic model. *J Neurosci* **25**: 2803–2810.

Fuentealba RA, Barria MI, Lee J, Cam J, Araya C, Escudero CA, Inestrosa NC, Bronfman FC, Bu G, Marzolo MP. 2007. ApoER2 expression increases Aβ production while decreasing Amyloid Precursor Protein (APP) endocytosis: Possible role in the partitioning of APP into lipid rafts and in the regulation of γ-secretase activity. *Mol Neurodegener* **2**: 14.

Gajera CR, Emich H, Lioubinski O, Christ A, Beckervordersandforth-Bonk R, Yoshikawa K, Bachmann S, Christensen EI, Gotz M, Kempermann G, et al. 2010. LRP2 in ependymal cells regulates BMP signaling in the adult neurogenic niche. *J Cell Sci* **123**: 1922–1930.

Gimbel DA, Nygaard HB, Coffey EE, Gunther EC, Lauren J, Gimbel ZA, Strittmatter SM. 2010. Memory impairment in transgenic Alzheimer mice requires cellular prion protein. *J Neurosci* **30**: 6367–6374.

Gong JS, Kobayashi M, Hayashi H, Zou K, Sawamura N, Fujita SC, Yanagisawa K, Michikawa M. 2002. Apolipoprotein E (ApoE) isoform-dependent lipid release from astrocytes prepared from human ApoE3 and ApoE4 knock-in mice. *J Biol Chem* **277**: 29919–29926.

Gotthardt M, Trommsdorff M, Nevitt MF, Shelton J, Richardson JA, Stockinger W, Nimpf J, Herz J. 2000. Interactions of the low density lipoprotein receptor gene family with cytosolic adaptor and scaffold proteins suggest diverse biological functions in cellular communication and signal transduction. *J Biol Chem* **275**: 25616–25624.

Greenberg SM, Rebeck GW, Vonsattel JPG, Gomez-Isla T, Hyman BT. 1995. Apolipoprotein E ε4 and cerebral hemorrhage associated with amyloid angiopathy. *Ann Neurol* **38**: 254–259.

Grehan S, Tse E, Taylor JM. 2001. Two distal downstream enhancers direct expression of the human apolipoprotein E gene to astrocytes in the brain. *J Neurosci* **21**: 812–822.

Groc L, Choquet D, Stephenson FA, Verrier D, Manzoni OJ, Chavis P. 2007. NMDA receptor surface trafficking and synaptic subunit composition are developmentally regulated by the extracellular matrix protein Reelin. *J Neurosci* **27**: 10165–10175.

Haass C, Selkoe DJ. 2007. Soluble protein oligomers in neurodegeneration: Lessons from the Alzheimer's amyloid β-peptide. *Nat Rev Mol Cell Biol* **8**: 101–112.

* Haass C, Kaether C, Sisodia S, Thinakaran G. 2011. Trafficking and proteolytic processing of APP. *Cold Spring Harb Perspect Med* doi: 10.1101/cshperspect.a006270.

Han X. 2007. Potential mechanisms contributing to sulfatide depletion at the earliest clinically recognizable stage of Alzheimer's disease: A tale of shotgun lipidomics. *J Neurochem* **103**: 171–179.

Hardingham GE, Fukunaga Y, Bading H. 2002. Extrasynaptic NMDARs oppose synaptic NMDARs by triggering CREB shut-off and cell death pathways. *Nat Neurosci* **5**: 405–414.

Harold D, Abraham R, Hollingworth P, Sims R, Gerrish A, Hamshere ML, Pahwa JS, Moskvina V, Dowzell K, Williams A, et al. 2009. Genome-wide association study

identifies variants at CLU and PICALM associated with Alzheimer's disease. *Nat Genet* **41**: 1088–1093.

Heinonen O, Lehtovirta M, Soininen H, Helisalmi S, Mannermaa A, Sorvari H, Kosunen O, Paljarvi L, Ryynanen M, Riekkinen PJ Sr. 1995. Alzheimer pathology of patients carrying apolipoprotein E ε4 allele. *Neurobiol Aging* **16**: 505–513.

Herz J. 2009. Apolipoprotein E receptors in the nervous system. *Curr Opin Lipidol* **20**: 190–196.

Herz J, Beffert U. 2000. Apolipoprotein E receptors: Linking brain development and Alzheimer's disease. *Nature Rev* **1**: 51–58.

Herz J, Chen Y. 2006. Reelin, lipoprotein receptors and synaptic plasticity. *Nat Rev Neurosci* **7**: 850–859.

Herz J, Clouthier DE, Hammer RE. 1992. LDL receptor-related protein internalizes and degrades uPA-PAI-1 complexes and is essential for embryo implantation. *Cell* **71**: 411–421.

Herz J, Chen Y, Masiulis I, Zhou L. 2009. Expanding functions of lipoprotein receptors. *J Lipid Res* **50**(Suppl): S287–S292.

Hiesberger T, Trommsdorff M, Howell BW, Goffinet A, Mumby MC, Cooper JA, Herz J. 1999. Direct binding of Reelin to VLDL receptor and ApoE receptor 2 induces tyrosine phosphorylation of disabled-1 and modulates tau phosphorylation. *Neuron* **24**: 481–489.

Hirsch-Reinshagen V, Zhou S, Burgess BL, Bernier L, McIsaac SA, Chan JY, Tansley GH, Cohn JS, Hayden MR, Wellington CL. 2004. Deficiency of ABCA1 impairs apolipoprotein E metabolism in brain. *J Biol Chem* **279**: 41197–41207.

Hirsch-Reinshagen V, Maia LF, Burgess BL, Blain JF, Naus KE, McIsaac SA, Parkinson PF, Chan JY, Tansley GH, Hayden MR, et al. 2005. The absence of ABCA1 decreases soluble ApoE levels but does not diminish amyloid deposition in two murine models of Alzheimer disease. *J Biol Chem* **280**: 43243–43256.

Hoe HS, Wessner D, Beffert U, Becker AG, Matsuoka Y, Rebeck GW. 2005. F-spondin interaction with the apolipoprotein E receptor ApoEr2 affects processing of amyloid precursor protein. *Mol Cell Biol* **25**: 9259–9268.

Hoe HS, Freeman J, Rebeck GW. 2006a. Apolipoprotein E decreases tau kinases and phospho-tau levels in primary neurons. *Mol Neurodegen* **1**: 18.

Hoe HS, Pocivavsek A, Chakraborty G, Fu Z, Vicini S, Ehlers MD, Rebeck GW. 2006b. Apolipoprotein E receptor 2 interactions with the N-methyl-D-aspartate receptor. *J Biol Chem* **281**: 3425–3431.

Hoe HS, Fu Z, Makarova A, Lee JY, Lu C, Feng L, Pajoohesh-Ganji A, Matsuoka Y, Hyman BT, Ehlers MD, et al. 2009. The effects of amyloid precursor protein on postsynaptic composition and activity. *J Biol Chem* **284**: 8495–8506.

Holtzman DM, Pitas RE, Kilbridge J, Nathan B, Mahley RW, Bu G, Schwartz AL. 1995. LRP mediates apolipoprotein E-dependent neurite outgrowth in a CNS-derived neuronal cell line. *Proc Natl Acad Sci* **92**: 9480–9484.

Holtzman DM, Bales KR, Tenkova T, Fagan AM, Parsadanian M, Sartorius LJ, Mackey B, Olney J, McKeel D, Wozniak D, et al. 2000a. Apolipoprotein E isoform-dependent amyloid deposition and neuritic degeneration in a mouse model of Alzheimer's disease. *Proc Natl Acad Sci* **97**: 2892–2897.

Holtzman DM, Fagan AM, Mackey B, Tenkova T, Sartorius L, Paul SM, Bales K, Ashe KH, Irizzary MC, Hyman BT. 2000b. ApoE facilitates neuritic and cerebrovascular plaque formation in the APPsw mouse model of Alzheimer's disease. *Ann Neurol* **47**: 739–747.

Hone E, Martins IJ, Jeoung M, Ji TH, Gandy SE, Martins RN. 2005. Alzheimer's disease amyloid-β peptide modulates apolipoprotein E isoform specific receptor binding. *J Alzheimers Dis* **7**: 303–314.

Hoover BR, Reed MN, Su J, Penrod RD, Kotilinek LA, Grant MK, Pitstick R, Carlson GA, Lanier LM, Yuan LL, et al. 2010. Tau mislocalization to dendritic spines mediates synaptic dysfunction independently of neurodegeneration. *Neuron* **68**: 1067–1081.

Howell BW, Gertler FB, Cooper JA. 1997. Mouse disabled (mDab1): A Src binding protein implicated in neuronal development. *EMBO J* **16**: 121–132.

Hu X, Crick SL, Bu G, Frieden C, Pappu RV, Lee JM. 2009. Amyloid seeds formed by cellular uptake, concentration, and aggregation of the amyloid-β peptide. *Proc Natl Acad Sci* **106**: 20324–20329.

Huang SS, Ling TY, Tseng WF, Huang YH, Tang FM, Leal SM, Huang JS. 2003. Cellular growth inhibition by IGFBP-3 and TGF-β1 requires LRP-1. *FASEB J* **17**: 2068–2081.

Irizarry MC, Cheung BS, Rebeck GW, Paul SM, Bales KR, Hyman BT. 2000. Apolipoprotein E affects the amount, form, and anatomical distribution of amyloid β-peptide deposition in homozygous APP(V717F) transgenic mice. *Acta Neuropathol* **100**: 451–458.

Ito S, Ohtsuki S, Kamiie J, Nezu Y, Terasaki T. 2007. Cerebral clearance of human amyloid-β peptide (1–40) across the blood-brain barrier is reduced by self-aggregation and formation of low-density lipoprotein receptor-related protein-1 ligand complexes. *J Neurochem* **103**: 2482–2490.

Ittner LM, Ke YD, Delerue F, Bi M, Gladbach A, van Eersel J, Wolfing H, Chieng BC, Christie MJ, Napier IA, et al. 2010. Dendritic function of tau mediates amyloid-β toxicity in Alzheimer's disease mouse models. *Cell* **142**: 387–397.

Jiang Q, Lee CY, Mandrekar S, Wilkinson B, Cramer P, Zelcer N, Mann K, Lamb B, Willson TM, Collins JL, et al. 2008. ApoE promotes the proteolytic degradation of Aβ. *Neuron* **58**: 681–693.

Johnson EB, Hammer RE, Herz J. 2005. Abnormal development of the apical ectodermal ridge and polysyndactyly in Megf7-deficient mice. *Hum Mol Genet* **14**: 3523–3538.

Kanekiyo T, Bu G. 2009. Receptor-associated protein interacts with amyloid-β peptide and promotes its cellular uptake. *J Biol Chem* **284**: 33352–33359.

Karner CM, Dietrich MF, Johnson EB, Kappesser N, Tennert C, Percin F, Wollnik B, Carroll TJ, Herz J. 2010. Lrp4 regulates initiation of ureteric budding and is crucial for kidney formation—A mouse model for Cenani-Lenz syndrome. *PLoS One* **5**: e10418. doi: 10.1371/journal.pone.0010418.

Kim J, Basak JM, Holtzman DM. 2009a. The role of apolipoprotein E in Alzheimer's disease. *Neuron* **63**: 287–303.

Kim J, Castellano JM, Jiang H, Basak JM, Parsadanian M, Pham V, Mason SM, Paul SM, Holtzman DM. 2009b. Overexpression of low-density lipoprotein receptor in the brain markedly inhibits amyloid deposition and increases extracellular Aβ clearance. *Neuron* **64**: 632–644.

Kinoshita A, Whelan CM, Smith CJ, Mikhailenko I, Rebeck GW, Strickland DK, Hyman BT. 2001. Demonstration by fluorescence resonance energy transfer of two sites of interaction between the low-density lipoprotein receptor-related protein and the amyloid precursor protein: Role of the intracellular adapter protein Fe65. *J Neurosci* **21**: 8354–8361.

Kocherhans S, Madhusudan A, Doehner J, Breu KS, Nitsch RM, Fritschy JM, Knuesel I. 2010. Reduced Reelin expression accelerates amyloid-beta plaque formation and tau pathology in transgenic Alzheimer's disease mice. *J Neurosci* **30**: 9228–9240.

Koistinaho M, Lin S, Wu X, Esterman M, Koger D, Hanson J, Higgs R, Liu F, Malkani S, Bales KR, et al. 2004. Apolipoprotein E promotes astrocyte colocalization and degradation of deposited amyloid-β peptides. *Nat Med* **10**: 719–726.

Koldamova R, Staufenbiel M, Lefterov I. 2005a. Lack of ABCA1 considerably decreases brain ApoE level and increases amyloid deposition in APP23 mice. *J Biol Chem* **280**: 43224–43235.

Koldamova RP, Lefterov IM, Staufenbiel M, Wolfe D, Huang S, Glorioso JC, Walter M, Roth MG, Lazo JS. 2005b. The liver X receptor ligand T0901317 decreases amyloid β production in vitro and in a mouse model of Alzheimer's disease. *J Biol Chem* **280**: 4079–4088.

Korwek KM, Trotter JH, Ladu MJ, Sullivan PM, Weeber EJ. 2009. ApoE isoform-dependent changes in hippocampal synaptic function. *Molec Neurodegen* **4**: 21.

Kounnas MZ, Moir RD, Rebeck GW, Bush AI, Argraves WS, Tanzi RE, Hyman BT, Strickland DK. 1995. LDL-receptor-related protein, a multifunctional apoE receptor, binds secreted β-amyloid precursor protein and mediates its degradation. *Cell* **82**: 331–340.

Kowal RC, Herz J, Weisgraber KH, Mahley RW, Brown MS, Goldstein JL. 1990. Opposing effects of apolipoproteins E and C on lipoprotein binding to low density lipoprotein receptor-related protein. *J Biol Chem* **265**: 10771–10779.

Lacor PN, Buniel MC, Chang L, Fernandez SJ, Gong Y, Viola KL, Lambert MP, Velasco PT, Bigio EH, Finch CE, et al. 2004. Synaptic targeting by Alzheimer's-related amyloid β oligomers. *J Neurosci* **24**: 10191–10200.

LaDu MJ, Falduto MT, Manelli AM, Reardon CA, Getz GS, Frail DE. 1994. Isoform-specific binding of apolipoprotein E to β-amyloid. *J Biol Chem* **269**: 23404–23406.

LaDu MJ, Gilligan SM, Lukens JR, Cabana VG, Reardon CA, Van Eldik LJ, Holtzman DM. 1998. Nascent astrocyte particles differ from lipoproteins in CSF. *J Neurochem* **70**: 2070–2081.

Lambert MP, Barlow AK, Chromy BA, Edwards C, Freed R, Liosatos M, Morgan TE, Rozovsky I, Trommer B, Viola KL, et al. 1998. Diffusible, nonfibrillar ligands derived from Aβ1–42 are potent central nervous system neurotoxins. *Proc Natl Acad Sci* **95**: 6448–6453.

Lambert JC, Heath S, Even G, Campion D, Sleegers K, Hiltunen M, Combarros O, Zelenika D, Bullido MJ,

Tavernier B, et al. 2009. Genome-wide association study identifies variants at CLU and CR1 associated with Alzheimer's disease. *Nat Genet* **41:** 1094–1099.

Lesne S, Koh MT, Kotilinek L, Kayed R, Glabe CG, Yang A, Gallagher M, Ashe KH. 2006. A specific amyloid-β protein assembly in the brain impairs memory. *Nature* **440:** 352–357.

Lillis AP, Van Duyn LB, Murphy-Ullrich JE, Strickland DK. 2008. LDL receptor-related protein 1: Unique tissue-specific functions revealed by selective gene knockout studies. *Physiol Rev* **88:** 887–918.

Liu Q, Zerbinatti CV, Zhang J, Hoe HS, Wang B, Cole SL, Herz J, Muglia L, Bu G. 2007. Amyloid precursor protein regulates brain apolipoprotein E and cholesterol metabolism through lipoprotein receptor LRP1. *Neuron* **56:** 66–78.

Loukinova E, Ranganathan S, Kuznetsov S, Gorlatova N, Migliorini MM, Loukinov D, Ulery PG, Mikhailenko I, Lawrence DA, Strickland DK. 2002. Platelet-derived growth factor (PDGF)-induced tyrosine phosphorylation of the low density lipoprotein receptor-related protein (LRP). Evidence for integrated co-receptor function between LRP and the PDGF. *J Biol Chem* **277:** 15499–15506.

Ma J, Yee A, Brewer HB, Das S, Potter H. 1994. Amyloid-associated proteins α-1-antichymotrypsin and apolipoprotein E promote assembly of Alzheimer beta-protein into filaments. *Nature* **372:** 92–94.

Mahley RW. 1988. Apolipoprotein E: Cholesterol transport protein with expanding role in cell biology. *Science* **240:** 622–630.

Mahley RW, Rall SC Jr. 2000. Apolipoprotein E: Far more than a lipid transport protein. *Annu Rev Genomics Hum Genet* **1:** 507–537.

Mahley RW, Huang Y, Weisgraber KH. 2006. Putting cholesterol in its place: ApoE and reverse cholesterol transport. *J Clin Invest* **116:** 1226–1229.

Mandrekar S, Jiang Q, Lee CY, Koenigsknecht-Talboo J, Holtzman DM, Landreth GE. 2009. Microglia mediate the clearance of soluble Aβ through fluid phase macropinocytosis. *J Neurosci* **29:** 4252–4262.

Masiulis I, Quill TA, Burk RF, Herz J. 2009. Differential functions of the Apoer2 intracellular domain in selenium uptake and cell signaling. *Biol Chem* **390:** 67–73.

Masliah E, Mallory M, Ge N, Alford M, Veinbergs I, Roses AD. 1995. Neurodegeneration in the central nervous system of apoE-deficient mice. *Exp Neurol* **136:** 107–122.

Matsuki T, Pramatarova A, Howell BW. 2008. Reduction of Crk and CrkL expression blocks reelin-induced dendritogenesis. *J Cell Sci* **121:** 1869–1875.

Mauch DH, Nagler K, Schumacher S, Goritz C, Muller EC, Otto A, Pfrieger FW. 2001. CNS synaptogenesis promoted by glia-derived cholesterol. *Science* **294:** 1354–1357.

May P, Rohlmann A, Bock HH, Zurhove K, Marth JD, Schomburg ED, Noebels JL, Beffert U, Sweatt JD, Weeber EJ, et al. 2004. Neuronal LRP1 functionally associates with postsynaptic proteins and is required for normal motor function in mice. *Mol Cell Biol* **24:** 8872–8883.

McLaughlin L, Zhu G, Mistry M, Ley-Ebert C, Stuart WD, Florio CJ, Groen PA, Witt SA, Kimball TR, Witte DP, et al. 2000. Apolipoprotein J/clusterin limits the severity of murine autoimmune myocarditis. *J Clin Invest* **106:** 1105–1113.

Michikawa M, Fan QW, Isobe I, Yanagisawa K. 2000. Apolipoprotein E exhibits isoform-specific promotion of lipid efflux from astrocytes and neurons in culture. *J Neurochem* **74:** 1008–1016.

Morris JC, Roe CM, Xiong C, Fagan AM, Goate AM, Holtzman DM, Mintun MA. 2010. APOE predicts amyloid-beta but not tau Alzheimer pathology in cognitively normal aging. *Ann Neurol* **67:** 122–131.

* Mucke L, Selkoe DJ. 2011. Neurotoxicity of amyloid β-protein: Synaptic and network dysfunction. *Cold Spring Harb Perspect Med* doi: 10.1101/cshperspect.a006338.

Mudher A, Shepherd D, Newman TA, Mildren P, Jukes JP, Squire A, Mears A, Drummond JA, Berg S, MacKay D, et al. 2004. GSK-3β inhibition reverses axonal transport defects and behavioural phenotypes in *Drosophila*. *Mol Psychiatry* **9:** 522–530.

Namba Y, Tomonaga M, Kawasaki H, Otomo E, Ikeda K. 1991. Apolipoprotein E immunoreactivity in cerebral amyloid deposits and neurofibrillary tangles in Alzheimer's disease kuru plaque amyloid in Creutzfeldt-Jacob disease. *Brain Res* **541:** 163–166.

Narita N, Holtzman DM, Schwartz AL, Bu G. 1997. α₂-Macroglobulin complexes with and mediates the endocytosis of β-amyloid peptide via cell surface low-density lipoprotein receptor-related protein. *J Neurochem* **69:** 1904–1911.

Narita M, Holtzman DM, Fagan AM, LaDu MJ, Yu L, Han X, Gross RW, Bu G, Schwartz AL. 2002. Cellular catabolism of lipid poor apolipoprotein E via cell surface LDL receptor-related protein. *J Biochem* **132:** 743–749.

Nathan BP, Bellosta S, Sanan DA, Weisgraber KH, Mahley RW, Pitas RE. 1994. Differential effects of apolipoproteins E3 and E4 on neuronal growth in vitro. *Science* **264:** 850–852.

Nickerson DA, Taylor SL, Fullerton SM, Weiss KM, Clark AG, Stengard JH, Salomaa V, Boerwinkle E, Sing CF. 2000. Sequence diversity and large-scale typing of SNPs in the human apolipoprotein E gene. *Genome Res* **10:** 1532–1545.

Niu S, Renfro A, Quattrocchi CC, Sheldon M, D'Arcangelo G. 2004. Reelin promotes hippocampal dendrite development through the VLDLR/ApoER2-Dab1 pathway. *Neuron* **41:** 71–84.

Niu S, Yabut O, D'Arcangelo G. 2008. The Reelin signaling pathway promotes dendritic spine development in hippocampal neurons. *J Neurosci* **28:** 10339–10348.

Nygaard HB, Strittmatter SM. 2009. Cellular prion protein mediates the toxicity of β-amyloid oligomers: Implications for Alzheimer disease. *Arch Neurol* **66:** 1325–1328.

Ohkubo N, Lee YD, Morishima A, Terashima T, Kikkawa S, Tohyama M, Sakanaka M, Tanaka J, Maeda N, Vitek MP, et al. 2003. Apolipoprotein E and Reelin ligands modulate tau phosphorylation through an apolipoprotein E receptor/disabled-1/glycogen synthase kinase-3β cascade. *FASEB J* **17:** 295–297.

Palop JJ, Mucke L. 2010. Amyloid-β-induced neuronal dysfunction in Alzheimer's disease: From synapses toward neural networks. *Nat Neurosci* **13:** 812–818.

Palop JJ, Chin J, Roberson ED, Wang J, Thwin MT, Bien-Ly N, Yoo J, Ho KO, Yu GQ, Kreitzer A, et al. 2007. Aberrant excitatory neuronal activity and compensatory remodeling of inhibitory hippocampal circuits in mouse models of Alzheimer's disease. *Neuron* **55:** 697–711.

Peters MM, Hill KE, Burk RF, Weeber EJ. 2006. Altered hippocampus synaptic function in selenoprotein P deficient mice. *Mol Neurodegener* **1:** 12.

Pfrieger FW. 2003. Cholesterol homeostasis and function in neurons of the central nervous system. *Cell Mol Life Sci* **60:** 1158–1171.

Pietrzik CU, Yoon IS, Jaeger S, Busse T, Weggen S, Koo EH. 2004. FE65 constitutes the functional link between the low-density lipoprotein receptor-related protein and the amyloid precursor protein. *J Neurosci* **24:** 4259–4265.

Pitas RE, Boyles JK, Lee SH, Foss D, Mahley RW. 1987. Astrocytes synthesize apolipoprotein E and metabolize apolipoprotein E-containing lipoproteins. *Biochim Biophys Acta* **917:** 148–161.

Poirier J. 2003. Apolipoprotein E and cholesterol metabolism in the pathogenesis and treatment of Alzheimer's disease. *Trends Mol Med* **9:** 94–101.

Pujadas L, Gruart A, Bosch C, Delgado L, Teixeira CM, Rossi D, de Lecea L, Martinez A, Delgado-Garcia JM, Soriano E. 2010. Reelin regulates postnatal neurogenesis and enhances spine hypertrophy and long-term potentiation. *J Neurosci* **30:** 4636–4649.

Puzzo D, Privitera L, Leznik E, Fa M, Staniszewski A, Palmeri A, Arancio O. 2008. Picomolar amyloid-β positively modulates synaptic plasticity and memory in hippocampus. *J Neurosci* **28:** 14537–14545.

Qiu S, Zhao LF, Korwek KM, Weeber EJ. 2006. Differential reelin-induced enhancement of NMDA and AMPA receptor activity in the adult hippocampus. *J Neurosci* **26:** 12943–12955.

Rapp A, Gmeiner B, Huttinger M. 2006. Implication of apoE isoforms in cholesterol metabolism by primary rat hippocampal neurons and astrocytes. *Biochimie* **88:** 473–483.

Rebeck GW, Reiter JS, Strickland DK, Hyman BT. 1993. Apolipoprotein E in sporadic Alzheimer's disease: Allelic variation and receptor interactions. *Neuron* **11:** 575–580.

Rebeck GW, Harr SD, Strickland DK, Hyman BT. 1995. Multiple, diverse senile plaque-associated proteins are ligands of an apolipoprotein receptor, the α2-macroglobulin receptor/low-density-lipoprotein receptor-related protein. *Ann Neurol* **37:** 211–217.

Reiman EM, Chen K, Liu X, Bandy D, Yu M, Lee W, Ayutyanont N, Keppler J, Reeder SA, Langbaum JB, et al. 2009. Fibrillar amyloid-β burden in cognitively normal people at 3 levels of genetic risk for Alzheimer's disease. *Proc Natl Acad Sci* **106:** 6820–6825.

Renner M, Lacor PN, Velasco PT, Xu J, Contractor A, Klein WL, Triller A. 2010. Deleterious effects of amyloid β oligomers acting as an extracellular scaffold for mGluR5. *Neuron* **66:** 739–754.

Roberson ED, Scearce-Levie K, Palop JJ, Yan F, Cheng IH, Wu T, Gerstein H, Yu GQ, Mucke L. 2007. Reducing endogenous tau ameliorates amyloid β-induced deficits in an Alzheimer's disease mouse model. *Science* **316:** 750–754.

Roberson ED, Halabisky B, Yoo JW, Yao J, Chin J, Yan F, Wu T, Hamto P, Devidze N, Yu GQ, et al. 2011. Amyloid-β/Fyn-induced synaptic, network, and cognitive impairments depend on tau levels in multiple mouse models of Alzheimer's disease. *J Neurosci* **31:** 700–711.

Rogaeva E, Meng Y, Lee JH, Gu Y, Kawarai T, Zou F, Katayama T, Baldwin CT, Cheng R, Hasegawa H, et al. 2007. The neuronal sortilin-related receptor SORL1 is genetically associated with Alzheimer disease. *Nat Genet* **39:** 168–177.

Ronicke R, Mikhaylova M, Ronicke S, Meinhardt J, Schroder UH, Fandrich M, Reiser G, Kreutz MR, Reymann KG. 2010. Early neuronal dysfunction by amyloid β oligomers depends on activation of NR2B-containing NMDA receptors. *Neurobiol Aging* doi: 10.1016/j.neurobiolaging.2010.01.011.

Rust MB, Gurniak CB, Renner M, Vara H, Morando L, Gorlich A, Sassoe-Pognetto M, Banchaabouchi MA, Giustetto M, Triller A, et al. 2010. Learning, AMPA receptor mobility and synaptic plasticity depend on n-cofilin-mediated actin dynamics. *EMBO J* **29:** 1889–1902.

Sadowski MJ, Pankiewicz J, Scholtzova H, Mehta PD, Prelli F, Quartermain D, Wisniewski T. 2006. Blocking the apolipoprotein E/amyloid-β interaction as a potential therapeutic approach for Alzheimer's disease. *Proc Natl Acad Sci* **103:** 18787–18792.

Sagare A, Deane R, Bell RD, Johnson B, Hamm K, Pendu R, Marky A, Lenting PJ, Wu Z, Zarcone T, et al. 2007. Clearance of amyloid-β by circulating lipoprotein receptors. *Nat Med* **13:** 1029–1031.

* Saido T, Leissring MA. 2011. Proteolytic degradation of amyloid β-protein. *Cold Spring Harb Perspect Med* doi: 10.1011/cshperspect.a006379.

Salter MW, Kalia LV. 2004. Src kinases: A hub for NMDA receptor regulation. *Nat Rev Neurosci* **5:** 317–328.

Sanan DA, Weisgraber KH, Russel SJ, Mahley RW, Huang D, Saunders A, Schmechel D, Wisniewski T, Frangione B, Roses B, et al. 1994. Apolipoprotein E associates with β amyloid peptide of Alzheimer's disease to form novel monofibrils. *J Clin Invest* **94:** 860–869.

Schaefer EJ, Heaton WH, Wetzel MG, Brewer HB Jr. 1982. Plasma apolipoprotein A-1 absence associated with a marked reduction of high density lipoproteins and premature coronary artery disease. *Arteriosclerosis* **2:** 16–26.

Scherzer CR, Offe K, Gearing M, Rees HD, Fang G, Heilman CJ, Schaller C, Bujo H, Levey AI, Lah JJ. 2004. Loss of apolipoprotein E receptor LR11 in Alzheimer disease. *Arch Neurol* **61:** 1200–1205.

Schmechel DE, Saunders AM, Strittmatter WJ, Crain BJ, Hulette CM, Joo SH, Pericak-Vance MA, Goldgaber D, Roses AD. 1993. Increased amyloid β-peptide deposition in cerebral cortex as a consequence of apolipoprotein genotype in late-onset Alzheimer disease. *Proc Natl Acad Sci* **90:** 9649–9653.

Shankar GM, Bloodgood BL, Townsend M, Walsh DM, Selkoe DJ, Sabatini BL. 2007. Natural oligomers of the Alzheimer amyloid-β protein induce reversible synapse loss by modulating an NMDA-type glutamate receptor-dependent signaling pathway. *J Neurosci* **27:** 2866–2875.

Shankar GM, Li S, Mehta TH, Garcia-Munoz A, Shepardson NE, Smith I, Brett FM, Farrell MA, Rowan MJ, Lemere CA, et al. 2008. Amyloid-β protein dimers isolated directly from Alzheimer's brains impair synaptic plasticity and memory. *Nat Med* **14:** 837–842.

Sheldon M, Rice DS, D'Arcangelo G, Yoneshima H, Nakajima K, Mikoshiba K, Howell BW, Cooper JA, Goldowitz D, Curran T. 1997. Scrambler and yotari disrupt the disabled gene and produce a reeler-like phenotype in mice. *Nature* **389:** 730–733.

Shibata M, Yamada S, Kumar SR, Calero M, Bading J, Frangione B, Holtzman DM, Miller CA, Strickland DK, Ghiso J, et al. 2000. Clearance of Alzheimer's amyloid-β1–40 peptide from brain by LDL receptor-related protein-1 at the blood-brain barrier. *J Clin Invest* **106:** 1489–1499.

Shu T, Ayala R, Nguyen MD, Xie Z, Gleeson JG, Tsai LH. 2004. Ndel1 operates in a common pathway with LIS1 and cytoplasmic dynein to regulate cortical neuronal positioning. *Neuron* **44:** 263–277.

Sinagra M, Verrier D, Frankova D, Korwek KM, Blahos J, Weeber EJ, Manzoni OJ, Chavis P. 2005. Reelin, very-low-density lipoprotein receptor, and apolipoprotein E receptor 2 control somatic NMDA receptor composition during hippocampal maturation in vitro. *J Neurosci* **25:** 6127–6136.

Snyder EM, Nong Y, Almeida CG, Paul S, Moran T, Choi EY, Nairn AC, Salter MW, Lombroso PJ, Gouras GK, et al. 2005. Regulation of NMDA receptor trafficking by amyloid-β. *Nat Neurosci* **8:** 1051–1058.

Sorci-Thomas M, Prack MM, Dashti N, Johnson F, Rudel LL, Williams DL. 1988. Apolipoprotein (apo) A-I production and mRNA abundance explain plasma apoA-I and high density lipoprotein differences between two nonhuman primate species with high and low susceptibilities to diet-induced hypercholesterolemia. *J Biol Chem* **263:** 5183–5189.

Stockinger W, Brandes C, Fasching D, Hermann M, Gotthardt M, Herz J, Schneider WJ, Nimpf J. 2000. The reelin receptor ApoER2 recruits JNK-interacting proteins-1 and -2. *J Biol Chem* **275:** 25625–25632.

Stolt PC, Chen Y, Liu P, Bock HH, Blacklow SC, Herz J. 2005. Phosphoinositide binding by the disabled-1 PTB domain is necessary for membrane localization and Reelin signal transduction. *J Biol Chem* **280:** 9671–9677.

Strasser V, Fasching D, Hauser C, Mayer H, Bock HH, Hiesberger T, Herz J, Weeber EJ, Sweatt JD, Pramatarova A, et al. 2004. Receptor clustering is involved in Reelin signaling. *Mol Cell Biol* **24:** 1378–1386.

Strittmatter WJ, Saunders AM, Schmechel D, Pericak-Vance M, Enghild J, Salvesen GS, Roses AD. 1993a. Apolipoprotein E: High avidity binding to β-amyloid and increased frequency of type 4 allele in late-onset familial Alzheimer disease. *Proc Natl Acad Sci* **90:** 1977–1981.

Strittmatter WJ, Weisgraber KH, Huang DY, Dong L-Y, Salvesen GS, Pericak-Vance M, Schmechel D, Saunders AM, Goldgaber D, Roses AD. 1993b. Binding of human apolipoprotein E to synthetic amyloid β peptide: Isoform-specific effects and implications for late-onset Alzheimer disease. *Proc Natl Acad Sci* **90:** 8098–8102.

Sunderland T, Mirza N, Putnam KT, Linker G, Bhupali D, Durham R, Soares H, Kimmel L, Friedman D, Bergeson J, et al. 2004. Cerebrospinal fluid β-amyloid₁₋₄₂ and tau in control subjects at risk for Alzheimer's disease: The effect of APOE ε4 allele. *Biol Psychiatry* **56:** 670–676.

Sydow A, Van der Jeugd A, Zheng F, Ahmed T, Balschun D, Petrova O, Drexler D, Zhou L, Rune G, Mandelkow E, et al. 2011. Tau-induced defects in synaptic plasticity, learning, and memory are reversible in transgenic mice after switching off the toxic tau mutant. *J Neurosci* **31:** 2511–2525.

Tamamizu-Kato S, Cohen JK, Drake CB, Kosaraju MG, Drury J, Narayanaswami V. 2008. Interaction with amyloid β peptide compromises the lipid binding function of apolipoprotein E. *Biochemistry* **47:** 5225–5234.

Terrand J, Bruban V, Zhou L, Gong W, El Asmar Z, May P, Zurhove K, Haffner P, Philippe C, Woldt E, et al. 2009. LRP1 controls intracellular cholesterol storage and fatty acid synthesis through modulation of Wnt signaling. *J Biol Chem* **284:** 381–388.

Tiraboschi P, Hansen LA, Masliah E, Alford M, Thal LJ, Corey-Bloom J. 2004. Impact of APOE genotype on neuropathologic and neurochemical markers of Alzheimer disease. *Neurology* **62:** 1977–1983.

Tissir F, Goffinet AM. 2003. Reelin and brain development. *Nat Rev Neurosci* **4:** 496–505.

Tokuda T, Calero M, Matsubara E, Vidal R, Kumar A, Permanne B, Zlokovic B, Smith JD, Ladu MJ, Rostagno A, et al. 2000. Lipidation of apolipoprotein E influences its isoform-specific interaction with Alzheimer's amyloid β peptides. *Biochem J* **348:** 359–365.

Townsend M, Shankar GM, Mehta T, Walsh DM, Selkoe DJ. 2006. Effects of secreted oligomers of amyloid β-protein on hippocampal synaptic plasticity: A potent role for trimers. *J Physiol* **572:** 477–492.

Trommsdorff M, Borg JP, Margolis B, Herz J. 1998. Interaction of cytosolic adaptor proteins with neuronal apolipoprotein E receptors and the amyloid precursor protein. *J Biol Chem* **273:** 33556–33560.

Trommsdorff M, Gotthardt M, Hiesberger T, Shelton J, Stockinger W, Nimpf J, Hammer RE, Richardson JA, Herz J. 1999. Reeler/Disabled-like disruption of neuronal migration in knockout mice lacking the VLDL receptor and ApoE receptor 2. *Cell* **97:** 689–701.

Ulery PG, Beers J, Mikhailenko I, Tanzi RE, Rebeck GW, Hyman BT, Strickland DK. 2000. Modulation of β-amyloid precursor protein processing by the low density lipoprotein receptor-related protein (LRP). Evidence that LRP contributes to the pathogenesis of Alzheimer's disease. *J Biol Chem* **275:** 7410–7415.

Van Uden E, Mallory M, Ieinbergs I, Alford M, Rockenstein E, Masliah E. 2002. Increased extracellular amyloid deposition and neurodegeneration in human amyloid precursor protein transgenic mice deficient in receptor-associated protein. *J Neurosci* **22:** 9298–9304.

Vazquez-Higuera JL, Mateo I, Sanchez-Juan P, Rodriguez-Rodriguez E, Pozueta A, Infante J, Berciano J, Combarros O. 2009. Genetic interaction between tau and the apolipoprotein E receptor LRP1 Increases Alzheimer's disease risk. *Dement Geriat Cogn Disord* **28:** 116–120.

Wahrle SE, Jiang H, Parsadanian M, Hartman RE, Bales KR, Paul SM, Holtzman DM. 2005. Deletion of Abca1 increases Aβ deposition in the PDAPP transgenic mouse model of Alzheimer disease. *J Biol Chem* **280:** 43236–43242.

Wahrle SE, Jiang H, Parsadanian M, Kim J, Li A, Knoten A, Jain S, Hirsch-Reinshagen V, Wellington CL, Bales KR, et al. 2008. Overexpression of ABCA1 reduces amyloid deposition in the PDAPP mouse model of Alzheimer disease. *J Clin Invest* **118:** 671–682.

Walsh DM, Klyubin I, Fadeeva JV, Cullen WK, Anwyl R, Wolfe MS, Rowan MJ, Selkoe DJ. 2002. Naturally secreted oligomers of amyloid β protein potently inhibit hippocampal long-term potentiation in vivo. *Nature* **416:** 535–539.

Weeber EJ, Beffert U, Jones C, Christian JM, Forster E, Sweatt JD, Herz J. 2002. Reelin and ApoE receptors cooperate to enhance hippocampal synaptic plasticity and learning. *J Biol Chem* **277:** 39944–39952.

Willnow TE, Hilpert J, Armstrong SA, Rohlmann A, Hammer RE, Burns DK, Herz J. 1996. Defective forebrain development in mice lacking gp330/megalin. *Proc Natl Acad Sci* **93:** 8460–8464.

Wisniewski T, Frangione B. 1992. Apolipoprotein E: A pathological chaperone protein in patients with cerebral and systemic amyloid. *Neurosci Lett* **135:** 235–238.

Wisniewski T, Castano EM, Golabek A, Vogel T, Frangione B. 1994. Acceleration of Alzheimer's fibril formation by apolipoprotein E in vitro. *Am J Pathol* **145:** 1030–1035.

Wood SJ, Chan W, Wetzel R. 1996. Seeding of Aβ fibril formation is inhibited by all three isotypes of apolipoprotein E. *Biochemistry* **35:** 12623–12628.

Xu P-T, Schmechel D, Qiu H-L, Herbstreith M, Rothrock-Christian T, Eyster M, Roses AD, Gilbert JR. 1999. Sialylated human apolipoprotein E (apoEs) is preferentially associated with neuron-enriched cultures from APOE transgenic mice. *Neurobiol Dis* **6:** 63–75.

Xu Q, Bernardo A, Walker D, Kanegawa T, Mahley RW, Huang Y. 2006. Profile and regulation of apolipoprotein E (ApoE) expression in the CNS in mice with targeting of green fluorescent protein gene to the ApoE locus. *J Neurosci* **26:** 4985–4994.

Yang D-S, Smith JD, Zhou Z, Gandy S, Martins RN. 1997. Characterization of the binding of amyloid-β peptide to cell culture-derived native apolipoprotein E2, E3, and E4 isoforms and to isoforms from human plasma. *J Neurochem* **68:** 721–725.

Yang DS, Small DH, Seydel U, Smith JD, Hallmayer J, Gandy SE, Martins RN. 1999. Apolipoprotein E promotes the binding and uptake of β-amyloid into Chinese hamster ovary cells in an isoform-specific manner. *Neuroscience* **90:** 1217–1226.

Zerbinatti CV, Wozniak DF, Cirrito J, Cam JA, Osaka H, Bales KR, Zhuo M, Paul SM, Holtzman DM, Bu G. 2004. Increased soluble amyloid-β peptide and memory deficits in amyloid model mice overexpressing the low-density lipoprotein receptor-related protein. *Proc Natl Acad Sci* **101:** 1075–1080.

Zerbinatti CV, Wahrle SE, Kim H, Cam JA, Bales K, Paul SM, Holtzman DM, Bu G. 2006. Apolipoprotein E and low density lipoprotein receptor-related protein facilitate intraneuronal Aβ42 accumulation in amyloid model mice. *J Biol Chem* **281:** 36180–36186.

Zhuo M, Holtzman DM, Li Y, Osaka H, DeMaro J, Jacquin M, Bu G. 2000. Role of tissue plasminogen activator receptor LRP in hippocampal long-term potentiation. *J Neurosci* **20:** 542–549.

Zlokovic BV. 2008. The blood-brain barrier in health and chronic neurodegenerative disorders. *Neuron* **57:** 178–201.

Zurhove K, Nakajima C, Herz J, Bock HH, May P. 2008. γ-secretase limits the inflammatory response through the processing of LRP1. *Sci Signal* **1:** ra15.

Animal Models of Alzheimer Disease

Frank M. LaFerla and Kim N. Green

Institute for Memory Impairments and Neurological Disorders, Department of Neurobiology and Behavior, University of California, Irvine, Irvine, California 92697-4545

Correspondence: laferla@uci.edu

Significant insights into the function of genes associated with Alzheimer disease and related dementias have occurred through studying genetically modified animals. Although none of the existing models fully reproduces the complete spectrum of this insidious human disease, critical aspects of Alzheimer pathology and disease processes can be experimentally recapitulated. Genetically modified animal models have helped advance our understanding of the underlying mechanisms of disease and have proven to be invaluable in the preclinical evaluation of potential therapeutic interventions. Continuing refinement and evolution to yield the next generation of animal models will facilitate successes in producing greater translational concordance between preclinical studies and human clinical trials and eventually lead to the introduction of novel therapies into clinical practice.

Alzheimer disease (AD), the most common cause of dementia, accounts for approximately two-thirds of all dementia cases and afflicts more than 35 million individuals worldwide, including more than 5.4 million Americans. It is a relentlessly progressive disorder that typically manifests initially by severe loss of memory, particularly of episodic memory. At present, the disorder is not curable, thereby increasing the urgency of developing and characterizing relevant animal models to facilitate translational research and preclinical drug development.

Research progress over the past two decades, including the elucidation of AD susceptibility and causative genes as well as other proteins involved in the pathogenic process, has profoundly facilitated the development of genetically altered mouse models (see http://www.alzforum.org/res/com/tra for a listing of cur-

rently available models). Animal models have played a major role in defining critical disease-related mechanisms and have been at the forefront of evaluating novel therapeutic approaches, with many treatments currently in clinical trial owing their origins to studies initially performed in mice. Nevertheless, there are significant translational issues that have been raised of late, as there has been some potential discordance between preclinical drug studies and human clinical trials.

ASPECTS OF HUMAN AD MODELED IN TRANSGENIC MICE

The vast majority of AD cases are sporadic (sAD), and the causes underlying these cases remain unknown. Neuropathologically, AD is characterized by the accumulation of amyloid-β (Aβ) plaques and neurofibrillary tangles, in addition to widespread synaptic loss, inflammation and oxidative damage, and neuronal death. Notably, the neuropathology and clinical phenotype are generally indistinguishable in the early-onset familial versus the sporadic form of the disease, with the biggest difference being the age of onset (Selkoe 2002). Because the etiology of idiopathic AD is unknown, animal models have relied on the utilization of genetic mutations associated with familial AD (fAD), with the rationale that the events downstream of the initial trigger are quite similar. These genetic models have still been invaluable in determining the molecular mechanisms of disease progression and for testing potential therapeutics. Although no single mouse model recapitulates all of the aspects of the disease spectrum, each model allows for in-depth analysis of one or two components of the disease, which is not readily possible or ethical with human patients or samples.

Transgenic mice overproducing mutant APP develop pathology that is similar to that found in the human brain; importantly, $A\beta$ accumulation into extracellular plaques occurs and is age-dependent—in other words, despite constant $A\beta$ production, plaques only occur in mid to late adulthood in the majority of these animals. Notably, plaque formation is accelerated when the longer $A\beta_{42}$ is preferentially cleaved from APP, as this peptide is more prone to aggregation than $A\beta_{40}$ and leads to earlier and more severe cognitive decline (reviewed in Findeis 2007). The importance of $A\beta_{42}$ to disease progression was highlighted by showing that elevated levels of $A\beta_{40}$, the shorter, more common form of $A\beta$, actually prevented the formation of $A\beta$ pathology in the widely used Tg2576 mouse model (McGowan et al. 2005). On the contrary, elevated levels of $A\beta_{42}$ markedly exacerbated pathology in the same mouse model.

$A\beta$ plaques found in the brains of AD transgenic mice are structurally similar to those found in the human brain; they initiate as diffuse plaques consisting mainly of $A\beta_{42}$, develop a dense $A\beta_{42}$ core, and then incorporate $A\beta_{40}$, as well as numerous other non-$A\beta$ components such as ubiquitin and α-synuclein (Yang et al. 2000). As in the human brain, these plaques stain positive with both thioflavin and Congo red, and show similar fibrillar structures by microscopy (Fig. 1).

Work in transgenic mice has highlighted the dynamic nature of extracellular plaques and has also aided in the clarification of important elements in both the brain environment and the $A\beta$ peptide needed for aggregation of $A\beta$ into plaques. Although formation of plaques in AD transgenic mice is typically age-dependent (as is AD pathology in humans), plaque formation occurs very quickly in the brains of older AD

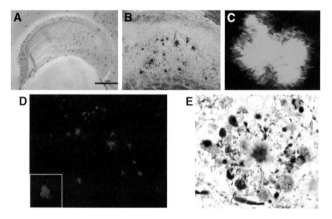

Figure 1. Visualization of amyloid plaques in 3xTg-AD mice with classical stains. 3xTg-AD mice develop diffuse and fibrillar plaques, as detected with antibody 6E10 (*A* and *B*), thioflavin-S (*C*), Congo red (*D*), and Gallyas stain (*E*).

 Cite this article as *Cold Spring Harb Perspect Med* doi: 10.1101/cshperspect.a006320

transgenic mice. This has been shown using a window in the skull of APP transgenic mice (Meyer-Luehmann et al. 2008) and further supported by data that plaque volume in aged AD transgenic mice rapidly returns to high levels within 30 days following plaque removal by immunotherapy (Oddo et al. 2004), in grafts of wild-type tissue into AD transgenic mouse brains (Meyer-Luehmann et al. 2003), and in the brains of prepathologic AD transgenic mice following injection with brain extracts from human AD brain or aged AD transgenic mouse (Meyer-Luehmann et al. 2006). These data indicate that the adult AD transgenic mouse brain is ripe for the development of Aβ pathology and the latter study also suggests that the ability of Aβ to act as a seed for aggregation is dependent on its source.

Most AD transgenic models exhibit memory impairments, with the cognitive deficits appearing to occur earlier than the appearance of extracellular plaques. These observations led to a search for earlier pathological species of Aβ that could be mediating cognitive decline. Research shifted to identifying the precursors to plaque formation and identifying how aggregation of Aβ was crucial to its toxicity. This led to the focus on soluble oligomeric Aβ species—low-molecular-weight aggregates up to ~150 kDa consisting of two to 30 Aβ peptides. As in AD transgenic mice, cognitive decline in humans is not proportional to Aβ plaque load (Terry et al. 1991), but does correlate with soluble Aβ species (Wang et al. 1999). However, in humans, unlike AD transgenic mice, cognitive decline does not begin until there is a large quantity of Aβ accumulation in the brain, including large amounts of amyloid plaques and probably oligomers. The latest data now indicate that soluble oligomeric species play a critical role in the pathogenicity of AD (for reviews, see Haass and Selkoe 2007; Walsh and Selkoe 2007). Evidence supporting involvement of soluble Aβ oligomers in AD is present in human postmortem brain tissue (Naslund et al. 2000; Kokubo et al. 2005); however, much of the evidence for the toxicity of oligomeric Aβ and its central part in AD has come directly from the use of transgenic mouse models of AD.

Intraneuronal Aβ has also gained experimental support in recent years (LaFerla et al. 2007). As in human AD and Down syndrome patients (who develop AD-like pathology by the fifth decade), many APP AD transgenic mice exhibit intraneuronal amyloid accumulation. The accumulation of intracellular Aβ has been shown to precede extracellular deposition in both human (Gyure et al. 2001; Mori et al. 2002) and some mouse studies (Oddo et al. 2003b). In fact, it was found in transgenic mice that intraneuronal Aβ strongly correlates with initial deficits on a hippocampal-based memory task (Billings et al. 2005). Data from transgenic AD mice also indicate that intraneuronal Aβ is more neurotoxic than extracellular Aβ (Casas et al. 2004).

The other hallmark pathology of human AD are the intraneuronal aggregates of hyperphosphorylated tau known as neurofibrillary tangles (NFTs) (Fig. 2). The amyloid cascade hypothesis predicts that tau hyperphosphorylation occurs as a downstream consequence of Aβ accumulation. APP-overexpressing transgenic mice have provided evidence both for and against this. Unlike humans with AD, these mouse models do not develop NFTs, yet many do show increased tau hyperphosphorylation (reviewed in Gotz et al. 2007). This could be because (1) human Aβ accumulation is not sufficient to cause NFT formation; (2) rodent tau has a different structure and sequence that may not be prone to aggregate formation; (3) the life span of mice is not prolonged enough to allow for enough hyperphosphorylation/aggregation as these pathologies develop over decades in humans; or (4) a combination of these. So whereas Aβ accumulation in APP overexpressing mice does not lead to NFT formation, it should be remembered that these animals still develop robust cognitive decline and also undergo more subtle alterations in tau that resemble the precursors to NFTs in the human brain (most notably hyperphosphorylated tau).

To model the NFTs seen in human AD it has been necessary to develop transgenic mice that express further gene alterations in addition to mutated APP such as mutated human tau (Lewis et al. 2001; Oddo et al. 2003b) or removal

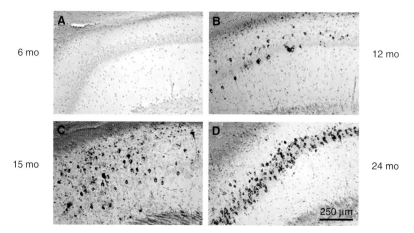

Figure 2. 3xTg-AD mice develop Gallyas-positive intraneuronal tangles. Age-dependent accumulation of Gallyas-positive aggregates within hippocampal neurons are observed in 3xTg-AD mice.

of nitric oxide synthase 2 (Wilcock et al. 2008). These multigenic AD transgenic models do develop NFTs similar to those seen in human brain and have aided the explication of the relationship between Aβ and tau (reviewed in Blurton-Jones and LaFerla 2006) with Aβ pathology seeming to precede the onset of tau pathology (Fig. 3), consistent with the amyloid cascade hypothesis. In addition to providing evidence that Aβ accumulation occurs proximal to the onset of tau pathology, multigenic models of AD have also allowed us to determine how

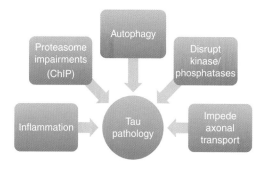

Figure 3. Pathways by which Aβ facilitates tau pathology. Several pathways have been implicated in the hyperphosphorylation and aggregation of tau in neurons. These include inflammation, proteasome impairments, impairments in autophagy, increased kinase activity, and decreased phosphatase activity, as well as impeded axonal transport.

manipulation of Aβ affects tau and vice versa. Some of the strongest data supporting tau pathology as a downstream event of Aβ accumulation have come from the study of these mice. For example, in the 3xTg-AD mice, which contain human APP, PS1, and tau mutant transgenes, appearance of intraneuronal Aβ precedes somatodendritic accumulation of tau (Oddo et al. 2003a). Furthermore, removal of intraneuronal Aβ via immunotherapy leads to the removal of somatodendritic tau shortly afterward, providing the tau is not aggregated (Oddo et al. 2004). It was also found that Aβ oligomers inhibit proteasome function, which normally serves to degrade excess tau proteins, leading to tau accumulation (reviewed in (Oddo 2008). Such impairments in proteasome activity have been shown in human AD as well (Keller et al. 2000).

A further connection between Aβ aggregation and downstream pathologies, such as tau, exists in the inflammatory response present in AD. Inflammation in AD is not exactly modeled in mice, as there are differences between humans and AD transgenic mice with respect to the nature and severity of the inflammation (Webster et al. 1999; Mehlhorn et al. 2000), yet AD transgenic mice are still valuable for revealing which aspects of inflammation may be key for the development or elimination of downstream pathologies. Data from AD transgenic

Cite this article as *Cold Spring Harb Perspect Med* doi: 10.1101/cshperspect.a006320

mice indicate that inflammation, including activation of complement and various cytokines, occurs downstream from the aggregation of Aβ (reviewed in Akiyama et al. 2000), and more specifically, in association with fibrillar Aβ (Kitazawa et al. 2005). Many of these inflammatory mediators that are up-regulated by Aβ can serve to increase tau pathology (reviewed in Blurton-Jones and LaFerla 2006). For example, activation of Cdk5 following an inflammatory response leads to tau hyperphosphorylation (Kitazawa et al. 2005). There is also production of reactive oxygen species as a result of this inflammatory response (Steele et al. 2007), which is damaging to cell membranes and may further exacerbate the inflammatory response. In both humans and AD transgenic mice, Aβ plaques are surrounded by activated microglia and astrocytes; thus even as the activation of the inflammatory response in AD can lead to the detrimental effects discussed above, activated microglia act in a beneficial manner by attempting to phagocytose Aβ plaques (Wyss-Coray and Mucke 2002). In support of the hypothesis that inflammation may have favorable effects in AD, acute inflammation, as brought about by treatment with lipopolysaccharide (LPS), has been shown to clear Aβ plaques (DiCarlo et al. 2001) in AD transgenic mice, whereas more chronic LPS treatment potentiates tau pathology (Kitazawa et al. 2005). Active and passive immunotherapy strategies using Aβ or antibodies against Aβ, respectively, have also proven useful in reducing plaque and, subsequently, tangle pathology as well as cognitive deficits in AD transgenic mice. The stimulation of microglia is one mechanism that appears to be involved in the reduction of plaque burden (reviewed in Morgan 2006) and further supports the idea that an inflammatory response in the AD brain has some positive effects.

MODELS BASED ON GENE ABLATION

In addition to transgenic mouse models, which overproduce and recapitulate the Aβ and tau pathologies that are associated with AD, numerous genetically modified mice have been produced that lack genes associated with this disorder. Although these mice do not recapitulate the human pathological phenotype per se, they have proven useful in elucidating the molecular mechanisms underlying the pathology, as well as identifying some of the other pathways that are the targets of crucial drugs. Specifically, knockout mice have been made of the APP secretases (BACE, presenilin [1 and 2], and ADAM 10 and 17; Shen et al. 1997; Herreman et al. 1999; Luo et al. 2001; Hartmann et al. 2002; Lee et al. 2003). In addition, both APP and tau knockout mice have proven invaluable in understanding disease progression, as well as in identifying physiological roles for the APP protein (Zheng et al. 1996; Takei et al. 2000).

The presenilins were identified as being a crucial component of γ-secretase in 1995, and their presence necessary for the production of Aβ. As such, the presenilins and the γ-secretase complex quickly became the primary small molecular drug target for AD. Presenilin 1 knockout mice were produced in 1997, and it was shown that homozygous knockout of PS1 was lethal, with developmental defects in both the central nervous system (CNS) and skeletal systems (Shen et al. 1997). Hence, the production of these mice were the first indications that presenilin, and the γ-secretase complex, had vital roles outside of the production of Aβ, and that inhibiting it may lead to undesirable off-target effects. Despite these early indications, and a wealth of subsequent publications showing numerous substrates for the γ-secretase complex (Beel and Sanders 2008), regulating many signaling pathways—including suppression of skin cancer (Zhang et al. 2007), as well as roles in calcium dyshomeostasis (Green and LaFerla 2008) and autophagy (Lee et al. 2010; Neely et al. 2011)—efforts progressed toward developing γ-secretase inhibitors and a great number of highly specific compounds were identified. These inhibitors have recently been tested in phase III clinical trials, and consistent with the wealth of data obtained from presenilin knockout mice, one of these was found to cause increased cognitive decline, and increased the incidence of skin cancer (Schor 2011). As such these inhibitor programs have largely been abandoned in preference for more APP selective γ-secretase inhibitors, or γ-secretase modulators, which do not inhibit the γ-secretase complex, but alter where it cleaves APP to generate less aggregate-prone species of Aβ.

BACE1 is the sole β-secretase enzyme, and its activity is also crucial for the production of Aβ. Several groups first identified it in 1999 (Hussain et al. 1999; Sinha et al. 1999; Vassar et al. 1999), but its physiological functions were unclear. As with presenilin and the γ-secretase complex, its cloning and identification made the creation of BACE inhibitor programs a primary target for the treatment of AD. Contrary to presenilin-deficient mice, BACE1 knockout mice were found to be healthy and viable with no obvious defects (Luo et al. 2001; Roberds et al. 2001) and, importantly, no longer produced any Aβ. Thus, BACE1 appears a much more attractive drug target that the γ-secretase complex owing to a lack of obvious deficits when its activity is ablated. As proof of concept that targeting of BACE1 for the treatment of AD would be effective, BACE1 knockout mice were crossed with the Tg2576 mice. The absence of BACE1 prevented cognitive decline in these animals and markedly reduced Aβ levels (Ohno et al. 2004). These BACE1 knockout mice have also been used to identify substrates other than APP and have highlighted β subunits of voltage-gated sodium channels (Dominguez et al. 2005; Wong et al. 2005; Kim et al. 2011), klotho (Bloch et al. 2009), and neuregulin-1 (Hu et al. 2006; Willem et al. 2006), which is essential for myelination of both peripheral and central neurons. Hence, BACE1 appears to have a role in the developmental myelination of the nervous system, with BACE1 knockout mice showing significantly reduced levels of myelination and myelin thickness (Hu et al. 2006; Willem et al. 2006). Further analyses revealed that BACE1 knockout mice had increased pain sensitivity and reduced grip strength (Hu et al. 2006). However, these deficits may be due to developmental issues that do not arise when BACE1 is ablated or inhibited in the developed/aged organism, and thus far, no conditional BACE1 knockout mice

exist to test this issue. Peripheral remyelination has been investigated in mature BACE1 knockout mice and has been shown to be impaired (Hu et al. 2008), yet axonal regeneration is enhanced following axotomy (Farah et al. 2011), suggesting a possible unwanted side effect of systemically administered BACE1 inhibitors.

Related to these deficits in myelination in BACE1 knockout a mouse, careful reanalysis has revealed subtle deficits in prepulse inhibition, hypersensitivity to a glutamatergic psychostimulant, cognitive impairments, and reduced dendritic spine densities (Laird et al. 2005; Savonenko et al. 2008). Collectively, BACE1 knockout mice have established BACE1 as a primary target for the treatment of AD with minimal off-target effects, but have highlighted its role in both myelination and regulation of the levels of voltage-gated sodium channels, suggesting that there could be some deleterious side effects from inhibiting BACE1 in the mature body/CNS. Regardless, inhibiting BACE1 in the adult brain appears to be far less problematic than inhibiting the presenilins and the γ-secretase complex, and remains a far safer target.

Given the information gleaned from BACE1 knockout mice, why is it that a γ-secretase inhibitor has been through a phase III clinical trial, whereas no BACE1 inhibitor results have come to light? This appears to be due to limitations of the compounds discovered thus far. BACE1 has a large active site, and it has been challenging to find compounds that cross the blood–brain barrier and are large enough to inhibit the active site without being broken down by endopeptidases (Huang et al. 2009). However, some promising compounds have been reported to lower Aβ levels in transgenic mice (Chang et al. 2004; Hussain et al. 2007; Fukumoto et al. 2010; Lerchner et al. 2010) and primates (Sankaranarayanan et al. 2009), and human clinical trials are ensuing.

Tau knockout mice have shed light on the mechanism by which Aβ induces cognitive deficits in APP transgenic models. Curiously, plaque load does not correlate well with cognitive decline in AD patients (Nagy et al. 1995), whereas cognitive deficits are detected in most APP transgenic mice prior to plaque deposition

(Billings et al. 2005). Furthermore, the involvement of tau in the pathogenesis of AD has never been fully understood—mutations in APP or presenilin lead to AD, but mutations in tau lead to their own neurodegenerative diseases. Tau becomes hyperphosphorylated during the AD process, and aggregates into NFTs. Many lines of evidence indicate that the presence of Aβ pathologies can activate kinases, down-regulate phosphatases, and impair degradation of tau, leading to tau pathology (Blurton-Jones and LaFerla 2006). However, what is the consequence of these tau pathologies on cognition and neuronal/synaptic loss, compared with the consequences of Aβ pathology alone? Notably, it has been shown that crossing APP transgenic mice onto a tau knockout background prevents all cognitive deficits associated with the presence of APP and Aβ (Roberson et al. 2007), including reduced spontaneous seizures (Palop et al. 2007) and long-term potentiation (LTP; Shipton et al. 2011). The absence of tau has no effect on the development of Aβ pathologies, including plaque load. Hence, endogenous murine tau is necessary for APP and Aβ to mediate its effects on cognition, LTP and hyperexcitibility of neurons. These exciting discoveries have shed light on the crucial role that tau may play in directly mediating the effects of Aβ on cognition and other adverse effects. Notably, APP transgenic mice do not develop extensive tau pathologies on their own—some hyperphosphorylation is seen, but the tau remains soluble and does not resemble the NTFs found in the human disease. Hence, soluble tau may be more important to the disease process than tau that has aggregated into NFTs. During the disease process, the axonal protein tau becomes mislocalized to the soma and dendrites. Accumulation of tau within the dendritic spines impairs synaptic function (Hoover et al. 2010), but only when the tau is phosphorylated. It has been shown that tau present in the dendrites can target the protein kinase Fyn to the postsynaptic membranes (Ittner et al. 2010). Once there, it phosphorylates the NR2b subunit of the NMDA (N-methyl-D-aspartate) receptor, causing it to stabilize with PSD-95. This stabilization leads to a greater influx of calcium through the NMDA receptor and can be synaptotoxic. Notably, Aβ oligomers can interact with NMDA receptors and so it may be the combined effects of both Aβ and tau that drive the effects at the synapse and lead to impaired cognition, LTP, hyperexcitibility, and changes in dendritic spine morphology and density. Hence, the use of tau knockout mice, if the effects seen are relevant to human AD, has radically changed our understanding of the role of tau in disease progression, and the nature of the relationship between Aβ and tau and their effects on cognition. Importantly, these studies and mice have highlighted an important role for tau outside of AD, but more generally in excitotoxicity.

TRANSLATIONAL ISSUES

More than 15 years have passed since the first transgenic models were derived that recapitulated aspects of AD pathology. Somewhat surprisingly, since that time, no new therapies for AD have been approved and introduced into the clinic, and the two currently approved drug classes (acetylcholinesterase inhibitors and memantine) were not tested in these transgenic mice prior to the clinic. This stark reality begs the question of how useful have these animal models actually been for the field? Have they been a distraction to the real issues facing an AD patient, or will their continued use bear fruits over the coming years? Why have so many therapies and interventions been successful in these models, but have universally failed when evaluated in clinic trials? Although an in-depth discussion of these questions is beyond the scope of this review, we will touch on some of the translational issues (Box 1).

The most widely used animal models in the field are in fact models based on the genetics of familial AD. Less than 1% of AD cases are due to autosomal-dominant AD, rather than sporadic AD, so the obvious initial question is whether fAD and sAD are the same phenotypical disease or are there subtle differences between the pathologies that would allow a treatment to work in one but not the other. By all pathological counts, they are essentially

---

BOX 1. TRANSLATIONAL CONCERNS WITH ANIMAL MODELS

- There is lack of concordance between preclinical models and human clinical trials.
  - Potential reasons: wrong targets, incomplete models, lack of variability among individuals in the models, patients enrolled too late, comorbidities
- Humans enrolled in clinical trials are heterogenous, whereas most models utilize in-bred stains on mice.
  - Potential solution: evaluating novel treatments in multiple lines may help address this point
- There is lack of substantial cell and synaptic loss in the majority of rodent models, suggesting the models better represent the prodromal phase of the disease.
- Models are of familial AD, and most people have sporadic AD.

---

the same disease, with abundant plaque and tangle accumulations in the same brain areas as well as high levels of synaptic and neuronal loss. The differences appear to be what causes the buildup of the pathologies in the first place. In fAD, a mutation in APP or PS1/2 causes the accumulation of Aβ, whereas the causes of Aβ accumulation in sAD are unclear, but likely to be a combination of genetic and environmental factors. Both are highly influenced by aging, with fAD manifesting at younger ages, and being more aggressive in its progression. A priori, one could postulate that fAD might be harder to treat than sAD, because of the aggressiveness of the pathology. Hence, transgenic mice that model fAD, and do so in a very short time frame (1–2 years) should be the hardest to treat, and should therefore translate to sAD very effectively. Obviously, the plethora of numerous failed clinical trials indicates that this is not the case, and so why do so many treatments show success in these aggressive mouse models of fAD and then fail in patients with sAD?

Although there are numerous hypotheses that may account for the discordance in results between preclinical animal models and human clinical trials, no doubt one of the most significant may be that many AD models do not recapitulate the extensive neuronal loss observed in the human condition. Human imaging studies and clinical–pathological studies show that patients with mild–moderate AD already have not only brain atrophy but also extensive neuronal loss in several brain regions. The therapies

that are being pioneered in mouse models are primarily targeting the pathologies modeled and not dealing with the issue of extensive neuronal loss. Hence, many of these therapies may be effective at preventing or clearing the pathology, and hence the disease, but are ineffective in people in which the pathology has already destroyed a huge proportion of the neurons that they need for memories and cognition. The acetylcholinesterase inhibitors were developed following studies identifying cholinergic loss as being a highly important factor in AD cognitive decline.

This raises two pertinent questions: First, why do mice not recapitulate the neuronal loss seen in the disease, and, second, can we develop models that do develop similar loss in which therapeutics can be evaluated? We believe that the fundamental reason why transgenic mice do not develop extensive neuronal loss, like human AD patients, is the amount of time needed. In human AD, disease progresses over decades. During this time synaptic disturbances, such as those measured in transgenic mice, could eventually lead to neuronal death. The two years during which we keep most transgenic APP mice may not be long enough for this to occur. Other issues also clearly play a role, such as background strains, such as the widely used C57/Bl6, which may be more resistant to excitotoxicity and heterogeneity of humans versus inbred mouse strains, as well as fundamental differences between mice and humans. For example, it is well established that APP transgenic mice have cognitive decline prior to plaques, and prior to any measurable neuronal loss. Furthermore, Aβ oligomers have been universally shown to impair LTP in countless studies, and it is easy to then connect this to the cognitive impairments seen in these mice. Yet there is no evidence that Aβ causes cognitive decline in humans prior to plaques (and neuronal loss). If Aβ impairs LTP in the human brain in the same, robust, fashion that it does in the rodent brain then presumably humans would experience cognitive decline in the absence of both plaques and neuronal loss whenever Aβ oligomers could first be detected (Kuo et al. 1996; Tomic et al. 2009; Woltjer et al. 2009), and this cannot be explained by cognitive reserve. This has not yet been shown to occur, suggesting that it is possible that Aβ may have different modes of action in the rodent brain compared with that of a human.

So how do we develop therapies that target the neuronal loss and how do we then test and validate them in vivo, prior to the clinic? Clinical trials for AD are expensive—upward of $10–20 million for a well-powered phase II/III trial. Hence, only the most promising compounds can be brought into the clinic, and every failure is costly and discouraging to alternative future trials. It should be noted that prevention trials have not yet been feasible, in part owing to a lack of biomarkers and the extreme expense associated with the numbers of people needed and the amount of time for which they would have to be evaluated, and therefore trials have only used cognitive outcome measures in usually mild–moderate AD patients—which means they already have extensive plaque and tangle loads, and that these have already caused extensive neuronal damage and loss, which in turn causes dementia. We have developed a novel approach to this problem by using an inducible transgenic mouse model of neuronal loss (Yamasaki et al. 2007). We use the tetracycline-off system to drive expression of diptheria toxin A chains in neurons under control of the Calmodulin Kinase II promoter. By withdrawing doxycycline from the diet, we can specifically ablate neurons in regions of the brain that are impacted in AD, and we can titrate that loss to levels seen in the AD brain. Mice show cognitive impairments, as expected, and can then be used to identify treatments that can improve cognition in the presence of extensive neuronal loss, such as that seen in AD patients. We are taking the approach of combining therapy testing in this model alongside a traditional APP/tau transgenic mouse, such as the 3xTg-AD, to identify treatments that can improve cognition in the presence of Aβ and tau pathologies, but also neuronal loss. This ensures that only the best therapies will be selected and proposed as clinical candidates.

If 15 years of using transgenic mouse models of AD have yielded no positive clinical results, then have these mice been a failure or even a distraction from the real problems with AD? The answer is unequivocally no—many novel approaches to reducing AD pathology have been discovered and developed in these transgenic mice, and will probably progress into successful clinical trials when we find ways to target prodromal stages of the disease through biomarkers, or attempt prevention. It is through these approaches that we will one day be able to prevent the occurrence of the disease as we age. For example, immunotherapy was developed in APP transgenic mice and could not have been proven to clear pathology without them. Immunotherapy has progressed into numerous clinical trials and has been shown to reduce both Aβ and tau levels in patients (Boche et al. 2010), as shown in mouse models (Schenk et al. 1999; Oddo et al. 2004). The effects on cognition have been mixed—benefits have been seen in patients without the apoε4 allele, but not in those with apoε4—which accounts for ~60% of patients. As targeting the plaques does nothing to address the extensive neuronal loss that has occurred in these patients, hints of effects on cognition are extremely promising. We would predict, from this, that immunization as an AD preventative may be effective. Furthermore, encephalitis caused by immunotherapy in a small cohort of patients may not occur before abundant Aβ deposits are found throughout the brain.

Other potential therapeutics developed in AD transgenic mice may yet show clinical success, either as preventatives or as treatments.

Some promising approaches include the copper/zinc chelator PBT2 (Adlard et al. 2008), which has shown efficacy in phase II clinical trials (Faux et al. 2010), and *scyllo*-inositol (McLaurin et al. 2006), which breaks up Aβ oligomers. Many companies are now exploring potential cognitive enhancers in AD transgenics, such as α7 agonists (Marighetto et al. 2008), phosphodiesterase inhibitors (Puzzo et al. 2009; Verhoest et al. 2009), H3 antagonists (Medhurst et al. 2007), and other approaches. Perhaps targeting cognitive decline in the presence of pathology will be more successful than targeting the pathology alone, which has been the trend of the past decade, or using a combination approach.

CONCLUSIONS

What will the next generation of transgenic models of AD bring, and how can they be developed to help develop therapeutics and preventatives for sporadic AD? A new era will be ushered in as other types of animal models are produced. For example, there may be advantages to moving away from mice and rats and genetically modifying other smaller animal species, particularly those in which the endogenous Aβ sequence is identical to humans and those in which processing of tau is more closely aligned to humans. In addition, we need to find ways to model sporadic AD, rather than familial AD. This means that the animals will need to develop pathology because they age, rather than because their genes program them to do so. Once such an animal is produced we will be able to study which aspects of the aging process drive the pathology in the first place, and then target them for prevention. We have already proposed using alternative models of neuronal loss to supplement AD pathology models, and think that this is also a good approach. Making such models will be challenging and will require a great deal of investment, both time and financial, and not all approaches will work. However, we need to improve on the current batch of AD transgenics and look to future so that we will be able to treat and prevent this insidious disease.

REFERENCES

Adlard PA, Cherny RA, Finkelstein DI, Gautier E, Robb E, Cortes M, Volitakis I, Liu X, Smith JP, Perez K, et al. 2008. Rapid restoration of cognition in Alzheimer's transgenic mice with 8-hydroxy quinoline analogs is associated with decreased interstitial Aβ. *Neuron* **59**: 43–55.

Akiyama H, Barger S, Barnum S, Bradt B, Bauer J, Cole GM, Cooper NR, Eikelenboom P, Emmerling M, Fiebich BL, et al. 2000. Inflammation and Alzheimer's disease. *Neurobiol Aging* **21**: 383–421.

Beel AJ, Sanders CR. 2008. Substrate specificity of γ-secretase and other intramembrane proteases. *Cell Mol Life Sci* **65**: 1311–1334.

Billings LM, Oddo S, Green KN, McGaugh JL, LaFerla FM. 2005. Intraneuronal Aβ causes the onset of early Alzheimer's disease-related cognitive deficits in transgenic mice. *Neuron* **45**: 675–688.

Bloch L, Sineshchekova O, Reichenbach D, Reiss K, Saftig P, Kuro-o M, Kaether C. 2009. Klotho is a substrate for α-, β- and γ-secretase. *FEBS Lett* **583**: 3221–3224.

Blurton-Jones M, LaFerla FM. 2006. Pathways by which Aβ facilitates tau pathology. *Curr Alzheimer Res* **3**: 437–448.

Boche D, Denham N, Holmes C, Nicoll JA. 2010. Neuropathology after active Aβ42 immunotherapy: Implications for Alzheimer's disease pathogenesis. *Acta Neuropathol* **120**: 369–384.

Casas C, Sergeant N, Itier JM, Blanchard V, Wirths O, van der Kolk N, Vingtdeux V, van de Steeg E, Ret G, Canton T, et al. 2004. Massive CA1/2 neuronal loss with intraneuronal and N-terminal truncated Aβ42 accumulation in a novel Alzheimer transgenic model. *Am J Pathol* **165**: 1289–1300.

Chang WP, Koelsch G, Wong S, Downs D, Da H, Weerasena V, Gordon B, Devasamudram T, Bilcer G, Ghosh AK, et al. 2004. In vivo inhibition of Aβ production by memapsin 2 (β-secretase) inhibitors. *J Neurochem* **89**: 1409–1416.

DiCarlo G, Wilcock D, Henderson D, Gordon M, Morgan D. 2001. Intrahippocampal LPS injections reduce Aβ load in APP + PS1 transgenic mice. *Neurobiol Aging* **22**: 1007–1012.

Dominguez D, Tournoy J, Hartmann D, Huth T, Cryns K, Deforce S, Serneels L, Camacho IE, Marjaux E, Craessaerts K, et al. 2005. Phenotypic and biochemical analyses of BACE1- and BACE2-deficient mice. *J Biol Chem* **280**: 30797–30806.

Farah MH, Pan BH, Hoffman PN, Ferraris D, Tsukamoto T, Nguyen T, Wong PC, Price DL, Slusher BS, Griffin JW. 2011. Reduced BACE1 activity enhances clearance of myelin debris and regeneration of axons in the injured peripheral nervous system. *J Neurosci* **31**: 5744–5754.

Faux NG, Ritchie CW, Gunn A, Rembach A, Tsatsanis A, Bedo J, Harrison J, Lannfelt L, Blennow K, Zetterberg H, et al. 2010. PBT2 rapidly improves cognition in Alzheimer's disease: Additional phase II analyses. *J Alzheimers Dis* **20**: 509–516.

Findeis MA. 2007. The role of amyloid β peptide 42 in Alzheimer's disease. *Pharmacol Ther* **116**: 266–286.

Fukumoto H, Takahashi H, Tarui N, Matsui J, Tomita T, Hirode M, Sagayama M, Maeda R, Kawamoto M, Hirai K, et al. 2010. A noncompetitive BACE1 inhibitor TAK-070 ameliorates Aβ pathology and behavioral deficits in a mouse model of Alzheimer's disease. *J Neurosci* **30:** 11157–11166.

Gotz J, Deters N, Doldissen A, Bokhari L, Ke Y, Wiesner A, Schonrock N, Ittner LM. 2007. A decade of tau transgenic animal models and beyond. *Brain Pathol* **17:** 91–103.

Green KN, LaFerla FM. 2008. Linking calcium to Aβ and Alzheimer's disease. *Neuron* **59:** 190–194.

Gyure KA, Durham R, Stewart WF, Smialek JE, Troncoso JC. 2001. Intraneuronal aβ-amyloid precedes development of amyloid plaques in Down syndrome. *Arch Pathol Lab Med* **125:** 489–492.

Haass C, Selkoe DJ. 2007. Soluble protein oligomers in neurodegeneration: Lessons from the Alzheimer's amyloid β-peptide. *Nat Rev Mol Cell Biol* **8:** 101–112.

Hartmann D, de Strooper B, Serneels L, Craessaerts K, Herreman A, Annaert W, Umans L, Lubke T, Lena Illert A, von Figura K, et al. 2002. The disintegrin/metalloprotease ADAM 10 is essential for Notch signalling but not for α-secretase activity in fibroblasts. *Human Mol Genet* **11:** 2615–2624.

Herreman A, Hartmann D, Annaert W, Saftig P, Craessaerts K, Serneels L, Umans L, Schrijvers V, Checler F, Vanderstichele H, et al. 1999. Presenilin 2 deficiency causes a mild pulmonary phenotype and no changes in amyloid precursor protein processing but enhances the embryonic lethal phenotype of presenilin 1 deficiency. *Proc Natl Acad Sci* **96:** 11872–11877.

Hoover BR, Reed MN, Su J, Penrod RD, Kotilinek LA, Grant MK, Pitstick R, Carlson GA, Lanier LM, Yuan LL, et al. 2010. Tau mislocalization to dendritic spines mediates synaptic dysfunction independently of neurodegeneration. *Neuron* **68:** 1067–1081.

Hu X, Hicks CW, He W, Wong P, Macklin WB, Trapp BD, Yan R. 2006. Bace1 modulates myelination in the central and peripheral nervous system. *Nat Neurosci* **9:** 1520–1525.

Hu X, He W, Diaconu C, Tang X, Kidd GJ, Macklin WB, Trapp BD, Yan R. 2008. Genetic deletion of BACE1 in mice affects remyelination of sciatic nerves. *FASEB J* **22:** 2970–2980.

Huang WH, Sheng R, Hu YZ. 2009. Progress in the development of nonpeptidomimetic BACE 1 inhibitors for Alzheimer's disease. *Curr Med Chem* **16:** 1806–1820.

Hussain I, Powell D, Howlett DR, Tew DG, Meek TD, Chapman C, Gloger IS, Murphy KE, Southan CD, Ryan DM, et al. 1999. Identification of a novel aspartic protease (Asp 2) as β-secretase. *Mol Cell Neurosci* **14:** 419–427.

Hussain I, Hawkins J, Harrison D, Hille C, Wayne G, Cutler L, Buck T, Walter D, Demont E, Howes C, et al. 2007. Oral administration of a potent and selective non-peptidic BACE-1 inhibitor decreases β-cleavage of amyloid precursor protein and amyloid-β production in vivo. *J Neurochem* **100:** 802–809.

Ittner LM, Ke YD, Delerue F, Bi M, Gladbach A, van Eersel J, Wolfing H, Chieng BC, Christie MJ, Napier IA, et al. 2010. Dendritic function of tau mediates amyloid-β toxicity in Alzheimer's disease mouse models. *Cell* **142:** 387–397.

Keller JN, Hanni KB, Markesbery WR. 2000. Impaired proteasome function in Alzheimer's disease. *J Neurochem* **75:** 436–439.

Kim DY, Gersbacher MT, Inquimbert P, Kovacs DM. 2011. Reduced sodium channel Na$_v$1.1 levels in BACE1-null mice. *J Biol Chem* **286:** 8106–8116.

Kitazawa M, Oddo S, Yamasaki TR, Green KN, LaFerla FM. 2005. Lipopolysaccharide-induced inflammation exacerbates tau pathology by a cyclin-dependent kinase 5-mediated pathway in a transgenic model of Alzheimer's disease. *J Neurosci* **25:** 8843–8853.

Kokubo H, Kayed R, Glabe CG, Yamaguchi H. 2005. Soluble Aβ oligomers ultrastructurally localize to cell processes and might be related to synaptic dysfunction in Alzheimer's disease brain. *Brain Res* **1031:** 222–228.

Kuo YM, Emmerling MR, Vigo-Pelfrey C, Kasunic TC, Kirkpatrick JB, Murdoch GH, Ball MJ, Roher AE. 1996. Water-soluble Aβ (N-40, N-42) oligomers in normal and Alzheimer disease brains. *J Biol Chem* **271:** 4077–4081.

LaFerla FM, Green KN, Oddo S. 2007. Intracellular amyloid-β in Alzheimer's disease. *Nat Rev Neurosci* **8:** 499–509.

Laird FM, Cai H, Savonenko AV, Farah MH, He K, Melnikova T, Wen H, Chiang HC, Xu G, Koliatsos VE, et al. 2005. BACE1, a major determinant of selective vulnerability of the brain to amyloid-β amyloidogenesis, is essential for cognitive, emotional, and synaptic functions. *J Neurosci* **25:** 11693–11709.

Lee DC, Sunnarborg SW, Hinkle CL, Myers TJ, Stevenson MY, Russell WE, Castner BJ, Gerhart MJ, Paxton RJ, Black RA, et al. 2003. TACE/ADAM17 processing of EGFR ligands indicates a role as a physiological convertase. *Ann NY Acad Sci* **995:** 22–38.

Lee JH, Yu WH, Kumar A, Lee S, Mohan PS, Peterhoff CM, Wolfe DM, Martinez-Vicente M, Massey AC, Sovak G, et al. 2010. Lysosomal proteolysis and autophagy require presenilin 1 and are disrupted by Alzheimer-related PS1 mutations. *Cell* **141:** 1146–1158.

Lerchner A, Machauer R, Betschart C, Veenstra S, Rueeger H, McCarthy C, Tintelnot-Blomley M, Jaton AL, Rabe S, Desrayaud S, et al. 2010. Macrocyclic BACE-1 inhibitors acutely reduce Aβ in brain after po application. *Bioorg Med Chem Lett* **20:** 603–607.

Lewis J, Dickson DW, Lin WL, Chisholm L, Corral A, Jones G, Yen SH, Sahara N, Skipper L, Yager D, et al. 2001. Enhanced neurofibrillary degeneration in transgenic mice expressing mutant tau and APP. *Science* **293:** 1487–1491.

Luo Y, Bolon B, Kahn S, Bennett BD, Babu-Khan S, Denis P, Fan W, Kha H, Zhang J, Gong Y, et al. 2001. Mice deficient in BACE1, the Alzheimer's β-secretase, have normal phenotype and abolished β-amyloid generation. *Nature Neurosci* **4:** 231–232.

Marighetto A, Valerio S, Desmedt A, Philippin JN, Trocme-Thibierge C, Morain P. 2008. Comparative effects of the α7 nicotinic partial agonist, S 24795, and the cholinesterase inhibitor, donepezil, against aging-related deficits in declarative and working memory in mice. *Psychopharmacol (Berl)* **197:** 499–508.

McGowan E, Pickford F, Kim J, Onstead L, Eriksen J, Yu C, Skipper L, Murphy MP, Beard J, Das P, et al. 2005. Aβ42 is essential for parenchymal and vascular amyloid deposition in mice. *Neuron* **47:** 191–199.

McLaurin J, Kierstead ME, Brown ME, Hawkes CA, Lambermon MH, Phinney AL, Darabie AA, Cousins JE, French

JE, Lan MF, et al. 2006. Cyclohexanehexol inhibitors of Aβ aggregation prevent and reverse Alzheimer phenotype in a mouse model. *Nature Med* **12:** 801–808.

Medhurst AD, Atkins AR, Beresford IJ, Brackenborough K, Briggs MA, Calver AR, Cilia J, Cluderay JE, Crook B, Davis JB, et al. 2007. GSK189254, a novel H3 receptor antagonist that binds to histamine H3 receptors in Alzheimer's disease brain and improves cognitive performance in preclinical models. *J Pharmacol Exp Ther* **321:** 1032–1045.

Mehlhorn G, Hollborn M, Schliebs R. 2000. Induction of cytokines in glial cells surrounding cortical β-amyloid plaques in transgenic Tg2576 mice with Alzheimer pathology. *Int J Dev Neurosci* **18:** 423–431.

Meyer-Luehmann M, Stalder M, Herzig MC, Kaeser SA, Kohler E, Pfeifer M, Boncristiano S, Mathews PM, Mercken M, Abramowski D, et al. 2003. Extracellular amyloid formation and associated pathology in neural grafts. *Nat Neurosci* **6:** 370–377.

Meyer-Luehmann M, Coomaraswamy J, Bolmont T, Kaeser S, Schaefer C, Kilger E, Neuenschwander A, Abramowski D, Frey P, Jaton AL, et al. 2006. Exogenous induction of cerebral β-amyloidogenesis is governed by agent and host. *Science* **313:** 1781–1784.

Meyer-Luehmann M, Spires-Jones TL, Prada C, Garcia-Alloza M, de Calignon A, Rozkalne A, Koenigsknecht-Talboo J, Holtzman DM, Bacskai BJ, Hyman BT. 2008. Rapid appearance and local toxicity of amyloid-β plaques in a mouse model of Alzheimer's disease. *Nature* **451:** 720–724.

Morgan D. 2006. Immunotherapy for Alzheimer's disease. *J Alzheimers Dis* **9:** 425–432.

Mori C, Spooner ET, Wisniewsk KE, Wisniewski TM, Yamaguch H, Saido TC, Tolan DR, Selkoe DJ, Lemere CA. 2002. Intraneuronal Aβ42 accumulation in Down syndrome brain. *Amyloid* **9:** 88–102.

Nagy Z, Esiri MM, Jobst KA, Morris JH, King EM, McDonald B, Litchfield S, Smith A, Barnetson L, Smith AD. 1995. Relative roles of plaques and tangles in the dementia of Alzheimer's disease: Correlations using three sets of neuropathological criteria. *Dementia* **6:** 21–31.

Naslund J, Haroutunian V, Mohs R, Davis KL, Davies P, Greengard P, Buxbaum JD. 2000. Correlation between elevated levels of amyloid β-peptide in the brain and cognitive decline. *JAMA* **283:** 1571–1577.

Neely KM, Green KN, LaFerla FM. 2011. Presenilin is necessary for efficient proteolysis through the autophagy-lysosome system in a γ-secretase-independent manner. *J Neurosci* **31:** 2781–2791.

Oddo S. 2008. The ubiquitin–proteasome system in Alzheimer's disease. *J Cell Mol Med* **12:** 363–373.

Oddo S, Caccamo A, Kitazawa M, Tseng BP, LaFerla FM. 2003a. Amyloid deposition precedes tangle formation in a triple transgenic model of Alzheimer's disease. *Neurobiol Aging* **24:** 1063–1070.

Oddo S, Caccamo A, Shepherd JD, Murphy MP, Golde TE, Kayed R, Metherate R, Mattson MP, Akbari Y, LaFerla FM. 2003b. Triple-transgenic model of Alzheimer's disease with plaques and tangles: Intracellular Aβ and synaptic dysfunction. *Neuron* **39:** 409–421.

Oddo S, Billings L, Kesslak JP, Cribbs DH, LaFerla FM. 2004. Aβ immunotherapy leads to clearance of early, but not late, hyperphosphorylated tau aggregates via the proteasome. *Neuron* **43:** 321–332.

Ohno M, Sametsky EA, Younkin LH, Oakley H, Younkin SG, Citron M, Vassar R, Disterhoft JF. 2004. BACE1 deficiency rescues memory deficits and cholinergic dysfunction in a mouse model of Alzheimer's disease. *Neuron* **41:** 27–33.

Palop JJ, Chin J, Roberson ED, Wang J, Thwin MT, Bien-Ly N, Yoo J, Ho KO, Yu GQ, Kreitzer A, et al. 2007. Aberrant excitatory neuronal activity and compensatory remodeling of inhibitory hippocampal circuits in mouse models of Alzheimer's disease. *Neuron* **55:** 697–711.

Puzzo D, Staniszewski A, Deng SX, Privitera L, Leznik E, Liu S, Zhang H, Feng Y, Palmeri A, Landry DW, et al. 2009. Phosphodiesterase 5 inhibition improves synaptic function, memory, and amyloid-β load in an Alzheimer's disease mouse model. *J Neurosci* **29:** 8075–8086.

Roberds SL, Anderson J, Basi G, Bienkowski MJ, Branstetter DG, Chen KS, Freedman SB, Frigon NL, Games D, Hu K, et al. 2001. BACE knockout mice are healthy despite lacking the primary β-secretase activity in brain: Implications for Alzheimer's disease therapeutics. *Human Mol Genet* **10:** 1317–1324.

Roberson ED, Scearce-Levie K, Palop JJ, Yan F, Cheng IH, Wu T, Gerstein H, Yu GQ, Mucke L. 2007. Reducing endogenous tau ameliorates amyloid β-induced deficits in an Alzheimer's disease mouse model. *Science* **316:** 750–754.

Sankaranarayanan S, Holahan MA, Colussi D, Crouthamel MC, Devanarayan V, Ellis J, Espeseth A, Gates AT, Graham SL, Gregro AR, et al. 2009. First demonstration of cerebrospinal fluid and plasma A β lowering with oral administration of a β-site amyloid precursor protein-cleaving enzyme 1 inhibitor in nonhuman primates. *J Pharmacol Exp Ther* **328:** 131–140.

Savonenko AV, Melnikova T, Laird FM, Stewart KA, Price DL, Wong PC. 2008. Alteration of BACE1-dependent NRG1/ErbB4 signaling and schizophrenia-like phenotypes in BACE1-null mice. *Proc Natl Acad Sci* **105:** 5585–5590.

Schenk D, Barbour R, Dunn W, Gordon G, Grajeda H, Guido T, Hu K, Huang J, Johnson-Wood K, Khan K, et al. 1999. Immunization with amyloid-β attenuates Alzheimer-disease-like pathology in the PDAPP mouse. *Nature* **400:** 173–177.

Schor NF. 2011. What the halted phase III γ-secretase inhibitor trial may (or may not) be telling us. *Ann Neurol* **69:** 237–239.

Shen J, Bronson RT, Chen DF, Xia W, Selkoe DJ, Tonegawa S. 1997. Skeletal and CNS defects in Presenilin-1-deficient mice. *Cell* **89:** 629–639.

Shipton OA, Leitz JR, Dworzak J, Acton CE, Tunbridge EM, Denk F, Dawson HN, Vitek MP, Wade-Martins R, Paulsen O, et al. 2011. Tau protein is required for amyloid β-induced impairment of hippocampal long-term potentiation. *J Neurosci* **31:** 1688–1692.

Sinha S, Anderson JP, Barbour R, Basi GS, Caccavello R, Davis D, Doan M, Dovey HF, Frigon N, Hong J, et al. 1999. Purification and cloning of amyloid precursor protein β-secretase from human brain. *Nature* **402:** 537–540.

Steele M, Stuchbury G, Munch G. 2007. The molecular basis of the prevention of Alzheimer's disease through healthy nutrition. *Exp Gerontol* **42:** 28–36.

Takei Y, Teng J, Harada A, Hirokawa N. 2000. Defects in axonal elongation and neuronal migration in mice with disrupted tau and map1b genes. *J Cell Biol* **150:** 989–1000.

Terry RD, Masliah E, Salmon DP, Butters N, DeTeresa R, Hill R, Hansen LA, Katzman R. 1991. Physical basis of cognitive alterations in Alzheimer's disease: Synapse loss is the major correlate of cognitive impairment. *Ann Neurol* **30:** 572–580.

Tomic JL, Pensalfini A, Head E, Glabe CG. 2009. Soluble fibrillar oligomer levels are elevated in Alzheimer's disease brain and correlate with cognitive dysfunction. *Neurobiol Dis* **35:** 352–358.

Vassar R, Bennett BD, Babu-Khan S, Kahn S, Mendiaz EA, Denis P, Teplow DB, Ross S, Amarante P, Loeloff R, et al. 1999. β-Secretase cleavage of Alzheimer's amyloid precursor protein by the transmembrane aspartic protease BACE. *Science* **286:** 735–741.

Verhoest PR, Proulx-Lafrance C, Corman M, Chenard L, Helal CJ, Hou X, Kleiman R, Liu S, Marr E, Menniti FS, et al. 2009. Identification of a brain penetrant PDE9A inhibitor utilizing prospective design and chemical enablement as a rapid lead optimization strategy. *J Med Chem* **52:** 7946–7949.

Walsh DM, Selkoe DJ. 2007. A β oligomers—A decade of discovery. *J Neurochem* **101:** 1172–1184.

Wang J, Dickson DW, Trojanowski JQ, Lee VM. 1999. The levels of soluble versus insoluble brain Aβ distinguish Alzheimer's disease from normal and pathologic aging. *Exp Neurol* **158:** 328–337.

Webster SD, Tenner AJ, Poulos TL, Cribbs DH. 1999. The mouse C1q A-chain sequence alters β-amyloid-induced complement activation. *Neurobiol Aging* **20:** 297–304.

Wilcock DM, Lewis MR, Van Nostrand WE, Davis J, Previti ML, Gharkholonarehe N, Vitek MP, Colton CA. 2008. Progression of amyloid pathology to Alzheimer's disease pathology in an amyloid precursor protein transgenic mouse model by removal of nitric oxide synthase 2. *J Neurosci* **28:** 1537–1545.

Willem M, Garratt AN, Novak B, Citron M, Kaufmann S, Rittger A, DeStrooper B, Saftig P, Birchmeier C, Haass C. 2006. Control of peripheral nerve myelination by the β-secretase BACE1. *Science* **314:** 664–666.

Woltjer RL, Sonnen JA, Sokal I, Rung LG, Yang W, Kjerulf JD, Klingert D, Johnson C, Rhew I, Tsuang D, et al. 2009. Quantitation and mapping of cerebral detergent-insoluble proteins in the elderly. *Brain Pathol* **19:** 365–374.

Wong HK, Sakurai T, Oyama F, Kaneko K, Wada K, Miyazaki H, Kurosawa M, De Strooper B, Saftig P, Nukina N. 2005. β Subunits of voltage-gated sodium channels are novel substrates of β-site amyloid precursor protein-cleaving enzyme (BACE1) and γ-secretase. *J Biol Chem* **280:** 23009–23017.

Wyss-Coray T, Mucke L. 2002. Inflammation in neurodegenerative disease—A double-edged sword. *Neuron* **35:** 419–432.

Yamasaki TR, Blurton Jones M, Morrissette DA, Kitazawa M, Oddo S, LaFerla FM. 2007. Neural stem cells improve memory in an inducible mouse model of neuronal loss. *J Neurosci* **27:** 11925–11933.

Yang F, Ueda K, Chen P, Ashe KH, Cole GM. 2000. Plaque-associated α-synuclein (NACP) pathology in aged transgenic mice expressing amyloid precursor protein. *Brain Res* **853:** 381–383.

Zhang YW, Wang R, Liu Q, Zhang H, Liao FF, Xu H. 2007. Presenilin/γ-secretase-dependent processing of β-amyloid precursor protein regulates EGF receptor expression. *Proc Natl Acad Sci* **104:** 10613–10618.

Zheng H, Jiang M, Trumbauer ME, Hopkins R, Sirinathsinghji DJ, Stevens KA, Conner MW, Slunt HH, Sisodia SS, Chen HY, et al. 1996. Mice deficient for the amyloid precursor protein gene. *Ann NY Acad Sci* **777:** 421–426.

Neurotoxicity of Amyloid β-Protein: Synaptic and Network Dysfunction

Lennart Mucke[1] and Dennis J. Selkoe[2]

[1]Gladstone Institute of Neurological Disease and University of California, San Francisco, San Francisco, California 94102

[2]Center for Neurologic Diseases, Harvard Medical School and Brigham and Women's Hospital, Boston, Massachusetts 02115

Correspondence: lmucke@gladstone.ucsf.edu, dselkoe@rics.bwh.harvard.edu

Evidence for an ever-expanding variety of molecular mediators of amyloid β-protein neurotoxicity (membrane lipids, receptor proteins, channel proteins, second messengers and related signaling cascades, cytoskeletal proteins, inflammatory mediators, etc.) has led to the notion that the binding of hydrophobic Aβ assemblies to cellular membranes triggers multiple effects affecting diverse pathways. It appears unlikely that there are only one or two cognate receptors for neurotoxic forms of Aβ and also that there are just one or two assembly forms of the peptide that induce neuronal dysfunction. Rather, various soluble (diffusible) oligomers of Aβ that may be in dynamic equilibrium with insoluble, fibrillar deposits (amyloid plaques) and that can bind to different components of neuronal and non-neuronal plasma membranes appear to induce complex patterns of synaptic dysfunction and network disorganization that underlie the intermittent but gradually progressive cognitive manifestations of the clinical disorder. Modern analyses of this problem utilize electrophysiology coupled with synaptic biochemistry and behavioral phenotyping of animal models to elucidate the affected circuits and assess the effects of potential therapeutic interventions.

A quarter of a century of research on amyloid β-protein (Aβ) has produced a wealth of evidence that its accumulation in brain regions serving memory and cognition contributes strongly to the development of Alzheimer disease (AD). Support has come from neuropathological, genetic, biochemical, animal modeling, biomarker and, recently, therapeutic studies. There is now little doubt that the accumulation of certain forms of Aβ is associated with, and probably induces, profound neuronal changes in the brain. Cells other than neurons, including microglia, astrocytes, and the endothelial and smooth muscle cells of cerebral blood vessels, can also be altered functionally and structurally by excessive Aβ levels. However, it is generally assumed that adverse effects of Aβ specifically on neurons and their processes help initiate the cardinal memory and cognitive deficits that define AD. The precise biochemical mechanisms by which various assembly forms of the peptide cause neuronal dysfunction and ultimately death remain to be defined.

Our focus in this chapter is the neuron and, in particular, the synapse. We emphasize that numerous synaptic and nonsynaptic neuronal changes, as well as effects on cells other than neurons, are likely to occur virtually simultaneously as the disease develops and progresses. Accordingly, it is simplistic to think about the actions of Aβ on neurons—both individually and in networks—in the absence of the non-neuronal events (e.g., microgliosis, astrocytosis, microvascular injury) that could contribute to altered neuronal integrity and function secondarily. Nevertheless, we will dissect this remarkably complex scenario in a reductionist fashion, focusing first and foremost on synaptic/neuronal changes induced by Aβ; these changes must ultimately be integrated with the effects on other cell types described in other articles in this collection.

MONOMERS, OLIGOMERS, AND FIBRILS: CHANGING IDEAS ABOUT WHICH FORMS OF Aβ IMPAIR NEURONAL FUNCTION AND HOW THEY DO SO

Early versions of the amyloid cascade hypothesis of AD posited adverse effects of amyloid plaques on surrounding dendrites, axons and glia, based in part on the light microscopic appearance of neuritic plaques (Selkoe 1991; Hardy and Higgins 1992). However, the recognition of buffer-soluble bioactive oligomers (e.g., dimers, trimers, tetramers, dodecamers, higher oligomers) in synthetic Aβ peptide preparations (Lambert et al. 1998; Bitan et al. 2001; Kayed et al. 2003), in cell culture media (Podlisny et al. 1995; Walsh et al. 2002), in amyloid precursor protein (APP) transgenic mouse brains (Kawarabayashi et al. 2001; Lesne et al. 2006; Shankar et al. 2009), and in AD brain tissue (Roher et al. 1996; McLean et al. 1999; Gong et al. 2003; Shankar et al. 2008) gave rise to the concept that the insoluble amyloid fibrils comprising the plaques might themselves be relatively inactive but serve as reservoirs of these smaller, potentially neurotoxic assemblies. Similarly, protofibrils of synthetic Aβ that were

thinner than classical 8 nm amyloid fibrils could be generated from synthetic Aβ peptide under certain in vitro conditions and also induce neurotoxic effects (Harper et al. 1997; Walsh et al. 1997; Hartley et al. 1999). These biochemical findings, coupled with analogous experimental observations for other pathogenic neuronal proteins (e.g., huntingtin and α-synuclein), have increasingly led the field to consider small, readily diffusible assemblies as principal cytotoxic forms of misfolded, self-aggregating proteins. The concept is consistent with—and emerged in part from—the demonstration that APP transgenic mice show electrophysiological, neuroanatomical and behavioral abnormalities well before the appearance of microscopically visible Aβ deposits (Holcomb et al. 1999; Hsia et al. 1999; Mucke et al. 2000).

This modification of the so-called "amyloid hypothesis" based on new findings does not rule out a neurotoxic role for amyloid plaques themselves. Indeed, there is abundant evidence of neuritic alteration in the immediate vicinity of AD plaques, such as local distortion and curvature of normally rather straight cortical dendrites around plaques, raising the possibility of decreased efficiency of neurotransmission along them (Hyman et al. 1995). Moreover, in APP transgenic mice, array tomography has revealed a striking penumbra of excitatory synapse loss and neuritic dystrophy that is greatest immediately adjacent to a plaque and lessens in a radial fashion, becoming virtually normal approximately 30–50 µm away from the plaque core edge (Spires-Jones et al. 2007; Koffie et al. 2009). Somewhat analogous findings have been described in sections of AD cortex (Serrano-Pozo et al. 2010). In mice, this penumbra is reactive with antibodies (e.g., Nab61) that are relatively specific for Aβ oligomers, at least in immunochemical assays. Although it is possible that such antibodies do not retain their oligomer specificity in the complex epitope environment of brain sections, such morphological analyses suggest that plaques confer synaptic and neuritic effects in part by acting as local reservoirs of diffusible oligomers. Independent experiments in which soluble oligomers and insoluble amyloid plaque cores were biochemically isolated from the same AD cortices and assayed electrophysiologically on wild-type mouse brain slices showed that soluble oligomers potently blocked LTP, whereas washed amyloid cores did not, unless they were first dissolved in harsh solvents (e.g., formic acid) to release their constituent oligomers (Shankar et al. 2008). In this context, it has been found that lipids can convert inert Aβ amyloid fibrils into neurotoxic protofibrils that can then alter learning in mice (Martins et al. 2008). Taken together, these and other experimental approaches suggest that plaques may confer local neurotoxicity because they are in equilibrium with surrounding oligomers and protofibrils. In principle, it makes biophysical sense that small oligomers would be more synaptotoxic than plaques, as the former collectively provide a much greater surface area for interaction with neurons (and glia) and their processes than do the large, nondiffusible plaques.

EARLY VERSUS LATE: REFOCUSING THE INVESTIGATIVE EMPHASIS FROM FRANK NEURODEGENERATION ONTO EARLIER SYNAPTIC PERTURBATIONS CAUSED BY Aβ

Most mouse lines transgenic for human (h) APP do not show overt neuronal loss, and this aspect of their phenotype is often criticized as a weakness of these models. However, it is unknown whether the loss of neurons in AD brains is directly caused by Aβ accumulation and, even if it is, whether it takes Aβ less than 2–3 years (the typical lifetime of a mouse) to kill neurons in the human brain. The notion that hAPP transgenic mice do not undergo neurodegeneration is a misunderstanding, in that they do develop substantial neuritic dystrophy and synapse loss, which are clear signs of a neuronal degenerative process, even if counts of cell bodies are not significantly decreased. Thus, hAPP mice are good models of Aβ-induced synaptic dysfunction. For the following reasons, this feature alone makes them directly relevant to the human condition.

Some two decades ago, quantitative neuropathological analyses revealed strong associations between the degrees of cognitive impairment and

synaptic alteration in AD subjects (DeKosky and Scheff 1990; Terry et al. 1991). Subsequent studies in hAPP transgenic mice and other experimental systems demonstrated that Aβ oligomers modulate both pre- and postsynaptic structures and functions in a dose- and assembly-dependent manner (for reviews, see Selkoe 2002; Palop and Mucke 2010). In hAPP mice, manipulations that prevent or reverse synaptic deficits also prevent or reverse cognitive impairment (e.g., McLaurin et al. 2006; Cisse et al. 2011a; Roberson et al. 2011), supporting the hypothesis that Aβ causes cognitive deficits in part by interfering with synaptic functions. Because these hAPP mice have little overt neuronal loss and develop their synaptic and cognitive impairments before forming amyloid plaques, it is likely that their synaptic deficits are caused by soluble Aβ assemblies rather than by plaques per se, and that these deficits reflect primary synaptotoxicity rather than secondary consequences of neuronal degeneration. Consistent with this notion, synthetic Aβ oligomers and soluble Aβ oligomers isolated from cell culture media or AD brain extracts acutely impair synaptic functions when added to hippocampal slices or slice cultures (e.g., Gong et al. 2003; Shankar et al. 2007, 2008; Li et al. 2009). Collectively, these and many other studies in the last few years have refocused the experimental approach to Aβ neurotoxicity from frank cell death to more subtle structural and functional deficits of synapses and neurites.

MODULATION OF SYNAPTIC TRANSMISSION BY Aβ: A NEGATIVE REGULATOR OF NEURONAL ACTIVITY POSTSYNAPTICALLY, BUT A POTENTIAL POSITIVE REGULATOR PRESYNAPTICALLY

In vivo and in vitro studies have demonstrated that high levels of Aβ, particularly in oligomeric forms, alter glutamatergic synaptic transmission and cause synapse loss (Hsia et al. 1999; Mucke et al. 2000; Walsh et al. 2002; Kamenetz et al. 2003; Shankar et al. 2007; Li et al. 2009). On the other hand, the production of Aβ and its secretion into the extracellular space are regulated in part by neuronal activity in vitro (Kamenetz et al. 2003) and in vivo (Cirrito et al. 2005). Increased neuronal activity enhances Aβ generation and blocking neuronal activity has the opposite effect (Kamenetz et al. 2003). This synaptic regulation of Aβ production is mediated, at least in part, by clathrin-dependent endocytosis of surface APP at presynaptic terminals, endosomal proteolytic cleavage of APP, and Aβ release at synaptic terminals (Cirrito et al. 2005). In addition, pathogenic Aβ species can also be released from dendrites (Wei et al. 2010). This neuronal activity-dependent regulation of Aβ secretion has been observed during pathological events, such as epileptiform activity induced by electrical stimulation (Cirrito et al. 2005), as well as during normal physiological processes, such as the sleep−wake cycle (Kang et al. 2009). Such experimental findings support the concept that APP, and its Aβ fragment in particular, are part of a feedback loop controlling neuronal excitability (Kamenetz et al. 2003). In this paradigm, Aβ production is enhanced by action potential-dependent synaptic activity, leading to increased levels of extracellular Aβ at and near synapses and reduction of excitatory transmission postsynaptically (Fig. 1). Pathologically elevated levels of Aβ would be expected to put this negative feedback regulator into overdrive, suppressing excitatory synaptic activity at the postsynaptic level. However, a caveat about some of the experimental observations just cited that underlie this model is that the investigators could not always be sure what assembly state the Aβ being detected was in, that is, soluble monomers and/or soluble oligomers. Because these assemblies are likely to exist in a dynamic equilibrium, it can be difficult to assign the neurophysiological effects of Aβ to a particular assembly form, depending on exactly how an experiment was conducted.

Some work suggests that Aβ could also act as a positive regulator at the presynaptic level. For example, relatively small increases in endogenous Aβ levels ($\sim$1.5$\times$), induced by inhibition of extracellular Aβ degradation in otherwise unmanipulated wild-type neurons, enhanced the release probability of synaptic vesicles and increased neuronal activity in neuronal culture (Abramov et al. 2009). In this

study, enhanced extracellular Aβ increased spontaneous excitatory postsynaptic currents without significantly altering inhibitory currents. Importantly, all these effects were exclusively presynaptic and dependent on firing rates, with lower facilitation seen in neurons with higher firing rates. Thus, small increases of Aβ may facilitate presynaptic glutamatergic release in neurons with low activity but not in neurons with high activity. Generally consistent with the above findings, another study reported that application of low concentrations of synthetic Aβ42 (picomolar range) markedly potentiated synaptic transmission, whereas higher concentrations of Aβ42 (low nanomolar range) caused the expected synaptic depression (Puzzo et al. 2008). In this study, the potentiating effect of Aβ did not affect postsynaptic N-methyl D-aspartate receptor (NMDAR) and α-amino-3-hydroxy-5-methyl-4-isoxazolepropionic acid receptor (AMPAR) currents but was dependent on α7-nAChR activation, suggesting a presynaptic mechanism mediated by build-up of Ca^{2+} in presynaptic terminals. Thus, Aβ may directly act on presynaptic α7-nAChR (Dineley et al. 2002) and be part of a positive feedback loop that increases presynaptic Ca^{2+} levels and Aβ secretion. Consistent with this model, blocking nAChRs or removing α7-nAChRs decreased Aβ secretion and blocked Aβ-induced facilitation (Wei et al. 2010).

It should be pointed out that the interpretation of physiological experiments examining synthetic Aβ42 is difficult, because its two extra hydrophobic residues (alanine and isoleucine) give it a remarkable propensity to aggregate, even at low concentrations. Oligomers of Aβ42 should have different biological properties than monomers of Aβ42 given their different structures. Consequently, in vitro studies of the normal function of Aβ should instead focus on the Aβ40 peptide, as this is by far (tenfold) the most abundant Aβ monomer under physiological conditions in young mammals. Studies that attribute normal biological functions to low levels of Aβ42 must confirm these findings using Aβ40.

Another emerging lesson is that Aβ-induced presynaptic effects depend on an optimal

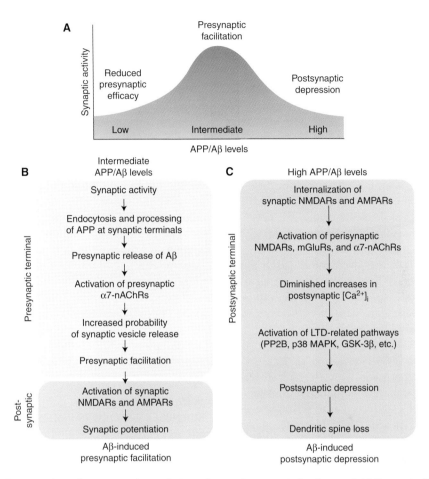

Figure 1. Presynaptic and postsynaptic regulation of synaptic transmission by amyloid β-protein (Aβ). (*A*) Hypothetical relationship between Aβ level and synaptic activity. Intermediate levels of Aβ enhance synaptic activity presynaptically, whereas abnormally high or low levels of Aβ impair synaptic activity by inducing postsynaptic depression or reducing presynaptic efficacy, respectively. (*B*) Within a physiological range, small increases in Aβ primarily facilitate presynaptic functions, resulting in synaptic potentiation. (*C*) At abnormally high levels, Aβ enhances long-term depression (LTD)-related mechanisms, resulting in postsynaptic depression and loss of dendritic spines (modified from Palop and Mucke 2010).

Aβ concentration (Fig. 1), with higher or lower concentrations potentially impairing synaptic transmission (Abramov et al. 2009). A positive modulatory effect of Aβ on synaptic transmission is further supported indirectly by the finding that abnormally low levels of Aβ in mice deficient for APP (Seabrook et al. 1999), PS1 (Saura et al. 2004), or BACE1 (Laird et al. 2005) are associated with synaptic transmission deficits. Overall, these and other data suggest an apparent bell-shaped relationship between extracellular Aβ and synaptic transmission in

which intermediate levels of Aβ potentiate presynaptic terminals, low levels reduce presynaptic efficacy, and high levels depress postsynaptic transmission.

Elevated Levels of Aβ Impair Synaptic Transmission by Enhancing Synaptic Depression

Excitatory synaptic transmission is tightly regulated by the number of active NMDARs and AMPARs at the synapse. NMDAR activation plays a central role, because it can induce either long-term potentiation (LTP) or long-term depression (LTD), depending on the extent of the resultant $[Ca^{2+}]_i$ rise in the dendritic spines and the downstream activation of specific intracellular cascades (Kullmann and Lamsa 2007). Activation of synaptic NMDARs and large increases in $[Ca^{2+}]_i$ are required for LTP, whereas internalization of synaptic NMDARs, activation of perisynaptic NMDARs, and lower increases in $[Ca^{2+}]_i$ are necessary for LTD. LTP induction promotes recruitment of AMPARs and growth of dendritic spines, whereas LTD induces spine shrinkage and synaptic loss (Kullmann and Lamsa 2007).

Pathological Aβ levels and assembly forms (e.g., oligomers) may indirectly cause a partial block of NMDARs and shift the activation of NMDAR-dependent signaling cascades toward pathways involved in the induction of LTD and synaptic loss (Fig. 1; Kamenetz et al. 2003; Hsieh et al. 2006; Shankar et al. 2007). This model is consistent with the fact that Aβ oligomers (but not monomers) impair LTP (Walsh et al. 2002; Shankar et al. 2008; Li et al. 2011) and enhance LTD (Fig. 1; Kim et al. 2001; Hsieh et al. 2006; Li et al. 2009). Although the mechanisms underlying Aβ-facilitated LTD have not yet been fully elucidated, they may involve receptor internalization (Snyder et al. 2005; Hsieh et al. 2006) or desensitization (Liu et al. 2004) and subsequent collapse of dendritic spines (Snyder et al. 2005; Hsieh et al. 2006). Aβ-dependent effects on synaptic function may be mediated by postsynaptic activation of α7-nAChR (Snyder et al. 2005), activation of extrasynaptic NMDA receptors (Shankar et al. 2007; Li et al. 2009), and downstream effects on calcineurin/STEP/cofilin, p38 MAPK, and GSK-3β signaling pathways, among others (Wang et al. 2004; Shankar et al. 2007; Li et al. 2009; Tackenberg and Brandt 2009).

Another way in which soluble Aβ oligomers may enhance LTD is by blocking neuronal glutamate uptake at synapses, leading to increased glutamate levels at the synaptic cleft (Fig. 2; Li et al. 2009). A resultant rise in glutamate levels would initially activate synaptic NMDARs followed by desensitization of the receptors and, ultimately, synaptic depression. Another effect of increased glutamate levels would be a spillover and activation of extra- or perisynaptic NR2B-enriched NMDARs, which play a major role in LTD induction (Liu et al. 2004) and have also been shown to help mediate the inhibition of LTP by soluble Aβ oligomers (Li et al. 2011). The activation of perisynaptic receptors may thus be involved in the facilitation of LTD by Aβ and the inhibition of LTP (Hsieh et al. 2006; Li et al. 2009, 2011). Thus, Aβ-induced synaptic depression may result from an initial increase in synaptic activation of NMDARs by glutamate, followed by synaptic NMDAR desensitization, NMDAR/AMPAR internalization, and activation of extrasynaptic NMDARs and mGluRs. Aβ-induced LTD-like processes may underlie Aβ-induced LTP deficits, as blocking LTD-related signaling cascades, such as mGluR or p38 MAPK, can prevent Aβ-dependent inhibition of LTP (Wang et al. 2004).

WHAT ARE THE RECEPTORS BY WHICH SOLUBLE OLIGOMERS PERTURB SYNAPTIC FUNCTION?

Although the many studies reviewed so far in this chapter have suggested some of the pathways through which elevated extracellular Aβ levels particularly in the form of soluble oligomers can alter synaptic transmission, precisely how soluble Aβ oligomers *initiate* effects on synaptic structure and function remains to be determined. Diverse lines of evidence suggest that extracellular oligomers can bind to pre- and postsynaptic elements on cultured neurons and in the AD cortex. Cellular and animal studies that have attempted to identify the molecular targets of the oligomers have yielded an array of candidates. Aβ has been reported to interact functionally—and sometimes also structurally—with several distinct types of plasma membrane–anchored receptors, including α7 nicotinic acetylcholine receptors, NMDA and AMPA receptors, insulin receptors, RAGE (the receptor for advanced glycation end-products), the prion protein, and the Ephrin-type B2 receptor (EphB2) (Yan et al. 1999; Lacor et al.

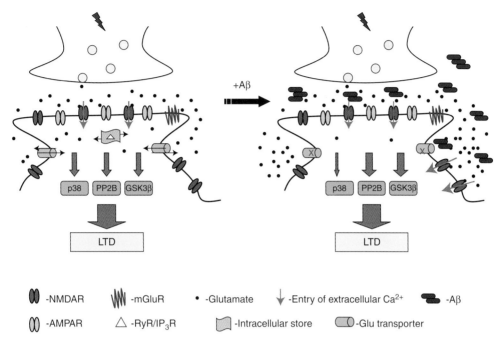

Figure 2. Schematic of the principal pathways implicated by this study in conventional LTD and in LTD facilitated by soluble Aβ oligomers (*left* panel). Conventional LTD requires NMDAR-mediated influx of extracellular calcium and liberation of intracellular calcium stores. This ultimately activates PP2B, GSK-3b, or p38 MAPK signaling pathways that induce LTD. (*Right* panel) Soluble Aβ oligomers lead to activation of more NMDAR, leading to extracellular calcium influx and activation of PP2B and GSK-3b pathways to facilitate LTD. Our data suggest that Aβ oligomers decrease glutamate uptake by neuronal transporters (red ×'s), resulting in the enhanced activation of NMDARs and thus facilitation of LTD-inducing pathways.

2004; Verdier et al. 2004; Lacor et al. 2007; Simakova and Arispe 2007; Koffie et al. 2009; Lauren et al. 2009; Gimbel et al. 2010; Cisse et al. 2011a).

Several key questions should be considered in interpreting such studies. Have the investigators rigorously specified the form of Aβ that is binding to cultured neurons or brain sections and performed the binding studies under physiologically relevant Aβ concentrations and conditions? Many studies have used synthetic Aβ peptides of a single defined length (e.g., Aβ1–40) at potentially supraphysiological concentrations (e.g., 0.1–10 μM). Physiological concentrations of Aβ peptides in human brain, interstitial fluid and cerebrospinal fluid are in the low nanomolar range or below, although concentrations in the most pathobiologically relevant sites of the AD brain, for example,

within and around synaptic clefts, are unknown and might be higher. Are the receptor interactions the authors report occurring with just the monomer (a physiological peptide in mammals), just certain soluble oligomers (e.g., dimers, trimers, dodecamers), and/or just protofibrils? Have the authors used biochemical methods such as size exclusion chromatography under entirely nondenaturing conditions to isolate and specify a particular assembly form, and can they assume that this form has not changed during the experiment (e.g., by recovering it intact after the exposure to neurons)?

These questions are relevant to the issue of whether secreted, soluble Aβ monomers have cognate physiological receptors, analogous, for example, to tachykinin receptors for substance P. If they do (and none has yet been confirmed unequivocally in multiple laboratories under physiological conditions), then are there entirely different receptors that bind soluble oligomers? One would think so, as the biochemical properties of oligomers are distinct from those of the secreted monomer; for example, they are folded differently. However, preferential binding to Aβ oligomers (as opposed to monomers) may not be required for a receptor to be a mediator of Aβ oligomer-induced neuronal dysfunction, because interactions of the receptor with these different Aβ species could elicit distinct signal transduction cascades. For example, dimerization of a particular receptor might be induced by Aβ oligomers but not monomers, despite comparable binding affinities. Ideally, interactions between Aβ oligomers and their receptor(s) would show classical ligand-receptor binding kinetics such as those of insulin and substance P with their cognate receptors. However, binding of Aβ oligomers to some putative receptors, for example, EphB2, triggers degradation of the receptor in the proteasome (Cisse et al. 2011a), which could result in more complex kinetics.

Because soluble oligomers (e.g., dimers, trimers, dodecamers) of Aβ42 have exposed hydrophobic residues that allow them to bind additional monomers and they are thus highly sticky, it seems probable from a biophysical perspective that Aβ42 interacts initially with other hydrophobic molecules, in particular membrane lipids, rather than relatively hydrophilic proteins like the ectodomains of the various candidate receptors mentioned above. Numerous studies using high levels of synthetic Aβ40 or Aβ42 indicate that such preparations can bind to membranes and perturb their structure, in some cases causing actual holes in the membrane that could conduct ions and thus induce cytotoxicity (Demuro et al. 2005; Lin et al. 2001). However, there is little evidence that such major membrane disruption occurs upon exposure of neurons to natural oligomers of secreted Aβ isolated from culture media or brain tissue and applied at nanomolar concentrations. More subtle but sustained (chronic) effects of Aβ oligomers on membrane lipids may well contribute to Aβ-induced neuronal

dysfunction (Sanchez-Mejia et al. 2008), which makes the further investigation of Aβ/lipid interactions an important objective.

Accordingly, we are in need of rigorous biochemical studies of fully purified natural monomers and oligomers isolated from AD brain tissue that are subsequently labeled, or else synthetic labeled oligomers with predetermined structures, allowing the performance of unbiased binding screens (e.g., using cross-linking) to identify which discrete surface molecules the monomers or the oligomers bind and what their binding kinetics are. Until such labor-intensive studies are performed by more than one laboratory, available data can only suggest that a particular receptor (e.g., the α7-nicotinic ACh receptor) plays a required role in membrane engagement and anchoring of Aβ and/or its downstream biological effects, not that they necessarily represent the initial binding receptor. In addition, the pathophysiological role(s) of putative Aβ oligomer receptors should be validated rigorously in relation to clinically relevant functional outcome measures in different experimental models and by independent groups, using genetic and pharmacological manipulations as well as electrophysiological, radiological, and behavioral outcome measures. For example, in independent studies, PrPc ablation either did (Lauren et al. 2009; Gimbel et al. 2010; Barry et al. 2011) or did not (Kessels and Malinow 2009; Balducci et al. 2010; Calella et al. 2010; Cisse et al. 2011b) prevent Aβ-induced neuronal dysfunction, leaving the functional significance of an Aβ/PrPc interaction uncertain at this writing.

EXTRACELLULAR VERSUS INTRANEURONAL Aβ: EVIDENCE FOR AND AGAINST AN ATTACK BY Aβ FROM WITHIN THE NEURON

The classical histopathology of AD brains is characterized by large numbers of extracellular deposits of Aβ in the cortical neuropil and in blood vessel walls (see Serrano-Pozo et al. 2011). This principally extracellular location is consistent with the fact that Aβ arises from the intraluminal/extracellular cleavage of APP by β-secretase followed by the intramembranous γ-secretase cleavages that release it from the membrane into the aqueous environment of the vesicle lumen or extracellular space (Haass et al. 1992, 2011; Shoji et al. 1992). Moreover, systemic amyloids are well known to occur in the extracellular space of various tissues, not intracellularly. The application to AD brain sections of monoclonal antibodies to epitopes that can only be on free Aβ (i.e., are not detectable in the Aβ sequence when it is within the APP molecule) generally reveals enormous amounts of extracellular Aβ-reactive material and little or no specific staining of cell bodies. However, some careful analyses have revealed the additional presence of intraneuronal Aβ immunoreactivity that appears to occur in the lumens of multivesicular bodies and some other types of intracellular vesicles (Takahashi et al. 2004, 2002; Gouras et al. 2005; Almeida et al. 2006). Such a locus is consistent with the cell biology of APP, as it has been shown in numerous studies that the proteolytic processing of APP to Aβ can occur in intracellular vesicles in the secretory and endosomal trafficking pathways. Uptake of Aβ42 through the endosomal/lysosomal pathway has been reported to cause lysosomal leakage (Yang et al. 1998), which could provide Aβ with access to the cytosol, although the normal occurrence of cytosolic Aβ has not been widely confirmed. The possible association of Aβ with mitochondria (Chen and Yan 2007) also suggests that Aβ can exist in these compartments. It is important to reiterate that intracellular Aβ can only be established using end-specific Aβ antibodies that are incapable of reacting with Aβ sequences within APP and its proteolytic products present abundantly inside neurons, as has recently been emphasized (Winton et al. 2011).

The interpretation of the intravesicular Aβ-reactive peptides reported in neurons is not entirely clear. These peptides could represent small amounts of Aβ produced by normal APP processing that is destined for secretion, or they may be in the process of being targeted for proteolytic degradation in the late endosomal/lysosomal system (see Ihara et al. 2011). It is also possible that they could represent previously secreted Aβ monomers and/or oligomers that have been taken back up into cells. In this regard, it is of interest that apparent dimers of Aβ have been detected by immunoprecipitation/western blotting in vesicles isolated from APP-expressing cells, including neurons (Walsh et al. 2000). The highly compact space of a vesicle lumen could afford the molecular crowding that Aβ monomers may need to enhance the chances of oligomer formation, compared with the relatively dilute state of the extracellular/interstitial fluid. Another topic for consideration is whether synaptic dysfunction and neurotoxicity arise principally from intracellular Aβ or from the far more abundant extracellular stores of monomers and oligomers found in AD brains or from both. Clearly, the extracellular application of biochemically isolated natural oligomers of Aβ at physiological concentrations has been shown to induce extensive neuronal changes, including altered synaptic plasticity and synapse form (Klyubin et al. 2005; Shankar et al. 2007, 2008; Li et al. 2009), abnormal tau phosphorylation progressing to neuritic dystrophy (Jin et al. 2011), and interference with memory (Cleary et al. 2005; Lesne et al. 2006; Shankar et al. 2008). One does not yet know whether a solely intraneuronal accumulation of such soluble oligomers is sufficient to induce these various AD-like phenotypes.

DISRUPTION OF COGNITIVE FUNCTIONS: FROM SYNAPSES TO NEURAL NETWORKS

The dynamic complexity of Aβ assembly forms is easily matched, if not outdone, by the complexity of the neural networks on which they act. Distributed networks such as the so-called "default network" comprise different brain regions, which, in turn, contain multiple interconnected circuits that are made up of distinct cell types and myriad synaptic contacts. A key unresolved question in the AD field is whether Aβ assemblies affect different neurons and synapses differentially. Answering this question is critical if one wants to predict the effects of Aβ on the output of neuronal circuits and the activity of networks (Palop et al. 2006; Palop

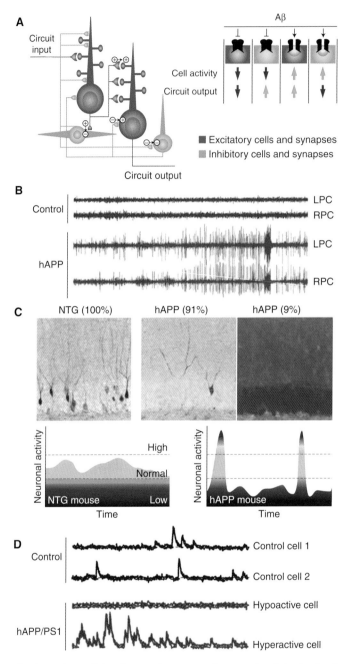

Figure 3. Pathologically elevated Aβ elicits abnormal patterns of neuronal activity in circuits and in wider networks in Alzheimer disease–related mouse models. (*A*) Neuronal circuits are formed by synaptic interactions between excitatory and inhibitory cells. Aβ might differentially affect excitatory (+) and inhibitory (−) synapses and cells, producing complex imbalances in circuit and network activity. (*B*) At the network level, high levels of Aβ increase network synchrony and elicit epileptiform activity, as illustrated here in EEG recordings from the left and right parietal cortex (LPC and RPC, respectively) of nontransgenic (NTG) controls (blue) and hAPP transgenic mice from line J20 (red). (*C*) hAPP mice show fluctuations in the neuronal expression of synaptic activity–dependent genes, suggesting network instability. (*See facing page for legend.*)

and Mucke 2010). For example, if Aβ impaired the synaptic function of inhibitory interneurons more than that of excitatory principal cells, it would be likely to cause disinhibition and overexcitation, rather than suppression, at the network level (Fig. 3). A similar effect would result if Aβ suppressed excitatory → inhibitory synapses more than excitatory → excitatory synapses.

Experimental evidence suggests that some GABAergic neurons may indeed be especially vulnerable to Aβ, which helps explain apparent discrepancies between results obtained in analyses of specific synapses versus circuits and networks. Early electrophysiological studies focused on two specific glutamatergic synapses in the hippocampus, the CA3 → Schaffer collateral → CA1 pyramidal cell synapse and the entorhinal cortex → perforant path → dentate gyrus granule cell synapse. At these synapses, Aβ has been reported in numerous studies to suppress transmission strength and/or long- and short-term plasticity (see Palop and Mucke 2010 for review). Based on just these two circuits, it might be expected that Aβ primarily suppresses network excitability, but this is not what actually happens in vivo.

Among the first clues suggesting that Aβ can elicit aberrant excitatory activity at the network level was the identification of anatomical and biochemical alterations in the dentate gyrus of hAPP mice that are typically seen in rodent models of epilepsy or other states of neuronal overexcitation. These alterations include reductions in calbindin and increases in neuropeptide Y (NPY; Palop et al. 2003; Palop et al. 2007). Video electroencephalogram (EEG) telemetry recordings in freely behaving hAPP mice have detected widespread cortical and hippocampal

epileptiform activity (Palop et al. 2007; Minkeviciene et al. 2009; Vogt et al. 2009; Roberson et al. 2011). Some of these EEG studies also documented intermittent, nonconvulsive seizures that were difficult or impossible to detect by visual observation. Although some lines of hAPP mice have frank convulsive seizures, such events appear to be rare in most hAPP mice. Convulsive seizures are also rare in sporadic AD, although this condition is clearly associated with an increased incidence of epilepsy (reviewed in Palop and Mucke 2009). Interestingly, clinically apparent seizures are much more common in cases with early-onset AD, particularly autosomal dominant pedigrees and AD associated with Down syndrome, suggesting a potentially causal role of high Aβ levels and aggressive cytopathology. The incidence of nonconvulsive (subclinical) seizure activity in familial and sporadic AD is unknown. Studies have recently been launched in multiple centers to address this intriguing issue.

Additional studies are also needed to elucidate the precise mechanisms by which Aβ elicits aberrant excitatory network activity. The possibilities include direct proexcitatory effects on principal glutamatergic neurons and impairments of inhibitory interneurons that therefore indirectly disinhibit the network (Palop et al. 2007; Busche et al. 2008; Palop and Mucke 2010). Acutely, exposure to synthetic or natural Aβ assemblies can increase neuronal activity in cell culture and cortical slices (Sanchez-Mejia et al. 2008; Supnet and Bezprozvanny 2010). The underlying mechanisms may involve increases in $[Ca^{2+}]_i$, activation of group IVA phospholipase A_2 (GIVA-PLA$_2$), increased release of arachidonic acid, and/or transient increases in surface levels of glutamate

Figure 3. (*Continued*) *Top*: Compared with NTG controls (*left*), hAPP-J20 mice show abnormally low (*middle*) or high (*right*) Arc expression in granule cells of the dentate gyrus (adapted, with permission, from Palop et al. 2005, 2007). Percentages indicate the proportion of mice showing the different patterns of Arc expression. Such marked increases in Arc expression are typically caused by seizure activity. *Bottom*: Interpretive diagram. Marked fluctuations in neuronal activity may directly impair cognition by reducing the time the network spends in activity patterns that promote normal cognitive functions. (*D*) In cortical circuits of mice monitored in vivo by calcium imaging, most neurons in NTG controls (blue traces) have an intermediate level of activity, whereas many neurons in hAPP/PS1 transgenic mice with high Aβ levels (red traces) are either hypoactive (*top*) or hyperactive (*bottom*). (Adapted, with permission, from Palop and Mucke 2010.)

receptors. Chronically, Aβ appears to interfere with neuronal glutamate transporters, resulting in increased levels of glutamate in and around the synaptic cleft, desensitization of glutamate receptors and engagement of LTD-related signaling pathways (Hsieh et al. 2006; Li et al. 2009; Wei et al. 2010). Pathogenic glial loops resulting in the production of excitotoxins may contribute as well. Aβ also increases met-enkaphalin levels in the hippocampus and entorhinal cortex, which could suppress the activity of inhibitory interneurons via stimulation of μ-opioid receptors. Indeed, pharmacological blockade of these receptors improved the performance of hAPP mice in the Morris water maze (Meilandt et al. 2008).

Overexcitation or hypersynchrony of neural networks triggers a multitude of compensatory responses, including extensive remodeling of neuronal circuits. This leads to a complex combination of decreased (probably primary) and increased (probably secondary) inhibitory pathways. For example, whereas hAPP mice show evidence for impaired function of GABAergic interneurons (Busche et al. 2008; Roberson et al. 2011), the outer molecular layers of their dentate gyri have extensive sprouting of GABAergic terminals, and their granule cells receive an increased number of inhibitory inputs (Palop et al. 2007). In addition, their mossy fiber collaterals contact basket cells, which would be expected to result in feed-forward inhibition of the granule cells from which the mossy fibers emanate. These alterations are consistent with the idea that the dentate gyrus, which epileptologists regard as the "gate" to the hippocampus, can activate mechanisms to block Aβ-induced aberrant excitatory activity. Much of this excess activity probably originates in cortical areas (Harris et al. 2010).

It is likely that, in AD and mouse models thereof, compensatory inhibitory mechanisms manage to delay and diminish excitotoxic processes that ultimately cause loss of synapses and neurons. However, these mechanisms may simultaneously constrain the agility of excitatory processes required for normal learning and memory. In addition, they probably contribute to a "yin and yang" between too much and too little neuronal activity, diminishing the amount of time networks spend in a physiological range of activity that is conducive to normal cognitive functions (Fig. 3C). Direct evidence for such fluctuations comes from studies monitoring neuronal expression of the activity-related gene product Arc in dentate granule cells or calcium fluxes in neocortical neurons of live hAPP mice (Palop et al. 2007; Busche et al. 2008).

THERAPEUTIC IMPLICATIONS OF THE CONCEPT THAT Aβ-MEDIATED NEUROTOXICITY OCCURS PRINCIPALLY AT THE LEVEL OF SYNAPTIC NETWORKS

What are the therapeutic implications of the complex synaptic and network alterations reviewed in this chapter? First, AD is a slowly progressive and highly dynamic process, with different mechanisms probably predominating at different stages of the disease. Supporting this notion, recent studies show that detrimental effects of Aβ on adult-born granule cells can be prevented by inhibiting GABA_A receptors during early stages of their development or by enhancing glutamatergic signaling during later stages of maturation (Sun et al. 2009). Second, if aberrant increases in network excitability or synchronization are indeed early/proximal events in the Aβ-triggered pathogenic cascade, identifying ways to block this process becomes a critical therapeutic objective. The effect of antiepileptic drugs has not yet been rigorously evaluated in patients with early AD, and the optimal drug to block Aβ-induced aberrant excitatory neuronal activity in experimental models has yet to be identified. It will probably have to target the specific mechanisms by which Aβ elicits aberrant excitatory neuronal activity, which also remain to be pinpointed.

A pragmatic way forward to deal with the complex cellular and network alterations that occur during AD is to lower the levels of Aβ itself by inhibiting its production or enhancing its removal (see Schenk et al. 2011). Several such strategies are currently being assessed in human trials. At this writing, it remains unsettled whether such strategies will be efficacious and safe (Golde et al. 2011; Selkoe 2011). For some of them, it is still uncertain whether they actually lower the levels of those Aβ assemblies that have the greatest impact on neuronal form and function. It therefore makes sense to complement these approaches with strategies that might make the brain more resistant to Aβ by targeting copathogenic factors or downstream mechanisms.

Examples of the latter strategies include reductions in the levels of the microtubule-associated protein tau (Roberson et al. 2007, 2011; Ittner et al. 2010; Jin et al. 2011; Morris et al. 2011) or of GIVA-PLA₂, (Sanchez-Mejia et al. 2008) or replacement of apoE4 function with apoE3-like function (Raber et al. 2000; Buttini et al. 2002; Mahley et al. 2006). Although the precise mechanisms by which these and similar interventions prevent Aβ-induced cognitive impairments without reducing Aβ levels remain to be determined, they may share a general effect of making the brain more resistant to aberrant excitatory synaptic activity. For example, even partial (50%) reduction of endogenous wild-type murine tau prevented synaptic and behavioral deficits in hAPP-J20 mice as well as evidence of neuronal over-excitation (Roberson et al. 2007; Morris et al. 2011; Roberson et al. 2011). Surprisingly, it did so without affecting Aβ levels, plaque formation or neuritic dystrophy. Similarly, knockdown of tau in cultured neurons made them markedly resistant to the cytoskeletal disruption and neuritic dystrophy induced by natural oligomers of Aβ isolated from AD cortex (Jin et al. 2011). Hippocampal slices from tau knockout mice were resistant to the LTP inhibition caused by synthetic Aβ peptide (Shipton et al. 2011). Tau reduction has also been shown to make mice with or without hAPP/Aβ overexpression more resistant to chemically induced seizures (Roberson et al. 2007; Ittner et al. 2010), suggesting a previously unrecognized role of tau in the regulation of neuronal activity. These various findings raise the intriguing possibility that nonaggregated wild-type tau fulfills a normal neuronal function that is required for Aβ and other excitotoxins to elicit aberrant excitatory activity.

Although the relative amounts of specific isoforms of tau and its exact amino acid sequence differ in mice and humans, the longest tau isoforms expressed in human and mouse brain are 88% identical and 92% similar. Proteins that are this highly conserved in amino acid sequence are likely to have conserved functions. Therefore, investigating the functions of mouse tau in transgenic models should provide clues regarding the roles of human tau in health and disease. This is particularly so because the enabling role of endogenous tau in Aβ-induced neuronal dysfunction probably does not depend on direct interactions between Aβ and tau, which are localized to separate compartments of the neuron. Instead, it may depend on permissive activities of tau, such as facilitation of neuronal excitability (Ittner et al. 2010), that are likely conserved in mice and humans. Such hypothetical tau functions could play a critical role in the pathogenesis of dementia and are not inconsistent with evidence that pathogenic tau aggregates cause neurodegeneration in AD and other tauopathies (Hoover et al. 2010; Zempel et al. 2010).

Intuitively, it makes sense that loss of neurons is a principal basis for cognitive decline in AD and other neurodegenerative dementias. However, several observations suggest that one should not view it as the *sine qua non* of functional decline, particularly early on in the syndrome. For example, the brain can compensate quite well for major losses of neurons, especially when these losses occur over prolonged periods of time. A striking example is a patient with long-standing communicating hydrocephalus who has only a rim of cortical ribbon left but functions quite well despite remarkably abnormal brain scans (Lewin 1980). Importantly, in APP transgenic mice, Aβ accumulation elicits severe synaptic impairments and unequivocal deficits in learning and memory without causing major neuronal loss, although neurites do degenerate. In tau transgenic mice, cognitive deficits are associated with neuronal loss, but these deficits can be reversed despite the persistence of the neuronal loss (SantaCruz et al. 2005).

Taken together, available data reviewed here and elsewhere raise the possibility that a significant proportion of the profound cognitive and behavioral deficits in AD patients are due to the dysfunction of synapses and neural networks (Selkoe 2002; Palop and Mucke 2010). This concept has far-reaching therapeutic implications. While the replacement and proper integration of whole neurons remains a very major challenge, the regeneration of neurites, the re-establishment of synaptic contacts and an improvement of network function appear within somewhat closer experimental reach. Fostering such restorative processes while also trying to diminish or block factors that fuel the progression of AD, such as Aβ and tau accumulation, should slow and ultimately even prevent cognitive dysfunction in this dauntingly complex syndrome.

REFERENCES

*Reference is also in this collection.

Abramov E, Dolev I, Fogel H, Ciccotosto GD, Ruff E, Slutsky I. 2009. Amyloid-β as a positive endogenous regulator of release probability at hippocampal synapses. *Nat Neurosci* **12:** 1567–1576.

Almeida CG, Takahashi RH, Gouras GK. 2006. β-Amyloid accumulation impairs multivesicular body sorting by inhibiting the ubiquitin-proteasome system. *J Neurosci* **26:** 4277–4288.

Balducci C, Beeg M, Stravalaci M, Bastone A, Sclip A, Biasini E, Tapella L, Colombo L, Manzoni C, Borsello T, et al. 2010. Synthetic amyloid-{β} oligomers impair long-term memory independently of cellular prion protein. *Proc Natl Acad Sci* **107:** 2295–2300.

Barry AE, Klyubin I, McDonald JM, Mably AJ, Farrell MA, Scott M, Walsh DM, Rowan MJ. 2011. Alzheimer's disease brain-derived amyloid-mediated inhibition of LTP in vivo is prevented by immunotargeting cellular prion protein. *J Neurosci* **31:** 7259–7263.

Bitan G, Lomakin A, Teplow DB. 2001. Amyloid β-protein oligomerization: Prenucleation interactions revealed by photo-induced cross-linking of unmodified proteins. *J Biol Chem* **276:** 35176–35184.

Busche MA, Eichhoff G, Adelsberger H, Abramowski D, Wiederhold KH, Haass C, Staufenbiel M, Konnerth A, Garaschuk O. 2008. Clusters of hyperactive neurons near amyloid plaques in a mouse model of Alzheimer's disease. *Science* **321:** 1686–1689.

Buttini M, Yu G-Q, Shockley K, Huang Y, Jones B, Masliah E, Mallory M, Yeo T, Longo FM, Mucke L. 2002. Modulation of Alzheimer-like synaptic and cholinergic deficits in transgenic mice by human apolipoprotein E depends on isoform, aging, and overexpression of amyloid β peptides but not on plaque formation. *J Neurosci* **22:** 10539–10548.

Calella AM, Farinelli M, Nuvolone M, Mirante O, Moos R, Falsig J, Mansuy IM, Aguzzi A. 2010. Prion protein and Aβ-related synaptic toxicity impairment. *EMBO Mol Med* **2:** 306–314.

Chen JX, Yan SD. 2007. Amyloid-β-induced mitochondrial dysfunction. *J Alzheimer's Dis* **12:** 177–184.

Cirrito JR, Yamada KA, Finn MB, Sloviter RS, Bales KR, May PC, Schoepp DD, Paul SM, Mennerick S, Holtzman DM. 2005. Synaptic activity regulates interstitial fluid amyloid-β levels in vivo. *Neuron* **48:** 913–922.

Cisse M, Halabisky B, Harris JA, Devidze N, Dubal D, Lotz G, Kim DH, Hamto T, Ho K, Yu G-Q, et al. 2011a. Reversing EphB2 depletion rescues cognitive functions in Alzheimer model. *Nature* **469:** 47–52.

Cisse M, Sanchez PE, Kim DH, Yu G-Q, Mucke L. 2011b. Ablation of cellular prion protein does not ameliorate abnormal neural network activity and cognitive dysfunction in the J20 line of human amyloid precursor protein transgenic mice. *J Neurosci* **31:** 10427–10431.

Cleary JP, Walsh DM, Hofmeister JJ, Shankar GM, Kuskowski MA, Selkoe DJ, Ashe KH. 2005. Natural oligomers of the amyloid-β protein specifically disrupt cognitive function. *Nat Neurosci* **8:** 79–84.

DeKosky ST, Scheff SW. 1990. Synapse loss in frontal cortex biopsies in Alzheimer's disease: Correlation with cognitive severity. *Ann Neurol* **27:** 457–464.

Demuro A, Mina E, Kayed R, Milton SC, Parker I, Glabe CG. 2005. Calcium dysregulation and membrane disruption as a ubiquitous neurotoxic mechanism of soluble amyloid oligomers. *J Biol Chem* **280:** 17294–17300.

Dineley KT, Bell KA, Bui D, Sweatt JD. 2002. β-Amyloid peptide activates α7 nicotinic acetylcholine receptors expressed in *Xenopus* oocytes. *J Biol Chem* **277:** 25056–25061.

Gimbel DA, Nygaard HB, Coffey EE, Gunther EC, Lauren J, Gimbel ZA, Strittmatter SM. 2010. Memory impairment in transgenic Alzheimer mice requires cellular prion protein. *J Neurosci* **30:** 6367–6374.

Golde TE, Schneider LS, Koo EH. 2011. Anti-aβ therapeutics in Alzheimer's disease: The need for a paradigm shift. *Neuron* **69:** 203–213.

Gong Y, Chang L, Viola KL, Lacor PN, Lambert MP, Finch CE, Krafft GA, Klein WL. 2003. Alzheimer's disease-affected brain: Presence of oligomeric Aβ ligands (ADDLs) suggests a molecular basis for reversible memory loss. *Proc Natl Acad Sci* **100:** 10417–10422.

Gouras GK, Almeida CG, Takahashi RH. 2005. Intraneuronal Aβ accumulation and origin of plaques in Alzheimer's disease. *Neurobiol Aging* **26:** 1235–1244.

Haass C, Schlossmacher M, Hung AY, Vigo-Pelfrey C, Mellon A, Ostaszewski B, Lieberburg I, Koo EH, Schenk D, Teplow D, et al. 1992. Amyloid β-peptide is produced by cultured cells during normal metabolism. *Nature* **359:** 322–325.

*Haass C, Kaether C, Sisodia S, Thinakaran G. 2011. Trafficking and proteolytic processing of APP. *Cold Spring Harb Perspect Med* doi: 10.1101/cshperspect.a006270.

Hardy JA, Higgins GA. 1992. Alzheimer's disease: The amyloid cascade hypothesis. *Science* **256:** 184–185.

Harper JD, Wong SS, Lieber CM, Lansbury PT Jr. 1997. Observation of metastable Ab amyloid protofibrils by atomic force microscopy. *Chem Biol* **4:** 119–125.

Harris JA, Devidze N, Verret L, Ho K, Hamto T, Lo I, Yu G-Q, Palop JJ, Masliah E, Mucke L. 2010. Transsynaptic progression of amyloid-β-induced neuronal dysfunction within the entorhinal–hippocampal network. *Neuron* **68:** 428–441.

Hartley D, Walsh DM, Ye CP, Diehl T, Vasquez S, Vassilev PM, Teplow DB, Selkoe DJ. 1999. Protofibrillar intermediates of amyloid β-protein induce acute electrophysiological changes and progressive neurotoxicity in cortical neurons. *J Neurosci* **19:** 8876–8884.

Holcomb LA, Gordon MN, Jantzen P, Hsiao K, Duff K, Morgan D. 1999. Behavioral changes in transgenic mice expressing both amyloid precursor protein and presenilin-1 mutations: Lack of association with amyloid deposits. *Behav Genet* **29:** 177–185.

Hoover BR, Reed MN, Su J, Penrod RD, Kotilinek LA, Grant MK, Pitstick R, Carlson GA, Lanier LM, Yuan LL, et al. 2010. Tau mislocalization to dendritic spines mediates synaptic dysfunction independently of neurodegeneration. *Neuron* **68:** 1067–1081.

Hsia AY, Masliah E, McConlogue L, Yu GQ, Tatsuno G, Hu K, Kholodenko D, Malenka RC, Nicoll RA, Mucke L. 1999. Plaque-independent disruption of neural circuits in Alzheimer's disease mouse models. *Proc Natl Acad Sci* **96:** 3228–3233.

Hsieh H, Boehm J, Sato C, Iwatsubo T, Tomita T, Sisodia S, Malinow R. 2006. AMPAR removal underlies Aβ-induced synaptic depression and dendritic spine loss. *Neuron* **52:** 831–843.

Hyman BT, West HL, Rebeck GW, Buldyrev SV, Mantegna RN, Ukleja M, Havlin S, Stanley HE. 1995. Quantitative analysis of senile plaques in Alzheimer's disease: Observation of log-normal size distribution and molecular epidemiology of differences associated with apolipoprotein E genotype and trisomy 21 (Down syndrome). *Proc Natl Acad Sci* **92:** 3586–3590.

* Ihara Y, Morishima-Kawashima M, Nixon R. 2011. The ubiquitin-proteasome system and the autophagic-lysosomal system in Alzheimer disease. *Cold Spring Harb Perspect Med* doi: 10.1101/cshperspect.a006361.

Ittner LM, Ke YD, Delerue F, Bi M, Gladbach A, van Eersel J, Wolfing H, Chieng BC, Christie MJ, Napier IA, et al. 2010. Dendritic function of tau mediates amyloid-β toxicity in Alzheimer's disease mouse models. *Cell* **142:** 387–397.

Jin M, Shepardson N, Yang T, Walsh D, Selkoe D. 2011. Soluble amyloid β-protein dimers isolated from Alzheimer cortex directly induce Tau hyperphosphorylation and neuritic degeneration. *Proc Natl Acad Sci* **108:** 5819–5824.

Kamenetz F, Tomita T, Hsieh H, Seabrook G, Borchelt D, Iwatsubo T, Sisodia S, Malinow R. 2003. APP processing and synaptic function. *Neuron* **37:** 925–937.

Kang JE, Lim MM, Bateman RJ, Lee JJ, Smyth LP, Cirrito JR, Fujiki N, Nishino S, Holtzman DM. 2009. Amyloid-β dynamics are regulated by orexin and the sleep–wake cycle. *Science* **326:** 1005–1007.

Kawarabayashi T, Younkin LH, Saido TC, Shoji M, Ashe KH, Younkin SG. 2001. Age-dependent changes in brain, CSF, and plasma amyloid (β) protein in the Tg2576 transgenic mouse model of Alzheimer's disease. *J Neurosci* **21:** 372–381.

Kayed R, Head E, Thompson JL, McIntire TM, Milton SC, Cotman CW, Glabe CG. 2003. Common structure of soluble amyloid oligomers implies common mechanism of pathogenesis. *Science* **300:** 486–489.

Kessels HW, Malinow R. 2009. Synaptic AMPA receptor plasticity and behavior. *Neuron* **61:** 340–350.

Kim JH, Anwyl R, Suh YH, Djamgoz MB, Rowan MJ. 2001. Use-dependent effects of amyloidogenic fragments of (β)-amyloid precursor protein on synaptic plasticity in rat hippocampus in vivo. *J Neurosci* **21** 1327–1333.

Klyubin I, Walsh DM, Lemere CA, Cullen WK, Shankar GM, Betts V, Spooner ET, Jiang L, Anwyl R, Selkoe DJ, et al. 2005. Amyloid β protein immunotherapy neutralizes Aβ oligomers that disrupt synaptic plasticity in vivo. *Nat Med* **11:** 556–561.

Koffie RM, Meyer-Luehmann M, Hashimoto T, Adams KW, Mielke ML, Garcia-Alloza M, Micheva KD, Smith SJ, Kim ML, Lee VM, et al. 2009. Oligomeric amyloid β associates with postsynaptic densities and correlates with excitatory synapse loss near senile plaques. *Proc Natl Acad Sci* **106:** 4012–4017.

Kullmann DM, Lamsa KP. 2007. Long-term synaptic plasticity in hippocampal interneurons. *Nat Rev Neurosci* **8:** 687–699.

Lacor PN, Buniel MC, Chang L, Fernandez SJ, Gong Y, Viola KL, Lambert MP, Velasco PT, Bigio EH, Finch CE, et al. 2004. Synaptic targeting by Alzheimer's-related amyloid β oligomers. *J Neurosci* **24:** 10191–10200.

Lacor PN, Buniel MC, Furlow PW, Clemente AS, Velasco PT, Wood M, Viola KL, Klein WL. 2007. Aβ oligomer-induced aberrations in synapse composition, shape, and density provide a molecular basis for loss of connectivity in Alzheimer's disease. *J Neurosci* **27:** 796–807.

Laird FM, Cai H, Savonenko AV, Farah MH, He K, Melnikova T, Wen H, Chiang HC, Xu G, Koliatsos VE, et al. 2005. BACE1, a major determinant of selective vulnerability of the brain to amyloid-β amyloidogenesis, is essential for cognitive, emotional, and synaptic functions. *J Neurosci* **25:** 11693–11709.

Lambert MP, Barlow AK, Chromy BA, Edwards C, Freed R, iosatos M, Morgan TE, Rozovsky I, Trommer B, Viola KL, et al. 1998. Diffusible, nonfibrillar ligands derived from Aβ$_{1-42}$ are potent central nervous system neurotoxins. *Proc Natl Acad Sci* **95:** 6448–6453.

Lauren J, Gimbel DA, Nygaard HB, Gilbert JW, Strittmatter SM. 2009. Cellular prion protein mediates impairment of synaptic plasticity by amyloid-β oligomers. *Nature* **457:** 1128–1132.

Lesne S, Koh MT, Kotilinek L, Kayed R, Glabe CG, Yang A, Gallagher M, Ashe KH. 2006. A specific amyloid-β protein assembly in the brain impairs memory. *Nature* **440:** 352–357.

Lewin R. 1980. Is your brain really necessary? *Science* **210:** 1232–1234.

Li S, Hong S, Shepardson NE, Walsh DM, Shankar GM, Selkoe D. 2009. Soluble oligomers of amyloid β protein facilitate hippocampal long-term depression by disrupting neuronal glutamate uptake. *Neuron* **62:** 788–801.

Li S, Jin M, Koeglsperger T, Shepardson NE, Shankar GM, Selkoe DJ. 2011. Soluble Aβ oligomers inhibit long-term potentiation through a mechanism involving excessive activation of extrasynaptic NR2B-containing NMDA receptors. *J Neurosci* **31:** 6627–6638.

Lin H, Bhatia R, Lal R. 2001. Amyloid β protein forms ion channels: Implications for Alzheimer's disease pathophysiology. *FASEB J* **15:** 2433–2444.

Liu L, Wong TP, Pozza MF, Lingenhoehl K, Wang Y, Sheng M, Auberson YP, Wang YT. 2004. Role of NMDA receptor subtypes in governing the direction of hippocampal synaptic plasticity. *Science* **304:** 1021–1024.

Mahley RW, Weisgraber KH, Huang Y. 2006. Apolipoprotein E4: A causative factor and therapeutic target in neuropathology, including Alzheimer's disease. *Proc Natl Acad Sci* **103:** 5644–5651.

Martins IC, Kuperstein I, Wilkinson H, Maes E, Vanbrabant M, Jonckheere W, Van Gelder P, Hartmann D, D'Hooge R, De Strooper B, et al. 2008. Lipids revert inert Aβ amyloid fibrils to neurotoxic protofibrils that affect learning in mice. *Embo J* **27:** 224–233.

McLaurin J, Kierstead ME, Brown ME, Hawkes CA, Lambermon MH, Phinney AL, Darabie AA, Cousins JE, French JE, Lan MF, et al. 2006. Cyclohexanehexol inhibitors of Aβ aggregation prevent and reverse Alzheimer phenotype in a mouse model. *Nat Med* **12:** 801–808.

McLean CA, Cherny RA, Fraser FW, Fuller SJ, Smith MJ, Beyreuther K, Bush AI, Masters CL. 1999. Soluble pool of Aβ amyloid as a determinant of severity of neurodegeneration in Alzheimer's disease. *Ann Neurol* **46:** 860–866.

Meilandt WJ, Yu G-Q, Chin J, Roberson ED, Palop JJ, Wu T, Scearce-Levie K, Mucke L. 2008. Enkephalin elevations contribute to neuronal and behavioral impairments in a transgenic mouse model of Alzheimer's disease. *J Neurosci* **28:** 5007–5017.

Minkeviciene R, Rheims S, Dobszay MB, Zilberter M, Hartikainen J, Fulop L, Penke B, Zilberter Y, Harkany T, Pitkanen A, et al. 2009. Amyloid β-induced neuronal hyperexcitability triggers progressive epilepsy. *J Neurosci* **29:** 3453–3462.

Morris M, Maeda S, Vossel K, Mucke L. 2011. The many faces of tau. *Neuron* **70:** 410–426.

Mucke L, Masliah E, Yu GQ, Mallory M, Rockenstein EM, Tatsuno G, Hu K, Kholodenko D, Johnson-Wood K, McConlogue L. 2000. High-level neuronal expression of aβ 1–42 in wild-type human amyloid protein precursor transgenic mice: Synaptotoxicity without plaque formation. *J Neurosci* **20:** 4050–4058.

Palop JJ, Mucke L. 2009. Epilepsy and cognitive impairments in Alzheimer disease. *Arch Neurol* **66:** 435–440.

Palop JJ, Mucke L. 2010. Amyloid-β-induced neuronal dysfunction in Alzheimer's disease: From synapses toward neural networks. *Nat Neurosci* **13:** 812–818.

Palop JJ, Jones B, Kekonius L, Chin J, Yu G-Q, Raber J, Masliah E, Mucke L. 2003. Neuronal depletion of calcium-dependent proteins in the dentate gyrus is tightly linked to Alzheimer's disease-related cognitive deficits. *Proc Natl Acad Sci* **100:** 9572–9577.

Palop JJ, Chin J, Bien-Ly N, Massaro C, Yeung BZ, Yu GQ, Mucke L. 2005. Vulnerability of dentate granule cells to disruption of arc expression in human amyloid precursor protein transgenic mice. *J Neurosci* **25:** 9686–9693.

Palop JJ, Chin J, Mucke L. 2006. A network dysfunction perspective on neurodegenerative diseases. *Nature* **443:** 768–773.

Palop JJ, Chin J, Roberson ED, Wang J, Thwin MT, Bien-Ly N, Yoo J, Ho KO, Yu G-Q, Kreitzer A, et al. 2007. Aberrant excitatory neuronal activity and compensatory remodeling of inhibitory hippocampal circuits in mouse models of Alzheimer's disease. *Neuron* **55:** 697–711.

Podlisny MB, Ostaszewski BL, Squazzo SL, Koo EH, Rydel RE, Teplow DB, Selkoe DJ. 1995a. Aggregation of secreted amyloid β-protein into SDS-stable oligomers in cell culture. *J Biol Chem* **270:** 9564–9570.

Puzzo D, Privitera L, Leznik E, Fa M, Staniszewski A, Palmeri A, Arancio O. 2008. Picomolar amyloid-β positively modulates synaptic plasticity and memory in hippocampus. *J Neurosci* **28:** 14537–14545.

Raber J, Wong D, Yu G-Q, Buttini M, Mahley RW, Pitas RE, Mucke L. 2000. Alzheimer's disease: Apolipoprotein E and cognitive performance. *Nature* **404:** 352–354.

Roberson ED, Halabisky B, Yoo JW, Yao J, Chin J, Yan F, Wu T, Hamto P, Devidze N, Yu G-Q, et al. 2011. Amyloid-β/Fyn-induced synaptic, network, and cognitive impairments depend on Tau levels in multiple mouse models of Alzheimer's disease. *J Neurosci* **31:** 700–711.

Roberson ED, Scearce-Levie K, Palop JJ, Yan F, Cheng IH, Wu T, Gerstein H, Yu G-Q, Mucke L. 2007. Reducing endogenous tau ameliorates Amyloid beta-induced deficits in an Alzheimer's disease mouse model. *Science* **316:** 750–754.

Roher AE, Chaney MO, Kuo Y-M, Webster SD, Stine WB, Haverkamp LJ, Woods AS, Cotter RJ, Tuohy JM, Krafft GA, et al. 1996. Morphology and toxicity of Aβ-(1–42) dimer derived from neuritic and vascular amyloid deposits of Alzheimer's disease. *J Biol Chem* **271:** 20631–20635.

Sanchez-Mejia RO, Newman JW, Toh S, G-Q Y, Zhou Y, Halabisky B, Cisse M, Scearce-Levie K, Cheng IH, Gan L, et al. 2008. Phospholipase A2 reduction ameliorates cognitve deficits in mouse model of Alzheimer's disease. *Nat Neurosci* **11:** 1311–1318.

SantaCruz K, Lewis J, Spires T, Paulson J, Kotilinek L, Ingelsson M, Guimaraes A, DeTure M, Ramsden M, McGowan E, et al. 2005. Tau suppression in a neurodegenerative mouse model improves memory function. *Science* **309:** 476–481.

Saura CA, Choi SY, Beglopoulos V, Malkani S, Zhang D, Shankaranarayana Rao BS, Chattarji S, Kelleher RJ, Kandel ER, Duff K, et al. 2004. Loss of presenilin function causes impairments of memory and synaptic plasticity followed by age-dependent neurodegeneration. *Neuron* **42:** 23–36.

* Schenk D, Basi GS, Pangalos MN. 2011. Treatment strategies targeting amyloid β-protein. *Cold Spring Harb Perspect Med* doi: 10.1101/cshperspect.a006387.

Seabrook GR, Smith DW, Bowery BJ, Easter A, Reynolds T, Fitzjohn SM, Morton RA, Zheng H, Dawson GR, Sirinathsinghji DJS, et al. 1999. Mechanisms contributing to the deficits in hippocampal synaptic plasticity in mice lacking amyloid precursor protein. *Neuropharmacology* **38:** 349–359.

Selkoe DJ. 1991. The molecular pathology of Alzheimer's disease. *Neuron* **6:** 487–498.

Selkoe DJ. 2002. Alzheimer's disease is a synaptic failure. *Science* **298:** 789–791.

Selkoe DJ. 2011. Resolving controversies on the path to Alzheimer's therapeutics. *Nat Med* **17:** 1060–1065.

* Serrano-Pozo A, Frosch MP, Masliah E, Hyman BT. 2011. Neuropathological alterations in Alzheimer disease. *Cold Spring Harb Pespect Med* doi: 10.1101/cshperspect.a006189.

Serrano-Pozo A, William CM, Ferrer I, Uro-Coste E, Delisle MB, Maurage CA, Hock C, Nitsch RM, Masliah E, Growdon JH, et al. 2010. Beneficial effect of human anti-amyloid-β active immunization on neurite morphology and tau pathology. *Brain* **133:** 1312–1327.

Shankar GM, Bloodgood BL, Townsend M, Walsh DM, Selkoe DJ, Sabatini BL. 2007. Natural oligomers of the Alzheimer amyloid-β protein induce reversible synapse loss by modulating an NMDA-type glutamate receptor-dependent signaling pathway. *J Neurosci* **27:** 2866–2875.

Shankar GM, Li S, Mehta TH, Garcia-Munoz A, Shepardson NE, Smith I, Brett FM, Farrell MA, Rowan MJ, Lemere CA, et al. 2008. Amyloid-β protein dimers isolated directly from Alzheimer's brains impair synaptic plasticity and memory. *Nat Med* **14:** 837–842.

Shankar GM, Leissring MA, Adame A, Sun X, Spooner E, Masliah E, Selkoe DJ, Lemere CA, Walsh DM. 2009. Biochemical and immunohistochemical analysis of an Alzheimer's disease mouse model reveals the presence of multiple cerebral Aβ assembly forms throughout life. *Neurobiol Dis* **36:** 293–302.

Shipton OA, Leitz JR, Dworzak J, Acton CE, Tunbridge EM, Denk F, Dawson HN, Vitek MP, Wade-Martins R, Paulsen O, et al. 2011. Tau protein is required for amyloid {β}-induced impairment of hippocampal long-term potentiation. *J Neurosci* **31:** 1688–1692.

Shoji M, Golde TE, Ghiso J, Cheung TT, Estus S, Shaffer LM, Cai X, McKay DM, Tintner R, Frangione B, et al. 1992. Production of the Alzheimer amyloid β protein by normal proteolytic processing. *Science* **258:** 126–129.

Simakova O, Arispe NJ. 2007. The cell-selective neurotoxicity of the Alzheimer's Aβ peptide is determined by surface phosphatidylserine and cytosolic ATP levels. Membrane binding is required for Aβ toxicity. *J Neurosci* **27:** 13719–13729.

Snyder EM, Nong Y, Almeida CG, Paul S, Moran T, Choi EY, Nairn AC, Salter MW, Lombroso PJ, Gouras GK, et al. 2005a. Regulation of NMDA receptor trafficking by amyloid-β. *Nat Neurosci* **8:** 1051–1058.

Spires-Jones TL, Meyer-Luehmann M, Osetek JD, Jones PB, Stern EA, Bacskai BJ, Hyman BT. 2007. Impaired spine stability underlies plaque-related spine loss in an Alzheimer's disease mouse model. *Am J Pathol* **171:** 1304–1311.

Sun B, Halabisky B, Zhou Y, Palop JJ, Yu GQ, Mucke L, Gan L. 2009. Imbalance between GABAergic and glutamatergic transmissions impairs adult neurogenesis in an animal model of Alzheimer's disease. *Cell Stem Cell* **5:** 624–633.

Supnet C, Bezprozvanny I. 2010. The dysregulation of intracellular calcium in Alzheimer disease. *Cell Calcium* **47:** 183–189.

Tackenberg C, Brandt R. 2009. Divergent pathways mediate spine alterations and cell death induced by amyloid-β, wild-type tau, and R406W tau. *J Neurosci* **29:** 14439–14450.

Takahashi RH, Milner TA, Li F, Nam EE, Edgar MA, Yamaguchi H, Beal MF, Xu H, Greengard P, Gouras GK. 2002.

Intraneuronal Alzheimer aβ42 accumulates in multivesicular bodies and is associated with synaptic pathology. *Am J Pathol* **161:** 1869–1879.

Takahashi RH, Almeida CG, Kearney PF, Yu F, Lin MT, Milner TA, Gouras GK. 2004. Oligomerization of Alzheimer's β-amyloid within processes and synapses of cultured neurons and brain. *J Neurosci* **24:** 3592–3599.

Terry RD, Masliah E, Salmon DP, Butters N, DeTeresa R, Hill R, Hansen LA, Katzman R. 1991. Physical basis of cognitive alterations in Alzheimer's disease: Synapse loss is the major correlate of cognitive impairment. *Ann Neurol* **30:** 572–580.

Verdier Y, Zarándi M, Penke B. 2004. Amyloid β-peptide interactions with neuronal and glial cell plasma membrane: Binding sites and implications for Alzheimer's disease. *J Pept Sci* **10:** 229–248.

Vogt DL, Thomas D, Galvan V, Bredesen DE, Lamb BT, Pimplikar SW. 2009. Abnormal neuronal networks and seizure susceptibility in mice overexpressing the APP intracellular domain. *Neurobiol Aging* **32:** 1725–1729.

Walsh DM, Lomakin A, Benedek GB, Maggio JE, Condron MM, Teplow DB. 1997. Amyloid b-protein fibrillogenesis: Detection of a protofibrillar intermediate. *J Biol Chem* **272:** 22364–22374.

Walsh DM, Tseng BP, Rydel RE, Podlisny MB, Selkoe DJ. 2000. Detection of intracellular oligomers of amyloid β-protein in cells derived from human brain. *Biochemistry* **39:** 10831–10839.

Walsh D, Klyubin I, Fadeeva J, William K. Cullen W, Anwyl R, Wolfe M, Rowan M, Selkoe D. 2002. Naturally secreted oligomers of the Alzheimer amyloid β-protein potently inhibit hippocampal long-term potentiation in vivo. *Nature* **416:** 535–539.

Wang Q, Walsh DM, Rowan MJ, Selkoe DJ, Anwyl R. 2004. Block of long-term potentiation by naturally secreted and synthetic amyloid β-peptide in hippocampal slices is mediated via activation of the kinases c-Jun N-terminal kinase, cyclin-dependent kinase 5, and pp38 mitogen-activated protein kinase as well as metabotropic glutamate receptor type 5. *J Neurosci* **24:** 3370–3378.

Wei W, Nguyen LN, Kessels HW, Hagiwara H, Sisodia S, Malinow R. 2010. Amyloid β from axons and dendrites reduces local spine number and plasticity. *Nat Neurosci* **13:** 190–196.

Winton MJ, Lee EB, Sun E, Wong MM, Leight S, Zhang B, Trojanowski JQ, Lee VM. 2011. Intraneuronal APP, not free Aβ peptides in 3xTg-AD mice: Implications for tau versus Aβ-mediated Alzheimer neurodegeneration. *J Neurosci* **31:** 7691–7699.

Yan SD, Roher A, Schmidt AM, Stern DM. 1999. Cellular cofactors for amyloid β-peptide-induced cell stress. Moving from cell culture to in vivo. *Am J Pathol* **155:** 1403–1411.

Yang AJ, Chandswangbhuvana D, Margol L, Glabe CG. 1998. Loss of endosomal/lysosomal membrane impermeability is an early event in amyloid Aβ1–42 pathogenesis. *J Neurosci Res* **52:** 691–698.

Zempel H, Thies E, Mandelkow E, Mandelkow EM. 2010. A {β} oligomers cause localized Ca^{2+} elevation, missorting of endogenous tau into dendrites, tau phosphorylation, and destruction of microtubules and spines. *J Neurosci* **30:** 11938–11950.

Inflammation in Alzheimer Disease—A Brief Review of the Basic Science and Clinical Literature

Tony Wyss-Coray[1,2] and Joseph Rogers[3]

[1]Department of Neurology and Neurological Sciences, Stanford University School of Medicine, Stanford, California 94305-5235

[2]Geriatric Research Education and Clinical Center, Veterans Affairs Palo Alto Health Care System, Palo Alto, California 94304

[3]Banner Sun Health Research Institute, Sun City, Arizona 85372

Correspondence: joseph.rogers@bannerhealth.com

Biochemical and neuropathological studies of brains from individuals with Alzheimer disease (AD) provide clear evidence for an activation of inflammatory pathways, and long-term use of anti-inflammatory drugs is linked with reduced risk to develop the disease. As cause and effect relationships between inflammation and AD are being worked out, there is a realization that some components of this complex molecular and cellular machinery are most likely promoting pathological processes leading to AD, whereas other components serve to do the opposite. The challenge will be to find ways of fine tuning inflammation to delay, prevent, or treat AD.

A recent PubMed search using the key word "Alzheimer's," the Boolean connector "AND," and several key words related to inflammation (e.g., cytokine, chemokine, complement) returned some 6114 different citations. Although that is less than a third of the 20,452 citations for "Alzheimer's AND amyloid," it is 423 citations more than the 5691 for "Alzheimer's AND tau." Clearly, inflammatory mechanisms in Alzheimer disease (AD) are a mainstream area of research.

Whether they are also an important area of research is a different question. As with virtually all the other mechanisms under investigation in AD, it still cannot be definitively stated whether inflammation is a cause, contributor, or secondary phenomenon in the disorder. Treatment trials have been a major disappointment, as they have been for virtually all other therapeutics that have attempted to address the underlying pathogenesis of AD rather than ameliorate its symptoms.

Much has been learned, nonetheless, at both basic science and clinical levels. Here, we review this literature and attempt to address, in as balanced and objective a manner as we can, some of the major controversies in the field. If nothing else, the burgeoning number of papers on inflammation and AD that are summarized in this review make plain the remarkable complexity of inflammatory mechanisms in AD and the many challenges that such complexity imposes with respect to selecting or developing appropriate therapeutics.

CELLULAR MEDIATORS

Microglia

In the mid-1980s it was discovered that microglia in the AD cortex could be labeled with antibodies to major histocompatibility complex type II cell surface glycoprotein (MHCII), a classic marker for activated immune cells (Luber-Narod and Rogers 1988; McGeer et al. 1988; Rogers et al. 1988). This not only created a much more convenient way to identify microglia compared to previous silver methods, but also opened the possibility that the brain might not be quite so immunologically privileged as previously supposed. Today, microglia are generally recognized as the brain's resident macrophages, and are considered to be pivotal players in innate immune/inflammatory responses in multiple neurologic disorders, including Parkinson's disease (Rogers et al. 2007), HIV dementia (Garden 2002), multiple sclerosis (Muzio et al. 2007), amyotrophic lateral sclerosis (Dewil et al. 2007), AD (Mandrekar-Colucci and Landreth 2010), and others. There is also general consensus on mechanisms of microglial actions in both the normal and diseased CNS, from the remarkable ability of these cells to survey vast extents of the brain (Davalos et al. 2005; Nimmerjahn et al. 2005; Wake et al. 2009) to their expression of classic pro- and anti-inflammatory mediators and receptors (Lue et al. 2001a,b; Wyss-Coray 2006; Cameron and Landreth 2010). Important advances beyond this basic body of knowledge, however, continue to be made, particularly with regard to intermediate states of microglial activation (reviewed in Colton and Willcock 2010) and microglial interactions with amyloid β peptide (Aβ) (reviewed in Combs 2009; Lee and Landreth 2010). For other recent and thorough reviews of microglia, the reader is referred to the excellent summaries by Colton (2009), Mandrekar-Colucci and Landreth (2010), and El Khoury and Luster (2008).

Microglia in the developing brain ultimately derive from the mesenchyme, in which myeloid progenitors give rise to cells that migrate to the CNS and proliferate as microglia (Rezaie and Male 2002). Migration of blood-derived macrophages into the CNS has also been suggested to occur later in fetal development (reviewed in Chan et al. 2007). Throughout development, microglia may play an important role in remodeling of the brain by removing presumably redundant, apoptotic neurons (Bessis et al. 2007; Caldero et al. 2009). In vivo activity of microglia has recently been visualized using two photon microscopy techniques (Davalos et al. 2005; Nimmerjahn et al. 2005; Wake et al. 2009). The extraordinary, dynamic images from these studies reveal that microglia constantly sample their immediate environment, including neighboring glia, blood vessels, and neurons, by extending and retracting their processes for distances up to some 80 μm (Nimmerjahn et al. 2005). In this manner, it has been estimated that the microglial population may survey the entire brain every few hours. Loss of synapses encountered by microglial processes has been reported using in vivo microscopy (Wake et al. 2009), supporting the potential role of microglia in normal synaptic remodeling. Microglia also contribute to a healthy CNS by attacking and removing potential pathogens and detritus, and by secreting tissue rebuilding factors (Wyss-Coray 2006). These essential, supportive mechanisms have been emphasized by Streit and Xue (2009), who have contended that "the only 'bad' microglial cell is a dead microglial cell."

Alternatively, several hundred reports of microglial attack mechanisms in neurologic disease suggest a more complex view. For example, in vitro, these cells secrete a wide range of inflammatory factors, many of which have the potential to automodulate microglial phenotype (see below) and to impact bystander neurons and their processes. These include reactive oxygen species (Coraci et al. 2002); Th1 cytokines such as IL-1β, IL-6, TNF-α, and interferon γ (INF-γ) (Lue et al. 2001a); chemokines such as macrophage inflammatory protein 1α (MIP1α), MIP1β, CXCL8, RANTES, and monocyte chemotactic protein 1 (MCP1) (El Khoury et al. 2003, 2007 2008); growth factors such as macrophage colony stimulating factor (Lue et al. 2001a); and complement components such as C1q, C3, C4, and C9 (Walker et al. 1995, 2001). They also express receptors associated with inflammatory activation, attack, and phagocytosis, including cytokine receptors (reviewed in Akiyama et al. 2000; John et al. 2003), chemokine receptors (Cartier et al. 2005; El Khoury et al. 2008), complement receptor 3 (Sedgwick et al. 1991), the receptor for advanced glycation endproducts (RAGE) (Walker and Lue 2005), Fc receptors (Okun et al. 2010), CD40 (Tan et al. 1999), formyl peptide (FP) receptors (Chen et al. 2007a; Brandenburg et al. 2008), various scavenger receptors (El Khoury et al. 1998; El Khoury and Luster 2008), and toll-like receptors (TLRs) (Landreth and Reed-Geaghan 2009). Elevation of these factors in culture and animal models typically results in neurodegeneration, and all have been reported to be elevated in pathologically-vulnerable regions of the AD brain (reviewed in Akiyama et al. 2000; Rogers et al. 2007; Landreth and Reed-Geaghan 2009). Similarly, signal transduction and transcription factor (e.g., NF-κB, PPARγ, Sp1) alterations associated with inflammation have been observed in microglial cultures and AD brain (Citron et al. 2008; Jiang et al. 2008; Granic et al. 2009; Mandrekar-Colucci and Landreth 2010). Not surprisingly, microglia are also capable of secreting anti-inflammatory mediators and growth factors such as IL-4, IL-10, IL-13, and TGF-β (reviewed in Wyss-Coray 2006; Colton 2009), just as peripheral monocytes do in the tissue-rebuilding phase that follows inflammatory attack.

Although there are likely to be multiple stimuli for the inflammatory responses of microglia in the AD brain, including simple detritus from other pathogenic reactions, aggregated Aβ deposits appear to be especially potent, as indicated by the dense accumulations of microglia expressing MHCII and other markers of activation within and around such deposits (Luber-Narod and Rogers 1988; McGeer et al. 1988; Rogers et al. 1988). Consistent with these histologic findings in situ, human elderly microglia in culture have been shown to migrate to aggregated Aβ spots dried down to the well floor, and to internalize portions of the Aβ (Lue et al. 2001b; Walker and Lue 2005). Similarly, microglia cultured on sections of AD cortex accumulate on Aβ deposits and appear to remove them (Bard et al. 2000). Additional studies have suggested, however, that microglia may not be able to degrade the Aβ they have taken up (Paresce et al. 1997; Walker and Lue 2005; Majumdar et al. 2007, 2008), potentially leading to a state of "frustrated phagocytosis" and to phenotypic and functional changes in the microglia.

Two-photon microscopy has clarified the anatomic relationships of microglia to Aβ by showing that microglial processes sample and react to Aβ deposits in transgenic mouse models. Recruitment of microglia to newly-formed plaques occurred within a few days in one study (Meyer-Luehmann et al. 2008), and was followed, in several studies, by establishment of a dynamic interface between microglial processes and Aβ deposits (Bolmont et al. 2008; Koenigsknecht-Talboo et al. 2008; Yan et al. 2009). Internalization and lysosome colocalization of Aβ was observed by Bolmont and colleagues (2008), and damage to neighboring neurons, coincident with the arrival of microglia, has also been reported (Meyer-Luehmann et al. 2008). Alternatively, Meyer-Luehmann and coworkers (2008) did not observe resolution of plaques over "days to weeks," and it remains to be shown whether or not the neurodegeneration following microglial recruitment to plaques is directly caused by the microglia. Positron emission tomography (PET) using benzodiazepine ligands for activated microglia has shown increasing signal for these cells in living AD versus control subjects (Cagnin et al. 2001; Edison et al. 2008), and an inverse correlation between benzodiazepine-positive microglial load and cognitive status scores (Edison et al. 2008). Notably, however, microglial load did not correlate with Aβ burden in the same subjects (Edison et al. 2008), and Wiley et al. (2009) were unable to confirm elevated microglial signal in AD subjects. Given repeated histologic findings of dense accumulations of microglia labeled with other activation markers (e.g., MHCII, IL-1) at sites of Aβ deposition, it may be that benzodiazepine binding, which also marks at least some astrocytes (Ji et al. 2008), may be labeling a microglial phenotype that is less engaged in interactions with Aβ. In addition, Aβ is unlikely to be the only stimulus for microglial activation in the AD brain. New studies with potentially more specific microglial ligands may help resolve these issues.

Mechanistic studies of the inflammatory factors and receptors mediating microglial localization and responses to Aβ have also been fruitful. In vitro, Aβ has been shown to stimulate expression of nearly all the proinflammatory mediators discussed earlier (c.f., Lue et al. 2001a; Walker et al. 2001), and many of the previously mentioned innate immune response receptors found on microglia have Aβ either as a direct or indirect ligand. For example, direct RAGE/Aβ binding helps guide microglia to Aβ deposits, an effect that is inhibited by treatment with anti-RAGE antibodies (Walker and Lue 2005; Chen et al. 2007b). Complement opsonization of Aβ (Rogers et al. 1992) and/ or binding to anti-Aβ antibodies (Bard et al. 2000) may also permit indirect interactions via microglial expression of complement receptor 3 (Sedgwick et al. 1991) and Fc receptors (Okun et al. 2010).

Over the last two decades, controversies have arisen as to whether microglia should be regarded as friend or foe to the nervous system (reviewed in Wyss-Coray 2006). This is perhaps natural given a cell type that is neuroprotective primarily by virtue of its capacity for attack. Microglia do not prevent apoptosis, neurodegenerative debris, bacterial invasion, or Aβ deposits; they attempt to remove such pathologies before further damage is performed. They also secrete anti-inflammatory mediators and growth factors. For these and other reasons, microglia are certainly vital to promoting a healthy CNS. Alternatively, many studies have shown that microglia are capable of killing or damaging neurons and, indeed, multiple mechanisms and mediators in brain appear to be devoted to keeping such toxicity in check, including CD22 (Mott et al. 2004), CD200

(Walker et al. 2009), fractalkine (Ransohoff 2007), TREM2 (Hsieh et al. 2009), and the complement defense protein CD59 (Singhrao et al. 1999; Yang et al. 2000).

A more balanced and sophisticated view of these issues is emerging from new research showing a continuum of microglial activation states that parallel similar phenotypic changes in peripheral macrophages (reviewed in Gordon and Taylor 2005; Colton 2009). Mediated primarily by the Th2 cytokines, IL-4, IL-10, IL-13, and TGF-β, deactivating alterations to macrophage and microglial morphology, antigenicity, and function appear to occur as coordinated, restorative sequelae after initial proinflammatory responses to pathogens and injury, and may be invoked in a long term fashion under conditions in which small amounts of the offending agent persist after an inflammatory attack (Bogdan 2008). Frustrated phagocytosis of Aβ may qualify as such an event. Several activation state nomenclatures have been suggested. Some are based on peripheral macrophage responses (M1, M2a, M2b, M2c) and reflect macrophage populations that are induced by specific Th2 cytokines and other factors (e.g., immune complexes, apoptotic cells) (Gordon and Taylor 2005). Colton (2009), has summarized an activation nomenclature that embraces many of the findings that have been reported for macrophages but works particularly well for microglia. Here, three activation states are proposed: 1) classical activation, which is stimulated by IFN-γ and characterized functionally by attack mechanisms; 2) alternative activation, which is stimulated by IL-4 and IL-13 and characterized functionally by tissue restorative, anti-inflammatory mechanisms; and 3) acquired deactivation, which is stimulated by TGF-β, IL-10, and apoptotic cells and characterized functionally by immunosuppression (but with a retained ability to phagocytose apoptotic cells). A mixture of classical activation, acquired deactivation, and increasing alternative activation is observed in AD (Colton 2009), and may ultimately further our understanding of the complex roles that microglia may play in neurodegenerative diseases, as well as how to manipulate them therapeutically.

For example, agents that drive microglia to a phenotype that favors attack on potential pathogens rather than bystander neurons should be an appealing target.

Astrocytes

Astrocytes are an essential neurosupportive cell type in brain. Their well-known interactions with neurons include secretion and recycling of transmitters, ion homeostasis, regulation of energy metabolism, synaptic remodeling, and modulation of oxidative stress. Tiling the entire brain in contiguous, orderly fashion, each single gray matter astrocyte has been estimated to envelope as many as 100,000 synapses (Halassa et al. 2007). As such, perturbation of the many neurosupportive astrocyte functions can have extremely deleterious consequences for the CNS (reviewed in Belanger and Magistretti 2009). Moreover, like microglia, astrocytes respond quickly to pathology with changes in their morphology, antigenicity, and function, and, like microglia, these reactive states have been increasingly recognized as a continuum with potentially beneficial and destructive consequences (reviewed in Sofroniew and Vinters 2010).

In brain of AD patients (Sofroniew and Vinters 2010) and AD transgenic mouse models (Rodriguez et al. 2009), reactive astrocytes occupy peri-plaque positions, encircling Aβ deposits in a manner reminiscent of glial scarring, a mechanism by which the cells may provide a barrier between healthy tissue and areas of injury or infection (Sofroniew and Vinters 2010). MCP1, which is highly concentrated in Aβ plaques, is chemotactic for adult astrocytes, and astrocytes express receptors that bind Aβ, including RAGE, low density lipoprotein receptor-like protein, membrane-associated proteoglycans, and scavenger receptor-like receptors. Collectively, these mechanisms may therefore account for the dense accumulation of reactive astrocytes at sites of aggregated Aβ deposition (Wyss-Coray et al. 2003). Several studies suggest that plaque-localized, reactive astrocytes take up and degrade Aβ (Nagele et al. 2003; Wyss-Coray et al. 2003; Koistinaho

et al. 2004). In Tg2576 transgenic mice such effects may be linked to insulin degrading enzyme (IDE), which appears to play a key role in Aβ degradation. Astrocyte expression of IDE is increased after Aβ exposure and is pronounced within glial fibrillary acidic protein (GFAP) immunoreactive astrocytes surrounding Aβ deposits (Leal et al. 2006). Extracellular clearance of Aβ may also occur via astrocyte secretion of matrix metalloproteinases (Yin et al. 2006). Exposure to Aβ, in turn, appears to disrupt astrocyte calcium homeostasis (Abramov et al. 2004; Chow et al. 2010), with subsequent increases in GFAP (Chow et al. 2010), a typical marker of astrocyte reactivity, as well as degeneration of neurons in astrocyte-neuron cocultures (Abramov et al. 2004).

Reactive astrocytes may provoke neuropathology through expression or overexpression of a number of inflammation-related factors. For example, S100β, a neurotropin that induces neurite proliferation, is overexpressed in AD brain and its levels are correlated with numbers of dystrophic neurites within Aβ deposits (Mrak et al. 1996). A similar correlation is found In APPV717F transgenic mouse brain, wherein astrocyte S100β overexpression increases with age to a point just prior to Aβ deposition (Sheng et al. 2000). In S100β overexpressing transgenic mice, inflammatory responses to intracerebroventricularly-infused Aβ are significantly augmented compared to wild-type and S100β knockout mice (Craft et al. 2005). After intracerebroventricular administration of lipopolysaccharide (LPS) or brain injury, both of which induce brain inflammation, astrocytes become more reactive and begin to show immunoreactivity for the γ-secretase components presenilin-1 and nicastrin (Nadler et al. 2008). Presenilin-2 expression also appears in AD but not nondemented control (ND) astrocytes (Takami et al. 1997). Exposure of cultured astrocytes to Aβ significantly increases IL-1β, TNF-α, iNOS, and NO production, with differential temporal effects depending on whether the Aβ is in fibrillar or oligomeric, nonfibrillar form (White et al. 2005). Transcripts for INF-γ and IL-12 are also increased in Tg2576 transgenic mouse astrocytes (and microglia) in an age-dependent manner (Abbas et al. 2002).

Many of these effects may trace back to alterations in astrocyte transcription factors. For example, the proinflammatory cytokines IL-1β, IL-6, and TNF-α are regulated by NF-κB and C/EBP transcription factor mechanisms. Astrocyte CEBPδ is dramatically upregulated in AD cortex (Li et al. 2004), and astrocyte NF-κB is activated on exposure to Aβ, leading to increased expression of IL-1β and IL-6 (Bales et al. 1998). NF-κB mechanisms in astrocytes also control secretion of chemokines and adhesion molecules that might permit invasion by peripheral leukocytes, further fueling the inflammatory response (Moynagh 2005). Calcineurin, a calcium-dependent phosphatase that helps mediate a wide range of inflammatory and calcium-dysregulatory responses, is increased in reactive AD astrocytes. In culture, adenoviral transfer of activated calcineurin results in astrocyte morphologic and gene expression profiles that closely parallel those observed in AD and AD transgenic mouse models (Norris et al. 2005). In turn, calcineurin actions induce activation and translocation of the transcription factor nuclear factor of activated T-cells (NFAT). Exposure of cultured astrocytes to Aβ activates NFAT, leading to decreases in excitatory amino acid transporter 2, increases in glutamate, and death of cocultured neurons (Abdul et al. 2009).

Oligodendrocytes

Oligodendrocytes and the myelin sheath they produce envelope axons and are critical for neurotransmission. Oligodendrocytes and myelin are also well known targets of immune reactions in other neurolgic disorders, particularly multiple sclerosis. Although AD research lags far behind in this area, histologic, molecular, electrophysiologic, and imaging data have revealed lesions and myelin abnormalities in AD white matter (reviewed in Roth et al. 2005), and focal demyelination of axons associated with Aβ deposits in gray matter has been convincingly shown in familial and sporadic AD, as well as in transgenic mouse models of AD (Mitew

et al. 2010). Stereotaxic injection of nM quantities of Aβ into the corpus callosum induces microglial proliferation, with attendent damage to myelin and losses of oligodendrocytes (Jantaratnotai et al. 2003). In vitro, oligodendrocyte toxicity has been reported for Aβ25-35 (Xu et al. 2001), Aβ40 (Xu et al. 2001; Lee et al. 2004), and Aβ42 (Roth et al. 2005). Perhaps because of their low glutathione and high iron content, oligodendroglia are also extremely vulnerable to oxidative stress (Juurlink 1997), one of the main weapons of inflammatory attack. Finally, oligodendrocytes have been reported to express mRNAs and to be immunoreactive for complement components C1q, C1s, C2, C3, C4, C5, C6, C7, C8, and C9, leading to the suggestion that they may be primary sources for the significantly increased levels of complement in pathologically-vulnerable regions of the AD brain (Hosokawa et al. 2003). Complement activation occurs on oligodendrocytes via C1q binding to myelin oligodendrocyte protein (Johns and Bernard 1997), and is likely to be enhanced by the low levels of C1 inhibitor and membrane cofactor protein expressed by the cells (Hosokawa et al. 2004). Given these conditions, it is not surprising that complement-activated oligodendroglia are observed in many neurodegenerative conditions in which inflammation has been identified, particularly AD (Yamada et al. 1990).

As with all the other cell types in this review, inflammation may play dual roles with respect to the oligodendrocyte. For example, several multiple sclerosis studies have suggested that an active, acute inflammatory response may be necessary for remyelination of demyelinated axons (Arnett et al. 2003; Foote and Blakemore 2005; Setzu et al. 2006). Likewise, Roth et al. (2005) have reported that Aβ42-mediated oligodendrocyte toxicity is actually reduced by prior exposure to LPS or INF-γ.

Neurons

As previously noted, neurons express a wide range of molecules that are designed to protect against inflammatory attack. These include CD22 (Mott et al. 2004), CD200 (Walker et al.

2009), fractalkine (Ransohoff 2007), TREM2 (Hsieh 2009), and the complement defense protein CD59 (Singhrao et al. 1999). Some of these protective mechanisms have been found to be deficient in AD. For example, neuronal expression of CD59 (Yang et al. 2000), and CD200 (Walker et al. 2009) is selectively decreased in pathologically-vulnerable regions of the AD brain. Fractalkine is also decreased in APP transgenic mouse cortex and hippocampus at ages in which these animals begin to show AD pathology (Duan et al. 2008). In fact, neither AD nor ND neurons express the complement regulators decay accelerating factor and complement receptor 1, and only weakly express membrane cofactor protein, suggesting that neurons should be particularly vulnerable to complement reactions (Singhrao et al. 1999).

MOLECULAR MEDIATORS

The Complement System

The complement system represents a key inflammatory pathway for the activation and execution of immune responses (Holers 1996). Because complement appears to be activated in neurodegenerative diseases and complement proteins are associated with plaques and tangles in AD, this pathway may hold clues to AD inflammation in general.

The complement system is capable of recognizing molecular patterns on pathogens or molecular patterns associated with injured tissues and dying cells. Recognition may be through C1q or mannose binding proteins, which contain collagen-like receptor binding domains (Tenner 1999), or through interactions with the multifunctional protein C3 (Sahu and Lambris 2001). Once activated, a diverse array of almost 30 proteins in the complement pathway can attract and activate immune cells, amplify antigen-specific immune responses, promote phagocytosis, facilitate complement-mediated cytolysis by the membrane attack complex (MAC), and regulate cell proliferation and differentiation (Fig. 1) (Holers 1996). Antigen-antibody complexes or antibodies bound to solid surfaces activate the

classical pathway of complement by binding C1q and then activating C1r and C1s, followed by C4, C2, and C3. Bacteria and various molecular patterns present, for example, on DNA or certain sugars can activate the alternative pathway by binding C3b and Factor B. Finally, mannose moieties on bacteria are recognized by mannan binding lectin in the lectin pathway (not shown in figure). All pathways result in the formation of multiprotein catalytic activities, the C3 convertases, generating two proteolytic C3 fragments: C3a, which is released in the fluid phase and involved in the chemotaxis of phagocytes, and C3b, which can bind covalently to acceptor molecules in solution or on cellular surfaces (Carroll 1998). C3b binding may activate the lytic pathway involving C5, C6, C7, C8, and C9, which culminates in the formation of the MAC, C5b-9, and may lead to cytotoxicity. This pathway also leads to the formation of C5a, another small proinflammatory peptide. Alternatively, C3b binding to targeted molecules, in a process called opsonization, mediates phagocytosis by a number of cells through their surface expression of complement receptors (Carroll 1998). In addition, bound C3b can be cleaved into smaller fragments, including iC3b, C3dg, and C3d, that can mediate binding of opsonized fragments to distinct complement receptors (CRs) (Holers 1996; Sahu and Lambris 2001). The CRs include C3aR, CR1 (CD35), CR2 (CD21), CR3 (CD11b/CD18), and CR4 (CD11c/CD18).

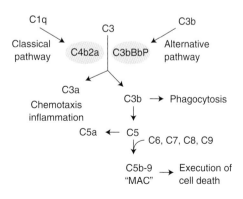

Figure 1. Brief schematic of the complement system (see text for details).

Complement proteins are produced mostly in the liver and are present at high levels in serum. However, glial cells and neurons in the CNS can synthesize these proteins as well, and their production is increased in brain injury and neurodegeneration (D'Ambrosio et al. 2001; Gasque 2004), including AD (Rogers et al. 1996; McGeer and McGeer 1999; Akiyama et al. 2000; Emmerling et al. 2000; Gasque et al. 2000). C1q and the MAC colocalize with amyloid plaques and tangle-bearing neurons (Eikelenboom and Stam 1982; Eikelenboom et al. 1989; Itagaki et al. 1994; Webster et al. 1997; Shen et al. 2001; Fonseca et al. 2004a). More recent support for activation of complement in AD comes from a number of transcriptome studies showing that complement gene expression is increased in the disease (Blalock et al. 2004; Katsel et al. 2009).

Assuming an absence of microbial pathogens, what might be the cause for activation of complement? Aggregated Aβ activates the complement system in vitro through the classical pathway by binding C1q and through the alternative pathway by binding C3b (Rogers et al. 1992; Jiang et al. 1994). Isolated tangles or tau aggregates can also activate the classical pathway by binding C1q (Shen et al. 2001). The accumulation of Aβ and tau may therefore promote the activation of complement and possibly neuroinflammation. Others have hypothesized that CNS antigen-specific autoantibodies can reach the CNS and, similar to glutamate receptor specific antibodies in Rasmussen's encephalitis, bind to neurons and other cells and activate the classical pathway of complement (D'Andrea 2003).

As mentioned earlier, complement can recognize degenerating or dying cells and fulfills an important role in the clearance of dead or degenerating cells in various tissues (Botto et al. 1998; Taylor et al. 2000). Although there is no direct support for this mechanism in AD, C1q has been shown to tag apoptotic neurons or neuronal blebs and promote their uptake by microglia in cell culture (Fraser et al. 2010). Moreover, C1q and C3 have recently been shown to mediate synaptic pruning during development and in a model of glaucoma, opening the possibility that complement factors may contribute to elimination of synapses in neurodegenerative diseases (Stevens et al. 2007).

Although none of the above observations can answer whether complement activation is beneficial or detrimental in AD, a number of studies have begun to address this question. APP mouse models in which C3 activation is inhibited by the overexpression of soluble complement receptor-related protein y (sCrry) show an increase in Aβ deposition and an accumulation of degenerating neurons (Wyss-Coray et al. 2002). Consistent with these findings, APP mice with a complete knockout of C3 also show increased Aβ and neuronal degeneration, accompanied by changes in microglial activation (Maier et al. 2008). These data suggest that C3 may work with microglia to help clear Aβ. Other studies have additionally shown that APP mice lacking complement C1q have less neuronal damage and glial cell activation than complement-sufficient mice, suggesting a role for C1q in neuronal integrity (Fonseca et al. 2004b). Alternatively, the "peripheral sink" hypothesis of DeMattos and colleagues (2001), involving binding of circulating Aβ to Aβ autoantibodies, may also apply to C3-opsonized Aβ in the peripheral circulation. In particular, a well-established mechanism for clearance of circulating pathogens, immune adherence (reviewed in Atkinson et al. 1994; Birmingham and Hebert 2001), appears to be operative with respect to circulating Aβ. Here, C3-dependent binding of Aβ to human erythrocyte CR1 has been shown, and is reported to be significantly deficient in the vast majority of AD patients, as well as many mild cognitive impairment (MCI) subjects (Rogers et al. 2006). Notably, subprimates do not express erythrocyte CR1, so that this pathway would not be evident in AD transgenic mouse models. Because previous transgenic mouse manipulations of the complement system (Wyss-Coray et al. 2002; Maier et al. 2008) were systemic and not restricted to brain, it is also possible that the effects observed on Aβ loads and neurodegeneration might have been mediated by alterations in peripheral complement mechanisms, alterations in brain complement mechanisms, or both.

In summary, complement is activated in AD, where it may exert regulatory functions and aid in the clearance of degenerating cells and protein aggregates. However, it is likely also to promote unwanted inflammation. Genetic susceptibility studies have recently linked single nucleotide polymorphisms in clusterin (ApoJ), a potent regulator of complement activation, and CR1 as relatively strong susceptibility genes for AD (Harold et al. 2009; Lambert et al. 2009). How these polymorphisms affect complement activity is unknown.

Cytokines and Other Soluble Signaling Proteins

Cytokines, chemokines, and related immune proteins are part of a soluble network of communication factors between cells. Although many of these proteins were discovered as potent regulators of inflammation and immune function, it is well accepted now that they have pleiotropic effects in many tissues, including the CNS, and regulate diverse cellular processes such as proliferation, survival, and differentiation. Numerous cytokines and chemokines have also been linked to CNS development. It is therefore not surprising that many of these proteins have altered levels in AD (Akiyama et al. 2000). Cytokine or chemokine changes in the brain parenchyma are frequently accompanied by parallel changes in protein levels in the CSF, and some of these proteins appear to be dysregulated in the periphery as well (Ray et al. 2007; Zhang et al. 2008; Soares et al. 2009; Hu et al. 2010b). The consequences of cytokine or chemokine changes on brain function and neurodegeneration relevant to AD are unknown, but a growing number of genetic studies in mice show that these immune proteins have potent effects on amyloidosis, neurodegeneration, and cognition (Wyss-Coray and Mucke 2002; Wyss-Coray 2006). Tumor necrosis factor (TNF)-α is one such factor that has received much attention because of its ability to promote Parkinson's disease (PD) progression (McCoy et al. 2006), whereas TNF receptor 1 knockout protects against AD- and PD-like disease in mice (Sriram et al. 2002; He

et al. 2007). Similarly potent effects are exerted by transforming growth factor (TGF)-β1, which is increased in human AD brains at the transcript and protein level, whereas TGF receptor expression is decreased (Wyss-Coray et al. 1997; Tesseur et al. 2006). TGF-β1 promotes cerebrovascular amyloidosis but delays parenchymal Aβ accumulation in APP mice that also overproduce this cytokine from astrocytes (Wyss-Coray et al. 2001). Interestingly, although APP mice with deficient TGF-β signaling in neurons show more neurodegeneration and amyloid accumulation (Tesseur et al. 2006), other APP mice expressing the same receptor in myeloid cells have reduced disease (Town et al. 2008). These studies on TGF-β provide a good example of the complexity of cytokine biology and how targeting such pathways in disease may be very challenging. Likewise, the chemokine CCL2 and its receptor CCR2, which play a key role in regulating the infiltration of peripheral monocytes into the brain (Charo and Ransohoff 2006), show a complex role in AD. Lack of CCR2 in mice results in reduced accumulation of microglia/monocytes in the brain and accelerates disease progression and Aβ deposition in a mouse model of AD (El Khoury et al. 2007). Because microglia from CCR2 knockout mice do not show aberrant proliferation (El Khoury et al. 2007), it has been postulated that changes in microglia accumulation are a consequence of monocyte infiltration. Conversely, overexpressing CCL2 in the brain results in increased microglial accumulation (Yamamoto et al. 2005). However, overexpressing CCL2 also results in increased Aβ accumulation, which may be due to a prominent increase in mouse ApoE (Yamamoto et al. 2005), a factor known to independently enhance Aβ deposition (Bales et al. 1999).

Several other cytokine mRNAs or proteins are expressed at increased or decreased levels in AD brain or periphery (Wyss-Coray 2006). A number of these have also been studied in AD mouse models, including IL-1β and IL-6, which surprisingly both appear to have beneficial effects on amyloidosis. Thus, using an inducible expression cassette, O'Banion's group showed that short-term expression of IL-1β in adult APP mice resulted in strong activation of glial cells, induction of various inflammatory factors, and reduced amyloid pathology (Shaftel et al. 2007). Similarly, viral overexpression of IL-6 in the hippocampus led to massive gliosis and neuroinflammation, reduced amyloidosis, and amelioration of cognitive deficits in APP mice (Chakrabarty et al. 2010). Interestingly, lifelong stable overexpression of IL-1 receptor antagonist or IL-6 had no effect on pathogenesis in another APP mouse model consistent with the concept that acute but not chronic activation of certain types of immune responses in the brain may be beneficial (Wyss-Coray 2006). Treatment of APP mice with macrophage-colony stimulating factor (M-CSF) (Boissonneault et al. 2009) or granulocyte-colony stimulating factor (G-CSF) (Sanchez-Ramos et al. 2009) in the periphery also had ameliorating effects on cognition and disease progression in these mice.

In summary, many cytokines and chemokines are clearly expressed at abnormal levels in AD. Although these proteins can strongly activate glial cells and induce neuroinflammation, they have surprisingly beneficial effects in mouse models of AD. Whether therapies based on these findings may be efficient in humans is unknown.

Toll-Like and Other Pattern Recognition Receptors

The immune system uses a large number of highly conserved pattern recognition receptors to detect either exogenous molecules associated with pathogens or endogenous molecules generated in response to cell and tissue injury (Janeway and Medzhitov 2002; Seong and Matzinger 2004). In addition to the complement recognition proteins discussed earlier, toll-like receptors (TLRs) have received particular attention with respect to their role in the injured CNS and possibly in AD (Landreth and Reed-Geaghan 2009). Stimulation of TLRs, of which there are at least 13 distinct members to date (Iwasaki and Medzhitov 2004), induces activation of NF-κB and subsequent transcriptional activation of numerous proinflammatory genes (Nguyen et al. 2002). In the CNS, TLRs are expressed prominently on microglia, but other cells express certain TLRs as well (Aravalli et al. 2007). CNS microinjections of the TLR 2 or 4 ligands zymosan and lipopolysaccharide (LPS), respectively, cause robust glial activation and elicit substantial neurodegeneration (Popovich et al. 2002; Lehnardt et al. 2003). Consistent with these findings, TLR4-deficient mice have smaller infarct volumes and better functional outcomes than control mice in a sterile model of experimental stroke (Caso et al. 2007). One well-known TLR activator is Aβ, which binds the TLR4 coreceptor CD14 (Fassbender et al. 2004; Liu et al. 2005) and can trigger microglia to secrete nitric oxide, IL-6, and other neurotoxic factors (Walter et al. 2007). Microglia lacking CD14, TLR2, or TLR4 appear to be unable to activate NF-κB or p38 MAP kinase signaling or phagocytosis in response to fibrillar Aβ (Reed-Geaghan et al. 2009). Perhaps as a result, levels of TNF-α and MIP-1β are significantly higher in the brains of AD mice with wild-type TLR4 than their mutant TLR4 AD mouse counterparts (Jin et al. 2008). On the other hand, TLR-mediated activation of microglia may also aid in the clearance of Aβ. Studies in AD mouse models with mutant TLR2 or TLR4 suggest that deficiencies in TLR signaling may cause cognitive impairments with a concomitant increase in Aβ deposition (Tahara et al. 2006; Richard et al. 2008). Likewise, acute administration of the TLR4 ligand LPS can promote Aβ clearance (DiCarlo et al. 2001). Whether these receptors normally exacerbate neurodegeneration or guide the clearance of protein aggregates is still largely unknown. In addition, it may be noteworthy that many studies, particularly with Aβ, have not considered the aggregation state of the peptide. The TLRs, however, are likely to be differentially engaged by monomers, oligomers, or fibrillar assemblies of Aβ and other amyloidogenic peptides, eliciting different types of responses in microglia (and other cells).

The receptor for advanced glycation endproducts (RAGE) is yet another pattern recognition receptor that has been linked to AD and has a critical role in inflammation. RAGE ligand binding results in the activation of Jak/Stat and NF-κB signaling, is up-regulated in AD brains, and functions as a receptor for Aβ (Schmidt et al. 2009). Using double transgenic PDAPP-J20 mice overproducing either wild-type RAGE (APP/RAGE) or a mutant RAGE protein that inhibits the endogenous receptor function (i.e., a dominant negative RAGE receptor, APP/dnRAGE), Arancio and colleagues showed a detrimental role for RAGE signaling in Aβ dependent neuronal perturbation that appears to involve NF-κB and MAPK signaling and results in increased synaptic transmission deficits, as well as cognitive impairment (Arancio et al. 2004). In a more aggressive mouse model of amyloidosis, expressing APP with an arctic mutation deletion of the RAGE gene did not have an effect on amyloid deposition or cognition in 12-month-old mice, although it dramatically reduced fibrillar Aβ deposits in 6-month-old mice (Vodopivec et al. 2009). Thus, although RAGE seems to be sufficient to mediate detrimental effects of Aβ, it may not be necessary.

Cyclooxygenases and Arachidonic Acid Metabolites

Cyclooxygenases (COX) convert arachidonic acid to prostaglandinH2 (PGH2), the first step in the synthesis of numerous prostanoids with different functions. Although COX-1 is constitutively expressed in many cell types and tissues and may be involved in the physiological production of prostanoids, COX-2 is increased during inflammation, resulting in proinflammatory prostanoid synthesis (Warner and Mitchell 2004). As one of the key targets of non-steroidal anti-inflammatory drugs (NSAIDs), cyclooxygenases were first strongly implicated in AD by a meta-analysis of 17 epidemiologic studies of long term NSAID use, wherein such long term use reduced AD risk by half (McGeer et al. 1996). These findings have been confirmed in a number of subsequent reports, but have not led to successful treatment trials thus far (see Clinical Studies below).

One possible reason for this failure may be that, like many other inflammatory mediators, prostaglandins are janus-faced, exerting beneficial or toxic functions depending on the setting. For example, COX-2, which is localized to post-synaptic sites, is involved in modulating physiological synaptic transmission, but excessive activation in pathological conditions or genetic overexpression in neurons in transgenic mice induces neuronal apoptosis and cognitive deficits (Andreasson et al. 2001; Liang et al. 2007). Transgenic overexpression of COX-2 in neurons has also been shown to lead to a two-fold increase in Aβ plaque formation in one APP mouse model (Xiang et al. 2002) and cognitive deficits in another model (Melnikova et al. 2006), supporting a detrimental role for COX-2 and its downstream products in neurodegeneration and AD. To characterize the function of the various prostanoids in CNS function and in AD, the Andreasson laboratory has studied mouse models with deficiencies in specific prostanoid receptors. Mice lacking PGE2 receptor EP2 have electrophysiological defects in the hippocampus and are cognitively impaired (Savonenko et al. 2009), but deletion of this receptor in APP mice results in less amyloidosis. Compared to APP mice without EP2 deletion, APP/EP2 knockout mice also show half the levels of F2-isoprostanes and F4-neuroprostanes, both of which are indicators of lipid peroxidation (Liang et al. 2005). On the other hand, EP4, another PGE2 receptor, seems to strongly inhibit inflammatory activation of microglia in vivo based on selective deletion experiments using the cre-lox system in mice (Shi et al. 2010). Together, these studies show that EP2 is necessary for normal physiological function in the CNS, but has detrimental effects in the inflammatory setting present in APP mouse brains, whereas EP4 functions as an inhibitor of inflammation. New therapeutic strategies targeting specific prostanoid receptors may therefore provide better tools to regulate inflammation in AD than conventional NSAIDs.

MOLECULAR GENETICS

Technologies to interrogate ever-larger numbers of biological molecules from complex fluids or tissues have become more generally available to researchers, and many studies have taken advantage of these tools to characterize vast numbers of genetic polymorphisms in the human genome, the complete transcriptome, or subsets of the proteome in AD. Perhaps not surprisingly, many of the "hits" or final lists of factors from these studies include molecules involved in immune and inflammatory responses. Future studies will nonetheless be necessary to determine whether any of them do indeed have a role in AD or could be used as biomarkers.

For example, two genome-wide association studies that interrogated several hundred thousand polymorphisms in the human genome in thousands of patients and controls have recently identified clusterin and CR1 as genetically linked to sporadic AD (Harold et al. 2009; Lambert et al. 2009). A similarly-scaled study from the Mayo Clinic confirmed these findings with a surprising congruency in effect size and probability (Jun et al. 2010), although odds ratios for both genes were rather small. The biological significance or functional involvement of clusterin and CR1 in AD are unknown, but it is intriguing that both genes point to the complement system (see above). In addition, significant genetic linkages of single nucleotide polymorphisms or haplotypes in case-control or population-based studies have been described for cytokines, chemokines, and acute phase proteins. These genes show typically very modest effects on AD risk and their biological significance is unknown. A ranking of polymorphisms based on meta-analyses of multiple association studies is available at AlzGene.org (http://www.alz-gene.org) (Bertram et al. 2007).

Changes in inflammatory pathways have also been noted in several microarray studies of gene expression profiles in AD brains or peripheral blood cells compared with those from healthy controls. In a review comparing several such transcriptome studies of the aging brain with those in AD, Blalock and colleagues (2005) noted that genes associated with inflammation are increased in aging, and that this is accentuated in AD. In agreement with this conclusion, a recent study in people above or below age 86 with or without AD reported a striking increase in transcripts related to major histocompatibility complex (MHC) genes, the complement cascade, and phagocytosis in the cognitively normal oldest-old compared to the other groups (Katsel et al. 2009), supporting the concept that a gain in brain immunity may be protective and that a failure to adapt to aging underlies neurodegeneration. Gene expression studies in blood cells from AD patients have also found many changes associated with immune and inflammatory pathways when compared to age-matched controls (Kalman et al. 2005; Fiala et al. 2007; Maes et al. 2007).

Consistent with transcriptional changes in immune-related factors in brain and blood, differences in levels of soluble immune mediators and other communication factors in cerebrospinal fluid or plasma have been linked to AD in antibody-based proteomic studies (Ray et al. 2007; Soares et al. 2009; Hu et al. 2010a,b). In addition, several reports have found complement proteins as well as clusterin to be among the most significant proteins discriminating AD from healthy control plasma using two-dimensional gel electrophoresis and mass spectrometry-based unbiased approaches (Hye et al. 2006; Sheta et al. 2006; Thambisetty et al. 2010). Whether these systemic changes directly relate to the neuropathology and cognitive impairment in AD is unknown and it remains to be seen whether they have diagnostic utility.

CLINICAL STUDIES

Epidemiology

Over 30 epidemiologic studies, including nine prospective studies, have evaluated the possibility that anti-inflammatory drug use might reduce risk or delay onset of AD, with the vast majority reporting beneficial effects. Many caveats have been given, however, for both the positive and negative findings. With respect to negative results, for example, many of the earliest surveys (e.g., Heyman et al. 1984) simply included anti-inflammatory drugs as one of many potential risk or protective factors for

AD, and may therefore have had an insufficient number of drug users to detect an effect. Other early studies, both positive and negative, were somewhat indirect, examining risk for AD given the presence of other disorders such as rheumatoid arthritis (reviewed as a meta-analysis by McGeer et al. 1996) and leprosy (McGeer et al. 1992), in which chronic and substantial use of anti-inflammatory drugs would be expected. The timing and duration of drug administration might also have been a complicating factor, as suggested by two early observational reports (in 't Veld et al. 2001; Zandi et al. 2002). Here, NSAID reduction of AD risk appeared to require the completion of a 2- to 3-year period of prior NSAID use. During that period of use, however, there was no reduction of AD risk (Zandi et al. 2002) or even a nonsignificant increase in AD risk (in 't Veld et al. 2001), suggesting that there may be a critical period and minimum duration for NSAID administration. Finally, lack of detail about the amount, duration, and, especially, type of anti-inflammatory drug taken by subjects was a common problem among early observational reports.

More recent, prospective studies have circumvented many of these challenges, typically evaluating a thousand or more subjects, categorizing anti-inflammatory drug classes, and sometimes obtaining explicit data on drug amounts and durations of use from pharamacy and computer records. In general, seven of these nine studies (Stewart et al. 1997; in 't Veld et al. 2001; Lindsay et al. 2002; Zandi et al. 2002; Cornelius et al. 2004; Szekely et al. 2008; Vlad et al. 2008) found that NSAID use was associated with a significantly decreased risk for AD. Moreover, a meta-analysis of a subset of these reports in which duration of use data were available showed that longer periods of NSAID use decreased risk in a duration-dependent manner (Szekely et al. 2007), a finding confirmed in a subsequent study with >200,000 AD and control cases (Vlad et al. 2008). Of the two remaining prospective studies (Arvanitakis et al. 2008; Breitner et al. 2009), Breitner and colleagues (2009) have argued that their discrepant, negative findings may be due to the possibility that NSAID use does not simply decrease AD risk,

but rather delays AD onset to later ages. If so, then one would expect a higher incidence of AD among very old NSAID users and a lower incidence among younger NSAID users. Subjects in the two discrepant studies were, in fact, markedly older than those in the seven positive studies.

Treatment Trials

Given the epidemiologic results, treatment trials with anti-inflammatory drugs have been disappointing. Again, however, many caveats can be given. A large-scale treatment trial with an enantiomer of flurbiprofen, for example, is often lumped into summaries of the negative results of anti-inflammatory drug treatment despite the fact that, by design, the enantiomer had little to no anti-inflammatory activity (Green et al. 2009). Rather, the drug was designed to modulate γ-secretase, a property shared by ibuprofen, which also failed in a recent clinical trial—albeit with only 132 subjects and a 12-month duration (Pasqualetti et al. 2009).

Cyclooxygenase-2 (COX-2) inhibitors have also been employed, without success, in AD treatment trials (Aisen et al. 2003; Reines et al. 2004), and one such study with rofecoxib in MCI patients actually reported an increased hazard ratio (Thal et al. 2005). Alternatively, COX-2 is expressed in brain primarily by neurons (Yasojima et al. 1999), and may be neuroprotective (reviewed in McGeer 2000). Moreover, COX-2 inhibition increases Aβ42 secretion in vitro (Kukar et al. 2005). It has therefore been argued that inhibition of COX-2 mechanisms would likely have null or deleterious consequences in AD treatment trials (McGeer et al. 2006). COX-1, by contrast, is highly expressed by microglia, and has been suggested to be a more appropriate target (McGeer et al. 2006). Although the lone positive NSAID treatment trial for AD did, in fact, employ a potent COX-1 inhibitor, indomethacin, it should be noted that the study only evaluated 44 total subjects and used pooled data across multiple cognitive status tests (Rogers et al. 1993).

Finally, the steroid anti-inflammatory, prednisone, has been partially investigated in one pilot trial (Rogers et al. 1993) and explored specifically in a larger, randomized, multicenter trial (Aisen et al. 2000) with no positive outcome and with some notable adverse reactions. In the pilot trial, Rogers and colleagues (1993) anecdotally reported increased agitation and wandering in several AD patients treated with prednisone. Aisen and coinvestigators (2000) also observed behavioral abnormalities in such subjects.

Prevention Trials

Aside from the MCI treatment trial with rofecoxib cited earlier (Thal et al. 2005), no large-scale clinical trial of the ability of NSAIDs to prevent or delay onset of AD has ever been completed. The ADAPT Research Group (Lyketsos et al. 2007) attempted such a study, administering the nonselective COX-1 inhibitor naproxen, the selective COX-2 inhibitor celecoxib, or placebo to nearly 3000 cognitively normal individuals who were at elevated risk for AD by virtue of their age (≥ 70 years old) and possession of a first-degree relative with dementia. However, the study was halted early on because of newly emerging cardiovascular concerns about celecoxib (e.g., Mukherjee et al. 2001), as well as adverse reactions observed in the trial itself (ADAPT Research Group 2006). Among subjects who completed at least one cognitive assessment and were included in an interim analysis, a significant increase in AD risk ratios was observed for both celecoxib and naproxen, but only when 46 patients qualifying for a diagnosis of MCI or prodromal AD and erroneously entered into the study as cognitively normal were included. Excluding these participants, as well as seven others with AD who were also erroneously enrolled, revealed no significant change in the hazard ratio for either celecoxib ($P = 0.24$) or naproxen ($P = 0.30$). Several other caveats may obtain as well. For example, median durations of celecoxib and naproxen exposure were 1.54 and 1.53 years, respectively, whereas previous epidemiologic studies have generally observed duration-dependent effects of NSAIDs (e.g., the meta-analysis of Szekely et al. 2007), with a likely minimum duration of 2–3 years exposure before beneficial outcomes are observed (in 't Veld et al. 2001; Zandi et al. 2002). It is also worth noting that instances of conversion to AD were quite few in the trial, such that the results actually appear to rest almost wholly on nine conversions in the placebo group, 11 in the celecoxib group, and 12 in the naproxen group. Finally, anecdotal reports of presentations at international symposia by the study authors have suggested that further follow up of the study participants has shown at least a trend to a beneficial effect of treatment.

CONCLUSIONS

The genetic, cellular, and molecular changes associated with AD provide ever-stronger support for an activation of immune and inflammatory processes in the disease. Together with the epidemiological studies, which show a strong benefit of long-term use of NSAIDs, it is tempting to conclude that AD is an inflammatory disease and that inhibiting inflammation would be beneficial. However, there are several observations that indicate a more complex view, as well as the difficulties inherent in targeting inflammation in AD.

It is clear, most notably from animal models for AD, that many classical inflammatory proteins and cytokines have double-edged functions and that simply suppressing them may cause more harm than good. It is also puzzling that—at least in one study (Katsel et al. 2009), but not another (Blalock et al. 2004)—brains from the oldest-old, cognitively normal humans showed stronger expression of complement factors and other immune molecules than brains from age-matched AD patients or younger people, suggesting protective functions of molecules typically seen as deleterious. Lastly, the observation that inflammatory pathways are altered in the periphery in AD, together with evidence that increased peripheral inflammation leads to more neurodegeneration and accelerated disease progression in animal models (Nguyen et al. 2004; Cunningham et al. 2005; Frank-Cannon et al. 2008; Godoy et al. 2008;

Palin et al. 2008) and possibly in AD (Holmes et al. 2003), argue for caution in deciding where inflammation should be therapeutically targeted.

In their balanced, cogent synthesis of the clinical literature on anti-inflammatory drugs and AD, Szekely and Zandi (2010) conclude with several arguments for why AD clinical trials with anti-inflammatory drugs should not be disbanded because of the generally negative treatment trial results to date, but rather should continue to be explored. They note, for example, that some 30% of elderly adults take NSAIDs for indications other than AD. If nothing else, would it not be prudent to know what effect the drugs are having on cognition in this very large population, especially in view of reports that NSAIDs might actually increase AD risk under certain conditions (Thal et al. 2005; Breitner et al. 2009)? Moreover, even if all the positive results from the dozens of epidemiologic studies on inflammation and AD risk are spurious, these widely-obtained, statistically significant results are unlikely to have derived simply from chance. If associations of inflammation with other factors account for the data, would it not be useful to know what those other factors are? Much has also been made of the potential risks of NSAID use in the elderly, and these risks certainly exist—particularly gastrointestinal and nephrologic complications. However, at least for prevention trials, how can one make rational risk-benefit comparisons when the only data with respect to benefit derive from a handful of patients who converted to AD in a single, disbanded study (ADAPT Research Group 2006; Lyketsos et al. 2007)?

Finally, it may be worth considering that virtually no large-scale treatment trial of any drug has successfully halted, much less reversed, the pathological or cognitive decline of AD, perhaps because so much irremediable damage has been done to the brain in the already-afflicted patients employed in treatment trials. Such caveats may apply in double measure to anti-inflammatory drugs, which are typically employed not to redress existing damage, but to address additional, subsequent damage that may be caused by the inflammatory response

itself. Moreover, as covered in this review, inflammation encompasses dozens of highly interactive molecular mediators and mechanisms, some potentially helpful and some potentially harmful. Likewise, the different anti-inflammatory drug classes target different sets of mediators and mechanisms. If the new data on microglial activation states (reviewed in Colton 2009; Colton and Wilcock 2010) tell us nothing else, it is that more selectively targeted NSAIDs need to be developed or explored so as to encourage beneficial phenotypes and mechanisms while discouraging harmful phenotypes and mechanisms. Given the continuing stream of basic science and epidemiologic publications on inflammation and AD, prevention trials with rationally selected anti-inflammatory drugs may continue to warrant consideration.

ACKNOWLEDGMENTS

This work was supported by the Department of Veterans Affairs (T.W.C.), NIH grant AG27505 (T.W.C.), the Arizona Alzheimer's Consortium (J.R.), and NIH grant AGO7367 (J.R.).

REFERENCES

Abbas N, Bednar I, Mix E, Marie S, Paterson D, Ljungberg A, Morris C, Winblad B, Nordberg A, Zhu J. 2002. Up-regulation of the inflammatory cytokines IFN-γ and IL-12 and down-regulation of IL-4 in cerebral cortex regions of APP(SWE) transgenic mice. *J Neuroimmunol* **126:** 50–57.

Abdul HM, Sama MA, Furman JL, Mathis DM, Beckett TL, Weidner AM, Patel ES, Baig I, Murphy MP, LeVine H III, et al. 2009. Cognitive decline in Alzheimer's disease is associated with selective changes in calcineurin/NFAT signaling. *J Neurosci* **29:** 12957–12969.

Abramov AY, Canevari L, Duchen MR. 2004. β-amyloid peptides induce mitochondrial dysfunction and oxidative stress in astrocytes and death of neurons through activation of NADPH oxidase. *J Neurosci* **24:** 565–575.

ADAPT Research Group. 2006. Cardiovascular and cerebrovascular events in the randomized, controlled Alzheimer's disease anti-inflammatory prevention trial (ADAPT). *PLoS Clin Trials* **1:** e33.

Aisen PS, Davis KL, Berg JD, Schafer K, Campbell K, Thomas RG, Weiner MF, Farlow MR, Sano M, Grundman M, et al. 2000. A randomized controlled trial of prednisone in Alzheimer's disease. *Neurology* **54:** 588–593.

Aisen PS, Schafer KA, Grundman M, Pfeiffer E, Sano M, Davis KL, Farlow MR, Jin S, Thomas RG, Thal LJ. 2003. Effects of rofecoxib or naproxen vs placebo on

Alzheimer disease progression: A randomized controlled trial. *JAMA* **289:** 2819–2826.

Akiyama H, Barger S, Barnum S, Bradt B, Bauer J, Cole GM, Cooper NR, Eikelenboom P, Emmerling M, Fiebich BL, et al. 2000. Inflammation and Alzheimer's disease. Neuroinflammation Working Group. *Neurobiol Aging* **21:** 383–421.

Andersen K, Launer LJ, Ott A, Hoes AW, Breteler MM, Hofman A. 1995. Do nonsteroidal anti-inflammatory drugs decrease the risk for Alzheimer's disease? The Rotterdam Study. *Neurology* **45:** 1441–1445.

Andreasson KI, Savonenko A, Vidensky S, Goellner JJ, Zhang Y, Shaffer A, Kaufmann WE, Worley PF, Isakson P, Markowska AL. 2001. Age-dependent cognitive deficits and neuronal apoptosis in cyclooxygenase-2 transgenic mice. *J Neurosci* **21:** 8198–8209.

Anthony JC, Breitner JC, Zandi PP, Meyer MR, Jurasova I, Norton MC, Stone SV. 2000. Reduced prevalence of AD in users of NSAIDs and H2 receptor antagonists: The Cache County study. *Neurology* **54:** 2066–2071.

Arancio O, Zhang HP, Chen X, Lin C, Trinchese F, Puzzo D, Liu S, Hegde A, Yan SF, Stern A, et al. 2004. RAGE potentiates Aβ-induced perturbation of neuronal function in transgenic mice. *Embo J* **23:** 4096–4105.

Aravalli RN, Peterson PK, Lokensgard JR. 2007. Toll-like receptors in defense and damage of the central nervous system. *J Neuroimmune Pharmacol* **2:** 297–312.

Arnett HA, Wang Y, Matsushima GK, Suzuki K, Ting JP. 2003. Functional genomic analysis of remyelination reveals importance of inflammation in oligodendrocyte regeneration. *J Neurosci* **23:** 9824–9832.

Arvanitakis Z, Grodstein F, Bienias JL, Schneider JA, Wilson RS, Kelly JF, Evans DA, Bennett DA. 2008. Relation of NSAIDs to incident AD, change in cognitive function, and AD pathology. *Neurology* **70:** 2219–2225.

Atkinson JP, Krych M, Nickells M, Birmingham D, Subramanian VB, Clemenza L, Alvarez J, Liszewski K. 1994. Complement receptors and regulatory proteins: Immune adherence revisited and abuse by microorganisms. *Clin Exp Immunol* **97:** 1–3.

Bales KR, Du Y, Dodel RC, Yan GM, Hamilton-Byrd E, Paul SM. 1998. The NF-κB/Rel family of proteins mediates Aβ-induced neurotoxicity and glial activation. *Brain Res Mol Brain Res* **57:** 63–72.

Bales KR, Verina T, Cummins DJ, Du Y, Dodel RC, Saura J, Fishman CE, DeLong CA, Piccardo P, Petegnief V, et al. 1999. Apolipoprotein E is essential for amyloid deposition in the APP(V717F) transgenic mouse model of Alzheimer's disease. *Proc Natl Acad Sci* **96:** 15233–15238.

Bard F, Cannon C, Barbour R, Burke RL, Games D, Grajeda H, Guido T, Hu K, Huang J, Johnson-Wood K, et al. 2000. Peripherally administered antibodies against amyloid β-peptide enter the central nervous system and reduce pathology in a mouse model of Alzheimer disease. *Nat Med* **6:** 916–919.

Beard CM, Kokman E, Kurland LT. 1991. Rheumatoid arthritis and susceptibility to Alzheimer's disease. *Lancet* **337.**

Beard CM, Waring SC, O'Brien PC, Kurland LT, Kokmen E. 1998. Nonsteroidal anti-inflammatory drug use and Alzheimer's disease: A case-control study in Rochester, Minnesota, 1980 through 1984. *Mayo Clin Proc* **73:** 951–955.

Belanger M, Magistretti PJ. 2009. The role of astroglia in neuroprotection. *Dialogues Clin Neurosci* **11:** 281–295.

Bertram L, McQueen MB, Mullin K, Blacker D, Tanzi RE. 2007. Systematic meta-analyses of Alzheimer disease genetic association studies: The AlzGene database. *Nat Genet* **39:** 17–23.

Bessis A, Bechade C, Bernard D, Roumier A. 2007. Microglial control of neuronal death and synaptic properties. *Glia* **55:** 233–238.

Birmingham DJ, Hebert LA. 2001. CR1 and CR1-like: The primate immune adherence receptors. *Immunol Rev* **180:** 100–111.

Blalock EM, Geddes JW, Chen KC, Porter NM, Markesbery WR, Landfield PW. 2004. Incipient Alzheimer's disease: Microarray correlation analyses reveal major transcriptional and tumor suppressor responses. *Proc Natl Acad Sci* **101:** 2173–2178.

Blalock EM, Chen KC, Stromberg AJ, Norris CM, Kadish I, Kraner SD, Porter NM, Landfield PW. 2005. Harnessing the power of gene microarrays for the study of brain aging and Alzheimer's disease: Statistical reliability and functional correlation. *Ageing Res Rev* **4:** 481–512.

Bogdan C. 2008. Mechanisms and consequences of persistence of intracellular pathogens: Leishmaniasis as an example. *Cell Microbiol* **10:** 1221–1234.

Boissonneault V, Filali M, Lessard M, Relton J, Wong G, Rivest S. 2009. Powerful beneficial effects of macrophage colony-stimulating factor on β-amyloid deposition and cognitive impairment in Alzheimer's disease. *Brain* **132:** 1078–1092.

Bolmont T, Haiss F, Eicke D, Radde R, Mathis CA, Klunk WE, Kohsaka S, Jucker M, Calhoun ME. 2008. Dynamics of the microglial/amyloid interaction indicate a role in plaque maintenance. *J Neurosci* **28:** 4283–4292.

Botto M, Dell'Agnola C, Bygrave AE, Thompson EM, Cook HT, Petry F, Loos M, Pandolfi PP, Walport MJ. 1998. Homozygous C1q deficiency causes glomerulonephritis associated with multiple apoptotic bodies. *Nat Genet* **19:** 56–59.

Brandenburg LO, Konrad M, Wruck C, Koch T, Pufe T, Lucius R. 2008. Involvement of formyl-peptide-receptor-like-1 and phospholipase D in the internalization and signal transduction of amyloid β 1–42 in glial cells. *Neuroscience* **156:** 266–276.

Breitner JC, Gau BA, Welsh KA, Plassman BL, McDonald WM, Helms MJ, Anthony JC. 1994. Inverse association of anti-inflammatory treatments and Alzheimer's disease: Initial results of a co-twin control study. *Neurology* **44:** 227–232.

Breitner JC, Welsh KA, Helms MJ, Gaskell PC, Gau BA, Roses AD, Pericak-Vance MA, Saunders AM. 1995. Delayed onset of Alzheimer's disease with nonsteroidal anti-inflammatory and histamine H2 blocking drugs. *Neurobiol Aging* **16:** 523–530.

Breitner JC, Haneuse SJ, Walker R, Dublin S, Crane PK, Gray SL, Larson EB. 2009. Risk of dementia and AD with prior exposure to NSAIDs in an elderly community-based cohort. *Neurology* **72:** 1899–1905.

Broe GA, Henderson AS, Creasey H, McCusker E, Korten AE, Jorm AF, Longley W, Anthony JC. 1990. A case-control study of Alzheimer's disease in Australia. *Neurology* **40:** 1698–1707.

Cite this article as *Cold Spring Harb Perspect Med* doi: 10.1101/cshperspect.a006346

Broe GA, Grayson DA, Creasey HM, Waite LM, Casey BJ, Bennett HP, Brooks WS, Halliday GM. 2000. Anti-inflammatory drugs protect against Alzheimer disease at low doses. *Arch Neurol* **57:** 1586–1591.

Cagnin A, Brooks DJ, Kennedy AM, Gunn RN, Myers R, Turkheimer FE, Jones T, Banati RB. 2001. In-vivo measurement of activated microglia in dementia. *Lancet* **358:** 461–467.

Caldero J, Brunet N, Ciutat D, Hereu M, Esquerda JE. 2009. Development of microglia in the chick embryo spinal cord: Implications in the regulation of motoneuronal survival and death. *J Neurosci Res* **87:** 2447–2466.

Cameron B, Landreth GE. 2010. Inflammation microglia, and Alzheimer's disease. *Neurobiol Dis* **37:** 503–509.

Canadian Study of Health and Aging. 1994. The Canadian Study of Health and Aging: Risk factors for Alzheimer's disease in Canada. *Neurology* **44:** 2073–2080.

Carroll MC. 1998. The role of complement and complement receptors in induction and regulation of immunity. *Annu Rev Immunol* **16:** 545–568.

Cartier L, Hartley O, Dubois-Dauphin M, Krause KH. 2005. Chemokine receptors in the central nervous system: Role in brain inflammation and neurodegenerative diseases. *Brain Res Brain Res Rev* **48:** 16–42.

Caso JR, Pradillo JM, Hurtado O, Lorenzo P, Moro MA, Lizasoain I. 2007. Toll-like receptor 4 is involved in brain damage and inflammation after experimental stroke. *Circulation* **115:** 1599–1608.

Chakrabarty P, Jansen-West K, Beccard A, Ceballos-Diaz C, Levites Y, Verbeeck C, Zubair AC, Dickson D, Golde TE, Das P. 2010. Massive gliosis induced by interleukin-6 suppresses Aβ deposition in vivo: Evidence against inflammation as a driving force for amyloid deposition. *FASEB J* **24:** 548–559.

Chan WY, Kohsaka S, Rezaie P. 2007. The origin and cell lineage of microglia: New concepts. *Brain Res Rev* **53:** 344–354.

Charo IF, Ransohoff RM. 2006. The many roles of chemokines and chemokine receptors in inflammation. *N Engl J Med* **354:** 610–621.

Chen K, Iribarren P, Huang J, Zhang L, Gong W, Cho EH, Lockett S, Dunlop NM, Wang JM. 2007a. Induction of the formyl peptide receptor 2 in microglia by IFN-γ and synergy with CD40 ligand. *J Immunol* **178:** 1759–1766.

Chen X, Walker DG, Schmidt AM, Arancio O, Lue LF, Yan SD. 2007b. RAGE: A potential target for Aβ-mediated cellular perturbation in Alzheimer's disease. *Curr Mol Med* **7:** 735–742.

Chow SK, Yu D, Macdonald CL, Buibas M, Silva GA. 2010. Amyloid β-peptide directly induces spontaneous calcium transients, delayed intercellular calcium waves and gliosis in rat cortical astrocytes. *ASN Neuro* **2:** e00026.

Citron BA, Dennis JS, Zeitlin RS, Echeverria V. 2008. Transcription factor Sp1 dysregulation in Alzheimer's disease. *J Neurosci Res* **86:** 2499–2504.

Colton CA. 2009. Heterogeneity of microglial activation in the innate immune response in the brain. *J Neuroimmune Pharmacol* **4:** 399–418.

Colton CA, Wilcock DM. 2010. Assessing activation states in microglia. *CNS Neurol Disord Drug Targets* **9:** 174–191.

Combs CK. 2009. Inflammation and microglia actions in Alzheimer's disease. *J Neuroimmune Pharmacol* **4:** 380–388.

Coraci IS, Husemann J, Berman JW, Hulette C, Dufour JH, Campanella GK, Luster AD, Silverstein SC, El-Khoury JB. 2002. CD36, a class B scavenger receptor, is expressed on microglia in Alzheimer's disease brains and can mediate production of reactive oxygen species in response to β-amyloid fibrils. *Am J Pathol* **160:** 101–112.

Cornelius C, Fastbom J, Winblad B, Viitanen M. 2004. Aspirin, NSAIDs, risk of dementia, and influence of the apolipoprotein E ε4 allele in an elderly population. *Neuroepidemiology* **23:** 135–143.

Craft JM, Watterson DM, Marks A, Van Eldik LJ. 2005. Enhanced susceptibility of S-100B transgenic mice to neuroinflammation and neuronal dysfunction induced by intracerebroventricular infusion of human β-amyloid. *Glia* **51:** 209–216.

Cunningham C, Wilcockson DC, Campion S, Lunnon K, Perry VH. 2005. Central and systemic endotoxin challenges exacerbate the local inflammatory response and increase neuronal death during chronic neurodegeneration. *J Neurosci* **25:** 9275–9284.

D'Ambrosio AL, Pinsky DJ, Connolly ES. 2001. The role of the complement cascade in ischemia/reperfusion injury: Implications for neuroprotection. *Mol Med* **7:** 367–382.

D'Andrea MR. 2003. Evidence linking neuronal cell death to autoimmunity in Alzheimer's disease. *Brain Res* **982:** 19–30.

Davalos D, Grutzendler J, Yang G, Kim JV, Zuo Y, Jung S, Littman DR, Dustin ML, Gan WB. 2005. ATP mediates rapid microglial response to local brain injury in vivo. *Nat Neurosci* **8:** 752–758.

DeMattos RB, Bales KR, Cummins DJ, Dodart J-C, Paul SM, Holtzman DM. 2001. Peripheral anti-Ab antibody alters CNS and plasma Ab clearance and decreases brain Ab burden in a mouse model of Alzheimer's disease. *Proc Natl Acad Sci* **98:** 8850–8855.

Dewil M, Van Den Bosch L, Robberecht W. 2007. Microglia in amyotrophic lateral sclerosis. *Acta Neurol Belg* **107:** 63–70.

DiCarlo G, Wilcock D, Henderson D, Gordon M, Morgan D. 2001. Intrahippocampal LPS injections reduce Ab load in APP+PS1 transgenic mice. *Neurobiol Aging* **22:** 1007–1012.

Duan RS, Yang X, Chen ZG, Lu MO, Morris C, Winblad B, Zhu J. 2008. Decreased fractalkine and increased IP-10 expression in aged brain of APP(swe) transgenic mice. *Neurochem Res* **33:** 1085–1089.

Edison P, Archer HA, Gerhard A, Hinz R, Pavese N, Turkheimer FE, Hammers A, Tai YF, Fox N, Kennedy A, et al. 2008. Microglia, amyloid, and cognition in Alzheimer's disease: An [11C](R)PK11195-PET and [11C]PIB-PET study. *Neurobiol Dis* **32:** 412–419.

Eikelenboom P, Stam FC. 1982. Immunoglobulins and complement factors in senile plaques. An immunoperoxidase study. *Acta Neuropathol (Berl)* **57:** 239–242.

Eikelenboom P, Hack CE, Rozemuller JM, Stam FC. 1989. Complement activation in amyloid plaques in Alzheimer's dementia. *Virchows Arch B Cell Pathol* **56:** 259–262.

El Khoury J, Luster AD. 2008. Mechanisms of microglia accumulation in Alzheimer's disease: Therapeutic implications. *Trends Pharmacol Sci* **29:** 626–632.

El Khoury J, Hickman SE, Thomas CA, Loike JD, Silverstein SC. 1998. Microglia, scavenger receptors, and the pathogenesis of Alzheimer's disease. *Neurobiol Aging* **19:** S81–S84.

El Khoury J, Moore KJ, Means TK, Leung J, Terada K, Toft M, Freeman MW, Luster AD. 2003. CD36 mediates the innate host response to β-amyloid. *J Exp Med* **197:** 1657–1666.

El Khoury J, Toft M, Hickman SE, Means TK, Terada K, Geula C, Luster AD. 2007. Ccr2 deficiency impairs microglial accumulation and accelerates progression of Alzheimer-like disease. *Nat Med* **13:** 432–438.

Emmerling MR, Watson MD, Raby CA, Spiegel K. 2000. The role of complement in Alzheimer's disease pathology. *Biochim Biophys Acta* **1502:** 158–171.

Fassbender K, Walter S, Kuhl S, Landmann R, Ishii K, Bertsch T, Stalder AK, Muehlhauser F, Liu Y, Ulmer AJ, et al. 2004. The LPS receptor (CD14) links innate immunity with Alzheimer's disease. *FASEB J* **18:** 203–205.

Fiala M, Liu PT, Espinosa-Jeffrey A, Rosenthal MJ, Bernard G, Ringman JM, Sayre J, Zhang L, Zaghi J, Dejbakhsh S, et al. 2007. Innate immunity and transcription of MGAT-III and Toll-like receptors in Alzheimer's disease patients are improved by bisdemethoxycurcumin. *Proc Natl Acad Sci* **104:** 12849–12854.

Fonseca MI, Kawas CH, Troncoso JC, Tenner AJ. 2004a. Neuronal localization of C1q in preclinical Alzheimer's disease. *Neurobiol Dis* **15:** 40–46.

Fonseca MI, Zhou J, Botto M, Tenner AJ. 2004b. Absence of C1q leads to less neuropathology in transgenic mouse models of Alzheimer's disease. *J Neurosci* **24:** 6457–6465.

Foote AK, Blakemore WF. 2005. Inflammation stimulates remyelination in areas of chronic demyelination. *Brain* **128:** 528–539.

Frank-Cannon TC, Tran T, Ruhn KA, Martinez TN, Hong J, Marvin M, Hartley M, Trevino I, O'Brien DE, Casey B, et al. 2008. Parkin deficiency increases vulnerability to inflammation-related nigral degeneration. *J Neurosci* **28:** 10825–10834.

Fraser DA, Pisalyaput K, Tenner AJ. 2010. C1q enhances microglial clearance of apoptotic neurons and neuronal blebs, and modulates subsequent inflammatory cytokine production. *J Neurochem* **112:** 733–743.

French LR, Schuman LM, Mortimer JA, Hutton JT, Boatman RA, Christians B. 1985. A case-control study of dementia of the Alzheimer type. *Am J Epidemiol* **121:** 414–421.

Garden GA. 2002. Microglia in human immunodeficiency virus-associated neurodegeneration. *Glia* **40:** 240–251.

Gasque P. 2004. Complement: A unique innate immune sensor for danger signals. *Mol Immunol* **41:** 1089–1098.

Gasque P, Dean YD, McGreal EP, Beek JV, Morgan BP. 2000. Complement components of the innate immune system in health and disease in the CNS. *Immunopharmacology* **49:** 171–186.

Godoy MC, Tarelli R, Ferrari CC, Sarchi MI, Pitossi FJ. 2008. Central and systemic IL-1 exacerbates neurodegeneration

and motor symptoms in a model of Parkinson's disease. *Brain* **131:** 1880–1894.

Gordon S, Taylor PR. 2005. Monocyte and macrophage heterogeneity. *Nat Rev Immunol* **5:** 953–964.

Granic I, Dolga AM, Nijholt IM, van Dijk G, Eisel UL. 2009. Inflammation and NF-κB in Alzheimer's disease and diabetes. *J Alzheimers Dis* **16:** 809–821.

Graves AB, White E, Koepsell TD, Reifler BV, van Belle G, Larson EB, Raskind M. 1990. A case-control study of Alzheimer's disease. *Ann Neurol* **28:** 766–774.

Green RC, Schneider LS, Amato DA, Beelen AP, Wilcock G, Swabb EA, Zavitz KH. 2009. Effect of tarenflurbil on cognitive decline and activities of daily living in patients with mild Alzheimer disease: A randomized controlled trial. *JAMA* **302:** 2557–2564.

Halassa MM, Fellin T, Takano H, Dong JH, Haydon PG. 2007. Synaptic islands defined by the territory of a single astrocyte. *J Neurosci* **27:** 6473–6477.

Harold D, Abraham R, Hollingworth P, Sims R, Gerrish A, Hamshere ML, Pahwa JS, Moskvina V, Dowzell K, Williams A, et al. 2009. Genome-wide association study identifies variants at CLU and PICALM associated with Alzheimer's disease. *Nat Genet* **41:** 1088–1093.

He P, Zhong Z, Lindholm K, Berning L, Lee W, Lemere C, Staufenbiel M, Li R, Shen Y. 2007. Deletion of tumor necrosis factor death receptor inhibits amyloid β generation and prevents learning and memory deficits in Alzheimer's mice. *J Cell Biol* **178:** 829–841.

Heyman A, Wilkinson WE, Stafford JA, Helms MJ, Sigmon AH, Weinberg T. 1984. Alzheimer's disease: A study of epidemiological aspects. *Ann Neurol* **15:** 335–341.

Holers VM. 1996. Complement. In *Clinical immunology principles and practice* (ed. Rich RR), pp. 363–391. Mosby–Year Book, St. Louis, MO.

Holmes C, El-Okl M, Williams AL, Cunningham C, Wilcockson D, Perry VH. 2003. Systemic infection, interleukin 1β, and cognitive decline in Alzheimer's disease. *J Neurol Neurosurg Psychiatry* **74:** 788–789.

Hosokawa M, Klegeris A, Maguire J, McGeer PL. 2003. Expression of complement messenger RNAs and proteins by human oligodendroglial cells. *Glia* **42:** 417–423.

Hosokawa M, Klegeris A, McGeer PL. 2004. Human oligodendroglial cells express low levels of C1 inhibitor and membrane cofactor protein mRNAs. *J Neuroinflammation* **1.**

Hsieh CL, Koike M, Spusta SC, Niemi EC, Yenari M, Nakamura MC, Seaman WE. 2009. A role for TREM2 ligands in the phagocytosis of apoptotic neuronal cells by microglia. *J Neurochem* **109:** 1144–1156.

Hu WT, Chen-Plotkin A, Arnold SE, Grossman M, Clark CM, Shaw LM, McCluskey L, Elman L, Karlawish J, Hurtig HI, et al. 2010a. Biomarker discovery for Alzheimer's disease, frontotemporal lobar degeneration, and Parkinson's disease. *Acta Neuropathol* **120:** 385–399.

Hu WT, Chen-Plotkin A, Arnold SE, Grossman M, Clark CM, Shaw LM, Pickering E, Kuhn M, Chen Y, McCluskey L, et al. 2010b. Novel CSF biomarkers for Alzheimer's disease and mild cognitive impairment. *Acta Neuropathol* **119:** 669–678.

Hye A, Lynham S, Thambisetty M, Causevic M, Campbell J, Byers HL, Hooper C, Rijsdijk F, Tabrizi SJ, Banner S, et al.

2006. Proteome-based plasma biomarkers for Alzheimer's disease. *Brain* 129: 3042–3050.

in 't Veld BA, Launer LJ, Hoes AW, Ott A, Hofman A, Breteler MM, Stricker BH. 1998. NSAIDs and incident Alzheimer's disease. The Rotterdam Study. *Neurobiol Aging* 19: 607–611.

in 't Veld BA, Ruitenberg A, Hofman A, Launer LJ, van Duijn CM, Stijnen T, Breteler MM, Stricker BH. 2001. Nonsteroidal antiinflammatory drugs and the risk of Alzheimer's disease. *N Engl J Med* 345: 1515–1521.

Itagaki S, Akiyama H, Saito H, McGeer PL. 1994. Ultrastructural localization of complement membrane attack complex (MAC)-like immunoreactivity in brains of patients with Alzheimer's disease. *Brain Res* 645: 78–84.

Iwasaki A, Medzhitov R. 2004. Toll-like receptor control of the adaptive immune responses. *Nat Immunol* 5: 987–995.

Janeway CA Jr, Medzhitov R. 2002. Innate immune recognition. *Annu Rev Immunol* 20: 197–216.

Jantaratnotai N, Ryu JK, Kim SU, McLarnon JG. 2003. Amyloid β peptide-induced corpus callosum damage and glial activation in vivo. *Neuroreport* 14: 1429–1433.

Jenkinson ML, Bliss MR, Brain AT, Scott DL. 1989. Rheumatoid arthritis and senile dementia of the Alzheimer's type. *Br J Rheumatol* 28: 86–88.

Ji B, Maeda J, Sawada M, Ono M, Okauchi T, Inaji M, Zhang MR, Suzuki K, Ando K, Staufenbiel M, et al. 2008. Imaging of peripheral benzodiazepine receptor expression as biomarkers of detrimental versus beneficial glial responses in mouse models of Alzheimer's and other CNS pathologies. *J Neurosci* 28: 12255–12267.

Jiang H, Burdick D, Glabe CG, Cotman CW, Tenner AJ. 1994. b-Amyloid activates complement by binding to a specific region of the collagen-like domain of the C1q A chain. *J Immunol* 152: 5050–5059.

Jiang Q, Heneka M, Landreth GE. 2008. The role of peroxisome proliferator-activated receptor-γ (PPARγ) in Alzheimer's disease: Therapeutic implications. *CNS Drugs* 22: 1–14.

Jin JJ, Kim HD, Maxwell JA, Li L, Fukuchi K. 2008. Toll-like receptor 4-dependent upregulation of cytokines in a transgenic mouse model of Alzheimer's disease. *J Neuroinflammation* 5: 23.

John GR, Lee SC, Brosnan CF. 2003. Cytokines: Powerful regulators of glial cell activation. *Neuroscientist* 9: 10–22.

Johns TG, Bernard CC. 1997. Binding of complement component C1q to myelin oligodendrocyte glycoprotein: A novel mechanism for regulating CNS inflammation. *Mol Immunol* 34: 33–38.

Jun G, Naj AC, Beecham GW, Wang LS, Buros J, Gallins PJ, Buxbaum JD, Ertekin-Taner N, Fallin MD, Friedland R, et al. 2010. Meta-analysis confirms CR1, CLU, and PICALM as Alzheimer disease risk loci and reveals interactions with APOE genotypes. *Arch Neurol* 67: 1473–1484.

Juurlink BH. 1997. Response of glial cells to ischemia: Roles of reactive oxygen species and glutathione. *Neurosci Biobehav Rev* 21: 151–166.

Kalman J, Kitajka K, Pakaski M, Zvara A, Juhasz A, Vincze G, Janka Z, Puskas LG. 2005. Gene expression profile analysis of lymphocytes from Alzheimer's patients. *Psychiatr Genet* 15: 1–6.

Katsel P, Tan W, Haroutunian V. 2009. Gain in brain immunity in the oldest-old differentiates cognitively normal from demented individuals. *PLoS One* 4: e7642.

Koenigsknecht-Talboo J, Meyer-Luehmann M, Parsadanian M, Garcia-Alloza M, Finn MB, Hyman BT, Bacskai BJ, Holtzman DM. 2008. Rapid microglial response around amyloid pathology after systemic anti-Aβ antibody administration in PDAPP mice. *J Neurosci* 28: 14156–14164.

Koistinaho M, Lin S, Wu X, Esterman M, Koger D, Hanson J, Higgs R, Liu F, Malkani S, Bales KR, et al. 2004. Apolipoprotein E promotes astrocyte colocalization and degradation of deposited amyloid-β peptides. *Nat Med* 10: 719–726.

Kukar T, Murphy MP, Eriksen JL, Sagi SA, Weggen S, Smith TE, Ladd T, Khan MA, Kache R, Beard J, et al. 2005. Diverse compounds mimic Alzheimer disease-causing mutations by augmenting Aβ42 production. *Nat Med* 11: 545–550.

Lambert JC, Heath S, Even G, Campion D, Sleegers K, Hiltunen M, Combarros O, Zelenika D, Bullido MJ, Tavernier B, et al. 2009. Genome-wide association study identifies variants at CLU and CR1 associated with Alzheimer's disease. *Nat Genet* 41: 1094–1099.

Landi F, Cesari M, Onder G, Russo A, Torre S, Bernabei R. 2003. Non-steroidal anti-inflammatory drug (NSAID) use and Alzheimer disease in community-dwelling elderly patients. *Am J Geriatr Psychiatry* 11: 179–185.

Landreth GE, Reed-Geaghan EG. 2009. Toll-like receptors in Alzheimer's disease. *Curr Top Microbiol Immunol* 336: 137–153.

Leal MC, Dorfman VB, Gamba AF, Frangione B, Wisniewski T, Castano EM, Sigurdsson EM, Morelli L. 2006. Plaque-associated overexpression of insulin-degrading enzyme in the cerebral cortex of aged transgenic tg2576 mice with Alzheimer pathology. *J Neuropathol Exp Neurol* 65: 976–987.

Lee CY, Landreth GE. 2010. The role of microglia in amyloid clearance from the AD brain. *J Neural Transm* 117: 949–960.

Lee JT, Xu J, Lee JM, Ku G, Han X, Yang DI, Chen S, Hsu CY. 2004. Amyloid-β peptide induces oligodendrocyte death by activating the neutral sphingomyelinase-ceramide pathway. *J Cell Biol* 164: 123–131.

Lehnardt S, Massillon L, Follett P, Jensen FE, Ratan R, Rosenberg PA, Volpe JJ, Vartanian T. 2003. Activation of innate immunity in the CNS triggers neurodegeneration through a Toll-like receptor 4-dependent pathway. *Proc Natl Acad Sci* 100: 8514–8519.

Li G, Shen YC, Li YT, Chen CH, Zhau YW, Silverman JM. 1992. A case-control study of Alzheimer's disease in China. *Neurology* 42: 1481–1488.

Li R, Strohmeyer R, Liang Z, Lue LF, Rogers J. 2004. CCAAT/enhancer binding protein delta (C/EBPdelta) expression and elevation in Alzheimer s disease. *Neurobiol Aging* 25: 991–999.

Liang X, Wang Q, Hand T, Wu L, Breyer RM, Montine TJ, Andreasson K. 2005. Deletion of the prostaglandin E2 EP2 receptor reduces oxidative damage and amyloid burden in a model of Alzheimer's disease. *J Neurosci* 25: 10180–10187.

Liang X, Wu L, Wang Q, Hand T, Bilak M, McCullough L, Andreasson K. 2007. Function of COX-2 and prostaglandins in neurological disease. *J Mol Neurosci* **33:** 94–99.

Lindsay J, Laurin D, Verreault R, Hebert R, Helliwell B, Hill GB, McDowell I. 2002. Risk factors for Alzheimer's disease: A prospective analysis from the Canadian Study of Health and Aging. *Am J Epidemiol* **156:** 445–453.

Liu Y, Walter S, Stagi M, Cherny D, Letiembre M, Schulz-Schaeffer W, Heine H, Penke B, Neumann H, Fassbender K. 2005. LPS receptor (CD14): A receptor for phagocytosis of Alzheimer's amyloid peptide. *Brain* **128:** 1778–1789.

Luber-Narod J, Rogers J. 1988. Immune system associated antigens expressed by cells of the human central nervous system. *Neurosci Lett* **94:** 17–22.

Lue LF, Rydel R, Brigham EF, Yang LB, Hampel H, Murphy GM, Brachova L, Yan SD, Walker DG, Shen Y, et al. 2001a. Inflammatory repertoire of Alzheimer's disease and nondemented elderly microglia in vitro. *Glia* **35:** 72–79.

Lue LF, Walker DG, Rogers J. 2001b. Modeling microglial activation in Alzheimer's disease with human postmortem microglial cultures. *Neurobiol Aging* **22:** 945–956.

Lyketsos CG, Breitner JC, Green RC, Martin BK, Meinert C, Piantadosi S, Sabbagh M. 2007. Naproxen and celecoxib do not prevent AD in early results from a randomized controlled trial. *Neurology* **68:** 1800–1808.

Maes OC, Xu S, Yu B, Chertkow HM, Wang E, Schipper HM. 2007. Transcriptional profiling of Alzheimer blood mononuclear cells by microarray. *Neurobiol Aging* **28:** 1795–1809.

Maier M, Peng Y, Jiang L, Seabrook TJ, Carroll MC, Lemere CA. 2008. Complement C3 deficiency leads to accelerated amyloid β plaque deposition and neurodegeneration and modulation of the microglia/macrophage phenotype in amyloid precursor protein transgenic mice. *J Neurosci* **28:** 6333–6341.

Majumdar A, Cruz D, Asamoah N, Buxbaum A, Sohar I, Lobel P, Maxfield FR. 2007. Activation of microglia acidifies lysosomes and leads to degradation of Alzheimer amyloid fibrils. *Mol Biol Cell* **18:** 1490–1496.

Majumdar A, Chung H, Dolios G, Wang R, Asamoah N, Lobel P, Maxfield FR. 2008. Degradation of fibrillar forms of Alzheimer's amyloid β-peptide by macrophages. *Neurobiol Aging* **29:** 707–715.

Mandrekar-Colucci S, Landreth GE. 2010. Microglia and inflammation in Alzheimer's disease. *CNS Neurol Disord Drug Targets* **9:** 156–167.

McCoy MK, Martinez TN, Ruhn KA, Szymkowski DE, Smith CG, Botterman BR, Tansey KE, Tansey MG. 2006. Blocking soluble tumor necrosis factor signaling with dominant-negative tumor necrosis factor inhibitor attenuates loss of dopaminergic neurons in models of Parkinson's disease. *J Neurosci* **26:** 9365–9375.

McGeer PL. 2000. Cyclo-oxygenase-2 inhibitors: Rationale and therapeutic potential for Alzheimer's disease. *Drugs Aging* **17:** 1–11.

McGeer PL, McGeer EG. 1999. Inflammation of the brain in Alzheimer's disease: Implications for therapy. *J Leukoc Biol* **65:** 409–415.

McGeer PL, Itagaki S, McGeer EG. 1988. Expression of the histocompatibility glycoprotein HLA-DR in neurological disease. *Acta Neuropathol* **76:** 550–557.

McGeer PL, McGeer E, Rogers J, Sibley J. 1990. Anti-inflammatory drugs and Alzheimer disease. *Lancet* **335:** 1037.

McGeer PL, Harada N, Kimura H, McGeer EG, Schulzer M. 1992. Prevalence of dementia amongst elderly Japanese with leprosy: Apparent effect of chronic drug therapy. *Dementia* **3:** 146–149.

McGeer PL, Schulzer M, McGeer EG. 1996. Arthritis and anti-inflammatory agents as possible protective factors for Alzheimer's disease: A review of 17 epidemiologic studies. *Neurology* **47:** 425–432.

McGeer PL, Rogers J, McGeer EG. 2006. Inflammation, anti-inflammatory agents and Alzheimer disease: The last 12 years. *J Alzheimers Dis* **9:** 271–276.

Melnikova T, Savonenko A, Wang Q, Liang X, Hand T, Wu L, Kaufmann WE, Vehmas A, Andreasson KI. 2006. Cycloxygenase-2 activity promotes cognitive deficits but not increased amyloid burden in a model of Alzheimer's disease in a sex-dimorphic pattern. *Neuroscience* **141:** 1149–1162.

Meyer-Luehmann M, Spires-Jones TL, Prada C, Garcia-Alloza M, de Calignon A, Rozkalne A, Koenigsknecht-Talboo J, Holtzman DM, Bacskai BJ, Hyman BT. 2008. Rapid appearance and local toxicity of amyloid-β plaques in a mouse model of Alzheimer's disease. *Nature* **451:** 720–724.

Mitew S, Kirkcaldie MT, Halliday GM, Shepherd CE, Vickers JC, Dickson TC. 2010. Focal demyelination in Alzheimer's disease and transgenic mouse models. *Acta Neuropathol* **119:** 567–577.

Mott RT, Ait-Ghezala G, Town T, Mori T, Vendrame M, Zeng J, Ehrhart J, Mullan M, Tan J. 2004. Neuronal expression of CD22: Novel mechanism for inhibiting microglial proinflammatory cytokine production. *Glia* **46:** 369–379.

Moynagh PN. 2005. The interleukin-1 signalling pathway in astrocytes: A key contributor to inflammation in the brain. *J Anat* **207:** 265–269.

Mrak RE, Sheng JG, Griffin WS. 1996. Correlation of astrocytic S100 β expression with dystrophic neurites in amyloid plaques of Alzheimer's disease. *J Neuropathol Exp Neurol* **55:** 273–279.

Mukherjee D, Nissen SE, Topol EJ. 2001. Risk of cardiovascular events associated with selective COX-2 inhibitors. *JAMA* **286:** 954–959.

Muzio L, Martino G, Furlan R. 2007. Multifaceted aspects of inflammation in multiple sclerosis: The role of microglia. *J Neuroimmunol* **191:** 39–44.

Myllykangas-Luosujarvi R, Isomaki H. 1994. Alzheimer's disease and rheumatoid arthritis. *Br J Rheumatol* **33:** 501–502.

Nadler Y, Alexandrovich A, Grigoriadis N, Hartmann T, Rao KS, Shohami E, Stein R. 2008. Increased expression of the γ-secretase components presenilin-1 and nicastrin in activated astrocytes and microglia following traumatic brain injury. *Glia* **56:** 552–567.

Nagele RG, D'Andrea MR, Lee H, Venkataraman V, Wang HY. 2003. Astrocytes accumulate A β 42 and give rise to astrocytic amyloid plaques in Alzheimer disease brains. *Brain Res* **971:** 197–209.

Nguyen MD, Julien JP, Rivest S. 2002. Innate immunity: The missing link in neuroprotection and neurodegeneration? *Nat Rev Neurosci* **3:** 216–227.

Nguyen MD, D'Aigle T, Gowing G, Julien JP, Rivest S. 2004. Exacerbation of motor neuron disease by chronic stimulation of innate immunity in a mouse model of amyotrophic lateral sclerosis. *J Neurosci* **24:** 1340–1349.

Nilsson SE, Johansson B, Takkinen S, Berg S, Zarit S, McClearn G, Melander A. 2003. Does aspirin protect against Alzheimer's dementia? A study in a Swedish population-based sample aged > or =80 years. *Eur J Clin Pharmacol* **59:** 313–319.

Nimmerjahn A, Kirchhoff F, Helmchen F. 2005. Resting microglial cells are highly dynamic surveillants of brain parenchyma in vivo. *Science* **308:** 1314–1318.

Norris CM, Kadish I, Blalock EM, Chen KC, Thibault V, Porter NM, Landfield PW, Kraner SD. 2005. Calcineurin triggers reactive/inflammatory processes in astrocytes and is upregulated in aging and Alzheimer's models. *J Neurosci* **25:** 4649–4658.

Okun E, Mattson MP, Arumugam TV. 2010. Involvement of Fc receptors in disorders of the central nervous system. *Neuromolecular Med* **12:** 164–178.

Palin K, Cunningham C, Forse P, Perry VH, Platt N. 2008. Systemic inflammation switches the inflammatory cytokine profile in CNS Wallerian degeneration. *Neurobiol Dis* **30:** 19–29.

Paresce DM, Chung H, Maxfield FR. 1997. Slow degradation of aggregates of the Alzheimer's disease amyloid β-protein by microglial cells. *J Biol Chem* **272:** 29390–29397.

Pasqualetti P, Bonomini C, Dal Forno G, Paulon L, Sinforiani E, Marra C, Zanetti O, Rossini PM. 2009. A randomized controlled study on effects of ibuprofen on cognitive progression of Alzheimer's disease. *Aging Clin Exp Res* **21:** 102–110.

Popovich PG, Guan Z, McGaughy V, Fisher L, Hickey WF, Basso DM. 2002. The neuropathological and behavioral consequences of intraspinal microglial/macrophage activation. *J Neuropathol Exp Neurol* **61:** 623–633.

Ransohoff RM. 2007. The MHP36 line of murine neural stem cells expresses functional CXCR1 chemokine receptors that initiate chemotaxis in vitro. *J Neuroimmunol* **186:** 199–200.

Ray S, Britschgi M, Herbert C, Takeda-Uchimura Y, Boxer A, Blennow K, Friedman LF, Galasko DR, Jutel M, Karydas A, et al. 2007. Classification and prediction of clinical Alzheimer's diagnosis based on plasma signaling proteins. *Nat Med* **13:** 1369–1362.

Reed-Geaghan EG, Savage JC, Hise AG, Landreth GE. 2009. CD14 and toll-like receptors 2 and 4 are required for fibrillar A{β}-stimulated microglial activation. *J Neurosci* **29:** 11982–11992.

Reines SA, Block GA, Morris JC, Liu G, Nessly ML, Lines CR, Norman BA, Baranak CC. 2004. Rofecoxib: No effect on Alzheimer's disease in a 1-year, randomized, blinded, controlled study. *Neurology* **62:** 66–71.

Rezaie P, Male D. 2002. Mesoglia & microglia–a historical review of the concept of mononuclear phagocytes within the central nervous system. *J Hist Neurosci* **11:** 325–374.

Rich JB, Rasmusson DX, Folstein MF, Carson KA, Kawas C, Brandt J. 1995. Nonsteroidal anti-inflammatory drugs in Alzheimer's disease. *Neurology* **45:** 51–55.

Richard KL, Filali M, Prefontaine P, Rivest S. 2008. Toll-like receptor 2 acts as a natural innate immune receptor to clear amyloid β 1–42 and delay the cognitive decline in a mouse model of Alzheimer's disease. *J Neurosci* **28:** 5784–5793.

Rodriguez JJ, Olabarria M, Chvatal A, Verkhratsky A. 2009. Astroglia in dementia and Alzheimer's disease. *Cell Death Differ* **16:** 378–385.

Rogers J, Luber-Narod J, Styren SD, Civin WH. 1988. Expression of immune system-associated antigens by cells of the human central nervous system: Relationship to the pathology of Alzheimer's disease. *Neurobiol Aging* **9:** 339–349.

Rogers J, Cooper NR, Webster S, Schultz J, McGeer PL, Styren SD, Civin WH, Brachova L, Bradt B, Ward P, et al. 1992. Complement activation by b-amyloid in Alzheimer disease. *Proc Natl Acad Sci* **89:** 10016–10020.

Rogers J, Kirby LC, Hempelman SR, Berry DL, McGeer PL, Kaszniak AW, Zalinski J, Cofield M, Mansukhani L, Willson P, et al. 1993. Clinical trial of indomethacin in Alzheimer's disease. *Neurology* **43:** 1609–1611.

Rogers J, Webster S, Lue LF, Brachova L, Civin WH, Emmerling M, Shivers B, Walker D, McGeer P. 1996. Inflammation and Alzheimer's disease pathogenesis. *Neurobiol Aging* **17:** 681–686.

Rogers J, Li R, Mastroeni D, Grover A, Leonard B, Ahern G, Cao P, Kolody H, Vedders L, Kolb WP, et al. 2006. Peripheral clearance of amyloid beta peptide by complement C3-dependent adherence to erythrocytes. *Neurobiol Aging* **27:** 1733–1739.

Rogers J, Mastroeni D, Leonard B, Joyce J, Grover A. 2007. Neuroinflammation in Alzheimer's disease and Parkinson's disease: Are microglia pathogenic in either disorder? *Int Rev Neurobiol* **82:** 235–246.

Roth AD, Ramirez G, Alarcon R, Von Bernhardi R. 2005. Oligodendrocytes damage in Alzheimer's disease: β amyloid toxicity and inflammation. *Biol Res* **38:** 381–387.

Sahu A, Lambris J. 2001. Structure and biology of complement protein C3, a connecting link between innate and acquired immunity. *Immunol Rev* **180:** 35–48.

Sanchez-Ramos J, Song S, Sava V, Catlow B, Lin X, Mori T, Cao C, Arendash GW. 2009. Granulocyte colony stimulating factor decreases brain amyloid burden and reverses cognitive impairment in Alzheimer's mice. *Neuroscience* **163:** 55–72.

Savonenko A, Munoz P, Melnikova T, Wang Q, Liang X, Breyer RM, Montine TJ, Kirkwood A, Andreasson K. 2009. Impaired cognition, sensorimotor gating, and hippocampal long-term depression in mice lacking the prostaglandin E2 EP2 receptor. *Exp Neurol* **217:** 63–73.

Schmidt AM, Sahagan B, Nelson RB, Selmer J, Rothlein R, Bell JM. 2009. The role of RAGE in amyloid-β peptide-mediated pathology in Alzheimer's disease. *Curr Opin Investig Drugs* **10:** 672–680.

Sedgwick JD, Schwender S, Imrich H, Dorries R, Butcher GW, ter Meulen V. 1991. Isolation and direct characterization of resident microglial cells from the normal and inflamed central nervous system. *Proc Natl Acad Sci* **88:** 7438–7442.

Seong SY, Matzinger P. 2004. Hydrophobicity: An ancient damage-associated molecular pattern that initiates innate immune responses. *Nat Rev Immunol* **4:** 469–478.

Setzu A, Lathia JD, Zhao C, Wells K, Rao MS, French-Constant C, Franklin RJ. 2006. Inflammation stimulates myelination by transplanted oligodendrocyte precursor cells. *Glia* **54:** 297–303.

Shaftel SS, Kyrkanides S, Olschowka JA, Miller JN, Johnson RE, O'Banion MK. 2007. Sustained hippocampal IL-1 β overexpression mediates chronic neuroinflammation and ameliorates Alzheimer plaque pathology. *J Clin Invest* **117:** 1595–1604.

Shen Y, Lue L-F, Yang L-B, Roher A, Kuo Y-M, Strohhmeyer R, Goux WJ, Lee V, Johnson GVW, Webster SD, et al. 2001. Complement activation by neurofibrillary tangles in Alzheimer's disease. *Neurosci Lett* **305:** 165–168.

Sheng JG, Mrak RE, Bales KR, Cordell B, Paul SM, Jones RA, Woodward S, Zhou XQ, McGinness JM, Griffin WS. 2000. Overexpression of the neuritotrophic cytokine S100 beta precedes the appearance of neuritic beta-amyloid plaques in APPV717F mice. *J Neurochem* **74:** 295–301.

Sheta EA, Appel SH, Goldknopf IL. 2006. 2D gel blood serum biomarkers reveal differential clinical proteomics of the neurodegenerative diseases. *Expert Rev Proteomics* **3:** 45–62.

Shi J, Johansson J, Woodling NS, Wang Q, Montine TJ, Andreasson K. 2010. The prostaglandin E2 E-prostanoid 4 receptor exerts anti-inflammatory effects in brain innate immunity. *J Immunol* **184:** 7207–7218.

Singhrao SK, Neal JW, Rushmere NK, Morgan BP, Gasque P. 1999. Differential expression of individual complement regulators in the brain and choroid plexus. *Lab Invest* **79:** 1247–1259.

Soares HD, Chen Y, Sabbagh M, Roher A, Schrijvers E, Breteler M. 2009. Identifying early markers of Alzheimer's disease using quantitative multiplex proteomic immunoassay panels. *Ann NY Acad Sci* **1180:** 56–67.

Sofroniew MV, Vinters HV. 2010. Astrocytes: Biology and pathology. *Acta Neuropathol* **119:** 7–35.

Sriram K, Matheson JM, Benkovic SA, Miller DB, Luster MI, O'Callaghan JP. 2002. Mice deficient in TNF receptors are protected against dopaminergic neurotoxicity: Implications for Parkinson's disease. *FASEB J* **16:** 1474–1476.

Stevens B, Allen NJ, Vazquez LE, Howell GR, Christopherson KS, Nouri N, Micheva KD, Mehalow AK, Huberman AD, Stafford B, et al. 2007. The classical complement cascade mediates CNS synapse elimination. *Cell* **131:** 1164–1178.

Stewart WF, Kawas C, Corrada M, Metter EJ. 1997. Risk of Alzheimer's disease and duration of NSAID use. *Neurology* **48:** 626–632.

Streit WJ, Xue QS. 2009. Life and death of microglia. *J Neuroimmune Pharmacol* **4:** 371–379.

Szekely CA, Zandi PP. 2010. Non-steroidal anti-inflammatory drugs and Alzheimer's disease: The epidemiological evidence. *CNS Neurol Disord Drug Targets* **9:** 132–139.

Szekely CA, Town T, Zandi PP. 2007. NSAIDs for the chemoprevention of Alzheimer's disease. *Subcell Biochem* **42:** 229–248.

Szekely CA, Breitner JC, Fitzpatrick AL, Rea TD, Psaty BM, Kuller LH, Zandi PP. 2008. NSAID use and dementia risk in the Cardiovascular Health Study: Role of APOE and NSAID type. *Neurology* **70:** 17–24.

Tahara K, Kim HD, Jin JJ, Maxwell JA, Li L, Fukuchi K. 2006. Role of toll-like receptor signalling in Aβ uptake and clearance. *Brain* **129:** 3006–3019.

Takami K, Terai K, Matsuo A, Walker DG, McGeer PL. 1997. Expression of presenilin-1 and -2 mRNAs in rat and Alzheimer's disease brains. *Brain Res* **748:** 122–130.

Tan J, Town T, Paris D, Mori T, Suo Z, Crawford F, Mattson MP, Flavell RA, Mullan M. 1999. Microglial activation resulting from CD40-CD40L interaction after β-amyloid stimulation. *Science* **286:** 2352–2355.

Taylor PR, Carugati A, Fadok VA, Cook HT, Andrews M, Carroll MC, Savill JS, Henson PM, Botto M, Walport MJ. 2000. A hierarchical role for classical pathway complement proteins in the clearance of apoptotic cells *in vivo*. *J Exp Med* **192:** 359–366.

Tenner AJ. 1999. Membrane receptors for soluble defense collagens. *Curr Opin Immunol* **11:** 34–41.

Tesseur I, Zou K, Esposito L, Bard F, Berber E, Can JV, Lin AH, Crews L, Tremblay P, Mathews P, et al. 2006. Deficiency in neuronal TGF-β signaling promotes neurodegeneration and Alzheimer's pathology. *J Clin Invest* **116:** 3060–3069.

Thal LJ, Ferris SH, Kirby L, Block GA, Lines CR, Yuen E, Assaid C, Nessly ML, Norman BA, Baranak CC, et al. 2005. A randomized, double-blind, study of rofecoxib in patients with mild cognitive impairment. *Neuropsychopharmacology* **30:** 1204–1215.

Thambisetty M, Simmons A, Velayudhan L, Hye A, Campbell J, Zhang Y, Wahlund LO, Westman E, Kinsey A, Gunert A, et al. 2010. Association of plasma clusterin concentration with severity, pathology, and progression in Alzheimer disease. *Arch Gen Psychiatry* **67:** 739–748.

Town T, Laouar Y, Pittenger C, Mori T, Szekely CA, Tan J, Duman RS, Flavell RA. 2008. Blocking TGF-β-Smad2/3 innate immune signaling mitigates Alzheimer-like pathology. *Nat Med* **14:** 681–687.

Vlad SC, Miller DR, Kowall NW, Felson DT. 2008. Protective effects of NSAIDs on the development of Alzheimer disease. *Neurology* **70:** 1672–1677.

Vodopivec I, Galichet A, Knobloch M, Bierhaus A, Heizmann CW, Nitsch RM. 2009. RAGE does not affect amyloid pathology in transgenic ArcAβ mice. *Neurodegener Dis* **6:** 270–280.

Wake H, Moorhouse AJ, Jinno S, Kohsaka S, Nabekura J. 2009. Resting microglia directly monitor the functional state of synapses in vivo and determine the fate of ischemic terminals. *J Neurosci* **29:** 3974–3980.

Walker DG, Lue LF. 2005. Investigations with cultured human microglia on pathogenic mechanisms of Alzheimer's disease and other neurodegenerative diseases. *J Neurosci Res* **81:** 412–425.

Walker DG, Kim SU, McGeer PL. 1995. Complement and cytokine gene expression in cultured microglial derived from postmortem human brains. *J Neurosci Res* **40:** 478–493.

Walker DG, Lue LF, Beach TG. 2001. Gene expression profiling of amyloid β peptide-stimulated human post-mortem brain microglia. *Neurobiol Aging* **22:** 957–966.

Walker DG, Dalsing-Hernandez JE, Campbell NA, Lue LF. 2009. Decreased expression of CD200 and CD200 receptor in Alzheimer's disease: A potential mechanism leading to chronic inflammation. *Exp Neurol* **215:** 5–19.

Walter S, Letiembre M, Liu Y, Heine H, Penke B, Hao W, Bode B, Manietta N, Walter J, Schulz-Schuffer W, et al. 2007. Role of the toll-like receptor 4 in neuroinflammation in Alzheimer's disease. *Cell Physiol Biochem* **20:** 947–956.

Warner TD, Mitchell JA. 2004. Cyclooxygenases: New forms, new inhibitors, and lessons from the clinic. *FASEB J* **18:** 790–804.

Webster S, Lue L-F, Brachova L, Tenner AJ, McGeer PL, Terai K, Walker DG, Bradt B, Cooper NR, Rogers J. 1997. Molecular and cellular characterization of the membrane attack complex, C5b-9, in Alzheimer's disease. *Neurobiol Aging* **18:** 415–421.

White JA, Manelli AM, Holmberg KH, Van Eldik LJ, Ladu MJ. 2005. Differential effects of oligomeric and fibrillar amyloid-β 1–42 on astrocyte-mediated inflammation. *Neurobiol Dis* **18:** 459–465.

Wiley CA, Lopresti BJ, Venneti S, Price J, Klunk WE, DeKosky ST, Mathis CA. 2009. Carbon 11-labeled Pittsburgh Compound B and carbon 11-labeled (R)-PK11195 positron emission tomographic imaging in Alzheimer disease. *Arch Neurol* **66:** 60–67.

Wolfson C, Perrault A, Moride Y, Esdaile JM, Abenhaim L, Momoli F. 2002. A case-control analysis of nonsteroidal anti-inflammatory drugs and Alzheimer's disease: Are they protective? *Neuroepidemiology* **21:** 81–86.

Wyss-Coray T. 2006. Inflammation in Alzheimer disease: Driving force, bystander or beneficial response? *Nat Med* **12:** 1005–1015.

Wyss-Coray T, Mucke L. 2002. Inflammation in neurodegenerative disease: A double-edged sword. *Neuron* **35:** 419–432.

Wyss-Coray T, Masliah E, Mallory M, McConlogue L, Johnson-Wood K, Lin C, Mucke L. 1997. Amyloidogenic role of cytokine TGF-b1 in transgenic mice and Alzheimer's disease. *Nature* **389:** 603–606.

Wyss-Coray T, Lin C, Yan F, Yu G, Rohde M, McConlogue L, Masliah E, Mucke L. 2001. TGF-b1 promotes microglial amyloid-b clearance and reduces plaque burden in transgenic mice. *Nat Med* **7:** 612–618.

Wyss-Coray T, Yan F, Lin AH, Lambris JD, Alexander JJ, Quigg RJ, Masliah E. 2002. Prominent neurodegeneration and increased plaque formation in complement-inhibited Alzheimer's mice. *Proc Natl Acad Sci* **99:** 10837–10842.

Wyss-Coray T, Loike JD, Brionne TC, Lu E, Anankov R, Yan F, Silverstein SC, Husemann J. 2003. Adult mouse astrocytes degrade amyloid-β in vitro and in situ. *Nat Med* **9:** 453–457.

Xiang Z, Ho L, Yemul S, Zhao Z, Qing W, Pompl P, Kelley K, Dang A, Teplow D, Pasinetti GM. 2002. Cyclooxygenase-2 promotes amyloid plaque deposition in a mouse model of Alzheimer's disease neuropathology. *Gene Expr* **10:** 271–278.

Xu J, Chen S, Ahmed SH, Chen H, Ku G, Goldberg MP, Hsu CY. 2001. Amyloid-β peptides are cytotoxic to oligodendrocytes. *J Neurosci* **21:** RC118.

Yamada T, Akiyama H, McGeer PL. 1990. Complement-activated oligodendroglia: A new pathogenic entity identified by immunostaining with antibodies to human complement proteins C3d and C4d. *Neurosci Lett* **112:** 161–166.

Yamamoto M, Horiba M, Buescher JL, Huang D, Gendelman HE, Ransohoff RM, Ikezu T. 2005. Overexpression of monocyte chemotactic protein-1/CCL2 in β-amyloid precursor protein transgenic mice show accelerated diffuse β-amyloid deposition. *Am J Pathol* **166:** 1475–1485.

Yan P, Bero AW, Cirrito JR, Xiao Q, Hu X, Wang Y, Gonzales E, Holtzman DM, Lee JM. 2009. Characterizing the appearance and growth of amyloid plaques in APP/PS1 mice. *J Neurosci* **29:** 10706–10714.

Yang LB, Li R, Meri S, Rogers J, Shen Y. 2000. Deficiency of complement defense protein CD59 may contribute to neurodegeneration in Alzheimer's disease. *J Neurosci* **20:** 7505–7509.

Yasojima K, Schwab C, McGeer EG, McGeer PL. 1999. Distribution of cyclooxygenase-1 and cyclooxygenase-2 mRNAs and proteins in human brain and peripheral organs. *Brain Res* **830:** 226–236.

Yin KJ, Cirrito JR, Yan P, Hu X, Xiao Q, Pan X, Bateman R, Song H, Hsu FF, Turk J, et al. 2006. Matrix metalloproteinases expressed by astrocytes mediate extracellular amyloid-β peptide catabolism. *J Neurosci* **26:** 10939–10948.

Zandi PP, Anthony JC, Hayden KM, Mehta K, Mayer L, Breitner JC. 2002. Reduced incidence of AD with NSAID but not H2 receptor antagonists: The Cache County Study. *Neurology* **59:** 880–886.

Zhang J, Sokal I, Peskind ER, Quinn JF, Jankovic J, Kenney C, Chung KA, Millard SP, Nutt JG, Montine TJ. 2008. CSF multianalyte profile distinguishes Alzheimer and Parkinson diseases. *Am J Clin Pathol* **129:** 526–529.

The Ubiquitin–Proteasome System and the Autophagic–Lysosomal System in Alzheimer Disease

Yasuo Ihara[1], Maho Morishima-Kawashima[2], and Ralph Nixon[3,4]

[1]Department of Neuropathology, Faculty of Life and Medical Science, Doshisha University, Kyoto 619-0225, Japan

[2]Department of Molecular Neuropathology, Graduate School of Pharmaceutical Sciences, Hokkaido University, Sapporo 060-0812, Japan

[3]Center for Dementia Research, Nathan Kline Institute, Orangeburg, New York 10962

[4]Departments of Psychiatry and Cell Biology, New York University Langone Medical Center, New York, New York 10016

Correspondence: yihara@mail.doshisha.ac.jp; nixon@nki.rfmh.org

As neurons age, their survival depends on eliminating a growing burden of damaged, potentially toxic proteins and organelles—a capability that declines owing to aging and disease factors. Here, we review the two proteolytic systems principally responsible for protein quality control in neurons and their important contributions to Alzheimer disease pathogenesis. In the first section, the discovery of paired helical filament ubiquitination is described as a backdrop for discussing the importance of the ubiquitin–proteasome system in Alzheimer disease. In the second section, we review the prominent involvement of the lysosomal system beginning with pathological endosomal–lysosomal activation and signaling at the very earliest stages of Alzheimer disease followed by the progressive failure of autophagy. These abnormalities, which result in part from Alzheimer-related genes acting directly on these lysosomal pathways, contribute to the development of each of the Alzheimer neuropathological hallmarks and represent a promising therapeutic target.

Cellular aging, the sine qua non for Alzheimer disease development, is associated with cumulative oxidative damage to proteins and membranes, translational errors leading to the synthesis of defective proteins, and various genetic and environmental insults to organelles and proteins (Terman 2001; Roy et al. 2002; Sohal et al. 2002; Troen 2003; Levine et al. 2004). In some aging-related neurodegenerative diseases, mutations of the pathogenic gene(s) may also cause anomalous conformations of the encoded protein or its metabolites, leading to increased proteolytic resistance and accumulation of these potentially toxic proteins (Soto 2003). A neuron's ability to function in the face of these mounting aging- and disease-related insults is determined in significant part by the efficiency with which it can eliminate this burden of damaged cellular constituents. An array of proteases regulates cell function, but two proteolytic systems are mainly responsible for the turnover of proteins and organelles—the proteasome and lysosomal systems (Grune et al. 2001; Berke et al. 2003; Goldberg 2003; Levine et al. 2004). The proteasome selectively degrades normal proteins (mainly those with short half-lives) and abnormal proteins, which are earmarked for elimination by a process involving their conjugation to ubiquitin (Ub; Goldberg 2003). The lysosomal system, and specifically the autophagic pathway, is the principal mechanism for degrading proteins with long half-lives and is the only system in cells for degrading organelles and large protein aggregates or inclusions. A second route to lysosomes, the endocytic pathway, delivers extracellular material and plasma membrane constituents to lysosomes under the direction of specific targeting signals (Nixon 2004).

Not surprisingly, protein quality control and proteostasis—the appropriate balance of protein synthesis, folding, and turnover in the cell—involve interdependent regulation of these two proteolytic systems. This interdependence is best exemplified by the regulatory influences of the protein ubiquitin. It has recently become appreciated that ubiquitination of proteins by covalent modification tags them for elimination not only through the proteasome (the ubiquitin–proteasome system or UPS) but also through the lysosomal system. Endocytosed receptors are targeted for lysosomal degradation, in part, by ubiquination in late endosomes/multivesicular bodies (MVBs). Recently, protein aggregates and certain organelles have been shown to be tagged with ubiquination for selective removal by autophagy (Narendra et al. 2009; Dikic et al. 2010; Youle et al. 2011), a degradative process previously believed to be only nonselective. In selective autophagy, an adaptor molecule with a ubiquitin-binding domain engages the ubiquitinated structure and couples it to the pre-autophagosomal isolation membrane for subsequent sequestration. The exact types of ubiquitin motifs recognized by the UPS and autophagy may differ and the degree to which ubiquitination drives autophagic protein turnover relative to that by proteasomes is still unclear. Nevertheless, the role of ubiquitin as a tag for targeting substrates for elimination is more universal than earlier imagined, implying that changes in ubiquitin balance may be one way that disease-related perturbations of one proteolytic system are likely to influence the other.

Interdependence of the proteasome and lysosomal system is also suggested by observations that, when proteasome activity is inhibited, proteins accumulate that become substrates for autophagy (Fortun et al. 2003). Inhibiting autophagy by genetically deleting components of the sequestration machinery causes ubiquitinated protein aggregates to appear in neurons, reflecting additional negative effects on the UPS (Korolchuk et al. 2009a,b). Besides ubiquitin, proteins identified to play regulatory roles in the UPS and autophagy are being increasingly identified (Zhao et al. 2007). For example, p62, an adaptor protein for autophagy, also influences proteasomal degradation, whereas VCP/p97 acting through p62 and ubiquitin regulates both the proteasome-dependent endoplasmic reticulum–associated degradation (ERAD) pathway and aspects of autophagosome maturation (Tresse et al. 2010). The E3 ligase Parkin, a protein implicated in Parkinson's disease, creates an autophagy signal on mitochondria and also tags proteins elsewhere for proteasomal degradation (Yoshii et al. 2011). Interestingly, proteasomal subunits may be degraded by lysosomes (Cuervo et al. 1995), hinting at an additional level of cross talk between these proteolytic systems.

Proteolysis has been an active area of Alzheimer disease research over the past two decades mainly in relation to the processing of specific proteins, like the β-amyloid precursor protein. A broader appreciation is emerging, however, of the roles of proteolytic systems in other crucial aspects of Alzheimer disease (AD) pathogenesis related to protein clearance, neural plasticity, and neurodegenerative mechanisms. In this article, we focus on the involvement of the UPS and the lysosomal system (endosomal–lysosomal pathway and autophagy) in AD, their contributions to disease development and progression, and the possibilities for targeting these systems in the design of innovative therapies for AD.

PART I: THE UBIQUITIN–PROTEASOME SYSTEM IN AD

Discovery of Ubiquitin in Paired Helical Filaments: A Personal Retrospective
by Yasuo Ihara

Polyclonal antibodies to the classical paired helical filaments (PHFs) found in the neurofibrillary tangles and dystrophic neurites of AD were first raised in about 1982, allowing exploration of the component(s) of PHFs using immunochemical approaches (Ihara et al. 1983). This strategy was useful because PHFs were resistant to conventional protease digestion, and it was difficult to obtain reproducible and distinct limited-digest protein fragments of PHFs for sequencing. Sodium dodecyl sulfate (SDS)-insoluble material was extracted from typical AD brains, and PHFs were partially purified from the SDS-insoluble material by differential centrifugation and sucrose density gradient centrifugation (Ihara et al. 1983). The PHFs obtained by these procedures were not yet sufficiently pure, as shown later by sequencing of fragments of PHF proteins (Kondo et al. 1988). The polyclonal PHF antisera that were initially raised also reacted with lipofuscin-like granules and other SDS-insoluble materials in the PHF-rich immunogen. A major frustration with the antisera was that, although they intensely stained neurofibrillary tangles (NFTs), dystrophic neurites, and neuropil threads in AD brain sections, they did not label a distinct band(s) on immunoblots of AD brain homogenates, instead giving peculiar smears running from very high to low molecular mass (Ihara et al. 1983). These immunoreactive smears were highly characteristic of AD brain homogenates and never seen in control brain homogenates. Thus, the indirect immunochemical approach to identify the PHF component proteins seemed unsuccessful at first. However, it

succeeded a few years later when fetal or neonatal brain homogenates were probed with anti-PHF antisera: A somewhat diffuse band around 50 kDa was intensely labeled in immunoblots of fetal brain homogenates. This protein reactive with the initial anti-PHF sera was soon identified as tau, a microtubule-associated protein (MAP), based on its molecular weight, isoform change during development, microtubule-binding activity, and heat stability (Kosik et al. 1986; Nukina and Ihara 1986; see also Brion et al. 1985; Grundke-Iqbal et al. 1986; Wood et al. 1986; discovery of tau in PHF is reviewed in Mandelkow and Mandelkow 2011).

In contrast to our initial PHF antisera, we assumed that a monoclonal antibody that recognizes a highly defined epitope on PHF would not give rise to the smearing pattern on immunoblots that greatly puzzled us. In 1985, we became aware of a hybrid system (Pike et al. 1982) for raising monoclonal antibodies to glycolipids. Lewis rats responded well to immunizations with partially purified PHF preparations, yielding high titers of antisera to PHFs. These rats provided splenocytes for fusion with mouse myeloma cells. We (Hiroshi Mori and Yasuo Ihara) employed a two-step screening procedure to identify monoclonals in the resultant hybridoma supernatants: first by enzyme-linked immunosorbent assay (ELISA) using plates coated with partially purified PHFs, and second by immunostaining of NFTs that were prepared from AD brains under nondenaturing conditions. Only two confirmed and stable cell lines emerged, the antibodies from which had very similar specificities on the blots: Besides the characteristic "PHF smear," they also labeled a very small protein of ∼8 kDa. Hiroshi Mori named these monoclonal antibodies DF (Dementia Filament) 1 and 2, of which the latter (DF2) was used for subsequent characterization (Mori et al. 1987).

In contrast to our PHF antisera, DF2 produced immunoreactive smears even in control brain homogenates (presumably representing Ub-conjugated proteins). In addition, DF2 gave a distinct band at 8 kDa on blots of aged human brain homogenates, whereas the PHF antisera had not given distinct bands. We were puzzled as to why the two antibodies labeled different bands, but hypothesized that they recognized different components of PHFs. Optical diffraction analyses carried out by Wischik et al. (1985) had suggested that the core of the PHF may be composed of a subunit around ∼100 kDa. We reasoned that one protein might make up the core framework of PHFs, whereas another might occur on a peripheral portion.

In AD cortical sections, we observed that NFTs and dystrophic neurites (Fig. 1) and, unexpectedly, granulovacuolar changes (Fig. 1, inset) were intensely immunolabeled by the DF2 monoclonal. When mild fixation conditions were used, innumerable neuropil threads were also detected. (One peculiar characteristic was an apparent "background" staining of AD brain sections, whereas widely used Ub polyclonal antibodies [Haas and Bright 1985] gave almost no background staining. This discrepancy was resolved in 1996: DF2 is specific for the conjugated form of Ub, whereas the Ub polyclonal antibodies are specific for free Ub [Morimoto et al. 1996].)

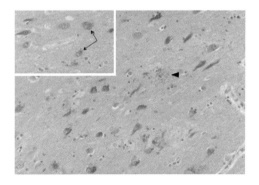

Figure 1. DF2 immunostaining of a tissue section from Alzheimer disease (AD) hippocampus. Neurofibrillary tangles and dystrophic neurites (arrowhead) are intensely labeled, whereas the neuropil (background) is uniformly stained, simulating nonspecific background staining. However, this was found to be true staining of ubiquitin-conjugated proteins in the neuropil (Morimoto et al. 1996). (*Inset*) Some neurons in CA1 undergo granulovacuolar changes (arrows) and are also intensely stained with DF2.

What was the small protein at 8 kDa that was strongly labeled by DF2? Purifying the protein was not difficult with high-performance liquid chromatography (HPLC), which was beginning to be used for protein fractionation. The sequence of the DF2-reactive protein up to approximately 30 residues exactly corresponded to that of ubiquitin (Mori et al. 1987). This was probably the first description of Ub protein modification in the field of neuropathology. Two seminal papers describing the significance of protein ubiquitination had recently been published by the Varshavsky laboratory (Ciechanover et al. 1984; Finley et al. 1984). Despite reading these papers, we could not understand why Ub is present on PHFs. Our understanding was that Ub is a tag for protein degradation: A Ub-tagged protein should be recognized and degraded by the proteasome, an unusually large cytoplasmic protease. However, Ub was found to have other functional roles; for example, a proportion of histone (H)2B is ubiquitinated in a way that has a role in the transcription.

Ubiquitin appeared to represent a novel constituent of PHFs; DF2 strongly stained SDS-stripped NFTs, suggesting that Ub was an integral component. Nevertheless, we felt that the immunochemical identification of the component was not sufficient to fully confirm the presence of the molecule on PHFs. At the time, there was some confusion about the PHF protein constituents. Using well-characterized antibodies to various MAPs as well as PHF polyclonal antibodies, tau had recently been established as a major component of PHFs (see above and Mandelkow and Mandelkow 2011). However, monoclonal antibodies to neurofilament (NF) proteins also strongly immunolabeled PHF (Anderton et al. 1982), and these were widely applied to AD brain sections. This confusion about PHF components was clarified when Nobuyuki Nukina and coworkers found significant cross-reactivities of certain NF monoclonal antibodies with phosphorylated epitopes of tau (Nukina et al. 1987). In light of such observations, it became essential to show unambiguously that Ub was a component of PHF. In 1987, we finally obtained definitive evidence using protein chemical techniques that Ub was integral to the PHF (Mori et al. 1987).

Ubiquitinated Tau in PHFs: K48-Linked Mono- and Polyubiquitin Modification

In the mid 1980s, the distinction between mono- and polyubiquitination was not yet clear, and the role of the multiubiquitin chain as a strong degradative signal was just emerging. A fraction of H2B was shown to be monoubiquitinated, and lymphocyte homing receptor was similarly found to be ubiquitinated, but the significance of monoubiquitination was entirely unclear. In our research on Ub in PHFs, we were unable to identify the Ub-conjugated protein by direct sequencing. It was most likely to be tau, but we had no definitive evidence. In the period 1989–1992, the Ihara laboratory was mostly involved in determining the phosphorylation sites on tau proteins in PHFs. We became aware that ion spray mass spectroscopy (MS) was an excellent method for determining phosphorylation sites on PHF-tau (Hasegawa et al. 1992). This provided an opportunity to reanalyze purified PHFs from AD cortex and identify the Ub-targeted protein.

We had previously raised antibodies to the carboxy-terminal region (Gly-76) of Ub, which was predicted to be conjugated with ε-amino groups of lysines of other proteins targeted for proteasomal degradation. However, despite repeated trials using these antibodies, we were unable to identify a particular HPLC peak containing the Ub carboxyl terminus. In our hands, Ub reactivity was detected exclusively in the insoluble AD brain fractions displaying so-called "PHF smears" on immunoblots. However, Ub itself was not responsible for this smear pattern, because we also observed Ub-negative/tau-positive smears, in addition to Ub-positive/tau-positive smears (Morishima-Kawashima et al. 1993). The guanidine HCl-solubilized, Ub- and tau-reactive material purified from AD cortex by HPLC was subjected to peptide mapping using *Achromobacter lyticus* protease I (AP1), which is highly specific for Lys-X bonds. This yielded peaks corresponding to API-generated fragments of Ub (Fig. 2), in addition to carboxy-terminal fragments of tau, whereas virtually no fragments derived from the amino-terminal portion of tau were recovered. As expected, fragments U1–U7 (see Fig. 2) were found in our digests, but U8 (the carboxy-terminal portion of Ub) was undetectable at the expected position of the nonconjugated U8. Instead, we observed several unusual HPLC peaks that neither corresponded to U1–U8 nor occurred in the digests of Ub-negative/tau-positive smears. By protein sequencing and MS, we identified four Ub-conjugated sites on tau (Fig. 3) and further identified K48-linked Ub chains (Morishima-Kawashima et al. 1993). Crude estimates suggested that most of the products were derived from monoubiquitination and only a minority from polyubiquitination.

These Ub- and tau-reactive smears were recovered exclusively from the buffer-insoluble fraction of AD cortex, suggesting that ubiquitination might occur after tau deposits into

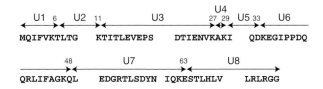

Figure 2. Schematic illustration of 76-residue ubiquitin. Ubiquitin has seven lysine residues and *Achromobacter lyticus* protease 1 (AP1) cleaves ubiquitin into eight fragments, U1–U8. G76 is conjugated with ε-amino groups of lysine in the target protein. K48-linked ubiquitin chain is a strong degradation signal. Besides this, K6-, 11-, 27-, 29-, and 63-linked multiubiquitin chains are found in the cell (Xu and Peng 2006). It is likely that each type of chain has a distinct role in the cellular metabolism.

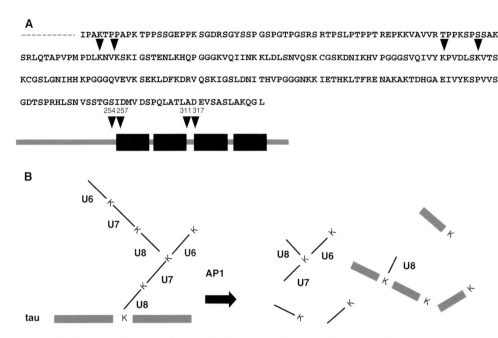

Figure 3. Ubiquitination sites on amino terminally processed tau. As shown in *A*, four ubiquitin conjugation sites were identified. These are located close to and in the microtubule-binding domain, K254, 257, 311, and 317 according to the numbering of the 441 amino acid human tau isoform. A size exclusion–purified paired helical filament PHF smear was further purified by reverse-phase HPLC, giving three broad (overlapped) peaks that existed only in smear fractions from AD brain. The last-eluting fraction contained a ubiquitin (Ub)-positive, tau-positive smear, which was subjected to AP1 digestion and reverse HPLC fractionation, followed by amino acid sequencing and mass spectrometric analysis. Several late-eluting peaks were found to contain branched fragments, mostly consisting of tau fragments and U8; a minority of U8 conjugated with Lys-48 of U6–U7, derived from the polyubiquitin chain (Morishima-Kawashima et al. 1993). Dysfunction of autophagic and endocytic pathways to lysosomes driven by relevant genes and other risk factors in Alzheimer disease (expressed on the *left* side of the diagram) causes or promotes pathophysiology critical to the development and progression of the disease (outlined on the *right* side of the diagram). See the text for further details.

aggregates. At that time, a simple model showed that cells conjugated Ub to abnormal proteins that were to be selectively degraded by the proteasome. If this was correct, minute amounts of abnormal PHF proteins tagged by Ub and targeted for the proteasome might be observed in the buffer-soluble fraction of cytoplasm, but we were unable to confirm this. However, recent work by Cripps et al. (2006) successfully used MC1 (a monoclonal specific for an abnormal PHF-like conformation of tau) to affinity purify soluble full-length tau from PHF-rich extracts of AD cortex and subject it to liquid chromatography–tandem MS (LC–MS/MS) analysis. The presence of K6, K11, and K48- linked polyubiquitinations—in

addition to monoubiquitination—was observed. Among these polyubiquitination sites, the K48-linked site was predominant. It is thus possible that a portion of MC1-reactive PHF-tau is in the soluble fraction and exists as free molecules in the cytoplasm, but this has not yet been confirmed.

Interestingly, immunocytochemical staining suggests that Ub exists in the mid-portion of neuropil threads (the largest source of PHF in the AD brain), whereas both ends of the threads are reactive for only tau, not Ub (Iwatsubo et al. 1992). This finding suggests that neuropil threads may extend at both ends: Tau may aggregate and deposit first, followed by its ubiquitination.

Ubiquitination of Other Neuropathological Inclusions

Following the discoveries about Ub and PHFs reviewed above, a variety of types of Ub–protein conjugates were detected in other neurodegenerative diseases. Although such findings were initially based solely on immunocytochemical evidence, we and others postulated that ubiquitination may be widely involved in the degradation of cytoplasmic proteins accumulating during aging and in a number of neurodegenerative diseases. Therefore, ubiquitinated inclusions may represent a failure of degradation by the Ub–proteasome system of neurons or glia. Early on, it was thought that Ub was associated with intermediate (10-nm) filaments in cells, because many inclusions seemed to consist of "altered" intermediate filaments (Lowe et al. 1988).

With the knowledge that DF2 recognizes Ub, we investigated whether DF2 stains other types of known intracellular inclusions. In the cortex, DF2 revealed fine dot-like stainings that had not been described before, and larger dot-like stainings were seen in the white matter, possibly derived from multivesicular and lysosome-related bodies. In addition, DF2 intensely labeled the classical granulovacuolar changes in the hippocampus in AD and other neurodegenerative disorders (Fig. 1, inset). We soon found that DF2 strongly stained cortical and brain stem Lewy bodies in brain sections from "diffuse Lewy body disease" (Kuzuhara et al. 1988), as originally described by Kenji Kosaka (1978), who proposed that some elderly subjects dying with dementia had many cortical Lewy bodies. In this dementia, Lewy bodies are abundant in cortical neurons, especially in the cingulate gyrus, in addition to their presence in the substantia nigra and locus ceruleus, their prototypical loci in Parkinson's disease. The eosinophilic round bodies with clear margins in brainstem neurons and the somewhat indistinct, smaller round bodies in cortical neurons are sometimes difficult to recognize with conventional hematoxylin–eosin stains, but anti-Ub antibodies such as DF2 labeled them well. Furthermore, DF2 revealed a possible evolution of Lewy bodies: Diffuse cytoplasmic accumulation of Ub-positive material might be followed by its gradual coalescence into an amorphous perinuclear inclusion (Kuzuhara et al. 1988). DF2 and other Ub antibodies also labeled elongated neurites (now known as Lewy neurites) in and near the sites of Lewy bodies. Because Lewy bodies did not stain for tau, the target protein of ubiquitination had to be distinct. In 1997, α-synuclein was shown to be the principal component of Lewy bodies (Spillantini et al. 1997). The accumulated α-synuclein was then shown to be ubiquitinated (Hasegawa et al. 2002).

The DF2 immunoreactivity of Lewy bodies led us to search for similar DF2-positive inclusions, and we found that Lewy-like bodies in motor neurons in amyotrophic lateral sclerosis (ALS; Murayama et al. 1990a) and Pick bodies in Pick's disease (Murayama et al. 1990b) were strongly reactive; the latter stained also for tau, whereas the former stained neither for tau nor α-synuclein. In this regard, the entity of frontotemporal lobar degeneration (FTLD) with Ub-positive/tau-negative inclusions was described later, and TDP43 was identified as the ubiquitinated protein in both this disorder and ALS (Neuman et al. 2006). It is noteworthy that the specific protein targets of ubiquitination that accumulate in insoluble deposits in distinct disorders have apparent major roles in the respective neurodegenerative processes: In AD, tau is ubiquitinated, in Parkinson's disease and dementia with Lewy bodies, it is α-synuclein, and in ALS and FTLD-U, it is TDP-43.

Significance of Ubiquitinated Neurofibrillary Tangles

The discovery of tau ubiqutination in PHFs suggested that living (but presumably injured) neurons may mount an attempt to remove the abnormal inclusions (NFTs) by Ub tagging, although this apparently fails to efficiently remove the tangles. The UPS was believed to be involved principally in the turnover of short-lived proteins (cytosolic, nuclear, and endoplasmic reticulum [ER]), and especially tightly regulated transcription factors; for this process, the proteolytic system requires adenosine triphosphate (ATP). There was initially a view that long-lived proteins, including tau, may be degraded principally by lysosomes, the other major protein degradation machinery of the cell.

Ubiquitination occurs in three steps. The first step is activation of the carboxyl terminus of Ub by an E1 protein (i.e., a Ub-activating enzyme), which consumes ATP. Second, there is conjugation of the ATP-activated Ub to an E2 protein (i.e., a Ub-conjugating enzyme). Third, there is ligation of Ub with an ε-amino group of lysine in the target protein by an E3 ligase. E3 ligase binds both the target protein and the E2–Ub complex; thousands of substrate-specific E3s ensure selective protein tagging and degradation. An E4 enzyme catalyzes the polyubiquitination of the target substrate that is bound to the E2–E3 complexes. Proteins tagged with chains of four or more K48-linked multiubiquitins provide the strongest signal for degradation by the 26S proteasome, because a chain of at least four Ub moieties is required for substrate recognition by the 26S proteasome complex. Ubiquitinated target proteins bind

to the 19S cap (RP), which has a Ub binding site and ATPase activity, and this leads to cleavage of Ub moieties from the target by deubiquitinating enzymes, unfolds the polypeptides and sends them to the narrow channel of the 20S core particle. The narrow canal of 20S proteasome ($\sim$700 kDa) consists of heptameric stacks of four rings, with the inner two being composed of β subunits and the outer two of α subunits (Gallastegui and Groll 2010). Thus, the general structure of the 20S core particle is $\alpha_{1-7}\beta_{1-7}\beta_{1-7}\alpha_{1-7}$ (Fig. 4). These subunits have activities as trypsin-like, chymotrypsin-like, and peptidyl–glutaminyl hydrolyzing activities. The catalytic portions face the interior surface; during its passage, the target protein is processed to short peptides, mostly between six and 10 amino acids. Deubiquitinating activity attached to the 19S cap is essential for complete degradation; if this is blocked, degradation is inhibited, and ubiquitinated substrates accumulate in the cytoplasm.

The 26S proteasome is primarily a cytosolic enzyme, but it is also found in ER membranes and localized to nuclei. The former activity is known as ER-associated degradation. The latter (nuclear) activity is thought to be involved in

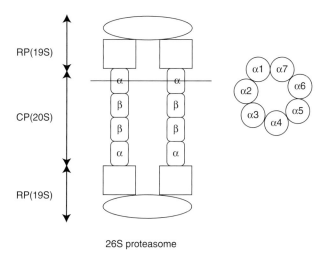

Figure 4. Schematic illustration of 26S proteasome. It consists of 19S regulatory particle (RP) and 20S core particle (CP). The narrow canal of CP consists of heptameric stacks of four rings, with the inner two being composed of β subunits and the outer two of α subunits. The image on the *right* shows a cross section at an indicated line (*left*). These subunits have trypsin-like, chymotrypsin-like, and peptidyl glutaminyl hydrolyzing activities. (Modified from Gallastegui and Groll 2010.)

the development of the ubiquitinated nuclear inclusions found in Huntington's disease and some types of spinocerebellar ataxia.

The question arises whether a fundamental impairment of proteasome function is involved in the formation of intracellular aggregates, in particular the NFT of AD. AD is the most common of numerous age-associated brain diseases, and the activity of brain proteasomes appears to decline with age (Keller et al. 2002). PHF have been associated with inhibition of the activity of the proteasome in a brain region–specific manner (Keller et al. 2000). That is, in areas where NFTs formed abundantly, including hippocampus and parahippocampal gyrus and superior and middle temporal gyri, proteasome activity (as assessed by chymortrypsin-like and postglutamyl peptidases) appeared to be most affected, whereas occipital gyri and cerebellum, which often have few or no NFTs, were least affected (Keller et al. 2000). Despite the decreased proteasomal enzymatic activity observed in AD brains, the levels of the α and β subunits were not decreased. This suggests that posttranslational modifications could cause the decreases in the activities of proteasome. Another study of AD brain tissues showed that hyperphosphorylated tau was bound to the proteasome, presumably to the 19S cap portion, and the more tau that was bound, the more that proteasomes appeared to be inhibited (Keck et al. 2003). In vitro experiments further showed that aggregated (recombinant) tau—but not nonaggregated (monomeric) tau—can inhibit the proteasome activity. The hyperphosphorylation of tau may not be related to suppression of proteasomes. Based on these various findings, it has been speculated that small aggregates of PHFs may bind to the cap portion of the 26S proteasome and inhibit its activity. This hypothesis is consistent with related observations made in other cell model systems (Bence et al. 2001). Taken together, the available evidence suggests that PHF-bearing neurons have defective activity of some of their proteasomes, which may contribute to the neurodegeneration. On the other hand, it seems unlikely that the decreasing activity of the proteasome leads to NFT formation. Aggregate formation itself may be a protective

event in AD neurons and help extend their life spans, as compared with neurons not bearing NFTs (Gomez-Isla et al. 1997).

The currently prevailing view of the temporal involvement of Ub in PHF evolution is that the aggregation of hyperphosphorylated tau is followed by ubiquitination. This is consistent with previous immunocytochemical observations (Bancher et al. 1991) and also with confocal microscopy reconstructions, suggesting that, in the neuropil threads of AD cortex, both growing ends of the threads contain full-length tau, whereas Ub is present at the mid portion, where the amino-terminal region of tau may have been processed (Iwatsubo et al. 1992). Similarly, in our biochemical studies, ubiquitinated tau was undetectable in the soluble fraction of cortex (but see Cripps et al. 2006), and only a portion of amino-terminally processed tau in the insoluble fraction was ubiquitinated (Morishima-Kawashima et al. 1993). The question remains why only a minority of the ubiquitin tagged to the processed tau in PHF is in the form of polyubiquitin chains, and what the significance is of the monoubiquitination that appears to represent the majority of ubiquitin found in PHFs (Morishima-Kawashima et al. 1993).

The Ubiquitin–Proteasome System in AD

Since ubiquitin immunoreactivity has been documented in a range of inclusion bodies, a role of the UPS in the pathogenesis of a number of neurodegenerative diseases, especially in AD, has been considered. Several molecules that are relevant to the UPS have been shown to be associated with AD. Let us first discuss UBB^{+1}, a mutant form of ubiquitin extending 19 amino acids at its carboxyl terminus which is generated owing to dinucleotide deletions of the ubiquitin mRNA through "molecular misreading" (van Leeuwen et al. 1998). UBB^{+1} protein accumulates in brains affected by AD and other diseases such as Pick's disease and Huntington's disease (Fischer et al. 2003). Because of the absence of the carboxy-terminal Gly-76, UBB^{+1} cannot ubiquitinate other proteins, but it is itself ubiquitinated efficiently. The resulting polyubiquitinated UBB^{+1} cannot be degraded by proteasomes and impairs the UPS (Lam et al. 2000), which may induce neurotoxicity. Indeed, transgenic mice expressing UBB^{+1} have an impaired UPS and show contextual memory deficits in both water maze and fear conditioning paradigms, without specific neuropathological findings (Fischer et al. 2009). Further, UBB^{+1} can enhance the susceptibility of yeast to the toxicity of protein aggregates (Tank et al. 2009).

Ubiquitin carboxy-terminal hydrolase L1 (UCH-L1), which was originally identified as a deubiquinating enzyme, has multiple functions, including as a ubiquitin ligase and a stabilizer of monoubiquitinated proteins (Setsuie and Wada 2007). Although UCH-L1 is genetically associated with Parkinson's disease (i.e., it is the PARK5 gene; Belin and Westerlund 2008), it has also been implicated in the pathogenesis of AD. A proteomic analysis has shown down-regulation and oxidative modification of UCH-L1 in the AD brain, and the levels of soluble UCH-L1 were inversely proportional to the number of NFTs (Choi et al. 2004). Moreover, administration of UCH-L1 can reverse the amyloid β-protein–induced synaptic dysfunction and memory loss in transgenic mice overexpressing APP and PS1 (Gong et al. 2006).

Next, ubiquilin-1 has been reported to be genetically linked to AD. Ubiquilin-1 interacts with both proteasomes and ubiquitinated proteins and regulates the proteasomal degradation of various proteins, including presenilin 1 (Haapasalo et al. 2010). An intronic polymorphism involving alternative splicing of exon 8 in the ubiquilin 1 gene (*UBQLN1*), which is genetically located near a well-established linkage peak for AD on chromosome 9q22, has been associated with increased risk for late-onset AD (Bertram et al. 2005). However, this finding has not been replicated by others (Smemo et al. 2006).

The earliest symptoms of AD are believed to be due to synaptic dysfunction, and in this context, numerous studies have established a significant role of the UPS in the regulation of synaptic plasticity. Although ubiquitin tagging was originally identified as a signal for protein destruction by the proteasome system, ubiquitination is now known to be a posttranslational modification in which ubiquitins can serve as signals for protein localization and sorting in various physiological phenomena such as signal transduction, the cell cycle, transcription, DNA repair, and endocytosis. In particular, the critical role of the UPS in synaptic plasticity, learning and memory formation needs to be emphasized (Bingol and Sheng 2011). The role of the UPS in synaptic plasticity was first highlighted in *Aplysia*. During the induction of long-term facilitation in the snail, the regulatory subunit of cAMP-dependent protein kinase (PKA) is ubiquitinated and degraded by the proteasome, generating persistently activated PKA (Hegde et al. 1993). Activated PKA induces transcription of ApUCH (UCH-L1 in mammals), a deubiquitinating enzyme, which has been found to be critical for the induction of long-term facilitation (Hegde et al. 1997). It is now known that the UPS also regulates turnover of neurotransmitter receptors, protein kinases, synaptic proteins, transcription factors, and other molecules critical for proper synaptic plasticity, thus controlling synaptic strength and connections during brain development in mammals (Bingol and Sheng 2011). The UPS is also critically involved in learning and memory. Bilateral injection of lactacystin, a specific proteasome inhibitor, into the CA1 region of the rat hippocampus blocks long-term memory formation (Lopez-Salon et al. 2001). This and numerous related findings suggest that degradation of certain critical proteins by the UPS is required during long-term memory formation. One of these proteins is arc, a negative regulator of synaptic strength that promotes the internalization of AMPA receptors and is degraded via the E3 ligase, UBE3A (Greer et al. 2010).

Synaptic loss has long been documented in AD brain (Gonatas et al. 1967) and, as expected, is strongly correlated with the degree of cognitive impairment (Terry et al. 1991). In transgenic mouse models of AD, synaptic deficits have been detected prior to the formation of amyloid plaques (Hsia et al. 1999). Among the various molecular species of Aβ present in the brain, soluble oligomeric forms of Aβ are arguably the most plausible candidates to impair synaptic function (reviewed in Walsh and Selkoe 2004). Soluble Aβ oligomers inhibit hippocampal long-term potentiation and alter memory and learning performance. They also facilitate long-term depression by, among other effects, disrupting synaptic glutamate uptake (Li et al. 2009). Recently, it has been shown that soluble Aβ oligomers isolated from AD cortex can induce tau hyperphosphorylation at AD-relevant epitopes and subsequent neuritic degeneration (Jin et al. 2011). Beyond an age-related reduction (Keller et al. 2002), proteasome activities decrease in AD in a brain region–specific manner, particularly in hippocampus, parahippocampal gyrus, superior and middle temporal gyri, and the inferior parietal lobule (Keller et al. 2000), areas that are especially critical for long-term memory formation. Moreover, soluble Aβ oligomers themselves can inhibit proteasomal activity (Tseng et al. 2008). Thus, it is possible that additive effects of Aβ oligomers and reduced proteasome activities in AD may accelerate synaptic dysfunction.

It is still unsettled how the degradation of tau is regulated under physiological conditions. It has been reported that tau is degraded by several major cellular degradation systems, including calpain, caspases, lysosomes, and proteasomes. As regards the proteasome, both the ATP-dependent 26S proteasome and the ATP-independent 20S proteasome have been reported to degrade normal, soluble tau (Cardozo et al. 2002; Zhang et al. 2005). However, administration of inhibitors of the proteasome has provided conflicting results: Treatment with lactacystin either did or did not suppress the degradation of tau (David et al. 2002; Brown et al. 2005a). On the other hand, it has been reported that the E3 ligase CHIP (carboxyl terminus of the Hsc70-interacting protein) binds to tau and is involved in the degradation of abnormal forms of tau, including insoluble tau and hyperphosphorylated tau, coordinately with Hsp70 (Petrucelli et al. 2004; Dickey et al. 2006). As described above, it has also been found that the 20S proteasome interacts with tau aggregates (Keck et al. 2003). Collectively, such findings suggest that the UPS may be implicated more in the degradation of abnormal forms of tau than of normal, soluble tau.

As in the case of tau, an impairment of proteasome activity by protein aggregates is observed for other proteins, such as polyglutamine-expanded proteins, the prion protein, and Aβ (Bence et al. 2001). Notably, immunotherapy against Aβ in the 3xTg-AD mice, which reduces Aβ oligomers, reverses the proteasome deficits of these transgenic mice (Tseng et al. 2008). Thus, the accumulation of tau and of Aβ, forming the two major protein lesions of AD, impairs proteasome activity in vivo.

Despite the substantial indirect evidence just reviewed that associates UPS dysfunction with key features of AD, it remains unclear whether aberration in the UPS plays a causative or only a secondary role. Besides its key role in the UPS, ubiquitin is now known to function as a signal tag in the lysosome–autophagy system (see below). Indeed, many recent studies suggest the involvement of autophagy in the pathogenesis of AD. For example, immunocytochemistry showing the presence of K63-linked polyubiquitin in a fraction of the NFTs in AD cortex (Paine et al. 2009) suggests an active involvement of autophagy in the mechanism of AD.

PART II: THE AUTOPHAGY AND THE ENDOSOMAL–LYSOSOMAL SYSTEM IN AD

The Lysosomal Network

The endocytic and autophagic pathways share in common the role of delivering unneeded cellular materials to lysosomes for degradation and recycling to provide energy and new synthesis. Vesicular compartments in these pathways actively cross-talk and have common points of regulation (Simonsen et al. 2009; Settembre et al. 2011). Under pathological conditions, a deficit in one pathway often impedes functioning of the other. Therefore, it is reasonable to view these two pathways, which intersect at the lysosome, as comprising a lysosomal network (Fig. 5).

Although key to the survival of all cells, *endocytosis* supports unique neuronal functions, including aspects of synaptic transmission and

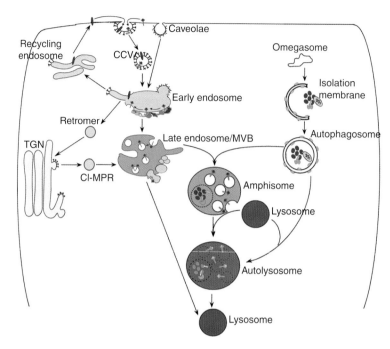

Figure 5. Schematic illustrating the endocytic and the autophagic pathways to the lysosome. See the text for details.

plasticity underlying memory and learning. Also, extracellular signals (e.g., growth factors) activate surface receptor complexes that, upon internalization, undergo retrograde axonal transport within "signaling endosomes" to promote neuronal survival and differentiation (Delcroix et al. 2003). That these vital processes are initiated in synaptic terminals at great distances from the perikaryon renders neurons particularly vulnerable to impairments of endocytic function and vesicular transport.

During the initiation of endocytosis, the invagination of plasma membranes into vesicles is mediated most often by the clathrin/adaptor protein complex, but also via caveolae or bulk macropinocytosis (Lim et al. 2011). Cargoes are delivered to early sorting endosomes through fusion mediated by the small GTPase Rab5 and additional Rab5 effector proteins (Fig. 5). Many cell surface proteins and lipids are returned to the plasma membrane via recycling endosomes, whereas other components are delivered to the Golgi by the retromer complex (Kelly et al. 2011). Still other cargoes reach

late endosomes when Rab7 and its effectors replace Rab5 and initiate further endosomal maturation (Poteryaev et al. 2010). An MVB is then created by inward budding of the surface membrane (Piper et al. 2001), thereby sorting cargoes into intraluminal vesicles. Ubiquitin, the crucial signal for efficient sorting of proteins into the MVB (Babst et al. 1997), initiates this process, which is mediated by a group of ESCRT complexes (endosomal sorting complex required for transport; Hurley 2010). Acid hydrolases, including cathepsins, are delivered from the trans-Golgi network (TGN) to MVBs/ late endosomes by either of two mannose-6-phosphate receptors: cation-dependent 46 kDa MPR (CD-MPR) and cation-independent 215 kDa MPR (CI-MPR; Mullins et al. 2001). Proteolysis begins in late endosomes/MVBs but accelerates upon fusion with lysosomes, where cathepsins are activated by the highly acidic (pH 4.5–5.5) intraluminal environment. The acidic pH is achieved mainly through the ATP-dependent proton pump, vacuolar ATPase (Nishi et al. 2002), but is also modulated by a group of chloride, sodium, calcium, and potassium transporters (Pillay et al. 2002).

Autophagy is the cell's principal degradative pathway for eliminating unwanted organelles and long-lived proteins and for clearing damaged, aggregated, or obsolete proteins (Wong et al. 2010). Autophagy refers to at least three processes by which intracellular constituents reach the lumen of MVBs or lysosomes for degradation: chaperone-mediated autophagy (CMA), microautophagy, and macroautophagy (Cuervo 2004; Levine et al. 2011). In CMA, cytosolic proteins containing a KFERQ motif (including proteins pathogenic in some neurodegenerative diseases) are selectively targeted by certain chaperones to the lysosomal lumen for degradation (Arias et al. 2011). Microautophagy involves the nonselective entry of small quantities of cytoplasm into lysosomes or late endosomes/MVBs when the limiting membranes of these compartments invaginate and pinch off small vesicles for digestion within the lumen (Sahu et al. 2011). Finally, macroautophagy mediates bulk or targeted degradation of cytoplasmic constituents. During macroautophagy, an elongated "isolation" membrane created from a preautophagosomal structure sequesters a region of cytoplasm to form a double-membrane-limited autophagosome (Fig. 5). Two ubiquitin-like protein conjugation pathways are known to coordinate this process (Ohsumi 2001). Sequestered material within autophagosomes is digested when lysosomes or late endosomes fuse with the outer membrane of the autophagosome (Gordon et al. 1988). Amphisomes formed by the fusion of autophagosomes with early endosomes or MVBs/late endosomes are especially important in neurons, where a considerable proportion of endocytosed cargo is directed to the autophagic pathway prior to being degraded by lysosomes (Larsen et al. 2002). This is especially true in axons (Lee et al. 2011). Induction of autophagy is generally controlled by the mTOR kinase (mammalian Target of Rapamycin), which is regulated by growth factors (especially insulin) and nutrient levels. Autophagy is constitutively active in neurons and is nonselective under nutrient deprivation conditions but may be selective when damage uncovers a molecular target on an organelle such as a mitochondrion (Youle et al. 2011), which initiates signaling and a ubiquitin-ligase-mediated chain of events that triggers selective sequestration of the organelle (Dikic et al. 2010; Weidberg et al. 2011).

Molecular Pathology of the Lysosomal Network

A continuum of pathological changes of the lysosomal network unfolds in neurons as Alzheimer disease progresses, including dysregulation of endocytosis, increased lysosome biogenesis and, later, progressive failure of lysosomal clearance mechanisms (Fig. 6; Nixon et al. 2006). These changes can be driven by known AD genetic and environmental risk factors, as discussed later. Endosome anomalies are the earliest specific pathology reported in AD brain tissue. Neuronal endosome enlargement, which is not characteristically observed in other major neurodegenerative diseases, develops in pyramidal neurons of the neocortex at a stage when plaques and tangles are restricted only to the hippocampus (Braak stage 2) and not in brains of similarly aged individuals free of AD-like hippocampal pathology (Cataldo et al. 1997, 2000). Similar endosomal anomalies develop gradually in Down syndrome brain, beginning decades before the appearance of classical AD pathology (Cataldo et al. 2000). Genes related to endocytosis, such as Rab5, Rab7, and Rab4, are among the earliest groups to show up-regulated transcription in AD (Ginsberg et al. 2010), and their corresponding proteins are abnormally recruited to endosomes, where they promote fusion and abnormal enlargement of early and late endosomes (Cataldo et al. 1997, 2008). This pattern is not seen in normal aging brain and is specific for AD among aging-related neurodegenerative diseases that have been studied (Cataldo et al. 2000).

As neuronal endosomes begin to enlarge, lysosomal biogenesis rises, as evidenced by lysosome proliferation and increased expression of acid hydrolases and other lysosome-related proteins (Nixon et al. 2006). Lysosome proliferation is followed by progressive enlargement

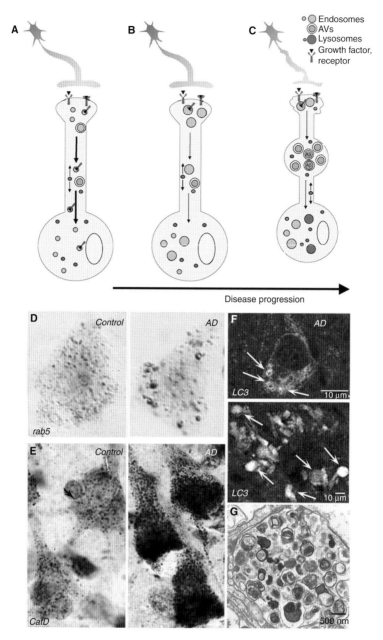

Figure 6. Progression of pathological changes in the lysosomal network in Alzheimer disease (AD). A normal neuron is depicted in *A*. At the earliest stages of AD (*B*), accelerated endocytosis, mediated in part by βCTF and/or by pathological activation of rab5, causes endosome enlargement (*D*; rab5 immunocytochemistry), defective retrograde transport of endosomes and their neurotrophin cargoes, proapoptotic pathway activation, and cholinergic neurodegeneration. Initial up-regulation of lysosome biogenesis (*E*; cathepsin D immunocyto-chemistry) is followed by progressive failure of lysosomal proteolysis (*C*), which impedes autophagy and the axonal transport of late endosomes/MVBs and autophagy-related vesicular compartments. These compart-ments, containing incompletely digested protein substrates, selectively accumulate within neurons and espe-cially dystrophic neurites (*C*), as depicted in *F* (LC3 immunocytochemistry) and *G* (ultrastructure of AVs in a dystrophic neurite). Failure of lysosomal proteolysis and autophagy in AD is caused by PS1 mutations in early-onset FAD and is also promoted by normal aging, oxidative stress, ApoE ε4, intracellular Aβ, and other AD-related genetic and environmental risk factors.

and distortion of these compartments. Cathepsin-positive vacuoles massively accumulate within swellings of dystrophic neurites throughout the neuropil and in senile plaques as they develop (Cataldo et al. 1990, 1991). Ultrastructural investigations of AD brain biopsies have revealed that the most prevalent organelles by far within dystrophic swellings are autophagic vacuoles (AVs), representing all stages of the macroautophagic process (Nixon et al. 2005), including autophagosomes. This implies that the progression of autophagy is delayed or impaired, because AVs are relatively rare in normal brain. AV accumulations are not specific to the degenerative phenomena of AD; however, in AD brain, the extensive numbers of dystrophic neurites (Masliah et al. 1993; Schmidt et al. 1994), their characteristic marked distension, and the fact that they are predominantly filled with AVs distinguish the pattern and magnitude of this pathology from that of other aging-related neurodegenerative diseases (Benzing et al. 1993). In non-AD neurodegenerative disorders, many types of vesicles and cytoskeletal elements are relatively abundant, suggesting general axonal transport failure distinct from the selective transport deficits seen in AD (Lee et al. 2011a,b).

The profuse and selective accumulation of AVs in neurons in AD reflects a defect in the clearance of AVs by lysosomes rather than an abnormally elevated induction of autophagy. The accumulating AVs are mainly electron-dense autolysosomes, indicating that autophagosome–lysosome fusion is relatively competent. Similar autophagy pathology is observed when lysosomal proteolysis is inhibited (Ivy et al. 1984; Koike et al. 2005; Yang et al. 2008). That presenilin 1 mutations, which are a cause of early-onset familial AD, impede lysosome proteolysis and accelerate neuritic dystrophy also supports a primary role for failure of proteolytic clearance (Lee et al. 2010). Increased autophagy induction in AD could, however, compound the defect in AV clearance in AD. Transcription of many lysosomal genes and factors promoting autophagy is up-regulated, whereas negative regulators of autophagy are down-regulated (Lipinski et al. 2010), although

not all studies support enhanced autophagy induction in AD (Pickford et al. 2008; Nixon et al. 2011).

AD Genetics Implicates the Lysosomal Network in Pathogenesis

Genetic factors that represent the strongest support for the amyloid/Aβ cascade hypothesis also act directly through Aβ-independent mechanisms to dysregulate the lysosomal network and contribute not only to Aβ accumulation but also to other critical aspects of AD pathogenesis (Fig. 7). Beyond its role as a component of γ-secretase, Presenilin 1 (PS1) is required for lysosome acidification, which is needed to activate cathepsins and other hydrolases that carry out digestion during autophagy (Lee et al. 2010). In the absence of PS1, the V0a1 subunit of v-ATPase is not N-glycosylated in the ER and is degraded before sufficient amounts can be delivered to autolysosomes/lysosomes to support lysosomal acidification. This function of PS1 is independent of the aspartyl protease activity of the molecule because proteolytically inactive PS1 mutated at one or both catalytic aspartates is able to restore normal lysosome acidification in PS1-deleted cells (Lee et al. 2010). Importantly, PS1 mutations also inhibit this process in fibroblasts from patients with familial AD (Lee et al. 2010), providing a basis for defective autophagy and the potentiation of autophagic–lysosomal and amyloid pathology and accelerated neuronal cell death observed in PS-FAD (Cataldo et al. 2004).

An additional copy of the *App* gene (genomic duplication) is sufficient to cause another form of early-onset FAD (Rovelet-Lecrux et al. 2006; Sleegers et al. 2006). *App* promoter polymorphisms that increase APP expression are also associated with early-onset AD (Athan et al. 2002). These findings support a longstanding hypothesis that the *App* gene on the trisomic copy of human chromosome 21 (HSA21) in Down syndrome (DS) is principally responsible for the invariant early development of AD in DS individuals (Margallo-Lana et al. 2004). In DS, the extra copy of *App* causes endocytic up-regulation and endosome pathology similar

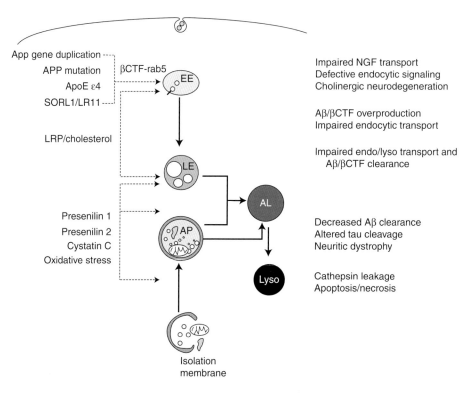

Figure 7. Dysfunction of autophagic and endocytic pathways to lysosomes driven by relevant genes and other risk factors in Alzheimer disease (*left* side of the diagram) causes or promotes pathophysiology critical to the development and progression of Alzheimer disease (*right* side of the diagram). See the text for further details.

to that seen at the earliest stages of sporadic AD, but beginning even earlier. Recently, these effects of increased *App* dosage were shown to be mediated specifically by the β-cleaved carboxy-terminal fragment of APP, βCTF (Jiang et al. 2010), which binds to a complex of signaling molecules on endosomes that pathologically activates rab5 (S Kim and RA Nixon, unpubl.). It is this abnormal rab5 activation that causes protein and lipid accumulation in endosomes, slowed lysosomal degradation of endocytic cargoes, endosome swelling (Cataldo et al. 2008), and disrupted retrograde transport of endosomes (S Kim and RA Nixon, unpubl.). Interactions between FAD-mutant forms of APP and APP binding protein (APP-BP1) on endosomes also initiate pathological rab5 activation, which was shown to promote a neuronal apoptosis cascade (Laifenfeld et al. 2007).

Acceleration of endosome pathology is also seen in individuals who inherit the ε4 allele of

APOE, a key mediator of neuronal cholesterol transport and the major genetic risk factor for late-onset AD (Cataldo et al. 2000). Moreover, among a very few additional pathological conditions associated with AD-like endosomal pathology are APP transgenic mice fed elevated dietary cholesterol and individuals with Niemann–Pick type C (NPC), a disorder of cholesterol homeostasis. High dietary LDL-cholesterol and overexpression of its receptor ApoE (particularly ApoE ε4) elevate βCTF levels (Ji et al. 2006; Cossec et al. 2010), and these levels are also elevated in NPC, DS, and AD, particularly in early-onset forms of AD caused by certain mutations of APP. The downstream consequences of βCTF-mediated rab5 activation and abnormal endosomal signaling for AD progression are many, as discussed later. Although less well characterized, a growing number of AD risk genes for late-onset AD identified through genome-wide screens and association studies have direct links to endocytic regulation (Seshadri et al. 2010; Hollingworth et al. 2011; Hu et al. 2011).

The genetics of other neurological diseases further support a close connection between disruption of lysosomal network function and selective vulnerability to neurodegeneration (Nixon et al. 2008). Lysosomal storage disorders involving primary defects in lysosome function commonly exhibit prominent neurodegenerative phenotypes, including neuritic dystrophies closely resembling the ultrastructural morphologies of dystrophic neurites in AD and, in some of these disorders, neurofibrillary tangles as well as increased amyloidogenic processing of APP and diffuse β-amyloid deposits (Ryazantsev et al. 2007; Ohmi et al. 2009; Bellettato et al. 2010). Inherited defects in the endocytic pathway are also associated with neurodegenerative disorders at a high frequency (Nixon 2004; Nixon et al. 2008; Rusten et al. 2008; Zhang 2008).

Biology of Lysosomal Network Dysregulation in AD and Its Pathological Consequences

Neuritic Dystrophy

Endocytosis and autophagy are highly active at synaptic terminals and axons and generate large numbers of endosomes and autophagosomes, representing a considerable burden of retrograde organelle trafficking to the perikaryon (Overly et al. 1996). Transport and autophagy must, therefore, be especially efficient to prevent "traffic jams." In healthy neurons, these mechanisms are, in fact, exceptionally efficient, as evidenced by a scarcity of autophagy-related intermediates, a high autophagic clearance capacity, and the rapidity with which axonal AVs accumulate when their clearance is impeded (Nixon et al. 2011), but they are also highly vulnerable to disruption (Boland et al. 2008; Cai et al. 2010; Lee et al. 2011a).

AVs and lysosomes constitute more than 95% of the organelles in dystrophic neuritic swellings in AD and AD mouse models, implying a cargo-specific defect in axonal transport, rather than a global one. Indeed, when lysosomal proteolysis is inhibited by blocking

acidification or directly inhibiting cathepsins, axonal transport of autophagy-related compartments is selectively slowed and intermittently interrupted. These organelles then accumulate selectively within axon swellings that acquire additional AD-like features, including local cytoskeletal protein hyperphosphorylation and ubiquitin immunolabeling (Lee et al. 2011a). These observations suggest how PS1 mutations, which impede lysosomal acidification (Lee et al. 2010), may markedly accelerate and amplify neuritic dystrophy in AD.

Similar neuritic dystrophy eventually develops in all forms of AD and in mouse AD models where only FAD-causing mutant APP is overexpressed. In these cases, the mechanism is not yet clear. Aβ administered directly into brains of wild-type rodents does not induce neuritic dystrophy, despite diffuse amyloid deposition (Frautschy et al. 1996, 1998), raising the possibility that other APP metabolites within neuronal compartments besides or in addition to Aβ could be important to the development of neuritic dystrophy. In this regard, elevated βCTF levels induced by APP overexpression, elevated dietary cholesterol, or overexpression of its receptor ApoE (particularly ApoE ε4) can upregulate endocytosis and enlarge endosomes (Laifenfeld et al. 2007; Chen et al. 2010; Cossec et al. 2010), leading to impaired endosome retrograde transport (S Kim and RA Nixon, unpubl.). Accelerated endocytosis also increases protein and lipid accumulation in endosomes and slows lysosomal degradation of endocytic cargoes (Cataldo et al. 2008), leading to lysosomal instability and neurodegeneration, as discussed below.

Protein Clearance Failure and Amyloidogenesis

In APP transgenic mouse models of AD, undigested autophagy substrates including LC3-II, p62, and ubiquitinated proteins accumulate in neuronal AVs, establishing that autophagic protein turnover in lysosomes is impeded (Yang et al. 2011). This general failure to clear autophagy substrates affects clearance of various proteins relevant to AD pathogenesis, including

Aβ, tau, and other factors, such as damaged mitochondria and activated caspases, that promote cell death (Yang et al. 2008).

Autophagy sequesters and digests unneeded or damaged organelles, some of which are APP-rich (Pickford et al. 2008). AVs are also enriched in APP substrates and secretases and, during autophagy, Aβ peptide is generated from APP (Yu et al. 2005), although it is subsequently degraded in lysosomes under normal circumstances (Heinrich et al. 1999; Bahr et al. 2002; Florez-McClure et al. 2007). Although less well studied as "Aβ degrading proteases" than the zinc metallopeptidase family (Guenette 2003; Eckman et al. 2005), cathepsins are considered an important route for Aβ/amyloid clearance (Mueller-Steiner et al. 2006; Nixon 2007; Butler et al. 2011) and human neurons may be particularly dependent on this mechanism (LeBlanc et al. 1999; reviewed in Saido and Leissring 2011). Chronic low-level stimulation of autophagy through peripheral administration of rapamycin or other agents (Tian et al. 2011), or enhancing lysosomal proteolysis selectively (Sun et al. 2008; Yang et al. 2011), can markedly diminish Aβ levels and amyloid load in APP transgenic mice, underscoring the importance of lysosomal clearance of Aβ.

Endocytic pathway up-regulation in AD stemming in part from pathological rab 5 activation generates higher levels of Aβ (Mathews et al. 2002; Grbovic et al. 2003) that must be cleared in part by lysosomes. Pathological rab5 activation, which in Down syndrome is dependent on βCTF generation (Jiang et al. 2010), can up-regulate endocytosis in a manner functionally equivalent to the elevated endocytosis associated with increased synaptic activity, which is considered a source of Aβ generation (Cirrito et al. 2008). An unknown amount of Aβ produced in endosomes reaches lysosomes directly or via production during autophagy (Nixon 2007), and accumulated AVs and MVBs appear to be the major intracellular reservoirs of Aβ immunoreactivity in AD brain (Takahashi et al. 2002; Yu et al. 2005). The acidic environment in lysosomes is particularly favorable for the initial stages of Aβ oligomerization (Peralvarez-Marin et al. 2008).

Tauopathy

Neurofibrillary tangles composed of tau proteins in a hyperphosphorylated state are rarely observed in abundance except in AD and a limited number of aging-related tauopathies. However, they are a prominent feature in at least two lysosomal disorders, NPC and mucopolysaccharidosis type IIB (MPS IIB; Ohmi et al. 2009), and in a mouse model of MPS IIB (Ryazantsev et al. 2007). In NPC, which arises from a defect in endosomal trafficking of cholesterol and the accumulation of unesterified cholesterol in late endosomes/lysosomes, additional features associated with AD are seen, including allele-selective influences of the APOE genotype on pathology and increased amyloidogenic processing of APP (Nixon 2004). The mechanisms explaining this connection are unclear, but tau has been found to be an autophagy substrate, at least when overexpressed (Berger et al. 2006). Incomplete charperone-mediated autophagy of tau generates fragments that aggregate and are cleared by macroautophagy (Wang et al. 2009). Moreover, autophagy preferentially degrades a caspase-cleaved fragment of tau implicated in tau neurotoxicity (Dolan et al. 2010). Consistent with these findings, rapamycin induction of autophagy reduces tau pathology in the triple transgenic AD mouse model (Caccamo et al. 2010), whereas in other models, autophagic–lysosomal dysfunction amplifies tau pathology and tau neurotoxicity (Hamano et al. 2008; Khurana et al. 2010).

Synaptic Dysfunction

Pathological Rab5 activation driving endocytic dysfunction in AD may negatively impact long-term potentiation (LTP) and long-term depression (LTD) aspects of synaptic plasticity closely associated with learning and memory (Kessels et al. 2009). LTD induction requires surface removal of AMPA receptors driven by their Rab5-dependent internalization (Brown et al. 2005b). Conversely, deletion of the neuronal rab5 GEF, rin1, reduces rab5 activation, increases LTP induction in the amygdala, and enhances fear learning and memory, most likely by increasing surface levels of AMPA receptors

(Dhaka et al. 2003). Autophagy may also modulate synaptic plasticity, which involves structural remodeling of nerve terminals (Boland et al. 2006) and the trafficking and degradation of receptors and other synaptic proteins (Leil et al. 2004; Rowland et al. 2006).

Neurodegeneration

A close connection between lysosomal network dysfunction and mechanisms of neurodegeneration is well documented (McCray et al. 2008; Nixon et al. 2008; Bellettato et al. 2010; Cherra et al. 2010). Deprived of the cytoprotective functions of autophagy, neurons, which cannot dilute toxic protein buildup by cell division, are particularly vulnerable to potentially toxic mutant, oxidized and aggregated proteins and peptide fragments. An important possible outcome of the accumulation of the latter in lysosomes is increased membrane permeability and release of hydrolases into the cytoplasm, even from otherwise intact lysosomes (Kroemer et al. 2005). Cataclysmic disruption of lysosomal membranes releases hydrolases that act as both the trigger and executioner in rapid necrosis (Syntichaki et al. 2003; Kroemer et al. 2005), whereas slow release of cathepsins more likely operates through signaling pathways to trigger apoptosis (Kroemer et al. 2005).

By up-regulating endocytosis, high dietary LDL-cholesterol and overexpression of its receptor ApoE (particularly ApoE ε4) elevate βCTF levels and increase delivery of Aβ1–42 to lysosomes in cellular model systems (Ji et al. 2006; Cossec et al. 2010). Accumulation of Aβ1–42, which is less efficiently degraded than Aβ1–40 owing to its strong propensity to aggregate, causes leakage of lysosomal enzymes into the cytosol prior to other morphological signs of cellular toxicity in vitro (Yang et al. 1998; Glabe 2001). Consistent with these findings, strong overexpression of human Aβ42, but not Aβ40, in *Drosophila* neurons induces age-related accumulation of Aβ in autolysosomes and neurotoxicity (Ling et al. 2009). Aβ42-induced neurotoxicity is further enhanced by autophagy activation and is partially rescued by autophagy inhibition. Expression of

the ApoE ε4 allele, but not ApoE ε3, in mice administered a neprilysin inhibitor increases Aβ immunoreactivity in lysosomes and causes neurodegeneration of hippocampal CA1, entorhinal, and septal neurons (Belinson et al. 2008). ApoE ε4 that traffics to lysosomes more readily than ApoE ε3, promotes leakage of acid hydrolases, and induces apoptosis in cultured neuronal cells by forming membrane-damaging intermediates in the low-pH environment (Ji et al. 2002).

Beyond influencing Aβ generation and toxicity, defective endosome functioning plays a crucial Aβ-independent role in the failure of retrograde NGF signaling that leads to basal forebrain cholinergic neuron degeneration in the Ts65Dn mouse model of DS (Cooper et al. 2001; Delcroix et al. 2004). Proteins known to play roles in both endocytosis regulation and cell survival decisions link the endosome dysregulation seen in AD to cell death cascade signaling (Vito et al. 1996, 1999; Missotten et al. 1999; Chen et al. 2000; Gout et al. 2000).

Remediating Lysosomal Network Dysfunction as AD Therapy

Recent evidence supports the value of targeting autophagy efficiency as a possible therapeutic strategy for AD. Peripheral administration of rapamycin to strongly stimulate autophagy substantially reduces amyloid deposition and tau pathology in both APP and triple transgenic mouse models of AD pathology (Caccamo et al. 2010; Spilman et al. 2010; Tian et al. 2011). Autophagy induction also has beneficial effects in transgenic models of several aging-related neurodegenerative diseases (Garcia-Arencibia et al. 2010). Stimulating lysosomal proteolytic efficiency in the TgCRND8 APP mouse model by deleting an endogenous inhibitor of lysosomal cysteine proteases (cystatin B) rescues lysosomal pathology, eliminates abnormal autolysosomal accumulation of autophagy substrates, including Aβ, decreases Aβ and amyloid deposition, and ameliorates learning and memory deficits (Yang et al. 2011). Similar therapeutic effects, including restoration of synaptic functions, are seen in APP mouse models after deleting cystatin C (Sun et al. 2008), by overexpressing cathepsin B (Mueller-Steiner et al. 2006), or by enhancing its activity (Butler et al. 2011). Collectively, these observations support the pathogenic significance of autophagic–lysosomal dysfunction in AD and specifically the importance of deficient lysosomal proteolysis.

CONCLUSION

As postmitotic cells, neurons are especially reliant on the lysosomal network to sort and clear normal and damaged proteins and support vital signaling functions. Not surprisingly, a defective endosomal–lysosomal pathway and certain autophagy-related genes are being linked with an unusually high frequency to neurodegenerative diseases, and the mechanistic relationship to neurodegeneration is becoming increasingly well established. Driven by the same genetic and environmental risk factors implicated in the Aβ/amyloid cascade hypothesis, a continuum of highly characteristic pathological changes in the lysosomal network evolves during AD, including dysregulation of endocytosis, increased lysosome biogenesis, and progressive failure of lysosomal proteolysis and autophagy. These deficits cripple neuronal functions critical for synaptic plasticity and neuron survival, lead to the hallmark neuritic dystrophy of AD, promote accumulation of toxic proteins—including Aβ, tau, activated caspases, and other cell death-promoting proteins—and initiate multiple neurodegenerative cascades. Remediation of lysosomal network dysfunction by several different approaches has been shown to have significant ameliorative effects on pathological and cognitive deficits in animal models of AD, underscoring the pathogenic significance of this dysfunction and the promise of therapeutic strategies targeting the lysosomal network in AD and other neurodegenerative disorders.

ACKNOWLEDGMENTS

The work of the Ihara laboratory on ubiquitin and PHF was carried out from 1985 to 1993, and Dr. Ihara thanks all laboratory members from that period (Department of Clinical Physiology, Tokyo Metropolitan Institute of Gerontology; Department of Neuropathology, Faculty of Medicine, University of Tokyo). In particular, the preparation of the DF2 antibody and identification of ubiquitin in PHF was performed collaboratively with Dr Hiroshi Mori, Department of Neuroscience, Osaka City University Graduate School of Medicine. For the introduction and section on autophagy and the lysosomal system, the assistance of Nicole Piorkowski and Corrinne Peterhoff in manuscript and figure preparation is gratefully acknowledged. Research from the Nixon laboratories is supported by the National Institute on Aging.

REFERENCES

*Reference is also in this collection.

Anderton BH, Breinburg D, Downes MJ, Green PJ, Tomlinson BE, Ulrich J, Wood JN, Kahn J. 1982. Monoclonal antibodies show that neurofibrillary tangles and neurofilaments share antigenic determinants. *Nature* **298:** 84–86.

Arias E, Cuervo AM. 2011. Chaperone-mediated autophagy in protein quality control. *Curr Opin Cell Biol* **23:** 184–189.

Athan ES, Lee JH, Arriaga A, Mayeux RP, Tycko B. 2002. Polymorphisms in the promoter of the human APP gene: Functional evaluation and allele frequencies in Alzheimer disease. *Arch Neurol* **59:** 1793–1799.

Babst M, Sato TK, Banta LM, Emr SD. 1997. Endosomal transport function in yeast requires a novel AAA-type ATPase, Vps4p. *EMBO J* **16:** 1820–1831.

Bahr BA, Bendiske J. 2002. The neuropathogenic contributions of lysosomal dysfunction. *J Neurochem* **83:** 481–489.

Bancher C, Grundke-Iqbal I, Iqbal K, Fried VA, Smith HT, Wisniewski HM. 1991. Abnormal phosphorylation of tau precedes ubiquitination in neurofibrillary pathology of Alzheimer disease. *Brain Res* **539:** 11–18.

Belin AC, Westerlund M. 2008. Parkinson's disease: A genetic perspective. *FEBS J* **275:** 1377–1383.

Belinson H, Lev D, Masliah E, Michaelson DM. 2008. Activation of the amyloid cascade in apolipoprotein E4 transgenic mice induces lysosomal activation and neurodegeneration resulting in marked cognitive deficits. *J Neurosci* **28:** 4690–701.

Bellettato CM, Scarpa M. 2010. Pathophysiology of neuropathic lysosomal storage disorders. *J Inherit Metab Dis* **33:** 347–362.

Bence NF, Sampat RM, Kopito RR. 2001. Impairment of the ubiquitin–proteasome system by protein aggregation. *Science* **292:** 1552–1555.

Benzing WC, Mufson EJ, Armstrong DM. 1993. Alzheimer's disease-like dystrophic neurites characteristically associated with senile plaques are not found within other neurodegenerative diseases unless amyloid β-protein deposition is present. *Brain Res* **606:** 10–18.

Berger Z, Ravikumar B, Menzies FM, Oroz LG, Underwood BR, Pangalos MN, Schmitt I, Wullner U, Evert BO, O'Kane CJ, et al. 2006. Rapamycin alleviates toxicity of different aggregate-prone proteins. *Hum Mol Genet* **15:** 433–442.

Berke SJ, Paulson HL. 2003. Protein aggregation and the ubiquitin proteasome pathway: Gaining the UPPer hand on neurodegeneration. *Curr Opin Genet Dev* **13:** 253–261.

Bertram L, Hiltunen M, Parkinson M, Ingelsson M, Lange C, Ramasamy K, Mullin K, Menon R, Sampson AJ, Hsiao MY, et al. 2005. Family-based association between Alzheimer's disease and variants in UBQLN1. *New Engl J Med* **352:** 884–894.

Bingol B, Sheng M. 2011. Deconstruction for reconstruction: The role of proteolysis in neural plasticity and disease. *Neuron* **69:** 22–32.

Boland B, Nixon RA. 2006. Neuronal macroautophagy: From development to degeneration. *Mol Aspects Med* **27:** 503–519.

Boland B, Kumar A, Lee S, Platt FM, Wegiel J, Yu WH, Nixon RA. 2008. Autophagy induction and autophagosome clearance in neurons: Relationship to autophagic pathology in Alzheimer's disease. *J Neurosci* **28:** 6926–6937.

Brion JP, Couck AM, Passareiro E, Flament-Durand J. 1985. Neurofibrillary tangles of Alzheimer's disease: An immunohistochemical study. *J Submicrosc Cytol* **17:** 89–96.

Brown MR, Bondada V, Keller JN, Thorpe J, Geddes JW. 2005a. Proteasome or calpain inhibition does not alter cellular tau levels in neuroblastoma cells or primary neurons. *J Alzheimer's Dis* **7:** 15–24.

Brown TC, Tran IC, Backos DS, Esteban JA. 2005b. NMDA receptor-dependent activation of the small GTPase Rab5 drives the removal of synaptic AMPA receptors during hippocampal LTD. *Neuron* **45:** 81–94.

Butler D, Hwang J, Estick C, Nishiyama A, Kumar SS, Baveghems C, Young-Oxendine HB, Wisniewski ML, Charalambides A, Bahr BA. 2011. Protective effects of positive lysosomal modulation in Alzheimer's disease transgenic mouse models. *PLoS One* **6:** e20501.

Caccamo A, Majumder S, Richardson A, Strong R, Oddo S. 2010. Molecular interplay between mammalian target of rapamycin (mTOR), amyloid-β, and Tau: Effects on cognitive impairments. *J Biol Chem* **285:** 13107–13120.

Cai Q, Lu L, Tian JH, Zhu YB, Qiao H, Sheng ZH. 2010. Snapin-regulated late endosomal transport is critical for efficient autophagy–lysosomal function in neurons. *Neuron* **68:** 73–86.

Cardozo C, Michaud C. 2002. Proteasome-mediated degradation of tau proteins occurs independently of the chymotrypsin-like activity by a nonprocessive pathway. *Arch Biochem Biophys* **408:** 103–110.

Cataldo AM, Nixon RA. 1990. Enzymatically active lysosomal proteases are associated with amyloid deposits in Alzheimer brain. *Proc Natl Acad Sci* **87:** 3861–3865.

Cataldo AM, Paskevich PA, Kominami E, Nixon RA. 1991. Lysosomal hydrolases of different classes are abnormally distributed in brains of patients with Alzheimer disease. *Proc Natl Acad Sci* **88:** 10998–11002.

Cataldo AM, Barnett JL, Pieroni C, Nixon RA. 1997. Increased neuronal endocytosis and protease delivery to early endosomes in sporadic Alzheimer's disease: Neuropathologic evidence for a mechanism of increased β-amyloidogenesis. *J Neurosci* **17:** 6142–6151.

Cataldo AM, Peterhoff CM, Troncoso JC, Gomez-Isla T, Hyman BT, Nixon RA. 2000. Endocytic pathway abnormalities precede amyloid β deposition in sporadic Alzheimer's disease and Down syndrome: Differential effects of APOE genotype and presenilin mutations. *Am J Pathol* **157:** 277–286.

Cataldo AM, Peterhoff CM, Schmidt SD, Terio NB, Duff K, Beard M, Mathews PM, Nixon RA. 2004. Presenilin mutations in familial Alzheimer disease and transgenic mouse models accelerate neuronal lysosomal pathology. *J Neuropathol Exp Neurol* **63:** 821–830.

Cataldo AM, Mathews PM, Boiteau AB, Hassinger LC, Peterhoff CM, Jiang Y, Mullaney K, Neve RL, Gruenberg J, Nixon RA. 2008. Down syndrome fibroblast model of Alzheimer-related endosome pathology. Accelerated endocytosis promotes late endocytic defects. *Am J Pathol* **173:** 370–384.

Chen B, Borinstein SC, Gillis J, Sykes VW, Bogler O. 2000. The glioma-associated protein SETA interacts with AIP1/Alix and ALG-2 and modulates apoptosis in astrocytes. *J Biol Chem* **275:** 19275–19281.

Chen X, Wagener JF, Morgan DH, Hui L, Ghribi O, Geiger JD. 2010. Endolysosome mechanisms associated with Alzheimer's disease-like pathology in rabbits ingesting cholesterol-enriched diet. *J Alzheimer's Dis* **22:** 1289–1303.

Cherra SJ 3rd, Dagda RK, Chu CT. 2010. Review: Autophagy and neurodegeneration: Survival at a cost? *Neuropathol Appl Neurobiol* **36:** 125–132.

Choi J, Levey AI, Weintraub ST, Rees HD, Gearing M, Chin LS, Li L. 2004. Oxidative modifications and downregulation of ubiquitin carboxyl-terminal hydrolase L1 associated with idiopathic Parkinson's and Alzheimer's diseases. *J Biol Chem* **279:** 13256–13264.

Ciechanover A, Finley D, Varshavsky A. 1984. Ubiquitin dependence of selective protein degradation demonstrated in the mammalian cell cycle mutant ts85. *Cell* **37:** 57–66.

Cirrito JR, Kang J-E, Lee J, Stewart FR, Verges DK, Silverio LM, Bu G, Mennerick S, Holtzman DM. 2008. Endocytosis is required for synaptic activity-dependent release of amyloid-β in vivo. *Neuron* **58:** 42–51.

Cooper JD, Salehi A, Delcroix JD, Howe CL, Belichenko PV, Chua-Couzens J, Kilbridge JF, Carlson EJ, Epstein CJ, Mobley WC. 2001. Failed retrograde transport of NGF in a mouse model of Down's syndrome: Reversal of cholinergic neurodegenerative phenotypes following NGF infusion. *Proc Natl Acad Sci* **98:** 10439–10444.

Cossec JC, Simon A, Marquer C, Moldrich RX, Leterrier C, Rossier J, Duyckaerts C, Lenkei Z, Potier MC. 2010. Clathrin-dependent APP endocytosis and Aβ secretion are highly sensitive to the level of plasma membrane cholesterol. *Biochim Biophys Acta* **1801:** 846–852.

Cripps D, Thomas SN, Jeng Y, Yang F, Davies P, Yang AJ. 2006. Alzheimer disease-specific conformation of hyperphosphorylated paired helical filament-Tau is polyubiquitinated through Lys-48, Lys-11, and Lys-6 ubiquitin conjugation. *J Biol Chem* **281:** 10825–10838.

Cuervo AM. 2004. Autophagy: Many paths to the same end. *Mol Cell Biochem* **263:** 55–72.

Cuervo AM, Palmer A, Rivett AJ, Knecht E. 1995. Degradation of proteasomes by lysosomes in rat liver. *Eur J Biochem* **227:** 792–800.

David DC, Layfield R, Serpell L, Narain Y, Goedert M, Spillantini MG. 2002. Proteasomal degradation of tau protein. *J Neurochem* **83:** 176–185.

Delcroix JD, Valletta JS, Wu C, Hunt SJ, Kowal AS, Mobley WC. 2003. NGF signaling in sensory neurons: Evidence that early endosomes carry NGF retrograde signals. *Neuron* **39:** 69–84.

Delcroix JD, Valletta J, Wu C, Howe CL, Lai CF, Cooper JD, Belichenko PV, Salehi A, Mobley WC. 2004. Trafficking the NGF signal: Implications for normal and degenerating neurons. *Prog Brain Res* **146:** 3–23.

Dhaka A, Costa RM, Hu H, Irvin DK, Patel A, Kornblum HI, Silva AJ, O'Dell TJ, Colicelli J. 2003. The RAS effector RIN1 modulates the formation of aversive memories. *J Neurosci* **23:** 748–757.

Dickey CA, Yue M, Lin WL, Dickson DW, Dunmore JH, Lee WC, Zehr C, West G, Cao S, Clark AM, et al. 2006. Deletion of the ubiquitin ligase CHIP leads to the accumulation, but not the aggregation, of both endogenous phospho- and caspase-3-cleaved tau species. *J Neurosci* **26:** 6985–6996.

Dikic I, Johansen T, Kirkin V. 2010. Selective autophagy in cancer development and therapy. *Cancer Res* **70:** 3431–3434.

Dolan PJ, Johnson GV. 2010. A caspase cleaved form of tau is preferentially degraded through the autophagy pathway. *J Biol Chem* **285:** 21978–21987.

Eckman EA, Eckman CB. 2005. Aβ-degrading enzymes: Modulators of Alzheimer's disease pathogenesis and targets for therapeutic intervention. *Biochem Soc Trans* **33:** 1101–1105.

Finley D, Ciechanover A, Varshavsky A. 1984. Thermolability of ubiquitin-activating enzyme from the mammalian cell cycle mutant ts85. *Cell* **37:** 43–55.

Fischer DF, De Vos RA, Van Dijk R, De Vrij FM, Proper EA, Sonnemans MA, Verhage MC, Sluijs JA, Hobo B, Zouambia M, et al. 2003. Disease-specific accumulation of mutant ubiquitin as a marker for proteasomal dysfunction in the brain. *FASEB J* **17:** 2014–2024.

Fischer DF, van Dijk R, van Tijn P, Hobo B, Verhage MC, van der Schors RC, Li KW, van Minnen J, Hol EM, van Leeuwen FW. 2009. Long-term proteasome dysfunction in the mouse brain by expression of aberrant ubiquitin. *Neurobiol Aging* **30:** 847–863.

Florez-McClure ML, Hohsfield LA, Fonte G, Bealor MT, Link CD. 2007. Decreased insulin-receptor signaling promotes the autophagic degradation of β-amyloid peptide in C. elegans. *Autophagy* **3:** 569–580.

Fortun J, Dunn WA Jr, Joy S, Li J, Notterpek L. 2003. Emerging role for autophagy in the removal of aggresomes in Schwann cells. *J Neurosci* **23:** 10672–10680.

Frautschy SA, Yang F, Calderon L, Cole GM. 1996. Rodent models of Alzheimer's disease: Rat A β infusion approaches to amyloid deposits. *Neurobiol Aging* **17:** 311–321.

Frautschy SA, Horn DL, Sigel JJ, Harris-White ME, Mendoza JJ, Yang F, Saido TC, Cole GM. 1998. Protease inhibitor coinfusion with amyloid β-protein results in enhanced deposition and toxicity in rat brain. *J Neurosci* **18:** 8311–8321.

Gallastegui N, Groll M. 2010. The 26S proteasome: Assembly and function of a destructive machine. *Trends Biochem Sci* **35:** 634–642.

Garcia-Arencibia M, Hochfeld WE, Toh PP, Rubinsztein DC. 2010. Autophagy, a guardian against neurodegeneration. *Semin Cell Dev Biol* **21:** 691–698.

Ginsberg SD, Alldred MJ, Counts SE, Cataldo AM, Neve RL, Jiang Y, Wuu J, Chao MV, Mufson EJ, Nixon RA, et al. 2010. Microarray analysis of hippocampal CA1 neurons implicates early endosomal dysfunction during Alzheimer's disease progression. *Biol Psychiat* **68:** 885–893.

Glabe C. 2001. Intracellular mechanisms of amyloid accumulation and pathogenesis in Alzheimer's disease. *J Mol Neurosci* **17:** 137–145.

Goldberg AL. 2003. Protein degradation and protection against misfolded or damaged proteins. *Nature* **426:** 895–899.

Gómez-Isla T, Hollister R, West H, Mui S, Growdon JH, Petersen RC, Parisi JE, Hyman BT. 1997. Neuronal loss correlates with but exceeds neurofibrillary tangles in Alzheimer's disease. *Ann Neurol* **41:** 17–24.

Gonatas NK. 1967. Neocortical synapses in a presenile dementia. *J Neuropathol Exp Neurol* **26:** 150–151.

Gong B, Cao Z, Zheng P, Vitolo OV, Liu S, Staniszewski A, Moolman D, Zhang H, Shelanski M, Arancio O. 2006. Ubiquitin hydrolase Uch-L1 rescues β-amyloid-induced decreases in synaptic function and contextual memory. *Cell* **126:** 775–788.

Gordon PB, Seglen PO. 1988. Prelysosomal convergence of autophagic and endocytic pathways. *Biochem Biophys Res Commun* **151:** 40–47.

Gout I, Middleton G, Adu J, Ninkina NN, Drobot LB, Filonenko V, Matsuka G, Davies AM, Waterfield M, Buchman VL. 2000. Negative regulation of PI 3-kinase by Ruk, a novel adaptor protein. *EMBO J* **19:** 4015–4025.

Grbovic OM, Mathews PM, Jiang Y, Schmidt SD, Dinakar R, Summers-Terio NB, Ceresa BP, Nixon RA, Cataldo AM. 2003. Rab5-stimulated up-regulation of the endocytic pathway increases intracellular β-cleaved amyloid precursor protein carboxyl-terminal fragment levels and Aβ production. *J Biol Chem* **278:** 31261–31268.

Greer PL, Hanayama R, Bloodgood BL, Mardinly AR, Lipton DM, Flavell SW, Kim TK, Griffith EC, Waldon Z, Maehr R, et al. 2010. The Angelman syndrome protein Ube3A regulates synapse development by ubiquitinating arc. *Cell* **140:** 704–716.

Grundke-Iqbal I, Iqbal K, Quinlan M, Tung YC, Zaidi MS, Wisniewski HM. 1986. Microtubule-associated protein tau. A component of Alzheimer paired helical filaments. *J Biol Chem* **261:** 6084–6089.

Grune T, Shringarpure R, Sitte N, Davies K. 2001. Age-related changes in protein oxidation and proteolysis in mammalian cells. *J Gerontol A Biol Sci Med Sci* **56:** B459–B467.

Guenette SY. 2003. Mechanisms of Aβ clearance and catabolism. *Neuromol Med* **4:** 147–160.

Haapasalo A, Viswanathan J, Bertram L, Soininen H, Tanzi RE, Hiltunen M. 2010. Emerging role of Alzheimer's disease-associated ubiquilin-1 in protein aggregation. *Biochem Soc Trans* **38:** 150–155.

Haas AL, Bright PM. 1985. The immunochemical detection and quantitation of intracellular ubiquitin–protein conjugates. *J Biol Chem* **260:** 12464–12473.

Hamano T, Gendron TF, Causevic E, Yen SH, Lin WL, Isidoro C, Deture M, Ko LW. 2008. Autophagic–lysosomal perturbation enhances tau aggregation in transfectants with induced wild-type tau expression. *Eur J Neurosci* **27:** 1119–30.

Hasegawa M, Morishima-Kawashima M, Takio K, Suzuki M, Titani K, Ihara Y. 1992. Protein sequence and mass spectrometric analyses of tau in the Alzheimer's disease brain. *J Biol Chem* **267:** 17047–17054.

Hasegawa M, Fujiwara H, Nonaka T, Wakabayashi K, Takahashi H, Lee VM, Trojanowski JQ, Mann D, Iwatsubo T. 2002. Phosphorylated α-synuclein is ubiquitinated in α-synucleinopathy lesions. *J Biol Chem* **277:** 49071–49076.

Hegde AN, Goldberg AL, Schwartz JH. 1993. Regulatory subunits of cAMP-dependent protein kinases are degraded after conjugation to ubiquitin: A molecular mechanism underlying long-term synaptic plasticity. *Proc Natl Acad Sci* **90:** 7436–7440.

Hegde AN, Inokuchi K, Pei W, Casadio A, Ghirardi M, Chain DG, Martin KC, Kandel ER, Schwartz JH. 1997. Ubiquitin C-terminal hydrolase is an immediate-early gene essential for long-term facilitation in Aplysia. *Cell* **89:** 115–126.

Heinrich M, Wickel M, Schneider-Brachert W, Sandberg C, Gahr J, Schwandner R, Weber T, Saftig P, Peters C, Brunner J, et al. 1999. Cathepsin D targeted by acid sphingomyelinase-derived ceramide. *EMBO J* **18:** 5252–5263.

Hollingworth P, Harold D, Jones L, Owen MJ, Williams J. 2011. Alzheimer's disease genetics: Current knowledge and future challenges. *Int J Geriatr Psychiat* **26:** 793–802.

Hsia AY, Masliah E, McConlogue L, Yu GQ, Tatsuno G, Hu K, Kholodenko D, Malenka RC, Nicoll RA, Mucke L. 1999. Plaque-independent disruption of neural circuits in Alzheimer's disease mouse models. *Proc Natl Acad Sci* **96:** 3228–3233.

Hu X, Pickering E, Liu YC, Hall S, Fournier H, Katz E, Dechairo B, John S, Van Eerdewegh P, Soares H. 2011. Meta-analysis for genome-wide association study identifies multiple variants at the BIN1 locus associated with late-onset Alzheimer's disease. *PLoS One* **6:** e16616.

Hurley JH. 2010. The ESCRT complexes. *Crit Rev Biochem Mol Biol* **45:** 463–487.

Ihara Y, Abraham C, Selkoe DJ. 1983. Antibodies to paired helical filaments in Alzheimer's disease do not recognize normal brain proteins. *Nature* **304:** 727–729.

Ivy GO, Schottler F, Wenzel J, Baudry M, Lynch G. 1984. Inhibitors of lysosomal enzymes: Accumulation of lipofuscin-like dense bodies in the brain. *Science* **226:** 985–987.

Iwatsubo T, Hasegawa M, Esaki Y, Ihara Y. 1992. Lack of ubiquitin immunoreactivities at both ends of neuropil threads—Possible bidirectional growth of neuropil threads. *Am J Pathol* **140:** 277–282.

Ji ZS, Miranda RD, Newhouse YM, Weisgraber KH, Huang Y, Mahley RW. 2002. Apolipoprotein E4 potentiates amyloid β peptide-induced lysosomal leakage and apoptosis in neuronal cells. *J Biol Chem* **277:** 21821–21828.

Ji ZS, Mullendorff K, Cheng IH, Miranda RD, Huang Y, Mahley RW. 2006. Reactivity of apolipoprotein E4 and amyloid β peptide: Lysosomal stability and neurodegeneration. *J Biol Chem* **281:** 2683–2692.

Jiang Y, Mullaney KA, Peterhoff CM, Che S, Schmidt SD, Boyer-Boiteau A, Ginsberg SD, Cataldo AM, Mathews PM, Nixon RA. 2010. Alzheimer's-related endosome dysfunction in Down syndrome is Aβ-independent but requires APP and is reversed by BACE-1 inhibition. *Proc Natl Acad Sci* **107:** 1630–1635.

Jin M, Shepardson N, Yang T, Chen G, Walsh D, Selkoe DJ. 2011. Soluble amyloid β-protein dimers isolated from Alzheimer cortex directly induce Tau hyperphosphorylation and neuritic degeneration. *Proc Natl Acad Sci* **108:** 5819–5824.

Keck S, Nitsch R, Grune T, Ullrich O. 2003. Proteasome inhibition by paired helical filament-tau in brains of patients with Alzheimer's disease. *J Neurochem* **85:** 115–122.

Keller JN, Hanni KB, Markesbery WR. 2000. Impaired proteasome function in Alzheimer's disease. *J Neurochem* **75:** 436–439.

Keller JN, Gee J, Ding Q. 2002. The proteasome in brain aging. *Ageing Res Rev* **1:** 279–293.

Kelly BT, Owen DJ. 2011. Endocytic sorting of transmembrane protein cargo. *Curr Opin Cell Biol* **23:** 404–412.

Kessels HW, Malinow R. 2009. Synaptic AMPA receptor plasticity and behavior. *Neuron* **61:** 340–350.

Khurana V, Elson-Schwab I, Fulga TA, Sharp KA, Loewen CA, Mulkearns E, Tyynela J, Scherzer CR, Feany MB. 2010. Lysosomal dysfunction promotes cleavage and neurotoxicity of tau in vivo. *PLoS Genet* **6:** e1001026.

Koike M, Shibata M, Waguri S, Yoshimura K, Tanida I, Kominami E, Gotow T, Peters C, von Figura K, Mizushima N, et al. 2005. Participation of autophagy in storage of lysosomes in neurons from mouse models of neuronal ceroid-lipofuscinoses (Batten disease). *Am J Pathol* **167:** 1713–1728.

Kondo J, Honda T, Mori H, Hamada Y, Miura R, Ogawara M, Ihara Y. 1988. The carboxyl third of tau is tightly bound to paired helical filaments. *Neuron* **1:** 827–834.

Korolchuk VI, Mansilla A, Menzies FM, Rubinsztein DC. 2009a. Autophagy inhibition compromises degradation of ubiquitin–proteasome pathway substrates. *Mol Cell* **33:** 517–527.

Korolchuk VI, Menzies FM, Rubinsztein DC. 2009b. A novel link between autophagy and the ubiquitin–proteasome system. *Autophagy* **5:** 862–863.

Kosaka K. 1978. Lewy bodies in cerebral cortex, report of three cases. *Acta Neuropathol* **42:** 127–134.

Kosik KS, Joachim CL, Selkoe DJ. 1986. Microtubule-associated protein tau (tau) is a major antigenic component of paired helical fragments in Alzheimer disease. *Proc Natl Acad Sci* **83:** 4044–4048.

Kroemer G, Jaattela M. 2005. Lysosomes and autophagy in cell death control. *Nat Rev Cancer* **5:** 886–97.

Kuzuhara S, Mori H, Izumiyama N, Yoshimura M, Ihara Y. 1988. Lewy bodies are ubiquitinated. A light and electron microscopic immunocytochemical study. *Acta Neuropathol* **75:** 345–353.

Laifenfeld D, Patzek LJ, McPhie DL, Chen Y, Levites Y, Cataldo AM, Neve RL. 2007. Rab5 mediates an amyloid precursor protein signaling pathway that leads to apoptosis. *J Neurosci* **27:** 7141–7153.

Lam YA, Pickart CM, Alban A, Landon M, Jamieson C, Ramage R, Mayer RJ, Layfield R. 2000. Inhibition of the ubiquitin–proteasome system in Alzheimer's disease. *Proc Natl Acad Sci* **97:** 9902–9906.

Larsen KE, Sulzer D. 2002. Autophagy in neurons: A review. *Histol Histopathol* **17:** 897–908.

LeBlanc AC, Goodyer CG. 1999. Role of endoplasmic reticulum, endosomal–lysosomal compartments, and microtubules in amyloid precursor protein metabolism of human neurons. *J Neurochem* **72:** 1832–42.

Lee JH, Yu WH, Kumar A, Lee S, Mohan PS, Peterhoff CM, Marinez-Vicente M, Massey AG, Sovak G, Uchiyama Y, et al. 2010. Presenilin 1 (PS1) is required for v-ATPase targeting and autolysosome acidification: PS1 mutations in Alzheimer's disease disrupt lysosomal proteolysis and autophagy. *Cell* **141:** 1146–1158.

Lee S, Sato Y, Nixon RA. 2011a. Lysosomal proteolysis inhibition selectively disrupts axonal transport of degradative organelles and causes an Alzheimer's-like axonal dystrophy. *J Neurosci* **31:** 7817–7830.

Lee S, Saito Y, Nixon RA. 2011b. Primary lysosomal dysfunction causes cargo-specific deficits of axonal transport leading to Alzheimer's-like neuritic dystrophy. *Autophagy* **7:** in press.

Leil TA, Chen ZW, Chang CS, Olsen RW. 2004. GABAA receptor-associated protein traffics GABA$_A$ receptors to the plasma membrane in neurons. *J Neurosci* **24:** 11429–11438.

Levine B, Klionsky DJ. 2004. Development by self-digestion; molecular mechanisms and biological functions of autophagy. *Dev Cell* **6:** 463–477.

Levine B, Mizushima N, Virgin HW. 2011. Autophagy in immunity and inflammation. *Nature* **469:** 323–335.

Li S, Hong S, Shepardson NE, Walsh DM, Shankar GM, Selkoe D. 2009. Soluble oligomers of amyloid β protein facilitate hippocampal long-term depression by disrupting neuronal glutamate uptake. *Neuron* **62:** 788–801.

Lim JP, Gleeson PA. 2011. Macropinocytosis: An endocytic pathway for internalising large gulps. *Immunol Cell Biol* doi: 10.1038/icb.2011.20.

Ling D, Song HJ, Garza D, Neufeld TP, Salvaterra PM. 2009. Aβ42-induced neurodegeneration via an age-dependent autophagic–lysosomal injury in *Drosophila*. *PLoS One* **4:** e4201.

Lipinski MM, Zheng B, Lu T, Yan Z, Py BF, Ng A, Xavier RJ, Li C, Yankner BA, Scherzer CR, et al. 2010. Genome-wide analysis reveals mechanisms modulating autophagy in normal brain aging and in Alzheimer's disease. *Proc Natl Acad Sci* **107:** 14164–14169.

Lopez-Salon M, Alonso M, Vianna MR, Viola H, Mello e Souza T, Izquierdo I, Pasquini JM, Medina JH. 2001. The ubiquitin–proteasome cascade is required for mammalian long-term memory formation. *Eur J Neurosci* **4:** 1820–1826.

Lowe J, Blanchard A, Morrell K, Lennox G, Reynolds L, Billett M, Landon M, Mayer RJ. 1988. Ubiquitin is a common factor in intermediate filament inclusion bodies of diverse type in man, including those of Parkinson's disease, Pick's disease, and Alzheimer's disease, as well as Rosenthal fibres in cerebellar astrocytomas, cytoplasmic bodies in muscle, and mallory bodies in alcoholic liver disease. *J Pathol* **155:** 9–15.

* Mandelkow E-M, Mandelkow E. 2011. Biochemistry and cell biology of tau protein in neurofibrillary degeneration. *Cold Spring Harb Perspect Med* doi: 10.1101/cshperspect.a006247.

Margallo-Lana M, Morris CM, Gibson AM, Tan AL, Kay DW, Tyrer SP, Moore BP, Ballard CG. 2004. Influence of the amyloid precursor protein locus on dementia in Down syndrome. *Neurology* **62:** 1996–1998.

Masliah E, Mallory M, Deerinck T, DeTeresa R, Lamont S, Miller A, Terry RD, Carragher B, Ellisman M. 1993. Re-evaluation of the structural organization of the neuritic plaques in Alzheimer's disease. *J Neuropathol Exp Neurol* **52:** 619–632.

Mathews PM, Guerra CB, Jiang Y, Grbovic OM, Kao BH, Schmidt SD, Dinakar R, Mercken M, Hille-Rehfeld A, Rohrer J, et al. 2002. Alzheimer's disease-related overexpression of the cation-dependent mannose 6-phosphate receptor increases Aβ secretion: Role for altered lysosomal hydrolase distribution in β-amyloidogenesis. *J Biol Chem* **277:** 5299–5307.

McCray BA, Taylor JP. 2008. The role of autophagy in age-related neurodegeneration. *Neurosignals* **16:** 75–84.

Missotten M, Nichols A, Rieger K, Sadoul R. 1999. Alix, a novel mouse protein undergoing calcium-dependent interaction with the apoptosis-linked-gene 2 (ALG-2) protein. *Cell Death Differ* **6:** 124–129.

Mori H, Kondo J, Ihara Y. 1987. Ubiquitin is a component of paired helical filaments in Alzheimer's disease. *Science* **235:** 1641–1644.

Morimoto T, Ide T, Ihara Y, Tamura A, Kirino T. 1996. Transient ischemia depletes free ubiquitin in the gerbil hippocampal CA1 neurons. *Am J Pathol* **148:** 249–257.

Morishima-Kawashima M, Hasegawa M, Takio K, Suzuki M, Titani K, Ihara Y. 1993. Ubiquitin is conjugated with amino-terminally processed tau in paired helical filaments. *Neuron* **10:** 1151–1160.

Mueller-Steiner S, Zhou Y, Arai H, Roberson ED, Sun B, Chen J, Wang X, Yu G, Esposito L, Mucke L, et al. 2006. Antiamyloidogenic and neuroprotective functions of cathepsin B: Implications for Alzheimer's disease. *Neuron* **51:** 703–714.

Mullins C, Bonifacino JS. 2001. The molecular machinery for lysosome biogenesis. *Bioessays* **23:** 333–343.

Murayama S, Mori H, Ihara Y, Bouldin TW, Suzuki K, Tomonaga M. 1990a. Immunocytochemical and ultrastructural studies of lower motor neurons in amyotrophic lateral sclerosis. *Ann Neurol* **27:** 137–148.

Murayama S, Mori H, Ihara Y, Tomonaga M. 1990b. Immunocytochemical and ultrastructural studies of Pick's disease. *Ann Neurol* **27:** 394–405.

Narendra D, Tanaka A, Suen DF, Youle RJ. 2009. Parkin-induced mitophagy in the pathogenesis of Parkinson disease. *Autophagy* **5:** 706–708.

Neumann M, Sampathu DM, Kwong LK, Truax AC, Micsenyi MC, Chou TT, Bruce J, Schuck T, Grossman M, Clark CM, et al. 2006. Ubiquitinated TDP-43 in frontotemporal lobar degeneration and amyotrophic lateral sclerosis. *Science* **314:** 130–133.

Nishi T, Forgac M. 2002. The vacuolar (H$^+$)-ATPases-nature's most versatile proton pumps. *Nat Rev Mol Cell Biol* **3:** 94–103.

Nixon RA. 2004. Niemann–Pick Type C disease and Alzheimer's disease: The APP-endosome connection fattens up. *Am J Pathol* **164:** 757–761.

Nixon RA. 2007. Autophagy, amyloidogenesis and Alzheimer disease. *J Cell Sci* **120:** 4081–4091.

Nixon RA, Cataldo AM. 2006. Lysosomal system pathways: Genes to neurodegeneration in Alzheimer's disease. *J Alzheimer's Dis* **9:** 277–289.

Nixon RA, Yang DS. 2011. Autophagy failure in Alzheimer's disease—Locating the primary defect. *Neurobiol Dis* **43:** 38–45.

Nixon RA, Wegiel J, Kumar A, Yu WH, Peterhoff C, Cataldo A, Cuervo AM. 2005. Extensive involvement of autophagy in Alzheimer disease: An immuno-electron microscopy study. *J Neuropathol Exp Neurol* **64:** 113–122.

Nixon RA, Yang DS, Lee JH. 2008. Neurodegenerative lysosomal disorders: A continuum from development to late age. *Autophagy* **4:** 590–599.

Nukina N, Ihara Y. 1986. One of the antigenic determinants of paired helical filaments is related to tau protein. *J Biochem* **99:** 1541–1544.

Nukina N, Kosik KS, Selkoe DJ. 1987. Recognition of Alzheimer paired helical filaments by monoclonal neurofilament antibodies is due to crossreaction with tau protein. *Proc Natl Acad Sci* **84:** 3415–3419.

Ohmi K, Kudo LC, Ryazantsev S, Zhao HZ, Karsten SL, Neufeld EF. 2009. Sanfilippo syndrome type B, a lysosomal storage disease, is also a tauopathy. *Proc Natl Acad Sci* **106:** 8332–8337.

Ohsumi Y. 2001. Molecular dissection of autophagy: Two ubiquitin-like systems. *Nat Rev Mol Cell Biol* **2:** 211–216.

Overly CC, Hollenbeck PJ. 1996. Dynamic organization of endocytic pathways in axons of cultured sympathetic neurons. *J Neurosci* **16:** 6056–6064.

Paine S, Bedford L, Thorpe JR, Mayer RJ, Cavey JR, Bajaj N, Sheppard PW, Lowe J, Layfield R. 2009. Immunoreactivity to Lys63-linked polyubiquitin is a feature of neurodegeneration. *Neurosci Lett* **460:** 205–208.

Peralvarez-Marin A, Barth A, Graslund A. 2008. Time-resolved infrared spectroscopy of pH-induced aggregation of the Alzheimer Aβ_{1-28} peptide. *J Mol Biol* **379:** 589–596.

Petrucelli L, Dickson D, Kehoe K, Taylor J, Snyder H, Grover A, De Lucia M, McGowan E, Lewis J, Prihar G, et al. 2004. CHIP and Hsp70 regulate tau ubiquitination, degradation and aggregation. *Hum Mol Genet* **13:** 703–714.

Pickford F, Masliah E, Britschgi M, Lucin K, Narasimhan R, Jaeger PA, Small S, Spencer B, Rockenstein E, Levine B, et al. 2008. The autophagy-related protein beclin 1 shows reduced expression in early Alzheimer disease and regulates amyloid β accumulation in mice. *J Clin Invest* **118:** 2190–2199.

Pike JW, Donaldson CA, Marion SL, Haussler MR. 1982. Development of hybridomas secreting monoclonal antibodies to the chicken intestinal 1 α,25-dihydroxyvitamin D3 receptor. *Proc Natl Acad Sci* **79:** 7719–7723.

Pillay CS, Elliott E, Dennison C. 2002. Endolysosomal proteolysis and its regulation. *Biochem J* **363:** 417–429.

Piper RC, Luzio JP. 2001. Late endosomes: Sorting and partitioning in multivesicular bodies. *Traffic* **2:** 612–621.

Poteryaev D, Datta S, Ackema K, Zerial M, Spang A. 2010. Identification of the switch in early-to-late endosome transition. *Cell* **141:** 497–508.

Rovelet-Lecrux A, Hannequin D, Raux G, Le Meur N, Laquerriere A, Vital A, Dumanchin C, Feuillette S, Brice A, Vercelletto M, et al. 2006. APP locus duplication causes autosomal dominant early-onset Alzheimer disease with cerebral amyloid angiopathy. *Nat Genet* **38:** 24–26.

Rowland AM, Richmond JE, Olsen JG, Hall DH, Bamber BA. 2006. Presynaptic terminals independently regulate synaptic clustering and autophagy of GABAA receptors in *Caenorhabditis elegans*. *J Neurosci* **26:** 1711–1720.

Roy AK, Oh T, Rivera O, Mubiru J, Song CS, Chatterjee B. 2002. Impacts of transcriptional regulation on aging and senescence. *Ageing Res Rev* **1:** 367–380.

Rusten TE, Simonsen A. 2008. ESCRT functions in autophagy and associated disease. *Cell Cycle* **7:** 1166–1172.

Ryazantsev S, Yu WH, Zhao HZ, Neufeld EF, Ohmi K. 2007. Lysosomal accumulation of SCMAS (subunit c of mitochondrial ATP synthase) in neurons of the mouse model of mucopolysaccharidosis III B. *Mol Genet Metab* **90:** 393–401.

Sahu R, Kaushik S, Clement CC, Cannizzo ES, Scharf B, Follenzi A, Potolicchio I, Nieves E, Cuervo AM, Santambrogio L. 2011. Microautophagy of cytosolic proteins by late endosomes. *Dev Cell* **20:** 131–139.

* Saido T, Leissring MA. 2011. Proteolytic degradation of amyloid β-protein. *Cold Spring Harb Perspect* doi: 10.1101.cshperspect.a006379.

Schmidt ML, DiDario AG, Lee VM, Trojanowski JQ. 1994. An extensive network of PHF tau-rich dystrophic neurites permeates neocortex and nearly all neuritic and diffuse amyloid plaques in Alzheimer disease. *FEBS Lett* **344:** 69–73.

Seshadri S, Fitzpatrick AL, Ikram MA, DeStefano AL, Gudnason V, Boada M, Bis JC, Smith AV, Carassquillo MM, Lambert JC, et al. 2010. Genome-wide analysis of genetic loci associated with Alzheimer disease. *JAMA* **303:** 1832–1840.

Setsuie R, Wada K. 2007. The functions of UCH-L1 and its relation to neurodegenerative diseases. *Neurochem Int* **51:** 105–111.

Settembre C, Di Malta C, Polito VA, Garcia Arencibia M, Vetrini F, Erdin S, Erdin SU, Huynh T, Medina D, Colella P, et al. 2011. TFEB links autophagy to lysosomal biogenesis. *Science* **332:** 1429–1433.

Simonsen A, Tooze SA. 2009. Coordination of membrane events during autophagy by multiple class III PI3-kinase complexes. *J Cell Biol* **186:** 773–782.

Sleegers K, Brouwers N, Gijselinck I, Theuns J, Goossens D, Wauters J, Del-Favero J, Cruts M, van Duijn CM, Van Broeckhoven C. 2006. APP duplication is sufficient to cause early onset Alzheimer's dementia with cerebral amyloid angiopathy. *Brain* **129:** 2977–2983.

Smemo S, Nowotny P, Hinrichs AL, Kauwe JS, Cherny S, Erickson K, Myers AJ, Kaleem M, Marlowe L, Gibson AM, et al. 2006. Ubiquilin 1 polymorphisms are not associated with late-onset Alzheimer's disease. *Ann Neurol* **59:** 21–26.

Sohal RS, Mockett RJ, Orr WC. 2002. Mechanisms of aging: An appraisal of the oxidative stress hypothesis. *Free Radic Biol Med* **33:** 575–586.

Soto C. 2003. Unfolding the role of protein misfolding in neurodegenerative diseases. *Nat Rev Neurosci* **4:** 49–60.

Spillantini MG, Schmidt ML, Lee VM, Trojanowski JQ, Jakes R, Goedert M. 1997. Alpha-synuclein in Lewy bodies. *Nature* **388:** 839–840.

Spilman P, Podlutskaya N, Hart MJ, Debnath J, Gorostiza O, Bredesen D, Richardson A, Strong R, Galvan V. 2010. Inhibition of mTOR by rapamycin abolishes cognitive deficits and reduces amyloid-β levels in a mouse model of Alzheimer's disease. *PLoS One* **5:** e9979.

Sun B, Zhou Y, Halabisky B, Lo I, Cho SH, Mueller-Steiner S, Devidze N, Wang X, Grubb A, Gan L. 2008. Cystatin C-cathepsin B axis regulates amyloid β levels and associated neuronal deficits in an animal model of Alzheimer's disease. *Neuron* **60:** 247–257.

Syntichaki P, Tavernarakis N. 2003. The biochemistry of neuronal necrosis: Rogue biology? *Nat Rev Neurosci* **4:** 672–684.

Takahashi RH, Milner TA, Li F, Nam EE, Edgar MA, Yamaguchi H, Beal MF, Xu H, Greengard P, Gouras GK. 2002. Intraneuronal Alzheimer aβ42 accumulates in multivesicular bodies and is associated with synaptic pathology. *Am J Pathol* **161:** 1869–1879.

Tank EM, True HL. 2009. Disease-associated mutant ubiquitin causes proteasomal impairment and enhances the toxicity of protein aggregates. *PLoS Genet* **5:** e1000382.

Terman A. 2001. Garbage catastrophe theory of aging: Imperfect removal of oxidative damage? *Redox Rep* **6:** 15–26.

Terry RD, Masliah E, Salmon DP, Butters N, DeTeresa R, Hill R, Hansen LA, Katzman R. 1991. Physical basis of cognitive alterations in Alzheimer's disease: Synapse loss is the major correlate of cognitive impairment. *Ann Neurol* **30:** 572–580.

Tian Y, Bustos V, Flajolet M, Greengard P. 2011. A small-molecule enhancer of autophagy decreases levels of A{β} and APP-CTF via Atg5-dependent autophagy pathway. *FASEB J* **25:** 1934–1942.

Tresse E, Salomons FA, Vesa J, Bott LC, Kimonis V, Yao TP, Dantuma NP, Taylor JP. 2010. VCP/p97 is essential for maturation of ubiquitin-containing autophagosomes and this function is impaired by mutations that cause IBMPFD. *Autophagy* **6:** 217–227.

Troen BR. 2003. The biology of aging. *Mt Sinai J Med* **70:** 3–22.

Tseng BP, Green KN, Chan JL, Blurton-Jones M, LaFerla FM. 2008. Aβ inhibits the proteasome and enhances amyloid and tau accumulation. *Neurobiol Aging* **29:** 1607–1618.

van Leeuwen FW, de Kleijn DP, van den Hurk HH, Neubauer A, Sonnemans MA, et al. 1998. Frameshift mutants of β amyloid precursor protein and ubiquitin-B in Alzheimer's and Down patients. *Science* **279:** 242–247.

Vito P, Lacana E, D'Adamio L. 1996. Interfering with apoptosis: Ca²⁺-binding protein ALG-2 and Alzheimer's disease gene ALG-3. *Science* **271:** 521–525.

Vito P, Pellegrini L, Guiet C, D'Adamio L. 1999. Cloning of AIP1, a novel protein that associates with the apoptosis-linked gene ALG-2 in a Ca²⁺-dependent reaction. *J Biol Chem* **274:** 1533–1540.

Walsh DM, Selkoe DJ. 2004. Deciphering the molecular basis of memory failure in Alzheimer's disease. *Neuron* **44:** 181–189.

Wang Y, Martinez-Vicente M, Kruger U, Kaushik S, Wong E, Mandelkow EM, Cuervo AM, Mandelkow E. 2009. Tau fragmentation, aggregation and clearance: The dual role of lysosomal processing. *Hum Mol Genet* **18:** 4153–4170.

Weidberg H, Shvets E, Elazar Z. 2011. Biogenesis and cargo selectivity of autophagosomes. *Annu Rev Biochem* **80:** 125–156.

Wischik CM, Crowther RA, Stewart M, Roth M. 1985. Subunit structure of paired helical filaments in Alzheimer's disease. *J Cell Biol* **100:** 1905–1912.

Wong E, Cuervo AM. 2010. Autophagy gone awry in neurodegenerative diseases. *Nat Neurosci* **13:** 805–811.

Wood JG, Mirra SS, Pollock NJ, Binder LI. 1986. Neurofibrillary tangles of Alzheimer disease share antigenic determinants with the axonal microtubule-associated protein tau (tau). *Proc Natl Acad Sci* **83:** 4040–4043.

Xu P, Peng J. 2006. Dissecting the ubiquitin pathway by mass spectrometry. *Biochim Biophys Acta* **1764:** 1940–1947.

Xu P, Peng J. 2008. Characterization of polyubiquitin chain structure by middle-down mass spectrometry. *Anal Chem* **80:** 3438–3444.

Yang AJ, Chandswangbhuvana D, Margol L, Glabe CG. 1998. Loss of endosomal/lysosomal membrane impermeability is an early event in amyloid Aβ1–42 pathogenesis. *J Neurosci Res* **52:** 691–698.

Yang DS, Kumar A, Stavrides P, Peterson J, Peterhoff CM, Pawlik M, Levy E, Cataldo AM, Nixon RA. 2008. Neuronal apoptosis and autophagy cross talk in aging PS/APP mice, a model of Alzheimer's disease. *Am J Pathol* **173:** 665–681.

Yang DS, Stavrides P, Mohan PS, Kaushik S, Kumar A, Ohno M, Schmidt SD, Wesson D, Bandyopadhyay U, Jiang Y, et al. 2011. Reversal of autophagy dysfunction in the TgCRND8 mouse model of Alzheimer's disease ameliorates amyloid pathologies and memory deficits. *Brain* **134:** 258–277.

Yoshii SR, Kishi C, Ishihara N, Mizushima N. 2011. Parkin mediates proteasome-dependent protein degradation and rupture of the outer mitochondrial membrane. *J Biol Chem* **286:** 19630–19640.

Youle RJ, Narendra DP. 2011. Mechanisms of mitophagy. *Nat Rev Mol Cell Biol* **12:** 9–14.

Yu WH, Cuervo AM, Kumar A, Peterhoff CM, Schmidt SD, Lee J-H, Mohan PS, Mercken M, Farmery MR, Tjernberg

I.O, et al. 2005. Macroautophagy—A novel β-amyloid peptide-generating pathway activated in Alzheimer's disease. *J Cell Biol* **171:** 87–98.

Zhang M. 2008. Endocytic mechanisms and drug discovery in neurodegenerative diseases. *Front Biosci* **13:** 6086–6105.

Zhang JY, Liu SJ, Li HL, Wang JZ. 2005. Microtubule-associated protein tau is a substrate of ATP/Mg^{2+}-dependent proteasome protease system. *J Neural Transm* **112:** 547–555.

Zhao J, Brault JJ, Schild A, Cao P, Sandri M, Schiaffino S, Lecker SH, Goldberg AL. 2007. FoxO3 coordinately activates protein degradation by the autophagic/lysosomal and proteasomal pathways in atrophying muscle cells. *Cell Metab* **6:** 472–483.

Proteolytic Degradation of Amyloid β-Protein

Takaomi Saido[1] and Malcolm A. Leissring[2]

[1]Riken Brain Science Institute, Saitamo 351-0198, Japan
[2]Department of Neuroscience, Mayo Clinic Florida, Jacksonville, Florida 32224

Correspondence: leissring@mayo.edu

The amyloid β-protein (Aβ) is subject to proteolytic degradation by a diverse array of peptidases and proteinases, known collectively as Aβ-degrading proteases (AβDPs). A growing number of AβDPs have been identified, which, under physiological and/or pathophysiological conditions, contribute significantly to the determination of endogenous cerebral Aβ levels. Despite more than a decade of investigation, the complete set of AβDPs remains to be established, and our understanding of even well-established AβDPs is incomplete. Nevertheless, the study of known AβDPs has contributed importantly to our understanding of the molecular pathogenesis of Alzheimer disease (AD) and has inspired the development of several novel therapeutic approaches to the regulation of cerebral Aβ levels. In this article, we discuss the general features of Aβ degradation and introduce the best-characterized AβDPs, focusing on their diverse properties and the numerous conceptual insights that have emerged from the study of each.

Amyloid β-protein (Aβ) is a normal product of cellular metabolism (Haass et al. 1993) derived from the amyloid precursor protein (APP) by the successive action of the β- and γ-secretases (see Haass et al. 2011). As is true for any other peptide, the production of Aβ is normally counterbalanced by its elimination via any of several processes operating in parallel, including proteolytic degradation, cell-mediated clearance, passive and active transport, and the aggregation and deposition of Aβ into insoluble aggregates. Although the relative importance of these different pathways remains to be established, a growing body of evidence suggests that proteolytic degradation is a particularly significant determinant of cerebral Aβ levels and, by extension, Alzheimer disease (AD) pathogenesis.

It has long been hypothesized that sporadic forms of AD may be attributable to defective clearance of Aβ (Selkoe 2001; Tanzi et al. 2004). Nevertheless, despite the obvious appeal of this simple idea, it had remained little more than a theoretic possibility. Recently, using newly developed techniques for quantifying the rates of Aβ production and clearance within the cerebrospinal fluid (CSF) in humans (Bateman et al. 2006), it was confirmed that sporadic AD patients do indeed exhibit significant defects in the clearance of CSF Aβ (Mawuenyega et al. 2010). Although these experiments cannot distinguish precisely which clearance mechanisms are impaired in these patients, these findings—together with the evidence reviewed in this article—lend strong support to the idea that defective Aβ degradation may be operative in AD.

Widespread interest in Aβ degradation did not take hold until the turn of the 21st century. A key turning point in the field came with the first study that was explicitly designed to examine Aβ degradation in the living animal (Iwata et al. 2000). In addition to identifying neprilysin (NEP) as one of the principal Aβ-degrading proteases (AβDPs), this study highlighted the pathophysiological significance of Aβ degradation to AD pathogenesis generally, thereby igniting interest in this previously underappreciated aspect of Aβ metabolism. A growing list of AβDPs have been identified which, by virtue of their diverse features, contribute in unique ways to the overall economy of brain Aβ. In this article, we provide an overview of the general features of Aβ degradation followed by a brief description of the some of the best characterized AβDPs and their diverse properties. We conclude with a discussion of the feasibility of developing therapies targeting Aβ proteolysis.

GENERAL FEATURES

Aβ Levels Are Potently Regulated by Proteolytic Degradation

Aβ is degraded by a large set of proteases with diverse characteristics (Table 1). Abundant evidence shows that AβDPs, both collectively and in many cases individually, contribute substantially to the determination of cerebral Aβ levels (Eckman and Eckman 2005; Leissring 2008;

Table 1. Proteases implicated in the degradation of Aβ

Type	Protease	Max. relative brain Aβ levels in KO[a]		Aβ substrates[b]		Subcellular localization[c]
		Aβ40	Aβ42	Oligos	Fibrils	
Metallo	NEP	2.0	2.0	Synth	No	Ex, ER, G
	NEP2	1.3	1.6			Ex, ER, G
	hMMEL					Ex, ER, G
	ECE1	1.3[d]	1.3[d]			Ex, ER, G, Endo
	ECE2	1.3	1.3			Ex, ER, G, Endo
	ACE	N.S.	N.S.			Ex, ER, G
	MMP2	1.2	1.3		Yes	Ex, ER, G
	MMP9	N.S.	1.3		Yes	Ex, ER, G
	MMP14/MT1-MMP				Yes	Ex, ER, G
	CD147/EMMPRIN					Ex, ER, G, Endo
	IDE	1.6	1.4	No	No	Ex, ER, Endo, Lyso, Mito
Serine	Plasmin	N.S.	N.S.	Natural	Yes	Ex, ER, G
	Acylpeptide hydrolase			Natural		Ex, Cyto
	Myelin basic protein				Yes	Ex, ER, G
Aspartyl	Cathepsin D	N.S.	3.0		Yes	Endo, Lyso
	BACE1	0.0	0.0			Endo, Lyso
	BACE2	N.S.	N.S.		No	Endo, Lyso
Cysteine	Cathepsin B	N.S.	N.S.		Yes	Ex, Endo, Lyso
Threonine	Proteasome					Cyto
Other	Catalytic antibodies					–

[a]Data reflect the maximum published values for endogenous cerebral Aβ levels in mice lacking both copies of individual AβDPs, expressed relative to wild-type controls. KO, knockout; N.S., no significant difference.

[b]Aggregated forms of Aβ known to be degraded by individual AβDPs. Synth, synthetic Aβ oligomers; Natural, naturally secreted Aβ oligomers.

[c]Ex, extracellular space; ER, endoplasmic reticulum; Endo, endosomes; Lyso, lysosomes; Mito, mitochondria; Cyto, cytosol.

[d]Effect induced by deletion of one copy of ECE1.

Leissring and Saido 2007; Turner and Nalivaeva 2007). In an illustrative study, the half-life of Aβ in brain interstitial fluid (ISF) was quantified in APP transgenic mice lacking or expressing NEP (Fig. 1A; Farris et al. 2007). This was accomplished by using in vivo microdialysis to quantify interstitial Aβ levels as a function of time before and after pharmacologic blockade of Aβ production (Farris et al. 2007). Genetic deletion of NEP resulted in a doubling of steady-state Aβ levels and, notably, a significant increase in the half-life of ISF Aβ (Fig. 1B). Conversely, transgenic overexpression of NEP in neurons by eightfold in an APP mouse model lowered Aβ levels by around 90% and, notably, prevented the development of any amyloid

plaques or downstream cytopathology when examined up to 14 months of age (Fig. 1C; Leissring et al. 2003). These and many other findings strongly suggest that AβDPs occupy an "upstream" position within the amyloid cascade that may be surpassed only by the proteases involved in Aβ production itself.

Net Aβ Levels Reflect the Balance between Rates of Production and Clearance

Aβ is generated and eliminated continuously, and the absolute concentration of Aβ, within a given compartment and at a given instant, is determined jointly by these opposing forces. An instructive analogy is that of a balance

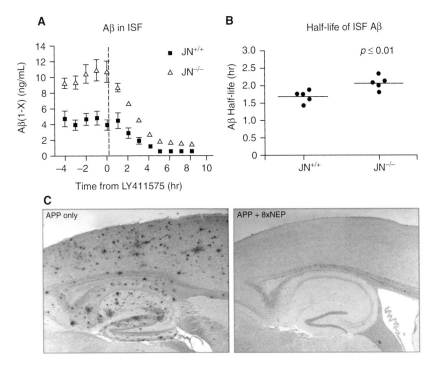

Figure 1. Aβ degradation is a potent determinant of brain Aβ levels and amyloid pathology. (A) Effects of genetic deletion of NEP on Aβ levels in the interstitial fluid (ISF) of the J9 line of APP transgenic mice monitored by in vivo microdialysis before and after blockade of Aβ production with the γ-secretase inhibitor, LY411575. Note that steady-state levels of Aβ are approximately doubled in J9 mice lacking NEP (JN$^{-/-}$). (Panel A is adapted from Farris et al. 2007; reprinted, with permission, from the authors.) (B) The half-life of ISF Aβ determined from the data in (A). Note that deletion of NEP results in a statistically significant (P < 0.01) 23% increase in the half-life of ISF Aβ, from 1.7 to 2.1 hours. (C) Transgenic overexpression of NEP by eightfold results in the complete prevention of amyloid plaque formation in the J20 line of APP transgenic mice up to 14 months of age. (Panel B is adapted from Leissring et al. 2003; reprinted, with permission, from the author.)

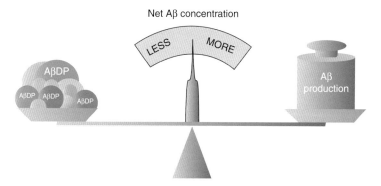

Figure 2. The balance analogy illustrates the relationship between AβDPs and net Aβ levels. By analogy with a balance, net Aβ concentrations (represented by the position of the pointer on the scale) are determined by the rate of Aβ production (represented by a single weight on one arm) relative to the overall rate of Aβ clearance (represented by a collection of counterweights on the other). Aβ clearance is performed by a collection of AβDPs (dark gray counterweights) working jointly with each other and with other eliminative processes (light gray counterweights). See text for additional details.

(Fig. 2), wherein the absolute rate of Aβ production, represented by a weight on one arm, is *counterbalanced* by the overall rate of Aβ clearance, represented by a large collection of diverse counterweights on the other arm.

The balance analogy serves to illustrate several general features of Aβ degradation:

1. *Net Aβ levels are determined by the relative, rather than absolute, rates of Aβ production and elimination.*

    Net Aβ concentrations can be elevated either by an increase in Aβ production or by a decrease in the overall rate of its elimination, and the converse is also true. However, no change in net Aβ levels will occur if these opposing forces vary in indirect proportion to one another—only if one changes with respect to the other.

2. *AβDPs work cooperatively with each other and with other catabolic processes to eliminate Aβ.*

    The catabolism of Aβ is mediated not only by multiple AβDPs but also by a diverse array of eliminative processes, including diffusion, passive and active transport, protein–protein interactions, aggregation, and deposition. These processes all operate simultaneously, in complex combinations that vary regionally and by subcellular compartment.

3. *Net Aβ levels are determined by the sum total of all catabolic processes.*

    Despite the complexity of Aβ catabolism, assuming production to be constant, the parameter most relevant to the determination of Aβ levels is the *overall rate* of Aβ catabolism, determined by the totality of all contributing processes. As a consequence, AβDPs and other Aβ-eliminating processes are *functionally interchangeable*, at least with respect to their influence determining net concentrations of Aβ.

4. *Proteolytic degradation of Aβ normally operates at or near its functional capacity.*

    In mice, genetic deletion of any one of several, markedly different AβDPs can result in significant elevations in endogenous cerebral Aβ (Table 1). These increases in net Aβ levels occur in a gene dosage-dependent manner, and simultaneous deletion of two different AβDPs has also been shown to produce roughly additive effects. Taken together, these findings show that multiple AβDPs exist, each of which is *rate limiting* in the determination of cerebral Aβ concentrations. More significantly, these findings suggest that there is *little or no reserve capacity* in the overall catabolism of cerebral Aβ.

5. *The mechanistic relationship between Aβ and AβDPs is bidirectional.*

Not only do AβDPs regulate Aβ via proteolytic degradation, but Aβ itself can also disrupt the function of AβDPs, either directly, via *competitive inhibition*, or indirectly, via a wide range of secondary processes triggered by Aβ accumulation, such as oxidative damage. Conversely, aggregated Aβ can also stimulate the production or activation of certain AβDPs. In these and other ways, AβDPs and Aβ interact *bidirectionally.*

Aβ Production and Degradation Are Asymmetric

The balance analogy, although illustrative of the mutual interdependence of Aβ production and degradation, fails to completely capture several fundamental asymmetries between the two processes. Collectively, these asymmetries offer important insights into the contribution of AβDPs to the normal regulation of cerebral Aβ levels and, by extension, the pathogenesis and potential treatment of AD.

Few Sources versus Many Diverse Sinks

Perhaps the most fundamental asymmetry is the difference in sheer complexity between Aβ production and degradation. Full-length Aβ peptides are produced by just two proteases, which act within a comparatively limited subset of subcellular compartments, primarily within neuronal cells. Aβ degradation, in contrast, is mediated by a considerably larger number of proteases, each with unique Aβ avidities, pH optima and, perhaps most critically, different regional, cellular, and subcellular localizations.

AβDPs Define Different Pools of Aβ

Proteolytic degradation of Aβ is the terminal event that defines the lifespan of a substantial portion of all Aβ peptides produced. By determining the temporal lifetime of individual Aβ molecules, proteolytic degradation also indirectly determines the spatial extent to which each molecule can be transported away from its site of production. As illustrated in Figure 3, AβDPs thus help to define specific *pools* of Aβ, the temporal and spatial extent of which is defined jointly by production and degradation. In light of the substantial variety in the regional and subcellular localization of many AβDPs (Table 1), it is evident that many different pools of Aβ exist, each contributing differently to overall Aβ levels and, potentially, to AD pathogenesis (Fig. 3). As such, functionally or spatially distinct AβDPs represent experimental probes for establishing the relative

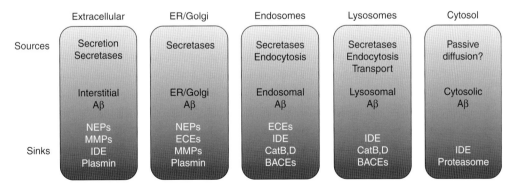

Figure 3. AβDPs regulate and help define distinct pools of Aβ. Aβ can be conceptualized as existing in distinct *pools* localized to different subcellular compartments (rounded rectangles). Each pool is characterized by different "sources" of Aβ (e.g., secretases, secretion) and different combinations of AβDPs. Because AβDPs vary considerably in terms of their subcellular localization, pH optima and other properties, Aβ within different subcellular compartments is regulated by diverse combinations of AβDPs.

importance of individual pools of Aβ, which might then be more selectively targeted for therapeutic benefit.

Aβ Degradation Is Catalytic and Irreversible

Proteolytic degradation is *catalytic* and *irreversible*, meaning that a single AβDP molecule can effect the permanent elimination of a large number of Aβ molecules, while itself remaining unchanged. Although it is true that Aβ production is also mediated by catalytic processes that can be rate limiting, in practice, Aβ production appears to be *substrate limited*. This can be seen from the fact that increases in APP expression—for instance, in Down's syndrome or in APP transgenic mice—result in roughly proportional increases in net Aβ production, both in the brain and in the periphery. Because small changes in the activities of multiple AβDPs can result in large changes in net Aβ levels, the catalytic nature of AβDPs suggests they are important both for the etiology and the potential treatment of AD.

Aβ Degradation Is Prone to a Range of Environmental and Age-Associated Insults

The pathogenesis of AD is known to be influenced by a range of environmental insults, whereas aging itself is known to be characterized by the accrual of oxidative damage (Zhu et al. 2007), as well as a general decrease in the expression of many proteins (Lu et al. 2004). AβDPs, in turn, are known to be vulnerable to a range of potentially damaging exogenous influences, including pharmacological inhibition, environmental insults, and age-related oxidative damage (Wang et al. 2003; Caccamo et al. 2005; Shinall et al. 2005; Neant-Fery et al. 2008). Given that age is the principle risk factor for AD, these considerations suggest that defective clearance of Aβ is likely to be operative not only in sporadic forms of AD, as was recently confirmed experimentally (Mawuenyega et al. 2010), but even in those cases attributable to increased production of Aβ due to genetic disturbances.

Aβ Degradation Can Take Place Distal to Sites of Production

The study of AβDPs has confirmed other evidence suggesting that Aβ exists in a dynamic equilibrium between various compartments, such as the secretory pathway, the endolysosomal system, the interstitial space, CSF, and even compartments outside the brain such as the circulatory system. Because these compartments are interconnected, either through physical contiguity or through active and passive Aβ transport, the degradation of Aβ in one compartment can result in the lowering of Aβ in the others. As a consequence, AβDPs can regulate net Aβ levels at sites distal to its production. This principle has an important therapeutic corollary. Whereas therapies aimed at blocking Aβ production must necessarily act locally, within Aβ-producing cells, therapies aimed at increasing Aβ catabolism are capable of exerting their effect in multiple compartments, including compartments outside the blood–brain barrier. In a striking demonstration of this principle, overexpression of NEP exclusively in the periphery (in skeletal muscle) was recently shown to lower steady-state Aβ levels and amyloid plaque deposition in brain (Liu et al. 2009).

SPECIFIC Aβ-DEGRADING PROTEASES

A large number of AβDPs have been identified to date (Table 1), but the state of our knowledge about each varies considerably. AβDPs can be classified by enzymological type (e.g., metalloproteases, cysteine proteases, etc.), by the assembly state of the Aβ substrates they hydrolyze (e.g., peptidases, oligopeptidases, or fibrillases), and by their subcellular localization (Table 1). There is a further, functional distinction between *endogenous regulators*, which regulate brain Aβ levels under physiological conditions, and *pathogenic regulators*, which are operative under pathological conditions, and these categories need not be mutually exclusive. In principle, a third functional category of AβDPs might be termed *therapeutic regulators*, which, it is important to emphasize, do not necessarily need to belong to either of the former categories to be effective.

In the following subsections, we briefly introduce the best characterized AβDPs, together with catalytic antibodies and endogenous protease inhibitors, focusing on the distinguishing features of each and the principles that have been learned from their study. Experimental evidence strongly suggests that additional AβDPs remain to be identified. For instance, simultaneous inhibition of multiple zinc-metalloproteases by i.c.v. infusion of the broad-spectrum metalloprotease inhibitor, phosphoramidon, resulted in a remarkable >fivefold increase in endogenous cerebral Aβ levels (Eckman et al. 2006). The magnitude of this increase is far greater than that seen by genetic deletion of any single AβDP (Table 1) or even from simultaneous deletion of multiple AβDPs (Eckman et al. 2006). In a similar finding, i.c.v. infusion of thiorphan in mice lacking both NEP and a related protease NEP2, nevertheless resulted in large increases in cerebral Aβ (Hafez et al. 2011). These and other findings strongly suggest that additional AβDPs remain to be identified that normally participate in Aβ catabolism and/or that might be used therapeutically.

Zinc-Metalloproteases

Neprilysin

The most extensively investigated and best characterized AβDP is NEP, a member of the M13 clan of zinc-metalloproteases (Howell et al. 1995; Hersh and Rodgers 2008). NEP was once termed "enkephalinase" because enkephalin is one of its best substrates in vitro (Turner 1998). However, enkephalin levels in the cerebral cortex were unchanged in NEP knockout (KO) mice (Saria et al. 1997; Iwata and Saido, unpubl. data), suggesting that NEP alone does not determine the steady-state levels of enkephalin in vivo. This is probably because there exist redundant catabolic mechanism(s) that involve exopeptidase(s), other endopeptidase(s), or both. In contrast, levels of both Aβ40 and Aβ42 are twofold higher in NEP KO mice than the levels in wild-type controls (Table 1; Iwata

et al. 2001), suggesting that NEP is an important endogenous regulator of Aβ.

NEP was first identified as an important AβDP in an experimental paradigm in which the degradation of radiolabeled Aβ42 injected into rat hippocampus was monitored in the presence or absence of different protease inhibitors (Iwata et al. 2000; Saido and Iwata 2006). NEP is a type II membrane-associated peptidase, the active site of which faces the lumenal or extracellular side of membranes (Roques et al. 1993; Turner 2004; Turner et al. 2001), a topology that is ideally suited for the degradation of largely extracytoplasmic peptides such as Aβ. NEP is almost exclusively expressed in neurons, not in glia, and the peptidase, after synthesis in the soma, is axonally transported to presynaptic terminals (Fukami et al. 2002), presumably in a manner similar to that in which APP is transported. Therefore, presynaptic terminals and nearby intracellular (lumenal) locations are likely to be the sites of Aβ degradation by NEP (Iwata et al. 2004). Importantly, the levels of Aβ inversely correlate with the gene dosage of NEP and thus with its enzymatic activity. These observations suggest that even partial loss of NEP expression/activity can cause the elevation of Aβ levels and could therefore induce amyloidosis on a long-term basis, in a similar manner to familial AD-causing gene mutations. The results also suggest that the rate constant for the intraparenchymal degradation of Aβ by NEP could account for as much as 50% of the total clearance activity (Saito et al., 2003).

Several insights have emerged from the study of NEP in APP transgenic mice. As discussed above, genetic deletion leads to an approximate doubling of steady-state levels of cerebral Aβ while accelerating amyloid deposition (see Fig. 1A). Qualitative pathological differences have emerged, as well. For example, deletion of NEP in the J9 line of transgenic mice led to the emergence of cerebral amyloid angiopathy that was not present in mice expressing two functional copies of NEP (Farris et al. 2007).

The therapeutic value of overexpressing NEP has also been investigated in APP transgenic mouse models. For example, as mentioned above, a cross between the J20 line of APP transgenic mice and a transgenic mouse that expresses eightfold higher levels of NEP (8xNEP) resulted in up to a 90% reduction in steady-state Aβ levels and the complete prevention of amyloid plaque formation and associated cytopathology when examined at up to 14 months of age (Fig. 1C; Leissring et al. 2003). NEP has been reported to degrade Aβ oligomers that impair neuronal plasticity and cognitive function in APP-Tg mice (Huang et al. 2006), although a different study saw no decrease in oligomers (Meilandt et al. 2009) (discussed below). As another potential therapeutic benefit, neuropeptide Y fragments generated by NEP-catalyzed proteolysis have been shown to be neuroprotective (Rose et al. 2009). Although these and other findings illustrate the potential benefits of therapeutic overexpression of NEP, there may also be risks. For example, the 8xNEP transgenic line has been shown to alternatively prevent or promote premature lethality in a strain-dependent manner (Leissring et al. 2003; Meilandt et al. 2009).

Like all known AβDPs, NEP degrades monomeric Aβ. Interestingly, some of the pathogenic APP mutations that reside within the Aβ sequence render Aβ monomers more resistant to NEP-catalyzed proteolysis (Tsubuki et al. 2003; Betts et al. 2008). It is less clear whether NEP can directly degrade oligomeric Aβ species. In vitro, NEP was reported to degrade oligomeric forms of synthetic Aβ (Kanemitsu et al. 2003), but it was incapable of degrading naturally secreted Aβ oligomers isolated from cultured cells (Leissring et al. 2003), suggesting that differences in the Aβ oligomer preparation might matter. Two findings in APP transgenic mice raise additional questions. On the one hand, deletion of NEP in 2 different mouse models was found to increase the concentration of Aβ oligomers (Huang et al. 2006; Farris et al. 2007). On the other hand, a cross between the 8xNEP line and the J20 line of APP transgenic mice resulted in dramatic decreases in monomeric Aβ levels and prevented all plaque formation (as reported previously by Leissring et al.

2003), yet oligomeric Aβ levels were unchanged (Meilandt et al. 2009). Moreover, in the latter study, NEP overexpression failed to reverse the learning and memory deficits present in the J20 line (Meilandt et al. 2009). Because different promoters were used, the extent to which the NEP and APP transgenes were coexpressed in the same population of neurons is not clear. Nevertheless, whether coexpressed appreciably or not, this result implies that NEP might not be capable of clearing at least some naturally produced Aβ oligomers.

NEP-Like Peptidases

Several close homologs of NEP are also implicated as candidate AβDPs (Table 1; Shirotani et al. 2001). For example, genetic ablation of NEP2 produces net increases in cerebral Aβ levels that are additive with those produced by deletion of NEP (Hafez et al. 2011). Another phosphoramidon-sensitive NEP homolog, human membrane metalloendopeptidase-like protein (hMMEL), was recently found to degrade Aβ in cultured cells (Huang et al. 2008). Although the exact contribution of each is still under investigation, it seems likely that the *collective* action of these and other NEP-like peptidases contribute significantly to the determination of cerebral Aβ levels.

Endothelin-Converting Enzymes

Two additional members of the M13 family of zinc metalloproteases, endothelin-converting enzymes 1 and 2 (ECE1, ECE2), are also known to be endogenous regulators of Aβ (Table 1; Eckman et al. 2001, 2003). In contrast to NEP and NEP-like peptidases, which are most active at neutral pH, ECEs have an acidic pH optimum and are therefore active primarily within acidic subcellular compartments (Table 1). As a consequence, ECEs primarily degrade Aβ at intracellular sites (Eckman et al. 2003). This point is important, because, together with other evidence (Leissring 2008), it serves to show that the vast majority of Aβ degradation likely occurs *before* the secretion of the monomer into the extracellular space.

Angiotensin-Converting Enzyme

Another important vasopeptidase implicated in the degradation of Aβ is angiotensin-converting enzyme (ACE) (Carvalho et al. 1997; Hu et al. 2001). Because pharmaceutical ACE inhibitors are widely used to treat hypertension, the question of whether ACE is an endogenous regulator of Aβ is a critical one. At present, the balance of the evidence suggests that it is not. Oral administration of the widely used ACE inhibitor, captopril, to APP transgenic mice resulted in no significant elevation in cerebral Aβ levels (Hemming et al. 2007b). Moreover, genetic deletion of ACE failed to produce any significant elevation in steady-state levels of endogenous Aβ (Table 1; Eckman et al. 2006). Nevertheless, because there is also genetic evidence that variants in the *Ace* gene are associated with the risk for late-onset AD (Bertram et al. 2007), it will be important to gain further clarity about the exact role of ACE in the degradation of Aβ under physiological and pathophysiological conditions.

Matrix-Metalloproteinases

Matrix-metalloproteinases (MMPs) represent another important group of AβDPs that can be distinguished, in part, by their ability to degrade both monomeric and fibrillar forms of Aβ (Table 1; Yan et al. 2006a). Multiple MMPs have been implicated in the degradation of Aβ, including MMP2 (Roher et al. 1994), MMP9 (Yan et al. 2006a) and MMP14 (a.k.a. MT1-MMP) (Liao and Van Nostrand 2010) but only a subset have been investigated in vivo. Relative to other AβDPs, MMPs are comparatively weak endogenous regulators of Aβ. For example, deletion of MMP2 or MMP9 in mice resulted in modest but statically significant increases in endogenous cortical and hippocampal Aβ (Yin et al. 2006) (Table 1). However, some special properties of MMPs suggest they are likely to be of considerably greater importance in a pathological context. First, MMPs normally exist as latent pro-enzymes that can be proteolytically processed to become fully active (Van Wart and Birkedal-Hansen 1990).

Interestingly, extracellular matrix metalloproteinase inducer (EMMPRIN; CD147), one of the proteases responsible for activating MMPs by this mechanism, was found to lower Aβ levels in cultured cells by inducing multiple MMPs (Vetrivel et al. 2008). Second, basal expression of MMPs is low but can be stimulated by pathological insults, including Aβ itself (Deb and Gottschall 1996). Consistent with these features, in APP transgenic mice, MMPs were found to be up-regulated in astrocytes adjacent to amyloid deposits (Yin et al. 2006). Moreover, in the same mice, i.c.v. infusion of the broad-spectrum MMP inhibitor, GM6001, resulted in significant increases (~50%) in both the steady-state levels and the half-life of ISF Aβ (Yin et al. 2006).

Insulin-Degrading Enzyme

Insulin-degrading enzyme (IDE) is another well-established AβDP that has been extensively investigated for its role in Aβ degradation using a wide array of experimental approaches, ranging from enzymological analyses to human molecular genetics (Hersh 2006). Although IDE is a zinc-metalloprotease, it belongs to a separate superfamily with distinct evolutionary origins, referred to as "inverzincins" because they feature a zinc-binding motif (HxxEH) that is inverted with respect to the canonical one (HExxH) present in most known zinc-metalloproteases (Becker and Roth 1992). The crystal structure of IDE is unusual, resembling a clam shell, with a large internal chamber formed from two bowl-shaped halves connected by a flexible linker (Shen et al. 2006). Because oligomeric and fibrillar forms of Aβ are too large to fit completely into its internal chamber, IDE is strictly a peptidase, i.e., it exclusively degrades monomeric Aβ.

Although functionally similar to vasopeptidases (e.g., ACE) in showing a preference for monomeric Aβ, IDE differs substantially in terms of its subcellular localization. It is well established that IDE is most abundant in the cytosol (Falkevall et al. 2006) and also present within mitochondria (Leissring et al. 2004; Farris et al. 2005), but there is less certainty about its presence in other subcellular compartments (Leissring et al. 2004), with various studies reporting its presence in peroxisomes (Kuo et al. 1994), endosomes (Hamel et al. 1991), the endoplasmic reticulum (Carpenter et al. 2010), and lysosomes (MA Leissring, unpubl.). Like most other AβDPs, IDE is also present in the extracellular space (Table 1), both in secreted (Qiu et al. 1998) and cell-associated (Vekrellis et al. 2000) forms. IDE lacks a canonical signal peptide sequence (Leissring et al. 2004) and it is exported independent of the classical secretory pathway (Zhao et al. 2009). The precise nature of the underlying secretion mechanism remains obscure, but accruing evidence suggests that it is mediated at least partly by exosomes (Bulloj et al. 2010; Tamboli et al. 2010).

Abundant evidence suggests that IDE is the major AβDP secreted into the medium of cultured cells (Qiu et al. 1998). For example, in cultured primary neurons, genetic deletion of IDE resulted in >90% decrease in the initial degradation rate of physiological levels of exogenous Aβ monomers (Farris et al. 2003), and similar results are seen with a wide variety of different cultured cells (MA Leissring, unpubl.). However, in vivo, genetic deletion of IDE resulted in elevations in cerebral Aβ levels which, although comparable to those induced by many AβDPs, are smaller than might be expected from results in cultured cells (Table 1; Farris et al. 2003). Two factors may contribute to this interesting disparity. First, although IDE is present in CSF (Qiu et al. 1998), it is likely that IDE accumulates in the medium of cultured cells to a greater extent than it does in extracellular fluids in vivo. Second, IDE KO mice suffer from chronic hyperinsulinemia (Farris et al. 2003; Abdul-Hay et al. 2011), which triggers age-dependent compensatory adaptations, including severe insulin and glucose intolerance (Abdul-Hay et al. 2011). The secondary consequences of IDE ablation thus obscure the impact of this important AβDP on brain Aβ levels. New pharmacologic inhibitors of IDE (Leissring et al. 2010) should make it possible to circumvent these compensatory changes and determine the direct contribution of IDE to cerebral brain Aβ levels.

Serine Proteases

Plasmin

Three functionally related serine proteases have been linked directly and indirectly to Aβ degradation: plasmin and urokinase-type and tissue-type plasminogen activators (uPA and tPA, respectively). Of these, only plasmin has been shown to directly degrade Aβ; like MMPs, it can degrade both monomeric and fibrillar forms (Table 1; Van Nostrand and Porter 1999; Tucker et al. 2000). tPA and uPA, however, are responsible for converting the inactive zymogen of plasmin (plasminogen) into its active form. The latter process is normally inhibited by the endogenous inhibitor, plasminogen activator inhibitor1 (PAI1; Myohanen and Vaheri 2004), and it is of great interest that pharmaceuticals which disrupt PAI1 have been developed that effectively lower brain Aβ in APP transgenic mice (Jacobsen et al. 2008). tPA is an excellent example of a pathologic regulator of Aβ, because it is stimulated by fibrillar proteins including Aβ (Van Nostrand and Porter 1999). uPA is of interest because of evidence linking variability around the gene for uPA (PLAU) to late-onset AD (Serretti et al. 2007).

Acylpeptide Hydrolase

A second serine protease implicated in the degradation of Aβ is acylpeptide hydrolase (APH), a predominantly cytosolic enzyme that catalyzes the hydrolysis of amino-terminally acetylated amino acids from small peptides (Table 1; Yamin et al. 2007). Intriguingly, APH has been reported to show a preference for degrading naturally secreted Aβ dimers and trimers (Yamin et al. 2009).

Myelin Basic Protein

In rather remarkable discovery, myelin basic protein (MBP), which is known to possesses endogenous serine protease activity, was recently identified as a bona fide AβDP (Liao et al. 2009). As is true for plasmin and APH, MBP can degrade both monomeric and fibrillar forms of Aβ (Table 1; Liao et al. 2009).

Cysteine Proteases

Cathepsin B

Cysteine proteases were initially implicated in Aβ degradation by in vivo pharmacological studies (Frautschy et al. 1998). However, only one cysteine protease, cathepsin B (CatB), has so far been specifically implicated in the degradation of Aβ in vivo (Mueller-Steiner et al. 2006). Interestingly, CatB is predominantly present within the endolysosomal protein degradation pathway (Mort and Buttle 1997), which is known to degrade Aβ and which is compromised in AD (Glabe 2001). CatB is secreted by exocytosis in certain pathological conditions (Mort and Buttle 1997) and has also been found to be present within extracellular amyloid plaques in AD (Mueller-Steiner et al. 2006). However, it is unclear whether CatB is operative in these compartments, because it exhibits optimal activity at pH 5–6 (Koga et al. 1991). Unlike most other known AβDPs, CatB is an endoprotease (Mort and Buttle 1997), but it is unusual for also having dipeptidyl carboxypeptidase activity (Mueller-Steiner et al. 2006).

Aspartyl Proteases

Cathepsin D

A second lysosomal protease implicated in Aβ degradation is the aspartyl protease, cathepsin D (CatD) (Leissring and Saido 2007). This role for CatD was initially discovered from analysis of brain homogenates, where it was shown to be the principal protease responsible for Aβ degradation at acidic pH (Hamazaki 1996; McDermott and Gibson 1996). Confirming its physiological relevance, CatD KO mice were recently found to have significant elevations in steady-state endogenous brain Aβ (Leissring et al. 2009). Consistent with its high activity in brain homogenates, deletion of CatD resulted in cerebral brain Aβ42 levels threefold higher than those in wild-type littermates, the largest increase observed in any AβDP KO mouse model (Table 1). Intriguingly, Aβ40 levels were unaffected in these mice, resulting in increases in the Aβ42/40 ratio that are comparable to those induced by presenilin mutations

(Leissring et al. 2009). Consistent with an effect on the critical Aβ42/40 ratio, deletion of CatD, unlike that of any other known AβDP, accelerates the onset of plaque formation. In the TgCRND8 APP transgenic mice, which normally develop amyloid plaques beginning at 3 months of age, deletion of CatD elicits plaque formation by just 3 weeks of age (MA Leissring, unpubl.). The differential increase in Aβ42 seen in the CatD KO mice has an intriguing mechanistic basis. Unlike CatB, CatD does not convert Aβ42 to Aβ40. Rather, CatD degrades Aβ42 and Aβ40 in a highly differential manner, with the affinity for Aβ42 and Aβ40 CatD being in the low nanomolar and low micromolar range, respectively, a factor that may drive preferential degradation of Aβ42 at low concentrations. At the same time, the turnover rate of Aβ42 is very slow, around 100-fold lower than that of Aβ40. Quite interestingly, the strong affinity of Aβ42 together with its slow turnover rate render Aβ42 a potent competitive inhibitor of CatD, even at relatively low (midnanomolar) concentrations (Leissring et al. 2009). Together with accumulating human molecular genetic evidence linking CatD to late-onset AD (Bertram et al. 2007), these findings suggest that CatD is a physiological and pathological regulator of Aβ, and they further suggest that CatD might be a downstream target of Aβ42 itself.

BACE1

Ironically, the major protease implicated in β-secretase activity, β-site APP cleaving enzyme 1 (BACE1; a.k.a. memapsin 2), is also capable of directly degrading Aβ (Fluhrer et al. 2003). Given BACE1's key role in Aβ production, the physiological relevance of this finding is difficult to assess but may explain the finding that transgenic overexpression of very high levels of BACE1 paradoxically resulted in reduced Aβ deposition in vivo (Lee et al. 2005).

BACE2

BACE2, a close homolog of BACE1, also avidly degrades Aβ in vitro, exhibiting a catalytic efficiency that is around 50-fold greater than

BACE1 (Abdul-Hay and Leissring 2011), higher in fact than the published values for any other known AβDP. Nevertheless, BACE2 KO mice show no net elevation in endogenous cerebral Aβ levels (Table 1; MA Leissring and SO Abdul-Hay, unpubl.). This is likely because BACE2 is expressed in astrocytes and other glia but not in neurons, which carry out the majority of Aβ production (Dominguez et al. 2005). Although these results suggest that BACE2 is not a physiologic regulator of Aβ, BACE2 might play some role in a pathological context because adult astrocytes are known to avidly degrade Aβ (Wyss-Coray et al. 2003).

The Proteasome

Aβ is also degraded by the proteasome (a.k.a., multicatalytic proteinase) by as-yet undetermined catalytic subunits (Lopez Salon et al. 2003). The proteasome is localized to the cytosol (Table 1) and, given that Aβ is produced in lumenal compartments, might therefore be assumed to play no physiologic role in Aβ degradation. However, some experimental evidence suggests that Aβ42 can diffuse passively from the lumen of the ER into the cytosol, where it is degraded jointly by the proteasome and IDE (Fig. 3; Schmitz et al. 2004). These and other findings—including evidence that Aβ accumulates within other intracellular organelles such as mitochondria (Yan et al. 2006b)—suggest that ill-defined pools of Aβ may exist that are degraded by certain AβDPs.

Aβ-Degrading Catalytic Antibodies

As is true for the secretases involved in Aβ production, the therapeutic targeting of AβDPs is complicated by the fact that each degrades multiple substrates besides Aβ. Catalytic antibodies have been suggested as an alternative that, by virtue of their higher specificity for particular antigenic targets, might improve the selectivity for Aβ. A surprisingly large number of Aβ-degrading immunoglobulins (Igs) and Ig-fragments have been discovered or engineered (Taguchi et al. 2008a). Although the catalytic efficiencies of most Aβ-degrading antibodies

is currently orders of magnitude slower than AβDPs, the technology exists to engineer existing antibodies or select new ones with improved properties (Taguchi et al. 2008b). Interestingly, Aβ-degrading antibodies are present in the sera of normal subjects and, notably, are increased in AD patients (Paul et al. 2010). Such antibodies can be harvested and may have therapeutic potential (Taguchi et al. 2008a). The exciting potential of catalytic Aβ-degrading antibodies makes this a topic worthy of continued investigation.

ENDOGENOUS INHIBITORS OF Aβ DEGRADATION

Several endogenous protease inhibitors have also been implicated in the regulation of Aβ degradation. Certainly the most interesting example is the nonneuronal isoform of APP itself (APP$_{751}$), which was in fact identified initially as a serine protease inhibitor (protease nexin II; Van Nostrand and Cunningham 1987; Van Nostrand et al. 1989) due to the presence of a Kunitz-type serine protease inhibitor (KPI) domain present in the longer APP isoforms (Ponte et al. 1988). The KPI domain inhibits Aβ degradation in cell culture by as-yet undetermined serine proteases (Naidu et al. 1995) and, intriguingly, transgenic mice overexpressing KPI-containing APP isoforms were found to have more severe amyloid pathology than mice expressing equivalent levels of APP lacking this domain (Higgins et al. 1993). It was later discovered that a second inhibitor domain exists within all isoforms of APP (Miyazaki et al. 1993), which has been mapped (to residues 579–601 of APP$_{770}$; Higashi and Miyazaki 2003) and shown to potently and selectively inhibit MMP2 (Higashi and Miyazaki 2008). Another serine protease inhibitor, alpha-1 antichymotrypsin, which was identified as a constituent of amyloid plaques (Abraham et al. 1988), has also been shown to inhibit the degradation of Aβ in vitro and in vivo (Abraham et al. 2000). The cysteine protease inhibitor cystatin C, which has been genetically linked to late-onset AD (Bertram et al. 2007), also regulates Aβ degradation by inhibiting CatB (Sun et al. 2008), although other mechanisms may also contribute to cystatin C's overall effect on amyloid plaque formation (Gauthier et al. 2011). Finally, as noted already, pharmacologic inhibitors of PAI1, which normally blocks that conversion of plasminogen to plasmin by tPA and uPA, have been shown to attenuate amyloid deposition in APP transgenic mice (Jacobsen et al. 2008).

THERAPEUTIC APPROACHES BASED ON Aβ DEGRADATION

One strategy for the treatment of chronically elevated Aβ levels in AD would be gene therapy using an AβDP. The introduction of NEP into the brains of APP transgenic mice using viral vectors has been shown to attenuate Aβ pathology, leading to improved cognitive function (Marr et al. 2003; Iwata et al. 2004; El-Amouri et al. 2008; Spencer et al. 2008). Although gene therapy for the treatment of Parkinson's disease in humans has already gained substantial momentum (Feng and Maguire-Zeiss 2010), its application to AD has not been as prominent, presumably due to the difference in the size and extent of the affected brain regions. However, in the very early stage of disease development, introduction of the NEP gene into the entorhinal cortex, which leads to expression of NEP in the hippocampus (Iwata et al. 2004), might generate a useful therapeutic effect. On the other hand, a significant reduction in cerebral Aβ levels and plaque formation has been achieved by expression of NEP in transplanted astrocytes (Hemming et al. 2007a), suggesting that neurons do not necessarily need to be directly infected with AβDPs to be effective. Substantial advances in gene therapy technology are anticipated in the coming years. IDE, ECEs, MMPs, BACE2, or other AβDPs could also be used in a similar manner to NEP, whereas the plasmin system should be more cautiously considered due to potential adverse side effects caused by hemorrhages (Murray et al. 2011).

AβDPs can be targeted by pharmacological therapies as well. Compared to the approach of inhibiting Aβ production, the notion that drugs could be developed which chronically stimulate Aβ degradation would seem to be impractical. However, because many AβDPs are regulated at least in part by endogenous inhibitors, it is feasible to enhance Aβ degradation via drugs that disrupt protease–inhibitor interactions. Indeed, this approach has been pursued preclinically, as illustrated by the development of PAI1 inhibitors that effectively promote Aβ degradation by plasmin (Jacobsen et al. 2008). Pharmacologic enhancement of the expression of AβDPs is another potential strategy. For example, neuronal NEP activity has been shown to be controlled by a neuropeptide, somatostatin (Saito et al. 2005), likely involving the phosphorylation status of the cytoplasmic domain of NEP (Kakiya R, Saito T, and Saido T, unpubl.). It should be feasible to develop synthetic small-molecule agonists that stimulate NEP by activating somatostatin receptors, such as the type four receptor, which is present exclusively in brain. Finally, for certain AβDPs, it may be feasible to develop compounds that directly activate proteolytic degradation. Consistent with this, compound screening has identified drug-like molecules that increase Aβ degradation by IDE several-fold (Cabrol et al. 2009).

CONCLUSIONS

Perhaps the most fundamental question yet to be answered is why Aβ is deposited in sporadic AD, which accounts for >99% of AD cases. It should be noted that the number of sporadic AD patients will grow as the average life expectancy increases, whereas the number of early-onset familial AD patients should remain proportional to the total population. The hypothesis that Aβ accumulation results at least in part from an age-dependent decline of Aβ degradation provides a plausible mechanism that may account for a substantial portion of AD cases. Virtually all humans accumulate Aβ in the brain as they age (Funato et al. 1998; Morishima-Kawashima et al. 2000), suggesting that Aβ deposition may be an unavoidable consequence of aging which may in turn place fundamental limits on the health of the brain. Because the conversion of "normal aging" to

AD via mild cognitive impairment appears to be a continuous process caused primarily by the gradual acceleration of Aβ accumulation, we may ultimately be able to implement presymptomatic interventions which include Aβ-reducing strategies utilizing degradation and clearance mechanisms to maintain lower Aβ levels during later life (Saito et al. 2003).

ACKNOWLEDGMENTS

This work is supported by grants from the American Health Assistance Foundation and the CART Fund (to M.A.L.).

REFERENCES

*Reference is also in this collection.

Abdul-Hay SO, Leissring MA. 2011. Functional cDNA screening identifies BACE-2 as a principal beta-amyloid-degrading protease. In *Alzheimer's Association International Conference on Alzheimer's Disease*, Proposal No. 17630. AAIC, Paris.

Abdul-Hay SO, Kang D, McBride M, Li L, Zhao J, Leissring MA. 2011. Deletion of insulin-degrading enzyme elicits antipodal, age-dependent effects on glucose and insulin tolerance. *PLoS One* **6:** e20818.

Abraham CR, Selkoe DJ, Potter H. 1988. Immunochemical identification of the serine protease inhibitor alpha 1-antichymotrypsin in the brain amyloid deposits of Alzheimer's disease. *Cell* **52:** 487–501.

Abraham CR, McGraw WT, Slot F, Yamin R. 2000. Alpha 1-antichymotrypsin inhibits A beta degradation in vitro and in vivo. *Ann NY Acad Sci* **920:** 245–248.

Bateman RJ, Munsell LY, Morris JC, Swarm R, Yarasheski KE, Holtzman DM. 2006. Human amyloid-beta synthesis and clearance rates as measured in cerebrospinal fluid in vivo. *Nat Med* **12:** 856–861.

Becker AB, Roth RA. 1992. An unusual active site identified in a family of zinc metalloendopeptidases. *Proc Natl Acad Sci* **89:** 3835–3839.

Bertram L, McQueen MB, Mullin K, Blacker D, Tanzi RE. 2007. Systematic meta-analyses of Alzheimer disease genetic association studies: The AlzGene database. *Nat Genet* **39:** 17–23.

Betts V, Leissring MA, Dolios G, Wang R, Selkoe DJ, Walsh DM. 2008. Aggregation catabolism of disease-associated intra-Abeta mutations: Reduced proteolysis of Abeta A21G by neprilysin. *Neurobiol Dis* **31:** 442–450.

Bulloj A, Leal MC, Xu H, Castano EM, Morelli L. 2010. Insulin-degrading enzyme sorting in exosomes: A secretory pathway for a key brain amyloid-beta degrading protease. *J Alzheimers Dis* **19:** 79–95.

Cabrol C, Huzarska MA, Dinolfo C, Rodriguez MC, Reinstatler L, Ni J, Yeh L-A, Cuny GD, Stein RL, Selkoe DJ, et al. 2009. Small-molecule activators of insulin-degrading enzyme discovered through high-throughput compound screening. *PLoS One* **4:** e5274.

Caccamo A, Oddo S, Sugarman MC, Akbari Y, LaFerla FM. 2005. Age- and region-dependent alterations in Abeta-degrading enzymes: Implications for Abeta-induced disorders. *Neurobiol Aging* **26:** 645–654.

Carpenter JE, Jackson W, de Souza GA, Haarr L, Grose C. 2010. Insulin-degrading enzyme binds to the nonglycosylated precursor of varicella-zoster virus gE protein found in the endoplasmic reticulum. *J Virol* **84:** 847–855.

Carvalho KM, Franca MS, Camarao GC, Ruchon AF. 1997. A new brain metalloendopeptidase which degrades the Alzheimer beta-amyloid 1–40 peptide producing soluble fragments without neurotoxic effects. *Braz J Med Biol Res* **30:** 1153–1156.

Deb S, Gottschall PE. 1996. Increased production of matrix metalloproteinases in enriched astrocyte and mixed hippocampal cultures treated with beta-amyloid peptides. *J Neurochem* **66:** 1641–1647.

Dominguez D, Tournoy J, Hartmann D, Huth T, Cryns K, Deforce S, Serneels L, Camacho IE, Marjaux E, Craesaerts K, et al. 2005. Phenotypic and biochemical analyses of BACE1- and BACE2-deficient mice. *J Biol Chem* **280:** 30797–30806.

Eckman EA, Eckman CB. 2005. Abeta-degrading enzymes: Modulators of Alzheimer's disease pathogenesis and targets for therapeutic intervention. *Biochem Soc Trans* **33:** 1101–1105.

Eckman EA, Reed DK, Eckman CB. 2001. Degradation of the Alzheimer's amyloid beta peptide by endothelin-converting enzyme. *J Biol Chem* **276:** 24540–24548.

Eckman EA, Watson M, Marlow L, Sambamurti K, Eckman CB. 2003. Alzheimer's disease beta-amyloid peptide is increased in mice deficient in endothelin-converting enzyme. *J Biol Chem* **278:** 2081–2084.

Eckman EA, Adams SK, Troendle FJ, Stodola BA, Kahn MA, Fauq AH, Xiao HD, Bernstein KE, Eckman CB. 2006. Regulation of steady-state beta-amyloid levels in the brain by neprilysin and endothelin-converting enzyme but not angiotensin-converting enzyme. *J Biol Chem* **281:** 30471–30478.

El-Amouri SS, Zhu H, Yu J, Marr R, Verma IM, Kindy MS. 2008. Neprilysin: An enzyme candidate to slow the progression of Alzheimer's disease. *Am J Pathol* **172:** 1342–1354.

Falkevall A, Alikhani N, Bhushan S, Pavlov PF, Busch K, Johnson KA, Eneqvist T, Tjernberg L, Ankarcrona M, Glaser E. 2006. Degradation of the amyloid beta-protein by the novel mitochondrial peptidasome, PreP. *J Biol Chem* **281:** 29096–29104.

Farris W, Mansourian S, Chang Y, Lindsley L, Eckman EA, Frosch MP, Eckman CB, Tanzi RE, Selkoe DJ, Guenette S. 2003. Insulin-degrading enzyme regulates the levels of insulin, amyloid beta-protein, and the beta-amyloid precursor protein intracellular domain in vivo. *Proc Natl Acad Sci* **100:** 4162–4167.

Farris W, Leissring MA, Hemming ML, Chang AY, Selkoe DJ. 2005. Alternative splicing of human insulin-degrading enzyme yields a novel isoform with a decreased ability to degrade insulin and amyloid beta-protein. *Biochemistry* **44:** 6513–6525.

Farris W, Schutz SG, Cirrito JR, Shankar GM, Sun X, George A, Leissring MA, Walsh DM, Qiu WQ, Holtzman DM, et al. 2007. Loss of neprilysin function promotes amyloid plaque formation and causes cerebral amyloid angiopathy. *Am J Pathol* **171:** 241–251.

Feng LR, Maguire-Zeiss KA. 2010. Gene therapy in Parkinson's disease: Rationale and current status. *CNS Drugs* **24:** 177–192.

Fluhrer R, Multhaup G, Schlicksupp A, Okochi M, Takeda M, Lammich S, Willem M, Westmeyer G, Bode W, Walter J, et al. 2003. Identification of a beta-secretase activity, which truncates amyloid beta-peptide after its presenilin-dependent generation. *J Biol Chem* **278:** 5531–5538.

Frautschy SA, Horn DL, Sigel JJ, Harris-White ME, Mendoza JJ, Yang F, Saido TC, Cole GM. 1998. Protease inhibitor coinfusion with amyloid beta-protein results in enhanced deposition and toxicity in rat brain. *J Neurosci* **18:** 8311–8321.

Fukami S, Watanabe K, Iwata N, Haraoka J, Lu B, Gerard NP, Gerard C, Fraser P, Westaway D, St George-Hyslop P, et al. 2002. Abeta-degrading endopeptidase, neprilysin, in mouse brain: Synaptic and axonal localization inversely correlating with Abeta pathology. *Neurosci Res* **43:** 39–56.

Funato H, Yoshimura M, Kusui K, Tamaoka A, Ishikawa K, Ohkoshi N, Namekata K, Okeda R, Ihara Y. 1998. Quantitation of amyloid beta-protein (A beta) in the cortex during aging and in Alzheimer's disease. *Am J Pathol* **152:** 1633–1640.

Gauthier S, Kaur G, Mi W, Tizon B, Levy E. 2011. Protective mechanisms by cystatin C in neurodegenerative diseases. *Front Biosci (Schol Ed)* **3:** 541–554.

Glabe C. 2001. Intracellular mechanisms of amyloid accumulation and pathogenesis in Alzheimer's disease. *J Mol Neurosci* **17:** 137–145.

Haass C, Hung AY, Schlossmacher MG, Oltersdorf T, Teplow DB, Selkoe DJ. 1993. Normal cellular processing of the beta-amyloid precursor protein results in the secretion of the amyloid beta peptide and related molecules. *Ann NY Acad Sci* **695:** 109–116.

* Haass C, Kaether C, Sisodia S, Thinakaran G. 2011. Trafficking and proteolytic processing of APP. *Cold Spring Harb Perspect Med* doi: 10.1101/cshperspect.a006270.

Hafez D, Huang JY, Huynh AM, Valtierra S, Rockenstein E, Bruno AM, Lu B, DesGroseillers L, Masliah E, Marr RA. 2011. Neprilysin-2 is an important beta-amyloid degrading enzyme. *Am J Pathol* **178:** 306–312.

Hamazaki H. 1996. Cathepsin D is involved in the clearance of Alzheimer's beta-amyloid protein. *FEBS Lett* **396:** 139–142.

Hamel FG, Mahoney MJ, Duckworth WC. 1991. Degradation of intraendosomal insulin by insulin-degrading enzyme without acidification. *Diabetes* **40:** 436–443.

Hemming ML, Patterson M, Reske-Nielsen C, Lin L, Isacson O, Selkoe DJ. 2007a. Reducing amyloid plaque burden via ex vivo gene delivery of an Aβ-degrading protease: A novel therapeutic approach to Alzheimer disease. *PLoS Med* **4:** e262.

Hemming ML, Selkoe DJ, Farris W. 2007b. Effects of prolonged angiotensin-converting enzyme inhibitor treatment on amyloid beta-protein metabolism in mouse models of Alzheimer disease. *Neurobiol Dis* **26:** 273–281.

Hersh LB. 2006. The insulysin (insulin degrading enzyme) enigma. *Cell Mol Life Sci* **63:** 2432–2434.

Hersh LB, Rodgers DW. 2008. Neprilysin and amyloid beta peptide degradation. *Curr Alzheimer Res* **5:** 225–231.

Higashi S, Miyazaki K. 2003. Identification of a region of beta-amyloid precursor protein essential for its gelatinase A inhibitory activity. *J Biol Chem* **278:** 14020–14028.

Higashi S, Miyazaki K. 2008. Identification of amino acid residues of the matrix metalloproteinase-2 essential for its selective inhibition by beta-amyloid precursor protein-derived inhibitor. *J Biol Chem* **283:** 10068–10078.

Higgins LS, Catalano R, Quon D, Cordell B. 1993. Transgenic mice expressing human β-APP751, but not mice expressing β-APP695, display early Alzheimer's disease-like histopathology. *Ann NY Acad Sci* **695:** 224–227.

Howell S, Nalbantoglu J, Crine P. 1995. Neutral endopeptidase can hydrolyze β-amyloid(1–40) but shows no effect on β-amyloid precursor protein metabolism. *Peptides* **16:** 647–652.

Hu J, Igarashi A, Kamata M, Nakagawa H. 2001. Angiotensin-converting enzyme degrades Alzheimer amyloid β-peptide (Aβ); retards Aβ aggregation, deposition, fibril formation; and inhibits cytotoxicity. *J Biol Chem* **276:** 47863–47868.

Huang SM, Mouri A, Kokubo H, Nakajima R, Suemoto T, Higuchi M, Staufenbiel M, Noda Y, Yamaguchi H, Nabeshima T, et al. 2006. Neprilysin-sensitive synapse-associated amyloid-β peptide oligomers impair neuronal plasticity and cognitive function. *J Biol Chem* **281:** 17941–17951.

Huang JY, Bruno AM, Patel CA, Huynh AM, Philibert KD, Glucksman MJ, Marr RA. 2008. Human membrane metallo-endopeptidase-like protein degrades both beta-amyloid 42 and beta-amyloid 40. *Neuroscience* **155:** 258–262.

Iwata N, Tsubuki S, Takaki Y, Watanabe K, Sekiguchi M, Hosoki E, Kawashima-Morishima M, Lee HJ, Hama E, Sekine-Aizawa Y, et al. 2000. Identification of the major Abeta1–42-degrading catabolic pathway in brain parenchyma: Suppression leads to biochemical and pathological deposition. *Nat Med* **6:** 143–150.

Iwata N, Tsubuki S, Takaki Y, Shirotani K, Lu B, Gerard NP, Gerard C, Hama E, Lee HJ, Saido TC. 2001. Metabolic regulation of brain Abeta by neprilysin. *Science* **292:** 1550–1552.

Iwata N, Mizukami H, Shirotani K, Takaki Y, Muramatsu S, Lu B, Gerard NP, Gerard C, Ozawa K, Saido TC. 2004. Presynaptic localization of neprilysin contributes to efficient clearance of amyloid-beta peptide in mouse brain. *J Neurosci* **24:** 991–998.

Jacobsen JS, Comery TA, Martone RL, Elokdah H, Crandall DL, Oganesian A, Aschmies S, Kirksey Y, Gonzales C, Xu J, et al. 2008. Enhanced clearance of Abeta in brain by sustaining the plasmin proteolysis cascade. *Proc Natl Acad Sci* **105:** 8754–8759.

Kanemitsu H, Tomiyama T, Mori H. 2003. Human neprilysin is capable of degrading amyloid beta peptide not only in the monomeric form but also the pathological oligomeric form. *Neurosci Lett* **350:** 113–116.

Koga H, Yamada H, Nishimura Y, Kato K, Imoto T. 1991. Multiple proteolytic action of rat liver cathepsin B: Specificities and pH-dependences of the endo- and exopeptidase activities. *J Biochem* **110**: 179–188.

Kuo WL, Gehm BD, Rosner MR, Li W, Keller G. 1994. Inducible expression and cellular localization of insulin-degrading enzyme in a stably transfected cell line. *J Biol Chem* **269**: 22599–22606.

Lee EB, Zhang B, Liu K, Greenbaum EA, Doms RW, Trojanowski JQ, Lee VM. 2005. BACE overexpression alters the subcellular processing of APP and inhibits Abeta deposition in vivo. *J Cell Biol* **168**: 291–302.

Leissring MA. 2008. The AβCs of Aβ-cleaving proteases. *J Biol Chem* **283**: 29645–29649.

Leissring MA, Saido TC. 2007. Aβ degradation. In *Alzheimer's disease: Advances in genetics, molecular and cellular biology* (ed. Sisodia S, Tanzi R), pp. 157–178. Springer, New York.

Leissring MA, Farris W, Chang AY, Walsh DM, Wu X, Sun X, Frosch MP, Selkoe DJ. 2003. Enhanced proteolysis of beta-amyloid in APP transgenic mice prevents plaque formation, secondary pathology, and premature death. *Neuron* **40**: 1087–1093.

Leissring MA, Farris W, Wu X, Christodoulou DC, Haigis MC, Guarente L, Selkoe DJ. 2004. Alternative translation initiation generates a novel isoform of insulin-degrading enzyme targeted to mitochondria. *Biochem J* **383**: 439–446.

Leissring MA, Reinstatler L, Sahara T, Roman R, Sevlever D, Saftig P, Levites Y, Golde TE, Burgess JD, Ertekin-Taner N, et al. 2009. Cathepsin D selectively degrades Aβ42 and tau: Implications for Alzheimer disease pathogenesis. In *Society for Neuroscience*, Program No. 139108. Society for Neuroscience, Chicago.

Leissring MA, Malito E, Hedouin S, Reinstatler L, Sahara T, Abdul-Hay SO, Choudhry S, Maharvi GM, Fauq AH, Huzarska M, May PS, Choi S, et al. 2010. Designed inhibitors of insulin-degrading enzyme regulate the catabolism and activity of insulin. *PLoS One* **5**: e10504.

Liao MC, Van Nostrand WE. 2010. Degradation of soluble and fibrillar amyloid β-protein by matrix metalloproteinase (MT1-MMP) in vitro. *Biochemistry* **49**: 1127–1136.

Liao MC, Ahmed M, Smith SO, Van Nostrand WE. 2009. Degradation of amyloid β protein by purified myelin basic protein. *J Biol Chem* **284**: 28917–28925.

Liu Y, Studzinski C, Beckett T, Guan H, Hersh MA, Murphy MP, Klein R, Hersh LB. 2009. Expression of neprilysin in skeletal muscle reduces amyloid burden in a transgenic mouse model of Alzheimer disease. *Mol Ther* **17**: 1381–1386.

Lopez Salon M, Pasquini L, Besio Moreno M, Pasquini JM, Soto E. 2003. Relationship between beta-amyloid degradation and the 26S proteasome in neural cells. *Exp Neurol* **180**: 131–143.

Lu T, Pan Y, Kao SY, Li C, Kohane I, Chan J, Yankner BA. 2004. Gene regulation and DNA damage in the ageing human brain. *Nature* **429**: 883–891.

Marr RA, Rockenstein E, Mukherjee A, Kindy MS, Hersh LB, Gage FH, Verma IM, Masliah E. 2003. Neprilysin gene transfer reduces human amyloid pathology in transgenic mice. *J Neurosci* **23**: 1992–1996.

Mawuenyega KG, Sigurdson W, Ovod V, Munsell L, Kasten T, Morris JC, Yarasheski KE, Bateman RJ. 2010. Decreased clearance of CNS beta-amyloid in Alzheimer's disease. *Science* **330**.

McDermott JR, Gibson AM. 1996. Degradation of Alzheimer's beta-amyloid protein by human cathepsin D. *Neuroreport* **7**: 2163–2166.

Meilandt WJ, Cisse M, Ho K, Wu T, Esposito LA, Scearce-Levie K, Cheng IH, Yu GQ, Mucke L. 2009. Neprilysin overexpression inhibits plaque formation but fails to reduce pathogenic Abeta oligomers and associated cognitive deficits in human amyloid precursor protein transgenic mice. *J Neurosci* **29**: 1977–1986.

Miyazaki K, Hasegawa M, Funahashi K, Umeda M. 1993. A metalloproteinase inhibitor domain in Alzheimer amyloid protein precursor. *Nature* **362**: 839–841.

Morishima-Kawashima M, Oshima N, Ogata H, Yamaguchi H, Yoshimura M, Sugihara S, Ihara Y. 2000. Effect of *apolipoprotein* E allele ε4 on the initial phase of amyloid β-protein accumulation in the human brain. *Am J Pathol* **157**: 2093–2099.

Mort JS, Buttle DJ. 1997. Cathepsin B. *Int J Biochem Cell Biol* **29**: 715–720.

Mueller-Steiner S, Zhou Y, Arai H, Roberson ED, Sun B, Chen J, Wang X, Yu G, Esposito L, Mucke L, et al. 2006. Antiamyloidogenic and neuroprotective functions of cathepsin B: Implications for Alzheimer's disease. *Neuron* **51**: 703–714.

Murray IV, Proza JF, Sohrabji F, Lawler JM. 2011. Vascular metabolic dysfunction in Alzheimer's disease: A review. *Exp Biol Med* **236**: 772–782.

Myohanen H, Vaheri A. 2004. Regulation and interactions in the activation of cell-associated plasminogen. *Cell Mol Life Sci* **61**: 2840–2858.

Naidu A, Quon D, Cordell B. 1995. Beta-amyloid peptide produced in vitro is degraded by proteinases released by cultured cells. *J Biol Chem* **270**: 1369–1374.

Neant-Fery M, Garcia-Ordonez RD, Logan TP, Selkoe DJ, Li L, Reinstatler L, Leissring MA. 2008. Molecular basis for the thiol sensitivity of insulin-degrading enzyme. *Proc Natl Acad Sci* **105**: 9582–9587.

Paul S, Planque S, Nishiyama Y. 2010. Immunological origin and functional properties of catalytic autoantibodies to amyloid beta peptide. *J Clin Immunol* **30** (Suppl 1): S43–S49.

Ponte P, Gonzalez-DeWhitt P, Schilling J, Miller J, Hsu D, Greenberg B, Davis K, Wallace W, Lieberburg I, Fuller F. 1988. A new A4 amyloid mRNA contains a domain homologous to serine proteinase inhibitors. *Nature* **331**: 525–527.

Qiu WQ, Walsh DM, Ye Z, Vekrellis K, Zhang J, Podlisny MB, Rosner MR, Safavi A, Hersh LB, Selkoe DJ. 1998. Insulin-degrading enzyme regulates extracellular levels of amyloid beta-protein by degradation. *J Biol Chem* **273**: 32730–32738.

Roques BP, Noble F, Dauge V, Fournie-Zaluski MC, Beaumont A. 1993. Neutral endopeptidase 24.11: Structure, inhibition, and experimental and clinical pharmacology. *Pharmacol Rev* **45**: 87–146.

Rose JB, Crews L, Rockenstein E, Adame A, Mante M, Hersh LB, Gage FH, Spencer B, Potkar R, Marr RA, Masliah E.

2009. Neuropeptide Y fragments derived from neprilysin processing are neuroprotective in a transgenic model of Alzheimer's disease. *J Neurosci* **29:** 1115–25.

Saido TC, Iwata N. 2006. Metabolism of amyloid β peptide and pathogenesis of Alzheimer's disease. Towards presymptomatic diagnosis, prevention and therapy. *Neurosci Res* **54:** 235–253.

Saito T, Iwata N, Tsubuki S, Takaki Y, Takano J, Huang SM, Suemoto T, Higuchi M, Saido TC. 2005. Somatostatin regulates brain amyloid β-peptide Aβ42 through modulation of proteolytic degradation. *Nat Med* **11:** 434–439.

Saito T, Takaki Y, Iwata N, Trojanowski J, Saido TC. 2006. Alzheimer's disease, neuropeptides, neuropeptidase, amyloid-beta peptide metabolism. *Sci Aging Knowledge Environ* **2003:** PE1.

Saria A, Hauser KF, Traurig HH, Turbek CS, Hersh L, Gerard C. 1997. Opioid-related changes in nociceptive threshold and in tissue levels of enkephalins after target disruption of the gene for neutral endopeptidase (EC 3.4.24.11) in mice. *Neurosci Lett* **234:** 27–30.

Schmitz A, Schneider A, Kummer MP, Herzog V. 2004. Endoplasmic reticulum-localized amyloid beta-peptide is degraded in the cytosol by two distinct degradation pathways. *Traffic* **5:** 89–101.

Selkoe D. 2001. Clearing the brain's amyloid cobwebs. *Neuron* **32:** 177–180.

Serretti A, Olgiati P, De Ronchi D. 2007. Genetics of Alzheimer's disease. A rapidly evolving field. *J Alzheimers Dis* **12:** 73–92.

Shen Y, Joachimiak A, Rosner MR, Tang W-J. 2006. Structures of human insulin-degrading enzyme reveal a new substrate mechanism. *Nature* **443:** 870–874.

Shinall H, Song ES, Hersh LB. 2005. Susceptibility of amyloid beta peptide degrading enzymes to oxidative damage: A potential Alzheimer's disease spiral. *Biochemistry* **44:** 15345–15350.

Shirotani K, Tsubuki S, Iwata N, Takaki Y, Harigaya W, Maruyama K, Kiryu-Seo S, Kiyama H, Iwata H, Tomita T, et al. 2001. Neprilysin degrades both amyloid beta peptides 1–40 and 1–42 most rapidly and efficiently among thiorphan- and phosphoramidon-sensitive endopeptidases. *J Biol Chem* **276:** 21895–21901.

Spencer B, Marr RA, Rockenstein E, Crews L, Adame A, Potkar R, Patrick C, Gage FH, Verma IM, Masliah E. 2008. Long-term neprilysin gene transfer is associated with reduced levels of intracellular Abeta and behavioral improvement in APP transgenic mice. *BMC Neurosci* **9:** 109.

Sun B, Zhou Y, Halabisky B, Lo I, Cho SH, Mueller-Steiner S, Devidze N, Wang X, Grubb A, Gan L. 2008. Cystatin C-cathepsin B axis regulates amyloid beta levels and associated neuronal deficits in an animal model of Alzheimer's disease. *Neuron* **60:** 247–257.

Taguchi H, Planque S, Nishiyama Y, Szabo P, Weksler ME, Friedland RP, Paul S. 2008a. Catalytic antibodies to amyloid beta peptide in defense against Alzheimer disease. *Autoimmun Rev* **7:** 391–397.

Taguchi H, Planque S, Sapparapu G, Boivin S, Hara M, Nishiyama Y, Paul S. 2008b. Exceptional amyloid beta peptide hydrolyzing activity of nonphysiological

immunoglobulin variable domain scaffolds. *J Biol Chem* **283:** 36724–36733.

Tamboli IY, Barth E, Christian L, Siepmann M, Kumar S, Singh S, Tolksdorf K, Heneka MT, Lutjohann D, Wunderlich P, et al. 2010. Statins promote the degradation of extracellular amyloid β-peptide by microglia via stimulation of exosome-associated insulin-degrading enzyme (IDE) secretion. *J Biol Chem* **285:** 37405–37414.

Tanzi RE, Moir RD, Wagner SL. 2004. Clearance of Alzheimer's Abeta peptide: The many roads to perdition. *Neuron* **43:** 605–608.

Tsubuki S, Takaki Y, Saido TC. 2003. Dutch, Flemish, Italian, Arctic mutations of APP and resistance of Abeta to physiologically relevant proteolytic degradation. *Lancet* **361:** 1957–1958.

Tucker HM, Kihiko-Ehmann M, Wright S, Rydel RE, Estus S. 2000. Tissue plasminogen activator requires plasminogen to modulate amyloid-beta neurotoxicity and deposition. *J Neurochem* **75:** 2172–2177.

Turner AJ. 1998. Neprilysin. In *Handbook of proteolytic enzymes* (ed. Barret AJ, Rawlings ND, Woessner JF), pp. 1080–1085. Academic, San Diego.

Turner AJ. 2004. Neprilysin. In *Handbook of proteolytic enzymes* (ed. Barret AJ, Rawlings ND, Woessner JF), pp. 419–426. Academic, London.

Turner AJ, Nalivaeva NN. 2007. New insights into the roles of metalloproteinases in neurodegeneration and neuroprotection. *Int Rev Neurobiol* **82:** 113–135.

Turner AJ, Isaac RE, Coates D. 2001. The neprilysin (NEP) family of zinc metalloendopeptidases: Genomics and function. *Bioessays* **23:** 261–269.

Van Nostrand WE, Cunningham DD. 1987. Purification of protease nexin II from human fibroblasts. *J Biol Chem* **262:** 8508–8514.

Van Nostrand WE, Porter M. 1999. Plasmin cleavage of the amyloid beta-protein: Alteration of secondary structure and stimulation of tissue plasminogen activator activity. *Biochemistry* **38:** 11570–11576.

Van Nostrand WE, Wagner SL, Suzuki M, Choi BH, Farrow JS, Geddes JW, Cotman CW, Cunningham DD. 1989. Protease nexin-II, a potent antichymotrypsin, shows identity to amyloid beta-protein precursor. *Nature* **341:** 546–549.

Van Wart HE, Birkedal-Hansen H. 1990. The cysteine switch: A principle of regulation of metalloproteinase activity with potential applicability to the entire matrix metalloproteinase gene family. *Proc Natl Acad Sci* **87:** 5578–5582.

Vekrellis K, Ye Z, Qiu WQ, Walsh D, Hartley D, Chesneau V, Rosner MR, Selkoe DJ. 2000. Neurons regulate extracellular levels of amyloid beta-protein via proteolysis by insulin-degrading enzyme. *J Neurosci* **20:** 1657–1665.

Vetrivel KS, Zhang X, Meckler X, Cheng H, Lee S, Gong P, Lopes KO, Chen Y, Iwata N, Yin KJ, et al. 2008. Evidence that CD147 modulation of beta-amyloid (Abeta) levels is mediated by extracellular degradation of secreted Abeta. *J Biol Chem* **283:** 19489–19498.

Wang DS, Iwata N, Hama E, Saido TC, Dickson DW. 2003. Oxidized neprilysin in aging and Alzheimer's disease brains. *Biochem Biophys Res Commun* **310:** 236–241.

Wyss-Coray T, Loike JD, Brionne TC, Lu E, Anankov R, Yan F, Silverstein SC, Husemann J. 2003. Adult mouse astrocytes degrade amyloid-beta in vitro and in situ. *Nat Med* **9:** 453–457.

Yamin R, Bagchi S, Hildebrant R, Scaloni A, Widom RL, Abraham CR. 2007. Acyl peptide hydrolase, a serine proteinase isolated from conditioned medium of neuroblastoma cells, degrades the amyloid-beta peptide. *J Neurochem* **100:** 458–467.

Yamin R, Zhao C, O'Connor PB, McKee AC, Abraham CR. 2009. Acyl peptide hydrolase degrades monomeric and oligomeric amyloid-beta peptide. *Mol Neurodegener* **4:** 33.

Yan P, Hu X, Song H, Yin K, Bateman RJ, Cirrito JR, Xiao Q, Hsu FF, Turk JW, Xu J, et al. 2006a. Matrix metalloproteinase-9 degrades amyloid-β fibrils in vitro and compact plaques in situ. *J Biol Chem* **281:** 24566–24574.

Yan SD, Xiong WC, Stern DM. 2006b. Mitochondrial amyloid-β peptide: Pathogenesis or late-phase development? *J Alzheimers Dis* **9:** 127–137.

Yin KJ, Cirrito JR, Yan P, Hu X, Xiao Q, Pan X, Bateman R, Song H, Hsu FF, Turk J, et al. 2006. Matrix metalloproteinases expressed by astrocytes mediate extracellular amyloid-beta peptide catabolism. *J Neurosci* **26:** 10939–10948.

Zhao J, Li L, Leissring MA. 2009. Insulin-degrading enzyme is exported via an unconventional protein secretion pathway. *Mol Neurodegener* **4:** 4.

Zhu X, Lee HG, Perry G, Smith MA. 2007. Alzheimer disease, the two-hit hypothesis: An update. *Biochim Biophys Acta* **1772:** 494–502.

Neurovascular Dysfunction and Faulty Amyloid β-Peptide Clearance in Alzheimer Disease

Abhay P. Sagare, Robert D. Bell, and Berislav V. Zlokovic

Center for Neurodegenerative and Vascular Brain Disorders and Interdisciplinary Program in Dementia Research, Arthur Kornberg Medical Research Building, University of Rochester School of Medicine and Dentistry, Rochester, New York 14642

Correspondence: Berislav_Zlokovic@urmc.rochester.edu

Neurovascular dysfunction is an integral part of Alzheimer disease (AD). Changes in the brain vascular system may contribute in a significant way to the onset and progression of cognitive decline and the development of a chronic neurodegenerative process associated with accumulation of amyloid β-peptide (Aβ) in brain and cerebral vessels in AD individuals and AD animal models. Here, we review the role of the neurovascular unit and molecular mechanisms in cerebral vascular cells behind the pathogenesis of AD. In particular, we focus on blood–brain barrier (BBB) dysfunction, decreased cerebral blood flow, and impaired vascular clearance of Aβ from brain. The data reviewed here support an essential role of the neurovascular and BBB mechanisms in AD pathogenesis.

Alzheimer disease (AD) is a neurodegenerative disorder associated with neurovascular dysfunction (Zlokovic 2005, 2010; de la Torre 2010; Marchesi 2011), cognitive decline (Cummings 2004), and accumulation in brain of amyloid β peptide (Aβ; Querfurth and LaFerla 2010) and tau-related lesions in neurons termed neurofibrillary tangles (Ballatore et al. 2007; Ittner and Gotz 2011). Multiple epidemiological studies have demonstrated a remarkable overlap among risk factors for cerebrovascular disorder and sporadic, late-onset AD (de la Torre 2010; Jellinger 2010; Kalaria 2010). For example, mid-life diabetes (Luchsinger et al. 2007; Knopman and Roberts 2010), hypertension (Iadecola and Davisson 2008), and obesity (Whitmer et al. 2008) have all been shown to increase the risk for both AD and vascular dementia. It is now generally acknowledged that most AD cases have mixed vascular pathology and small-vessel disease (Jellinger 2010; Marchesi 2011). Moreover, reduced brain blood perfusion (Ruitenberg et al. 2005), silent infarcts (Vermeer et al. 2003), and the presence of one or more infarctions (Snowdon et al. 1997) all increase the risk of AD.

The amyloid hypothesis states that Aβ initiates a cascade of events leading to neuronal injury and loss (Hardy and Selkoe 2002) associated with cognitive decline (Cummings 2004). According to an alternative two-hit vascular hypothesis of AD (Zlokovic 2005, 2010; de la Torre 2010; Marchesi 2011), Aβ accumulation in the brain is a second insult (*hit 2*) that is initiated by vascular damage (*hit 1*; Fig. 1). Although the molecular and cellular events for

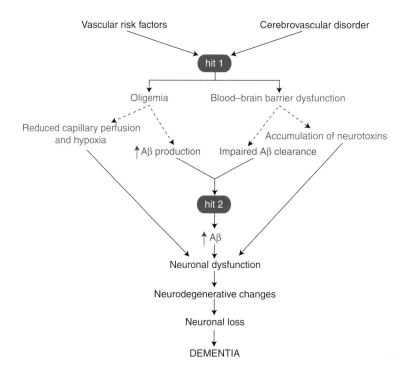

Figure 1. The vascular hypothesis of Alzheimer disease. Vascular risk factors (e.g., hypertension, diabetes, obesity, cardiac disease) and/or an initial vascular damage mediated by a cerebrovascular disorder (e.g., ischemia, stroke) lead to brain hypoperfusion (oligemia) and/or blood–brain barrier (BBB) dysfunction (*hit 1*), which is associated with a diminished brain capillary flow/hypoxia and accumulation of multiple neurotoxins in brain, respectively, that can impact neuronal function contributing to the development of neurodegenerative changes and cognitive decline (solid lines). In a parallel pathway, BBB dysfunction and hypoperfusion/hypoxia can reduce amyloid β peptide (Aβ) vascular clearance across the BBB and increase Aβ production from Aβ-precursor protein (APP), respectively, causing Aβ accumulation in brain (*hit 2*; dashed lines). Elevated Aβ levels lead to formation of neurotoxic Aβ oligomers, causing neuronal dysfunction, on the one hand, and self-aggregation, on the other, which leads to self-propagation of Aβ-mediated brain disorder and the development of cerebral β-amyloidosis. According to the vascular hypothesis, a pathogenic tau phosphorylation in neurons and the development of tau-related pathology including neurofibrillary tangles (not shown in the diagram) may be triggered independently or simultaneously by a hypoperfusion/hypoxia insult and/or direct Aβ neurotoxicity.

each step in the disease process and for each risk factor are not absolutely clear, all vascular factors might share a common final disease pathway, involving brain microvascular dysfunction and/or degeneration, as well as Aβ and tau pathology (Zlokovic 2011), as discussed below. The vascular hypothesis maintains that reduced cerebral blood flow (CBF) and hypoxia, from one end, and blood–brain barrier (BBB) dysfunction associated with accumulation of different vasculotoxic and neurotoxic macromolecules in the brain, from the other, can initiate neuronal dysfunction and

neurodegenerative changes independently and/or prior to Aβ deposition (Zlokovic 2005, 2010; Bell et al. 2010; de la Torre 2010; Marchesi 2011). Moreover, several studies have suggested that cerebrovascular dysfunction and injury lead to faulty Aβ clearance from brain (Deane et al. 2004; Zlokovic 2005), increased influx of peripheral Aβ across the BBB (Deane et al. 2003; Eisele et al. 2010), and/or elevated expression of β-amyloid precursor protein (APP; Atwood et al. 2002; Kumar-Singh et al. 2005; Cullen et al. 2006; Weller et al. 2008), resulting in Aβ accumulation in the brain and around cerebral blood vessels. Elevated levels of Aβ in brain may in turn accelerate neurovascular (Deane et al. 2003; Bell et al. 2009) and neuronal (Yan et al. 1996; Walsh et al. 2002; Takuma et al. 2009) dysfunction and promote self-propagation (Meyer-Luehmann et al. 2006, 2008; Eisele et al. 2010), as in prion diseases (Prusiner 1996), leading to cerebral β-amyloidosis (Zlokovic 2008).

Here we will review the role of the neurovascular unit and molecular mechanisms within cerebral vascular cells behind the pathogenesis of AD. In particular, we will focus on BBB dysfunction, decreased CBF, and impaired vascular clearance of Aβ from brain.

NEUROVASCULAR UNIT

The neurovascular unit (NVU) consists of different cell types, including (1) *vascular cells* such as brain endothelial cells, a site of the anatomical BBB in vivo, pericytes, and vascular smooth muscle cells (VSMCs), (2) *glial cells* such as astrocytes, microglia and oliogodendroglia, and (3) *neurons* (Fig. 2A; Zlokovic 2008; Guo and Lo 2009; Moskowitz et al. 2010). The close proximity of nonneuronal neighboring cells with each other and with neurons allows for effective cell-to-cell cross-communications that are critical for normal functions in the healthy central nervous system (CNS) and are

increasingly recognized as important in the disease process in multiple neurological disorders (Boillee et al. 2006; Zhong et al. 2008; Zlokovic 2008).

The NVU functions in the healthy brain include control of neurovascular coupling and BBB permeability, matrix interactions, inactivation of neurotransmitters, signaling through angioneurins (i.e., growth factors that have both the neurotrophic and vasculotrophic functions) (Zacchigna et al. 2008), and clearance of toxins from brain (Fig. 2B).

The BBB is a highly specialized, continuous endothelial cell membrane that normally prevents the entry of plasma components, red blood cells, and leukocytes into the brain. In addition, through specific transporters in brain endothelium, the BBB regulates delivery of energy metabolites and essential nutrients that are required for proper neuronal and synaptic functions. The BBB is responsible for maintaining the constant "chemical" composition of brain interstitial fluid required for optimal brain function. Under physiological conditions, the BBB and pericytes control entry from blood and promote clearance from brain of various potentially neurotoxic and vasculotoxic macromolecules (Zlokovic 2008).

Alzheimer disease is associated with microvascular dysfunction, defective BBB, and vascular factors (Bailey et al. 2004; Wu et al. 2005;

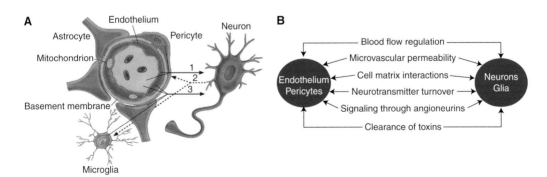

Figure 2. The neurovascular unit and neurovascular functions. (*A*) A schematic illustration of the neurovascular unit at the level of brain capillary consisting of brain endothelial cells, pericytes, astrocytes, microglia, and neurons. Endothelial cells and pericytes share a common basement membrane and form direct "peg and socket" contacts. Astrocyte end-feet processes ensheath the capillary wall made up of pericytes and endothelial cells. (*B*) Vascular cells (endothelium and pericytes), glia (e.g., astrocytes), and neurons regulate multiple neurovascular functions. (Modified from Zlokovic 2008.)

Zlokovic 2005, 2008; Paul et al. 2007; Zipser et al. 2007; Kalaria 2010; Knopman and Roberts 2010; Miyazaki et al. 2011; Neuwelt et al. 2011). Microvascular degeneration diminishes CBF, resulting in shortages in oxygen supply, energy substrates, and nutrients to the brain. On the other hand, microvascular defects compromise clearance of neurotoxic molecules from brain, resulting in accumulation of pathological deposits in brain interstitial fluid, nonneuronal cells, and neurons. According to the recent evidence, microvascular injury ultimately leads to neuronal dysfunction and development of neurodegenerative changes. Vascular damage may also contribute to the development of cerebral β-amyloidosis and cerebral amyloid angiopathy (CAA) caused by accumulation of Aβ in brain and the vessel wall, respectively (Zlokovic 2008).

CEREBRAL BLOOD FLOW DYSREGULATION AND REDUCTIONS

An adequate blood supply is ensured by a tight coupling between local tissue metabolic demands and blood perfusion of the active neuronal site. The link between regional synaptic activity and a CBF increase is known as functional hyperemia. Neurovascular coupling requires intact and effectively innervated pial and intracerebral arteries and normal responsiveness of brain endothelium, VSMCs, and pericytes to vasoactive stimuli (Iadecola 2004; Peppiatt et al. 2006; Bell et al. 2010). In addition to VSMCs, recent studies have shown that pericytes control brain capillary diameter by constricting the vessel wall (Peppiatt et al. 2006), which under ischemic conditions can completely obstructs capillary flow (Yemisci et al. 2009). Astrocytes have also been shown to regulate CBF responses by influencing contractile properties of small penetrating intracerebral arteries (Takano et al. 2007; Kuchibhotla et al. 2009).

Functional hyperemia is the basis for functional magnetic resonance imaging that has revolutionized our understanding of human brain in health and disease (Girouard and Iadecola 2006). Functional neuroimaging studies in AD

individuals have shown that neurovascular uncoupling or diminished CBF responses to brain activation may occur prior to neurodegenerative changes (Smith et al. 1999; Bookheimer et al. 2000; Ruitenberg et al. 2005; Knopman and Roberts 2010). In addition, it has been reported that cognitively normal individuals bearing the apolipoprotein E (APOE) ε4 allele, which is known to be the major genetic risk factor for late-onset AD (Bertram et al. 2007; Kim et al. 2009; Verghese et al. 2011), have reduced functional hyperemia response in the absence of brain atrophy or Aβ/amyloid accumulation (Sheline et al. 2010). Diminished resting CBF has been also shown in elderly individuals at risk to develop AD (Iadecola 2004; Knopman and Roberts 2010).

Studies in animal models have indicated that CBF reductions can induce and/or amplify neuronal dysfunction and/or neuropathological changes resembling AD pathology. For example, it has been shown that Aβ constricts cerebral arteries (Thomas et al. 1996), and that endothelium-dependent regulation of cortical microcirculation is diminished in a mouse model of AD before Aβ accumulation (Iadecola et al. 1999). Moreover, in AD mice, mild hypoperfusion increases neuronal Aβ levels and tau phosphophorylation at an epitope associated with AD-type paired helical filaments (Koike et al. 2010). Brain ischemia in rodents leads to accumulation of hyperphosphorylated tau in neurons and filament formation similar to that present in human AD tauopathy (Gordon-Krajcer et al. 2007). Arterial carotid occlusion in rats leads to memory impairment, neuronal dysfunction, synaptic changes and accumulation of neurotoxic Aβ oligomers (Wang et al. 2010). Mice expressing APP and transforming growth factor β develop neurovascular uncoupling, cholinergic denervation, accelerated Aβ deposition and age-dependent cognitive decline (Ongali et al. 2010).

It has been demonstrated that moderate CBF reductions, comparable to those as seen in the aging brain, are associated with diminished cerebral protein synthesis (Hossmann 1994; Iadecola 2004). CBF reductions >50% impair ATP synthesis and decrease the ability of neurons to fire action potentials. In addition, focal CBF reductions comparable to those as in chronic neurodegenerative disorders such as AD lead to shifts in intracellular pH, water and electrolytes that are attributed to a loss of activity of multiple energy-dependent ion pumps such as sodium/hydrogen exchanger and ATP-dependent sodium pump at the BBB (Zlokovic 2008). CBF reductions may also lead to accumulation of different toxins and glutamate in brain owing to a loss of activity at the BBB of ATP-binding cassette (ABC) efflux transporters (Dutheil et al. 2010; Elali and Hermann 2011) and Na-dependent transporters for the excitatory amino acids (O'Kane et al. 1999; Hardingham 2009), respectively. Severe reductions in CBF ($>80\%$), similar to those found after an ischemic stroke lead to neuronal death. It is of note that changes in the NVU including degeneration of brain capillaries and/or reductions in the resting CBF may be the first sign of the disease process prior to neuronal changes and neurodegeneration.

MICROVASCULAR DEGENERATION

Alzheimer disease individuals and other dementia patients frequently have focal degenerative changes in brain microcirculation including atrophy and reductions in capillary network, a rise in endothelial vacuolization and loss of mitochondria, accumulation of collagen and perlecans in the basement capillary membrane, loss of BBB tight junction proteins (Farkas and Luiten 2001; Bailey et al. 2004; Iadecola 2004; Wu et al. 2005; Zlokovic 2005; Kalaria 2010), and leakage of blood-derived molecules (Paul et al. 2007; Zipser et al. 2007; Kalaria 2010). Aβ accumulation and amyloid deposition in pial and intracerebral arteries lead to CAA, which according to some studies is present in $>80\%$ of AD patients (Jellinger 2010; Viswanathan and Greenberg 2011). AD patients with CAA frequently develop atrophy in the VSMC layer of small arteries, causing a rupture of the vessel wall and intracerebral bleeding in about 30% of patients, which in turn aggravates dementia (Ghiso and Frangione 2002; Cordonnier 2011). Patients with heredi-

tary cerebral β-amyloidosis with CAA in leptomeningeal and intracerebral arteries of the Dutch, Iowa, Arctic, Flemish, Italian, and Piedmont L34V type develop massive hemorrhagic strokes and dementia owing to VSMC degeneration in the vessel wall (Fossati et al. 2010). Similar, duplication of the APP gene results in AD dementia with CAA and intracerebral hemorrhage (Rovelet-Lecrux et al. 2006).

BBB DYSFUNCTION IN AD

Changes in the expression of several BBB transporters mediating nutrient transport, ion pumps, ABC transporters, and/or receptors mediating transport of peptides and proteins, including blood-to-brain and brain-to-blood exchanges of Aβ, have been described in AD and AD models (see below). Here we will focus on (1) glucose transporter 1 (GLUT1), which is a BBB-specific transporter that is of special importance because glucose is a key energy source for brain, (2) the receptor for advanced glycation end products (RAGE) that mediates Aβ reentry into the brain from circulation and the neurovascular inflammatory response, and (3) lipoprotein receptor-related protein 1 (LRP), which is a major Aβ clearance receptor at the BBB mediating Aβ efflux from brain and its systemic clearance.

GLUT1

GLUT1 expression at the BBB is diminished in AD individuals (Mooradian et al. 1997), suggesting a shortage in glucose supply to the brain. Positron emission tomography (PET) studies with ^{18}F-2-fluoro-2-deoxy-D-glucose (FDG), have demonstrated diminished glucose uptake by the brain in individuals at increased risk for dementia (Hunt et al. 2007; Herholz 2010). Several studies have suggested that reduced glucose uptake across the BBB as seen by FDG-PET can precede brain atrophy (Mosconi et al. 2006; Hunt et al. 2007; Samuraki et al. 2007; Mosconi et al. 2008; Herholz 2010) and may be used as a potential biomarker for AD (Miller 2009; Perrin et al. 2009).

RAGE

RAGE is a multiligand receptor of the immunoglobulin superfamily (Neeper et al. 1992). RAGE binds distinct classes of ligands including AGE proteins, S100/calgranulins, Aβ, amphoterin, and the family of crossed β-sheet macromolecules (Yan et al. 2010). RAGE interaction with ligands activates signal transduction pathways, leading to sustained cellular stress as shown in chronic diseases such as diabetes, inflammation, and AD (Bucciarelli et al. 2002; Bierhaus et al. 2005; Schmidt et al. 2009). The extracellular domain of RAGE contains one V-type and two C-type immunoglobulin domains (Yan et al. 2010). Most ligands bind to RAGE's V-domain. A single, transmembrane spanning domain is followed by a short, charged cytoplasmic domain-mediating signal transduction after ligand binding to RAGE (Yan et al. 2010). A recent crystal structure analysis of RAGE revealed a versatile structure, which explains the ability of RAGE to bind multiple, structurally distinct ligands (Koch et al. 2010; Park et al. 2010).

As a cell surface receptor for Aβ (Yan et al. 1996), RAGE binds monomeric and oligomeric Aβ via its V-domain and aggregated Aβ via its C1 domain (Sturchler et al. 2008; Yan et al. 2010). RAGE mediates Aβ-induced neurotoxicity directly by causing oxidant stress and indirectly by activating microglia (Yan et al. 1996). In addition, intraneuronal Aβ transport via RAGE leads to mitochondrial dysfunction (Takuma et al. 2009). Targeted expression of RAGE in neurons in *APP*-transgenic mice accelerates cognitive decline and Aβ-induced neuronal perturbation (Arancio et al. 2004).

Expression of RAGE is increased in cerebrovascular endothelial cells under pathological conditions, including those seen in AD models and AD (Yan et al. 1995, 1996; Deane et al. 2003). At the BBB RAGE mediates (1) transport of circulating Aβ into the brain (Mackic et al. 1998; Deane et al. 2003), (2) NF-κB-dependent endothelial cell activation resulting in neuroinflammatory response, and (3) generation of endothelin-1 suppressing the CBF (Fig. 3; Deane et al. 2003). In addition, expression of RAGE in brain endothelium initiates cellular signaling, leading to monocyte trafficking across the BBB (Giri et al. 2000). It is of note that RAGE expression is increased in both neurons and endothelium in an Aβ-rich or AGE-rich environment as in AD (Yan et al. 1995), which amplifies Aβ-mediated pathogenic responses.

The cellular events triggered by RAGE at the BBB, neurons, microglia, and VSMCs may be implicated in the onset and progression of disease in AD models and possibly in AD. Therefore, RAGE is a potential therapeutic target in AD and blocking RAGE might contribute to control of Aβ-mediated brain disorder.

LRP

LRP, a member of the LDL receptor family, has a dual role as a rapid cargo endocytotic cellular transporter and a transmembrane cell signaling receptor (Zlokovic et al. 2010). LRP regulates transport and metabolism of apoE-associated cholesterol (Herz 2001; Herz and Strickland 2001; Herz et al. 2009). Its extracellular heavy α-chain (515 kDa) is noncovalently linked to a transmembrane and cytoplasmic light β-chain domain (85 kDa). The α-chain has four ligand-binding domains (clusters I–IV; Obermoeller-McCormick et al. 2001; Meijer et al. 2007). Domains II and IV bind more than 40 structurally diverse ligands including, to name a few, apoE, α2-macroglobulin (α2M), tissue plasminogen activator (tPA), proteinase-inhibitors, blood coagulation factor VIII, receptor-associated protein (RAP), Aβ, prion protein, and aprotinin (Hussain et al. 1999; Neels et al. 1999; Herz 2001; Herz and Strickland 2001; Croy et al. 2003; Deane et al. 2004; Meijer et al. 2007; Demeule et al. 2008; Lillis et al. 2008; Parkyn et al. 2008; Herz et al. 2009; Zlokovic et al. 2010). LRP's cytoplasmic tail comprises two NPXY motifs, and one YXXL motif and two di-leucine motifs that both are required for rapid endocytosis of LRP ligands (Li et al. 2001; Deane et al. 2004, 2008). The cytoplasmic tail phosphorylated on serine and/or tyrosine residues (Bu et al. 1998; van der Geer 2002) interacts with different adaptor proteins associated with cell signaling such as disabled-1,

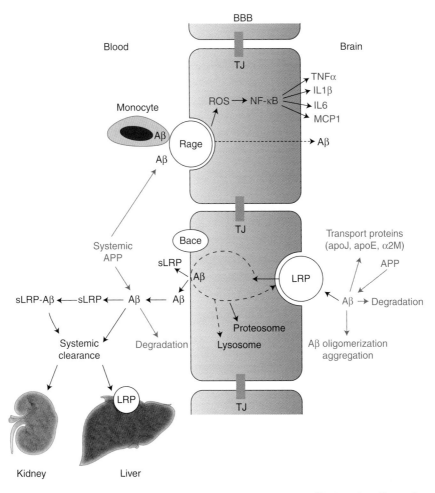

Figure 3. The role of blood–brain barrier (BBB) transport in homeostasis of brain Aβ. *Influx pathway*: RAGE, the receptor for advanced glycation end products, mediates influx and reentry of circulating Aβ across the BBB. RAGE-mediated Aβ influx is accompanied by generation of reactive oxygen species (ROS) and activation of nuclear factor-κB (NF-κB)-mediated inflammatory response in endothelium, that is, increased production of cytokines including tumor necrosis factor α (TNFα), interleukin (IL) 1β and 6, and monocyte chemotactic protein-1 (MCP1), as well as increased expression of several leukocyte adhesion molecules (not shown). RAGE also mediates transport of Aβ-laden monocytes across the BBB. *Efflux pathway*: LRP, the low-density lipoprotein receptor-related protein-1, mediates Aβ clearance from brain via transport of free Aβ and Aβ-bound to apoE2 and apoE3, but not apoE4, across the BBB. Other Aβ transport proteins in brain interstitial fluid such as apoJ and α-2 macroglobulin (α2M) influence Aβ clearance from brain. Aβ enzymatic clearance, oligomerization, and aggregation also control Aβ levels in brain. Soluble form of LRP (sLRP) in plasma is a major binding protein of plasma Aβ. sLRP is produced by the proteolytic cleavage from LRP mediated by β-secretase (BACE). Liver and kidneys mediate systemic clearance of free Aβ and of sLRP–Aβ complexes. APP, Aβ-precurosr protein. TJ, tight junctions. (Modified from Zlokovic 2008.)

FE65, and postsynaptic density protein 95 (Trommsdorff et al. 1998; Gotthardt et al. 2000; Herz et al. 2009).

Within the NVU, LRP is expressed in brain endothelium, VSMCs, pericytes, astrocytes, and neurons (Herz and Bock 2002; Polavarapu et al. 2007). LRP internalizes its ligands and directs them to lysosomes for proteolytic degradation. Recent studies have demonstrated that LRP also transports its ligands transcellularly across the BBB including Aβ (Shibata et al. 2000; Deane et al. 2004), RAP (Pan et al. 2004), tPA (Benchenane et al. 2005), lipid-free and lipidated apoE2 and apoE3, including their respective complexes with Aβ (Deane et al. 2008), and a family of Kunitz domain-derived peptides (Demeule et al. 2008).

Initial studies have suggested that LRP is linked genetically to AD and CAA (Kang et al. 1997; Lambert et al. 1998; Wavrant-DeVrieze et al. 1999; Christoforidis et al. 2005; Ballatore et al. 2007), but this has not been confirmed by later studies (Harold et al. 2009; Lambert et al. 2009). LRP and many of its ligands are normally deposited in senile plaques (Rebeck et al. 1995; Arelin et al. 2002). It has been shown that LRP interacts with APP, which influences Aβ generation (Pietrzik et al. 2004; Waldron et al. 2008). LRP also mediates Aβ neuronal uptake via α2M and apoE (Narita et al. 1997; Qiu et al. 1999; DeMattos et al. 2004; Zerbinatti et al. 2004; Zerbinatti and Bu 2005; Deane et al. 2008). The exact implication of these findings for the development of Aβ pathology remain, however, unclear. On another note, LRP interacts with γ-secretase, an APP processing enzyme, which results in inhibition of the inflammatory response, suggesting a potential for modulating inflammation (Zurhove et al. 2008).

As illustrated in Figure 3, several studies have demonstrated that LRP has a key role in a three-step serial clearance mechanism mediating Aβ elimination from brain and body (Zlokovic et al. 2010). In multiple animal models, binding of Aβ to LRP at the abluminal side of the BBB results in its rapid clearance into the blood (Shibata et al. 2000; Deane et al. 2004, 2008; Shiiki et al. 2004; Cirrito et al. 2005; Ito et al. 2006; Bell et al. 2007; Jaeger et al. 2009; Shinohara et al. 2010). A decreased expression of LRP in the choroid plexus epithelium (Johanson et al. 2006) leads to Aβ accumulation in the choroid plexus (Behl et al. 2009, 2010). Because RAP blocks apoE-dependent uptake of Aβ by astrocytes, it has been suggested that LRP and/or another member of the LDL receptor family are involved in astrocyte-mediated clearance of Aβ (Koistinaho et al. 2004). Studies

using in vitro BBB models (Nazer et al. 2008; Yamada et al. 2008) have confirmed the role of LRP in Aβ endothelial cellular uptake and endocytosis, respectively, resulting in clearance of Aβ.

Reduced LRP levels in brain microvessels correlate with endogenous Aβ deposition in a chronic hydrocephalus model in rats (Klinge et al. 2006) and Aβ cerebrovascular and brain accumulation in AD patients (Shibata et al. 2000; Donahue et al. 2006). Several studies have indicated that LRP expression in brain endothelium decreases with normal aging in rodents, nonhuman primates, and humans, as well as in AD models and AD patients (Kang et al. 2000; Shibata et al. 2000; Bading et al. 2002; Deane et al. 2004; Donahue et al. 2006; Bell and Zlokovic 2009). LRP reductions have been reported in cerebral VSMCs associated with Aβ accumulation in the wall of small pial and intracerebral arteries (Bell et al. 2009). Therefore, LRP down-regulation at the BBB and in vascular cells may contribute to cerebrovascular and focal parenchymal Aβ accumulations.

In blood, the circulating form of LRP (i.e., soluble LRP, sLRP) provides a key endogenous peripheral "sink" activity for Aβ, as shown in a mouse model of AD (Sagare et al. 2007). In neurologically healthy humans and mice, sLRP binds >70% of circulating Aβ, preventing free Aβ access to the brain (Fig. 3; Sagare et al. 2007). In AD patients and AD transgenic mice, Aβ binding to sLRP is compromised by oxidation, resulting in increased levels of oxidized sLRP, which does not bind Aβ (Sagare et al. 2007). This is associated with elevated levels of free Aβ40 and Aβ42 in plasma that can reenter the brain via RAGE-mediated transport across the BBB (Deane et al. 2003; Ujiie et al. 2003; Donahue et al. 2006; Sagare et al. 2007). Moreover, in the human hippocampus, an increased RAGE expression in brain endothelium of the BBB has been shown in advanced AD compared with early stage AD and/or individuals with mild cognitive impairment (MCI; Miller et al. 2008). This might further contribute to Aβ accumulation in brain via accelerated Aβ influx from blood. In one study, a diminished sLRP-Aβ peripheral binding has been shown to precede an increase in the tau/Aβ42 CSF ratio and a drop in global cognitive decline in individuals with MCI converting into AD (Sagare et al. 2011a). Importantly, recombinant LRP fragments can effectively replace oxidized sLRP and sequester free Aβ in plasma in AD patients and AD transgenic mice, ultimately reducing Aβ-related pathology in brain (Sagare et al. 2007). Consistent with these findings, it has been suggested that sLRP and anti-RAGE antibodies that are present in Baxter's intravenous immunoglobulin preparation Gammagard Liquid may contribute to the observed beneficial effects of Gammagard Liquid in AD patients (Relkin et al. 2009; Weber et al. 2009) by improving the peripheral Aβ sequestration and preventing entry of free Aβ into the brain (Dodel et al. 2010).

LRP in the liver mediates rapid peripheral clearance of Aβ (Tamaki et al. 2006, 2007). It is of note that reduced hepatic LRP levels have been shown to be associated with decreased peripheral Aβ clearance in the aged rats (Tamaki et al. 2006, 2007). Regulation of Aβ brain levels by the liver has been recently demonstrated in an independent study (Sagare et al. 2011b; Sutcliffe et al. 2011).

VASCULAR-SPECIFIC GENES

Recent findings suggest that unsuccessful vascular regeneration may lead to degeneration of brain endothelium in AD and AD models. It has been shown that brain endothelial cells in AD express extremely low levels of the mesenchyme homeobox gene 2 (*MEOX-2*; Wu et al. 2005), a transcription factor that regulates vascular cell differentiation and remodeling, and whose expression in the adult brain is restricted to the vascular system (Gorski and Walsh 2003). Low levels of MEOX-2 expression in AD brain endothelium have been shown to mediate an aberrant angiogenic response to vascular endothelial growth factor (Wu et al. 2005), ultimately resulting in vessel regression associated with reductions in the resting CBF (Fig. 4). Low levels of *MEOX-2* also promote proteasomal degradation of LRP in brain endothelium (Wu et al.

2005) that diminishes Aβ clearance at the BBB. On the other hand, accumulation of Aβ on the outer membrane of the blood vessels is anti-angiogenic per se (Paris et al. 2004a,b). Therefore, Aβ may act in concert with low expression of MEOX2 at the BBB to focally reduce brain capillary density in AD models and AD. Importantly, MEOX2 expression is diminished by hypoxia, suggesting that hypoxia may be upstream of MEOX2 depletion seen in AD brain endothelium (Wu et al. 2005).

Interestingly, mice with a single allele of *Meox2* develop a primary cerebral endothelial hypoplasia with an intact BBB, but a significant brain perfusion deficit (Wu et al. 2005), which has been shown to lead to secondary neurodegenerative changes prior to Aβ accumulation (Bell et al. 2010). Neurodegenerative changes in *Meox2*$^{+/-}$ mice were, however, significantly less pronounced than in pericyte-deficient mice, which have a comparable brain hypoperfusion to *Meox2*$^{+/-}$ mice but also a compromised BBB (Bell et al. 2010). These data indicate that chronic hypoperfusion alone can cause neuronal injury, but not to the same extent as when combined with BBB breakdown.

Recent studies have also shown that AD patients as well as mouse models with high cerebrovascular levels of serum response factor (SRF) and myocardin (MYOCD), the two transcription factors that control VSMC differentiation, develop a hypercontractile cerebral arterial phenotype, resulting in brain hypoperfusion, diminished functional hyperemia, and CAA (Chow et al. 2007; Bell et al. 2009). MYOCD, a SAF-A/B, Acinus, and PIAS domain family nuclear protein, is a VCMC-specific transcriptional co-activator that binds SRF to induce gene expression (Wang et al. 2001). SRF is a ubiquitously expressed transcription factor that binds to a ten-base pair *cis* element called a CArG box, which is located in the regulatory region of numerous target genes (Sun et al. 2006). MYOCD and SRF constitute a molecular switch for the VSMC differentiation program (Chen et al. 2002; Li et al. 2003). In addition, it has been shown that increased levels of MYOCD and SRF in AD VSMCs may suppress

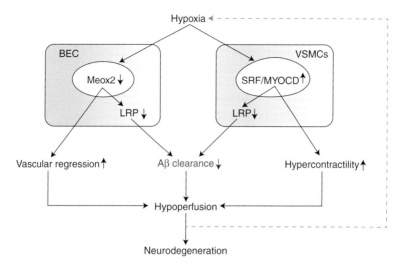

Figure 4. Alterations in vascular-specific gene expression mediating neurovascular dysfunction in AD. (*Left*) Hypoxia down-regulates mesenchyme homeobox gene-2 (MEOX2) in brain endothelial cells (BEC). Reduced levels of MEOX2 lead to unsuccessful vascular remodeling and vascular regression, resulting in a primary endothelial hypoplasia and brain hypoperfusion. On the other hand, reduced levels of MEOX2 stimulate proteosomal degradation of LRP, a major Aβ clearance receptor, leading to a loss of LRP from BEC and reduced Aβ clearance from brain. (*Right*) Hypoxia increases expression of myocardin (MYOCD) in vascular smooth muscle cells (VSMCs) resulting in elevated levels of MYOCD and serum response factor (SRF). Elevated SRF/MYOCD levels lead to increased expression of several contractile proteins and calcium-regulated channels in VSMCs, resulting in a hypercontractile phenotype of small cerebral arteries and brain hypoperfusion. On the other hand, increased SRF/MYOCD activity stimulates directed expression of the sterol binding protein-2, which is a major transcriptional suppressor of LRP. Loss of LRP from VSMCs diminishes Aβ clearance from small cerebral arteries, leading to deposition of Aβ and amyloid in the arterial wall known as CAA, cerebral amyloid angiopathy. It is of note that changes in the expression of vascular-restricted genes MEOX2 and MYCD can trigger both an Aβ-independent brain hypoperfusion and Aβ accumulation, mediating neuronal dysfunction. Interestingly, hypoxia seems to be upstream to both a diminished MEOX2 expression in BEC and an increased MYOCD expression in VSMCs.

Aβ clearance and thus exacerbate CAA (Bell et al. 2009). Namely, high levels of MYOCD and SRF in VSMCs lead to directed expression of sterol response element binding protein 2 (SREBP2), which is a major LRP transcriptional suppressor ultimately resulting in LRP depletion, which diminishes LRP-mediated Aβ clearance from the vessel wall (Fig. 4). Hypoxia increases MYOCD levels in VSMCs (Reynolds et al. 2004; Chow et al. 2007; Bell et al. 2009), and it has been shown that it is also upstream of elevated MYOCD/SRF expression in cerebral arterial VSMCs (Bell et al. 2009). More studies are needed, however, to establish the exact role of vascular-specific genes MEOX2 and MYOCD in the development of Alzheimer neurovascular dysfunction.

CONCLUDING REMARKS

Recent clinical observations provide strong evidence for the link between cerebrovascular disease and AD and the role of vascular risk factors in AD. In this chapter, we have briefly reviewed literature on dysregulated and diminished CBF, BBB dysfunction, and impaired vascular clearance of Aβ from brain, supporting an essential role of the neurovascular and BBB mechanisms in AD pathogenesis. Several studies in animal models of AD and more recently in AD patients (Mawuenyega et al. 2010) have demonstrated a diminished Aβ clearance from brain. The recognition of Aβ clearance pathways opens exciting new therapeutic opportunities for AD. It is now established that faulty clearance from brain and across the BBB leads to elevated Aβ levels in brain that in turn have been shown to contribute to the formation of neurotoxic Aβ oligomers (Walsh et al. 2002) and the development of Aβ-mediated brain storage disorder and cerebral β-amyloidosis (Zlokovic 2008).

The activation of neurovascular pathogenic pathways has been shown to compromise synaptic and neuronal functions prior to and/or in parallel with Aβ accumulation and development of intraneuronal tangles, neuronal loss, and dementia. Some early molecular targets within the neurovascular pathway include receptors RAGE and LRP at the BBB and possibly vascular-specific genes MEOX2 and MYOCD.

Focusing on comorbidity, vascular risk factors associated with AD such as hypoperfusion, hypertension, ministrokes, and/or diabetes might generate useful models of human dementia. The proposed neurovascular model of AD raises a set of new important questions that require further study, as recently discussed (Zlokovic 2011). For example, the molecular basis of the neurovascular link with neurodegenerative disorders is still poorly understood as well as the molecular cues underlying the cross talks between different cell types of the NVU, including vascular and glia cells, and how these cellular interactions influence neuronal activity. Addressing these questions will lead to better understanding of the neurovascular link with neurodegeneration process, which will lead to the development of novel neurovascular-based approaches for AD (Zlokovic 2011).

ACKNOWLEDGMENTS

B.V.Z. thanks the United States National Institutes of Health grants R37 AG023084 and R37 NS34467 and the Zilkha family for supporting his research.

REFERENCES

Arancio O, Zhang HP, Chen X, Lin C, Trinchese F, Puzzo D, Liu S, Hegde A, Yan SF, Stern A, et al. 2004. RAGE potentiates Aβ-induced perturbation of neuronal function in transgenic mice. *EMBO J* **23:** 4096–4105.

Arelin K, Kinoshita A, Whelan CM, Irizarry MC, Rebeck GW, Strickland DK, Hyman BT. 2002. LRP and senile plaques in Alzheimer's disease: Colocalization with apolipoprotein E and with activated astrocytes. *Brain Res Mol Brain Res* **104:** 38–46.

Atwood CS, Bishop GM, Perry G, Smith MA. 2002. Amyloid-β: A vascular sealant that protects against hemorrhage? *J Neurosci Res* **70:** 356.

Bading JR, Yamada S, Mackic JB, Kirkman L, Miller C, Calero M, Ghiso J, Frangione B, Zlokovic BV. 2002. Brain clearance of Alzheimer's amyloid-β40 in the squirrel monkey: A SPECT study in a primate model of cerebral amyloid angiopathy. *J Drug Target* **10:** 359–368.

Bailey TL, Rivara CB, Rocher AB, Hof PR. 2004. The nature and effects of cortical microvascular pathology in aging and Alzheimer's disease. *Neurol Res* **26:** 573–578.

Ballatore C, Lee VM, Trojanowski JQ. 2007. Tau-mediated neurodegeneration in Alzheimer's disease and related disorders. *Nat Rev Neurosci* **8:** 663–672.

Behl M, Zhang Y, Monnot AD, Jiang W, Zheng W. 2009. Increased β-amyloid levels in the choroid plexus following lead exposure and the involvement of low-density lipoprotein receptor protein-1. *Toxicol Appl Pharmacol* **240:** 245–254.

Behl M, Zhang Y, Shi Y, Cheng J, Du Y, Zheng W. 2010. Lead-induced accumulation of β-amyloid in the choroid plexus: Role of low density lipoprotein receptor protein-1 and protein kinase C. *Neurotoxicology* **31:** 524–532.

Bell RD, Zlokovic BV. 2009. Neurovascular mechanisms and blood–brain barrier disorder in Alzheimer's disease. *Acta Neuropathol* **118:** 103–113.

Bell RD, Sagare AP, Friedman AE, Bedi GS, Holtzman DM, Deane R, Zlokovic BV. 2007. Transport pathways for clearance of human Alzheimer's amyloid β-peptide and apolipoproteins E and J in the mouse central nervous system. *J Cereb Blood Flow Metab* **27:** 909–918.

Bell RD, Deane R, Chow N, Long X, Sagare A, Singh I, Streb JW, Guo H, Rubio A, Van Nostrand W, et al. 2009. SRF and myocardin regulate LRP-mediated amyloid-β clearance in brain vascular cells. *Nat Cell Biol* **11:** 143–153.

Bell RD, Winkler EA, Sagare AP, Singh I, LaRue B, Deane R, Zlokovic BV. 2010. Pericytes control key neurovascular functions and neuronal phenotype in the adult brain and during brain aging. *Neuron* **68:** 409–427.

Benchenane K, Berezowski V, Ali C, Fernandez-Monreal M, Lopez-Atalaya JP, Brillault J, Chuquet J, Nouvelot A, MacKenzie ET, Bu G, et al. 2005. Tissue-type plasminogen activator crosses the intact blood–brain barrier by low-density lipoprotein receptor-related protein-mediated transcytosis. *Circulation* **111:** 2241–2249.

Bertram L, McQueen MB, Mullin K, Blacker D, Tanzi RE. 2007. Systematic meta-analyses of Alzheimer disease genetic association studies: The AlzGene database. *Nat Genet* **39:** 17–23.

Bierhaus A, Humpert PM, Morcos M, Wendt T, Chavakis T, Arnold B, Stern DM, Nawroth PP. 2005. Understanding RAGE, the receptor for advanced glycation end products. *J Mol Med (Berl)* **83:** 876–886.

Boillee S, Yamanaka K, Lobsiger CS, Copeland NG, Jenkins NA, Kassiotis G, Kollias G, Cleveland DW. 2006. Onset and progression in inherited ALS determined by motor neurons and microglia. *Science* **312:** 1389–1392.

Bookheimer SY, Strojwas MH, Cohen MS, Saunders AM, Pericak-Vance MA, Mazziotta JC, Small GW. 2000. Patterns of brain activation in people at risk for Alzheimer's disease. *New Engl J Med* **343:** 450–456.

Bu G, Sun Y, Schwartz AL, Holtzman DM. 1998. Nerve growth factor induces rapid increases in functional cell surface low density lipoprotein receptor-related protein. *J Biol Chem* **273:** 13359–13365.

Bucciarelli LG, Wendt T, Qu W, Lu Y, Lalla E, Rong LL, Goova MT, Moser B, Kislinger T, Lee DC, et al. 2002. RAGE blockade stabilizes established atherosclerosis in diabetic apolipoprotein E-null mice. *Circulation* **106:** 2827–2835.

Chen J, Kitchen CM, Streb JW, Miano JM. 2002. Myocardin: A component of a molecular switch for smooth muscle differentiation. *J Mol Cell Cardiol* **34:** 1345–1356.

Chow N, Bell RD, Deane R, Streb JW, Chen J, Brooks A, Van Nostrand W, Miano JM, Zlokovic BV. 2007. Serum response factor and myocardin mediate arterial hypercontractility and cerebral blood flow dysregulation in Alzheimer's phenotype. *Proc Natl Acad Sci* **104:** 823–828.

Christoforidis M, Schober R, Krohn K. 2005. Genetic-morphologic association study: Association between the low density lipoprotein-receptor related protein (LRP) and cerebral amyloid angiopathy. *Neuropathol Appl Neurosci* **31:** 11–19.

Cirrito JR, Deane R, Fagan AM, Spinner ML, Parsadanian M, Finn MB, Jiang H, Prior JL, Sagare A, Bales KR, et al. 2005. P-glycoprotein deficiency at the blood–brain barrier increases amyloid-β deposition in an Alzheimer disease mouse model. *J Clin Invest* **115:** 3285–3290.

Cordonnier C. 2011. Brain microbleeds: More evidence, but still a clinical dilemma. *Curr Opin Neurol* **24:** 69–74.

Croy JE, Shin WD, Knauer MF, Knauer DJ, Komives EA. 2003. All three LDL receptor homology regions of the LDL receptor-related protein bind multiple ligands. *Biochemistry* **42:** 13049–13057.

Cullen KM, Kocsi Z, Stone J. 2006. Microvascular pathology in the aging human brain: Evidence that senile plaques are sites of microhaemorrhages. *Neurobiol Aging* **27:** 1786–1796.

Cummings JL. 2004. Alzheimer's disease. *New Engl J Med* **351:** 56–67.

Deane R, Du Yan S, Submamaryan RK, LaRue B, Jovanovic S, Hogg E, Welch D, Manness L, Lin C, Yu J, et al. 2003. RAGE mediates amyloid-β peptide transport across the blood–brain barrier and accumulation in brain. *Nat Med* **9:** 907–913.

Deane R, Wu Z, Sagare A, Davis J, Du Yan S, Hamm K, Xu F, Parisi M, LaRue B, Hu HW, et al. 2004. LRP/amyloid β-peptide interaction mediates differential brain efflux of Aβ isoforms. *Neuron* **43:** 333–344.

Deane R, Sagare A, Hamm K, Parisi M, Lane S, Finn MB, Holtzman DM, Zlokovic BV. 2008. apoE isoform-specific disruption of amyloid β peptide clearance from mouse brain. *J Clin Invest* **118:** 4002–4013.

de la Torre JC. 2010. Vascular risk factor detection and control may prevent Alzheimer's disease. *Aging Res Rev* **9:** 218–225.

DeMattos RB, Cirrito JR, Parsadanian M, May PC, O'Dell MA, Taylor JW, Harmony JA, Aronow BJ, Bales KR, Paul SM, et al. 2004. ApoE and clusterin cooperatively suppress Aβ levels and deposition: Evidence that ApoE regulates extracellular Aβ metabolism in vivo. *Neuron* **41:** 193–202.

Demeule M, Currie JC, Bertrand Y, Che C, Nguyen T, Regina A, Gabathuler R, Castaigne JP, Beliveau R. 2008. Involvement of the low-density lipoprotein receptor-related protein in the transcytosis of the brain delivery vector angiopep-2. *J Neurochem* **106:** 1534–1544.

Dodel R, Neff F, Noelker C, Pul R, Du Y, Bacher M, Oertel W. 2010. Intravenous immunoglobulins as a treatment for Alzheimer's disease: Rationale and current evidence. *Drugs* **70:** 513–528.

Donahue J, Flaherty S, Johanson C, Duncan J, Silverberg G, Miller M, Tavares R, Yang W, Wu Q, Sabo E, et al. 2006. RAGE, LRP-1, and amyloid-β protein in Alzheimer's disease. *Acta Neuropathol* **112:** 405–415.

Dutheil F, Jacob A, Dauchy S, Beaune P, Scherrmann JM, Decleves X, Loriot MA. 2010. ABC transporters and cytochromes P450 in the human central nervous system: Influence on brain pharmacokinetics and contribution to neurodegenerative disorders. *Expert Opin Drug Metab Toxicol* **6:** 1161–1174.

Eisele YS, Obermuller U, Heilbronner G, Baumann F, Kaeser SA, Wolburg H, Walker LC, Staufenbiel M, Heikenwalder M, Jucker M. 2010. Peripherally applied Aβ-containing inoculates induce cerebral β-amyloidosis. *Science* **330:** 980–982.

Elali A, Hermann DM. 2011. ATP-binding cassette transporters and their roles in protecting the brain. *Neuroscientist* **17:** 423–436.

Farkas E, Luiten PG. 2001. Cerebral microvascular pathology in aging and Alzheimer's disease. *Prog Neurobiol* **64:** 575–611.

Fossati S, Cam J, Meyerson J, Mezhericher E, Romero IA, Couraud PO, Weksler BB, Ghiso J, Frangione B. 2002. Amyloidosis and Alzheimer's disease. *Adv Drug Deliv Rev* **54:** 1539–1551.

Ghiso J, Rostagno A. 2010. Differential activation of mitochondrial apoptotic pathways by vasculotropic amyloid-β variants in cells composing the cerebral vessel walls. *FASEB* **24:** 229–241.

Giri R, Shen Y, Stins M, Du Yan S, Schmidt AM, Stern D, Kim KS, Zlokovic B, Kalra VK. 2000. β-Amyloid-induced migration of monocytes across human brain endothelial cells involves RAGE and PECAM-1. *Am J Physiol Cell Physiol* **279:** C1772–C1781.

Girouard H, Iadecola C. 2006. Neurovascular coupling in the normal brain and in hypertension, stroke, and Alzheimer disease. *J Appl Physiol* **100:** 328–335.

Gordon-Krajcer W, Kozniewska E, Lazarewicz JW, Ksiezak-Reding H. 2007. Differential changes in phosphorylation of tau at PHF-1 and 12E8 epitopes during brain ischemia and reperfusion in gerbils. *Neurochem Res* **32:** 729–737.

Gorski DH, Walsh K. 2003. Control of vascular cell differentiation by homeobox transcription factors. *Trends Cardiovasc Med* **13:** 213–220.

Gotthardt M, Trommsdorff M, Nevitt MF, Shelton J, Richardson JA, Stockinger W, Nimpf J, Herz J. 2000. Interactions of the low density lipoprotein receptor gene family with cytosolic adaptor and scaffold proteins suggest diverse biological functions in cellular communication and signal transduction. *J Biol Chem* **275:** 25616–25624.

Guo S, Lo EH. 2009. Dysfunctional cell–cell signaling in the neurovascular unit as a paradigm for central nervous system disease. *Stroke* **40:** S4–S7.

Hardingham GE. 2009. Coupling of the NMDA receptor to neuroprotective and neurodestructive events. *Biochem Soc Trans* **37:** 1147–1160.

Hardy J, Selkoe DJ. 2002. The amyloid hypothesis of Alzheimer's disease: Progress and problems on the road to therapeutics. *Science* **297:** 353–356.

Harold D, Abraham R, Hollingworth P, Sims R, Gerrish A, Hamshere ML, Pahwa JS, Moskvina V, Dowzell K, Williams A, et al. 2009. Genome-wide association study identifies variants at CLU and PICALM associated with Alzheimer's disease. *Nat Genet* **41:** 1088–1093.

Herholz K. 2010. Cerebral glucose metabolism in preclinical and prodromal Alzheimer's disease. *Expert Rev Neurother* **10:** 1667–1673.

Herz J. 2001. The LDL receptor gene family: (Un)expected signal transducers in the brain. *Neuron* **29:** 571–581.

Herz J, Bock HH. 2002. Lipoprotein receptors in the nervous system. *Annu Rev Biochem* **71:** 405–434.

Herz J, Strickland DK. 2001. LRP: A multifunctional scavenger and signaling receptor. *J Clin Invest* **108:** 779–784.

Herz J, Chen Y, Masiulis I, Zhou L. 2009. Expanding functions of lipoprotein receptors. *J Lip Res* **50:** S287–292.

Hossmann KA. 1994. Viability thresholds and the penumbra of focal ischemia. *Ann Neurol* **36:** 557–565.

Hunt A, Schonknecht P, Henze M, Seidl U, Haberkorn U, Schroder J. 2007. Reduced cerebral glucose metabolism in patients at risk for Alzheimer's disease. *Psychiat Res* **155:** 147–154.

Hussain MM, Strickland DK, Bakillah A. 1999. The mammalian low-density lipoprotein receptor family. *Annu Rev Nutr* **19:** 141–172.

Iadecola C. 2004. Neurovascular regulation in the normal brain and in Alzheimer's disease. *Nat Rev Neurosci* **5:** 347–360.

Iadecola C, Davisson RL. 2008. Hypertension and cerebrovascular dysfunction. *Cell Metab* **7:** 476–484.

Iadecola C, Zhang F, Niwa K, Eckman C, Turner SK, Fischer E, Younkin S, Borchelt DR, Hsiao KK, Carlson GA. 1999. SOD1 rescues cerebral endothelial dysfunction in mice overexpressing amyloid precursor protein. *Nat Neurosci* **2:** 157–161.

Ito S, Ohtsuki S, Terasaki T. 2006. Functional characterization of the brain-to-blood efflux clearance of human amyloid-β peptide (1–40) across the rat blood–brain barrier. *Neurosci Res* **56:** 246–252.

Ittner LM, Gotz J. 2011. Amyloid-β and tau—A toxic pas de deux in Alzheimer's disease. *Nat Rev Neurosci* **12:** 65–72.

Jaeger LB, Dohgu S, Hwang MC, Farr SA, Murphy MP, Fleegal-DeMotta MA, Lynch JL, Robinson SM, Niehoff ML, Johnson SN, et al. 2009. Testing the neurovascular hypothesis of Alzheimer's disease: LRP-1 antisense reduces blood–brain barrier clearance, increases brain levels of amyloid-β protein, and impairs cognition. *J Alzheimer's Dis* **17:** 553–570.

Jellinger KA. 2010. Prevalence and impact of cerebrovascular lesions in Alzheimer and lewy body diseases. *Neurodegen Dis* **7:** 112–115.

Johanson C, Flaherty S, Messier A, Duncan J III, Silverberg G. 2006. Expression of the β-amyloid transporter, LRP1, in aging choroid plexus: Implications for the CSF–brain systemin NPH and Alzheimer's disease. *Cerebrospinal Fluid Res* **3:** S29.

Kalaria RN. 2010. Vascular basis for brain degeneration: Faltering controls and risk factors for dementia. *Nutr Rev* **68:** S74–S87.

Kang DE, Saitoh T, Chen X, Xia Y, Masliah E, Hansen LA, Thomas RG, Thal LJ, Katzman R. 1997. Genetic association of the low-density lipoprotein receptor-related protein gene (LRP), an apolipoprotein E receptor, with late-onset Alzheimer's disease. *Neurology* **49:** 56–61.

Kang DE, Pietrzik CU, Baum L, Chevallier N, Merriam DE, Kounnas MZ, Wagner SL, Troncoso JC, Kawas CH, Katzman R, et al. 2000. Modulation of amyloid β-protein clearance and Alzheimer's disease susceptibility by the LDL receptor-related protein pathway. *J Clin Invest* **106:** 1159–1166.

Kim J, Basak JM, Holtzman DM. 2009. The role of apolipoprotein E in Alzheimer's disease. *Neuron* **63:** 287–303.

Klinge PM, Samii A, Niescken S, Brinker T, Silverberg GD. 2006. Brain amyloid accumulates in aged rats with kaolin-induced hydrocephalus. *Neuroreport* **17:** 657–660.

Knopman DS, Roberts R. 2010. Vascular risk factors: Imaging and neuropathologic correlates. *J Alzheimers Dis* **20:** 699–709.

Koch M, Chitayat S, Dattilo BM, Schiefner A, Diez J, Chazin WJ, Fritz G. 2010. Structural basis for ligand recognition and activation of RAGE. *Structure* **18:** 1342–1352.

Koike MA, Green KN, Blurton-Jones M, Laferla FM. 2010. Oligemic hypoperfusion differentially affects tau and amyloid-β. *Am J Pathol* **177:** 300–310.

Koistinaho M, Lin S, Wu X, Esterman M, Koger D, Hanson J, Higgs R, Liu F, Malkani S, Bales KR, et al. 2004. Apolipoprotein E promotes astrocyte colocalization and degradation of deposited amyloid-β peptides. *Nat Med* **10:** 719–726.

Kuchibhotla KV, Lattarulo CR, Hyman BT, Bacskai BJ. 2009. Synchronous hyperactivity and intercellular calcium waves in astrocytes in Alzheimer mice. *Science* **323:** 1211–1215.

Kumar-Singh S, Pirici D, McGowan E, Serneels S, Ceuterick C, Hardy J, Duff K, Dickson D, Van Broeckhoven C. 2005. Dense-core plaques in Tg2576 and PSAPP mouse models of Alzheimer's disease are centered on vessel walls. *Am J Pathol* **167:** 527–543.

Lambert JC, Wavrant-De Vrieze F, Amouyel P, Chartier-Harlin MC. 1998. Association at LRP gene locus with sporadic late-onset Alzheimer's disease. *Lancet* **351:** 1787–1788.

Lambert JC, Heath S, Even G, Campion D, Sleegers K, Hiltunen M, Combarros O, Zelenika D, Bullido MJ, Tavernier B, et al. 2009. Genome-wide association study identifies variants at CLU and CR1 associated with Alzheimer's disease. *Nat Genet* **41:** 1094–1099.

Li Y, Lu W, Marzolo MP, Bu G. 2001. Differential functions of members of the low density lipoprotein receptor family suggested by their distinct endocytosis rates. *J Biol Chem* **276**: 18000–18006.

Li S, Wang DZ, Wang Z, Richardson JA, Olson EN. 2003. The serum response factor coactivator myocardin is required for vascular smooth muscle development. *Proc Natl Acad Sci* **100**: 9366–9370.

Lillis AP, Van Duyn LB, Murphy-Ullrich JE, Strickland DK. 2008. LDL receptor-related protein 1: Unique tissue-specific functions revealed by selective gene knock-out studies. *Physiol Rev* **88**: 887–918.

Luchsinger JA, Reitz C, Patel B, Tang MX, Manly JJ, Mayeux R. 2007. Relation of diabetes to mild cognitive impairment. *Arch Neurol* **64**: 570–575.

Mackic JB, Stins M, McComb JG, Calero M, Ghiso J, Kim KS, Yan SD, Stern D, Schmidt AM, Frangione B, et al. 1998. Human blood–brain barrier receptors for Alzheimer's amyloid-β 1–40. Asymmetrical binding, endocytosis, and transcytosis at the apical side of brain microvascular endothelial cell monolayer. *J Clin Invest* **102**: 734–743.

Marchesi VT. 2011. Alzheimer's dementia begins as a disease of small blood vessels, damaged by oxidative-induced inflammation and dysregulated amyloid metabolism: Implications for early detection and therapy. *FASEB J* **25**: 5–13.

Mawuenyega KG, Sigurdson W, Ovod V, Munsell L, Kasten T, Morris JC, Yarasheski KE, Bateman RJ. 2010. Decreased clearance of CNS β-amyloid in Alzheimer's disease. *Science* **330**: 1774.

Meijer AB, Rohlena J, van der Zwaan C, van Zonneveld AJ, Boertjes RC, Lenting PJ, Mertens K. 2007. Functional duplication of ligand-binding domains within low-density lipoprotein receptor-related protein for interaction with receptor associated protein, α2-macroglobulin, factor IXa and factor VIII. *Biochim Biophys Acta* **1774**: 714–722.

Meyer-Luehmann M, Coomaraswamy J, Bolmont T, Kaeser S, Schaefer C, Kilger E, Neuenschwander A, Abramowski D, Frey P, Jaton AL, et al. 2006. Exogenous induction of cerebral β-amyloidogenesis is governed by agent and host. *Science* **313**: 1781–1784.

Meyer-Luehmann M, Spires-Jones TL, Prada C, Garcia-Alloza M, de Calignon A, Rozkalne A, Koenigsknecht-Talboo J, Holtzman DM, Bacskai BJ, Hyman BT. 2008. Rapid appearance and local toxicity of amyloid-β plaques in a mouse model of Alzheimer's disease. *Nature* **451**: 720–724.

Miller G. 2009. Alzheimer's biomarker initiative hits its stride. *Science* **326**: 386–389.

Miller MC, Tavares R, Johanson CE, Hovanesian V, Donahue JE, Gonzalez L, Silverberg GD, Stopa EG. 2008. Hippocampal RAGE immunoreactivity in early and advanced Alzheimer's disease. *Brain Res* **1230**: 273–280.

Miyazaki K, Ohta Y, Nagai M, Morimoto N, Kurata T, Takehisa Y, Ikeda Y, Matsuura T, Abe K. 2011. Disruption of neurovascular unit prior to motor neuron degeneration in amyotrophic lateral sclerosis. *J Neurosci Res* **89**: 718–728.

Mooradian AD, Chung HC, Shah GN. 1997. GLUT-1 expression in the cerebra of patients with Alzheimer's disease. *Neurobiol Aging* **18**: 469–474.

Mosconi L, Sorbi S, de Leon MJ, Li Y, Nacmias B, Myoung PS, Tsui W, Ginestroni A, Bessi V, Fayyazz M, et al. 2006. Hypometabolism exceeds atrophy in presymptomatic early-onset familial Alzheimer's disease. *J Nucl Med* **47**: 1778–1786.

Mosconi L, De Santi S, Li J, Tsui WH, Li Y, Boppana M, Laska E, Rusinek H, de Leon MJ. 2008. Hippocampal hypometabolism predicts cognitive decline from normal aging. *Neurobiol Aging* **29**: 676–692.

Moskowitz MA, Lo EH, Iadecola C. 2010. The science of stroke: Mechanisms in search of treatments. *Neuron* **67**: 181–198.

Narita M, Holtzman DM, Schwartz AL, Bu G. 1997. α2-Macroglobulin complexes with and mediates the endocytosis of β-amyloid peptide via cell surface low-density lipoprotein receptor-related protein. *J Neurochem* **69**: 1904–1911.

Nazer B, Hong S, Selkoe DJ. 2008. LRP promotes endocytosis and degradation, but not transcytosis, of the amyloid-β peptide in a blood–brain barrier in vitro model. *Neurobiol Dis* **30**: 94–102.

Neels JG, van Den Berg BM, Lookene A, Olivecrona G, Pannekoek H, van Zonneveld AJ. 1999. The second and fourth cluster of class A cysteine-rich repeats of the low density lipoprotein receptor-related protein share ligand-binding properties. *J Biol Chem* **274**: 31305–31311.

Neeper M, Schmidt AM, Brett J, Yan SD, Wang F, Pan YC, Elliston K, Stern D, Shaw A. 1992. Cloning and expression of a cell surface receptor for advanced glycosylation end products of proteins. *J Biol Chem* **267**: 14998–15004.

Neuwelt EA, Bauer B, Fahlke C, Fricker G, Iadecola C, Janigro D, Leybaert L, Molnar Z, O'Donnell ME, Povlishock JT, et al. 2011. Engaging neuroscience to advance translational research in brain barrier biology. *Nat Rev Neurosci* **12**: 169–182.

Obermoeller-McCormick LM, Li Y, Osaka H, FitzGerald DJ, Schwartz AL, Bu G. 2001. Dissection of receptor folding and ligand-binding property with functional minireceptors of LDL receptor-related protein. *J Cell Sci* **114**: 899–908.

O'Kane RL, Martinez-Lopez I, DeJoseph MR, Vina JR, Hawkins RA. 1999. Na(+)-dependent glutamate transporters (EAAT1, EAAT2, and EAAT3) of the blood–brain barrier. A mechanism for glutamate removal. *J Biol Chem* **274**: 31891–31895.

Ongali B, Nicolakakis N, Lecrux C, Aboulkassim T, Rosa-Neto P, Papadopoulos P, Tong XK, Hamel E. 2010. Transgenic mice overexpressing APP and transforming growth factor-β1 feature cognitive and vascular hallmarks of Alzheimer's disease. *Am J Pathol* **177**: 3071–3080.

Pan W, Kastin AJ, Zankel TC, van Kerkhof P, Terasaki T, Bu G. 2004. Efficient transfer of receptor-associated protein (RAP) across the blood–brain barrier. *J Cell Sci* **117**: 5071–5078.

Paris D, Patel N, DelleDonne A, Quadros A, Smeed R, Mullan M. 2004a. Impaired angiogenesis in a transgenic mouse model of cerebral amyloidosis. *Neurosci Lett* **366**: 80–85.

Paris D, Townsend K, Quadros A, Humphrey J, Sun J, Brem S, Wotoczek-Obadia M, DelleDonne A, Patel N, Obregon DF, et al. 2004b. Inhibition of angiogenesis by Aβ peptides. *Angiogenesis* **7**: 75–85.

Park H, Adsit FG, Boyington JC. 2010. The 1.5 Å crystal structure of human receptor for advanced glycation endproducts (RAGE) ectodomains reveals unique features determining ligand binding. *J Biol Chem* **285:** 40762–40770.

Parkyn CJ, Vermeulen EG, Mootoosamy RC, Sunyach C, Jacobsen C, Oxvig C, Moestrup S, Liu Q, Bu G, Jen A, et al. 2008. LRP1 controls biosynthetic and endocytic trafficking of neuronal prion protein. *J Cell Sci* **121:** 773–783.

Paul J, Strickland S, Melchor JP. 2007. Fibrin deposition accelerates neurovascular damage and neuroinflammation in mouse models of Alzheimer's disease. *J Exp Med* **204:** 1999–2008.

Peppiatt CM, Howarth C, Mobbs P, Attwell D. 2006. Bidirectional control of CNS capillary diameter by pericytes. *Nature* **443:** 700–704.

Perrin RJ, Fagan AM, Holtzman DM. 2009. Multimodal techniques for diagnosis and prognosis of Alzheimer's disease. *Nature* **461:** 916–922.

Pietrzik CU, Yoon IS, Jaeger S, Busse T, Weggen S, Koo EH. 2004. FE65 constitutes the functional link between the low-density lipoprotein receptor-related protein and the amyloid precursor protein. *J Neurosci* **24:** 4259–4265.

Polavarapu R, Gongora MC, Yi H, Ranganthan S, Lawrence DA, Strickland D, Yepes M. 2007. Tissue-type plasminogen activator-mediated shedding of astrocytic low-density lipoprotein receptor-related protein increases the permeability of the neurovascular unit. *Blood* **109:** 3270–3278.

Prusiner SB. 1996. Molecular biology and genetics of prion diseases. *Cold Spring Harb Sym* **61:** 473–493.

Qiu Z, Strickland DK, Hyman BT, Rebeck GW. 1999. Alpha2-macroglobulin enhances the clearance of endogenous soluble β-amyloid peptide via low-density lipoprotein receptor-related protein in cortical neurons. *J Neurochem* **73:** 1393–1398.

Querfurth HW, LaFerla FM. 2010. Alzheimer's disease. *New Engl J Med* **362:** 329–344.

Rebeck GW, Harr SD, Strickland DK, Hyman BT. 1995. Multiple, diverse senile plaque-associated proteins are ligands of an apolipoprotein E receptor, the α 2-macroglobulin receptor/low-density-lipoprotein receptor-related protein. *Ann Neurol* **37:** 211–217.

Relkin NR, Szabo P, Adamiak B, Burgut T, Monthe C, Lent RW, Younkin S, Younkin L, Schiff R, Weksler ME. 2009. 18-Month study of intravenous immunoglobulin for treatment of mild Alzheimer disease. *Neurobiol Aging* **30:** 1728–1736.

Reynolds PR, Mucenski ML, Le Cras TD, Nichols WC, Whitsett JA. 2004. Midkine is regulated by hypoxia and causes pulmonary vascular remodeling. *J Biol Chem* **279:** 37124–37132.

Rovelet-Lecrux A, Hannequin D, Raux G, Le Meur N, Laquerriere A, Vital A, Dumanchin C, Feuillette S, Brice A, Vercelletto M, et al. 2006. APP locus duplication causes autosomal dominant early-onset Alzheimer disease with cerebral amyloid angiopathy. *Nat Genet* **38:** 24–26.

Ruitenberg A, den Heijer T, Bakker SL, van Swieten JC, Koudstaal PJ, Hofman A, Breteler MM. 2005. Cerebral hypoperfusion and clinical onset of dementia: The Rotterdam Study. *Ann Neurol* **57:** 789–794.

Sagare A, Deane R, Bell RD, Johnson B, Hamm K, Pendu R, Marky A, Lenting PJ, Wu Z, Zarcone T, et al. 2007. Clearance of amyloid-β by circulating lipoprotein receptors. *Nat Med* **13:** 1029–1031.

Sagare AP, Deane R, Zetterberg H, Wallin A, Blennow K, Zlokovic BV. 2011a. Impaired lipoprotein receptor-mediated peripheral binding of plasma amyloid-β is an early biomarker for mild cognitive impairment preceding Alzheimer's disease. *J Alzheimer's Dis* **24:** 25–34.

Sagare AP, Winkler EA, Bell RD, Deane R, Zlokovic BV. 2011b. From the liver to the blood–brain barrier: An interconnected system regulating brain amyloid-β levels. *J Neurosci Res* **89:** 967–968.

Samuraki M, Matsunari I, Chen WP, Yajima K, Yanase D, Fujikawa A, Takeda N, Nishimura S, Matsuda H, Yamada M. 2007. Partial volume effect-corrected FDG PET and grey matter volume loss in patients with mild Alzheimer's disease. *Euro J Nucl Med Mol Imag* **34:** 1658–1669.

Schmidt AM, Sahagan B, Nelson RB, Selmer J, Rothlein R, Bell JM. 2009. The role of RAGE in amyloid-β peptide-mediated pathology in Alzheimer's disease. *Curr Opin Investig Drugs* **10:** 672–680.

Sheline YI, Morris JC, Snyder AZ, Price JL, Yan Z, D'Angelo G, Liu C, Dixit S, Benzinger T, Fagan A, et al. 2010. APOE4 allele disrupts resting state fMRI connectivity in the absence of amyloid plaques or decreased CSF Aβ42. *J Neurosci* **30:** 17035–17040.

Shibata M, Yamada S, Kumar SR, Calero M, Bading J, Frangione B, Holtzman DM, Miller CA, Strickland DK, Ghiso J, et al. 2000. Clearance of Alzheimer's amyloid-ss(1–40) peptide from brain by LDL receptor-related protein-1 at the blood–brain barrier. *J Clin Invest* **106:** 1489–1499.

Shiiki T, Ohtsuki S, Kurihara A, Naganuma H, Nishimura K, Tachikawa M, Hosoya K, Terasaki T. 2004. Brain insulin impairs amyloid-β(1–40) clearance from the brain. *J Neurosci* **24:** 9632–9637.

Shinohara M, Sato N, Kurinami H, Takeuchi D, Takeda S, Shimamura M, Yamashita T, Uchiyama Y, Rakugi H, Morishita R. 2010. Reduction of brain β-amyloid (Aβ) by fluvastatin, a hydroxymethylglutaryl-CoA reductase inhibitor, through increase in degradation of amyloid precursor protein C-terminal fragments (APP-CTFs) and Aβ clearance. *J Biol Chem* **285:** 22091–22102.

Smith CD, Andersen AH, Kryscio RJ, Schmitt FA, Kindy MS, Blonder LX, Avison MJ. 1999. Altered brain activation in cognitively intact individuals at high risk for Alzheimer's disease. *Neurology* **53:** 1391–1396.

Snowdon DA, Greiner LH, Mortimer JA, Riley KP, Greiner PA, Markesbery WR. 1997. Brain infarction and the clinical expression of Alzheimer disease. The Nun Study. *JAMA* **277:** 813–817.

Sturchler E, Galichet A, Weibel M, Leclerc E, Heizmann CW. 2008. Site-specific blockade of RAGE-Vd prevents amyloid-β oligomer neurotoxicity. *J Neurosci* **28:** 5149–5158.

Sun Q, Chen G, Streb JW, Long X, Yang Y, Stoeckert CJ Jr, Miano JM. 2006. Defining the mammalian CArGome. *Genome Res* **16:** 197–207.

Sutcliffe JG, Hedlund PB, Thomas EA, Bloom FE, Hilbush BS. 2011. Peripheral reduction of β-amyloid is sufficient to reduce brain β-amyloid: Implications for Alzheimer's disease. *J Neurosci Res* **89:** 808–814.

Takano T, Han X, Deane R, Zlokovic B, Nedergaard M. 2007. Two-photon imaging of astrocytic Ca^{2+} signaling and the microvasculature in experimental mice models of Alzheimer's disease. *Ann NY Acad Sci* **1097:** 40–50.

Takuma K, Fang F, Zhang W, Yan S, Fukuzaki E, Du H, Sosunov A, McKhann G, Funatsu Y, Nakamichi N, et al. 2009. RAGE-mediated signaling contributes to intraneuronal transport of amyloid-β and neuronal dysfunction. *Proc Natl Acad Sci* **106:** 20021–20026.

Tamaki C, Ohtsuki S, Iwatsubo T, Hashimoto T, Yamada K, Yabuki C, Terasaki T. 2006. Major involvement of low-density lipoprotein receptor-related protein 1 in the clearance of plasma free amyloid β-peptide by the liver. *Pharm Res* **23:** 1407–1416.

Tamaki C, Ohtsuki S, Terasaki T. 2007. Insulin facilitates the hepatic clearance of plasma amyloid β-peptide (1–40) by intracellular translocation of low-density lipoprotein receptor-related protein 1 (LRP-1) to the plasma membrane in hepatocytes. *Mol Pharm* **72:** 850–855.

Thomas T, Thomas G, McLendon C, Sutton T, Mullan M. 1996. β-Amyloid-mediated vasoactivity and vascular endothelial damage. *Nature* **380:** 168–171.

Trommsdorff M, Borg JP, Margolis B, Herz J. 1998. Interaction of cytosolic adaptor proteins with neuronal apolipoprotein E receptors and the amyloid precursor protein. *J Biol Chem* **273:** 33556–33560.

Ujiie M, Dickstein DL, Carlow DA, Jefferies WA. 2003. Blood–brain barrier permeability precedes senile plaque formation in an Alzheimer disease model. *Microcirculation* **10:** 463–470.

van der Geer P. 2002. Phosphorylation of LRP1: Regulation of transport and signal transduction. *Trends Cardiovasc Med* **12:** 160–165.

Verghese PB, Castellano JM, Holtzman DM. 2011. Apolipoprotein E in Alzheimer's disease and other neurological disorders. *Lancet Neurol* **10:** 241–252.

Vermeer SE, Prins ND, den Heijer T, Hofman A, Koudstaal PJ, Breteler MM. 2003. Silent brain infarcts and the risk of dementia and cognitive decline. *New Engl J Med* **348:** 1215–1222.

Viswanathan A, Greenberg SM. 2011. Cerebral amyloid angiopathy (CAA) in the elderly. *Ann Neurol* doi: 10.1002/ana.22516.

Waldron E, Heilig C, Schweitzer A, Nadella N, Jaeger S, Martin AM, Weggen S, Brix K, Pietrzik CU. 2008. LRP1 modulates APP trafficking along early compartments of the secretory pathway. *Neurobiol Dis* **31:** 188–197.

Walsh DM, Klyubin I, Fadeeva JV, Cullen WK, Anwyl R, Wolfe MS, Rowan MJ, Selkoe DJ. 2002. Naturally secreted oligomers of amyloid β protein potently inhibit hippocampal long-term potentiation in vivo. *Nature* **416:** 535–539.

Wang D, Chang PS, Wang Z, Sutherland L, Richardson JA, Small E, Krieg PA, Olson EN. 2001. Activation of cardiac gene expression by myocardin, a transcriptional cofactor for serum response factor. *Cell* **105:** 851–862.

Wang X, Xing A, Xu C, Cai Q, Liu H, Li L. 2010. Cerebrovascular hypoperfusion induces spatial memory impairment, synaptic changes, and amyloid-β oligomerization in rats. *J Alzheimers Dis* **21:** 813–822.

Wavrant-DeVrieze F, Lambert JC, Stas L, Crook R, Cottel D, Pasquier F, Frigard B, Lambrechts M, Thiry E, Amouyel P, et al. 1999. Association between coding variability in the LRP gene and the risk of late-onset Alzheimer's disease. *Hum Genet* **104:** 432–434.

Weber A, Engelmaier A, Teschner W, Ehrlich HJ, Schwarz HP. 2009. Intravenous immunoglobulin (IVIg) Gammagard Liquid contains anti-RAGE IgG and sLRP. *Alzheimer's Dement* **5:** P416.

Weller RO, Subash M, Preston SD, Mazanti I, Carare RO. 2008. Perivascular drainage of amyloid-β peptides from the brain and its failure in cerebral amyloid angiopathy and Alzheimer's disease. *Brain Pathol* **18:** 253–266.

Whitmer RA, Gustafson DR, Barrett-Connor E, Haan MN, Gunderson EP, Yaffe K. 2008. Central obesity and increased risk of dementia more than three decades later. *Neurology* **71:** 1057–1064.

Wu Z, Guo H, Chow N, Sallstrom J, Bell RD, Deane R, Brooks AI, Kanagala S, Rubio A, Sagare A, et al. 2005. Role of the MEOX2 homeobox gene in neurovascular dysfunction in Alzheimer disease. *Nat Med* **11:** 959–965.

Yamada K, Hashimoto T, Yabuki C, Nagae Y, Tachikawa M, Strickland DK, Liu Q, Bu G, Basak JM, Holtzman DM, et al. 2008. The low density lipoprotein receptor-related protein 1 mediates uptake of amyloid β peptides in an in vitro model of the blood–brain barrier cells. *J Biol Chem* **283:** 34554–34562.

Yan SD, Yan SF, Chen X, Fu J, Chen M, Kuppusamy P, Smith MA, Perry G, Godman GC, Nawroth P, et al. 1995. Nonenzymatically glycated tau in Alzheimer's disease induces neuronal oxidant stress resulting in cytokine gene expression and release of amyloid β-peptide. *Nat Med* **1:** 693–699.

Yan SD, Chen X, Fu J, Chen M, Zhu H, Roher A, Slattery T, Zhao L, Nagashima M, Morser J, et al. 1996. RAGE and amyloid-β peptide neurotoxicity in Alzheimer's disease. *Nature* **382:** 685–691.

Yan SF, Ramasamy R, Schmidt AM. 2010. The RAGE axis: A fundamental mechanism signaling danger to the vulnerable vasculature. *Circul Res* **106:** 842–853.

Yemisci M, Gursoy-Ozdemir Y, Vural A, Can A, Topalkara K, Dalkara T. 2009. Pericyte contraction induced by oxidative-nitrative stress impairs capillary reflow despite successful opening of an occluded cerebral artery. *Nat Med* **15:** 1031–1037.

Zacchigna S, Lambrechts D, Carmeliet P. 2008. Neurovascular signalling defects in neurodegeneration. *Nat Rev Neurosci* **9:**169–81.

Zerbinatti CV, Bu G. 2005. LRP and Alzheimer's disease. *Rev Neurosci* **16:** 123–135.

Zerbinatti CV, Wozniak DF, Cirrito J, Cam JA, Osaka H, Bales KR, Zhuo M, Paul SM, Holtzman DM, Bu G. 2004. Increased soluble amyloid-β peptide and memory deficits in amyloid model mice overexpressing the low-density lipoprotein receptor-related protein. *Proc Natl Acad Sci* **101:** 1075–1080.

Zhong Z, Deane R, Ali Z, Parisi M, Shapovalov Y, O'Banion MK, Stojanovic K, Sagare A, Boillee S, Cleveland DW, et al. 2008. ALS-causing SOD1 mutants generate vascular changes prior to motor neuron degeneration. *Nat Neurosci* **11:** 420–422.

Zipser BD, Johanson CE, Gonzalez L, Berzin TM, Tavares R, Hulette CM, Vitek MP, Hovanesian V, Stopa EG. 2007. Microvascular injury and blood–brain barrier leakage in Alzheimer's disease. *Neurobiol Aging* **28:** 977–986.

Zlokovic BV. 2005. Neurovascular mechanisms of Alzheimer's neurodegeneration. *Trends Neurosci* **28:** 202–208.

Zlokovic BV. 2008. The blood–brain barrier in health and chronic neurodegenerative disorders. *Neuron* **57:** 178–201.

Zlokovic BV. 2010. Neurodegeneration and the neurovascular unit. *Nat Med* **16:** 1370–1371.

Zlokovic BZ. 2011. Neurovascular pathways to neurodegeneration in Alzheimer's disease and other disorders. *Nat Rev Neurosci* (in press).

Zlokovic BV, Deane R, Sagare AP, Bell RD, Winkler EA. 2010. Low-density lipoprotein receptor-related protein-1: A serial clearance homeostatic mechanism controlling Alzheimer's amyloid β-peptide elimination from the brain. *J Neurochem* **115:** 1077–1089.

Zurhove K, Nakajima C, Herz J, Bock HH, May P. 2008. γ-Secretase limits the inflammatory response through the processing of LRP1. *Sci Signal* **1:** ra15.

Treatment Strategies Targeting Amyloid β-Protein

Dale Schenk[1], Guriqbal S. Basi[1], and Menelas N. Pangalos[2]

[1]Netotope Biosciences Inc., San Francisco, California 94080

[2]AstraZeneca, Mereside, Alderley Park SK10 4TG, United Kingdom

Correspondence: dale.schenk@elan.com

With the advent of the key discovery in the mid-1980s that the amyloid β-protein (Aβ) is the core constituent of the amyloid plaque pathology found in Alzheimer disease (AD), an intensive effort has been underway to attempt to mitigate its role in the hope of treating the disease. This effort fully matured when it was clarified that the Aβ is a normal product of cleavage of the amyloid precursor protein, and well-defined proteases for this process were identified. Further therapeutic options have been developed around the concept of anti-Aβ aggregation inhibitors and the surprising finding that immunization with Aβ itself leads to reduction of pathology in animal models of the disease. Here we review the progress in this field toward the goal of targeting Aβ for treatment and prevention of AD and identify some of the major challenges for the future of this area of medicine.

Treatment of Alzheimer disease (AD) through a biological and molecular understanding of the disease has been the cornerstone of research in the field for the past 20 years. In this article we will review some of the therapeutic efforts that are being pursued and have been attempted over this period during which the amyloid β (Aβ) peptide has been the primary target. These efforts can generally be divided into three areas: β- and γ-secretase inhibition, Aβ aggregation inhibitors, and active and passive Aβ immunotherapy approaches (Fig. 1).

β- AND γ-SECRETASE INHIBITORS FOR AD

The identification of Aβ as the primary constituent of amyloid plaques in Alzheimer brain presented a tangible target for developing therapies for the disease (Fig. 2). The three fundamental approaches currently in play targeting Aβ for treatment and prevention of AD involve inhibiting its production, preventing its aggregation (or promoting its disaggregation), and promoting its clearance. Therapeutic advances with the latter two approaches are discussed in the following sections of this article. The focus of this section is therapeutic advances on inhibiting production of Aβ.

The pathologic accumulation of Aβ in plaques is postulated to result from an imbalance between production and clearance during aging. Transgenic mouse models overexpressing human amyloid precursor protein (APP) bearing certain familial AD mutations have validated overproduction of Aβ as driving AD-type amyloid pathology. The mouse models have

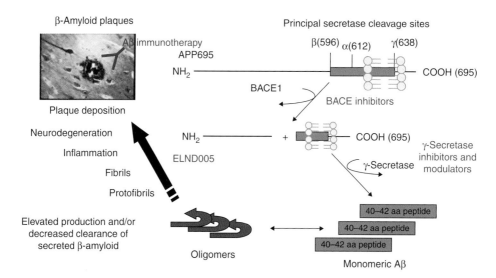

Figure 1. Amyloidogenic processing of amyloid precursor protein (APP) by BACE1 and γ-secretase. The figure depicts the principal proteolytic processing steps of APP leading to the production of 40–42-residue amyloid β (Aβ) peptide, the subsequent steps ultimately culminating in compaction and deposition of the peptide in β-amyloid plaques in brain of AD patients (and transgenic AD mouse models), and the primary point of intervention by the different therapeutic antiamyloid approaches discussed in this article.

also provided insights into the interrelationship between related pathologies characteristic of the disease, for example, tau, inflammatory end points (e.g., microgliosis, astrocytosis), neuritic dystrophy, and Aβ-related behavioral deficits (presumed preclinical surrogates of the cognitive deficits in patients). Nevertheless, the Aβ overproduction mouse models do not exhibit robust neuronal loss characteristic of the advanced human disease as judged postmortem. An additional caveat of current mouse models in the context of therapeutics targeting production of amyloid is that, in contrast to rare familial forms of AD (Scheuner et al. 1996), there is limited evidence that sporadic AD is a driven by overproduction of Aβ (Fukumoto et al. 2002; Holsinger et al. 2002; Yang et al. 2003; Li et al. 2004). Indeed, evidence in support of the alternative possibility—that accumulation of β amyloid in sporadic AD results from reduced clearance and/or turnover of the peptide—has been reported (Mawuenyega et al. 2010). Irrespective of whether overproduction or reduced clearance causes amyloid pathology in sporadic AD, clinical

evaluation of the benefits of inhibiting production as a therapeutic strategy for sporadic AD is still warranted from two perspectives. First is the ample evidence for pathology attributable to toxic effects of excess soluble Aβ (Gong et al. 2003; Kayed et al. 2003; Lacor et al. 2004; Cleary et al. 2005; Lesne et al. 2006; Townsend et al. 2006b; Cheng et al. 2007; Walsh and Selkoe 2007; Klyubin et al. 2008; Shankar et al. 2008) as well as pathology attributable to plaque-associated Aβ (Spires et al. 2005; Kuchibhotla et al. 2008; Meyer-Luehmann et al. 2008, 2009). Second, inhibiting production offers a logical approach for restoring homeostasis between production and clearance if retarded clearance mechanisms are a widespread contributor to sporadic AD. Interestingly, the findings of Mawuenyega et al. are consistent with the conclusion that a partial inhibition of production (common target ∼30%) could be therapeutically efficacious, as the observed in vivo clearance of Aβ40 and Aβ42 was reduced by ∼35% in sporadic AD patients in comparison with healthy controls.

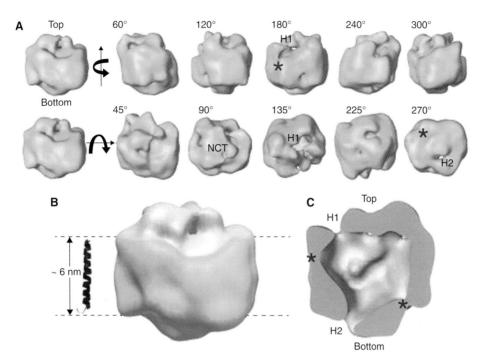

Figure 2. Electron micrograph based 3D structure of the γ-secretase complex. (*A*) Surface rendering of the 3D reconstruction. The first row displays side views generated by rotating the map around a vertical axis, and the second row shows tilted views by rotating around a horizontal axis. The rotation angles are shown within each view. Two openings at the top and bottom are labeled H1 and H2, respectively, where visible. The top density is labeled NCT because the lectin labeling showed that the NCT ectodomain is located at this surface. (*B*) The potential transmembrane segment with the belt-like structure is outlined in blue by two parallel dashed lines, 60 Å apart. For size comparison, a typical transmembrane α-helix, taken from the rhodopsin structure (Protein Data Bank ID code 1GZM), is shown to the left of the structure. (*C*) A cut-open view of the γ-secretase complex from the side, revealing a large central chamber and one opening (H1) at the top and one at the bottom (H2). Two weak-density lateral regions are labeled with asterisks. (Image is from Lazarov et al. 2006; printed with permission from D. Selkoe.)

The constitutive production of Aβ from APP, a type I transmembrane protein, revealed the central role of two distinct proteases, and provided a cornerstone for drug discovery efforts. The two primary amyloidogenic proteases are commonly referred to as BACE1 (β-site APP cleaving enzyme 1) and γ-secretase. The initial cleavage of APP leading to Aβ generation is mediated by BACE1 (Fig. 3), and results in two products, an amino-terminal fragment of APP termed sAPPβ that is released into the luminal/extracellular compartment, and a membrane embedded carboxy-terminal fragment, termed C99. C99 is the immediate substrate for a series of cleavages by γ-secretase.

The primary products of γ cleavage of C99 are the 40- or 42-residue β-amyloid peptide, and the APP intracellular domain (AICD). Detailed analyses of the cleavage events mediated by both enzymes on APP have revealed additional minor sites of cleavage by BACE1, as well as a complex processive proteolytic activity by γ-secretase (see Harrison et al. 2004; John 2006; Haass et al. 2011).

BACE1 and γ-secretase presented obvious drug targets for inhibiting production of Aβ, and they have been the subjects of intensive research. Properties distinguishing these enzymes from one another include the fact that BACE1 is a monomeric protein displaying relative

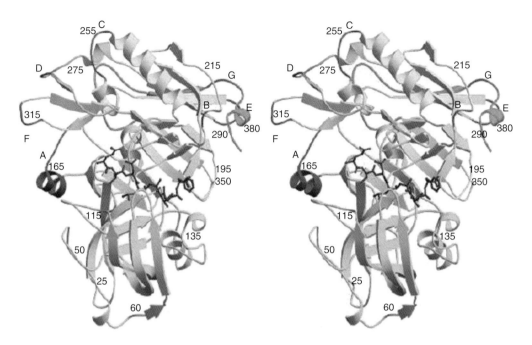

Figure 3. Crystal structure of BACE1 complexed with a small molecule inhibitor. The crystal structure of BACE1 complexed to inhibitor OM99-2. Stereo view of the polypeptide backbone of BACE1 is shown as a ribbon diagram. The amino-terminal and carboxy-terminal lobes are blue and yellow, respectively, insertion loops (relative to pepsin) designated A–G in the carboxy-terminal lobe are magenta, and the COOH-terminal extension unique to BACE is green. The inhibitor bound between the lobes is shown in red. (Modified from Hong et al. 2000.)

specificity for cleavage site sequence, and that it catalyzes substrate cleavage in an aqueous environment. In contrast, γ-secretase is a multisubunit protein complex comprising four subunits, with little apparent specificity for sequence, and it performs water-mediated catalysis of the transmembrane domains of substrates in the hydrophobic environment of the plasma membrane. Features in common between the two enzymes include the fact that both are membrane-bound aspartyl proteases, both have been demonstrated to process multiple substrates in addition to APP, and at least in the case of APP, both cleave the substrate at multiple sites (in common with most proteases).

These common properties have presented challenges for development of small-molecule inhibitors targeting either enzyme. In the case of γ-secretase, its many substrates, particularly Notch, have made clinical development of substrate-selective inhibitors difficult. In the case of BACE1, the conventional aspartyl protease nature of this target (i.e., an extended substrate binding groove) shows limited discovery of central nervous system (CNS)-permeable small molecule inhibitors. Nevertheless, progress has been made on both fronts, as we will now discuss.

γ-Secretase Inhibitors

Three principal classes of γ-secretase inhibitors (GSIs) have progressed into AD clinical trials: nonselective inhibitors, cleavage site modulators, and APP-selective/Notch-sparing inhibitors. Expert reviews of the rich medicinal chemistry underlying the three approaches have been published over the years (Josien 2002; Harrison et al. 2004; Churcher and Beher 2005; Pissarnitski 2007; Olson and Albright 2008; Garofalo 2009), and the interested reader is directed to those publications for further background, as this article will review clinical properties and results from GSIs in AD trials. Progress with, and limitations of, GSIs have been intertwined with the unfolding story of the complex biology of this target. To appreciate the rationale for testing each of these inhibitor classes, a review of the complex biology of γ-secretase accompanies the review of the progress with each inhibitor.

Biochemical identification of presenilin 1 (PS1) as the target of substrate-based transition state isosteres (Esler et al. 2000; Li et al. 2000), as well as inhibitors of Aβ production discovered from cell-based screens (Seiffert et al. 2000), provided conclusive evidence to settle the argument, based on reverse genetic approaches supporting PS1 and PS2 as a critical component of γ-secretase (De Strooper et al. 1998; Herreman et al. 1999, 2000; Steiner et al. 1999), that two transmembrane aspartyl residues in the presenilin amino-terminal fragment (NTF) and carboxy-terminal fragment (CTF) comprised the active site of γ-secretase (Wolfe et al. 1999). This discovery culminated in the recognition of γ-secretase as the first example of intramembrane cleaving aspartyl proteases (iClip). The recognition of PS as the catalytic subunit of γ-secretase established the molecular identity of the target of ongoing efforts toward clinical development of what subsequently came to be appreciated as nonselective γ-secretase inhibitors.

The most advanced nonselective GSI, Semagacestat (LY450139, IC$_{50}$ of ~60 nM for cellular Aβ; reviewed in Henley et al. 2009) progressed into phase 3 human testing by Eli Lilly and Co. before further development was halted (Eli Lilly 2010). Semagacestat's origins stemmed from a collaboration between Athena Neurosciences and Eli Lilly & Co. that provided two seminal demonstrations: first, that acute pharmacologic inhibition of γ-secretase by an early lead in the series (known as DAPT) could effectively lower brain Aβ production in PDAPP mice (a mutant APP transgenic model of AD pathology; Dovey et al. 2001); and second, that inhibition for 3 mo of γ-secretase in PDAPP with LY411575 (a picomolar optimized GSI lead derived from DAPT) decreased plaques and related amyloid pathologies (May et al. 2001). Single-dose studies explored the safety and tolerability of Semgacestat (i.e., LY450139) in healthy volunteers given 5–140 mg of the compound and revealed the pharmacokinetic–pharmacodynamic relationship of Aβ as a biomarker in plasma and cerebrospinal fluid (CSF; Siemers et al. 2005, 2007). Single doses of semagacestat were safe and well tolerated. Pharmacokinetic and pharmacodynamic characterization revealed a plasma $t_{1/2}$ of 2.5 h and a dose-dependent reduction of plasma Aβ over the first 6 h (ranging from 40% at 50 mg to 73% at 140 mg), followed by a well-documented transient increase in Aβ above baseline. Repeat-dose studies in AD patients explored safety and tolerability and Aβ biomarker effects as primary end points and clinical measures of cognition as secondary end points in patients dosed with 5–50 mg/d semagacestat for 2 or 6 wk (Siemers et al. 2006). A subsequent study explored doses ranging up to 140 mg in AD patients treated for a total of 14 wk in an ascending dose design (Fleisher et al. 2008). As in the single-dose studies, a dose-proportional increase in drug exposure with concomitant reduction of plasma Aβ was observed in the repeat dose studies, with good overall tolerability. No significant effects on the secondary clinical end points (ADAS-Cog and ADAS-ADL) were observed in the 14-wk study, which was not powered to see an effect on these end points. Although a reduction in steady-state CSF Aβ level (considered a more proximal biomarker of brain Aβ) was not observed in the studies cited above, a decline in the rate of synthesis of brain Aβ, monitored in CSF using a novel stable isotope labeling kinetic method, was effected by semagacestat in a dose-responsive manner in healthy volunteers given single doses of 100, 140, or 280 mg of drug (Bateman et al. 2009). Based on the cumulative evidence just reviewed, a phase 3 trial of semagacestat in AD was launched by Eli Lilly and Co. Although generally well tolerated in the single-dose studies, drug-related adverse events were noted in the repeat-dose studies, consistent with its mechanism of action for inhibition of Notch signaling in peripheral tissues (e.g., skin rash, hair color change, and gastrointestinal effects). These observations are consistent with the effects of nonselective GSIs reported in preclinical studies (Searfoss et al. 2003; Milano et al. 2004; Wong et al. 2004; Hyde et al. 2006). A decline in cognition of patients on drug relative to placebo, as well the emergence of skin neoplasms in the LY-450139 phase 3 study, noted in the press release announcing early termination of the trial, are reminiscent of phenotypes noted in partial or conditional PS loss of function models (Fig. 4; Saura et al. 2004; Tournoy et al. 2004; Li et al. 2007).

Other nonselective GSIs—for example, MK-0752 and PF-03084014 (Wei et al. 2010)—are being tested in certain cancer indications by Merck and Pfizer, respectively, based on the rationale that dysregulated Notch signaling leads to oncologic transformation. Limited data is available with MK-0752 from the perspective of AD: In phase 1 studies reported by Rosen et al. (2006), MK-0752 exhibited CSF concentrations equivalent to estimated free plasma concentrations, a 2 h delayed T_{max} in CSF relative to plasma, and a dose-related reduction of CSF Aβ40 over a 4–12-h period following single doses >300 mg. The highest dose tested, 1000 mg, produced a sustained reduction in CSF Aβ over 24 h. No clinical findings have been reported to date with PF-03084014, and as oncological testing of GSIs falls outside the scope of this article, MK-0752 and PF-03084014 will not be reviewed further here.

Owing to challenges associated with the inhibition of Notch signaling by nonselective GSIs, drug development targeting this enzyme branched into two parallel strategies, cleavage site modulators and APP-selective inhibitors. The discovery of the prototype γ-secretase cleavage site modulators such as Tarenflurbil (Flurizan, R-flurbiprofen) arose from cell culture experiments examining the effects of nonsteroidal anti-inflammatory drugs (NSAIDs) on APP processing (Weggen et al. 2001), which appeared to relate to epidemiological studies, suggesting a reduced prevalence of AD associated with prolonged use of select NSAIDs, particularly ibuprofen (Breitner et al. 1995; Stewart

et al. 1997; McGeer and McGeer 1998). Although preclinical studies with ibuprofen in transgenic mouse models of AD showed efficacy against β-amyloid and inflammatory endpoints (Lim et al. 2000), consistent with the epidemiological studies, prospective treatment studies of NSAIDs in mild–moderate AD failed to show benefit on primary outcome measures (Aisen et al. 2003; Thal et al. 2005). However, the in vitro studies investigating the mechanism of action revealed that certain NSAIDs, namely ibuprofen, indomethacin, and sulindac sulfide, selectively lowered secretion of Aβ42 (at concentrations of 100–250 μM) with a concomitant increase in Aβ38, without decreasing production of Aβ40 or the Notch intracellular domain, in a cyclooxygenase 1 (COX1)-independent manner (Weggen et al. 2001). This mechanistic insight into a possible effect of certain NSAIDs on γ-secretase, combined with an early recognition that the 42-residue isoform of Aβ conferred a higher risk of developing AD owing to its increased amyloidogenic potential versus shorter isoforms (e.g., Aβ40), provided support for clinical testing of these so-called γ-secretase modulators as AD therapeutics. The demonstration that R-enantiomers of ibuprofen and flurbiprofen retained Aβ42-lowering activity of the parent without inhibiting COX1 (Morihara et al. 2002; Eriksen 2003) suggested R-enantiomers as the preferred clinical candidate for testing in AD. However, the drug concentrations required to lower brain Aβ42 (100–250 μM, based on in vitro activity) are not achieved following typical daily oral dosing regimens of 10–50 mg/kg R-flurbiprofen (Eriksen et al. 2003). Hence, the observed reduction of brain Aβ42 in preclinical studies is difficult to extend to man.

R-Flurbiprofen represented the first selective Aβ-lowering agent/γ-secretase modulator advanced into clinical testing, namely by Myriad Genetics Inc. In a 21-d study in healthy elderly (55–80 year) volunteers given placebo, 400, 800, or 1600 mg/d in a twice-per-day regimen, R-flurbiprofen was safe and well tolerated, and displayed dose-dependent pharmacokinetics in brain and plasma with respect to C_{max}, whereas exposure in plasma appeared

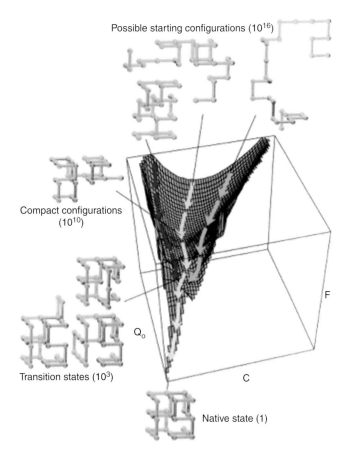

Figure 4. Spatial energy flow diagram of protein folding. The diagram depicts how, following immediate synthesis, a polypeptide initially has a very high level of possible folding and conformational states (10^{10}). The drive toward a lower energy state results in a reduced number, although still extremely high, of possible conformational states. Eventually with time, these various states, by different routes, converge toward a small number of possibilities, shown on the bottom of the figure. (Modified from Dinner et al. 2000.)

saturated at 800 mg/d dose and above, and had a 0.5%–1% CSF-to-plasma ratio (consistent with preclinical observations). Drug levels in plasma at C_{max} for the three dose groups (83, 158, and 185 μM, respectively) were in the range for lowering of plasma Aβ42 (Galasko et al. 2007). No changes from baseline to day 21 were observed in plasma Aβ42 (sampled at trough drug levels following last dose), CSF Aβ42 (sampled circa plasma T_{max}), or shorter species of Aβ. Bioinversion of the *R*- to *S*-enatiomer of drug was observed rarely in the treated population. Tarenflurbil was then tested at 400 or 800 mg on a twice-per-day schedule in a 12 mo (+12 mo extended treatment phase)

phase 2 double-blind placebo-controlled, multicenter study of mild–moderate AD patients (a curious dosing choice in light of the phase 1 data showing saturation at doses above 800 mg/d). A prespecified analysis showed a treatment effect, manifested as lower rates of decline in activities in daily living (ADAS-ADL) and global function (CDR-sb) just in mild AD patients (baseline Mini-Mental-State Exam, MMSE, 20–26) in the 800 mg b.i.d. dose group relative to placebo at 12 and 24 mo (Wilcock et al. 2008). The treatment effect of the 800 mg b.i.d. dose in mild AD patients at 24 mo was retained in benefits on activities of daily living and global function and also extended to include benefits in cognitive function (ADAS-cog), relative to placebo at 12 mo + 400 mg b.i.d. tarenflurbil 12 mo, or else placebo for 12 mo + 800 mg b.i.d. tarenflurbil for 12 mo. No benefits on primary outcome measures were noted for any time point in moderate AD patients (baseline MMSE 15–19) treated with either dose of tarenflurbil relative to placebo. In fact, moderate AD patients on 800 mg b.i.d. drug showed a faster rate of decline in CDR sum of boxes relative to placebo. No effects on the most proximal mechanistic biomarker, CSF Aβ42, nor drug exposures associated with the different treatment arms, were reported. Clinical testing in mild AD patients treated with 800 mg flurizan b.i.d. for 18 mo in a large multicenter pivotal phase 3 trial failed to meet primary endpoints (ADCS-ADL and ADAS-Cog; Green et al. 2009). Secondary analysis did not reveal any association between primary outcomes and drug pharamcokinetic parameters (C_{max} and AUC). Although further development of tarneflurbil was discontinued, subsequent preclinical progress with more potent NSAID-based GSMs is encouraging (Kounnas et al. 2010). Because tarenflurbil did not affect Aβ42 levels in the phase 3 patients as anticipated from its preclinical mechanism of action, the lack of clinical efficacy remains difficult to interpret.

Cinnamide-based compounds originating from Torrey Pines Therapeutics represent a second class of GSMs, now under development at Eisai Corp. Clinical development of the lead in this class, E2012, initially halted owing to a safety observation in a preclinical model, was resumed following satisfactory resolution of the findings (Nagy et al. 2011). No information regarding clinical or preclinical data with E2012 has been formally reported in a scientific forum by Eisai. However, Portelius et al. using IP-MALDI-TOF mass spectrometry, observed a dose-dependent increase in CSF Aβ37 in dogs over a 24-h period following a single dose treatment with 20 and 80 mg/kg E2012, along with a concomitant decrease in Aβ1–39, Aβ1–40, and Aβ1–42 (Portelius et al. 2010).

Systematic studies into the mechanism of substrate cleavage by γ-secretase indicate a processive activity of the enzyme, with an initiating cleavage near the cytosolic/membrane leaflet interface and subsequent cleavages every two or three residues into the transmembrane domain of the substrate (Takami et al. 2009; Xu 2009; Fukumori et al. 2010). These insights have bolstered the rationale underlying the cleavage site modulation by NSAIDs and hopefully will aid in the development of improved small molecules for clinical testing. Additional paths for modulating substrate cleavage by γ-secretase based on a nucleotide binding site (Feng et al. 2001; Netzer et al. 2003; Fraering et al. 2005) are in early stages of investigation. Hence, although the initial clinical outcome with cleavage site modulators has been disappointing, the mechanistic underpinning for continued efforts in this area has been strengthened in the interim.

Notch-sparing or APP substrate selective γ-secretase inhibitors represent the third class of compounds to have advanced to clinical testing in AD. As a class, all compounds in this category are based on a sulfonamide pharmacophore, demonstrate equipotent inhibition of Aβ40 and Aβ42, and display all the signatures of classic nonselective GSIs (Martone et al. 2009; Basi et al. 2010; Gillman et al. 2010). Clinical development of BMS-299897, a 7 nM inhibitor of Aβ production in cells that is a 15-fold less potent inhibitor of Notch cleavage in cells (Barten et al. 2005), was discontinued by Bristol-Myers Squib owing to a combination of pharmacokinetic liabilities (autoinduction of clearance mediated via pregnane X-receptor transactivation) and lack of Aβ reduction in man (Gillman et al. 2010).

The lack of Notch-associated gastrointestinal (GI) toxicity following repeated dosing with BMS-299897 in preclinical models (Milano et al. 2004; Barten et al. 2005) supported renewed efforts for discovery of improved analogs, and BMS-708163 is being advanced through clinical studies by Bristol-Myers Squib at the time of writing. BMS-708163, a 0.3 nM and 193-fold selective inhibitor of Aβ production versus Notch signaling in cells, lowers plasma and brain Aβ in rats in a dose-dependent manner, and a >25% reduction of

CSF and brain Aβ relative to baseline levels is sustained for >24 h following a single dose of 2 mg/kg in dogs (Gillman et al. 2010). Results from early clinical studies in healthy young and elderly volunteers as well as early AD/MCI patients indicated that BMS-708163 is generally safe and well tolerated in single doses up to 800 mg, and up to 200 mg following multiple doses for 28 d (Albright et al. 2008; Tong et al. 2010). Pharmacokinetic parameters of BMS-708163 revealed a T_{max} at 1–1.5 h, dose-related increases in C_{max} and AUC, and a plasma half-life of ∼40 h following a single dose. An approximately twofold accumulation in exposure was observed in subsequent multiple-dose studies. Pharmacodynamic analyses revealed a sustained (72-h) dose-dependent reduction of plasma Aβ following single oral doses ≥400 mg, and a reduction over the initial 6–8 h followed by an increase above baseline between 8 and 72 h at doses ≤200 mg. Serial monitoring of CSF on an hourly basis over 40 h following single oral doses of 50, 200, or 400 mg revealed dose-dependent reductions of all Aβ species measured (38, 40, and 42), with reductions of ∼25% at 24 h after single doses of 200 mg (40% reduction at nadir, 12 h) and 400 mg (55% reduction at nadir). A sustained reduction in CSF Aβ similar to that observed following a single 200-mg dose was also observed following 28 days of treatment with 100 mg. Phase 2 trials of BMS-708163 in patients with mild to moderate AD as well as prodromal AD are in progress (ClinicalTrials.gov, identifierNCT00890890).

Begacestat (GSI-953), discovered at Wyeth (Mayer et al. 2008; Cole et al. 2009; Pu et al. 2009) and currently undergoing clinical development by Pfizer, represents the third of four Notch-sparing GSIs to have advanced into clinical testing. In preclinical safety models (rat and dog), Begacestat, a 12 nM (IC_{50} for cellular Aβ) approximately 17-fold selective (Aβ < Notch) GSI, manifested histological evidence of slight to mild Notch inhibition-related changes in GI cell populations at doses well above the therapeutic dose (Martone et al. 2009). In man, target inhibition by begacestat was evidenced by a dose-dependent, transient (from 1 to 4 h postdose) reduction of plasma Aβ in healthy volunteers following a single dose at doses between 10 and 600 mg (Martone et al. 2009). The current status of clinical development of begacestat is not publicly known. ELND006, a fourth APP-selective GSI, was progressed into clinical development by Elan Pharmaceuticals. The compound was well tolerated in single-dose studies ranging from 3 to 100 mg in healthy volunteers, with a typical dose-dependent initial decrease followed by rebound above baseline of plasma Aβ (Liang et al. 2011a). A dose-limiting liver toxicity with ELND006 was observed at 30 mg following a daily 21-d oral dosing study investigating a range of daily doses between 3 and 30 mg. In this multidose study, Aβ1−x in plasma was reduced by 27% at 5 h after the last dose in the 30 mg cohort, whereas CSF Aβ1−x showed a linear dose-responsive decrease of ∼10% at 3 mg to ∼38% at 30 mg (Liang et al. 2011b). Further development of ELND006 has been halted.

BACE Inhibitors

The discovery of soluble Aβ peptide in biological fluids (Haass et al. 1992; Seubert et al. 1992) consistent with the constitutive processing of APP was followed by a nearly decade-long effort to molecularly identify the responsible enzyme. The simultaneous reports of cloning BACE1 (β-site APP cleaving enzyme) and its closely related homolog, BACE2, by a variety of approaches (Hussain et al. 1999, 2000; Saunders et al. 1999; Sinha et al. 1999; Vassar et al. 1999; Yan et al. 1999; Acquati et al. 2000; Bennett et al. 2000; Lin et al. 2000) delivered the second molecular target for discovery of drugs to inhibit amyloid production. Knockout mouse models provided in vivo validation of the long-suspected pivotal role for β-secretase in Aβ production and the apparent safety of this target based on the relatively benign phenotype of BACE1-deficient mice (Cai et al. 2001; Luo et al. 2001, 2003; Roberds et al. 2001). Beneficial effects of BACE inhibition modeled in knockout (KO) mice for rescuing Aβ-driven cholinergic dysfunction (Ohno et al. 2004) and memory deficits (Ohno et al. 2006) in APP transgenic mice were also reported. Subsequent characterization of BACE1, as well as BACE1/BACE2 double KO mice, however, revealed roles for this enzyme in cellular pathways involved in myelination and behavior (Harrison et al. 2003; Dominguez et al. 2005; Laird et al. 2005; Hu et al. 2006; Willem et al. 2006; Kobayashi et al. 2008; Savonenko et al. 2008). In addition, the appreciation of an expanded list of BACE1 substrates beyond APP (Kitazume et al. 2001, 2005; Lichtenthaler et al. 2003; Wong et al. 2005; Spoelgen et al. 2006; Kuhn et al. 2007; Woodard-Grice et al. 2008; Hemming et al. 2009; Kihara et al. 2010), many of which are consistent with in vivo phenotypes observed in BACE1-deficient mice, serve as cautionary notes regarding potential safety issues associated with BACE1 inhibitors. Delayed onset of AD pathology in APP × BACE1$^{+/-}$ mice suggest that, as with GSIs, partial inhibition of BACE1 may be a solution toward mitigating the potential safety issues associated with inhibiting this protease (Laird et al. 2005; McConlogue et al. 2007).

The reports of BACE1 cloning were followed in rapid succession by solution of the X-ray crystal structure of BACE1 in complex with a peptidic inhibitor (Hong et al. 2000), and provided a barometer of the industry-wide rational design-based approaches that were in progress to discover potent small molecule inhibitors. The crystal structure illuminated the challenge that lay ahead: reducing the peptidic inhibitor observed in the long substrate-binding grove of BACE1 into a CNS-active small (MW < 500) molecule with favorable drug-like properties. Furthermore, selectivity for inhibition of BACE1 over related aspartyl proteases, such as BACE2 and cathepsin-D, was an additional constraint imposed on potential clinical candidates, in light of the antagonistic amyloidogenic activity of BACE2 (Farzan et al. 2000; Yan et al. 2001; Fluhrer et al. 2002; Basi et al. 2003) and the essential role of cathepsin-D in lysosomal function (Saftig et al. 1996; Benes et al. 2008). The interested reader is directed to expert medicinal chemistry reviews for structure–activity relationship studies toward the objectives

of CNS-active, BACE1-selective, drug-like inhibitors (Hussain 2004; Thompson et al. 2005; Durham and Shepherd 2006; John 2006; Ziora et al. 2006; Ghosh et al. 2008; Silvestri 2008; Hamada and Kiso 2009; Stachel 2009). Incompatibility between MW constraints (imposed by potency requirements) and size (for CNS permeability) have proven to be significant challenges in overcoming the p-gylcoprotein-mediated efflux of BACE1 inhibitors from the CNS and has slowed advancement into the clinic of the many research efforts that were launched to discover and develop BACE inhibitors for treatment of AD. Nevertheless, progress to the clinic has been achieved, with several entrants from the pharmaceutical industry believed to be in or near the clinic, and some known examples are detailed below.

Whereas most investigators focused on solving the molecular weight versus potency and selectivity requirements of a BACE1 inhibitor using an iterative rational design approach combining medicinal chemistry and structural elucidation of inhibitor:BACE1 cocrystals, Chang et al. (2004) reported in vivo activity with a cell-penetrant carrier peptide conjugated to a potent peptidic isostere inhibitor. Their result provided a short cut around the limiting chemical properties and a path to clinical development by Comentis of an otherwise CNS incompatible molecule (reviewed in Ghosh et al. 2008). Thus, CTS-21166, arising from collaboration between the Ghosh group at University of Illinois, Chicago, and the Tang group at Oklahoma Medical Research Foundation, is in clinical development for AD at Comentis. Very little has been published on this molecule, and it is unclear if CTS-21116 is still in clinical development today.

As ongoing optimization of leads from rational design-based approaches continues, investigators from Eli Lilly have reported preclinical and clinical findings with a novel BACE inhibitor, LY2811376 (MW 320), discovered and optimized from a fragment-based approach (Boggs et al. 2010; May et al. 2010). The relatively modest in vitro potency of LY2811376 (~100 nM in primary neuronal cultures, 250 nM in a FRET in vitro BACE assay, and 300 nM in HEK293 cells), combined with ~10-fold selectivity over BACE2 and ~60-fold selectivity over cathepsin-D, delivered robust in vivo efficacy at relatively low doses. Dose-responsive and concordant acute reduction of cortical sAPPβ (lowered 33%–43%), C99 (lowered 56%–78%), and Aβ1–x (lowered 47%–68%) were observed following oral gavage of PDAPP mice with 10, 30, or 100 mg/kg LY2811476. A single oral dose of 10 mg produced a sustained effect on these same biomarkers in CSF, plasma, and hippocampus of PDAPP mice for 6–9 h, with a nonsignificant transient elevation of sAPPα in CSF at 3 h. In beagle dogs, a dose-related reduction in plasma Aβ was achieved following single oral doses of 0.5–5 mg/kg, followed by a gradual return to baseline over 36–48 h without a rebound above baseline (as seen with GSIs). Also in dogs, CSF Aβ1–x and Aβ1–42 were reduced from 3 to 24 h following a single oral dose of 5 mg/kg, with return to baseline by 48 h (May et al. 2010). The safety, pharmacokinetics, and pharmacodynamics of LY2811476 were studied in phase 1 single ascending dose (SAD) and a 14-d multiple ascending dose (MAD) studies investigating 10 and 25 mg doses in healthy volunteers (Martenyi et al. 2010). LY2811476 was generally safe and well tolerated in single-dose studies ranging between 5 and 90 mg. Treatment-emergent adverse events were mostly mild and manageable, with no clinically meaningful changes in vital signs or bioanalytes. In the SAD study, LY2811476 demonstrated dose-related increases in C_{max} and exposure, with a terminal $t_{1/2} > 24$ h. The $t_{1/2}$ based on two cohorts dosed in the MAD study was 66–81 h for the two doses (10 and 25 mg). Dose-dependent pharmacodynamic effects on Aβ in plasma ranging between 45% and 82% reduction at nadir (6–8 h postdose) were observed in individuals treated with 15–90 mg LY2811476, with sustained reduction at 120 h postdose and no rebound above baseline during this time period. In the 14-d MAD study, reduction of plasma Aβ1–40 reached steady state with 1 wk of daily dosing of both 10 and 25 mg. Similar dose-related biomarker changes in CSF (monitored via an indwelling catheter)

of Aβ species (reduction of Aβ1–40, 1–42) and APP metabolite (elevation in sAPPα and reduction in sAPPβ) were observed in the 30 and 90 mg cohorts of the SAD study at 36 h post- versus 4 h predose. Unfortunately, despite these encouraging biomarker effects, further clinical development of LY2811376 has been discontinued owing to preclinical toxicity, the nature of which as not yet been disclosed (Martenyi et al. 2010).

Summary and Prospects for β- and γ-Secretase Inhibitors

Inhibiting Aβ generation as a strategy for AD therapy has been a productive avenue of research. The key proteases mediating production of Aβ from APP, BACE1, and γ-secretase have been identified at the molecular level, and their study has revealed novel biology and mechanistic insights into the unique catalytic activities carried out by each enzyme. However, progress toward inhibiting their activity in man and achieving lowered Aβ production in AD patients remains an unrealized objective. The challenges associated with this ultimate objective have been detailed above, and future progress will benefit from rapid and timely dissemination of preclinical and clinical data associated with inhibition of each target, to the ultimate benefit of patients and family members affected. The emerging consensus for earlier treatment (Aisen et al. 2011; Golde et al. 2011) emphasizes the need for safer therapies, earlier diagnosis, and the further validation of preclinical biomarkers predictive of clinical conversion to AD. In the case of γ-secretase, research into the mechanism of activity of this enzyme suggests more potent cleavage site modulators (Kounnas et al. 2010) or perhaps subunit-selective inhibitors (Zhao et al. 2008; Serneels et al. 2009; He et al. 2010) could provide safer drugs for earlier treatment. In the case of BACE1, additional candidates are suspected to be advancing into or through clinical testing based on the patent literature; the publication of clinical findings with these additional BACE1 inhibitors is eagerly awaited. Furthermore, just as the GI toxicity of nonselective

GSIs highlighted the in vivo importance of Notch as a γ-substrate, disclosure of the preclinical toxicity observed with LY2811376 is awaited to better understand the limitations of BACE1 inhibitors. Looking forward, as with diseases such as cancer, hypertension, atherosclerosis, and HIV–AIDS, the treatment of AD will probably be best managed through combinatorial approaches, either multimodal anti-Aβ therapies (e.g., immunotherapy + secretase inhibitor; secretase inhibitor + aggregation inhibitor) or cross-modal (e.g., anti-Aβ + anti-tau).

Overview of Aβ Aggregation and Related Treatment Strategies

With the discovery of Aβ as the core constituent of vascular and plaque depositss (Glenner and Wong 1984), the search for Aβ aggregation inhibitors began. The hypothesis is that disaggregating amyloid plaques and/or preventing Aβ aggregation should have potential therapeutic benefits by reducing the pathology of the disease. Despite the simplicity of the hypothesis, turning this vision into a reality has been daunting. Reasons for the difficulties associated with this therapeutic approach range from biophysical challenges associated with the inherently extremely low energy state of amyloid fibrils to basic understanding of the process of Aβ aggregation. Added to these hurdles is the multitude of challenges associated with the development of orally bioavailable small molecules with the characteristic pharmaceutical qualities required for success.

Despite these difficulties, a number of compounds continue in clinical testing that have the potential to succeed as Aβ aggregation inhibitors. Lessons learned from this effort should prove invaluable for future therapeutic efforts aimed at AD as well as possible treatments for other diseases associated with amyloid formation, which are quite numerous.

The Biophysics of Aβ Aggregation

Amyloid is a generic term describing tissue deposits of an aggregated proteins with the common characteristic of ∼8–10 nm-diameter fibrils composed of polymers of β-pleated sheet conformation that exhibit birefringence under polarized light after staining with the dye Congo red. The β-pleated sheet structure is due to the amino acid backbone and not to the side-chains (R groups), although the latter do play a role in intermediate structures of amyloidogenic proteins prior to amyloid formation and hence are relevant. Although different amyloid fibrils vary somewhat in absolute width and length depending upon the subunit protein in question, they share the common feature of being extremely stable and resistant to disaggregation (Calamai et al. 2005). The stability of these structure in terms of ΔG can be enormous (Calamai et al. 2005). As an example of this stability, amyloid fibrils of Aβ isolated from the brains of patients who died with AD are insoluble to both heat and SDS detergent. It is only with extraordinary measures such as the utilization of highly chaotropic salts (e.g., guanidine HCl) or formic acid that they dissolve into their peptide subunits (Roher et al. 1993).

From a biophysical perspective, fibrillization of Aβ can be easily studied in vitro. At concentrations at or above low micromolar levels, the peptide will form stable fibrils. The kinetics of this process, although variable, are dependent upon the buffer conditions as well as the absolute concentrations of Aβ. The reaction can be easily monitored either by a change in the circular dichroism spectrum owing to the formation of β-pleated sheet-rich assemblies or by the fluorescence of thioflavin, which binds amyloid fibrils and increases as they accumulate. It is important to note that both of these methods provide little or no information about intermediate structures of potential relevance but rather inform the investigator about the final stage of the process, namely amyloid formation. This caveat is extremely important, because unique individual folding steps of diverse peptides must occur for amyloid fibril formation to ultimately take place, and each step can be biophysically unique. The early step is termed the latency phase (Lee et al. 2007). This describes a poorly understood process wherein a small number of amyloidogenic peptides of one type (e.g., Aβ1–42) come together to form tiny nuclei that are subsequently assembled into protofibrils (often ∼4 nm diameter) that will serve as the core of the mature amyloid fibril (∼8 nm). This nucleation step, fortunately for humans, is energetically extremely disfavored under normal circumstances and hence seldom occurs randomly in nature. One can view the process as having a high transition-state energy barrier. There are at least three ways of driving this process forward. One is by increasing the concentration of the amyloidogenic protein. The second is by introducing mutations into the protein that reduce its energy barrier to achieve a misfolded, β-rich conformer that can lead to the initiation of a fibril (Chiti et al. 2003). The third is. . .?

In Vitro Efforts to Identify Aβ Aggregation Inhibitors

A relatively simple approach to follow the fibrillization of Aβ was introduced in the mid-1990s by several groups that involved monitoring the fluorescence of thioflavin T (e.g., Wood et al. 1996). Thioflavin T has enhanced fluorescence when it binds to amyloid fibrils composed of many different amyloidogenic proteins. The precise reasons for this binding are not completely understood but probably have to do with interaction with the β-pleated sheet structure and intercalation into the growing fibrils. This assay ushered in a series of mechanistic publications as well as numerous screens for compounds by both academic and pharmaceutical laboratories. Indeed, proteins, peptides, herbs, natural products and a wide range of small molecules of both known and unknown activities have been shown to block Aβ fibrillization (see Table 1 and Lorenzo and Yankner 1994; Tomiyama et al. 1994; Bronfman et al. 1996; Higaki et al. 1997; Kihara et al. 1999; Reixach et al. 2000; Thomas et al. 2001; Ono et al. 2002, 2004; Khurana et al. 2003; Blanchard et al. 2004; Hirohata et al. 2005; Fujiwara et al. 2006; Kokkoni et al. 2006; Durairajan et al. 2008; Ryu et al. 2008; Wiesehan et al. 2008; Hong et al. 2009; Rodriguez-Rodriguez et al. 2009). The list of agents is clearly very diverse. Despite this structural diversity, there are some general properties shared by many of the compounds or small molecules that have been identified to inhibit Aβ fibrillization. First, their potency is typically low, with inhibitory activity seen only in the micromolar range. This suggested that stoichiometric amounts of these inhibitors were required to block Aβ fibrillization. Second, with only a few exceptions, these compounds are symmetrical and often planar, with large ring structures. Taken together, these facts have made them difficult starting points for classic medicinal chemistry lead optimization. As a second-tier experimental follow-up to in vitro aggregation assays such as with thioflavin T, a number of these putative Aβ aggregation inhibitors were tested in cellular assays of Aβ neurotoxicity to see if they could effectively block the biological effects. Some of the early compounds were indeed effective, although generally at micromolar concentrations (Blanchard et al. 2004), again making them difficult to progress toward in vivo drug studies. Despite these drawbacks, a few of the early compounds were pursued as far as animal testing in APP transgenic mice to examine whether they would have an effect on plaque burden. Unfortunately, all but a very few were not effective in reducing or retarding plaque pathology (Fig. 5; Yang et al. 2005). As a result of the largely negative outcome of these studies, the general approach of identifying useful Aβ aggregation inhibitors via thioflavin screens has fallen out of favor.

Research to better understand all aspects of the biophysics of amyloid formation of multiple proteins has progressed in the past 10 years in several directions. Most importantly, a more complete understanding of fibril formation and factors involved in the process began to emerge from the use of NMR analyses and calorimetric approaches. The conceptualization of intermediate structures, in particular, led to a refinement of hypotheses and models regarding amyloid formation in general (Lashuel et al. 2002). One significant step forward was the development of a model with high predictive value by Dobson and colleagues (Chiti et al. 2003). This model proposed that the likelihood of a given protein or peptide to form amyloid was dependent upon its charge, hydrophibicity,

A

Aβ immunized
PDAPP mice

B

AN 1792
(Aβ) immunized
patients

C

Passive anti-
Aβ treated
patient

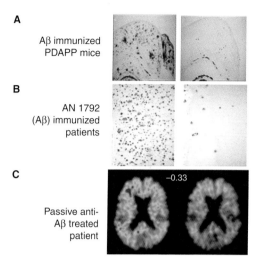

Figure 5. Reduction of Aβ plaque pathology by Aβ immunotherapy in mouse APP transgenic mice and patients suffering from Alzheimer disease. The *left* panel in each image illustrates amyloid pathology in control (*A*), in reference (*B*), or at a baseline (*C*) and the *right* panel in each image illustrates amyloid pathology following immunotherapy. (*A*) Mice immunized with full-length Aβ peptide at mid-age (when plaques are already present) 6 months later show an actual reduction in plaque burden relative to vehicle-treated controls. (From Schenk et al. 1999; reprinted with permission from the author.) (*B*) Patients who were immunized with AN 1792 (full-length Aβ peptide) from a phase 1 study who eventually died and went to autopsy exhibited low levels of absence of Aβ plaques. (Modified from Nicoll et al. 2006; reprinted with permission from the author.) (*C*) Living patients from a phase 2 study treated with bapinuezumab (a humanized monoclonal antibody directed to the amino-terminal region of Aβ) showed a reduced level of PET-PIB (positron-emission tomography-Pittsburgh compound B) retention following treatment, suggesting reduced Aβ plaque burden. (From Rinne et al. 2010; reprinted with permission from the author.)

and β-pleated sheet propensity. Testing of the model by insertion of novel amino acids to increase or decrease the kinetics of amyloid fibril formation was highly predictive. In addition, the model also predicted that a number of known pathogenic mutations in Aβ and other amyloid-forming proteins potentially did so by this mechanism. This concept, together with that of intermediate energy states predisposing

to amyloid formation, has changed our current thinking of how proteins become amyloidogenic. Specifically, rather than a few proteins with the capability of forming amyloid in our genome, an alternative view is that nearly all proteins can do so under the appropriate circumstances (Dobson 2003). The idea is that most proteins avoid amyloidogenesis by either never reaching high enough monomer concentrations or have a sufficiently high-energy barrier that amyloid formation is extraordinarily unlikely to occur. The inverse of this concept is that if unusual, adverse environments or circumstances exist, amyloid can form as a consequence.

With these new concepts in mind, alternative ideas and thoughts have arisen about what steps an inhibitor of fibrillization might be able to interfere with. For example, an inhibitor might be able to bind to or stabilize a nonamyloid form of Aβ, representing an intermediate, and in this way indirectly block fibril formation (Liu et al. 2006). Less binding stability of such an inhibitor would be required, because it would not be required to block an extremely highly favored forward reaction of fibril formation in the presence of micromolar levels of Aβ and thioflavin, as had been previously attempted. This general approach and insight has led to a renewed interest and effort in attempts to indirectly block Aβ aggregation—both in vitro and in vivo.

Animal Studies Exploring Aβ Aggregation Inhibitors

Tramiposate is an example of a small molecule that blocks Aβ fibrillization experimentally and was ultimately pursued both in animal models and through large-scale pivotal clinical trials in mild to moderate AD. Tramiposate is a derivative of proprionic acid and is thus nonsymmetrical and small. Biophysically, it is capable of blocking Aβ aggregation and fibrillization effectively at low micromolar concentrations. Whereas the exact form of Aβ that tramiposate interacts with is not known (Gervais et al. 2007), it is likely to be an oligomeric or protofibrillar form of the peptide. The consequence is that fibrils of the peptide are inhibited from forming in the presence of the compound. Atomic force microscopy also suggests that small, globular forms of the peptide are stabilized in its presence (Gervais et al. 2007). The compound was tested in APP transgenic mice to see if it would have any effects on Aβ plaque burden. Results from this study suggested that it does reduce amyloid burden in Tg2576 mice by about 50%, reaching statistical significance. In addition to these effects, the compound also reduced other Aβ-related pathologies in these mice (Gervais et al. 2007).

Recently, animal evidence for another molecule has suggested its potential role in blocking Aβ fibrillization and promoting its decrease in brain. In the early 1990s, McLaurin and colleagues at the Univerisity of Toronto became interested in the possibility that Aβ might interact with phospholipid moieties (McLaurin and Chakrabartty 1996). This work led to several publications that suggested that a key manipulable interaction might involve Aβ binding to inositol (McLaurin et al. 1998, 2000; Fung et al. 2005). Inositol exists in multiple isoforms biologically with the most common form being *myo*-inositol, a precursor used by all cells for a variety of other organic molecules. Notably, it was shown that *scyllo*-inositol but not most other inositol stereoisomers were very effective in blocking Aβ aggregation and fibrillization via a number of independent approaches. These findings led to a key series of experiments which demonstrated that *scyllo*-inositol, in particular, is effective in reducing amyloid burden and improving behavior and survival in the TgCRND8 transgenic mouse model (McLaurin et al. 2006). One interesting feature of the inositols is that they are actively taken up by glucose transporters at the blood–brain barrier, suggesting that, unlike many compounds emerging from medicinal chemistry, they can achieve relatively high concentrations within the brain following peripheral administration. At the neuronal level, *scyllo*-inositol has been demonstrated to prevent the inhibition of hippocampal LTP caused by cell-secreted oligomers of Aβ (Townsend et al. 2006a). This finding suggests that its mode of action is to impede or block the toxicity of oligomers—thought to be key neurotoxic forms of Aβ in the brain.

Clinical Studies Investigating Aβ Aggregation Inhibitors

As a result of the above findings, tramiposate entered phase 1 and 2 trials for mild to moderate AD. These studies showed that the agent was well tolerated and had a good safety profile that supported further clinical development. Exploratory clinical end points were also examined in the phase 2 study (Aisen et al. 2006). Although none of the prespecified endpoints demonstrated benefit, some secondary analyses suggested the possibility of improvement in some subgroups. The effects of tramiposate on CSF Aβ levels were also investigated; the compound appeared to increase CSF Aβ, although very modestly. Pharmacokinetic studies suggested that, whereas the compound could be found in the CSF of treated patients, the amounts were below those required to block Aβ fibrillization in vitro. Taken together, these findings resulted in tramiposate entering large phase 3 pivotal trials. Ultimately, the agent did not meet its primary end points of improvement in the ADAS-COG or Clinical Global Impression of Change. Although the study was not published, it was observed by the company that there was very high variability among the clinical sites in terms of extent of decline of patient groups, which resulted in higher than expected variance in the placebo group decline. No changes in biomarkers were described as a result of treatment. Unfortunately, because of the lack of change in biomarkers, the interpretation of the negative findings from the tramiposate phase 3 study are not interpretable. Did the compound even reach its brain target of Aβ in sufficient concentrations to have an effect? If it did, was it pharmacologically ineffective? Or was it potentially effective but the variance of the population was so great that this masked its benefits? This example of the inability to interpret the results of putatively disease-modifying agents emphasizes the critical requirement for biomarkers in all AD clinical trials. The need is twofold: first, for biomarkers that provide information on whether a given agent has reached its target and had the predicted molecular effect; second, for biomarkers that provide information on whether a downstream feature of the disease was affected. Without these types of data, clinical studies entailing enormous patient effort and risk, to say nothing of time and cost, are expended without any significant provision of knowledge and insight.

Based upon the preclinical studies reviewed in the previous section, *scyllo*-inositol appeared to be a reasonable candidate for clinical investigation of the effects of an Aβ aggregation inhibitor in mild to moderate AD. Multiple phase 1 studies were conducted, and the compound was found to be reasonably safe and well tolerated. These studies resulted in a phase 2 trial that was recently completed under the sponsorship of Elan Pharmaceuticals and Transition Therapeutics; it examined safety, tolerability and possible efficacy of three doses (0.25, 1, or 2 g b.i.d.) of ELND005 (*scyllo*-inositol) over an 18 month period. The study was amended by the sponsors to limit the active arm to only the 0.25 g b.i.d. dose, owing to possible safety and tolerability issues of the two higher doses. This amendment indicates that *scyllo*-inositol, like most investigational molecules, will need to be thoroughly tested clinically before a clear safety profile can be fully established. The 18 month study was completed in mid-2010 (Salloway et al. 2009).

Future Efforts for Aβ Aggregation Inhibitors

Aside from *scyllo*-inositol, few other molecules that block Aβ aggregation are currently in clinical development. From the perspective of medical hypothesis testing, because the molecule appears to capable of neutralizing Aβ oligomers cytotoxicity, if enough compound enters the brain, it will be a good test of whether toxic oligomers play a role in the clinical manifestations of AD. This is critical because, to date, almost all findings about Aβ oligomers are either in tissue culture or involve mouse models.

In summary, although antiaggregation is an intuitively logical target for neutralizing the effects of amyloid plaques and Aβ oligomer toxicity, only two such agents have progressed to advanced clinical testing in AD patients. Of these, one has failed in pivotal clinical trials for less than clear reasons, and the data for the second are in press at this writing. Nevertheless, our improved understanding of the biophysics and biology of Aβ fibrillization is likely to identify additional molecules worthy of human testing in the future.

Aβ IMMUNOTHERAPY

Crossing the blood–brain barrier remains one of the major obstacles in CNS drug discovery and has historically limited our efforts to targets amenable to medicinal chemistry-driven, small molecule drug discovery. The blood–brain barrier cannot, however, be solely blamed for this small molecule-centric view, and with hindsight, more thought was needed (and indeed is still needed) to be applied to non-small-molecule platforms, whether they be antibody-, peptide-, vaccine-, cell-, or oligonucleotide-based. In 1999, work from Schenk and colleagues at Elan Pharmaceuticals spurred this area of discovery with a potentially transformational approach. These investigators reported striking results following immunization of PDAPP transgenic mice with an intraperitoneal injection of aggregated Aβ once a month for nearly a year (Schenk et al. 1999). This immunization with Aβ1–42 peptide, subsequently referred to as "active immunization," generated a polyclonal antibody response to Aβ, resulting in significantly reduced amyloid plaque burden, neuritic dystrophy and associated inflammatory changes in the brains of these animals, even when active immunization was started in older animals with pre-existing amyloid pathology. These unexpected findings have since been replicated in hundreds of reports, expanding both our understanding of potential mechanisms and the biological responses that result. Importantly, this work has also spurred a new field of "active" and "passive" immunotherapy for neurodegenerative diseases aimed at slowing or perhaps even arresting the neurodegenerative process (Schenk 2002; Pangalos et al. 2005).

Preclinical Observations

Following the seminal 1999 paper on active Aβ immunization, the same group first demonstrated that one could circumvent the immune response (i.e., not rely on the animal's ability to generate anti-Aβ antibodies following active immunization) by direct administration of anti-Aβ antibodies into transgenic APP mice. This "passive immunization" approach was likewise very effective at clearing amyloid plaques and reversing neuritic and glial pathology (Bard et al. 2000), to a degree similar to that seen in the original active peptide immunization. Plaque lowering appeared to be dependent on the antibody being able to recognize and bind aggregated Aβ in the brain, as antibodies unable to bind to amyloid plaques in vitro had no significant impact on plaque pathology in vivo (Bard et al. 2000). It is important to note that immunotherapy has an impact on disease pathology beyond amyloid plaque clearance. Amino-terminal specific anti-Aβ antibodies reduce neuritic dystrophy as early as 4 days after treatment, with beneficial effects lasting for over a month (Lombardo et al. 2003; Brendza et al. 2005). Passive and active immunization have both been reported to reduce early tau hyperphosphorylation and cytopathology (Oddo et al. 2004; Wilcock et al. 2009), supporting human genetic evidence that Aβ pathology lies upstream of the alteration of (invariably wild-type) tau in AD. The benefits of immunotherapy on cognition in preclinical models have also been repeated in many studies since the original observations on this aspect (Janus et al. 2000; Morgan et al. 2000). Active and passive immunization which targets amino-terminal and central domains of Aβ have dramatically and sometimes very rapidly improved performance in a variety of cognition assays independent of plaque clearance, suggesting that mechanisms such as sequestration of toxic soluble Aβ species may be critical for improving behavioral deficits observed in transgenic mouse models of AD (Dodart et al. 2002; Kotilinek et al. 2002; Sigurdsson et al. 2004). Both approaches also rescue the abnormal hippocampal synaptic plasticity that occurs in rodents exposed to soluble Aβ oligomers (Klyubin et al. 2005).

Alternative modalities and routes of administration have also been investigated following the first active and passive immunotherapy studies. Intranasal administration of Aβ in a mouse model of AD significantly lowered Aβ and realted cytopathology in the mouse brain (Weiner et al. 2000; Leverone et al. 2003), and others have effectively treated mice with Aβ sequences either using phage display or expressed on adeno-associated virus (Zhang et al. 2003; Lavie et al. 2004). Irrespective of the approach taken, results have consistently demonstrated that active and passive immunization strategies, targeting specific sequences within the Aβ peptide, are able to slow or reverse disease pathology and reverse memory deficits in preclinical models of AD.

Potential Mechanisms of Action

There is generally good agreement as to the preclinical effectiveness of both active and passive immunization approaches in APP transgenic mice. In contrast, the precise mechanism(s) by which anti-Aβ antibodies elicit their beneficial effects in rodents are less well understood and ardently debated. Early mouse immunization studies reported a decrease in MAC-1 (CD11b) positive activated microglia around amyloid plaques but an increase in MHC class II cells associated with punctate Aβ staining around the walls or lumens of blood vessels. These cells phenotypically resembled activated microglia or monocytes (Schenk et al. 1999). Subsequent ex vivo experiments showed that microglia bound to and phagocytosed amyloid plaques decorated with anti-Aβ antibodies in an Fc-dependent manner. Furthermore, microglial-mediated phagocytosis of plaques required antibody binding to the amyloid plaque itself rather than to fibrillar or oligomeric Aβ species (Bard et al. 2000; Wilcock et al. 2003, 2004). Therefore, one proposed mechanism of action is that anti-Aβ antibodies enter the brain following treatment with either an active or passive immunization protocol, bind to parenchymal plaque-bound Aβ and recruit phagocytosing microglia via their cell surface expressed Fc-receptors. However, in contrast to these data, some studies have reported that amyloid plaque clearance can occur in a non-Fc-dependent manner. Anti-Aβ F(ab′)$_2$ fragments, that is, lacking an Fc-region, rapidly cleared amyloid plaques in vivo in a manner indistinguishable from the parental full-length antibody (Bacskai et al. 2002). In addition, two studies have demonstrated that immunotherapy can robustly clear amyloid plaque pathology either when Fc receptors are knocked out (Das et al. 2003) or when microglia have been ablated for four continuous weeks (Grathwohl et al. 2009). These contradictory data suggest at least two mechanisms of amyloid clearance, one that is microglia-dependent and one that is microglia-independent.

A second potential mechanism of action centers on the ability of anti-Aβ antibodies to bind and block the formation and/or neurotoxic activity of soluble Aβ species. This idea is supported by the experiments described above with anti-Aβ F(ab′)$_2$ fragments and suggest that antibodies binding to Aβ can shift an Aβ equilibrium away from more toxic aggregated states to less toxic monomeric states. This is further suggested by in vitro data in which anti-Aβ antibodies blocked the formation of Aβ fibrils and dissolved pre-existing fibrils (Solomon et al. 1997). Subsequent studies identified amino-terminal residues of Aβ (amino acids 3–6 [EFRH]) as the minimally effective epitope for this activity. In support of this, antibodies directed to residues 4–10 of Aβ inhibit decrease both fibril formation and Aβ-mediated neuronal death (McLaurin et al. 2002). More recently, Aβ neutralizing antibodies have been shown to reverse LTP and cognitive deficits by blocking the synaptotoxic activity of soluble Aβ oligomers, including those isolated directly from AD brain (Klyubin et al. 2005; Shankar et al. 2008). Taken together, these findings suggest immunotherapy can have a rapid effect on learning and memory through removal of a variety of soluble toxic Aβ species, independently of any effects on amyloid pathology, at least in APP transgenic models. This concept is consistent with data generated in our and

other laboratories in which treatments with a variety of amyloid-lowering drugs can rapidly and robustly reverse cognitive deficits in the absence of effects on plaque pathology (Comery et al. 2005).

The mechanisms described above would theoretically require anti-Aβ antibodies to enter the CNS. Although studies have demonstrated systemically administered antibodies do cross the blood–brain barrier and decorate a large portion of amyloid plaques, the level of central exposure is very low, with only 0.1%–0.5% of a systemically administered antibody reaching the brain (Bard et al. 2000; Choe et al. 2007). This observation raises questions as to how anti-Aβ immunotherapy has such dramatic and widespread effects in the CNS while antibody levels in the brain remain so low. The amyloid "sink" hypothesis is based on the finding that Aβ is actively transported out of the CNS by the low-density lipoprotein receptor (LRP-1; Deane et al. 2004) and actively pumped into the CNS by the receptor for advanced glycation end products (RAGE; Schmidt et al. 2009), among other mechanisms. These transport mechanisms are thought to keep Aβ in a complex equilibrium between the brain and periphery. Using m266, a high-affinity antibody binding to a central epitope of Aβ, De Mattos and colleagues were able to sequester peripheral pools of Aβ, prevent transport of Aβ back into the brain and shift the Aβ equilibrium to one of net Aβ clearance out of the brain (DeMattos et al. 2001, 2002a,b). Importantly, this antibody is highly specific for soluble Aβ and does not bind well to amyloid plaques. This "peripheral sink" hypothesis is obviously attractive, as it highlights a potential mechanism by which immunotherapy can enhance Aβ clearance without requiring central penetration of peripherally circulating antibodies. More recently, investigators have tried to elucidate the relative contribution of Aβ clearance via the periphery (Vasilevko et al. 2007). They used a transgenic mouse carrying Swedish, Dutch, and Iowa APP mutations. The "DI" Aβ peptide derived from these mice has negligible affinity for the LRP receptor and, as a result, undergoes little active transport across the blood–brain barrier.

Immunotherapy had no effect on parenchymal or vascular amyloid deposition in this mouse model, whereas central administration of antibodies into the brains of these mice produced a rapid and robust clearance of amyloid deposits. These results support a role for the "peripheral sink" hypothesis and suggest that intact Aβ transport mechanisms can enhance antibody-mediated clearance of Aβ. However, whereas some have noted that acute treatment with m266 is able to trap Aβ in the periphery and acutely reverse cognitive deficits in APP transgenic mice (Dodart et al. 2002), others have shown that chronic treatment with m266 has no impact on cortical plaque pathology (Seubert et al. 2008). Interestingly, a recent report has questioned the "peripheral sink" hypothesis by studying the dynamics and efflux of ^{125}I-labeled Aβ from the CNS and suggesting that peripherally administered m266 sequesters soluble Aβ in the brain, resulting in a reduced rather than enhanced Aβ efflux (Yamada et al. 2009).

At the end of the day, the robustness of the preclinical immunotherapy on Aβ-mediated physiology, behavior, and pathology are strong, and none of the mechanisms described above are mutually exclusive. It is possible and in fact likely that centrally and peripherally mediated effects work in tandem to help lower the levels of toxic Aβ species and, over time, enhance clearance of amyloid plaques in the CNS.

Learning from the First Clinical Trial (of AN1792) and Some Related Concerns

Based on the strong preclinical efficacy data described above and an IND enabling safety studies in mice, rabbits, guinea pigs, and non-human primates, an active immunization trial was initiated in patients using full-length Aβ1–42 in combination with a previously validated adjuvant, QS-21. This therapeutic mixture will be referred to as AN1792 for the remainder of this article. The initial single dose phase 1 trial in 24 patients demonstrated good tolerability, leading to the initiation of a larger, multidose phase 1 study with 64 patients given AN1792 and 16 given the adjuvant alone. Dosing intervals of this active immunization were 0, 4, 12,

and 24 wk. The study drug was reasonably well tolerated with treatment-related adverse events (AEs) reported in 23% of patients, but with no relationship between dose and AE incidence. One patient in the study had developed a meningoencephalitis, diagnosed after death. Approximately 20% of this elderly phase 1 patient population had an initially positive anti-Aβ antibody titer, increasing to nearly 60% with further immunizations. No treatment differences were observed across efficacy measures in this safety trial, apart from less decline on the Disability Assessment of Dementia scores in active versus placebo treated patients (Bayer et al. 2005).

Based on these two small phase 1 trials, a phase 2a trial was initiated in 372 mild to moderate AD patients to better understand the immunogenicity, safety, and tolerability profile of AN1792. The trial was not powered to show a treatment effect on cognitive decline. This trial was terminated early following four reports of acute meningoencephalitis that later were shown to have affected a total of 6% of all the actively immunized patients (18 out of 300; Orgogozo et al. 2003). Sixteen of the 18 patients who developed the sterile meningioencephalitis had received two doses of AN1792, and the median latency from the last injection to symptoms was 40 days. Almost all of the 18 patients who developed clinically diagnosed meningoencephalitis gradually improved to baseline, but at the time of autopsy patients were left with cerebrovascular lesions. Analysis of this interrupted trial (patients received between one and three of the six planned AN1792 immunizations) showed that ~20% of patients developed a good antibody response to Aβ, with no correlation between antibody titter and the development of meningoencephalitis.

The first efficacy report from the phase 2a trial with AN1792 came from a subset-analysis of 30 patients treated in Switzerland, and as the results are based on a single site only, any interpretation should be treated with caution. The data suggested a slowing in cognitive decline, as measured by ADAS-COG and MMSE, particularly in those patients generating the highest antibody titers (Hock et al.

2003). The full analysis of all patients treated in this phase 2a trial were reported in 2005 and yielded quite different results (Gilman et al. 2005). No significant effects were found between antibody responders and placebo groups on a number of exploratory measures of cognition or disability (including ADAS-Cog, Disability Assessment for Dementia [DAD], CDR, or MMSE). However in a nine-component neuropsychological test battery (NTB), antibody responders performed significantly better than placebo-treated patients. Furthermore, improvements in some memory components of the NTB, including immediate and delayed memory, were associated with an increased antibody response, suggesting a possible dose-dependent effect of the treatment. In a subset of patients, CSF tau, a potential measure of neurodegeneration, was significantly decreased in antibody responders compared with placebo treated patients, whereas Aβ42 levels remained unchanged. Volumetric MRI was also used to examine cerebral changes in patients treated with AN1792. Comparison of scans predosing and 12 mo after two or three AN1792 doses demonstrated that antibody responders had greater total brain volume loss, ventricular enlargement, and hippocampal volume loss. This apparent loss in brain and hippocampal volume was not associated with a worsening in cognitive function and indeed an improvement in NTB (Fox et al. 2005). A number of factors could explain this surprising finding. For example, increased removal of amyloid deposits, changes in plaque composition or changes in CSF dynamics resulting from increased Aβ outflow could each alter the water content of the brain, resulting in an apparent loss of brain volume (Fox et al. 2005). Another plausible explanation for this observed loss in brain volume could be an acceleration of neuronal degeneration. However, this is unlikely given that antibody responders with increased volume loss showed less cognitive decline on the NTB, and antibody responders had reduced rather than increased CSF tau (Gilman et al. 2005). Finally, the mean loss of cortical volume could have been related to the development of subclinical meningoencephalitis in some of

the AN1792-treated patients, associated with shifts in brain fluid and electrolyte balance.

Independent neuropathological assessments of trial subjects who died of unrelated causes many months or years after receiving AN1792 has yielded interesting findings. The first patient studied at autopsy came from the multidose phase 1 trial and was found to have had meningoencephalitis as detected by CD^{4+} T-cell infiltrates in the leptomeninges, most densely associated with amyloid laden blood vessels, as well as sparse lymphocyte infiltration in the cortex and perivascular spaces (Nicoll et al. 2003). Interestingly, however, there were areas of the neocortex with significant evidence of plaque removal, reduced neuritic dystrophy and reduced astrocyte clusters. Furthermore, in some areas devoid of amyloid deposits, there was evidence of Aβ immunoreactivity in microglia (Nicoll et al. 2003), resembling the microglial staining seen in preclinical mouse experiments. A second report of an AN1792-treated patient with meningoencephalitis also highlighted a decrease in diffuse and neuritic plaques with accompanying activated microglia immunoreactive for Aβ surrounding small "collapsed" plaques (Ferrer et al. 2004). Interestingly, this decrease in amyloid burden was accompanied by an attenuated local stress response, as measured by reduced levels of stress-activated kinase and c-jun amino-terminal kinase. Both enzymes have been implicated in the hyperphosphorylation of tau, and indeed, collapsed plaques were devoid of phospho-tau immunoreactivity. Finally, there was no apparent reduction in vascular Aβ in this patient, and there were multiple, small cortical hemorrhages that may or may not have been related to the presence of severe small vessel disease (Ferrer et al. 2004). Studies from three more AN1972 recipients examined at autopsy, two with meningoencephalitis and one without, corroborated the findings reported by Nicoll et al. and Ferrer et al. and highlight that cortical amyloid plaque pathology can be reduced following Aβ vaccination in the absence of meningoencephalitis (Masliah et al. 2005; Patton et al. 2006b). A more detailed analysis focusing on the cerebrovasculature of nine patients who died between 4 months and 5 years after their first AN1792 immunization showed that treated patients had significantly more Aβ40 and Aβ42 in their blood vessels and a higher density of cortical microhemorrhages (Boche et al. 2008). However, it should be noted that two of the longest survivors had an almost complete absence of vascular Aβ. This finding is consistent with a hypothesis in which Aβ immunization results in solublization of amyloid plaques and exit of Aβ via the perivascular space, leading to a transient increase in cerebrovascular Aβ that is ultimately cleared over time (Boche et al. 2008). Finally, immunohistochemistry of the Aβ species cleared from the brains of patients treated with AN1792 revealed that all major species were impacted (Aβ40, Aβ42, and amino-terminally truncated Aβ species; Nicoll et al. 2006; Patton et al. 2006a).

Long-term follow-up of 129 patients from the phase 2a trial at a mean of 4.6 yr after their AN1792 immunization revealed that numerous patients previously classified as antibody responders still had a low but detectable anti-Aβ antibody titer. Overall, the responder group had significantly less decline as measured on DAD and dependency scales. In addition, MRI brain volume measures now identified no differences between AN1792 and placebo-treated patients, in contrast to the original phase 2 trial findings reported by Fox and colleagues in 2005 (Vellas et al. 2009). In contrast to the above findings, a study of a subset of 15 U.K. patients treated with AN1792 followed to autopsy suggested continued disease progression and cognitive decline. In eight of these progressing subjects who were autopsied, two showed no apparent decrease in plaque burden, four had intermediate decreases, and two had marked decreases (Holmes et al. 2008). Although all AN1792 follow-up studies have shown variable reductions in amyloid plaque burden, data from these long-term follow-up studies reporting cognitive end points need to be treated with care. The phase 2 AN1792 study was halted early with most patients receiving only one or two doses of study drug and most never reaching an optimal or sustained anti-Aβ antibody titer.

Two of the major adverse events observed in the trials with AN1792 were meningoencephalitis and cerebral microhemorrhage. Examination of some of the encephalitis cases postmortem revealed a marked CD^{4+} T-cell infiltration suggestive of a T-cell response to Aβ (Nicoll et al. 2003; Ferrer et al. 2004; Masliah et al. 2005). The principal T-cell epitopes on Aβ have been mapped to its carboxyl terminus (Glaser et al. 1998; Monsonego et al. 2003) and can therefore be avoided by immunizing with Aβ sequences devoid of these T-cell epitopes in the next generation of active vaccines. Currently, a number of newer vaccines employing only a fragment of Aβ peptide to circumvent a T-cell response are in clinical development. Thus far, by employing this new strategy, no new reports from these follow-on vaccines of meningoencephalitis have been reported. Concerns have also been raised about the potential for active and passive immunotherapy to cause microhemorrhages, an event that has been reported to occur in AD patients as part of the natural history of the disease (Yates et al. 2011). Some efforts have been made to model these events in APP transgenic mice, although the results have been variable. Passive immunizations with antibodies recognizing a variety of Aβ epitopes in transgenic APP mice with CAA have resulted in an increased incidence of CAA-associated microhemorrhages (Pfeifer et al. 2002; Wilcock et al. 2004; Racke et al. 2005). The implications of these mouse findings remain unclear given that the doses of antibody used were sometimes high and the animals had very severe and pre-existing cerebral amyloid angiopathy. Furthermore, these findings have not been observed by others in clinical trials to date (Goni and Sigurdsson 2005).

Current Clinical Approaches to Immunotherapy

Passive Immunization

Although active immunization produces an oligoclonal response and is more convenient to administer, passive immunotherapy using humanized monoclonal anti-Aβ antibodies confers the potential advantage of being easier to stop should serious adverse events be observed during the course of a clinical trial. Two humanized monoclonal antibodies, bapineuzumab and LY2062430, are currently in late-stage clinical development in large multinational trials. Bapineuzumab is an amino-terminal specific antibody derived from the murine monoclonal antibody 3D6. 3D6 has been reported to enhance the clearance of amyloid plaques and significantly reduce total levels of brain Aβ, inflammation, neuritic dystrophy, and synapse loss in the brains of APP transgenic mice (Bard et al. 2000). LY2062430, which is derived from the murine antibody m266, is specific to amino acids 16–24 of Aβ. m266 has been shown to lower brain Aβ levels in the CNS, although there are conflicting data in regard to its ability to clear amyloid pathology from the brains of APP transgenic animals (DeMattos et al. 2001; Seubert et al. 2008). Both antibodies have been reported to acutely reverse memory deficits in APP transgenic mice, with m266 appearing more potent than 3D6 perhaps owing to its preferential binding to soluble Aβ species.

A 234 patient, phase 2a safety and tolerability trial with bapineuzumab has recently been reported. Patients were randomly assigned one of four bapineuzumab doses (0.15, 0.5, 1.0, or 2.0 mg/kg), with intravenous infusions spaced 13 wk apart and final patient assessment completed at week 78. No significant differences were found in primary efficacy endpoints, although post-hoc analyses suggested some cognitive and functional benefit in treatment completers and in non-ApoE4 carriers. No significant decreases were observed in exploratory biomarkers. MRI analyses showed no treatment differences in brain or ventricular volume and CSF Aβx-42 and total tau remained unchanged but with a trend toward decreased phopho-tau181 (Salloway et al. 2009). Twenty-eight patients in a separate phase 2 trail of bapineuzimab were assessed for cortical amyloid load using the ^{11}C-PiB PET tracer (19 patients were on study drug and seven on placebo). Treatment with bapineuzumab for 78 wk significantly reduced PiB retention across cortical brain areas compared with the patients' baseline

scans and to placebo. Patients on babpineuzumab had a decrease in PiB retention of 8.5% compared with an increase in PiB retention of 16.9% with placebo, suggesting that bapineuzumab can reduce cortical fibrillar Aβ by ∼25% over a 78-wk period (Rinne et al. 2010). These data are critically important, as they help establish that the ongoing phase 3 bapineuzumab trials will test whether amyloid plaque reduction over 78 wk has any impact on cognitive decline or disease progression in mild to moderate AD patients. The rate of AEs was higher for bapineuzumab than placebo at respective means of 7.5 events compared with 5.7 events, with more than 90% of AEs being mild to moderate in severity. Vasogenic edema (VE) was the only dose-dependent AE and was detected by brain MRI in 10% of treated patients (12/124) versus no placebo patients. VE incidence increased with dose (3.2% for 0.15 mg/kg compared with 26.7% for 2.0 mg/kg) and with ApoE4 gene dose (4.3% with no copies of ApoE4 compared with 33.3% with two copies of ApoE4; Salloway et al. 2009).

Data from clinical trials with LY2062430 patients have yet to be published, but recent data from the initial clinical trials has been orally presented by Ron DeMattos and Eric Siemers (http://www.quintiles.com/information-library/videos/icad-eric-siemers/). In a phase 2a trial, four doses of antibody were tested in patients with mild to moderate AD, with approximately 10 patients per dose arm (100 mg/wk, 400 mg/wk, 100 mg every 4 wk, and 400 mg every 4 wk). None of the 42 treated patients showed any evidence of VEs, microhemorrhage or inflammation, and four patients showed antibody titers against the LY2062430 antibody, although these did not appear to be neutralizing antibodies. Plasma and CSF Aβ levels were significantly elevated, and 0.1% of the antibody was detected in the CSF. No changes were reported in CSF tau. Interestingly, levels of free and unbound CSF Aβ40 appeared to go down, whereas free and unbound Aβ42 increased with rising antibody doses. These changes were suggested to reflect a "leaching" from the brain of plaque bound Aβ42. In addition, data were presented suggesting that amino-terminally truncated fragments of Aβ, probably derived from the brain, were also increased in the CSF following drug treatment. Two additional monoclonal antibodies, GSK933776A (GSK) and gantenerumab (Roche), are in early development, but no data are available in the public domain reporting clinical findings.

Another approach currently in mid-stage development and somewhat related to passive immunotherapy is infusion of intravenous immunoglobulin (IVIg) antibody, an FDA-approved purified immunoglobulin pool from normal donors used for the treatment of inflammatory diseases. In a small seven-patient study of mild to moderate AD patients, IVIg infusions once a month for 6 months resulted in increased plasma levels of Aβ and an improvement in cognitive function. These results mirror a previous report in five AD patients treated with IVIg in which decreased CSF Aβ and increased peripheral Aβ were observed. The latter study also reported stabilization of cognitive decline but no improvement (Dodel et al. 2004).

Active Immunization

Following on from the original AN1792 active immunization trial, three clinical trials are currently testing active immunization in mild to moderate AD patients. ACC-001 is a novel immunoconjugate being developed by Pfizer (formerly Wyeth) and Janssen AIP (J&J and Elan) that links an amino-terminal Aβ fragment to the carrier protein CRM, used for many years in pediatric vaccines such as Prevnar (http://www.theodora.com/drugs/prevnar_for_injection_wyeth.html). CAD-106 is being developed in a collaboration between Novartis and Cytos. Similar to ACC-001, this vaccine is devoid of any Aβ T-cell epitopes and is made up of the first six amino acids of Aβ conjugated to a virus like particle. V950 is an active immunization being developed by Merck, although no information on its design is currently available. Finally, a company called Affiris had developed an Affitope vaccine technology using short six-amino acid peptides that mimic the native Aβ sequence.

THE FUTURE: OPPORTUNITIES AND CHALLENGES

As active and passive immunization approaches continue to bring together investigators from two of the most complex and incompletely understood fields of science, neuroscience and immunology, there is real hope that further improvements to our mechanistic knowledge of AD will enable the successful clinical implementation of these approaches for the treatment of this devastating neurodegenerative disorder. If a safe and well-tolerated immunization strategy—whether active or passive—can be successfully developed, one can envisage a scenario where improving diagnosis of the disease will allow patients to be treated ever earlier, preventing progression of neuropathology and the development of progressive memory impairment.

ACKNOWLEDGMENTS

The authors wish to thank Dr. Patrick L. May for graciously sharing results with us prior to publication.

REFERENCES

Acquati F, Accarino M, Nucci C, Fumagalli P, Jovine L, Ottolenghi S, Taramelli R. 2000. The gene encoding DRAP (BACE2), a glycosylated transmembrane protein of the aspartic protease family, maps to the down critical region. *FEBS Lett* **468:** 59–64.

Aisen PS, Schafer KA, Grundman M, Pfeiffer E, Sano M, Davis KL, Farlow MR, Jin S, Thomas RG, Thal LJ. 2003. Effects of rofecoxib or naproxen vs placebo on Alzheimer disease progression: A randomized controlled trial. *JAMA* **289:** 2819–2826.

Aisen PS, Saumier D, Briand R, Laurin J, Gervais F, Tremblay P, Garceau D. 2006. A Phase II study targeting amyloid-β with 3APS in mild-to-moderate Alzheimer disease. *Neurology* **67:** 1757–1763.

Aisen PS, Andrieu S, Sampaio C, Carrillo M, Khachaturian ZS, Dubois B, Feldman HH, Petersen RC, Siemers E, Doody RS, et al. 2011. Report of the task force on designing clinical trials in early (predementia) AD. *Neurology* **76:** 280–286.

Albright CF, Dockens R, Olson RE, Meredith JE, Siemmon R, Lentz KJW, Denton R, Pilcher G, Zaczek R. 2008. BMS-708163, a potent and selective γ-secretase inhibitor, decreases CSF Ab at safe and tolerable doses in animals, and humans. In *International Conference on Alzheimer's Disease*, 2008, HT-01-05. Alzheimer's Association, Chicago.

Bacskai BJ, Kajdasz ST, McLellan ME, Games D, Seubert P, Schenk D, Hyman BT. 2002. Non-Fc-mediated mechanisms are involved in clearance of amyloid-β in vivo by immunotherapy. *J Neurosci* **22:** 7873–7878.

Bard F, Cannon C, Barbour R, Burke R-L, Games D, Grajeda H, Guido T, Hu K, Huang J, Johnson-Wood K, et al. 2000. Peripherally administered antibodies against amyloid β-peptide enter the central nervous system and reduce pathology in a mouse model of Alzheimer disease. *Nat Med* **6:** 916–919.

Barten DM, Guss VL, Corsa JA, Loo A, Hansel SB, Zheng M, Munoz B, Srinivasan K, Wang B, Robertson BJ, et al. 2005. Dynamics of β-amyloid reductions in brain, cerebrospinal fluid, and plasma of β-amyloid precursor protein transgenic mice treated with a γ-secretase inhibitor. *J Pharmacol Exp Ther* **312:** 635–643.

Basi G, Frigon N, Barbour R, Doan T, Gordon G, McConlogue L, Sinha S, Zeller M. 2003. Antagonistic effects of β-site amyloid precursor protein-cleaving enzymes 1 and 2 on β-amyloid peptide production in cells. *J Biol Chem* **278:** 31512–31520.

Basi GS, Hemphill S, Brigham EF, Liao A, Aubele DL, Baker J, Barbour R, Bova M, Chen XH, Dappen MS, et al. 2010. Amyloid precursor protein selective γ-secretase inhibitors for treatment of Alzheimer's disease. *Alzheimer's Res Ther* **2:** 36.

Bateman RJ, Siemers ER, Mawuenyega KG, Wen G, Browning KR, Sigurdson WC, Yarasheski KE, Friedrich SW, Demattos RB, May PC, et al. 2009. A γ-secretase inhibitor decreases amyloid-β production in the central nervous system. *Ann Neurol* **66:** 48–54.

Bayer AJ, Bullock R, Jones RW, Wilkinson D, Paterson KR, Jenkins L, Millais SB, Donoghue D. 2005. Evaluation of the safety and immunogenicity of synthetic Aβ42 (AN1792) in patients with AD. *Neurology* **64:** 94–101.

Benes P, Vetvicka V, Fusek M. 2008. Cathepsin D—Many functions of one aspartic protease. *Crit Rev Oncol Hematol* **68:** 12–28.

Bennett BD, Babu-Khan S, Loeloff R, Louis JC, Curran E, Citron M, Vassar R. 2000. Expression analysis of BACE2 in brain and peripheral tissues. *J Biol Chem* **275:** 20647–20651.

Blanchard BJ, Chen A, Rozeboom LM, Stafford KA, Weigele P, Ingram VM. 2004. Efficient reversal of Alzheimer's disease fibril formation and elimination of neurotoxicity by a small molecule. *Proc Natl Acad Sci* **101:** 14326–14332.

Boche D, Zotova E, Weller RO, Love S, Neal JW, Pickering RM, Wilkinson D, Holmes C, Nicoll JA. 2008. Consequence of Aβ immunization on the vasculature of human Alzheimer's disease brain. *Brain* **131:** 3299–3310.

Boggs LN, Lindstrom T, Watson B, Sheehan S, Audia JE, May PC. 2010. Proof-of-concept pharmacodynamic assessment of a prototypic BACE1 inhibitor at steady-state using IV infusion dosing in the PDAPP transgenic mouse model of Alzheimer's Disease. In *International Conference on Alzheimer's Disease*, P3–304, S541. Alzheimer's Association, Honolulu, HI.

Breitner JC, Welsh KA, Helms MJ, Gaskell PC, Gau BA, Roses AD, Pericak-Vance MA, Saunders AM. 1995. Delayed onset of Alzheimer's disease with nonsteroidal anti-inflammatory and histamine H2 blocking drugs. *Neurobiol Aging* **16:** 523–530.

Brendza RP, Bacskai BJ, Cirrito JR, Simmons KA, Skoch JM, Klunk WE, Mathis CA, Bales KR, Paul SM, Hyman BT, et al. 2005. Anti-Aβ antibody treatment promotes the rapid recovery of amyloid-associated neuritic dystrophy in PDAPP transgenic mice. *J Clin Invest* **115:** 428–433.

Bronfman FC, Garrido J, Alvarez A, Morgan C, Inestrosa NC. 1996. Laminin inhibits amyloid-β-peptide fibrillation. *Neurosci Lett* **218:** 201–203.

Cai H, Wang Y, McCarthy D, Wen H, Borchelt DR, Price DL, Wong PC. 2001. BACE1 is the major β-secretase for generation of Aβ peptides by neurons. *Nat Neurosci* **4:** 233–234.

Calamai M, Chiti F, Dobson CM. 2005. Amyloid fibril formation can proceed from different conformations of a partially unfolded protein. *Biophys J* **89:** 4201–4210.

Chang WP, Koelsch G, Wong S, Downs D, Da H, Weerasena V, Gordon B, Devasamudram T, Bilcer G, Ghosh AK, et al. 2004. In vivo inhibition of Aβ production by memapsin 2 (β-secretase) inhibitors. *J Neurochem* **89:** 1409–1416.

Cheng IH, Scearce-Levie K, Legleiter J, Palop JJ, Gerstein H, Bien-Ly N, Puolivali J, Lesne S, Ashe KH, Muchowski PJ, et al. 2007. Accelerating amyloid-β fibrillization reduces oligomer levels and functional deficits in Alzheimer disease mouse models. *J Biol Chem* **282:** 23818–23828.

Chiti F, Stefani M, Taddei N, Ramponi G, Dobson CM. 2003. Rationalization of the effects of mutations on peptide and protein aggregation rates. *Nature* **424:** 805–808.

Choe L, D'Ascenzo M, Relkin NR, Pappin D, Ross P, Williamson B, Guertin S, Pribil P, Lee KH. 2007. 8-Plex quantitation of changes in cerebrospinal fluid protein expression in subjects undergoing intravenous immunoglobulin treatment for Alzheimer's disease. *Proteomics* **7:** 3651–3660.

Churcher I, Beher D. 2005. γ-Secretase as a therapeutic target for the treatment of Alzheimer's disease. *Curr Pharm Des* **11:** 3363–3382.

Cleary JP, Walsh DM, Hofmeister JJ, Shankar GM, Kuskowski MA, Selkoe DJ, Ashe KH. 2005. Natural oligomers of the amyloid-β protein specifically disrupt cognitive function. *Nat Neurosci* **8:** 79–84.

ClinicalTrials.gov. A multicenter, double blind, placebo-controlled, safety and tolerability study of BMS-708163 in patients with prodromal Alzheimer's disease. Identifier NCT00890890. Last updated September 15, 2011.

Cole DC, Stock JR, Kreft AF, Antane M, Aschmies SH, Atchison KP, Casebier DS, Comery TA, Martone RL, Aschmies S, et al. 2005. Acute γ-secretase inhibition improves contextual fear conditioning in the Tg2576 mouse model of Alzheimer's disease. *J Neurosci* **25:** 8898–8902.

Das P, Chapoval S, Howard V, David CS, Golde TE. 2003. Immune responses against Aβ1–42 in HLA class II transgenic mice: Implications for Aβ1–42 immune-mediated therapies. *Neurobiol Aging* **24:** 969–976.

Deane R, Wu Z, Sagare A, Davis J, Du Yan S, Hamm K, Xu F, Parisi M, LaRue B, Hu HW, et al. 2004. LRP/amyloid β-peptide interaction mediates differential brain efflux of Aβ isoforms. *Neuron* **43:** 333–344.

DeMattos RB, Bales KR, Cummins DJ, Dodart JC, Paul SM, Holtzman DM. 2001. Peripheral anti-Aβ antibody alters CNS and plasma Aβ clearance and decreases brain Aβ burden in a mouse model of Alzheimer's disease. [See comment.] *Proc Natl Acad Sci* **98:** 8850–8855.

DeMattos RB, Bales KR, Cummins DJ, Paul SM, Holtzman DM. 2002a. Brain to plasma amyloid-β efflux: A measure of brain amyloid burden in a mouse model of Alzheimer's disease. *Science* **295:** 2264–2267.

DeMattos RB, Bales KR, Parsadanian M, O'Dell MA, Foss EM, Paul SM, Holtzman DM. 2002b. Plaque-associated disruption of CSF and plasma amyloid-β (Aβ) equilibrium in a mouse model of Alzheimer's disease. *J Neurochem* **81:** 229–236.

De Strooper B, Saftig P, Craessaerts K, Vanderstichele H, Guhde G, Annaert W, Von Figura K, Van Leuven F. 1998. Deficiency of presenilin-1 inhibits the normal cleavage of amyloid precursor protein. *Nature* **391:** 387–390.

Dinner AR, Sali A, Smith LJ, Dobson CM, Karplus M. 2000. Understanding protein folding via free-energy surfaces from theory and experiment. *Trends Biochem Sci* **25:** 331–339.

Dobson CM. 2003. Protein folding and misfolding. *Nature* **426:** 884–890.

Dodart JC, Bales KR, Gannon KS, Greene SJ, DeMattos RB, Mathis C, DeLong CA, Wu S, Wu X, Holtzman DM, et al. 2002. Immunization reverses memory deficits without reducing brain Aβ burden in Alzheimer's disease model. *Nat Neurosci* **5:** 452–457.

Dodel RC, Du Y, Depboylu C, Hampel H, Frolich L, Haag A, Hemmeter U, Paulsen S, Teipel SJ, Brettschneider S, et al. 2004. Intravenous immunoglobulins containing antibodies against β-amyloid for the treatment of Alzheimer's disease. *J Neurol Neurosurg Psychiat* **75:** 1472–1474.

Dominguez D, Tournoy J, Hartmann D, Huth T, Cryns K, Deforce S, Serneels L, Camacho IE, Marjaux E, Craessaerts K, et al. 2005. Phenotypic and biochemical analyses of BACE1- and BACE2-deficient mice. *J Biol Chem* **280:** 30797–30806.

Dovey HF, John V, Anderson JP, Chen LZ, de Saint Andrieu P, Fang LY, Freedman SB, Folmer B, Goldbach E, Holsztynska EJ, et al. 2001. Functional γ-secretase inhibitors reduce β-amyloid peptide levels in brain. *J Neurochem* **76:** 173–181.

Durairajan SS, Yuan Q, Xie L, Chan WS, Kum WF, Koo I, Liu C, Song Y, Huang JD, Klein WL, et al. 2008. Salvianolic acid B inhibits Aβ fibril formation and disaggregates preformed fibrils and protects against Aβ-induced cytotoxicity. *Neurochem Int* **52:** 741–750.

Durham TB, Shepherd TA. 2006. Progress toward the discovery and development of efficacious BACE inhibitors. *Curr Opin Drug Discov Devel* **9:** 776–791.

Eli Lilly. 2010. Lilly halts development of semagacestat for Alzheimer's disease based on preliminary results of phase III clinical trials. Press release, Eli Lilly, Indianapolis.

Eriksen JL, Sagi SA, Smith TE, Weggen S, Das P, McLendon DC, Ozols VV, Jessing KW, Zavitz KH, Koo EH, et al. 2003. NSAIDs and enantiomers of flurbiprofen target γ-secretase and lower Aβ 42 in vivo. *J Clin Invest* **112:** 440–449.

Esler WP, Kimberly WT, Ostaszewski BL, Diehl TS, Moore CL, Tsai JY, Rahmati T, Xia W, Selkoe DJ, Wolfe MS. 2000. Transition-state analogue inhibitors of γ-secretase bind directly to presenilin-1. *Nat Cell Biol* **2:** 428–434.

Farzan M, Schnitzler CE, Vasilieva N, Leung D, Choe H. 2000. BACE2, a β-secretase homolog, cleaves at the β site and within the amyloid-β region of the amyloid-β precursor protein. *Proc Natl Acad Sci* **97:** 9712–9717.

Feng R, Rampon C, Tang YP, Shrom D, Jin J, Kyin M, Sopher B, Miller MW, Ware CB, Martin GM, et al. 2001. Deficient neurogenesis in forebrain-specific presenilin-1 knockout mice is associated with reduced clearance of hippocampal memory traces. *Neuron* **32:** 911–926.

Ferrer I, Boada Rovira M, Sanchez Guerra ML, Rey MJ, Costa-Jussa F. 2004. Neuropathology and pathogenesis of encephalitis following amyloid-β immunization in Alzheimer's disease. *Brain Pathol* **14:** 11–20.

Fleisher AS, Raman R, Siemers ER, Becerra L, Clark CM, Dean RA, Farlow MR, Galvin JE, Peskind ER, Quinn JF, et al. 2008. Phase 2 safety trial targeting amyloid β production with a γ-secretase inhibitor in Alzheimer disease. *Arch Neurol* **65:** 1031–1038.

Fluhrer R, Capell A, Westmeyer G, Willem M, Hartung B, Condron MM, Teplow DB, Haass C, Walter J. 2002. A non-amyloidogenic function of BACE-2 in the secretory pathway. *J Neurochem* **81:** 1011–1020.

Fox NC, Black RS, Gilman S, Rossor MN, Griffith SG, Jenkins L, Koller M. 2005. Effects of Aβ immunization (AN1792) on MRI measures of cerebral volume in Alzheimer disease. *Neurology* **64:** 1563–1572.

Fraering PC, Ye W, LaVoie MJ, Ostaszewski BL, Selkoe DJ, Wolfe MS. 2005. γ-Secretase substrate selectivity can be modulated directly via interaction with a nucleotide-binding site. *J Biol Chem* **280:** 41987–41996.

Fujiwara H, Iwasaki K, Furukawa K, Seki T, He M, Maruyama M, Tomita N, Kudo Y, Higuchi M, Saido TC, et al. 2006. *Uncaria rhynchophylla*, a Chinese medicinal herb, has potent antiaggregation effects on Alzheimer's β-amyloid proteins. *J Neurosci Res* **84:** 427–433.

Fukumori A, Fluhrer R, Steiner H, Haass C. 2010. Three-amino acid spacing of presenilin endoproteolysis suggests a general stepwise cleavage of γ-secretase-mediated intramembrane proteolysis. *J Neurosci* **30:** 7853–7862.

Fukumoto H, Cheung BS, Hyman BT, Irizarry MC. 2002. β-Secretase protein and activity are increased in the neocortex in Alzheimer disease. *Arch Neurol* **59:** 1381–1389.

Fung J, Darabie AA, McLaurin J. 2005. Contribution of simple saccharides to the stabilization of amyloid structure. *Biochem Biophys Res Commun* **328:** 1067–1072.

Galasko DR, Graff-Radford N, May S, Hendrix S, Cottrell BA, Sagi SA, Mather G, Laughlin M, Zavitz KH, Swabb E, et al. 2007. Safety, tolerability, pharmacokinetics, and Aβ levels after short-term administration of *R*-flurbiprofen in healthy elderly individuals. *Alzheimer Dis Assoc Disord* **21:** 292–299.

Garofalo AW. 2009. Patents targeting γ-secretase inhibition and modulation for the treatment of Alzheimer's disease: 2004–2008. *Expert Opin Ther Patents* **187:** 639–703.

Gervais F, Paquette J, Morissette C, Krzywkowski P, Yu M, Azzi M, Lacombe D, Kong X, Aman A, Laurin J, et al. 2007. Targeting soluble Aβ peptide with Tramiprosate for the treatment of brain amyloidosis. *Neurobiol Aging* **28:** 537–547.

Ghosh AK, Kumaragurubaran N, Hong L, Koelsh G, Tang J. 2008. Memapsin 2 (β-secretase) inhibitors: Drug development. *Curr Alzheimer Res* **5:** 121–131.

Gillman KW, Starrett JE, Parker MF, Xie K, Bronson JJ, Marcin LR, McElhone KE, Bergstrom CP, Mate RA, Williams R, et al. 2010. Discovery and evaluation of BMS-708163, a potent, selective and orally bioavailable Î³-secretase inhibitor. *ACS Med Chem Lett* **1:** 120–124.

Gilman S, Koller M, Black RS, Jenkins L, Griffith SG, Fox NC, Eisner L, Kirby L, Rovira MB, Forette F, et al. 2005. Clinical effects of Aβ immunization (AN1792) in patients with AD in an interrupted trial. *Neurology* **64:** 1553–1562.

Glaser R, Kiecolt-Glaser JK, Malarkey WB, Sheridan JF. 1998. The influence of psychological stress on the immune response to vaccines. *Ann NY Acad Sci* **840:** 649–655.

Glenner GG, Wong CW. 1984. Alzheimer's disease: Initial report of the purification and characterization of a novel cerebrovascular amyloid protein. *Biochem Biophys Res Commun* **120:** 885–890.

Golde TE, Schneider LS, Koo EH. 2011. Anti-aβ therapeutics in Alzheimer's disease: The need for a paradigm shift. *Neuron* **69:** 203–213.

Gong Y, Chang L, Viola KL, Lacor PN, Lambert MP, Finch CE, Krafft GA, Klein WL. 2003. Alzheimer's disease-affected brain: Presence of oligomeric A β ligands (ADDLs) suggests a molecular basis for reversible memory loss. *Proc Natl Acad Sci* **100:** 10417–10422.

Goni F, Sigurdsson EM. 2005. New directions towards safer and effective vaccines for Alzheimer's disease. *Curr Opin Mol Ther* **7:** 17–23.

Grathwohl SA, Kalin RE, Bolmont T, Prokop S, Winkelmann G, Kaeser SA, Odenthal J, Radde R, Eldh T, Gandy S, et al. 2009. Formation and maintenance of Alzheimer's disease β-amyloid plaques in the absence of microglia. *Nat Neurosci* **12:** 1361–1363.

Green RC, Schneider LS, Amato DA, Beelen AP, Wilcock G, Swabb EA, Zavitz KH, Tarenflurbil Phase 3 Study G. 2009. Effect of tarenflurbil on cognitive decline and activities of daily living in patients with mild Alzheimer disease: A randomized controlled trial. *JAMA* **302:** 2557–2564.

Haass C, Schlossmacher MG, Hung AY, Vigo-Pelfrey C, Mellon A, Ostaszewski BL, Lieberburg I, Koo EH, Schenk D, Teplow DB, et al. 1992. Amyloid β-peptide is produced by cultured cells during normal metabolism. *Nature* **359:** 322–325.

Hamada Y, Kiso Y. 2009. Recent progress itne the discovery of non-peptidic BACE1 inhibitors. *Expert Opin Drug Discov* **4:** 391–416.

Harrison SM, Harper AJ, Hawkins J, Duddy G, Grau E, Pugh PL, Winter PH, Shilliam CS, Hughes ZA, Dawson LA, et al. 2003. BACE1 (β-secretase) transgenic and knockout mice: Identification of neurochemical deficits and behavioral changes. *Mol Cell Neurosci* **24:** 646–655.

Harrison T, Churcher I, Beher D. 2004. γ-Secretase as a target for drug intervention in Alzheimer's disease. *Curr Opin Drug Discov Devel* **7:** 709–719.

He G, Luo W, Li P, Remmers C, Netzer WJ, Hendrick J, Bettayeb K, Flajolet M, Gorelick F, Wennogle LP, et al. 2010.

Gamma-secretase activating protein is a therapeutic target for Alzheimer's disease. *Nature* **467:** 95–98.

Hemming ML, Elias JE, Gygi SP, Selkoe DJ. 2009. Identification of β-secretase (BACE1) substrates using quantitative proteomics. *PLoS One* **4:** e8477.

Henley DB, May PC, Dean RA, Siemers ER. 2009. Development of semagacestat (LY450139), a functional γ-secretase inhibitor, for the treatment of Alzheimer's disease. *Expert Opin Pharmacother* **10:** 1657–1664.

Herreman A, Hartmann D, Annaert W, Saftig P, Craessaerts K, Serneels L, Umans L, Schrijvers V, Checler F, Vanderstichele H, et al. 1999. Presenilin 2 deficiency causes a mild pulmonary phenotype and no changes in amyloid precursor protein processing but enhances the embryonic lethal phenotype of presenilin 1 deficiency. *Proc Natl Acad Sci* **96:** 11872–11877.

Herreman A, Serneels L, Annaert W, Collen D, Schoonjans L, De Strooper B. 2000. Total inactivation of γ-secretase activity in presenilin-deficient embryonic stem cells. *Nat Cell Biol* **2:** 461–462.

Higaki J, Murphy GM Jr, Cordell B. 1997. Inhibition of β-amyloid formation by haloperidol: A possible mechanism for reduced frequency of Alzheimer's disease pathology in schizophrenia. *J Neurochem* **68:** 333–336.

Hirohata M, Ono K, Naiki H, Yamada M. 2005. Non-steroidal anti-inflammatory drugs have anti-amyloidogenic effects for Alzheimer's β-amyloid fibrils in vitro. *Neuropharmacology* **49:** 1088–1099.

Hock C, Konietzko U, Streffer JR, Tracy J, Signorell A, Muller-Tillmanns B, Lemke U, Henke K, Moritz E, Garcia E, et al. 2003. Antibodies against β-amyloid slow cognitive decline in Alzheimer's disease. [See comment.] *Neuron* **38:** 547–554.

Holmes C, Boche D, Wilkinson D, Yadegarfar G, Hopkins V, Bayer A, Jones RW, Bullock R, Love S, Neal JW, et al. 2008. Long-term effects of Aβ42 immunisation in Alzheimer's disease: Follow-up of a randomised, placebo-controlled phase I trial. *Lancet* **372:** 216–223.

Holsinger RM, McLean CA, Beyreuther K, Masters CL, Evin G. 2002. Increased expression of the amyloid precursor β-secretase in Alzheimer's disease. *Ann Neurol* **51:** 783–786.

Hong L, Koelsch G, Lin X, Wu S, Terzyan S, Ghosh AK, Zhang XC, Tang J. 2000. Structure of the protease domain of memapsin 2 (β-secretase) complexed with inhibitor. *Science* **290:** 150–153.

Hong HS, Rana S, Barrigan L, Shi A, Zhang Y, Zhou F, Jin LW, Hua DH. 2009. Inhibition of Alzheimer's amyloid toxicity with a tricyclic pyrone molecule in vitro and in vivo. *J Neurochem* **108:** 1097–1108.

Hu X, Hicks CW, He W, Wong P, Macklin WB, Trapp BD, Yan R. 2006. Bace1 modulates myelination in the central and peripheral nervous system. *Nat Neurosci* **9:** 1520–1525.

Hussain I. 2004. The potential for BACE1 inhibitors in the treatment of Alzheimer's disease. *IDrugs* **7:** 653–658.

Hussain I, Powell D, Howlett DR, Tew DG, Meek TD, Chapman C, Gloger IS, Murphy KE, Southan CD, Ryan DM, et al. 1999. Identification of a novel aspartic protease (Asp 2) as β-secretase. *Mol Cell Neurosci* **14:** 419–427.

Hussain I, Powell DJ, Howlett DR, Chapman GA, Gilmour L, Murdock PR, Tew DG, Meek TD, Chapman C,

Schneider K, et al. 2000. ASP1 (BACE2) cleaves the amyloid precursor protein at the β-secretase site. *Mol Cell Neurosci* **16:** 609–619.

Hyde LA, McHugh NA, Chen J, Zhang Q, Manfra D, Nomeir AA, Josien H, Bara T, Clader JW, Zhang L, et al. 2006. Studies to investigate the in vivo therapeutic window of the γ-secretase inhibitor N^2-[(2S)-2-(3,5-difluorphenyl)-2-hydroxyethanoyl]-N^1-[(7S)-5-methyl-6-oxo-6,7-dihydro-5H-dibenzo[b,d]azepin-7-yl]-L-alaninamide (LY411,575) in the CRND8 mouse. *J Pharmacol Exp Ther* **319:** 1133–1143.

Janus C, Pearson J, McLaurin J, Mathews PM, Jiang Y, Schmidt SD, Chishti MA, Horne P, Heslin D, French J, et al. 2000. A β peptide immunization reduces behavioural impairment and plaques in a model of Alzheimer's disease. [See comment.] *Nature* **408:** 979–982.

John V. 2006. Human β-secretase (BACE) and BACE inhibitors: Progress report. *Curr Top Med Chem* **6:** 569–578.

Josien H. 2002. Recent advances in the development of γ-secretase inhibitors. *Curr Opin Drug Discov Devel* **5:** 513–525.

Kayed R, Head E, Thompson JL, McIntire TM, Milton SC, Cotman CW, Glabe CG. 2003. Common structure of soluble amyloid oligomers implies common mechanism of pathogenesis. *Science* **300:** 486–489.

Khurana R, Ionescu-Zanetti C, Pope M, Li J, Nielson L, Ramirez-Alvarado M, Regan L, Fink AL, Carter SA. 2003. A general model for amyloid fibril assembly based on morphological studies using atomic force microscopy. *Biophys J* **85:** 1135–1144.

Kihara T, Shimohama S, Akaike A. 1999. Effects of nicotinic receptor agonists on β-amyloid β-sheet formation. *Jpn J Pharmacol* **79:** 393–396.

Kihara T, Shimmyo Y, Akaike A, Niidome T, Sugimoto H. 2010. Aβ-induced BACE-1 cleaves N-terminal sequence of mPGES-2. *Biochem Biophys Res Commun* **393:** 728–733.

Kitazume S, Tachida Y, Oka R, Shirotani K, Saido TC, Hashimoto Y. 2001. Alzheimer's β-secretase, β-site amyloid precursor protein-cleaving enzyme, is responsible for cleavage secretion of a Golgi-resident sialyltransferase. *Proc Natl Acad Sci* **98:** 13554–13559.

Kitazume S, Nakagawa K, Oka R, Tachida Y, Ogawa K, Luo Y, Citron M, Shitara H, Taya C, Yonekawa H, et al. 2005. In vivo cleavage of α2,6-sialyltransferase by Alzheimer β-secretase. *J Biol Chem* **280:** 8589–8595.

Klyubin I, Walsh DM, Lemere CA, Cullen WK, Shankar GM, Betts V, Spooner ET, Jiang L, Anwyl R, Selkoe DJ, et al. 2005. Amyloid β protein immunotherapy neutralizes Aβ oligomers that disrupt synaptic plasticity in vivo. *Nat Med* **11:** 556–561.

Klyubin I, Betts V, Welzel AT, Blennow K, Zetterberg H, Wallin A, Lemere CA, Cullen WK, Peng Y, Wisniewski T, et al. 2008. Amyloid β protein dimer-containing human CSF disrupts synaptic plasticity: Prevention by systemic passive immunization. *J Neurosci* **28:** 4231–4237.

Kobayashi D, Zeller M, Cole T, Buttini M, McConlogue L, Sinha S, Freedman S, Morris RG, Chen KS. 2008. BACE1 gene deletion: Impact on behavioral function in a model of Alzheimer's disease. *Neurobiol Aging* **29:** 861–873.

Kokkoni N, Stott K, Amijee H, Mason JM, Doig AJ. 2006. N-Methylated peptide inhibitors of β-amyloid aggregation and toxicity. Optimization of the inhibitor structure. *Biochemistry* **45:** 9906–9918.

Kotilinek LA, Bacskai B, Westerman M, Kawarabayashi T, Younkin L, Hyman BT, Younkin S, Ashe KH. 2002. Reversible memory loss in a mouse transgenic model of Alzheimer's disease. *J Neurosci* **22:** 6331–6335.

Kounnas MZ, Danks AM, Cheng S, Tyree C, Ackerman E, Zhang X, Ahn K, Nguyen P, Comer D, Mao L, et al. 2010. Modulation of γ-secretase reduces β-amyloid deposition in a transgenic mouse model of Alzheimer's disease. *Neuron* **67:** 769–780.

Kuchibhotla KV, Goldman ST, Lattarulo CR, Wu HY, Hyman BT, Bacskai BJ. 2008. Aβ plaques lead to aberrant regulation of calcium homeostasis in vivo resulting in structural and functional disruption of neuronal networks. *Neuron* **59:** 214–225.

Kuhn PH, Marjaux E, Imhof A, De Strooper B, Haass C, Lichtenthaler SF. 2007. Regulated intramembrane proteolysis of the interleukin-1 receptor II by α-, β-, and γ-secretase. *J Biol Chem* **282:** 11982–11995.

Lacor PN, Buniel MC, Chang L, Fernandez SJ, Gong Y, Viola KL, Lambert MP, Velasco PT, Bigio EH, Finch CE, et al. 2004. Synaptic targeting by Alzheimer's-related amyloid β oligomers. *J Neurosci* **24:** 10191–10200.

Laird FM, Cai H, Savonenko AV, Farah MH, He K, Melnikova T, Wen H, Chiang HC, Xu G, Koliatsos VE, et al. 2005. BACE1, a major determinant of selective vulnerability of the brain to amyloid-β amyloidogenesis, is essential for cognitive, emotional, and synaptic functions. *J Neurosci* **25:** 11693–11709.

Lashuel HA, Hartley DM, Balakhaneh D, Aggarwal A, Teichberg S, Callaway DJ. 2002. New class of inhibitors of amyloid-β fibril formation. Implications for the mechanism of pathogenesis in Alzheimer's disease. *J Biol Chem* **277:** 42881–42890.

Lavie V, Becker M, Cohen-Kupiec R, Yacoby I, Koppel R, Wedenig M, Hutter-Paier B, Solomon B. 2004. EFRH-phage immunization of Alzheimer's disease animal model improves behavioral performance in Morris water maze trials. *J Mol Neurosci* **24:** 105–113.

Lazarov VK, Fraering PC, Ye W, Wolfe MS, Selkoe DJ, Li H. 2006. Electron microscopic structure of purified, active γ-secretase reveals an aqueous intramembrane chamber and two pores. *Proc Natl Acad Sci* **103:** 6889–6894.

Lee CC, Nayak A, Sethuraman A, Belfort G, McRae GJ. 2007. A three-stage kinetic model of amyloid fibrillation. *Biophys J* **92:** 3448–3458.

Lesne S, Koh MT, Kotilinek L, Kayed R, Glabe CG, Yang A, Gallagher M, Ashe KH. 2006. A specific amyloid-β protein assembly in the brain impairs memory. *Nature* **440:** 352–357.

Leverone JF, Spooner ET, Lehman HK, Clements JD, Lemere CA. 2003. Aβ1–15 is less immunogenic than Aβ1–40/42 for intranasal immunization of wild-type mice but may be effective for "boosting." *Vaccine* **21:** 2197–2206.

Li YM, Xu M, Lai MT, Huang Q, Castro JL, DiMuzio-Mower J, Harrison T, Lellis C, Nadin A, Neduvelil JG, et al. 2000. Photoactivated γ-secretase inhibitors directed to the active site covalently label presenilin 1. *Nature* **405:** 689–694.

Li R, Lindholm K, Yang LB, Yue X, Citron M, Yan R, Beach T, Sue L, Sabbagh M, Cai H, et al. 2004. Amyloid β peptide load is correlated with increased β-secretase activity in sporadic Alzheimer's disease patients. *Proc Natl Acad Sci* **101**: 3632–3637.

Li T, Wen H, Brayton C, Laird FM, Ma G, Peng S, Placanica L, Wu TC, Crain BJ, Price DL, et al. 2007. Moderate reduction of γ-secretase attenuates amyloid burden and limits mechanism-based liabilities. *J Neurosci* **27**: 10849–10859.

Liang E, Lohr L, Munson ML, Crans G, Cedarbaum J. 2011a. A phase 1 dose escalation study to evaluate the safety, tolerability, pharmacokinetics, and pharmacodynamics of single oral doses of ELND006 in healthy elderly subjects. In *International Conference on Alzheimer's Disease.* Alzheimer's Association, Paris.

Liang E, Wenzhong Liu, Lohr L, Nguyen V, Lin HH, Munson ML, Crans G, Cedarbaum J. 2011b. A phase 1, dose escalation study to evaluate the safety, tolerability, pharmacokinetics, and pharmacodynamics of multiple oral daily doses of ELND006 in healthy elderly subjects. In *International Conference on Alzheimer's Disease.* Alzheimer's Association, Paris.

Lichtenthaler SF, Dominguez DI, Westmeyer GG, Reiss K, Haass C, Saftig P, De Strooper B, Seed B. 2003. The cell adhesion protein P-selectin glycoprotein ligand-1 is a substrate for the aspartyl protease BACE1. *J Biol Chem* **278**: 48713–48719.

Lim GP, Yang F, Chu T, Chen P, Beech W, Teter B, Tran T, Ubeda O, Ashe KH, Frautschy SA, et al. 2000. Ibuprofen suppresses plaque pathology and inflammation in a mouse model for Alzheimer's disease. *J Neurosci* **20**: 5709–5714.

Lin X, Koelsch G, Wu S, Downs D, Dashti A, Tang J. 2000. Human aspartic protease memapsin 2 cleaves the β-secretase site of β-amyloid precursor protein. *Proc Natl Acad Sci* **97**: 1456–1460.

Liu D, Xu Y, Feng Y, Liu H, Shen X, Chen K, Ma J, Jiang H. 2006. Inhibitor discovery targeting the intermediate structure of β-amyloid peptide on the conformational transition pathway: Implications in the aggregation mechanism of β-amyloid peptide. *Biochemistry* **45**: 10963–10972.

Lombardo JA, Stern EA, McLellan ME, Kajdasz ST, Hickey GA, Bacskai BJ, Hyman BT. 2003. Amyloid-β antibody treatment leads to rapid normalization of plaque-induced neuritic alterations. *J Neurosci* **23**: 10879–10883.

Lorenzo A, Yankner BA. 1994. β-Amyloid neurotoxicity requires fibril formation and is inhibited by congo red. *Proc Natl Acad Sci* **91**: 12243–12247.

Luo Y, Bolon B, Kahn S, Bennett BD, Babu-Khan S, Denis P, Fan W, Kha H, Zhang J, Gong Y, et al. 2001. Mice deficient in BACE1, the Alzheimer's β-secretase, have normal phenotype and abolished β-amyloid generation. *Nat Neurosci* **4**: 231–232.

Luo Y, Bolon B, Damore MA, Fitzpatrick D, Liu H, Zhang J, Yan Q, Vassar R, Citron M. 2003. BACE1 (β-secretase) knockout mice do not acquire compensatory gene expression changes or develop neural lesions over time. *Neurobiol Dis* **14**: 81–88.

Martenyi F, Lowe S, Dean RA, Monk SA, Gonzales CR, Friedrich S, May PC, Audia JE, Citron M, LaBell ES, et al. 2010. Central and peripheral pharmacokinetic and pharmacodynamic effects of the β-site cleavage enzyme (BACE1) inhibitor LY2811376 in humans. In *International Conference on Alzheimer's Disease*, P4-008. Alzheimer's Association, Honolulu, HI.

Martone RL, Zhou H, Atchison K, Comery T, Xu JZ, Huang X, Gong X, Jin M, Kreft A, Harrison B, et al. 2009. Begacestat (GSI-953): A novel, selective thiophene sulfonamide inhibitor of amyloid precursor protein γ-secretase for the treatment of Alzheimer's disease. *J Pharmacol Exp Ther* **331**: 598–608.

Masliah E, Hansen L, Adame A, Crews L, Bard F, Lee C, Seubert P, Games D, Kirby L, Schenk D. 2005. Aβ vaccination effects on plaque pathology in the absence of encephalitis in Alzheimer disease. *Neurology* **64**: 129–131.

Mawuenyega KG, Sigurdson W, Ovod V, Munsell L, Kasten T, Morris JC, Yarasheski KE, Bateman RJ. 2010. Decreased clearance of CNS β-amyloid in Alzheimer's disease. *Science* **330**: 1774.

May PC, Altstiel LD, Bender MH, Boggs LN, Calligaro DO, Fuson KS, Gitter BD, Hyslop PA, Jordan WH, Li WY, et al. 2001. Marked reduction of Ab accumulation and b-amyloid plaque pathology in mice upon chronic treatment with a functional γ-secretase inhibitor. *Soc Neurosci Abstr* **27**: 1806.

May PC, Boggs LN, Yang Z, Lindstrom T, Calligaro D, Citron M, Sheehan S, Audia JE. 2010. Central and peripheral pharmacodynamiceffects of BACE1 inhibition following oral administration of LY2811376 to PDAPP mice and beagle dog. In *International Conference on Alzheimer's Disease*, P3-467, S590. Alzheimer's Associaiton, Honolulu, HI.

Mayer SC, Kreft AF, Harrison B, Abou-Gharbia M, Antane M, Aschmies S, Atchison K, Chlenov M, Cole DC, Comery T, et al. 2008. Discovery of begacestat, a Notch-1-sparing γ-secretase inhibitor for the treatment of Alzheimer's disease. *J Med Chem* **51**: 7348–7351.

McConlogue L, Buttini M, Anderson JP, Brigham EF, Chen KS, Freedman SB, Games D, Johnson-Wood K, Lee M, Zeller M, et al. 2007. Partial reduction of BACE1 has dramatic effects on Alzheimer plaque and synaptic pathology in APP Transgenic Mice. *J Biol Chem* **282**: 26326–26334.

McGeer EG, McGeer PL. 1998. The importance of inflammatory mechanisms in Alzheimer disease. *Exp Gerontol* **33**: 371–378.

McLaurin J, Chakrabartty A. 1996. Membrane disruption by Alzheimer β-amyloid peptides mediated through specific binding to either phospholipids or gangliosides. Implications for neurotoxicity. *J Biol Chem* **271**: 26482–26489.

McLaurin J, Franklin T, Chakrabartty A, Fraser PE. 1998. Phosphatidylinositol and inositol involvement in Alzheimer amyloid-β fibril growth and arrest. *J Mol Biol* **278**: 183–194.

McLaurin J, Golomb R, Jurewicz A, Antel JP, Fraser PE. 2000. Inositol stereoisomers stabilize an oligomeric aggregate of Alzheimer amyloid β peptide and inhibit aβ-induced toxicity. *J Biol Chem* **275**: 18495–18502.

McLaurin J, Cecal R, Kierstead ME, Tian X, Phinney AL, Manea M, French JE, Lambermon MH, Darabie AA, Brown ME, et al. 2002. Therapeutically effective antibodies against amyloid-β peptide target amyloid-β residues 4–10 and inhibit cytotoxicity and fibrillogenesis. [See comment.] *Nat Med* **8:** 1263–1269.

McLaurin J, Kierstead ME, Brown ME, Hawkes CA, Lambermon MH, Phinney AL, Darabie AA, Cousins JE, French JE, Lan MF, et al. 2006. Cyclohexanehexol inhibitors of Aβ aggregation prevent and reverse Alzheimer phenotype in a mouse model. *Nat Med* **12:** 801–808.

Meyer-Luehmann M, Spires-Jones TL, Prada C, Garcia-Alloza M, de Calignon A, Rozkalne A, Koenigsknecht-Talboo J, Holtzman DM, Bacskai BJ, Hyman BT. 2008. Rapid appearance and local toxicity of amyloid-β plaques in a mouse model of Alzheimer's disease. *Nature* **451:** 720–724.

Meyer-Luehmann M, Mielke M, Spires-Jones TL, Stoothoff W, Jones P, Bacskai BJ, Hyman BT. 2009. A reporter of local dendritic translocation shows plaque-related loss of neural system function in APP-transgenic mice. *J Neurosci* **29:** 12636–12640.

Milano J, McKay J, Dagenais C, Foster-Brown L, Pognan F, Gadient R, Jacobs RT, Zacco A, Greenberg B, Ciaccio PJ. 2004. Modulation of notch processing by γ-secretase inhibitors causes intestinal goblet cell metaplasia and induction of genes known to specify gut secretory lineage differentiation. *Toxicol Sci* **82:** 341–358.

Monsonego A, Zota V, Karni A, Krieger JI, Bar-Or A, Bitan G, Budson AE, Sperling R, Selkoe DJ, Weiner HL. 2003. Increased T cell reactivity to amyloid β protein in older humans and patients with Alzheimer disease. *J Clin Invest* **112:** 415–422.

Morgan D, Diamond DM, Gottschall PE, Ugen KE, Dickey C, Hardy J, Duff K, Jantzen P, DiCarlo G, Wilcock D, et al. 2000. A β peptide vaccination prevents memory loss in an animal model of Alzheimer's disease.[See comment.] [Erratum appears in *Nature* 2001; 412: 660.] *Nature* **408:** 982–985.

Morihara T, Chu T, Ubeda O, Beech W, Cole GM. 2002. Selective inhibition of Aβ42 production by NSAID R-enantiomers. *J Neurochem* **83:** 1009–1012.

Nagy C, Schuck E, Ishibashi A, Nakatini Y, Rege B, Logevinsky V. 2011. Neurodegenerative diseases. 10th International Conference, AD/PD: Advances, Concepts and Challenges. Barcelona, Spain.

Netzer WJ, Dou F, Cai D, Veach D, Jean S, Li Y, Bornmann WG, Clarkson B, Xu H, Greengard P. 2003. Gleevec inhibits β-amyloid production but not Notch cleavage. *Proc Natl Acad Sci* **100:** 12444–12449.

Nicoll JAR, Wilkinson D, Holmes C, Steart P, Markham H, Weller RO. 2003. Neuropathology of human Alzheimer disease after immunization with amyloid-β peptide: A case report. *Nat Med* **9:** 448–452.

Nicoll JA, Barton E, Boche D, Neal JW, Ferrer I, Thompson P, Vlachouli C, Wilkinson D, Bayer A, Games D, et al. 2006. Aβ species removal after aβ42 immunization. *J Neuropathol Exp Neurol* **65:** 1040–1048.

Oddo S, Billings L, Kesslak JP, Cribbs DH, LaFerla FM. 2004. Aβ immunotherapy leads to clearance of early, but not late, hyperphosphorylated tau aggregates via the proteasome. *Neuron* **43:** 321–332.

Ohno M, Sametsky EA, Younkin LH, Oakley H, Younkin SG, Citron M, Vassar R, Disterhoft JF. 2004. BACE1 deficiency rescues memory deficits and cholinergic dysfunction in a mouse model of Alzheimer's disease. *Neuron* **41:** 27–33.

Ohno M, Chang L, Tseng W, Oakley H, Citron M, Klein WL, Vassar R, Disterhoft JF. 2006. Temporal memory deficits in Alzheimer's mouse models: Rescue by genetic deletion of BACE1. *Eur J Neurosci* **23:** 251–260.

Olson RE, Albright CF. 2008. Recent progress in the medicinal chemistry of γ-secretase inhibitors. *Curr Top Med Chem* **8:** 17–33.

Ono K, Hasegawa K, Yamada M, Naiki H. 2002. Nicotine breaks down preformed Alzheimer's β-amyloid fibrils in vitro. *Biol Psychiat* **52:** 880–886.

Ono K, Yoshiike Y, Takashima A, Hasegawa K, Naiki H, Yamada M. 2004. Vitamin A exhibits potent antiamyloidogenic and fibril-destabilizing effects in vitro. *Exp Neurol* **189:** 380–392.

Orgogozo JM, Gilman S, Dartigues JF, Laurent B, Puel M, Kirby LC, Jouanny P, Dubois B, Eisner L, Flitman S, et al. 2003. Subacute meningoencephalitis in a subset of patients with AD after Aβ42 immunization. *Neurology* **61:** 46–54.

Pangalos MN, Jacobsen SJ, Reinhart PH. 2005. Disease modifying strategies for the treatment of Alzheimer's disease targeted at modulating levels of the β-amyloid peptide. *Biochem Soc Trans* **33:** 553–558.

Patton RL, Kalback WM, Esh CL, Kokjohn TA, Van Vickle GD, Luehrs DC, Kuo YM, Lopez J, Brune D, Ferrer I, et al. 2006a. Amyloid-β peptide remnants in AN-1792-immunized Alzheimer's disease patients: A biochemical analysis. *Am J Pathol* **169:** 1048–1063.

Patton RL, Kalback WM, Esh CL, Kokjohn TA, Van Vickle GD, Luehrs DC, Kuo YM, Lopez J, Brune D, Ferrer I, et al. 2006b. Amyloid-β peptide remnants in AN-1792-immunized Alzheimer's disease patients: A biochemical analysis. [See comment.] *Am J Pathol* **169:** 1048–1063.

Pfeifer M, Boncristiano S, Bondolfi L, Stalder A, Deller T, Staufenbiel M, Mathews PM, Jucker M. 2002. Cerebral hemorrhage after passive anti-Aβ immunotherapy. *Science* **298:** 1379.

Pissarnitski D. 2007. Advances in γ-secretase modulation. *Curr Opin Drug Discov Devel* **10:** 392–402.

Portelius E, Van Broeck B, Andreasson U, Gustavsson MK, Mercken M, Zetterberg H, Borghys H, Blennow K. 2010. Acute effect on the Aβ isoform pattern in CSF in response to γ-secretase modulator and inhibitor treatment in dogs. *J Alzheimer's Dis* **21:** 1005–1012.

Pu J, Kreft AF, Aschmies SH, Atchison KP, Berkowitz J, Caggiano TJ, Chlenov M, Diamantidis G, Harrison BL, Hu Y, et al. 2009. Synthesis and structure–activity relationship of a novel series of heterocyclic sulfonamide γ-secretase inhibitors. *Bioorg Med Chem* **17:** 4708–4717.

Racke MM, Boone LI, Hepburn DL, Parsadainian M, Bryan MT, Ness DK, Piroozi KS, Jordan WH, Brown DD, Hoffman WP, et al. 2005. Exacerbation of cerebral amyloid angiopathy-associated microhemorrhage in amyloid precursor protein transgenic mice by immunotherapy is dependent on antibody recognition of deposited forms of amyloid β. *J Neurosci* **25:** 629–636.

Reixach N, Crooks E, Ostresh JM, Houghten RA, Blondelle SE. 2000. Inhibition of β-amyloid-induced neurotoxicity by imidazopyridoindoles derived from a synthetic combinatorial library. *J Struct Biol* **130:** 247–258.

Rinne JO, Brooks DJ, Rossor MN, Fox NC, Bullock R, Klunk WE, Mathis CA, Blennow K, Barakos J, Okello AA, et al. 2010. ^{11}C-PiB PET assessment of change in fibrillar amyloid-β load in patients with Alzheimer's disease treated with bapineuzumab: A phase 2, double-blind, placebo-controlled, ascending-dose study. *Lancet Neurol* **9:** 363–372.

Roberds SL, Anderson J, Basi G, Bienkowski MJ, Branstetter DG, Chen KS, Freedman SB, Frigon NL, Games D, Hu K, et al. 2001. BACE knockout mice are healthy despite lacking the primary β-secretase activity in brain: Implications for Alzheimer's disease therapeutics. *Hum Mol Genet* **10:** 1317–1324.

Rodriguez-Rodriguez C, Sanchez de Groot N, Rimola A, Alvarez-Larena A, Lloveras V, Vidal-Gancedo J, Ventura S, Vendrell J, Sodupe M, Gonzalez-Duarte P. 2009. Design, selection, and characterization of thioflavin-based intercalation compounds with metal chelating properties for application in Alzheimer's disease. *J Am Chem Soc* **131:** 1436–1451.

Roher AE, Palmer KC, Yurewicz EC, Ball MJ, Greenberg BD. 1993. Morphological and biochemical analyses of amyloid plaque core proteins purified from Alzheimer disease brain tissue. *J Neurochem* **61:** 1916–1926.

Rosen LB, Stone JA, Plump A, Yuan J, Harrison T, Flynn M, Dallob A, Matthews C, Stevenson D, Schmidt D, et al. 2006. The γ secretase inhibitor MK-0752 acutely and significantly reduces CSF Aβ40 concentrations in humans. In *International Conference on Alzheimer's Disease,* S79, O74-p03-02. Alzheimer's Association, Madrid.

Ryu J, Kanapathipillai M, Lentzen G, Park CB. 2008. Inhibition of β-amyloid peptide aggregation and neurotoxicity by α-D-mannosylglycerate, a natural extremolyte. *Peptides* **29:** 578–584.

Saftig P, Peters C, von Figura K, Craessaerts K, Van Leuven F, De Strooper B. 1996. Amyloidogenic processing of human amyloid precursor protein in hippocampal neurons devoid of cathepsin D. *J Biol Chem* **271:** 27241–27244.

Salloway S, Sperling R, Gilman S, Fox NC, Blennow K, Raskind M, Sabbagh M, Honig LS, Doody R, van Dyck CH, et al. 2009. A phase 2 multiple ascending dose trial of bapineuzumab in mild to moderate Alzheimer disease. *Neurology* **73:** 2061–2070.

Saunders AJ, Kim T-W, Tanzi R. 1999. BACE maps to chromosome 11 and a BACE homolog, BACE2, reside in the obligate Down syndrome region of chromosome 21. *Science* **286:** 1255a.

Saura CA, Choi SY, Beglopoulos V, Malkani S, Zhang D, Shankaranarayana Rao BS, Chattarji S, Kelleher RJ 3rd, Kandel ER, Duff K, et al. 2004. Loss of presenilin function causes impairments of memory and synaptic plasticity followed by age-dependent neurodegeneration. *Neuron* **42:** 23–36.

Savonenko AV, Melnikova T, Laird FM, Stewart KA, Price DL, Wong PC. 2008. Alteration of BACE1-dependent NRG1/ErbB4 signaling and schizophrenia-like phenotypes in BACE1-null mice. *Proc Natl Acad Sci* **105:** 5585–5590.

Schenk D. 2002. Amyloid-β immunotherapy for Alzheimer's disease: The end of the beginning. *Nat Rev Neurosci* **3:** 824–828.

Schenk D, Barbour R, Dunn W, Gordon G, Grajeda H, Guido T, Hu K, Huang J, Johnson-Wood K, Khan K, et al. 1999. Immunization with amyloid-β attenuates Alzheimer disease-like pathology in the PDAPP mouse. *Nature* **400:** 173–177.

Scheuner D, Eckman C, Jensen M, Song X, Citron M, Suzuki N, Bird TD, Hardy J, Hutton M, Kukull W, et al. 1996. Secreted amyloid β-protein similar to that in the senile plaques of Alzheimer's disease is increased in vivo by the presenilin 1 and 2 and APP mutations linked to familial Alzheimer's disease. *Nat Med* **2:** 864–870.

Schmidt AM, Sahagan B, Nelson RB, Selmer J, Rothlein R, Bell JM. 2009. The role of RAGE in amyloid-β peptide-mediated pathology in Alzheimer's disease. *Curr Opin Investig Drugs* **10:** 672–680.

Searfoss GH, Jordan WH, Calligaro DO, Galbreath EJ, Schirtzinger LM, Berridge BR, Gao H, Higgins MA, May PC, Ryan TP. 2003. Adipsin, a biomarker of gastrointestinal toxicity mediated by a functional γ-secretase inhibitor. *J Biol Chem* **278:** 46107–46116.

Seiffert D, Bradley JD, Rominger CM, Rominger DH, Yang F, Meredith JE Jr, Wang Q, Roach AH, Thompson LA, Spitz SM, et al. 2000. Presenilin-1 and -2 are molecular targets for γ-secretase inhibitors. *J Biol Chem* **275:** 34086–34091.

Serneels L, Van Biervliet J, Craessaerts K, Dejaegere T, Horre K, Van Houtvin T, Esselmann H, Paul S, Schafer MK, Berezovska O, et al. 2009. γ-Secretase heterogeneity in the Aph1 subunit: Relevance for Alzheimer's disease. *Science* **324:** 639–642.

Seubert P, Vigo-Pelfrey C, Esch F, Lee M, Dovey H, Davis D, Sinha S, Schlossmacher M, Whaley J, Swindlehurst C, et al. 1992. Isolation and quantification of soluble Alzheimer's β-peptide from biological fluids. *Nature* **359:** 325–327.

Seubert P, Barbour R, Khan K, Motter R, Tang P, Kholodenko D, Kling K, Schenk D, Johnson-Wood K, Schroeter S, et al. 2008. Antibody capture of soluble Aβ does not reduce cortical Aβ amyloidosis in the PDAPP mouse. *Neurodegener Dis* **5:** 65–71.

Shankar GM, Li S, Mehta TH, Garcia-Munoz A, Shepardson NE, Smith I, Brett FM, Farrell MA, Rowan MJ, Lemere CA, et al. 2008. Amyloid-β protein dimers isolated directly from Alzheimer's brains impair synaptic plasticity and memory. *Nat Med* **14:** 837–842.

Siemers E, Skinner M, Dean RA, Gonzales C, Satterwhite J, Farlow M, Ness D, May PC. 2005. Safety, tolerability, and changes in amyloid β concentrations after administration of a γ-secretase inhibitor in volunteers. *Clin Neuropharmacol* **28:** 126–132.

Siemers ER, Quinn JF, Kaye J, Farlow MR, Porsteinsson A, Tariot P, Zoulnouni P, Galvin JE, Holtzman DM, Knopman DS, et al. 2006. Effects of a γ-secretase inhibitor in a randomized study of patients with Alzheimer disease. *Neurology* **66:** 602–604.

Siemers ER, Dean RA, Friedrich S, Ferguson-Sells L, Gonzales C, Farlow MR, May PC. 2007. Safety, tolerability, and effects on plasma and cerebrospinal fluid amyloid-β after inhibition of γ-secretase. *Clin Neuropharmacol* **30:** 317–325.

Sigurdsson EM, Knudsen E, Asuni A, Fitzer-Attas C, Sage D, Quartermain D, Goni F, Frangione B, Wisniewski T. 2004.

An attenuated immune response is sufficient to enhance cognition in an Alzheimer's disease mouse model immunized with amyloid-β derivatives. *J Neurosci* **24:** 6277–6282.

Silvestri R. 2008. Boom in the development of non-peptidic b-secretase (BACE1) inhibitors for the treatment of Alzheimer's Disease. *Med Res Rev* **29:** 295–338.

Sinha S, Anderson JP, Barbour R, Basi GS, Caccavello R, Davis D, Doan M, Dovey HF, Frigon N, Hong J, et al. 1999. Purification and cloning of amyloid precursor protein β-secretase from human brain. *Nature* **402:** 537–540.

Solomon B, Koppel R, Frankel D, Hanan-Aharon E. 1997. Disaggregation of Alzheimer β-amyloid by site-directed mAb. *Proc Natl Acad Sci* **94:** 4109–4112.

Spires TL, Meyer-Luehmann M, Stern EA, McLean PJ, Skoch J, Nguyen PT, Bacskai BJ, Hyman BT. 2005. Dendritic spine abnormalities in amyloid precursor protein transgenic mice demonstrated by gene transfer and intravital multiphoton microscopy. *J Neurosci* **25:** 7278–7287.

Spoelgen R, von Arnim CA, Thomas AV, Peltan ID, Koker M, Deng A, Irizarry MC, Andersen OM, Willnow TE, Hyman BT. 2006. Interaction of the cytosolic domains of sorLA/LR11 with the amyloid precursor protein (APP) and β-secretase β-site APP-cleaving enzyme. *J Neurosci* **26:** 418–428.

Stachel SJ. 2009. Progress toward the development of a viable BACE-1 inhibitor. *Drug Devl Res* **70:** 101–110.

Steiner H, Duff K, Capell A, Romig H, Grim MG, Lincoln S, Hardy J, Yu X, Picciano M, Fechteler K, et al. 1999. A loss of function mutation of presenilin-2 interferes with amyloid β-peptide production and notch signaling. *J Biol Chem* **274:** 28669–28673.

Stewart WF, Kawas C, Corrada M, Metter EJ. 1997. Risk of Alzheimer's disease and duration of NSAID use. *Neurology* **48:** 626–632.

Takami M, Nagashima Y, Sano Y, Ishihara S, Morishima-Kawashima M, Funamoto S, Ihara Y. 2009. γ-Secretase: Successive tripeptide and tetrapeptide release from the transmembrane domain of β-carboxyl terminal fragment. *J Neurosci* **29:** 13042–13052.

Thal LJ, Ferris SH, Kirby L, Block GA, Lines CR, Yuen E, Assaid C, Nessly ML, Norman BA, Baranak CC, et al. 2005. A randomized, double-blind, study of rofecoxib in patients with mild cognitive impairment. *Neuropsychopharmacology* **30:** 1204–1215.

Thomas T, Nadackal TG, Thomas K. 2001. Aspirin and nonsteroidal anti-inflammatory drugs inhibit amyloid-β aggregation. *Neuroreport* **12:** 3263–3267.

Thompson LA, Bronson JJ, Zusi FC. 2005. Progress in the discovery of BACE inhibitors. *Curr Pharm Des* **11:** 3383–3404.

Tomiyama T, Asano S, Suwa Y, Morita T, Kataoka K, Mori H, Endo N. 1994. Rifampicin prevents the aggregation and neurotoxicity of amyloid β protein in vitro. *Biochem Biophys Res Commun* **204:** 76–83.

Tong G, Castaneda L, Wang J-S, Sverdlov A, Huang S-P, Slemmnon R, Gu H, Wong O, Li H, Berman RM, et al. 2010. A study to evaluate the effects of single oral doses of BMS-708163 in the cerebrospinal fluid of healthy young men. In *Alzheimer's and Demential, Proceedings of International Conference on Alzheimer's Disease,* S143, O143-p107-107. Alzheimer's Associaiton, Honolulu, HI.

Tournoy J, Bossuyt X, Snellinx A, Regent M, Garmyn M, Serneels L, Saftig P, Craessaerts K, De Strooper B, Hartmann D. 2004. Partial loss of presenilins causes seborrheic keratosis and autoimmune disease in mice. *Hum Mol Genet* **13:** 1321–1331.

Townsend M, Cleary JP, Mehta T, Hofmeister J, Lesne S, O'Hare E, Walsh DM, Selkoe DJ. 2006a. Orally available compound prevents deficits in memory caused by the Alzheimer amyloid-β oligomers. *Ann Neurology* **60:** 668–676.

Townsend M, Shankar GM, Mehta T, Walsh DM, Selkoe DJ. 2006b. Effects of secreted oligomers of amyloid β-protein on hippocampal synaptic plasticity: A potent role for trimers. *J Physiol* **572:** 477–492.

Vasilevko V, Xu F, Previti ML, Van Nostrand WE, Cribbs DH. 2007. Experimental investigation of antibody-mediated clearance mechanisms of amyloid-β in CNS of Tg-SwDI transgenic mice. *J Neurosci* **27:** 13376–13383.

Vassar R, Bennett BD, Babu-Khan S, Kahn S, Mendiaz EA, Denis P, Teplow DB, Ross S, Amarante P, Loeloff R, et al. 1999. β-Secretase cleavage of Alzheimer's amyloid precursor protein by the transmembrane aspartic protease BACE. *Science* **286:** 735–741.

Vellas B, Black R, Thal LJ, Fox NC, Daniels M, McLennan G, Tompkins C, Leibman C, Pomfret M, Grundman M, et al. 2009. Long-term follow-up of patients immunized with AN1792: Reduced functional decline in antibody responders. *Curr Alzheimer Res* **6:** 144–151.

Walsh DM, Selkoe DJ. 2007. A β oligomers—A decade of discovery. *J Neurochem* **101:** 1172–1184.

Weggen S, Eriksen JL, Das P, Sagi SA, Wang R, Pietrzik CU, Findlay KA, Smith TE, Murphy MP, Bulter T, et al. 2001. A subset of NSAIDs lower amyloidogenic Aβ42 independently of cyclooxygenase activity. *Nature* **414:** 212–216.

Wei P, Walls M, Qiu M, Ding R, Denlinger RH, Wong A, Tsaparikos K, Jani JP, Hosea N, Sands M, et al. 2010. Evaluation of selective γ-secretase inhibitor PF-03084014 for its antitumor efficacy and gastrointestinal safety to guide optimal clinical trial design. *Mol Cancer Ther* **9:** 1618–1628.

Weiner HL, Lemere CA, Maron R, Spooner ET, Grenfell TJ, Mori C, Issazadeh S, Hancock WW, Selkoe DJ. 2000. Nasal administration of amyloid-β peptide decreases cerebral amyloid burden in a mouse model of Alzheimer's disease. *Ann Neurology* **48:** 567–579.

Wiesehan K, Stohr J, Nagel-Steger L, van Groen T, Riesner D, Willbold D. 2008. Inhibition of cytotoxicity and amyloid fibril formation by a D-amino acid peptide that specifically binds to Alzheimer's disease amyloid peptide. *Protein Eng Des Sel* **21:** 241–246.

Wilcock DM, DiCarlo G, Henderson D, Jackson J, Clarke K, Ugen KE, Gordon MN, Morgan D. 2003. Intracranially administered anti-Aβ antibodies reduce β-amyloid deposition by mechanisms both independent of and associated with microglial activation. *J Neurosci* **23:** 3745–3751.

Wilcock DM, Rojiani A, Rosenthal A, Subbarao S, Freeman MJ, Gordon MN, Morgan D. 2004. Passive immunotherapy against Aβ in aged APP-transgenic mice reverses cognitive deficits and depletes parenchymal amyloid deposits in spite of increased vascular amyloid and microhemorrhage. *J Neuroinflamm* **1:** 24.

Wilcock GK, Black SE, Hendrix SB, Zavitz KH, Swabb EA, Laughlin MA. 2008. Efficacy and safety of tarenflurbil in mild to moderate Alzheimer's disease: A randomised phase II trial. *Lancet Neurol* **7:** 483–493.

Wilcock DM, Gharkholonarehe N, Van Nostrand WE, Davis J, Vitek MP, Colton CA. 2009. Amyloid reduction by amyloid-β vaccination also reduces mouse tau pathology and protects from neuron loss in two mouse models of Alzheimer's disease. *J Neurosci* **29:** 7957–7965.

Willem M, Garratt AN, Novak B, Citron M, Kaufmann S, Rittger A, DeStrooper B, Saftig P, Birchmeier C, Haass C. 2006. Control of peripheral nerve myelination by the β-secretase BACE1. *Science* **314:** 664–666.

Wolfe MS, Xia W, Ostaszewski BL, Diehl TS, Kimberly WT, Selkoe DJ. 1999. Two transmembrane aspartates in presenilin-1 required for presenilin endoproteolysis and γ-secretase activity. *Nature* **398:** 513–517.

Wong GT, Manfra D, Poulet FM, Zhang Q, Josien H, Bara T, Engstrom L, Pinzon-Ortiz M, Fine JS, Lee HJ, et al. 2004. Chronic treatment with the γ-secretase inhibitor LY-411,575 inhibits β-amyloid peptide production and alters lymphopoiesis and intestinal cell differentiation. *J Biol Chem* **279:** 12876–12882.

Wong HK, Sakurai T, Oyama F, Kaneko K, Wada K, Miyazaki H, Kurosawa M, De Strooper B, Saftig P, Nukina N. 2005. β Subunits of voltage-gated sodium channels are novel substrates of β-site amyloid precursor protein-cleaving enzyme (BACE1) and γ-secretase. *J Biol Chem* **280:** 23009–23017.

Wood SJ, MacKenzie L, Maleeff B, Hurle MR, Wetzel R. 1996. Selective inhibition of Aβ fibril formation. *J Biol Chem* **271:** 4086–4092.

Woodard-Grice AV, McBrayer AC, Wakefield JK, Zhuo Y, Bellis SL. 2008. Proteolytic shedding of ST6Gal-I by BACE1 regulates the glycosylation and function of α4β1 integrins. *J Biol Chem* **283:** 26364–26373.

Xu X. 2009. Gamma-secretase catalyzes sequential cleavages of the AβPP transmembrane domain. *J Alzheimer's Dis* **16:** 211–224.

Yamada K, Yabuki C, Seubert P, Schenk D, Hori Y, Ohtsuki S, Terasaki T, Hashimoto T, Iwatsubo T. 2009. A β immunotherapy: Intracerebral sequestration of Aβ by an anti-Aβ monoclonal antibody 266 with high affinity to soluble Aβ. *J Neurosci* **29:** 11393–11398.

Yan R, Bienkowski MJ, Shuck ME, Miao H, Tory MC, Pauley AM, Brashier JR, Stratman NC, Mathews WR, Buhl AE, et al. 1999. Membrane-anchored aspartyl protease with Alzheimer's disease β-secretase activity. *Nature* **402:** 533–537.

Yan R, Munzner JB, Shuck ME, Bienkowski MJ. 2001. BACE2 functions as an alternative α-secretase in cells. *J Biol Chem* **276:** 34019–34027.

Yang LB, Lindholm K, Yan R, Citron M, Xia W, Yang XL, Beach T, Sue L, Wong P, Price D, et al. 2003. Elevated β-secretase expression and enzymatic activity detected in sporadic Alzheimer disease. *Nat Med* **9:** 3–4.

Yang F, Lim GP, Begum AN, Ubeda OJ, Simmons MR, Ambegaokar SS, Chen PP, Kayed R, Glabe CG, Frautschy SA, et al. 2005. Curcumin inhibits formation of amyloid β oligomers and fibrils, binds plaques, and reduces amyloid in vivo. *J Biol Chem* **280:** 5892–5901.

Yates PA, Sirisriro R, Villemagne VL, Farquharson S, Masters CL, Rowe CC, AIBL Research Group. 2011. Cerebral microhemorrhage and brain β-amyloid in aging and Alzheimer disease. *Neurology* **77:** 48–54.

Zhang J, Wu X, Qin C, Qi J, Ma S, Zhang H, Kong Q, Chen D, Ba D, He W. 2003. A novel recombinant adeno-associated virus vaccine reduces behavioral impairment and β-amyloid plaques in a mouse model of Alzheimer's disease. *Neurobiol Dis* **14:** 365–379.

Zhao B, Yu M, Neitzel M, Marugg J, Jagodzinski J, Lee M, Hu K, Schenk D, Yednock T, Basi G. 2008. Identification of γ-secretase inhibitor potency determinants on presenilin. *J Biol Chem* **283:** 2927–2938.

Ziora Z, Kimura T, Kiso Y. 2006. Small-sized BACE1 inhibitors. *Drugs Future* **31:** 53–63.

Developing Therapeutic Approaches to Tau, Selected Kinases, and Related Neuronal Protein Targets

Virginia M-Y. Lee[1], Kurt R. Brunden[1], Michael Hutton[2], and John Q. Trojanowski[1]

[1]Center for Neurodegenerative Disease Research, Institute on Aging, Department of Pathology and Laboratory Medicine, School of Medicine, University of Pennsylvania, Philadelphia, Pennsylvania 19104

[2]Eli Lilly and Co., Indianapolis, Indiana 46285

Correspondence: kbrunden@upenn.edu

A hallmark of the Alzheimer disease (AD) brain is the presence of inclusions within neurons that are comprised of fibrils formed from the microtubule-stabilizing protein tau. The formation of misfolded multimeric tau species is believed to contribute to the progressive neuron loss and cognitive impairments of AD. Moreover, mutations in tau have been shown to cause a form of frontotemporal lobar degeneration in which tau neuronal inclusions observed in the brain are similar to those seen in AD. Here we review the more compelling strategies that are designed to reduce the contribution of misfolded tau to AD neuropathology, including those directed at correcting a possible loss of tau function resulting from sequestration of cellular tau and to minimizing possible gain-of-function toxicities caused by multimeric tau species. Finally, we discuss the challenges and potential benefits of tau-directed drug discovery programs.

INTRODUCTION TO TAU PATHOLOGY AND GENETICS

The Alzheimer disease (AD) brain contains two key pathological features that are used to make a definitive diagnosis; extracellular deposits referred to as senile plaques, and neuronal intracellular inclusions called neurofibrillary tangles (NFTs). As discussed in detail in other articles of this volume, senile plaques are comprised of fibrils of amyloid β (Aβ) peptides (Glenner and Wong 1984) that are formed during proteolytic processing of the amyloid precursor protein (APP) (Kang et al. 1987). Here

we focus on the other hallmark of the Alzheimer disease (AD) brain, the NFTs that are formed from insoluble fibrils of tau protein (Kidd 1963; Lee et al. 1991). More specifically, we review the likely involvement of misfolded tau in the neurodegeneration and memory impairments observed in AD, and present possible therapeutic strategies to ameliorate tau-mediated pathology.

Tau is highly enriched within neurons of the central nervous system, in which it appears to play an important role in the formation and stabilization of microtubules (MTs) (Drechsel et al. 1992; Gustke et al. 1994). MTs are critical to neuronal function, serving as conduits on which key cellular components are transported along axons. In the human CNS, there are six major tau isoforms that are generated by differential splicing of exons 2, 3, and 10 of the tau transcript (Fig. 1) (Goedert et al. 1989; Andreadis et al. 1992). The inclusion or exclusion of exon 10 results in tau species that contain either four (4-R) or three (3-R) microtubule-binding repeats, respectively, with the ratio of 3-R-to-4-R tau being ~1 in the normal brain (Hong et al. 1998). In AD and other related neurodegenerative "tauopathies," which include Pick's disease, progressive supranuclear palsy (PSP), and corticobasal degeneration (CBD), misfolded and hyperphosphorylated tau accumulates as insoluble fibrils primarily within neuronal cell bodies (as NFTs) and in processes (as neuropil threads or dystrophic neurites), but

also as tau inclusions in astrocytes and microglia (Lee et al. 2001; Ballatore et al. 2007b). The presence of tau inclusions in AD and a large number of other neurodegenerative tauopathies suggests that these deposits somehow contribute to development of synaptic deficits and neuronal loss. In fact, cortical NFT density correlates well with cognitive decline in AD unlike senile plaque burden (Wilcock and Esiri 1982; Braak and Braak 1991; Arriagada et al. 1992; Gomez-Isla et al. 1997), which occurs early and appears to reach a plateau prior to the onset of clinical symptoms. Indeed, ~90% of the tau pathology burden in AD is in dystrophic neurites so that tangle counts underestimate the total burden of tau pathology (Mitchell et al. 2000). Proof that altered tau function and/or structure can cause neurodegeneration has

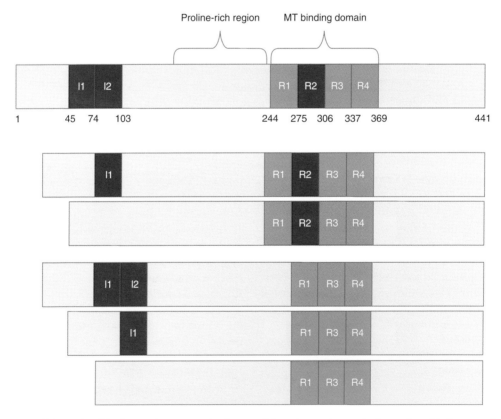

Figure 1. Schematic of the longest human tau isoform and the other major tau isoforms found in humans that are generated through posttranscriptional splicing of exons 2 (I1), 3 (I2), and 10 (R2). The inclusion or exclusion of exon 10 results in tau with four or three binding repeats within the MT binding domain (4R-tau or 3R-tau), respectively. Amino acid numbers are depicted along the bottom of the longest tau isoform.

been provided by the discovery that Frontotemporal Dementia with Parkinsonism linked to Chromosome 17 (FTDP-17) results from mutations in the *tau* gene (Hong et al. 1998; Hutton et al. 1998). Although there are no reported tau mutations in AD, the similarities in tau pathology observed in the various tauopathies suggests that tau plays a pivotal role mediating neurodegeneration in all of these diseases.

The tau mutations observed in FTDP-17 fall into two general classes; those that affect the splicing of exon 10, such that the 4-R-to-3-R tau ratio is increased, and those that alter tau structure and function. The latter are predominantly located within the MT-binding domains (Goedert and Jakes 2005). These FTDP-17 mutations offer an opportunity to understand how tau alterations might lead to neurodegeneration, and current tau gain-of-function and loss-of-function hypotheses, as discussed further below, have resulted largely from studies of mutated tau. For example, it is known that 4-R tau binds MTs more avidly than 3-R tau (Panda et al. 2003), and thus FTDP-17 mutations that result in increased 4-R tau because of altered splicing of exon 10 (Hong et al. 1998) might lead to an overstabilization of MTs with resulting axonal dysfunction. Conversely, FTDP-17 mutations within the MT-binding domains of tau generally reduce the binding of tau to MTs (Hasegawa et al. 1998; Hong et al. 1998; Dayanandan et al. 1999), perhaps leading to a destabilization of MTs. In addition, mutations that reduce tau binding to MTs could increase the concentration of unbound tau and thus promote the formation of tau multimers and fibrils that have been proposed to elicit a direct toxic effect on neurons. Many of the tau coding-region mutations in FTDP-17 also promote enhancement of tau oligomerization and fibrillization (Hong et al. 1998; Nacharaju et al. 1999; Barghorn et al. 2000; Avila et al. 2006). Finally, in vitro tau assembly studies have suggested that under reducing conditions, 4R tau forms fibrils more readily than 3R tau (Barghorn and Mandelkow 2002; Jeganathan et al. 2008). As a reducing environment is generally maintained in cells, the exon 10 splicing mutations that increase 4R tau may also accelerate

tau aggregation in patients. This observation may provide a simple explanation of why the two types of tau mutations that appear to have opposing effects on microtubule binding result in a broadly similar clinical and pathological syndrome.

Although the FTDP-17 mutations provide important evidence that tau misfolding and multimerization can lead to neurodegeneration, the absence of tau mutations in AD suggests that other tau changes and/or factor(s) are required to initiate tau pathogenesis in this disease. For example, posttranslational phosphorylation of tau appears to cause structural and functional changes that mimic those observed with FTDP-17 mutations and tau proteins isolated from paired helical filaments (PHFs) from AD brains do not bind to MTs unless they are dephosphorylated (Bramblett et al. 1993). The ability to recapture MT binding on dephosphorylation provides evidence that modulation of tau phosphorylation may be a viable therapeutic strategy. Tau is phosphorylated at multiple serine (ser) and threonine (thr) residues (Buee et al. 2000; Avila 2006), and increased phosphorylation at many of these sites results in reduced tau binding to MTs (Alonso et al. 1996; Wagner et al. 1996; Merrick et al. 1997) and/or a greater propensity for tau to assemble into fibrils (Alonso et al. 1996; Necula and Kuret 2004). However, phosphorylation at certain sites prevents tau fibrillization (Schneider et al. 1999), and there is thus greater consensus that the primary effect of tau hyperphosphorylation is to decrease MT binding and increase the cytosolic tau concentration (Ballatore et al. 2007b; Brunden et al. 2009). In general, the extent to which posttranslational phosphorylation contributes to the onset of tau pathology in AD is still uncertain, as tau hyperphosphorylation is also observed in FTDP-17, in which tau mutations are presumably responsible for the development of pathology.

Tau can also be modified through the addition of β-N-acetylglucosamine (O-GlcNac) at certain ser and thr phosphorylation sites, and there is evidence that increased O-GlcNac modification of tau results in a corresponding decrease in phosphorylation (Lefebvre et al. 2003; Liu et al. 2004). Tau can also undergo tyrosine phosphorylation (Lee et al. 2004), sumoylation, and nitration (Gong et al. 2005; Reynolds et al. 2006), although the consequences of these modifications are presently unclear. Finally, it has recently been shown that tau can undergo acetylation on multiple lysines (Min et al. 2010; Cohen et al. 2011), including lysine residues (K280/K281) within a MT binding repeat. The acetylation of tau at K280, much like phosphorylation at certain tau residues, impairs the ability of tau to bind MTs and increases its propensity to fibrillize (Cohen et al. 2011). Importantly, tau within NFTs are found to be acetylated at K280 in PSP, CBD, and other tau diseases with inclusions formed by 4-R tau, or in AD in which NFTs contain a mixture of 4-R and 3-R tau. Similarly, NFT-like inclusions within Tg mouse models of tauopathy are acetylated at K280. As discussed further below, this suggests that a new therapeutic strategy for AD and related tauopathies might be the inhibition of tau acetylation.

TAU AS A DRUG TARGET

The aforementioned studies have provided important information about how tau mutations and posttranslational modification can affect its microtubule binding and assembly into multimeric structures. These findings suggest potential therapeutic strategies to reduce the untoward effects of altered tau in neurodegenerative disease, and these approaches are generally directed to overcoming tau loss-of-function or reducing levels of potentially toxic tau species (Fig. 2). More specifically, there are ongoing research programs within academia and/or industry that are aimed at identifying prototype drug candidates, which will:

- Compensate for a loss of tau stabilization of MTs, given the importance of MTs in axonal transport and proper neuronal function.

- Attenuate tau hyperphosphorylation through the inhibition of key tau kinases, thereby restoring tau interaction with MTs and perhaps reducing tau aggregation.

- Prevent tau–tau interactions and resulting multimerization, thus mitigating the formation of potentially neurotoxic tau species.

- Increase degradation of misfolded or otherwise pathologically altered tau through an enhancement of cellular catabolic pathways, again with the objective of reducing the levels of toxic forms of tau.

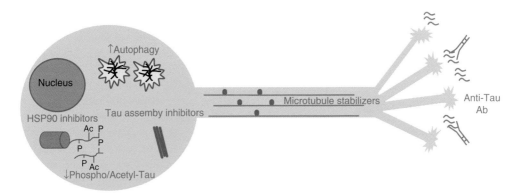

Figure 2. Possible tau-based therapeutic strategies in Alzheimer disease. A loss of tau function might be overcome with microtubule-stabilizing agents or inhibitors of tau hyperphosphorylation and/or acetylation. Potentially toxic tau oligomers or fibrils might be prevented by inhibitors of tau multimeric assembly. Inhibition of HSP90 and the resulting elevation of the chaperones HSP70/HSP40 may increase proteasomal degradation of hyperphosphorylated tau. Misfolded tau multimers might be cleared through enhancement of macroautophagy. Finally, misfolded tau species may be released from cells and internalized by nearby neurons, thereby "seeding" the formation of pathological tau in the recipient cell. If confirmed, this spreading of tau pathology might be inhibited by antibodies that bind misfolded tau in the brain interstitial fluid.

In addition to the above, there is new emerging evidence that tau pathology may spread in the brain through the release of tau species into the interstitial fluid that can be internalized by nearby neurons, thereby acting as "seeds" to foster the formation of additional pathologic tau (Clavaguera et al. 2009). Further validation of this mechanism of tau transmission would suggest additional therapeutic approaches, including passive immunotherapy strategies whereby tau-directed antibodies might prevent the spread of pathologic tau. In the following sections, we will discuss in detail these various tau-directed strategies for the treatment of AD and related pathologies, including the challenges associated with each approach.

COMPENSATION FOR TAU LOSS-OF-FUNCTION

As noted, a possible cause of the neurodegeneration observed in tauopathies is a loss of tau function with resulting MT destabilization. Support for this hypothesis is provided by the observed decrease within the AD brain of the stabilized MT marker, acetyl-tubulin (Hempen and Brion 1996). Likewise, pyramidal neurons in the AD brain have been reported to have reduced MT density (Cash et al. 2003). Finally, Tg mice that overexpress 3-R tau display an age-dependent formation of intraneuronal tau inclusions in the brainstem, spinal cord, and cortex that is accompanied by a reduction of MT density and deficiencies in fast axonal transport (Ishihara et al. 1999).

These data suggest that compensation for tau loss-of-function with MT-stabilizing drugs might be a therapeutic strategy for the treatment of AD and related tauopathies. Drugs of this type have been employed for some time in the treatment of cancer, as molecules such as paclitaxel and docetaxol (Saloustros et al. 2008) inhibit cancer cell division through alteration of the mitotic spindle. However, the potent antimitotic properties of these drugs come at the cost of severe side effects, including neutropenia and peripheral neuropathies (Bedard et al. 2010). Thus, it is unlikely that these chemotherapeutic agents could be used safely in

AD and other tauopathies using current cancer dosing regimens, as long-term dosing would likely be required in these neurodegenerative disorders. However, a complete loss of tau function is unlikely in tauopathies, and thus it may be possible to use doses of MT-stabilizing drugs that are lower than those currently employed in cancer chemotherapy to compensate for loss of tau activity. In fact, important proof-of-principle data have been obtained, which suggest that relatively low doses of a MT-stabilizing compound can improve neuronal deficits that result from tau misfolding. Utilizing the T44 tau Tg mouse model, which shows motor neuron MT deficits and functional impairments (Ishihara et al. 1999), Zhang et al. (2005) showed that weekly administration of 10 or 25 mg/m^2 of a paclitaxel formulation for a total of 12 weeks resulted in marked improvements in MT density, fast axonal transport, and motor performance. Furthermore, the drug-treated animals did not show any discernible signs of associated toxicities or side effects. The paclitaxel doses used in this study were much lower than the typical human doses of 135–175 mg/m^2, and thus provide hope that small molecule MT-stabilizing compounds can be used safely for the treatment of tauopathies.

Although these data provided important validation of the concept of compensating for tau loss-of-function, it is unlikely that paclitaxel will be suitable for the treatment of CNS disorders. The taxanes, including paclitaxel and docetaxel, have poor BBB permeability that is thought to result, at least in part, from these molecules being substrates for the P-glycoprotein (Pgp) transporter that prevents xenobiotics from accumulating in the brain (Sparreboom et al. 1997; Fellner et al. 2002). Improved taxanes have been synthesized that are not Pgp substrates (Cisternino et al. 2003; Ballatore et al. 2007a; Ojima et al. 2008; Metzger-Filho et al. 2009), but recent data from our laboratory suggest that such compounds still have poor brain penetration (Brunden et al. 2011). However, several examples from the epothilone class of MT-stabilizing compounds, some of which have progressed to clinical testing for cancer (Altmann 2005; Beer et al. 2007; Denduluri et al. 2007), partition readily across the BBB and one of these molecules, epothilone D, has a long-lasting pharmacodynamic effect in the brain (Brunden et al. 2011). Treatment of Tg mice that express mutant human tau, and which develop NFT-like tau pathology, with low doses of epothilone D resulted in an improvement of CNS MT density, a reduction of axonal dystrophy, and an improvement of cognitive performance relative to vehicle-treated littermates (Brunden et al. 2010b). Importantly, no side effects were noted in the epothilone D-treated mice in this proof-of-concept prevention study in tau Tg mice, including an absence of neutropenia or signs of peripheral neuropathy. These data suggest that a brain-penetrant MT-stabilizing agent such as epothilone D might be suitable for clinical evaluation in patients with AD or a related tauopathy.

A potential alternative to brain-penetrant small molecule MT-stabilizing drugs such as the epothilones is the octapeptide, NAP. This peptide is believed to interact with neuron-specific βIII-tubulin (Divinski et al. 2006; Matsuoka et al. 2007), and intranasal administration of NAP to Tg mice that develop both Aβ and tau pathology resulted in a reduction of hyperphosphorylated tau and diminution of Aβ peptide levels. Similarly, a recent study showed that intranasal dosing of NAP to Tg mice expressing mutated tau also led to a reduction of tau phosphorylation (Shiryaev et al. 2009). Although the mechanism(s) by which NAP stabilization of MTs leads to a decrease of tau phosphorylation and Aβ levels is unclear, these data nonetheless provide additional support for a therapeutic strategy of compensating for tau loss-of-function in AD. NAP (davunetide) has progressed to clinical testing, with a Phase IIa trial recently completed in AD patients (see http://www.allontherapeutics.com) and pivotal clinical trials underway.

Although the improvement in MT density observed in tau Tg mice on treatment with MT-stabilizing molecules suggests a compensation for tau loss-of-function, it is possible that these agents improve neuronal health through additional complementary mechanisms. For example, it has recently been shown that MT

stabilization with paclitaxel enhances regeneration after spinal cord injury in rats (Hellal et al. 2011). Injured CNS axons appear to have a collapse of MT integrity that results in the formation of retraction bulbs, and an enhancement of MT stabilization in such cells promotes axon regeneration (Erturk et al. 2007). Thus, it is possible that MT-stabilizing agents such as epothilone D attenuate axonal retraction/damage that arises from tau-mediated toxicity in tau Tg mouse models. MT-stabilizing compounds might also affect axonal transport by increasing the engagement of motor proteins with MTs. It is known that tau binding to MTs can have an inhibitory effect on kinesin-mediated anterograde axonal transport in cell culture systems in which tau is overexpressed (Stamer et al. 2002; Vershinin et al. 2007; Dixit et al. 2008), although this has not been shown in vivo. Because paclitaxel binding to tubulin has been shown to reduce the amount of tau incorporated into MTs (Kar et al. 2003), it is conceivable that paclitaxel and other MT-stabilizing agents, which share the paclitaxel binding site (such as the epothilones), reduce tau binding to MTs, thereby allowing greater kinesin engagement with MTs and improving anterograde axonal transport. However, this possibility has not yet been investigated in tau Tg mouse models.

INHIBITION OF TAU PHOSPHORYLATION

Another possible strategy to improve MT stabilization in AD and other tauopathies is to prevent the phosphorylation that reduces tau interaction with MTs (Alonso et al. 1994, 1996; Wagner et al. 1996; Merrick et al. 1997). Decreasing tau phosphorylation might also reduce levels of unbound tau that are available for the formation of potentially toxic oligomeric and fibrillar structures (Alonso et al. 1996; Necula and Kuret 2004). A therapeutic strategy based on inhibition of tau phosphorylation has practical appeal because protein kinases provide a proven, if extremely difficult, class of drug targets with which the pharmaceutical industry has considerable experience.

Although normal tau is phosphorylated at multiple sites, the extent of phosphorylation at these sites is relatively low. However, in AD brain tau phosphorylation is increased three- to fourfold (Ksiezak-Reding et al. 1992; Kopke et al. 1993; Matsuo et al. 1994), mostly through increased levels of phosphorylation on the tau that is incorporated into neurofibrillary inclusions. There are ~25 ser and thr residues within tau that appear to be sites of enhanced phosphorylation in AD (Morishima-Kawashima et al. 1995; Hanger et al. 1998), and these are found primarily in the proline-rich domain and the carboxy-terminal region (see Fig. 1), although a few sites also reside within the MT-binding domains (Hanger et al. 2009). A number of candidate kinases have been proposed to play a role in the posttranslational phosphorylation of tau (Mazanetz and Fischer 2007; Gong and Iqbal 2008; Hanger et al. 2009). Among these are kinases that modify ser/thr residues that precede a proline residue, including glycogen synthase kinase 3 (GSK-3) α and β, cyclin-dependent kinase 5 (CDK5), and mitogen-activated kinase 1 (MAPK1). In addition, nonproline directed kinases such as protein kinase A, p38 and microtubule-affinity regulated kinases (MARK1–4) (Drewes et al. 1997) have been implicated in tau phosphorylation. Of these various kinases, the existing data arguably support GSK-3β and CDK5 as being the best-validated tau kinase targets, and these enzymes will be the focus of further discussion here.

GSK-3 α and/or β, or more simply GSK-3 because available research tools generally do not discriminate between these closely related isoforms, colocalizes with NFT in the AD brain (Yamaguchi et al. 1996; Imahori and Uchida 1997). Similarly, CDK5 is also found in NFTs (Yamaguchi et al. 1996; Pei et al. 1998; Augustinack et al. 2002). CDK5 requires a regulatory subunit for activity and interacts with p35 and p39, or with their more stable proteolytic products, p25, and p29, respectively. Overexpression of p25 in Tg mice has been reported to result in tau hyperphosphorylation (Ahlijanian et al. 2000; Noble et al. 2003). Similarly, Tg mice expressing GSK-3β display increased tau phosphorylation, as well as learning and memory deficits (Spittaels et al. 2000; Lucas et al. 2001;

Hernandez et al. 2002). Interestingly, there is recent evidence of coordinated regulation of GSK-3 and CDK5, as mice that overexpress the p25 regulatory subunit of CDK5 have decreased GSK-3 activity that has been attributed to phosphorylation of an inhibitory ser[9] residue on GSK-3 (Wen et al. 2008). Moreover, inhibition of CDK5 resulted in an increase of tau phosphorylation by GSK-3 (Wen et al. 2008). Nonetheless, there are ongoing efforts by a number of industry and academic laboratories to identify inhibitors of both CDK5 and GSK-3.

In the case of GSK-3, these drug discovery activities have been further spurred by the observation that GSK-3 activity may affect Aβ production (Aplin et al. 1997; Phiel et al. 2003; Rockenstein et al. 2007) and by studies in tau Tg mice in which prototype inhibitors of GSK-3 have been reported to result in a diminution of both tau phosphorylation and intracellular tau inclusions. For example, daily administration of the GSK-3 inhibitor LiCl for 30 days to JNPL3 tau Tg mice, which overexpress P301L 4R-tau, resulted in the inhibition of GSK-3 activity, reductions of both phospho-tau and insoluble tau, and lessening of axonal degeneration (Noble et al. 2005). These authors also showed a similar effect on tau phosphorylation and insolubility using a somewhat selective small molecule GSK-3 inhibitor (Noble et al. 2005). Treatment of another Tg mouse line, which expresses tau harboring three missense mutations, with LiCl also resulted in a decrement of both tau phosphorylation and tau intracellular inclusions (Perez et al. 2003). Furthermore, treatment of young Tg mice that express 3R-tau with LiCl for 4 months resulted in a reduction of insoluble tau, although somewhat surprisingly there was not an apparent reduction of the assessed phospho-tau epitopes (Nakashima et al. 2005). Finally, a relatively nonspecific but brain-penetrant kinase inhibitor was shown to decrease total levels of hyperphosphorylated tau (migrating at 64kDa) and improve motor function in JNPL3 tau Tg mice, albeit without a reduction of NFTs, thereby suggesting that smaller tau assemblies might have caused neuronal dysfunction (Le Corre et al. 2006).

The various medicinal chemistry approaches that have been employed to develop tau kinase inhibitors have been reviewed elsewhere (Churcher 2006; Mazanetz and Fischer 2007). However, it is worth considering here the challenges associated with this therapeutic strategy. As noted above, a number of candidate kinases have been proposed to phosphorylate tau. However, it is still unclear which of these are important in AD or even whether the majority of the hyperphosphorylation occurs before or after initial tau assembly. It is possible and perhaps likely that multiple kinases act on tau in the brain, and thus selective inhibition of a single kinase may not prevent the detrimental effects associated with tau hyperphosphorylation. In this regard, it is difficult to develop exquisitely selective kinase inhibitors because most compounds are directed to the ATP-binding site that is common to all kinases. Although a nonselective ser/thr kinase inhibitor may have some advantages in AD because of the likely involvement of more than one kinase in tau hyperphosphorylation, a lack of selectivity could also lead to an increased likelihood of side effects. Finally, even highly selective inhibition of individual tau kinases implicated in AD may prove problematic, as these enzymes are known to modify other critical cellular proteins. Such "on-target" dose limiting toxicity is known to impact drug development for GSK-3, which plays an important role in the regulation of glycogen metabolism, cell proliferation, and oncogenesis (Rayasam et al. 2009). Likewise, CDK5 has been suggested to regulate axonal and synaptic function (Dhavan and Tsai 2001).

An alternative approach to decreasing tau hyperphosphorylation would be to increase phosphate removal. The dephosphorylation of tau appears to result primarily from the action of protein phosphatase 2A (PP2A) (Matsuo et al. 1994), and there is evidence that this enzyme is compromised in AD brain (Gong et al. 1995). One potential strategy to increase PP2A-mediated dephosphorylation of tau would be to decrease the binding of one or both of the inhibitory proteins that regulate PPA2 activity (Tanimukai et al. 2009).

Another possible alternative strategy to regulating tau phosphorylation has emerged that does not entail kinase inhibition. Tau is also modified through the addition of β-N-acetylglucosamine at ser/thr residues (O-GlcNAc), and there is evidence of an inverse relationship between the extent of O-GlcNAc modification and the degree of tau phosphorylation (Lefebvre et al. 2003; Liu et al. 2004). The O-GlcNAc modification can be reversed by O-GlcNAcase, and a prototype inhibitor of this enzyme caused a decrease of tau phosphorylation in normal rats (Yuzwa et al. 2008). These data suggest that inhibition of O-GlcNAcase may be a potential therapeutic approach for AD and other tauopathies, although many proteins undergo O-GlcNAc addition and there may therefore be as yet undefined detrimental consequences of sustained inhibition of O-GlcNAcase.

Finally, very recent data indicate that another tau posttranslational modification, acetylation, may impart changes that resemble those observed after phosphorylation (Min et al. 2010; Cohen et al. 2011). In particular, acetylation of lysine residues 280 within a MT binding repeat of tau decreases its ability to induce MT assembly and increases its propensity to fibrillize (Cohen et al. 2011). Tau acetylation has also been suggested to decrease proteasome-mediated degradation of phosphorylated tau (Min et al. 2010). Accordingly, inhibition of tau acetylation in AD and related 4-R tauopathies could increase tau binding to MTs, reduce tau aggregation, and enhance catabolism of phospho-tau species. The most straightforward approach to attenuating tau acetylation would be inhibition of the appropriate acetyl-transferase(s). However, these enzymes, like protein kinases, have multiple cellular substrates. For example, the p300/CBP acetyl-transferase implicated in tau acetylation (Min et al. 2010; Cohen et al. 2011) has more than 75 described protein substrates (Yang and Seto 2008; Bowers et al. 2010). Thus, it is unclear whether drugs can be developed that will decrease tau acetylation specifically without affecting other substrates that could induce side effects.

ENHANCEMENT OF TAU DEGRADATION

The hypothesis that tau oligomers or fibrils are harmful suggests that increased catabolism of pathological tau would be beneficial. Cells are equipped to degrade misfolded proteins by two general mechanisms; via the ubiquitin-proteasome system (UPS) and through autophagy (Fig. 2). In the former, proteins that are destined for catabolism are modified on lysine residues through the addition of ubiquitin molecules, with subsequent degradation by the proteasome. Because proteins must gain entry into a "pore" within the proteasome complex to undergo proteolysis, it is unlikely that large oligomeric tau species can be acted on by proteasomes. However, although normal tau is not believed to be degraded by the UPS, this pathway has been implicated in the turn-over of phosphorylated tau. The "carboxy terminus of HSP70-interacting protein" (CHIP) appears to regulate tau ubiquitination (Petrucelli et al. 2004; Shimura et al. 2004) and CHIP knockout mice display an accumulation of phospho-tau (Dickey et al. 2006b). CHIP can form a complex with the molecular chaperone HSP70 and target proteins to the proteasome, and increased HSP70 expression in cell culture models leads to a decrease in insoluble phospho-tau and an increase of soluble tau (Dou et al. 2003; Petrucelli et al. 2004). HSP90 is another molecular chaperone that assists in protein refolding, and inhibition of the ATPase function of HSP90 with compounds such as geldanamycin results in an increased expression of HSP70 and HSP40 (Zhang and Burrows 2004). HSP90 inhibition in cell culture leads to an increased degradation of phospho-tau (Dickey et al. 2006a) that appears to result from a change of HSP90 chaperone function such that phospho-tau is targeted to the CHIP/HSP70 complex, in which it is polyubiquinated and degraded by the proteasome (Dickey et al. 2007). Importantly, HSP90 inhibitors have been shown to reduce the amount of hyperphosphorylated tau in Tg mouse models. Both acute and subchronic dosing of JNPL3 tau Tg mice with the brain-penetrant HSP90 inhibitor PU-DZ8 led to a reduction of both soluble and hyperphosphorylated insoluble tau (Luo et al. 2007). Interestingly, PU-DZ8 treatment also caused a reduction of p35, the cofactor required for CDK5 activity. Thus, HSP90 inhibition may affect phosphorylated tau levels both through increased proteasomal degradation of tau and reduced CDK5-mediated tau phosphorylation. In another study, a 7-day administration of the HSP90 inhibitor EC102 to Tg mice that express all six isoforms of normal human tau and which develop tau inclusions, resulted in a reduction of phospho-tau species (Dickey et al. 2007).

As with all therapeutic strategies, the possible benefits of HSP90 inhibition will have to be weighed against potential safety risks. A priori, it would seem that prolonged HSP90 inhibition would be problematic, as this will lead to the degradation of other Hsp90 client proteins in addition to tau. Moreover, genetic knockout of HSP90 in mice is lethal. However, there appears to be some selectivity of HSP90 inhibitors for HSP90 found within cancer cells as opposed to normal cells (Solit and Chiosis 2008; Mahalingam et al. 2009). Although the reason for this selectivity is not fully understood, several hypotheses have been proposed (Chiosis and Neckers 2006; Solit and Chiosis 2008). These include the possibility of a preferential binding of inhibitors to HSP90 that is bound to multimeric chaperone complexes that are elevated in cancer cells (Kamal et al. 2003), or that HSP90 levels may be limiting in cancer cells because of an increased burden of misfolded proteins. Regardless of the explanation, it remains to be shown whether neurons harboring excessive hyperphosphorylated tau are also selectively affected by HSP90 inhibitors, although it appears that HSP90 inhibitors bind to cortical homogenates from AD brain with greater affinity than to those from control brain (Dickey et al. 2007).

As noted, misfolded and/or hyperphosphorylated tau that assembles into larger oligomers or fibrils is unlikely to be degraded by the UPS because of their exclusion from the proteasome pore. However, there is evidence that larger protein aggregates, including tau multimers, can be cleared through autophagy.

Multiple forms of autophagy have been described (Nixon 2006; Williams et al. 2006), but the degradation of large protein aggregates and defective cellular organelles is believed to occur via macroautophagy, whereby an autophagasome encapsulates the material to be degraded and subsequently fuses with a lysosome. Macroautophagy can be induced with the drug rapamycin, and treatment of flies expressing wild-type or mutant human tau with rapamycin led to a diminution of insoluble tau (Berger et al. 2006). Conversely, perturbation of lysosome function or inhibition of autophagy in neuroblastoma cells expressing human tau resulted in slower tau clearance (Hamano et al. 2008). More recent work has implicated the autophagy-lysosomal system in tau fragmentation and the clearance of tau aggregates (Wang et al. 2009). Thus, although there are still relatively few reports on the role of autophagy in the degradation of misfolded tau, it is possible that up-regulation of this cellular process might be beneficial in reducing pathological tau species. However, it is not entirely clear that an induction of autophagy will be beneficial in AD and other tauopathies, as it has been suggested that the autophagic deficits, which have been observed in AD brain result from impaired clearance of autophagic vesicles and not faulty initiation of autophagy (Boland et al. 2008).

If an up-regulation of autophagy is found to be an appropriate strategy for AD, it should be noted that the most characterized inducer of autophagy, rapamycin, alters the mTOR signaling pathway and has a variety of other biological effects, including immunosuppression (Delgoffe and Powell 2009). Moreover, there is evidence that rapamycin suppresses tau translation, which appears to be regulated by the mTOR effector 70-kDA ribosomal protein S6 kinase (Morita and Sobue 2009). Thus, although chronic treatment of WT mice with rapamycin extended their lifespan and reduced aging related diseases (Harrison et al. 2009; Miller et al. 2011), the potential complications of prolonged alteration of the mTOR signal transduction suggest that alternative autophagy enhancers will be required for the treatment of neurodegenerative disease. In this regard, LiCl has been suggested to induce autophagy through its inhibition of inositol monophosphatase (Sarkar et al. 2005) and, in fact, it is possible that the reduction in phosphorylated tau levels (Noble et al. 2005) and the reduction of tau lesions (Nakashima et al. 2005) observed on LiCl treatment discussed above were due both to effects both on GSK3 and autophagy.

In addition to up-regulating intracellular tau degradation, another potential approach to lowering misfolded tau in AD brain is via active or passive immunization (Fig. 2). A similar strategy is presently being pursued to lower senile plaque burden, as several active and passive Aβ immunization clinical trials have been completed or are ongoing (Orgogozo et al. 2003; Rinne et al. 2010; Wilcock 2010). Multiple hypotheses have been proposed to explain how Aβ antibodies could lead to plaque reductions. For example, it is possible that a low level of Aβ antibody enters the brain and binds to plaques, thereby invoking complement-mediated microglial clearance. Alternatively, a peripheral sink mechanism may exist whereby the formation of Aβ-antibody complexes in blood lowers free Aβ levels, altering the brain-blood Aβ equilibrium such that Aβ moves from the brain into the blood.

Regardless of how Aβ antibodies might reduce plaques, these data beg the question of whether tau immunization might reduce misfolded tau in the AD brain. It is important to point out that, unlike senile plaques, NFTs and tau neuropil threads are generally intracellular. Thus, tau inclusions would not likely be accessible at sufficient levels to extracellular antibody that enters the brain parenchyma from blood. Although these fundamental concerns suggest that tau immunization may not be a practical therapeutic approach for AD, recent data provide reason for cautious optimism. In particular, an interesting and provocative study (Clavaguera et al. 2009) showed that injection of brain-derived pathological tau from one tau Tg mouse line into the brains of another tau Tg mouse line that does not normally form intraneuronal inclusions led to the formation of pathological tau deposits in the recipient mice. These results suggest that mis-folded tau that is released into the brain inter-stitial fluid, perhaps from injured or dying neurons, might be internalized by nearby cells to "seed" further tau misfolding and accumula-tion. This hypothesis is further bolstered by studies, which indicate that aggregated tau can be transferred between cells in culture (Frost et al. 2009). If further confirmed, this mechanism of tau transmission may provide an explanation for the observed stereotypical spreading of tau pathology in AD (Braak et al. 1993), and suggests that an antitau antibody which recognizes the "seeding" tau species might prevent the transmission and further progres-sion of tau pathology. In this regard, there has been a report of tau immunotherapy in which JNPL3 tau Tg mice were vaccinated with a phospho-tau peptide (Asuni et al. 2007). Anti-antigen antibodies were generated by the mice, and there was a reduction of pathological tau as assessed by immunohistochemistry. Wheth-er this amelioration of tau pathology resulted from a slowing of tau transmission or through another mechanism is unknown, but additional studies of tau immunization in Tg models of AD are warranted. However, it should be noted that vaccination of wild-type mice with recombinant human tau led to the induction of NFT-like structures, axonal damage, and gliosis (Rosen-mann et al. 2006). Thus, certain tau immuno-gens may be detrimental and perhaps a passive immunization approach using antibodies di-rected to the misfolded tau species responsible for cell-to-cell transmission would have fewer side effects.

Finally, it should be noted that another ther-apeutic strategy that has recently been suggested for AD is to lower overall tau levels (i.e., not just hyperphosphorylated or misfolded tau). Initial support for this concept was provided by data demonstrating that hAPP (PDAPP) Tg mice, which develop Aβ plaques like those seen in AD, show reduced behavioral deficits when endogenous tau levels were lowered by crossing the hAPP mice with $tau^{-/-}$ mice (Roberson et al. 2007). This behavioral improvement was not caused by changes in Aβ or senile plaque levels in the $hAPP/tau^{-/-}$ mice relative to

$hAPP/tau^{+/+}$ counterparts. Interestingly, the reduction of tau also led to greater resistance to excitotoxic insults (Roberson et al. 2007). This observation may relate to recent data indi-cating that tau has a dendritic function in the postsynaptic targeting of the kinase Fyn (Ittner et al. 2010). Fyn-mediated phosphorylation of the NR2b subunit of the NMDA receptor strengthens its interaction with the postsynaptic protein, PSD95. Tau-deficient mice were shown to have reduced susceptibility to excitotoxic sei-zures because of impaired NMDA-PSD95 inter-action (Ittner et al. 2010). Moreover, hAPP $(APP23)/tau^{-/-}$ mice showed improved cog-nitive performance relative to tau-expressing hAPP controls, presumably because of a reduc-tion of Aβ-mediated excitotoxicity that was thought to be dependent on the presence of tau (Ittner et al. 2010).

Although these data suggest that there may be value in lowering total tau levels in AD, this perspective is not universally embraced, and caution should be exercised in the interpreta-tion of these results. First, there is another recent report, which suggests that a loss of tau is detri-mental and enhances degeneration in a another hAPP (A_{sw}) Tg mouse model (Dawson et al. 2010). In addition, the absence of a profound phenotype in $tau^{-/-}$ and $hAPP/tau^{-/-}$ mice might suggest that a loss of tau is well tolerated and does not greatly affect MT function. How-ever, these mice do develop some neurologi-cal impairments with age, including cognitive and motor deficits (Harada et al. 1994; Ikegami et al. 2000). In addition, there may well be com-pensatory changes during development that offset the loss of tau in these knockout mice. In this regard, it has been reported that $tau^{-/-}$ have increased expression of MAP1a (Harada et al. 1994). Although a therapeutic strategy based on the lowering of total tau levels merits further study, a "Goldilocks-like" bal-ance may be needed whereby tau concentrations are decreased enough to reduce Fyn targeting to dendrites but not so much as to compromise tau-mediated MT stabilization. In this regard, the combination of a tau-lowering agent and a MT-stabilizing compound might address both Aβ- and tau-mediated toxicities in AD.

INHIBITION OF TAU FIBRILLIZATION

The hypothesis that tau fibril formation may be spread by the internalization of misfolded extracellular tau seeds will require further study. However, it is generally accepted that tau fibrils are formed from a nucleation-elongation process in which a misfolded tau nucleating structure is formed that then promotes the further assembly of normal tau protein into oligomers and ultimately fibrils (Margittai and Langen 2004; Congdon et al. 2008). Thus, one conceptually straightforward strategy to prevent the formation of potentially harmful tau oligomers and/or fibrils would be to identify molecules that block the formation of tau nucleating structures and/or the elongation of nascent protofibrils (Fig. 3). Although simple in theory, this therapeutic approach is challenging from a drug development perspective because of the difficulty of disrupting protein–protein interactions that involve large surface areas. The search for inhibitors of tau assembly has been greatly aided by the discovery that bona fide fibrils with verisimilitude to those found in AD brain can be formed in vitro from isolated recombinant tau (Wille et al. 1992), with this assembly facilitated significantly by coincubation with anionic cofactors such as heparin or arachidonic acid (Goedert et al. 1996; Wilson and Binder 1997). This has led to efforts in several laboratories to identify inhibitors of tau fibril formation, and a number of molecules with differing chemical scaffolds have been described and discussed in several recent reviews (Brunden et al. 2009, 2010a; Ballatore et al. 2010b; Bulic et al. 2010). The chemical or biological properties of many of these compounds may preclude their use in animals or humans, although some may have potential for further development.

Interestingly, one of the first described tau fibrillization inhibitors has progressed to clinical testing in AD patients. Methylene blue was shown to block tau–tau interactions and alter tau fibril structure in 1996 (Wischik et al. 1996), and a Phase II AD clinical trial has recently been completed with this compound (trade name of Rember[TM]) (Staff et al. 2008). The clinical data suggest that the drug-treatment group had reduced cognitive decline relative to the placebo group, although interpretation of the data was complicated by problems with the formulation of the highest dose group that led to lower than expected exposures of the drug. These preliminary clinical data are encouraging, and further confirmation of efficacy in a pivotal Phase III trial could provide important validation of the use of tau fibrillization inhibitors for the treatment of AD. It should be noted that methylene blue is known to be a highly promiscuous molecule that can affect multiple protein targets (Gillman 2010; Oz et al. 2010). Therefore, effects in AD patients,

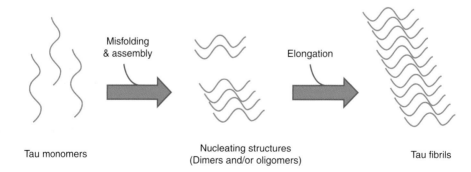

Figure 3. The assembly of tau into multimers and fibrils. Tau is normally unstructured in solution, and in axons the majority of tau is typically associated with MTs. In AD, tau can become misfolded and assemble into multimeric structures. Certain of these multimers can serve as nucleating structures to which additional tau can be added to yield classical amyloid-type fibrils.

even if confirmed in a Phase III study, may not be solely attributable to prevention of tau fibrillization.

To our knowledge, no other inhibitors of tau fibril assembly have progressed to efficacy testing in animal models of AD or tauopathy. Several inhibitors of tau fibrillization have been shown to inhibit tau inclusion formation in a cell-based model (Pickhardt et al. 2005, 2007; Khlistunova et al. 2006; Bulic et al. 2007), and one or more of these compounds may be suitable for testing in animals if they have appropriate pharmacokinetic properties and can cross the BBB. In this regard, example molecules from the aminothienopyridazine (ATPZ) class of tau fibrillization inhibitors have been identified that are absorbed orally in mice and which show good plasma half-lives along with equilibration across the BBB (Ballatore et al. 2010a). Thus, it is likely that one or more novel tau fibrillization inhibitors will be examined in a mouse model of tauopathy in the near future.

In most reports, the concentrations of compound required to inhibit tau fibrillization were nearly equimolar to the tau concentration used in the in vitro assays (Brunden et al. 2009, 2010a). This suggests that most of the described tau fibrillization inhibitors either have a relatively low affinity for tau, or that they form complexes with misfolded monomers or small multimers of tau to prevent fibrillization. It will therefore be important to show that the fibrillization inhibitors do not alter normal tau function. For example, the ATPZ class of tau fibril assembly inhibitors do not appear to affect the ability of tau to promote MT stabilization (Crowe et al. 2009; Ballatore et al. 2010a). A mechanism based on compound interaction with monomeric tau also raises the issue of whether sufficient brain drug levels can be achieved to bind the majority of tau monomers within neurons. In this regard, it has been estimated that under normal circumstances >99% of tau is bound to MTs (Congdon et al. 2008). Although the amount of tau bound to MTs is presumably reduced in tauopathies, even a 10-fold increase in free tau would still result in a sub-μM concentration of tau monomers if a total intraneuronal cytoplasmic tau level of $\sim$1 μM is assumed (Drubin et al. 1985). Thus, it should be feasible to attain effective brain concentrations of brain-penetrant tau fibril inhibitors. Moreover, tau aggregation inhibitors might also be expected to interfere with the extracellular transmission of aggregated tau nuclei, if this mechanism of pathology spreading plays a significant role, which would further increase the likely efficacy of stoichiometric inhibitors at feasible exposure levels.

UNIQUE CHALLENGES OF TAU-DIRECTED DRUG DISCOVERY AND DEVELOPMENT

Many of the complexities associated with tau-directed drug discovery approaches were mentioned in the previous sections. However, certain aspects of these challenges merit further discussion, particularly as they compare to therapeutic strategies focused on reducing Aβ levels in AD. As discussed in other articles within this volume, there have been significant advances in the development of inhibitors of the β- and γ-secretase enzymes that are responsible for the release of Aβ from APP. The pharmaceutical industry has considerable experience in developing enzyme inhibitors, and thus the APP-processing secretases are viewed as highly "druggable" targets. In contrast, the tau-based strategies discussed here are not focused on classical pharmaceutical drug targets, with the debatable exceptions of the tau kinases and HSP90. In fact, even the development of tau kinase and HSP90 inhibitors is rendered more difficult by the uncertainty of which kinase(s) are responsible for tau hyperphosphorylation, the challenges of developing kinase inhibitors with sufficient selectivity and the very real possibility of on-target toxicity linked to the critical functional role of the known tau kinases and Hsp90. The totality of these challenges to tau drug discovery has resulted in relatively modest industry efforts in this research area to date, although there are signs of increased interest in tau-directed therapeutic approaches.

Because of the complexities of tau drug discovery strategies, the academic community has an important role to play in validating these therapeutic methods. This is particularly true for the more unconventional pharmaceutical tactics, such as inhibition of tau multimer assembly, increasing tau degradation through up-regulation of autophagy, blocking tau spread in the brain with antibodies, or compensating for tau loss-of-function with MT stabilizing compounds. In each of these cases, the development of prototype reagents of sufficient quality to test the hypothesis and subsequent demonstration of proof-of-principle efficacy in established Tg mouse models of tauopathy will be critical to generating future industry investment in these therapeutic strategies. It is important that the design of these studies and the Tg models used be considered carefully. Previously published tau-based drug studies in Tg models have often suffered from underpowered group sizes, as well as a lack of information on drug exposure levels and target engagement. Moreover, there is a clear need for agreement on what constitutes robust efficacy endpoints linked to tau pathogenesis and associated neurodegeneration.

Although there are clear challenges to tau-based drug discovery, there may also be advantages relative to Aβ-targeted approaches. Emerging data suggest that Aβ deposition into senile plaques could occur years before the onset of cognitive deficits (Jack et al. 2010). Thus, it is possible that a drug designed to reduce Aβ levels and senile plaques would need to be administered well before the onset of AD clinical symptoms to be effective in slowing or preventing disease progression. Advancements in PET/MRI brain imaging and other biomarkers may eventually allow for the identification of nonsymptomatic individuals at risk for AD. However, demonstration of efficacy with an Aβ-directed drug in such a population may require multiple years of dosing unless a highly validated surrogate marker is identified and approved by regulatory agencies. In contrast, the development of tau inclusions appears to be more proximal to the onset of memory deficits (Jack et al. 2010). Thus, there may be a greater chance of demonstrating efficacy with a tau-directed agent in patients with MCI and early AD than with an Aβ-directed drug.

In conclusion, there are compelling reasons to attempt to identify drug candidates that can reduce the extent of tau-induced pathology in AD and related tauopathies. Although this area of drug discovery research is not as advanced as that directed to reducing Aβ and senile plaque levels in AD there is growing interest in tau-focused approaches as the central role of this pathology in the disease becomes more widely appreciated and the relevant research tools continue to improve.

ACKNOWLEDGMENTS

We thank our colleagues and collaborators for their contributions to the work summarized here, which has been supported by grants from the NIH (P01 AG09215, P30 AG10124, P01 AG11542, P01 AG14382, P01 AG14449, P01 AG17586, PO1 AG19724, P01 NS-044233, UO1 AG24904), the Nathan Bilger Alzheimer Initiative, and the Marian S. Ware Alzheimer Program. Finally, we are indebted to our patients and their families whose commitment to research has made our work possible.

REFERENCES

Ahlijanian MK, Barrezueta NX, Williams RD, Jakowski A, Kowsz KP, McCarthy S, Coskran T, Carlo A, Seymour PA, Burkhardt JE, et al. 2000. Hyperphosphorylated tan and neurofilament and cytoskeletal disruptions in mice overexpressing human p25, an activator of cdk5. *Proc Natl Acad Sci* **97**: 2910–2915.

Alonso AD, Zaidi T, Grundke-Iqbal I, Iqbal K. 1994. Role of abnormally phosphorylated tan in the breakdown of microtubules in Alzheimer-disease. *Proc Natl Acad Sci* **91**: 5562–5566.

Alonso AD, Grundke-Iqbal I, Iqbal K. 1996. Alzheimer's disease hyperphosphorylated tau sequesters normal tau into tangles of filaments and disassembles microtubules. *Nat Med* **2**: 783–787.

Altmann KH. 2005. Recent developments in the chemical biology of epothilones. *Curr Pharm Des* **11**: 1595–1613.

Andreadis A, Brown WM, Kosik KS. 1992. Structure and novel exons of the human-tau gene. *Biochemistry* **31**: 10626–10633.

Aplin AE, Jacobsen JS, Anderton BH, Gallo JM. 1997. Effect of increased glycogen synthase kinase-3 activity upon the maturation of the amyloid precursor protein in transfected cells. *Neuroreport* **8**: 639–643.

Arriagada PV, Growdon JH, Hedleywhyte ET, Hyman BT. 1992. Neurofibrillary tangles but not senile plaques parallel duration and severity of Alzheimers disease. *Neurology* **42:** 631–639.

Asuni AA, Boutajangout A, Quartermain D, Sigurdsson EM. 2007. Immunotherapy targeting pathological tau conformers in a tangle mouse model reduces brain pathology with associated functional improvements. *J Neurosci* **27:** 9115–9129.

Augustinack JC, Sanders JL, Tsai LH, Hyman BT. 2002. Colocalization and fluorescence resonance energy transfer between cdk5 and AT8 suggests a close association in pre-neurofibrillary tangles and neurofibrillary tangles. *J Neuropathol Exp Neurol* **61:** 557–564.

Avila J. 2006. Tau phosphorylation and aggregation in Alzheimer's disease pathology. *FEBS Lett* **580:** 2922–2927.

Avila J, Santa-Maria I, Perez M, Hernandez F, Moreno F. 2006. Tau phosphorylation, aggregation, and cell toxicity. *J Biomed Biotech* **2006:** 1–5.

Ballatore C, Hyde E, Deiches RF, Lee VMY, Trojanowski JQ, Huryn D, Smith AB. 2007a. Paclitaxel C-10 carbamates: Potential candidates for the treatment of neurodegenerative tauopathies. *Bioorg Med Chem Lett* **17:** 3642–3646.

Ballatore C, Lee VMY, Trojanowski JQ. 2007b. Tau-mediated neurodegeneration in Alzheimer's disease and related disorders. *Nat Rev Neurosci* **8:** 663–672.

Ballatore C, Brunden KR, Piscitelli F, James MJ, Crowe A, Yao Y, Hyde E, Trojanowsi JQ, Lee VM-Y, Smith AB III. 2010a. Discovery of brain-penetrant, orally bioavailable aminothienopyridazine inhibitors of tau aggregation. *J Med Chem* **53:** 3739–3747.

Ballatore C, Brunden KR, Trojanowski JQ, Lee VM-Y, Smith AB III, Huryn D. 2010b. Modulation of protein-protein interactions as a therpeutic strategy for the treatment of neurodegenerative tauopathies. *Curr Topics Med Chem* **11:** 317–330.

Barghorn S, Mandelkow E. 2002. Toward a unified scheme for the aggregation of tau into Alzheimer paired helical filaments. *Biochemistry* **41:** 14885–14896.

Barghorn S, Zheng-Fischhofer Q, Ackmann M, Biernat J, von Bergen M, Mandelkow EM, Mandelkow E. 2000. Structure, microtubule interactions, and paired helical filament aggregation by tau mutants of frontotemporal dementias. *Biochemistry* **39:** 11714–11721.

Bedard PL, Di Leo A, Piccart-Gebhart MJ. 2010. Taxanes: Optimizing adjuvant chemotherapy for early-stage breast cancer. *Nat Rev Clin Oncol* **7:** 22–36.

Beer TM, Higano CS, Saleh M, Dreicer R, Hudes G, Picus J, Rarick M, Fehrenbacher L, Hannah AL. 2007. Phase II study of KOS-862 in patients with metastatic androgen independent prostate cancer previously treated with docetaxel. *Invest New Drugs* **25:** 565–570.

Berger Z, Ravikumar B, Menzies FM, Oroz LG, Underwood BR, Pangalos MN, Schmitt I, Wullner U, Evert BO, O'Kane CJ, et al. 2006. Rapamycin alleviates toxicity of different aggregate-prone proteins. *Hum Mol Genet* **15:** 433–442.

Boland B, Kumar A, Lee S, Platt FM, Wegiel J, Yu WH, Nixon RA. 2008. Autophagy induction and autophagosome clearance in neurons: Relationship to autophagic pathology in Alzheimer's disease. *J Neurosci* **28:** 6926–6937.

Bowers EM, Yan G, Mukherjee C, Orry A, Wang L, Holbert MA, Crump NT, Hazzalin CA, Liszczak G, Yuan H, et al.

2010. Virtual ligand screening of the p300/CBP histone acetyltransferase: Identification of a selective small molecule inhibitor. *Chem Biol* **17:** 471–482.

Braak H, Braak E. 1991. Neuropathological staging of Alzheimer-related changes. *Acta Neuropathol* **82:** 239–259.

Braak H, Braak E, Bohl J. 1993. Staging of Alzheimer-related cortical destruction. *Eur Neurol* **33:** 403–408.

Bramblett GT, Goedert M, Jakes R, Merrick SE, Trojanowski JQ, Lee VMY. 1993. Abnormal tau-phosphorylation at Ser(396) in Alzheimers-disease recapitulates development and contributes to reduced microtubule-binding. *Neuron* **10:** 1089–1099.

Brunden KR, Trojanowski JQ, Lee VMY. 2009. Advances in tau-focused drug discovery for Alzheimer's disease and related tauopathies. *Nat Rev Drug Discov* **8:** 783–793.

Brunden KR, Ballatore C, Crowe A, Smith AB III, Lee VM-Y, Trojanowski JQ. 2010a. Tau-directed drug discovery for Alzheimer's disease and related tauopathies: A focus on tau assembly inhibitors. *Exp Neurol* **223:** 304–310.

Brunden KR, Zhang B, Carroll J, Yao Y, Potuzak JS, Hogan A-ML, Iba M, James MJ, Xie SX, Ballatore C, et al. 2010b. Epothilone D improves microtubule denstiry, axonal integrity and cognition in a transgenic mouse model of tauopathy. *J Neurosci* **30:** 13861–13866.

Brunden KR, Yao Y, Potuzak JS, Ferrar NI, Ballatore C, James MJ, Hogan AL, Trojanowski JQ, Smith AB3, Lee VMY. 2011. The characterization of microtubule-stabilizing drugs as possible therapeutic agents for Alzheimer's disease and related tauopathies. *Pharmacol Res* **63:** 341–351.

Buee L, Bussiere T, Buee-Scherrer V, Delacourte A, Hof PR. 2000. Tau protein isoforms, phosphorylation and role in neurodegenerative disorders. *Brain Res Rev* **33:** 95–130.

Bulic B, Pickhardt M, Khlistunova I, Biernat J, Mandelkow EM, Mandelkow E, Waldmann H. 2007. Rhodanine-based tau aggregation inhibitors in cell models of tauopathy. *Angewandte Chem-International Edition* **46:** 9215–9219.

Bulic B, Pickhardt M, Mandelkow EM, Mandelkow E. 2010. Tau protein and tau aggregation inhibitors. *Neuropharmacology* **59:** 276–289.

Cash AD, Aliev G, Siedlak SL, Nunomura A, Fujioka H, Zhu XW, Raina AK, Vinters HV, Tabaton M, Johnson AB, et al. 2003. Microtubule reduction in Alzheimer's disease and aging is independent of tau filament formation. *Am J Pathol* **162:** 1623–1627.

Chiosis G, Neckers L. 2006. Tumor selectivity of Hsp90 inhibitors: The explanation remains elusive. *ACS Chem Biol* **1:** 279–284.

Churcher I. 2006. Tau therapeutic strategies for the treatment of Alzheimer's disease. *Curr Topics Med Chem* **6:** 579–595.

Cisternino S, Bourasset F, Archimbaud Y, Semiond D, Sanderink G, Scherrmann JM. 2003. Nonlinear accumulation in the brain of the new taxoid TXD258 following saturation of P-glycoprotein at the blood-brain barrier in mice and rats. *Br J Pharmacol* **138:** 1367–1375.

Clavaguera F, Bolmont T, Crowther RA, Abramowski D, Frank S, Probst A, Fraser G, Stalder AK, Beibel M, Staufenbiel M, et al. 2009. Transmission and spreading of tauopathy in transgenic mouse brain. *Nature Cell Biol* **11**: 909–913.

Cohen TJ, Guo J, Hurtado DE, Kwong LK, Mills IP, Trojanowski JQ, Lee VMY. 2011. Tau acetylation inhibits its function and accelerates aggregation. *Nature Comm* **2**: 252.

Congdon EE, Kim S, Bonchak J, Songrug T, Matzavinos A, Kuret J. 2008. Nucleation-dependent tau filament formation—The importance of dimerization and an estimation of elementary rate constants. *J Biol Chem* **283**: 13806–13816.

Crowe A, Huang W, Ballatore C, Johnson R, Hogan A, Huang R, Wichtermann J, McCoy J, Huryn D, Auld D, et al. 2009. The identification of aminothienopyridazine inhibitors of tau assembly by quantitative high-throughput screening. *Biochemistry* **48**: 7732–7745.

Dawson HN, Cantillana V, Jansen M, Wang H, Vitek MP, Wilcock DM, Lynch JR, Laskowitz DT. 2010. Loss of tau elicits axonal degeneration in a mouse model of Alzheimer's Disease. *Neuroscience* **169**: 516–531.

Dayanandan R, Van Slegtenhorst M, Mack TGA, Ko L, Yen SH, Leroy K, Brion JP, Anderton BH, Hutton M, Lovestone S. 1999. Mutations in tau reduce its microtubule binding properties in intact cells and affect its phosphorylation. *FEBS Lett* **446**: 228–232.

Delgoffe GM, Powell JD. 2009. mTOR: Taking cues from the immune microenvironment. *Immunology* **127**: 459–465.

Denduluri N, Low JA, Lee JJ, Berman AW, Walshe JM, Vatas U, Chow CK, Steinberg SM, Yang SX, Swain SM. 2007. Phase II trial of ixabepilone, an epothilone B analog, in patients with metastatic breast cancer previously untreated with taxanes. *J Clin Oncol* **25**: 3421–3427.

Dhavan R, Tsai LH. 2001. A decade of CDK5. *Nature Rev Molec Cell Biol* **2**: 749–759.

Dickey CA, Dunmore J, Lu BW, Wang JW, Lee WC, Kamal A, Burrows F, Eckman C, Hutton M, Petrucelli L. 2006a. HSP induction mediates selective clearance of tau phosphorylated at proline-directed Ser/Thr sites but not KXGS (MARK) sites. *FASEB J* **20**: 753–755.

Dickey CA, Yue M, Lin WL, Dickson DW, Dunmore JH, Lee WC, Zehr C, West G, Cao S, Clark AMK, et al. 2006b. Deletion of the ubiquitin ligase CHIP leads to the accumulation, but not the aggregation, of both endogenous phospho- and caspase-3-cleaved tau species. *J Neurosci* **26**: 6985–6996.

Dickey CA, Kamal A, Lundgren K, Klosak N, Bailey RM, Dunmore J, Ash P, Shoraka S, Zlatkovic J, Eckman CB, et al. 2007. The high-affinity HSP90-CHIP complex recognizes and selectively degrades phosphorylated tau client proteins. *J Clin Invest* **117**: 648–658.

Divinski I, Holtser-Cochav M, Vulih-Schultzman I, Steingart RA, Gozes I. 2006. Peptide neuroprotection through specific interaction with brain tubulin. *J Neurochem* **98**: 973–984.

Dixit R, Ross JL, Goldman YE, Holzbaur ELF. 2008. Differential regulation of dynein and kinesin motor proteins by tau. *Science* **319**: 1086–1089.

Dou F, Netzer WJ, Tanemura K, Li F, Hartl FU, Takashima A, Gouras GK, Greengard P, Xu HX. 2003. Chaperones increase association of tau protein with microtubules. *Proc Natl Acad Sci* **100**: 721–726.

Drechsel DN, Hyman AA, Cobb MH, Kirschner MW. 1992. Modulation of the dynamic instability of tubulin assembly by the microtubule-associated protein tau. *Mol Biol Cell* **3**: 1141–1154.

Drewes G, Ebneth A, Preuss U, Mandelkow EM, Mandelkow E. 1997. MARK, a novel family of protein kinases that phosphorylate microtubule-associated proteins and trigger microtubule disruption. *Cell* **89**: 297–308.

Drubin DG, Feinstein SC, Shooter EM, Kirschner MW. 1985. Nerve growth-factor induced Neurite Outgrowth in Pc12 cells involves the coordinate induction of microtubule assembly and assembly-promoting factors. *J Cell Biol* **101**: 1799–1807.

Erturk A, Hellal F, Enes J, Bradke F. 2007. Disorganized microtubules underlie the formation of retraction bulbs and the failure of axonal regeneration. *J Neurosci* **27**: 9169–9180.

Fellner S, Bauer B, Miller DS, Schaffrik M, Fankhanel M, Spruss T, Bernhardt G, Graeff C, Farber L, Gschaidmeier H, et al. 2002. Transport of paclitaxel (Taxol) across the blood-brain barrier in vitro and in vivo. *J Clin Invest* **110**: 1309–1318.

Frost B, Jacks RL, Diamond MI. 2009. Propagation of tau misfolding from the outside to the inside of a cell. *J Biol Chem* **284**: 12845–12852.

Gillman PK. 2011. CNS toxicity involving methylene blue: The exempler for understanding and predicting drug interactions that precipitate serotonin toxicity. *J Psychopharmacol* **25**: 429–436.

Glenner GG, Wong CW. 1984. Alzheimers disease—initial report of the purification and characterization of a novel cerebrovascular amyloid protein. *Biochem Biophys Res Commun* **120**: 885–890.

Goedert M, Jakes R. 2005. Mutations causing neurodegenerative tauopathies. *Biochim Biophys Acta-Molecular Basis of Disease* **1739**: 240–250.

Goedert M, Spillantini MG, Jakes R, Rutherford D, Crowther RA. 1989. Multiple isoforms of human microtubule-associated protein-tau—sequences and localization in neurofibrillary tangles of Alzheimers-disease. *Neuron* **3**: 519–526.

Goedert M, Jakes R, Spillantini MG, Hasegawa M, Smith MJ, Crowther RA. 1996. Assembly of microtubule-associated protein tau into Alzheimer-like filaments induced by sulphated glycosaminoglycans. *Nature* **383**: 550–553.

Gomez-Isla T, Hollister R, West H, Mui S, Growdon JH, Petersen RC, Parisi JE, Hyman BT. 1997. Neuronal loss correlates with but exceeds neurofibrillary tangles in Alzheimer's disease. *Ann Neurol* **41**: 17–24.

Gong CX, Iqbal K. 2008. Hyperphosphorylation of microtubule-associated protein tau: A promising therapeutic target for Alzheimer disease. *Curr Med Chem* **15**: 2321–2328.

Gong CX, Shaikh S, Wang JZ, Zaidi T, Grundke-Iqbal I, Iqbal K. 1995. Phosphatase-activity toward abnormally phosphorylated-tau—decrease in Alzheimer-disease brain. *J Neurochem* **65**: 732–738.

Gong CX, Liu F, Grundke-Iqbal I, Iqbal K. 2005. Post-translational modifications of tau protein in Alzheimer's disease. *J Neural Transm* **112**: 813–838.

Gustke N, Trinczek B, Biernat J, Mandelkow EM, Mandelkow E. 1994. Domains of tau-protein and interactions with microtubules. *Biochemistry* **33**: 9511–9522.

Hamano T, Gendron TF, Causevic E, Yen SH, Lin WL, Isidoro C, DeTure M, Ko LW. 2008. Autophagic-lysosomal perturbation enhances tau aggregation in transfectants with induced wild-type tau expression. *Eur J Neurosci* **27**: 1119–1130.

Hanger DP, Betts JC, Loviny TLF, Blackstock WP, Anderton BH. 1998. New phosphorylation sites identified in hyperphosphorylated tau (paired helical filament-tau) from Alzheimer's disease brain using nanoelectrospray mass spectrometry. *J Neurochem* **71**: 2465–2476.

Hanger DP, Anderton BH, Noble W. 2009. Tau phosphorylation: The therapeutic challenge for neurodegenerative disease. *Trends Molec Med* **15**: 112–119.

Harada A, Oguchi K, Okabe S, Kuno J, Terada S, Ohshima T, Satoyoshitake R, Takei Y, Noda T, Hirokawa N. 1994. Altered microtubule organization in small-caliber axons of mice lacking tau-protein. *Nature* **369**: 488–491.

Harrison DE, Strong R, Sharp ZD, Nelson JF, Astle CM, Flurkey K, Nadon NL, Wilkinson JE, Frenkel K, Carter CS, et al. 2009. Rapamycin fed late in life extends lifespan in genetically heterogeneous mice. *Nature* **460**: 392–395.

Hasegawa M, Smith MJ, Goedert M. 1998. Tau proteins with FTDP-17 mutations have a reduced ability to promote microtubule assembly. *FEBS Lett* **437**: 207–210.

Hellal F, Hurtado A, Ruschel J, Flynn KC, Laskowski CJ, Umlauf M, Kapitein LC, Strikis D, Lemmon V, Bixby J, et al. 2011. Microtubule stabilization reduces scarring and causes axon regeneration after spinal cord injury. *Science* **331**: 928–931.

Hempen B, Brion JP. 1996. Reduction of acetylated α-tubulin immunoreactivity in neurofibrillary tangle-bearing neurons in Alzheimer's disease. *J Neuropathol Exp Neurol* **55**: 964–972.

Hernandez F, Borrell J, Guaza C, Avila J, Lucas JJ. 2002. Spatial learning deficit in transgenic mice that conditionally over-express GSK-3 beta in the brain but do not form tau filaments. *J Neurochem* **83**: 1529–1533.

Hong M, Zhukareva V, Vogelsberg-Ragaglia V, Wszolek Z, Reed L, Miller BI, Geschwind DH, Bird TD, McKeel D, Goate A, et al. 1998. Mutation-specific functional impairments in distinct Tau isoforms of hereditary FTDP-17. *Science* **282**: 1914–1917.

Hutton M, Lendon CL, Rizzu P, Baker M, Froelich S, Houlden H, Pickering-Brown S, Chakraverty S, Isaacs A, Grover A, et al. 1998. Association of missense and 5′-splice-site mutations in tau with the inherited dementia FTDP-17. *Nature* **393**: 702–705.

Ikegami S, Harada A, Hirokawa N. 2000. Muscle weakness, hyperactivity, and impairment in fear conditioning in tau-deficient mice. *Neurosci Lett* **279**: 129–132.

Imahori K, Uchida T. 1997. Physiology and pathology of tau protein kinases in relation to Alzheimer's disease. *J Biochem* **121**: 179–188.

Ishihara T, Hong M, Zhang B, Nakagawa Y, Lee MK, Trojanowski JQ, Lee VMY. 1999. Age-dependent emergence and progression of a tauopathy in transgenic mice over-expressing the shortest human tau isoform. *Neuron* **24**: 751–762.

Ittner LM, Ke YD, Delerue F, Bi MA, Gladbach A, van Eersel J, Wolfing H, Chieng BC, Christie MJ, Napier IA, et al. 2010. Dendritic function of tau mediates amyloid-beta toxicity in Alzheimer's disease mouse models. *Cell* **142**: 387–397.

Jack CR, Knopman DS, Jagust WJ, Shaw LM, Aisen PS, Weiner MW, Petersen RC, Trojanowski JQ. 2010. Hypothetical model of dynamic biomarkers of the Alzheimer's pathological cascade. *Lancet Neurol* **9**: 119–128.

Jeganathan S, von Bergen M, Mandelkow EM, Mandelkow E. 2008. The natively unfolded character of Tau and its aggregation to Alzheimer-like paired helical filaments. *Biochemistry* **47**: 10526–10539.

Kamal A, Thao L, Sensintaffar J, Zhang L, Boehm MF, Fritz LC, Burrows FJ. 2003. A high-affinity conformation of Hsp90 confers tumour selectivity on Hsp90 inhibitors. *Nature* **425**: 407–410.

Kang J, Lemaire HG, Unterbeck A, Salbaum JM, Masters CL, Grzeschik KH, Multhaup G, Beyreuther K, Mullerhill B. 1987. The precursor of alzheimers-disease amyloid-a4 protein resembles a cell-surface receptor. *Nature* **325**: 733–736.

Kar S, Fan J, Smith MJ, Goedert M, Amos LA. 2003. Repeat motifs of tau bind to the insides of microtubules in the absence of taxol. *EMBO J* **22**: 70–77.

Khlistunova I, Biernat J, Wang YP, Pickhardt M, von Bergen M, Gazova Z, Mandelkow E, Mandelkow M. 2006. Inducible expression of tau repeat domain in cell models of tauopathy—Aggregation is toxic to cells but can be reversed by inhibitor drugs. *J Biol Chem* **281**: 1205–1214.

Kidd M. 1963. Paired helical filaments in electron microscopy of alzheimers disease. *Nature* **197**: 192–193.

Kopke E, Tung YC, Shaikh S, Alonso AD, Iqbal K, Grundke-Iqbal I. 1993. Microtubule-associated protein-tau—abnormal phosphorylation of a non-paired helical filament pool in alzheimer-disease. *J Biol Chem* **268**: 24374–24384.

Ksiezak-Reding H, Liu WK, Yen SH. 1992. Phosphate analysis and dephosphorylation of modified tau associated with paired helical filaments. *Brain Res* **597**: 209–219.

Le Corre S, Klafki HW, Plesnila N, Hubinger G, Obermeier A, Sahagun H, Monse B, Seneci P, Lewis J, Eriksen J, et al. 2006. An inhibitor of tau hyperphosphorylation prevents severe motor impairments in tau transgenic mice. *Proc Natl Acad Sci* **103**: 9673–9678.

Lee VMY, Balin BJ, Otvos L, Trojanowski JQ. 1991. A68—A major subunit of paired helical filaments and derivatized forms of normal-tau. *Science* **251**: 675–678.

Lee VMY, Goedert M, Trojanowski JQ. 2001. Neurodegenerative tauopathies. *Annu Rev Neurosci* **24**: 1121–1159.

Lee G, Thangavel R, Sharma VM, Litersky JM, Bhaskar K, Fang SM, Do LH, Andreadis A, Van Hoesen G, Ksiezak-Reding H. 2004. Phosphorylation of tau by fyn: Implications for Alzheimer's disease. *J Neurosci* **24**: 2304–2312.

Lefebvre T, Ferreira S, Dupont-Wallois L, Bussiere T, Dupire MJ, Delacourte A, Michalski JC, Caillet-Boudin ML. 2003. Evidence of a balance between phosphorylation and O-GlcNAc glycosylation of Tau proteins—a role in nuclear localization. *Biochim Biophys Acta-General Subjects* **1619**: 167–176.

Liu F, Iqbal K, Grundke-Iqbal I, Hart GW, Gong CX. 2004. O-GlcNAcylation regulates phosphorylation of tau: A mechanism involved in Alzheimer's disease. *Proc Natl Acad Sci* **101:** 10804–10809.

Lucas JJ, Hernandez F, Gomez-Ramos P, Moran MA, Hen R, Avila J. 2001. Decreased nuclear beta-catenin, tau hyperphosphorylation and neurodegeneration in GSK-3 beta conditional transgenic mice. *EMBO J* **20:** 27–39.

Luo WJ, Dou F, Rodina A, Chip S, Kim J, Zhao Q, Moulick K, Aguirre J, Wu N, Greengard P, et al. 2007. Roles of heat-shock protein 90 in maintaining and facilitating the neurodegenerative phenotype in tauopathies. *Proc Natl Acad Sci* **104:** 9511–9516.

Mahalingam D, Swords R, Carew JS, Nawrocki ST, Bhalla K, Giles FJ. 2009. Targeting HSP90 for cancer therapy. *Br J Cancer* **100:** 1523–1529.

Margittai M, Langen R. 2004. Template-assisted filament growth by parallel stacking of tau. *Proc Natl Acad Sci* **101:** 10278–10283.

Matsuo ES, Shin RW, Billingsley ML, Vandevoorde A, O'Connor M, Trojanowski JQ, Lee VMY. 1994. Biopsy-derived adult human brain tau is phosphorylated at many of the same sites as Alzheimers-disease paired helical filament-tau. *Neuron* **13:** 989–1002.

Matsuoka Y, Gray AJ, Hirata-Fukae C, Minami SS, Waterhouse EG, Mattson MP, LaFerla FM, Gozes I, Aisen PS. 2007. Intranasal NAP administration reduces accumulation of amyloid peptide and tau hyperphosphorylation in a transgenic mouse model of Alzheimer's disease at early pathological stage. *J Mol Neurosci* **31:** 165–170.

Mazanetz MP, Fischer PM. 2007. Untangling tau hyperphosphorylation in drug design for neurodegenerative diseases. *Nat Rev Drug Discov* **6:** 464–479.

Merrick SE, Trojanowski JQ, Lee VMY. 1997. Selective destruction of stable microtubules and axons by inhibitors of protein serine/threonine phosphatases in cultured human neurons (NT2N cells). *J Neurosci* **17:** 5726–5737.

Metzger-Filho O, Moulin C, de Azambuja E, Ahmad A. 2009. Larotaxel: Broadening the road with new taxanes. *Expert Opin Investig Drugs* **18:** 1183–1189.

Miller RA, Harrison DE, Astle CM, Baur JA, Boyd AR, de Cabo R, Fernandez E, Flurkey K, Javors MA, Nelson JF, et al. 2011. Rapamycin, but not resveratrol or simvastatin, extends life span of genetically heterogeneous mice. *J Gerontol A Biol Sci Med Sci* **66:** 191–201.

Min SW, Cho SH, Zhou YG, Schroeder S, Haroutunian V, Seeley WW, Huang EJ, Shen Y, Masliah E, Mukherjee C, et al. 2010. Acetylation of tau inhibits its degradation and contributes to tauopathy. *Neuron* **67:** 953–966.

Mitchell TW, Nissanov J, Han LY, Mufson EJ, Schneider JA, Cochran EJ, Bennett DA, Lee VMY, Trojanowski JQ, Arnold SE. 2000. Novel method to quantify neuropil threads in brains from elders with or without cognitive impairment. *J Histochem Cytochem* **48:** 1627–1637.

Morishima-Kawashima M, Hasegawa M, Takio K, Suzuki M, Yoshida H, Titani K, Ihara Y. 1995. Proline-directed and non-proline-directed phosphorylation of Phf-Tau. *J Biol Chem* **270:** 823–829.

Morita T, Sobue K. 2009. Specification of neuronal polarity regulated by local translation of CRMP2 and tau via

the mTOR-p70S6K pathway. *J Biol Chem* **284:** 27734–27745.

Nacharaju P, Lewis J, Easson C, Yen S, Hackett J, Hutton M, Yen SH. 1999. Accelerated filament formation from tau protein with specific FTDP-17 missense mutations. *J Neuropathol Exp Neurol* **58:** 545.

Nakashima H, Ishihara T, Suguimoto P, Yokota O, Oshima E, Kugo A, Terada S, Hamamura T, Trojanowski JQ, Lee VMY, et al. 2005. Chronic lithium treatment decreases tau lesions by promoting ubiquitination in a mouse model of tauopathies. *Acta Neuropathol* **110:** 547–556.

Necula M, Kuret J. 2004. Pseudophosphorylation and glycation of tau protein enhance but do not trigger fibrillization in vitro. *J Biol Chem* **279:** 49694–49703.

Nixon RA. 2006. Autophagy in neurodegenerative disease: Friend, foe or turncoat? *Trends Neurosci* **29:** 528–535.

Noble W, Olm V, Takata K, Casey MO, Meyerson J, Gaynor K, LaFrancois J, Wang LL, Kondo T, Davies P, et al. 2003. Cdk5 is a key factor in tau aggregation and tangle formation in vivo. *Neuron* **38:** 555–565.

Noble W, Planel E, Zehr C, Olm V, Meyerson J, Suleman F, Gaynor K, Wang L, LaFrancois J, Feinstein B, et al. 2005. Inhibition of glycogen synthase kinase-3 by lithium correlates with reduced tauopathy and degeneration in vivo. *Proc Natl Acad Sci* **102:** 6990–6995.

Ojima I, Chen J, Sun L, Borella CP, Wang T, Miller ML, Lin SN, Geng XD, Kuznetsova LR, Qu CX, et al. 2008. Design, synthesis, and biological evaluation of new-generation taxoids. *J Med Chem* **51:** 3203–3221.

Orgogozo JM, Gilman S, Dartigues JF, Laurent B, Puel M, Kirby LC, Jouanny P, Dubois B, Eisner L, Flitman S, et al. 2003. Subacute meningoencephalitis in a subset of patients with AD after A beta 42 immunization. *Neurology* **61:** 46–54.

Oz M, Lorke DE, Hasan M, Petroianu GA. 2011. Cellular and molecular actions of methylene blue in the nervous system. *Med Res Rev* **31:** 93–117.

Panda D, Samuel JC, Massie M, Feinstein SC, Wilson L. 2003. Differential regulation of microtubule dynamics by three- and four-repeat tau: Implications for the onset of neurodegenerative disease. *Proc Natl Acad Sci* **100:** 9548–9553.

Pei JJ, Grundke-Iqbal I, Iqbal K, Bogdanovic N, Winblad B, Cowburn RF. 1998. Accumulation of cyclin-dependent kinase 5 (cdk5) in neurons with early stages of Alzheimer's disease neurofibrillary degeneration. *Brain Res* **797:** 267–277.

Perez M, Hernandez F, Lim F, Diaz-Nido J, Avila J. 2003. Chronic lithium treatment decreases mutant tau protein aggregation in a transgenic mouse model. *J Alzheimer's Disease* **5:** 301–308.

Petrucelli L, Dickson D, Kehoe K, Taylor J, Snyder H, Grover A, De Lucia M, McGowan E, Lewis J, Prihar G, et al. 2004. CHIP and Hsp70 regulate tau ubiquitination, degradation and aggregation. *Hum Mol Genet* **13:** 703–714.

Phiel CJ, Wilson CA, Lee VMY, Klein PS. 2003. GSK-3 α regulates production of Alzheimer's disease amyloid-beta peptides. *Nature* **423:** 435–439.

Pickhardt M, Gazova Z, von Bergen M, Khlistunova I, Wang YP, Hascher A, Mandelkow EM, Biernat J, Mandelkow E.

Cite this article as *Cold Spring Harb Perspect Med* doi: 10.1101/cshperspect.a006437

2005. Anthraquinones inhibit tau aggregation and dissolve Alzheimer's paired helical filaments in vitro and in cells. *J Biol Chem* **280:** 3628–3635.

Pickhardt M, Larbig G, Khlistunova I, Coksezen A, Meyer B, Mandelkow EM, Schmidt B, Mandelkow E. 2007. Phenylthiazolyl-hydrazide and its derivatives are potent inhibitors of tau aggregation and toxicity in vitro and in cells. *Biochemistry* **46:** 10016–10023.

Rayasam GV, Tulasi VK, Sodhi R, Davis JA, Ray A. 2009. Glycogen synthase kinase 3: More than a namesake. *Br J Pharmacol* **156:** 885–898.

Reynolds MR, Reyes JF, Fu YF, Bigio EH, Guillozet-Bongaarts AL, Berry RW, Binder LI. 2006. Tau nitration occurs at tyrosine 29 in the fibrillar lesions of Alzheimer's disease and other tauopathies. *J Neurosci* **26:** 10636–10645.

Rinne JO, Brooks DJ, Rossor MN, Fox NC, Bullock R, Klunk WE, Mathis CA, Blennow K, Barakos J, Okello AA, et al. 2010. C-11-PiB PET assessment of change in fibrillar amyloid-beta load in patients with Alzheimer's disease treated with bapineuzumab: A phase 2, double-blind, placebo-controlled, ascending-dose study. *Lancet Neurol* **9:** 363–372.

Roberson ED, Scearce-Levie K, Palop JJ, Yan FR, Cheng IH, Wu T, Gerstein H, Yu GQ, Mucke L. 2007. Reducing endogenous tau ameliorates amyloid beta-induced deficits in an Alzheimer's disease mouse model. *Science* **316:** 750–754.

Rockenstein E, Torrance M, Adame A, Mante M, Bar-on P, Rose JB, Crews L, Masliah E. 2007. Neuroprotective effects of regulators of the glycogen synthase kinase-3 beta signaling pathway in a transgenic model of Alzheimer's disease are associated with reduced amyloid precursor protein phosphorylation. *J Neurosci* **27:** 1981–1991.

Rosenmann H, Grigoriadis N, Karussis D, Boimel M, Touloumi O, Ovadia H, Abramsky O. 2006. Tauopathy-like abnormalities and neurologic deficits in mice immunized with neuronal tau protein. *Arch Neurol* **63:** 1459–1467.

Saloustros E, Mavroudis D, Georgoulias V. 2008. Paclitaxel and docetaxel in the treatment of breast cancer. *Expert Opin Pharmacother* **9:** 2603–2616.

Sarkar S, Floto RA, Berger Z, Imarisio S, Cordenier A, Pasco M, Cook LJ, Rubinsztein DC. 2005. Lithium induces autophagy by inhibiting inositol monophosphatase. *J Cell Biol* **170:** 1101–1111.

Schneider A, Biernat J, von Bergen M, Mandelkow E, Mandelkow EM. 1999. Phosphorylation that detaches tau from microtubules S262 and S214 protects it against aggregation into Alzheimer paired helical filaments. *J Neurochem* **73:** S26.

Shimura H, Schwartz D, Gygi SP, Kosik KS. 2004. CHIP-Hsc70 complex ubiquitinates phosphorylated tau and enhances cell survival. *J Biol Chem* **279:** 4869–4876.

Shiryaev N, Jouroukhin Y, Giladi E, Polyzoidou E, Grigoriadis NC, Rosenmann H, Gozes I. 2009. NAP protects memory, increases soluble tau and reduces tau hyperphosphorylation in a tauopathy model. *Neurobiol Dis* **34:** 381–388.

Solit DB, Chiosis G. 2008. Development and application of Hsp90 inhibitors. *Drug Discovery Today* **13:** 38–43.

Sparreboom A, vanAsperen J, Mayer U, Schinkel AH, Smit JW, Meijer DKF, Borst P, Nooijen WJ, Beijnen JH, vanTellingen O. 1997. Limited oral bioavailability and active epithelial excretion of paclitaxel (Taxol) caused by P-glycoprotein in the intestine. *Proc Natl Acad Sci* **94:** 2031–2035.

Spittaels K, Van Den Haute C, Van Dorpe J, Geerts H, Mercken M, Bruynseels K, Lasrado R, Vandezande K, Laenen I, Boon T, et al. 2000. Glycogen synthase kinase-3 beta phosphorylates protein tau and rescues the axonopathy in the central nervous system of human four-repeat tau transgenic mice. *J Biol Chem* **275:** 41340–41349.

Staff RT, Ahearn TS, Murray AD, Benthan P, Seng KM, Wischik C. 2008. Tau aggregation inhibitor (TAI) therapy with rember arrests the trajectory of rCBF decline in brain regions affected by tau pathology in mild to moderate Alzheimer's disease. *Alzheimer's Dementia* **4:** T775.

Stamer K, Vogel R, Thies E, Mandelkow E, Mandelkow EM. 2002. Tau blocks traffic of organelles, neurofilaments, and APP vesicles in neurons and enhances oxidative stress. *J Cell Biol* **156:** 1051–1063.

Tanimukai H, Kudo T, Tanaka T, Grundke-Iqbal I, Iqbal K, Takeda M. 2009. Novel therapeutic strategies for neurodegenerative disease. *Psychogeriatrics* **9:** 103–109.

Vershinin M, Carter BC, Razafsky DS, King SJ, Gross SP. 2007. Multiple-motor based transport and its regulation by Tau. *Proc Natl Acad Sci* **104:** 87–92.

Wagner U, Utton M, Gallo JM, Miller CCJ. 1996. Cellular phosphorylation of tau by GSK-3 beta influences tau binding to microtubules and microtubule organisation. *J Cell Sci* **109:** 1537–1543.

Wang YP, Martinez-Vicente M, Kruger U, Kaushik S, Wong E, Mandelkow EM, Cuervo AM, Mandelkow E. 2009. Tau fragmentation, aggregation and clearance: The dual role of lysosomal processing. *Hum Mol Genet* **18:** 4153–4170.

Wen Y, Planel E, Herman M, Figueroa HY, Wang LL, Liu L, Lau LF, Yu WH, Duff KE. 2008. Interplay between cyclin-dependent kinase 5 and glycogen synthase kinase 3 beta mediated by neuregulin signaling leads to differential effects on tau phosphorylation and amyloid precursor protein processing. *J Neurosci* **28:** 2624–2632.

Wilcock GK. 2010. Bapineuzumab in Alzheimer's disease: Where now? *Lancet Neurol* **9:** 134–136.

Wilcock GK, Esiri MM. 1982. Plaques, tangles and dementia—a quantitative study. *J Neurol Sci* **56:** 343–356.

Wille H, Drewes G, Biernat J, Mandelkow EM, Mandelkow E. 1992. Alzheimer-like paired helical filaments and antiparallel dimers formed from microtubule-associated protein-tau in vitro. *J Cell Biol* **118:** 573–584.

Williams A, Jahreiss L, Sarkar S, Saiki S, Menzies FM, Ravikumar B, Rubinsztein DC. 2006. Aggregate-prone proteins are cleared from the cytosol by autophagy: Therapeutic implications. *Curr Topics Dev Biol* **76:** 89–101.

Wilson DM, Binder LI. 1997. Free fatty acids stimulate the polymerization of tau and amyloid beta peptides—In vitro evidence for a common effector of pathogenesis in Alzheimer's disease. *Am J Pathol* **150:** 2181–2195.

Wischik CM, Edwards PC, Lai RYK, Roth M, Harrington CR. 1996. Selective inhibition of Alzheimer disease-like tau aggregation by phenothiazines. *Proc Natl Acad Sci* **93:** 11213–11218.

Yamaguchi H, Ishiguro K, Uchida T, Takashima A, Lemere CA, Imahori K. 1996. Preferential labeling of Alzheimer neurofibrillary tangles with antisera for tau protein kinase (TPK)I glycogen synthase kinase-3 beta and cyclin-dependent kinase 5, a component of TPK II. *Acta Neuropathol* **92:** 232–241.

Yang XJ, Seto E. 2008. Lysine acetylation: Codified crosstalk with other posttranslational modifications. *Mol Cell* **31:** 449–461.

Yuzwa SA, Macauley MS, Heinonen JE, Shan XY, Dennis RJ, He YA, Whitworth GE, Stubbs KA, McEachern EJ, Davies GJ, et al. 2008. A potent mechanism-inspired O-GlcNAcase inhibitor that blocks phosphorylation of tau in vivo. *Nat Chem Biol* **4:** 483–490.

Zhang B, Maiti A, Shively S, Lakhani F, McDonald-Jones G, Bruce J, Lee EB, Xie SX, Joyce S, Li C, et al. 2005. Microtubule-binding drugs offset tau sequestration by stabilizing microtubules and reversing fast axonal transport deficits in a tauopathy model. *Proc Natl Acad Sci* **102:** 227–231.

Zhang H, Burrows F. 2004. Targeting multiple signal transduction pathways through inhibition of Hsp90. *J Mol Med Jmmunol* **82:** 488–499.

Symptomatic and Nonamyloid/Tau Based Pharmacologic Treatment for Alzheimer Disease

Paul S. Aisen[1], Jeffrey Cummings[2], and Lon S. Schneider[3]

[1]University of California, San Diego, California 92093

[2]Cleveland Clinic, Cleveland, Ohio 44195

[3]University of Southern California, Los Angeles, California 90007

Correspondence: paisen@ucsd.edu

In this work we consider marketed drugs for Alzheimer disease (AD) including acetylcholinesterase inhibitors (AChE-Is) and antiglutamatergic treatment involving the *N*-methyl-D-aspartate (NMDA) receptor. We discuss medications and substances available for use as cognitive enhancers that are not approved for AD or cognitive impairment, and other neurotransmitter-related therapies in development or currently being researched. We also review putative therapies that aim to slow disease progression by mechanisms not directly related to amyloid or tau.

REGULATORY LANDSCAPE AND CLINICAL TRIALS

North American and European Union regulatory criteria for marketing approval of putative symptomatic and disease-modifying therapeutic agents for Alzheimer disease (AD) are based on a demonstration of efficacy supported by improvements compared to placebo treatment on cognitive function, activities of daily living (ADL), and often evidence of overall clinical improvement or less overall decline, accompanied by adequate evidence of safety (Schneider 2008b). In practice this has led to rather standardized protocols by sponsors of experimental drugs. For example, mild to moderate AD is indexed by a Mini-Mental State Examination (MMSE) score of 10–26 and standardized outcomes including the Alzheimer's Disease Assessment Scale—Cognitive Portion (ADAS-cog), the Alzheimer's Disease Cooperative Study Activities of Daily Living (ADCS-ADL) scale, or the Disability Assessment for Dementia (DAD). A clinician's global assessment (known as a Clinician Interview Based Impression of Change with caregiver input [CIBIC+] or ADCS Clinical Global Impression of Change [CGIC]) or the Clinical Dementia Rating (CDR), an interview-based overall dementia severity assessment, are the conventional outcomes measures. The trials are commonly 6–18 months in duration: 6 months for symptomatic and 12–18 months for disease-modifying trials. There is a current trend to include more mild patients with AD, operationalized as MMSE greater than 20, amnestic mild cognitive impairment (MCI), or MCI due to AD, prodromal or early AD (supported by a positive cerebrospinal fluid [CSF] or imaging biomarker) (Schneider 2008b; Albert et al. 2011).

Five cholinesterase inhibitors, memantine, the Ginkgo biloba extract EGb 761, and cerebrolysin have some level of marketing approval for the treatment of AD in the Western hemisphere, Europe, Australia/New Zealand, Japan, and many Asian countries. One antipsychotic, risperidone, is specifically approved in several countries, e.g., UK, Spain, and Canada for the treatment of agitation, psychosis, or the behavioral and psychological symptoms of dementia (BPSD) occurring in AD.

Considering Mechanisms of Action

Demonstration of a mechanism, pharmacodynamic effect, or target engagement either in preclinical in vitro or in animal models, or in humans does not establish the relevance of the mechanism to the effect the drug might have on clinical manifestations. Many agents, including various antioxidant and so-called antiaging cocktails, are marketed based on the chemical properties of ingredients rather than randomized controlled trials of safety and efficacy. Such products may not have established safety, and certainly have no evidence of efficacy. Moreover, most drug products have multiple actions. Thus, with the few exceptions of drugs and antibodies that clearly engage only one target, characterizing a particular drug as having a certain mechanism of action may be misleading; yet this is often done as a matter of convenience or for categorization.

ACETYLCHOLINESTERASE INHIBITORS

Acetylcholinesterase inhibitors (AChE-Is) are the first class of agents specifically approved by the US Food and Drug Administration (FDA) for the treatment of AD (Fig. 1). Tacrine (Cognex) was approved in 1993 followed by approval of donepezil (Aricept) in 1996, rivastigmine (Exelon) in 2000, and galantamine (Reminyl, Razadyne) in 2001. Memantine (Namenda)—an NMDA receptor antagonist—approval followed in 2004 (Fig. 1). Tacrine had a short half-life requiring administration every 4 hours and had substantial associated hepatotoxicity, requiring frequent monitoring of liver enzymes. These limitations were not present with later AChE-Is. Tacrine is rarely used, is no longer available in many countries, and will not be discussed here.

All AChE-Is share the characteristic of inhibiting acetylcholinesterase and each of these agents has additional distinctive pharmacologic aspects. AChE-Is are thought to bind acetylcholinesterase in the synaptic cleft so that acetylcholine released from the presynaptic cholinergic terminal has an increased residence time within the synapse and is more likely to interact with the postsynaptic cholinergic receptor. The enhanced postsynaptic activity renders more normal the function of the cholinergic system.

Donepezil is a selective AChE-I, rivastigmine is a mixed acetylcholinesterase and butyrylcholinesterase inhibitor, and galantamine is described as having an allosteric nicotinic modulating effect as well as being an AChE-I. The clinical consequences of the differential pharmacology of the AChE-Is, if any, are unknown.

For purposes of drug development, patients were identified for AChE-I clinical trials as having mild to moderate AD by requiring a MMSE (Folstein et al. 1975) score between ten and 26 in most trials. All AChE-Is are approved for treatment of mild to moderate AD. In the clinical development of donepezil, trials of patients with moderate to severe AD were conducted and established efficacy of this agent in patients with MMSE scores of 0–15. Donepezil is approved for mild, moderate, and severe AD.

To meet the criteria for approval by the FDA as a treatment for AD, an agent must be shown in two well-conducted trials to be statistically significantly superior to placebo on a test of cognition (regarded as the central feature of AD) and a global scale or an assessment of ADL (Schneider 2008) The usual measure of cognition in mild to moderate AD is the ADAS-Cog (Rosen et al. 1984). In patients with moderate to severe AD the cognitive measure most

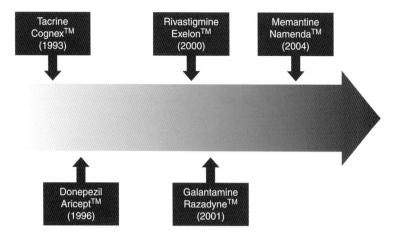

Figure 1. Timeline of approved treatments for Alzheimer disease.

commonly used is the Severe Impairment Battery (SIB) (Schmitt et al. 1997). The global outcome used in most AChE-I trials is the CIBIC+ (Schneider et al. 1997). ADL scales used in AChE-I trials include the ADCS ADL scale (Galasko et al. 1997) or the DAD (Gelinas et al. 1999). Changes in behavior are commonly measured as secondary outcomes in AChE-I clinical trials, and the most commonly used instrument is the Neuropsychiatric Inventory (NPI) (Cummings et al. 1994). Pharmacoeconomic data are collected in some trials using the Resource Utilization in Dementia (RUD) scale (Wimo and Winblad 2003). Most clinical trials of AChE-Is have been 6 months in duration; some have been as short as 3 months and some as long as 2 years (AD2000 Collaborative Group 2004).

The responses to treatment with different AChE-Is have overlapping confidence intervals (CI), and no individual cholinesterase inhibitor has been shown to be superior to others in terms of efficacy. The mean response on the ADAS-cog is approximately 2.0 points with CI of 1.5–2.5 points (Birks 2006). The response on the CIBIC+ is usually in the range of 1.9 (CI 1.3–3.0) on a scale in which 4 represents no change. 3, 2 and 1 represent mild, moderate and marked improvement, and 5, 6, and 7 represent mild, moderate, and marked worsening (Whitehead et al. 2004). A two-point (CI 0.5–

2.5) drug–placebo difference is common at trial conclusion on the ADCS ADL and a two-point (CI 0.5–4.0) drug–placebo difference on the NPI total score is common at trial conclusion. Approximately 25% of patients have a measurable improvement on the ADAS-Cog compared to 15% of patients on placebo. In addition to the drug–placebo difference in improvement, AChE-Is produce a delay in decline that affects as many as 80% of patients participating in a clinical trial (Geldmacher et al. 2006). Improvement on the ADAS-Cog is taken as an indication of improvement in the core clinical features of AD, whereas a drug–placebo difference in CIBIC+ or an ADL scale is accepted as a measure of clinically meaningful improvement. As noted, most clinical trials of AChE-Is are 6 months in duration and establish benefit for 6 months of therapy; some 1-year trials (Winblad et al. 2001) or 2-year trials (AD2000 Collaborative Group 2004) have been conducted and continued to show a drug–placebo difference at study conclusion. These observations support the long-term use of AChE-Is in the treatment of AD.

AD dementia is preceded by a period of cognitive impairment in which patients show decline in episodic memory and other cognitive abilities, but the changes are not sufficiently severe to reach the criteria for dementia. This clinical syndrome has been called mild cognitive impairment (MCI) (Petersen et al. 2001). Clinical trials of AChE-Is for the treatment of cognitive deficits of MCI have been uniformly negative (Jelic et al. 2006). It is now recognized that MCI is an etiologically heterogeneous state with only approximately 60–70% of patients having underlying AD (Jicha et al. 2006). The lack of response to AChE-Is in MCI may reflect the absence of an AD-type pathophysiology in a substantial number of patients included in the trial. In the ADCS MCI study, there was a drug–placebo benefit in favor of donepezil in MCI patients who were apolipoprotein E4 carriers, a group likely to have a high underlying rate of AD pathophysiology (Petersen et al. 2001). This suggests that prodromal AD may respond to treatment by AChE-Is. However, many of the patients enrolled in MCI trials could also have fulfilled criteria for AD.

Gastrointestinal side effects are common in patients placed on AChE-Is. Anorexia, nausea, vomiting, diarrhea, and weight loss may occur and should be monitored in patients treated with these agents. In addition, cholinergic influences may slow heart rate and bradycardia is a contraindication to use of AChE-Is. Occasional patients have experienced changes in urinary function. Muscle cramps have been reported with donepezil and abnormalities in dreaming also have been reported with donepezil.

In addition to the use of AChE-Is in AD, rivastigmine has been approved by the FDA for treatment of mild to moderate Parkinson's disease dementia (Emre et al. 2004). AChE-Is have also been assessed in clinical trials of vascular dementia (Black et al. 2003; Kavirajan and Schneider 2007), mixed AD and cerebrovascular disease (Erkinjuntti et al. 2002), and dementia with Lewy bodies (McKeith et al. 2000). None of these indications has been approved by the FDA and use of AChE-Is in these settings is off label.

Donepezil has a half-life of 70 hours and is administered once daily (Table 1). It is 96% protein bound with 100% bioavailability; it is metabolized by 2D6 and 3A4 cytochrome P450 enzymes. Treatment is begun with 5 mg/day and, if the patient shows no intolerance,

the dose is advanced to 10 mg/day usually after 1 month. A 23 mg once-daily dose has recently been approved for use in patients with moderate to severe AD (Okamura et al. 2008). Acetylcholinesterase positron emission tomography (PET) studies suggest that the 10 mg dose produces an approximately 60% inhibition of central acetylcholinesterase (Okamura et al. 2008). Rivastigmine has a peripheral half-life of 1.5 hours and a central half-life of 8 hours. The capsules are given twice daily and, when administered as the patch formulation, the patch is replaced once daily. Rivastigmine is not metabolized through the cytochrome P450 system; it is 40% protein bound and has 40% bioavailability. Rivastigmine is initiated in an oral dose of 1.5 mg orally twice daily and, as tolerance is determined, advanced to 3 mg, 4.5 mg, and 6 mg twice daily for a total target dose of 12 mg/day. Titration is typically at 1-month intervals and is determined by patient tolerance for the agent. The transdermal patch formulation of rivastigmine is initiated at a patch strength of 4.6 mg and advanced to 9.5 mg after 1 month if no intolerance is observed. Galantamine has a half-life of 7 hours and is given twice daily, unless the extended release formulation is used and administered once daily. Galantamine is initiated at a dose of 4 mg twice daily (8 mg/day in a single dose for the extended release formulation) and advanced to 16 and 24 mg/day at 1-month intervals. Galantamine is metabolized by the cytochrome P450 enzymes 2D6 and 3A4. It is 18% protein and has 90% bioavailability.

There are conflicting data as to whether AChE-Is have any disease-modifying properties with respect to AD. They affect disease course by improving symptoms and delaying decline as described above. Basic science observations suggest that enhancement of cholinergic function may reduce the generation of β-amyloid protein (Kimura et al. 2005). Some imaging studies have suggested less brain atrophy over time in patients treated with AChE-Is (Krishnan et al. 2003). In addition, some long-term observations suggest less decline in patients treated with AChE-Is or combination therapy of AChE-Is with memantine compared to

Table 1. Characteristics of cholinesterase inhibitors

Characteristic	Cholinesterase inhibitors		
	Donepezil	Rivastigmine	Galantamine
Trade name	Aricept (Aricet in some countries)	Exelon	Razadyne and Razadyne-ER
Indications	Mild to moderate and severe AD	Mild to moderate AD; Parkinson's disease dementia	Mild to moderate AD
Half-life	70 hours	1.5 hours (brain half-life is 8 hours)	7 hours
Administration schedule	q.d.	b.i.d. for capsules; q.d. for the patch	b.i.d. for the non-ER form: q.d. for the ER form
Metabolism by hepatic CYP enzymes	2D6, 3A4	No	2D6, 3A4
Protein binding	96%	40%	18%
Bioavailability	100%	40%	90%
Time to peak serum level	3–4 hours	1 hour	1 hour (2.5 hours with food); 4.5 hours for ER form
Absorption delayed by food	No	No	Yes (1 hour to 2.5 hours)
Titration	Begin with 5 mg and advance to 10 mg after 1 month	Oral form: 1.5 mg b.i.d. for 4 weeks; 3 mg b.i.d. for 4 weeks; 4.5 mg b.i.d. for 4 weeks; advance to 6 mg b.i.d. if tolerated. Patch form: begin the 5 cm^2 patch for 1 month then advance to 10 cm^2 patch	Non-ER form: begin 4 mg b.i.d.; advance to 8 mg b.i.d. after 1 month and to 12 mg b.i.d. after 1 month. ER form: begin at 8 mg q.d.; advance after 1 month to 16 mg DQ and after 1 month to 24 mg q.d.

Tacrine (Cognex) is now rarely used because of associated liver enzyme elevations and is not included in this chart.

patients not receiving therapy with these agents (Lopez et al. 2009; Rountree et al. 2009). Other clinical and imaging studies, however, suggest no disease-modifying benefit from treatment with AChE-Is (Jack et al. 2008; Schneider and Sano 2009). Disease-modifying effects, if present, must be small in magnitude.

Patients intolerant to one AChE-I may be able to tolerate an alternate cholinesterase inhibitor and the effort to keep patients on therapy should be made when intolerance occurs. Patients started on an oral medication might be switched to patch therapy or vice versa. Patients showing no efficacy in response to treatment with one cholinesterase inhibitor (uninterrupted continuing decline of cognition) may also be switched to another. Any benefit from switching in this circumstance however is not established.

Continuing benefit from use of AChE-Is has been shown in trials lasting up to 2 years, among patients followed over that length of time (AD2000 Collaborative Group 2004). In addition, patients with severe AD—not previously treated with AChE-Is—respond to treatment with AChE-Is, and donepezil is approved for treatment in this advanced phase of the disease. These observations suggest that long-term treatment with AChE-Is may continue to provide benefit. When AChE-Is are discontinued because the patient or the clinician believe that no further benefit is possible, patients should be observed for cognitive decline, loss of ADL, or emergent behavioral disturbances (Holmes et al. 2004). If adverse cognitive, functional, or behavioral changes occur soon after discontinuation then physicians and patients should consider whether the patient had been benefiting from treatment and whether to reinitiate medications at the starting doses.

MEMANTINE

Memantine was used in Germany for the treatment of Parkinson's disease prior to its approval in the USA and globally for treatment of AD. A key 12-week clinical trial of memantine for patients with dementia, mainly AD, residing in nursing homes was published in 1999 (Winblad and Poritis 1999) followed by publication of a monotherapy trial in 2000 (Reisberg et al. 2003a) and of a donepezil add-on trial in 2004 (Tariot et al. 2004). Memantine was approved by the FDA in the USA in 2004 for treatment of moderate to severe AD, meaning patients with MMSE scores less than 15. Memantine is an NMDA receptor antagonist that replaces potassium in the NMDA receptor channel to reduce entry of calcium into neurons and avoid calcium-stimulated apoptotic cell death cascades. It is uncertain if the neuroprotective activities observed consistently in in vitro studies account for the symptomatic benefit observed in clinical trials. In vitro experimental studies suggest reduced Aβ plaque deposition and reduced tau hyperphosphorylation following treatment with memantine (Martinez-Coria et al. 2010). Physiological studies establish a beneficial effect for long-term potentiation (LTP), the physiological correlate of memory (Frankiewicz and Parsons 1999). This latter observation provides a potential explanation for the symptomatic benefit observed with treatment with memantine.

Clinical trials of memantine have been very similar in design to those conducted with AChE-Is, but have involved patients with moderate to severe AD, rather than mild to moderate AD. Trials have typically been 6 months in duration with the SIB, CIBIC+, or ADCS-ADL as primary outcomes and ADL or behavior as secondary outcomes. The magnitude of benefit from treatment with memantine is similar to the magnitude observed for AChE-Is. Two of three moderate to severe AD trials with memantine showed statistical significance on their primary outcomes (Reisberg et al. 2003b; van Dyck et al. 2007), including an add-on trial, in which patients on long-term treatment with donepezil, randomized to receive either placebo or add-on memantine, showed that add-on therapy with memantine produced a statistically significant benefit compared to add-on therapy with placebo (Tariot et al. 2004).

Several clinical trials have been conducted with memantine patients with mild to moderate AD. One of these trials showed benefit on cognition, global assessment, and behavior (Peskind et al. 2006); two trials did not show significant drug–placebo differences (Bakchine and Loft 2008; Porsteinsson et al. 2008). Memantine is not approved by the FDA for patients with mild AD. European regulatory authorities extended the range of approval for use of memantine to patients with MMSE scores of 19 and below.

Memantine has a half-life of 60–80 hours, is 50% protein bound, is not metabolized by the cytochrome P450 hepatic enzymes, and its absorption is not delayed by food (Table 2). Memantine is subject to renal excretion and the dose should be decreased by 50% in AD patients with renal failure. Memantine is initiated at a dose of 5 mg per day for 1 week, it is then advanced to 5 mg twice daily for 1 week; the next dose is 10 mg in the morning and 5 mg in the evening for 1 week; and the final dose is 10 mg twice daily. This is the continuing permanent dose for patients who do not have evidence of intolerance. Adverse events reported with memantine therapy include headache, dizziness, and somnolence. There have been reports of confusion during the titration period and occasional reports of hallucinations.

Memantine is approved for moderate to severe AD and may be given either alone or in conjunction with an AChE-I. No adverse drug interactions have been reported with patients receiving AChE-Is plus memantine, and the drugs are safe when used together. Although some long-term open-label observations suggest that combination therapy with an ACHE-I and memantine may ameliorate the course of AD (Lopez et al. 2009; Rountree et al. 2009), other studies suggest otherwise (Schneider et al. 2011). Observations in the course of

Table 2. Characteristics of memantine

Trade name	Namenda (Ebixa or Axura in some countries)
Indications	Moderate to severe AD (USA) up to MMSE scores of 20 in Europe and Asia
Half-life	60–80 hours
Protein binding	50%
Metabolism by hepatic CYP enzymes	No
Absorption delayed by food	No
Time to peak serum level	3–7 hours
Adjustment in hepatic or renal disease	Decrease dose by 50% in patients with renal failure
Titration	5 q.d. for 1 week; 5 b.i.d. for 1 week; 10 mg in a.m. and 5 mg in p.m. for 1 week; 10 mg b.i.d. thereafter

double-blind placebo-controlled trials suggested that patients on therapy decline at equal rates when compared to patients not receiving therapy (Schneider and Sano 2009).

Patients are usually treated with memantine or a combination of an ACHE-I plus memantine until late in the course of AD. Pharmacotherapy may be continued until the patients succumbs or until their physicians and family conclude that the quality of life of the patient is sufficiently compromised that pharmacotherapy is futile.

Use of Psychotropic Agents to Treat Behavioral Disturbances in AD

Behavioral disturbances are common in AD, including depression, agitation, irritability, aberrant motor behaviors, and psychosis (Cummings 2003). There are no agents approved by the FDA specifically for treatment of behavioral disturbances in AD. Antipsychotics—both conventional and atypical—are associated with increased mortality and some antipsychotics are associated with increased risk for cerebrovascular accidents or stroke when administered to elderly patients with AD. The risk of death is increased from ~2.6% to ~4.5% during an average of 10 weeks of therapy. Long-term observations suggest that continuing therapy is associated with a continuing increased risk for mortality (Kales et al. 2007; Ballard et al. 2009). Several 1–12 week long clinical trials suggest that risperidone and

possibly other atypical antipsychotic agents in low doses are efficacious in reducing psychosis and agitation in mainly nursing home patients with AD (Ballard and Waite 2006; Schneider et al. 2006). Given the evidence of benefit and harm for the use of antipsychotics in AD, the clinician must exercise caution when prescribing these agents. Strategies for use of antipsychotics in patients with AD involve avoiding their use in patients with cardiovascular or pulmonary disease (the two most common causes of death in mortality studies), using these agents only in patients for whom nonpharmacologic interventions have failed and the behaviors are extreme, employing treatment for only the period required and attempting to eliminate the agents as soon as possible, and informing the patient and caregiver of the risks involved.

Clinical trials have been largely negative in showing benefit for treatment of depression in AD with antidepressant medications (Lyketsos et al. 2000; Olin et al. 2002; Rosenberg et al. 2010; Weintraub et al. 2010). There is no consistent evidence base for the use of antidepressants in AD. Individual practitioners may use practice-based evidence to guide their therapeutic decisions. Several recent trials suggest that use of valproate to treat agitation has no superiority over placebo and is associated with substantial toxicity (Tariot et al. 2005; Herrmann et al. 2007). Early trials suggested the benefit of carbamazepine as a treatment for agitation (Tariot et al. 1998). Anxiolytics and hypnotics are generally to be avoided in patients with AD as they may increase confusion. Short-term use of benzodiazepines such as lorazepam or clonazepam may be useful in patients with episodes of agitation.

There is an urgent need for effective, safe, psychotropic agents for treatment of behavioral disturbances in AD and other dementing disorders.

OTHER TREATMENTS MARKETED FOR AD IN SOME COUNTRIES

The following three substances are approved for use or widely used in some individual countries for cognitive impairment syndromes but are not FDA or EMA approved.

Ginkgo Biloba

Ginkgo biloba leaves and extracts are widely used in over-the-counter preparations marketed in the USA as food supplements or nutraceuticals and, as such, explicit health claims are not listed in their labeling (Schneider 2008a). In several countries *G. biloba* is advocated for the treatment of a broad range of medical conditions including, as examples, tinnitus and dizziness. The extract that is approved for use in some countries is Ginkgo biloba extract EGb 761 (Ipsen Pharma, and Schwabe Pharmaceuticals), standardized to contain two major constituents: 22–27% flavonoids and 5–7% terpene lactones (ginkgolides and bilobalide).

The flavonoids are active as antioxidants and appear neuroprotective. Ginkgolide B is a potent antagonist of the platelet-activating factor receptor. Ginkgolides A and J variously inhibit hippocampal neuron dysfunction and neuronal cell death caused by amyloid-β protein-42 (Aβ42). Ginkgolides A and J decrease Aβ42-induced pathological behaviors, enhance neurogenesis in animal models of AD, and inhibit Aβ aggregation, providing considerable rationale for *G. biloba* extracts as potential treatments for AD.

Trials in older and younger adults who do not have cognitive impairment show mixed results at best (Schneider 2008a). One meta-analysis of eight trials did not find evidence for cognitive benefits with *G. biloba* in noncognitively impaired participants younger than 60 years treated for up to 13 weeks. Two placebo-controlled trials reported contradictory effects in noncognitively impaired older adults, and the magnitude of the cognitive effects were small in the positive trial.

A systematic review that included 35 clinical trials and 4247 participants reported inconsistent evidence that *G. biloba* had clinically significant benefits for dementia or cognitive impairment (Birks and Grimley Evans 2009). One 6-month trial in mild to moderate AD sponsored by Schwabe Pharmaceuticals, conducted with the hope of gaining US FDA marketing approval, failed to demonstrate efficacy (Schneider et al. 2005), as did another 6-month trial performed at British primary care sites with 120 mg/day doses of EGb 761 (McCarney et al. 2008).

Perhaps because of its popularity and perceived safety there have been three prevention trials undertaken using EGb 761 at 240 mg daily doses. A trial involving 118 participants without MCI or dementia, all older than 85 years, randomized to receive *G. biloba* extract or placebo and followed up for 42 months, showed a nonsignificant effect for *G. biloba* to delay progression to MCI (Dodge et al. 2008). Of potential concern, however, was that more ischemic strokes and transient ischemic episodes occurred in the *G. biloba* group. The GEM trial randomized 3069 persons to *G. biloba* extract or placebo who had no cognitive impairment or MCI for a median duration of more than 6 years and found no clinical effects for the extract on cognition or time to dementia (DeKosky et al. 2008). A second prevention trial, GuidAge, conducted in France and involving 2854 participants with memory complaints or MCI, randomized to *G. biloba* or placebo and followed for more than 5 years, also failed to find effects for ginkgo on the primary outcome of time to onset of AD or other dementia (Ipsen press release, 22 June 2010). Thus, there is very little evidence for the efficacy of *G. biloba* either for improving symptoms or preventing AD.

Cerebrolysin

Cerebrolysin is a somewhat controversial approach to neurotrophic therapy for AD. This product is a parenterally administered digested peptide preparation derived from pig brain. In vitro studies suggest that this peptide mixture has neuroprotective effects. There is some evidence of brain penetration with peripheral administration. There have been a number of clinical studies of Cerebrolysin infusion therapy in AD, with some results suggesting symptomatic benefit (Okamura et al. 2008). As a result, it has being widely used in many countries. Skepticism arises from the poorly defined composition and mechanisms and inconsistencies in clinical findings, but some have called for more definitive trials.

Huperzine A

Huperzine A is a plant extract with potent, selective AchE1 inhibition used in China for the treatment of dementia. Preclinical studies suggest possible neuroprotective mechanisms. A recent Phase II trial in the USA failed to demonstrate efficacy of the usual dose used in China, 200 mcg twice daily, but did provide some evidence of cognitive enhancement at twice this dose (Rafii et al. 2011).

DIETARY SUPPLEMENTS, VITAMINS, NUTRICEUTICALS, MEDICAL FOODS

A dietary supplement is defined by US law as a product (other than tobacco) that is intended to supplement the diet; contains one or more dietary ingredients (including vitamins, minerals, herbs or other botanicals, amino acids, and other substances) or their constituents; is intended to be taken by mouth; and is labeled on the front panel as being a dietary supplement (United States Dietary Supplement Health and Education Act of 1994 (http://www.fda.gov/opacom/laws/dshea.html#sec3).

The word nutraceutical has no official meaning, but was coined to imply nontraditional products with pharmaceutical effects. A dietary supplement promoter cannot make a health-disease treatment claim for the substance.

Thus, for example, a supplement could be advertised as enhancing "brain power," brain cells or concentration, but not as a treatment for AD or attention deficit disorder, as the latter are health claims.

Several dietary supplements and vitamins have been used in clinical trials for AD, cognitive impairment, or age associated memory impairment (AAMI; older individuals who have cognitive test scores below the norms for young adults) and have been indirectly promoted by various interest groups as treatments for AD. Formulations of these substances vary, with no regulatory standard except that products must contain the substance advertised.

Docosahexaenoic Acid

Docosahexaenoic acid (DHA) is the primary constituent of membranes in the central nervous system (CNS). DHA levels in brain decline with age, but can be restored with dietary supplementation. Adding DHA to the diet of transgenic mice with amyloid deposition in brain reduces amyloid accumulation and improves cognitive performance. There is thus a reasonable rationale for studying DHA supplementation as a therapeutic intervention for cognitive aging and AD.

One trial conducted by a manufacturer of DHA, Martek, in individuals with AAMI did not yield significant results. Post-hoc analyses suggest possible benefits in measures of episodic memory (Okamura et al. 2008).

An NIA-funded trial of DHA for mild to moderate AD was, however, negative (Quinn et al. 2010). Treatment with DHA for 18 months increased CSF levels (in the subset who underwent lumbar punctures), but did not alter the decline in cognitive and functional assessments.

B Vitamins

Elevated homocysteine in blood is considered a risk factor for cardiovascular disease, vascular dementia, and AD. Plasma concentrations increase when homocysteine's metabolism to methionine or cysteine is impaired, which may occur under a number of circumstances, including natural aging. Increased blood levels of homocysteine are associated with damage to vascular endothelial cells through lipid peroxidation and release of endothelium-derived relaxing factor, and may increase the risk of vascular thrombosis. More relevant to AD, homocysteine potentiates the neurotoxic effects of β-amyloid peptides in vitro. Homocysteine plasma levels can be reduced by as much as 30% using regimens of B vitamins (e.g., B12 1 mg/day, B6 25 mg/day, and folic acid 5 mg/day). A placebo-controlled clinical trial of these vitamins over 18 months confirmed that substantial reduction in homocysteine could be achieved but did not slow the rate of cognitive decline in AD compared to placebo (Aisen et al. 2008; Okamura et al. 2008). A study of a similar regimen in individuals with MCI showed reduction of whole brain atrophy with vitamin use for 2 years (Smith et al. 2010). A fixed combination of B6, B12, and folate known as Cerefolin is marketed as a medical food (see below) for treatment of metabolic abnormalities associated with AD.

Vitamin E

The antioxidant effects of vitamin E (DL-α-tocopherol) might have an impact on reducing clinical progression. In the prototypical antioxidant trial, vitamin E (1000 IU twice a day) and selegiline (5 mg twice a day), each given alone to moderately impaired patients with AD, delayed the time until patients required nursing home placement, died, or lost ADL (Sano et al. 1997).

Overall, the delayed time to these end points was approximately 7 months compared to placebo. There were no effects on cognition in this group of patients, who were more severely impaired than in many other studies. Adverse effects included falls and syncope in selegiline patients (9 and 10%, respectively), α-tocopherol patients (14 and 7%, respectively), and the combination (22 and 16%, respectively).

A multicenter trial in MCI patients reported no significant delay in conversion to AD or dementia in cognitive effects with α-tocopherol (or donepezil) over 3 years of treatment (Petersen et al. 2005). Taken together, considering the absence of cognitive efficacy and the potential risks for treatment, vitamin E cannot be recommended as treatment.

Homotaurine

Originally synthesized and manufactured as a drug in development for AD under the name tramiprosate (3-amino-1-propanesulfonic acid) and the trade name Alzhemed, the amino acid homotaurine is now sold in Canada as a nutraceutical under the brand name Vivimind. The rationale for this is that, although the product is synthesized, homotaurine is also a natural component of certain seaweeds.

The rationale for its development as a prescription drug for AD was as an Aβ aggregation inhibitor. After a Phase II safety study in which CSF Aβ was decreased (Aisen et al. 2006), two 18-month Phase III trials (one of which was stopped early) did not show efficacy. The company currently advances its use without a specific health claim as a food supplement.

MEDICAL FOODS

A medical food is "a food which is formulated to be consumed or administered enterally (or orally) under the supervision of a physician, and which is intended for the specific dietary management of a disease or condition for which distinctive nutritional requirements, based on recognized scientific principles, are established by medical evaluation," under the Orphan Drug Amendments of 1988 and the Nutrition Labeling and Education Act of 1990 (see 21 U.S.C. sec. 360ee(b)(3), 21 C.F.R. sec. 101.9(j)(8), and "Guidance for Industry: Frequently Asked Questions About Medical Foods" (May 2007), FDA website).

In addition, the contents of a medical food must fulfill the Generally Recognized as Safe (GRAS) designation for foods.

Axona (Ketasyn; AC-1202)

A mixture of medium-chain triglycerides, brand named Axona, was marketed in March 2009 as a medical food for AD. The rationale is that AD or other cognitive impairment may be partly a consequence of impaired glucose metabolism (see below), and that this can be treated by using medium-chain triglycerides that are converted to ketones, raising ketone levels, which enhance mitochondrial electron transport that otherwise was impaired by the impaired glucose metabolism (Henderson et al. 2009). Separately, some studies show that a ketogenic diet reduces Aβ40 and 42 in transgenic mice.

In two 12-week placebo-controlled randomized trials for AD and AAMI there was no statistical evidence for cognitive or behavioral effects (Henderson et al. 2009). In the trial with 152 AD patients significant improvements on the ADAScog were noted at 6 weeks but not at 12 weeks, and post hoc the very few APOE4-negative patients in the trial seemed to improve at 12 weeks (Henderson et al. 2009). The 159-patient trial with AAMI patients was also not significant, showing two of the memory subscales to be significant in post hoc analyses.

Souvenaid

Another company, Danone, is developing and testing in clinical trials a brand name medical food, Souvenaid, that is comprised of a combination of food supplements, including uridine monophosphate, choline, omega-3 fatty acids (EPA, DHA), phospholipids, B vitamins, and antioxidants (Scheltens et al. 2010). The rationale is that this specific combination might synergistically enhance dendritic spine growth, synapse formation, neurotransmitter precursors, and neurotransmitter release, ultimately improving cognitive function. The company also claims the combination reduced amyloid production and toxicity in the preclinical models. Results of a 12-week, placebo-controlled trial in 225 patients with AD were nonsignificant on most of the outcomes (Scheltens et al. 2010). There are ongoing, longer, and larger trials in the USA and Europe.

Thus, there is no evidence for efficacy for these two medical foods and more studies are needed.

OTHER NEUROTRANSMITTER-BASED TREATMENTS

Cholinergic Agonists

A range of M1, muscarinic agonists with variable specificity for the M1 receptor subtype have been tested in 6-month symptomatic trials. Although some have shown distinct cognitive signals on standard clinical trials outcomes, they also produce considerable and troublesome cholinergic adverse effects such as gastrointestinal disturbances, diaphoresis, syncope, and hypersalivation. The M1 agonists also show salutary effects on Aβ in preclinical models. There have been no trials of lower doses over longer time periods to assess the potential for disease modification.

Neuronal Nicotinic Receptor Agonists

Neuronal nicotinic acetylcholine receptors (NNRs) are widespread throughout the central and peripheral nervous system. They mediate aspects of memory, attention, arousal, mood, anxiety, and sensory perception. NNR agonists can affect acetylcholine receptors through full and partial agonism or positive allosteric modulation. Receptor stimulation may increase release of several neurotransmitters implicated in CNS disorders including dopamine, serotonin, glycine, glutamate, and GABA. There may be a physiological inverted dose-response where low doses of NNR agonists enhance cognition and higher doses do not.

Two classes of NNRs may be involved in CNS disorders: (1) α7, and (2) α4/β2, and serve as targets. The α7 agonists predominate in areas more directly linked to memory and may also serve a neuroprotective function by reducing oxygen free radicals and nitric oxide. An α7 agonist in particular could be expected to be both symptomatic and have disease modifying properties as it enhances cognitive performance in behavioral models that capture domains of working memory, recognition memory, memory consolidation, and sensory gating deficit, increases the release of both presynaptic and postsynaptic calcium, and increases the release of Ach, glutamate, serotonin, and dopamine.

PDE Inhibition

A rational behind phosphdiesterase 4 (PDE4) inhibition is that it leads to CREB up-regulation, which should promote neurotrophin expression, and thus may have both cognition enhancing and neuroprotective effects. The molecules in development so far have not succeeded, having manifested significant cardiac and gastrointestinal adverse effects.

EHT0202 (etazolate HCl) shows both potential symptomatic and disease-modifying effects in AD, acting as a PDE-4 inhibitor and GABA-A receptor modulator, increasing α-secretase activity and sAPP α secretion, thus lowering Aβ. PDE inhibitors involving a variety of PDE enzymes are being tested in early-phase AD trials (Okamura et al. 2008).

AMPA Receptor Modulation

More challenging, in terms of safety, is the work being done on neurotrophically high-impact AMPA modulators. Lilly's high-impact LY451395 failed in an AD Phase II trial, but this trial used tiny doses (0.2 mg for 28 days, then 1.0 mg thereafter) which speaks to the low therapeutic index, probably related to seizure risk. Cortex believes they have achieved the necessary balance between trophic effect and seizure risk with CX-1837, but have not completed that molecule's preclinical testing.

H3 Antagonists

The H3 receptor has the highest affinity for histamine among the four histamine receptors and is predominantly expressed in the cerebral cortex, hippocampus, and hypothalamus in which it functions as a presynaptic autoreceptor to regulate histamine release and cholinergic and monoaminergic neurotransmitter release. H3 blockage results in the release of neurotransmitters and is associated with enhanced cognitive function in preclinical models. Several H3 receptor agonists are in early stage clinical trials for treatment of the cognitive or motivational aspects of AD.

OTHER APPROACHES TO AD TREATMENT

There are many drug development programs pursuing strategies not directly related to amyloid, tau, or neurotransmission. As discussed above, the putative mechanisms may be impossible to specify and may be multiple; there is generally no way to connect drug activity in experimental symptoms specific to clinical results in the management of AD. Many such agents are listed in Table 3, and examples are discussed below.

DRUGS WITH METABOLIC ACTIONS

There is evidence that diabetes may increase the risk of AD, and a variety of animal and human studies support the concept that insulin resistance in brain may play a role in AD (Craft 2007). Increasing attention is being paid to the possible interrelationship between AD and diabetes as epidemiologic studies suggest that people with Type 2 diabetes mellitus are twice as likely to develop AD as nondiabetics. Insulin may prevent the soluble toxic form of Aβ from damaging neurons. Insulin protection was enhanced by the presence of rosiglitazone. Intranasal or IV insulin has been shown to improve cognitive performance in small studies of individuals with AD. Additional studies of insulin therapy are planned.

PPARγ-Agonists

The peroxisome proliferator activated receptor γ (PPARγ) is activated by a variety of fatty acids and fatty acid derivatives, and regulates adipocyte differentiation and function. PPARγ-agonists such as rosiglitazone (Avandia) and pioglitazone (Actos) further mediate insulin actions and are marketed drugs for diabetes. They also may have actions relevant to AD, including anti-inflammatory effects. However, a study of a pioglitazone found mixed results, with no difference on most cognitive measures (Sato et al. 2009; Geldmacher et al. 2011). Six- and 12-month Phase III trials of rosiglitazone, a PPARγ agonist also targeting insulin resistance and related pathways failed to

Table 3. Selected drug development programs

Name	Sponsor	Proposed mechanism or therapeutic rationale	Target population	Supportive studies	Nonsupportive studies/issues	Current status
Insulin	NIA	Correction of insulin abnormalities that may contribute to pathology and synaptic dysfunction	MCI, AD	Small Phase II RCTs with some positive effects (Craft et al. 2011)		Additional Phase II trials planned
Rosiglitazone	GSK	Anti-inflammatory effect; improve brain insulin resistance	AD	Exploratory Phase II analyses (Risner et al. 2006)	Phase III	Not actively pursued
Dimebon	Medivation/Pfizer	Mitochondrial neuroprotectant	AD, HD	Phase II (Doody et al. 2008)	Phase III monotherapy	Phase III add-on study in progress
DHA	NIA, Martek	Restore membrane function	AD, AAMI	Epidemiology plus post-hoc analyses in cognitive aging trial	ADCS trial in AD	Additional studies in genetic subgroups and/or MCI are under discussion
Cerebrolysin	EBEWE	Neurotrophic activity	AD	Effect of some doses on cognition or global status in randomized trials	Inconsistent results	Marketed in many countries
Statins	NIA, Pfizer	Alter cholesterol/amyloid pathways	Normal, AD	Epidemiology; small randomized study	ADCS, LEADe	Not actively pursued for AD
Estrogen	NIA	Engage brain estrogen receptors	Normal, AD	Epidemiology; small randomized study	ADCS, WHI,	Not actively pursued for AD
NSAIDs	NIA, Merck	Reduce harmful brain inflammation	AD, MCI	Epidemiology	ADCS, Merck	Not actively pursued for AD
B vitamins	NIA	Reduce homocysteine	AD	Epidemiology	ADCS	?MCI
HGH, IGF-1	Merck, others	Normalize HGH-IGF-1 pathways	AD, aging	Epidemiology	MK-677 trial	Not actively pursued for AD
Lithium		Inhibit tau phosphorylation plus other neuroprotective mechanisms	AD, tauopathies	Preclinical data	Negative RCT	Not actively pursued for AD
Valproic acid	NIA	Inhibit tau phosphorylation plus other neuroprotective mechanisms	AD	Preclinical data	Negative RCT	Not actively pursued for AD

Table 3. *Continued*

Name	Sponsor	Proposed mechanism or therapeutic rationale	Target population	Supportive studies	Nonsupportive studies/issues	Current status
Resveratrol	NIA	SIRT-1	AD, normal aging	In vitro, animal studies	Limited brain penetration	RCT in AD beginning
Axona	Accera	Correct ketone body accumulation	AD	Post-hoc results	Negative RCT	Marketed as medical food
Souvenaid		Combination of vitamins to improve brain cell function	AD	Post-hoc results	Negative RCT	Marketed as medical food
Xaliproden	Sanofi-Aventis	Neuroprotection	AD	Preclinical data	Negative RCT	Not actively pursued for AD
Vitamin E	NIA	Antioxidant	Normal, MCI, AD	Positive AD trial	Negative MCI trial	Use limited by toxicity concerns
Ginkgo biloba	NIA, Schwabe, Ipsen	Antioxidant	Normal, AD	Some randomized trials in AD	Negative AD and prevention trials	Over-the-counter preparations widely used
Idebenone	Takeda	Antioxidant	AD	Preclinical data	Randomized trial	Not actively pursued for AD
Acetyl-L-carnitine	Sigma Tau	Antioxidant	AD	Preclinical data	Randomized trials	Two negative RCTs
Leuprolide	Curaxis	Gonadotropin pathways	AD	Preclinical studies, epidemiology	Randomized trial	Negative RCT
NGF gene delivery	NIA Ceregene	Neurotrophic	AD	Phase I open label study	Requires neurosurgical procedure	Phase II in progress

Cite this article as *Cold Spring Harb Perspect Med* doi: 10.1101/cshperspect.a006395

demonstrate significant benefit (Harrington et al. 2009; Gold et al. 2010), although post-hoc analysis in an early study suggested benefit in the APOE ε4 negative subgroup (Risner et al. 2006).

Dimebon (Latrepirdine)

The course of the dimebon development program includes a number of interesting lessons on the process of bringing new AD treatments forward (Doody 2009). Dimebon was initially identified by Russian scientists who screened compounds available for clinical use in that country for activity similar to that of the established AD treatments. They sought a single compound that would combine cholinesterase inhibition with NMDA antagonism. The lead compound to arise from this process was dimebon, a drug used as an antihistamine in Russia until the late 1980s. Following an 8-week open trial in 14 patients (Bachurin et al. 2001), dimebon was licensed by a US company, Medivation, and underwent a 6-month, placebo-controlled Phase II trial, conducted in Russia, in 183 individuals with mild to moderate AD, similar in design to standard trials used with cholinesterase inhibitors and memantine. The results were strikingly positive, with consistent favorable effects on both primary and secondary measures of cognition, function, and behavior (Doody et al. 2008). Further, a blinded extension of the trial to 12 months indicated that benefits of the drug in comparison to placebo appeared to increase with time. This trial suggested that dimebon might have benefits beyond the expectations for a combined cholinesterase inhibitor/NMDA antagonist, and indeed the very limited potency against those targets argued that dimebon must work by a novel mechanism. Activity in vitro against models of mitochondrial toxicity supported that dimebon may be a mitochondrial cytoprotectant. Thus, a drug identified using standard screens appeared to be highly effective based on an unexpected and novel mechanism.

An international Phase III trial was launched to replicate the Russian study findings but including nearly 600 patients, and several other studies were started to explore the efficacy of dimebon added onto donepezil treatment, and to evaluate efficacy in moderate to severe AD. However, the confirmatory study results showed no efficacy, with no apparent explanation for this inconsistency with the Russian Phase II trial. Another Phase III trial, assessing the addition of dimebon to standard therapy for 1 year, continues. Lessons from the dimebon program include the role of serendipity, and the unpredictability and inconsistency in Phase II and smaller sample size AD trials learned from other programs (Schneider 2008b), as well as reasons specific to this drug (Jones 2010).

Statins

Epidemiological evidence suggests that cholesterol lowering and the use of 3-hydroxy-3-methylglutaryl coenzyme A (HMG-CoA) reductase inhibitors ("statins") may modulate the enzymatic processing of amyloid precursor protein and consequently the production of β-amyloid, and impact the development or progression of AD. Furthermore, cholesterol-fed rabbits show increased Aβ in brain, and hypercholesterolemia induced by a high-cholesterol diet results in increased levels of Aβ in the CNS. Statin administration in vitro reduces intra- and extracellular Aβ levels in neuronal cultures. Observational studies of patient records showed a 60–73% lower prevalence of and markedly reduced risk for AD in lovastatin (Mevacor)- or pravastatin (Pravachol)-treated patients.

Clinical trials, however, have not supported the use of statins for AD. A randomized, placebo-controlled trial of pravastatin in 5804 subjects with risk factors for vascular disease reported favorable cardiovascular outcomes but no significant effect on cognitive function or disability during an approximately 3-year follow-up period (Trompet et al. 2010). In a randomized, placebo-controlled trial of the effect of simvastatin on cardiovascular outcomes in a subgroup of 5806 patients aged 70 or more years, there was no significant difference in the proportion of patients with cognitive impairment or in the incidence of dementia over the average 5-year follow-up period. Two large placebo-controlled trials, one with simvastatin and another with atorvastatin, over 18 months did not show positive effects for the drugs in slowing the clinical decline (McGuinness et al. 2009).

Estrogens

Preclinical evidence amply demonstrates that estrogens improve cognitive function through cholinergic neuroprotective and neurotrophic effects. Clinical evidence of a possible effect for estrogen replacement therapy (ERT) has included observations of an inverse relationship between ERT and death-certificate diagnoses of dementia, several case-control and cohort studies in which hormonal therapy reducing the risk of AD were reported, and small clinical reports suggesting that estradiol, estrone, or conjugated equine estrogens enhance cognitive function in AD (Henderson 2006). However, larger studies have not confirmed benefits (Mulnard et al. 2000). Indeed, the large Women's Health Initiative trial revealed an increased risk of dementia and cognitive impairment in women treated with hormone replacement therapy (Shumaker et al. 2003). It is possible but not proven that estrogen treatment in midlife around menopause could be neurotrophic and preventative of the onset of AD, but beyond a few epidemiological studies, evidence is lacking. Particularly in view of growing concerns about adverse health effects, the use of estrogen replacement late in life to prevent or treat MCI or AD cannot be recommended.

ANTI-INFLAMMATORY DRUGS

There has been enormous interest for more than two decades in the suppression of brain inflammatory activity as an approach to slowing disease progression in AD. Unfortunately, randomized trials of multiple anti-inflammatory regimens, including glucocorticoids (Aisen et al. 2000), nonsteroidal anti-inflammatory drugs (both nonselective and COX-2 selective) (Aisen et al. 2003; Lyketsos et al. 2007), hydroxychloroquine (Van Gool et al. 2001),

and dapsone have all failed to demonstrate efficacy.

Curcumin is the active ingredient of curry spicy and is widely used as a food additive in Asian cooking. It has antioxidant properties and has been shown in experimental models to have anti-inflammatory, antioxidant, and anti-amyloid effects (Ringman et al. 2005). There is concern about the brain bioavailability of curcumin, however, and improved formulations are being sought.

INHIBITOR OF THE RECEPTOR FOR ADVANCED GLYCATION ENDPRODUCTS

The receptor for advanced glycation endproducts (RAGE) is present on neurons, glia, and endothelial cells and is mainly of interest in diabetes and vascular disease in which there is an increased level of various ligands including advanced glycation endproducts that bind to it, effecting pro-inflammatory activity. It is of interest in AD because of a relationship of AD to diabetes and because the amyloid peptide is also a RAGE ligand, and this interaction may contribute to brain inflammation and accumulation of amyloid. The latter effect might result in increased CNS Aβ as well as inflammatory effects in AD patients. Thus RAGE blockers could be therapeutically useful in diabetes and AD. After a small Phase II trial indicated the tolerability of an oral inhibitor of RAGE in AD (Sabbagh et al. 2010), an 18-month trial was launched, with results expected soon.

NGF GENE DELIVERY

The most important component of the brain's capacity to protect the function of cholinergic neurons is nerve growth factor (NGF). Early attempts to utilize NGF to protect these neurons in AD were unsuccessful because of toxicity; NGF delivered into the CSF stimulates ependymal cell proliferation with resulting toxicity such as pain. The advance of gene delivery methods has led to a resurgence of interest in NGF; primate studies showed that NGF gene delivery to the cholinergic nucleus basalis

Cite this article as *Cold Spring Harb Perspect Med* doi: 10.1101/cshperspect.a006395

resulted in long-term gene expression with neurotrophic effects.

A Phase I study of stereotactic NGF gene delivery using transformed fibroblasts derived from skin biopsies showed that NGF expression could be induced in nucleus basalis cells in humans with AD, with some evidence of increased brain function by FDG-PET scanning (Tuszynski et al. 2005). An NIA-funded, randomized, sham-surgery controlled Phase II trial of NGF gene delivery using a viral vector is currently in progress.

SIRTUINS AND RESVERATROL

Modifications of DNA and post-translational nuclear proteins may produce lasting alterations in chromatin, alter patterns of gene expression, and may affect neuroplasticity. Dysregulation of such epigenetic mechanisms may affect aging brain and cognitive impairment. Histone deacetylation (HDAC) may contribute to pathologic transcriptional aberrations in brain disease and HDAC activation may have therapeutic potential. Sirtuins, a family of histone deacetylation compounds, may be important to epigenetic mechanisms, and may be involved in the cellular protection afforded by calorie restriction (Gan 2007). Targeting sirtuins represents a new approach to neurodegenerative disorders.

There is great interest in the potential benefits of polyphenolic compounds derived from various fruits, vegetables, and plants. Polyphenols are potent antioxidants in vitro, and have been studied as potential therapeutics in cardiovascular disease and cancer, in part based on epidemiological evidence. Similarly, there is interest in polyphenols to reduce the adverse effects of aging on the function of organs including brain; neuroprotective effects have been shown in vitro.

Resveratrol is a polyphenol particularly abundant in the skin of red grapes; it has been suggested that this may in part explain epidemiological links between red wine consumption and reduced risk of AD (Vingtdeux et al. 2008). In vivo data have clearly shown the neuroprotective properties of the naturally occurring polyphenol resveratrol in rodent models for stress and diseases. Furthermore, recent work in cell cultures and animal models has shed light on the molecular mechanisms potentially involved in the beneficial effects of resveratrol intake against the neurodegenerative process in AD. Laboratory studies indicate that resveratrol is an activator of sirtuins. Resveratrol and other sirtuin activators increase longevity and slow brain atrophy in a number of species including nonhuman primates.

Although brain penetration of resveratrol is limited, some studies suggest that it may have a peripheral action that reduces brain amyloid accumulation. A NIA-funded study of the impact of resveratrol on biomarkers of AD will be initiated in early 2011.

SUMMARY

AChE-Is and the NMDA receptor antagonist memantine are FDA approved for treatment of AD. Transmitter based therapies represent the only validated treatments of AD. Deficits in transmitters not addressed by current therapies suggest that manipulation of these transmitter systems are worthy targets for cognitive enhancement. A plethora of metabolic, intracellular, and neuroprotective approaches populate this potential therapeutic space and represent new and emerging treatments for AD. Particularly for drug development programs aiming to slow progression of underlying pathobiological mechanisms, clinical impact is likely to be greatest if treatment is initiated early, prior to the onset of dementia or even in the presymptomatic stage of the disease process.

ACKNOWLEDGMENTS

Dr. Aisen serves on a scientific advisory board for NeuroPhage and serves as a consultant to Elan Corporation, Wyeth, Eisai Inc., Schering-Plough Corp., Bristol-Myers Squibb, Eli Lilly and Company, NeuroPhage, Merck & Co., Roche, Amgen, Genentech, Inc., Abbott, Pfizer Inc, Novartis, Bayer, and Medivation, Inc. He receives research support from Pfizer Inc, Baxter International Inc., and the NIH [NIA

U01-AG10483 (PI), NIA U01-AG024904 (Coordinating Center Director), NIA R01-AG030048 (PI), and R01-AG16381 (Co-I)]; and he has received stock options from Medivation, Inc. and NeuroPhage.

Dr. Cummings has provided consultation to Abbott, Acadia, ADAMAS, Astellas, Baxter, Bayer, Bristol-Meyers Squibb, Eisai, EnVivo, Forest, Genentech, GlaxoSmithKline, Janssen, Lilly, Lundbeck, Medivation, Merck, Neurokos, Novartis, Pfizer, Prana, QR Pharma, reMYND, Signum, Sonexa, Takeda, and Toyama pharmaceutical companies. He has stock options in ADAMAS, Prana, Sonexa, and Neurokos. Dr. Cummings owns the copyright of the Neuropsychiatric Inventory.

Dr. Schneider reports being an editor on the Cochrane Collaboration Dementia and Cognitive Improvement Group, which oversees systematic reviews of drugs for cognitive impairment and dementia. He received a grant from the Alzheimer's Association for a registry for dementia and cognitive impairment trials; he is also in receipt of grant or research support from Baxter, Elan Pharmaceuticals, Johnson & Johnson, Eli Lilly, Myriad, Novartis, and Pfizer. He has served as a consultant for or received consulting fees from Abbott Laboratories, AC Immune, Allergan, Allon, Alzheimer Drug Discovery Foundation, AstraZeneca, Bristol-Myers Squibb, Elan, Eli Lilly, Exonhit, Forest, GlaxoSmithKline, Ipsen Pharmaceuticals, Johnson & Johnson, Lundbeck, Myriad, Medavante, Medivation, Merck, Merz, Novartis, Pfizer, Roche, Sanofi-Aventis, Schering-Plough, Schwabe, Toyama, and Transition Therapeutics.

REFERENCES

AD2000 Collaborative Group. 2004. Long-term donepezil treatment in 565 patients with Alzheimer's disease (AD2000): Randomised double-blind trial. *Lancet* **363:** 2105–2115.

Aisen PS, Davis KL, Berg JD, Schafer K, Campbell K, Thomas RG, Weiner MF, Farlow MR, Sano M, Grundman M, et al. 2000. A randomized controlled trial of prednisone in Alzheimer's disease. Alzheimer's Disease Cooperative Study. *Neurology* **54:** 588–593.

Aisen PS, Schafer KA, Grundman M, Pfeiffer E, Sano M, Davis KL, Farlow MR, Jin S, Thomas RG, Thal LJ. 2003. Effects of rofecoxib or naproxen vs placebo on Alzheimer disease progression: A randomized controlled trial. *J Am Med Assoc* **289:** 2819–2826.

Aisen PS, Saumier D, Briand R, Laurin J, Gervais F, Tremblay P, Garceau D. 2006. A Phase II study targeting amyloid-beta with 3APS in mild-to-moderate Alzheimer disease. *Neurology* **67:** 1757–1763.

Aisen PS, Schneider LS, Sano M, Diaz-Arrastia R, van Dyck CH, Weiner MF, Bottiglieri T, Jin S, Stokes KT, Thomas RG, et al. 2008. High-dose B vitamin supplementation and cognitive decline in Alzheimer disease: A randomized controlled trial [see comment]. *J Am Med Assoc* **300:** 1774–1783.

Albert MS, Dekosky ST, Dickson D, Dubois B, Feldman HH, Fox NC, Gamst A, Holtzman DM, Jagust WJ, Petersen RC, et al. 2011. The diagnosis of mild cognitive impairment due to Alzheimer's disease: Recommendations from the National Institute on Aging–Alzheimer's Association workgroups on diagnostic guidelines for Alzheimer's disease. *Alzheimers Dement* **7:** 270–279.

Bachurin S, Bukatina E, Lermontova N, Tkachenko S, Afanasiev A, Grigoriev V, Grigorieva I, Ivanov YU, Sablin S, Zefirov N. 2001. Antihistamine agent dimebon as a novel neuroprotector and a cognition enhancer. *Ann NY Acad Sci* **939:** 425–435.

Bakchine S, Loft H. 2008. Memantine treatment in patients with mild to moderate Alzheimer's disease: Results of a randomised, double-blind, placebo-controlled 6-month study. *J Alzheimers Dis* **13:** 97–107.

Ballard C, Waite J. 2006. The effectiveness of atypical antipsychotics for the treatment of aggression and psychosis in Alzheimer's disease. *Cochrane Database Syst Rev* CD003476.

Ballard C, Hanney ML, Theodoulou M, Douglas S, McShane R, Kossakowski K, Gill R, Juszczak E, Yu LM, Jacoby R. 2009. The dementia antipsychotic withdrawal trial (DART-AD): Long-term follow-up of a randomised placebo-controlled trial. *Lancet Neurol* **8:** 151–157.

Birks J. 2006. Cholinesterase inhibitors for Alzheimer's disease. *Cochrane Database Syst Rev* CD005593.

Birks J, Grimley Evans J. 2009. *Ginkgo biloba for cognitive impairment and dementia.* John Wiley, Chichester, UK.

Black S, Roman GC, Geldmacher DS, Salloway S, Hecker J, Burns A, Perdomo C, Kumar D, Pratt R. 2003. Efficacy and tolerability of donepezil in vascular dementia: Positive results of a 24-week, multicenter, international, randomized, placebo-controlled clinical trial. *Stroke* **34:** 2323–2330.

Craft S. 2007. Insulin resistance and Alzheimer's disease pathogenesis: Potential mechanisms and implications for treatment. *Curr Alzheimer Res* **4:** 147–152.

Craft S, Baker LD, Montine TJ, Minoshima S, Watson GS, Claxton A, Arbuckle M, Callaghan M, Tsai E, Plymate SR, et al. 2011. Intranasal insulin therapy for Alzheimer disease and amnestic mild cognitive impairment. *Arch Neurol* doi: 10.1001/archneurol.2011.233.

Cummings J. 2003. *Neuropsychiatry of Alzheimer's disease and related dementias.* Martin Dunitz, London.

Cummings JL, Mega M, Gray K, Rosenberg-Thompson S, Carusi DA, Gornbein J. 1994. The Neuropsychiatric Inventory: Comprehensive assessment of psychopathology in dementia. *Neurology* **44:** 2308–2314.

DeKosky ST, Williamson JD, Fitzpatrick AL, Kronmal RA, Ives DG, Saxton JA, Lopez OL, Burke G, Carlson MC, Fried LP, et al. 2008. Ginkgo biloba for prevention of dementia: A randomized controlled trial. *J Am Med Assoc* **300:** 2253–2262.

Dodge HH, Zitzelberger T, Oken BS, Howieson D, Kaye J. 2008. A randomized placebo-controlled trial of Ginkgo biloba for the prevention of cognitive decline. *Neurology* **70:** 1809–1817.

Doody RS. 2009. Dimebon as a potential therapy for Alzheimer's disease. *CNS Spectr* **14:** 16–18.

Doody RS, Gavrilova SI, Sano M, Thomas RG, Aisen PS, Bachurin SO, Seely L, Hung D. 2008. Effect of dimebon on cognition, activities of daily living, behaviour, and global function in patients with mild-to-moderate Alzheimer's disease: A randomised, double-blind, placebo-controlled study. *Lancet* **372:** 207–215.

Emre M, Aarsland D, Albanese A, Byrne EJ, Deuschl G, De Deyn PP, Durif F, Kulisevsky J, van Laar T, Lees A, et al. 2004. Rivastigmine for dementia associated with Parkinson's disease. *N Engl J Med* **351:** 2509–2518.

Erkinjuntti T, Kurz A, Gauthier S, Bullock R, Lilienfeld S, Damaraju CV. 2002. Efficacy of galantamine in probable vascular dementia and Alzheimer's disease combined with cerebrovascular disease: A randomised trial. *Lancet* **359:** 1283–1290.

Folstein MF, Folstein SE, McHugh PR. 1975. "Mini-mental state." A practical method for grading the cognitive state of patients for the clinician. *J Psychiatr Res* **12:** 189–198.

Frankiewicz T, Parsons CG. 1999. Memantine restores long term potentiation impaired by tonic N-methyl-D-aspartate (NMDA) receptor activation following reduction of Mg^{2+} in hippocampal slices. *Neuropharmacology* **38:** 1253–1259.

Galasko D, Bennett D, Sano M, Ernesto C, Thomas R, Grundman M, Ferris S. 1997. An inventory to assess activities of daily living for clinical trials in Alzheimer's disease. The Alzheimer's Disease Cooperative Study. *Alzheimer Dis Assoc Disord* **11** (Suppl 2): S33–S39.

Gan L. 2007. Therapeutic potential of sirtuin-activating compounds in Alzheimer's disease. *Drug News Perspect* **20:** 233–239.

Geldmacher DS, Frolich L, Doody RS, Erkinjuntti T, Vellas B, Jones RW, Banerjee S, Lin P, Sano M. 2006. Realistic expectations for treatment success in Alzheimer's disease. *J Nutr Health Aging* **10:** 417–429.

Geldmacher DS, Fritsch T, McClendon MJ, Landreth G. 2011. A randomized pilot clinical trial of the safety of pioglitazone in treatment of patients with Alzheimer's disease. *Arch Neurol* **68:** 45–50.

Gelinas I, Gauthier L, McIntyre M, Gauthier S. 1999. Development of a functional measure for persons with Alzheimer's disease: The disability assessment for dementia. *Am J Occup Ther* **53:** 471–481.

Gold M, Alderton C, Zvartau-Hind M, Egginton S, Saunders AM, Irizarry M, Craft S, Landreth G, Linnamägi Ü, Sawchak S. 2010. Rosiglitazone monotherapy in mild-to-moderate Alzheimer's disease: Results from a randomized, double-blind, placebo-controlled Phase III study. *Dement Geriatr Cogn Disord* **30:** 131–146.

Harrington C, Sawchak S, Chiang C, Davies J, Saunders A, Irizarry M, Zvartau-Hind M, van Dyck C, Gold M.

2009. Effects of rosiglitazone-extended release as adjunctive therapy to acetylcholinesterase inhibitors over 48 weeks on cognition in apoe4-stratified subjects with mild-to-moderate Alzheimer's disease. *Alzheimers Dement* **5:** e17–e18.

Henderson VW. 2006. Estrogen-containing hormone therapy and Alzheimer's disease risk: Understanding discrepant inferences from observational and experimental research. *Neuroscience* **138:** 1031–1039.

Henderson S, Vogel J, Barr L, Garvin F, Jones J, Costantini L. 2009. Study of the ketogenic agent AC-1202 in mild to moderate Alzheimer's disease: A randomized, double-blind, placebo-controlled, multicenter trial. *Nutr Metab* **6:** 31.

Herrmann N, Lanctot KL, Rothenburg LS, Eryavec G. 2007. A placebo-controlled trial of valproate for agitation and aggression in Alzheimer's disease. *Dement Geriatr Cogn Disord* **23:** 116–119.

Holmes C, Wilkinson D, Dean C, Vethanayagam S, Olivieri S, Langley A, Pandita-Gunawardena ND, Hogg F, Clare C, Damms J. 2004. The efficacy of donepezil in the treatment of neuropsychiatric symptoms in Alzheimer's disease. *Neurology* **63:** 214–219.

Jack CR Jr, Petersen RC, Grundman M, Jin S, Gamst A, Ward CP, Sencakova D, Doody RS, Thal LJ. 2008. Longitudinal MRI findings from the vitamin E and donepezil treatment study for MCI. *Neurobiol Aging* **29:** 1285–1295.

Jelic V, Kivipelto M, Winblad B. 2006. Clinical trials in mild cognitive impairment: Lessons for the future. *J Neurol Neurosurg Psychiatry* **77:** 429–438.

Jicha GA, Parisi JE, Dickson DW, Johnson K, Cha R, Ivnik RJ, Tangalos EG, Boeve BF, Knopman DS, Braak H, et al. 2006. Neuropathologic outcome of mild cognitive impairment following progression to clinical dementia. *Arch Neurol* **63:** 674–681.

Jones R. 2010. Dimebon disappointment. *Alzheimers Res Ther* **2:** 25.

Kales HC, Valenstein M, Kim HM, McCarthy JF, Ganoczy D, Cunningham F, Blow FC. 2007. Mortality risk in patients with dementia treated with antipsychotics versus other psychiatric medications. *Am J Psychiatry* **164:** 1568–1576.

Kavirajan H, Schneider LS. 2007. Efficacy and adverse effects of cholinesterase inhibitors and memantine in vascular dementia: A meta-analysis of randomised controlled trials [see comment]. *Lancet Neurol* **6:** 782–792.

Kimura M, Akasofu S, Ogura H, Sawada K. 2005. Protective effect of donepezil against Aβ (1–40) neurotoxicity in rat septal neurons. *Brain Res* **1047:** 72–84.

Krishnan KR, Charles HC, Doraiswamy PM, Mintzer J, Weisler R, Yu X, Perdomo C, Ieni JR, Rogers S. 2003. Randomized, placebo-controlled trial of the effects of donepezil on neuronal markers and hippocampal volumes in Alzheimer's disease. *Am J Psychiatry* **160:** 2003–2011.

Lopez OL, Becker JT, Wahed AS, Saxton J, Sweet RA, Wolk DA, Klunk W, Dekosky ST. 2009. Long-term effects of the concomitant use of memantine with cholinesterase inhibition in Alzheimer disease. *J Neurol Neurosurg Psychiatry* **80:** 600–607.

Lyketsos CG, Sheppard JM, Steele CD, Kopunek S, Steinberg M, Baker AS, Brandt J, Rabins PV. 2000. Randomized, placebo-controlled, double-blind clinical trial of sertraline in the treatment of depression complicating Alzheimer's disease: Initial results from the Depression in Alzheimer's Disease study. *Am J Psychiatry* **157:** 1686–1689.

Lyketsos CG, Breitner JC, Green RC, Martin BK, Meinert C, Piantadosi S, Sabbagh M. 2007. Naproxen and celecoxib do not prevent AD in early results from a randomized controlled trial. *Neurology* **68:** 1800–1808.

Martinez-Coria H, Green KN, Billings LM, Kitazawa M, Albrecht M, Rammes G, Parsons CG, Gupta S, Banerjee P, LaFerla FM. 2010. Memantine improves cognition and reduces Alzheimer's-like neuropathology in transgenic mice. *Am J Pathol* **176:** 870–880.

McCarney R, Fisher P, Iliffe S, van Haselen R, Griffin M, van der Meulen J, Warner J. 2008. Ginkgo biloba for mild to moderate dementia in a community setting: A pragmatic, randomised, parallel-group, double-blind, placebo-controlled trial. *Int J Geriatr Psychiatry* **23:** 1222–1230.

McGuinness B, Craig D, Bullock R, Passmore P. 2009. Statins for the prevention of dementia. *Cochrane Database Syst Rev* CD003160.

McKeith I, Del Ser T, Spano P, Emre M, Wesnes K, Anand R, Cicin-Sain A, Ferrara R, Spiegel R. 2000. Efficacy of rivastigmine in dementia with Lewy bodies: A randomised, double-blind, placebo-controlled international study. *Lancet* **356:** 2031–2036.

Mulnard RA, Cotman CW, Kawas C, van Dyck CH, Sano M, Doody R, Koss E, Pfeiffer E, Jin S, Gamst A, et al. 2000. Estrogen replacement therapy for treatment of mild to moderate Alzheimer disease: A randomized controlled trial. Alzheimer's Disease Cooperative Study. *J Am Med Assoc* **283:** 1007–1015.

Okamura N, Funaki Y, Tashiro M, Kato M, Ishikawa Y, Maruyama M, Ishikawa H, Meguro K, Iwata R, Yanai K. 2008. In vivo visualization of donepezil binding in the brain of patients with Alzheimer's disease. *Br J Clin Pharmacol* **65:** 472–479.

Olin JT, Katz IR, Meyers BS, Schneider LS, Lebowitz BD. 2002. Provisional diagnostic criteria for depression of Alzheimer disease: Rationale and background. *Am J Geriatr Psychiatry* **10:** 129–141.

Peskind ER, Potkin SG, Pomara N, Ott BR, Graham SM, Olin JT, McDonald S. 2006. Memantine treatment in mild to moderate Alzheimer disease: A 24-week randomized, controlled trial. *Am J Geriatr Psychiatry* **14:** 704–715.

Petersen RC, Doody R, Kurz A, Mohs RC, Morris JC, Rabins PV, Ritchie K, Rossor M, Thal L, Winblad B. 2001. Current concepts in mild cognitive impairment. *Arch Neurol* **58:** 1985–1992.

Petersen RC, Thomas RG, Grundman M, Bennett D, Doody R, Ferris S, Galasko D, Jin S, Kaye J, Levey A, et al. 2005. Vitamin E and donepezil for the treatment of mild cognitive impairment [see comment]. *New Engl J Med* **352:** 2379–2388.

Porsteinsson AP, Grossberg GT, Mintzer J, Olin JT. 2008. Memantine treatment in patients with mild to moderate Alzheimer's disease already receiving a cholinesterase inhibitor: A randomized, double-blind, placebo-controlled trial. *Curr Alzheimer Res* **5:** 83–89.

Quinn JF, Raman R, Thomas RG, Yurko-Mauro K, Nelson EB, Van Dyck C, Galvin JE, Emond J, Jack CR Jr, Weiner M, et al. 2010. Docosahexaenoic acid supplementation and cognitive decline in Alzheimer disease: A randomized trial. *J Am Med Assoc* **304:** 1903–1911.

Rafii MS, Walsh S, Little JT, Behan KE, Reynolds B, Ward CJ, Thomas R, Aisen PS. 2011. A phase II trial of huperzine A in mild to moderate Alzheimer disease. *Neurology* **76:** 1389–1394.

Reisberg B, Doody R, Stoffler A, Schmitt F, Ferris S, Mobius HJ. 2003a. Memantine in moderate-to-severe Alzheimer's disease. *N Engl J Med* **348:** 1333–1341.

Reisberg B, Doody R, Stoffler A, Schmitt F, Ferris S, Mobius HJ, Memantine Study Group. 2003b. Memantine in moderate-to-severe Alzheimer's disease [see comment]. *New Engl J Med* **348:** 1333–1341.

Ringman JM, Frautschy SA, Cole GM, Masterman DL, Cummings JL. 2005. A potential role of the curry spice curcumin in Alzheimer's disease. *Curr Alzheimer Res* **2:** 131–136.

Risner ME, Saunders AM, Altman JF, Ormandy GC, Craft S, Foley IM, Zvartau-Hind ME, Hosford DA, Roses AD. 2006. Efficacy of rosiglitazone in a genetically defined population with mild-to-moderate Alzheimer's disease. *Pharmacogenomics J* **6:** 246–254.

Rosen WG, Mohs RC, Davis KL. 1984. A new rating scale for Alzheimer's disease. *Am J Psychiatry* **141:** 1356–1364.

Rosenberg PB, Drye LT, Martin BK, Frangakis C, Mintzer JE, Weintraub D, Porsteinsson AP, Schneider LS, Rabins PV, Munro CA, et al. 2010. Sertraline for the treatment of depression in Alzheimer disease. *Am J Geriatr Psychiatry* **18:** 136–145.

Rountree SD, Chan W, Pavlik VN, Darby EJ, Siddiqui S, Doody RS. 2009. Persistent treatment with cholinesterase inhibitors and/or memantine slows clinical progression of Alzheimer disease. *Alzheimers Res Ther* **1:** 7.

Sabbagh MN, Agro A, Bell J, Aisen PS, Schweizer E, Galasko D. 2010. PF-04494700, an oral inhibitor of receptor for advanced glycation end products (RAGE), in Alzheimer disease. *Alzheimer Dis Assoc Disord* **25:** 206–212.

Sano M, Ernesto C, Thomas RG, Klauber MR, Schafer K, Grundman M, Woodbury P, Growdon J, Cotman CW, Pfeiffer E, et al. 1997. A controlled trial of selegiline, alpha-tocopherol, or both as treatment for Alzheimer's disease. The Alzheimer's Disease Cooperative Study [see comment]. *New Engl J Med* **336:** 1216–1222.

Sato T, Hanyu H, Hirao K, Kanetaka H, Sakurai H, Iwamoto T. 2011. Efficacy of PPAR-gamma agonist pioglitazone in mild Alzheimer disease. *Neurobiol Aging* **32:** 1626–1633.

Scheltens P, Kamphuis PJGH, Verhey FRJ, Olde Rikkert MGM, Wurtman RJ, Wilkinson D, Twisk JWR, Kurz A. 2010. Efficacy of a medical food in mild Alzheimer's disease: A randomized, controlled trial. *Alzheimers Dement* **6:** 1–10; e11.

Schmitt FA, Ashford W, Ernesto C, Saxton J, Schneider LS, Clark CM, Ferris SH, Mackell JA, Schafer K, Thal LJ. 1997. The severe impairment battery: Concurrent validity and the assessment of longitudinal change in Alzheimer's disease. The Alzheimer's Disease Cooperative Study. *Alzheimer Dis Assoc Disord* **11** (Suppl 2)**:** S51–S56.

Schneider LS. 2008a. Ginkgo biloba extract and preventing Alzheimer disease [comment]. *J Am Med Assoc* **300:** 2306–2308.

Schneider LS. 2008b. Issues in design and conduct of clinical trials for cognitive-enhancing drugs. In *Animal and translational models for CNS drug discovery* (ed. Robert AM, Franco B), pp. 21–76. Academic, San Diego.

Schneider LS, Sano M. 2009. Current Alzheimer's disease clinical trials: Methods and placebo outcomes. *Alzheimers Dement* **5:** 388–397.

Schneider LS, Olin JT, Doody RS, Clark CM, Morris JC, Reisberg B, Schmitt FA, Grundman M, Thomas RG, Ferris SH. 1997. Validity and reliability of the Alzheimer's Disease Cooperative Study—clinical global impression of change. The Alzheimer's Disease Cooperative Study. *Alzheimer Dis Assoc Disord* **11** (Suppl 2): S22–S32.

Schneider LS, DeKosky ST, Farlow MR, Tariot PN, Hoerr R, Kieser M. 2005. A randomized, double-blind, placebo-controlled trial of two doses of Ginkgo biloba extract in dementia of the Alzheimer's type [see comment]. *Curr Alzheimer Res* **2:** 541–551.

Schneider LS, Dagerman K, Insel PS. 2006. Efficacy and adverse effects of atypical antipsychotics for dementia: Meta-analysis of randomized, placebo-controlled trials. *Am J Geriatr Psychiatry* **14:** 191–210.

Schneider LS, Insel PS, Weiner MW, for the Alzheimer's Disease Neuroimaging Initiative. 2011. Treatment with cholinesterase inhibitors and memantine of patients in the Alzheimer's Disease Neuroimaging Initiative. *Arch Neurol* **68:** 58–66.

Shumaker SA, Legault C, Rapp SR, Thal L, Wallace RB, Ockene JK, Hendrix SL, Jones BN 3rd, Assaf AR, Jackson RD, et al. 2003. Estrogen plus progestin and the incidence of dementia and mild cognitive impairment in postmenopausal women: The Women's Health Initiative Memory Study: A randomized controlled trial. *J Am Med Assoc* **289:** 2651–2662.

Smith AD, Smith SM, de Jager CA, Whitbread P, Johnston C, Agacinski G, Oulhaj A, Bradley KM, Jacoby R, Refsum H. 2010. Homocysteine-lowering by B vitamins slows the rate of accelerated brain atrophy in mild cognitive impairment: A randomized controlled trial. *PLoS One* **5:** e12244.

Tariot PN, Erb R, Podgorski CA, Cox C, Patel S, Jakimovich L, Irvine C. 1998. Efficacy and tolerability of carbamazepine for agitation and aggression in dementia. *Am J Psychiatry* **155:** 54–61.

Tariot PN, Farlow MR, Grossberg GT, Graham SM, McDonald S, Gergel I. 2004. Memantine treatment in patients with moderate to severe Alzheimer disease already receiving donepezil: A randomized controlled trial. *J Am Med Assoc* **291:** 317–324.

Tariot PN, Raman R, Jakimovich L, Schneider L, Porsteinsson A, Thomas R, Mintzer J, Brenner R, Schafer K, Thal L. 2005. Divalproex sodium in nursing home residents with possible or probable Alzheimer Disease complicated by agitation: A randomized, controlled trial. *Am J Geriatr Psychiatry* **13:** 942–949.

Trompet S, van Vliet P, de Craen AJ, Jolles J, Buckley BM, Murphy MB, Ford I, Macfarlane PW, Sattar N, Packard CJ, et al. 2010. Pravastatin and cognitive function in the elderly. Results of the PROSPER study. *J Neurol* **257:** 85–90.

Tuszynski MH, Thal L, Pay M, Salmon DP, HS UBakay R, Patel P, Blesch A, Vahlsing HL, Ho G, et al. 2005. A phase 1 clinical trial of nerve growth factor gene therapy for Alzheimer disease. *Nat Med* **11:** 551–555.

van Dyck CH, Tariot PN, Meyers B, Resnick ME. 2007. A 24-week randomized, controlled trial of memantine in patients with moderate-to-severe Alzheimer disease. *Alzheimer Dis Assoc Disord* **21:** 136–143.

Van Gool WA, Weinstein HC, Scheltens P, Walstra GJ. 2001. Effect of hydroxychloroquine on progression of dementia in early Alzheimer's disease: An 18-month randomised, double-blind, placebo-controlled study. *Lancet* **358:** 455–460.

Vingtdeux V, Dreses-Werringloer U, Zhao H, Davies P, Marambaud P. 2008. Therapeutic potential of resveratrol in Alzheimer's disease. *BMC Neurosci* **9** (Suppl 2): S6.

Weintraub D, Rosenberg PB, Drye LT, Martin BK, Frangakis C, Mintzer JE, Porsteinsson AP, Schneider LS, Rabins PV, Munro CA, et al. 2010. Sertraline for the treatment of depression in Alzheimer disease: Week-24 outcomes. *Am J Geriatr Psychiatry* **18:** 332–340.

Whitehead A, Perdomo C, Pratt RD, Birks J, Wilcock GK, Evans JG. 2004. Donepezil for the symptomatic treatment of patients with mild to moderate Alzheimer's disease: A meta-analysis of individual patient data from randomised controlled trials. *Int J Geriatr Psychiatry* **19:** 624–633.

Wimo A, Winblad B. 2003. Resource utilisation in dementia: RUD Lite. *Brain Aging* **3:** 48–59.

Winblad B, Poritis N. 1999. Memantine in severe dementia: results of the 9M-Best Study (benefit and efficacy in severely demented patients during treatment with memantine). *Int J Geriatr Psychiatry* **14:** 135–146.

Winblad B, Engedal K, Soininen H, Verhey F, Waldemar G, Wimo A, Wetterholm AL, Zhang R, Haglund A, Subbiah P. 2001. A 1-year, randomized, placebo-controlled study of donepezil in patients with mild to moderate AD. *Neurology* **57:** 489–495.

Alzheimer Disease in 2020

David M. Holtzman[1], Eckhard Mandelkow[2], and Dennis J. Selkoe[3]

[1]Department of Neurology, Alzheimer's Disease Research Center, Hope Center for Neurological Disorders, Washington University School of Medicine, St. Louis, Missouri 63110

[2]Max-Planck Unit for Structural Molecular Biology, c/o DESY, 22607 Hamburg, Germany; and DZNE, German Center for Neurodegenerative Diseases, and CAESAR Research Center, 53175 Bonn, Germany

[3]Center for Neurologic Diseases, Harvard Medical School and Brigham and Women's Hospital, Boston, Massachusetts 02115

Correspondence: holtzman@neuro.wustl.edu

Remarkable advances in unraveling the biological underpinnings of Alzheimer disease (AD) have occurred during the last 25 years. Despite this, we have made only the smallest of dents in the development of truly disease-modifying treatments. What will change over the next 10 years? While the answer is not clear, we make several predictions on the state of the field in 2020, based on the rich knowledge described in the preceding chapters of this book. As such, our predictions represent some of the principal unresolved questions that we believe deserve special investigative attention in the coming decade.

It is a challenge to prognosticate in any field of science, and this is certainly the case in the enormously complex area of Alzheimer disease (AD). Nonetheless, both laboratory and clinical research in this field have moved forward at a rapid pace. Based on what we know in 2011, we make some predictions for what the landscape will look like in 2020 and just beyond.

GENETICS

Great progress has been made in identifying and mechanistically characterizing genes that cause autosomal-dominant, early-onset AD: *APP*, *PS1*, and *PS2*. Moreover, *APOE4* has been found to be by far the strongest genetic risk factor for late-onset AD. Single nucleotide polymorphisms in several other genes have recently been shown to be associated with increased or decreased risk for develping late-onset AD. Although their contributions to genetic risk are statistically significant in various populations, they have much smaller effect sizes than that of *APOE*. By 2020, with the advances in whole-genome and exome sequencing, a large percentage of all genes and DNA sequence variations contributing importantly to AD will probably have been identified. This will have occurred not just for genes that play a small role in overall risk, but also for genes that represent rare variants that actually cause AD. The genetic discoveries will increasingly be driven by the use of endophenotypes such as quantitative assessments of clinical variables, brain imaging, and cerebrospinal fluid (CSF) and plasma biomarkers, combined with advanced informatics methods. New genetic findings combined with molecular and systems biology approaches will have identified several signaling pathways contributing to AD for which targeted therapies will be in development.

PROTEIN AGGREGATION

It is increasingly clear that AD, like most other neurodegenerative diseases, is fundamentally a disorder of altered protein folding and aggregation. In the case of AD, the two primary culprits appear to be amyloid β-protein (Aβ) and tau. One of the difficulties in studying disorders of protein misfolding and misassembly relates to the tools available to study the proteins of interest. By 2020, it is likely that more sensitive and specific tools will be available to sense and detect monomers, oligomers, and fibrils of Aβ, tau, and other proteins that aggregate in neuro-degenerative diseases. It is likely that we will be able to distinguish these different assembly forms not only in vitro but also in intact cells and in vivo, in both animals and humans. The correlations between the presence of various protein conformations and cellular, synaptic, and brain network dysfunction will be much clearer than they are now. By 2020, the ability to monitor such protein forms will have enabled several new compounds targeting Aβ, tau, apoE, or other molecules strongly implicated in AD pathogenesis to be developed and to enter pre-vention or treatment trials. Mounting data sug-gest that the spreading of diffusible oligomers and other protein aggregates from cell to cell within the brain, probably through specific neuronal networks, may contribute to AD pro-gression. By 2020, we predict that it will be more clear whether a prion-like mechanism of spread, in particular for the tau protein, is an important pathogenic feature of AD, and therapies target-ing this spread may have been shown to have benefits in animal models and be ready to enter human trials. It has become apparent that a complex network of cell biological pathways and processes regulates both normal and abnor-mal protein folding, the so-called proteostasis network. How aggregates of Aβ and tau are related to this network and to autophagy, pro-teasome function, and cell signaling pathways that influence proteostasis will be better under-stood and used to develop novel treatments.

CELL BIOLOGY OF NEURODEGENERATION

Although quite a lot is known about the cell bio-logical underpinnings of AD, we may have only touched the tip of the iceberg. Although we do not expect things to be crystal clear by 2020, sev-eral advances are likely to have taken place. The sequence and time course of biochemical, cellu-lar, and neurovascular abnormalites that con-tribute to brain dysfunction in AD should be better understood, including at which AD stages synaptic dysfunction, inflammation, and frank neuronal death contribute to various clinical features of cognitive impairment. Importantly, we will have a better understanding of the na-ture of brain dysfunction at different stages of AD-type pathology in both animal models and humans, owing to the advent of more sophisti-cated tools to study micro- and macrolevel brain circuitry and synaptic transmission. These tools are already emerging in the area of basic neuro-biology, and the growing interplay between this field and the applied study of AD will be more intense than it is now. Importantly, by 2020, we will better understand Aβ and tau metabo-lism in vivo and how different factors both inside and outside of the central nervous system contribute to levels of these molecules in differ-ent cellular and bodily compartments. The rate-limiting steps in the biosynthetic and clearance pathways that regulate the levels of these pro-teins and are thus attractive for therapeutic tar-geting will become more apparent. The detailed mechanisms of how apoE influences Aβ aggre-gation and clearance as well as the molecules that mediate this process will be rapidly advanc-ing. Whether and how apoE4 also contributes to AD via non-Aβ-related mechanisms will be-come apparent, and apoE-based therapies will probably be entering clinical trials.

The issue of whether monomeric Aβ has a robust and specific normal function will have been clarified, and whether and how APP metabolites other than Aβ play a pathophysio-logical role in AD will have been better sorted out. The emerging linkage among brain energy metabolism, neuronal activity, and the regional vulnerability to AD pathology will be much better understood. Lifestyle factors and possible pharmacological manipulations to influence them will become a more active area of research in both animals and humans. Beyond Aβ and tau, how factors related to aging, bioenergetic stress, brain injury/ischemia, and newly identified genes contribute to the progression of neurodegeneration will be under study at the organismal and cellullar levels. Investigators will probe receptors, signaling pathways, and effectors that explain how Aβ accumulation leads gradually to tau alteration and the impaired function and structure of neuronal processes.

CELL–CELL INTERACTIONS AND INFLAMMATION

In several neurodegenerative diseases, there is now evidence of both cell-autonomous and non-cell-autonomous processes that contribute to pathogenesis. Considerable progress in this area should occur during the coming decade by studying genes recently implicated in AD, new stem cell technologies, novel approaches to neurogenesis, and improved rodent models of cell-autonomous and non-cell-autonomous processes, with attendent therapeutic implications. Integration of findings from cellular models with animal models to understand the impact of cellular changes on physiology and network function will provide new insights into what is important and what is not in AD pathogenesis in vivo. Importantly, integrating cellular studies with improved animal models that develop multiple features of AD without marked overexpression of AD genes will produce a better understanding of how Aβ accumulation is linked to downstream neurotoxicity, including, for example, how it leads in different individuals to exacerbation of principally tau or principally synuclein aggregation in tangle-rich AD versus the Lewy body variant of AD. This quest will be facilitated by novel methods that allow for quantitative assessment in animals and humans of synaptic function locally and in networks during the evolution of AD pathophysiology and following application

of agents targeting specific molecules/pathways. Whereas it is already clear that neuroinflammation is involved in AD pathogenesis, we will better understand by 2020 the roles of astrocytes, microglia, complement components, cytokines/chemokines, and the peripheral immune system in both contributing to neurodegeneration and protecting against it. Based on this information, both prevention and treatment trials with immunomodulatory drugs targeting specific pathways in the innate or adaptive immune systems will be in various stages of development.

CLINICAL TRIALS AND TREATMENT

At this writing, the only medications that have an impact, albeit modest and transient, on the cardinal symptoms of patients with mild to moderate AD dementia are acetylcholinesterase inhibitors and an NMDA receptor antagonist. It appears that the pathology of AD begins to develop 10–20 or more years prior to currently recognizable clinical signs of AD. By the time the clinical phenotype is recognized, substantial synaptic and neuronal degeneration and profound inflammatory changes have already occurred. For therapeutics to have a significant impact on delaying or actually preventing AD, it is likely that patients will need to be diagnosed at the stage of preclinical AD (i.e., presence of AD neuropathology but no clear clinical manifestations) or during early symptomatic AD, and then be given disease-modifying agents. By 2020, several trials of promising disease-modifying therapies will have been initiated and perhaps even completed through public–private consortiums in which asymptomatic subjects with early-onset familial AD or late-onset AD are identified via biomarkers as having a high risk to convert to the symptomatic stage over the following 3–5 years. All AD clinical trials, by the time they reach late phase 2, will use experimental treatments that have been shown by biomarker criteria to be hitting their intended target in man. It is very likely that one or more of these secondary prevention—or presymptomatic—trials will be in phase 3, and that phase 2 data will have strongly

Table 1. Alzheimerology in 2020

Risk assessment at around age 50 and then every 10 years:
  History (emphasizing family history) and neurological exam
  Brief cognitive screen and neuropsychological testing
  Gene screen on "AD risk chip" (+ other familial dementias)
  Imaging—Aβ scan, tau scan, MRI
  Blood "Aβ antibody challenge": basal and evoked Aβ levels
  CSF assays for Aβ, tau, and other biomarkers
Outcome: a numerical AD risk score

suggested that not only have biomarker levels improved, but also a slowing of the subtle decline in memory and executive function has occurred. It is also likely that, by 2020, one or more new symptomatic agents for AD will have been approved by regulatory agencies for those with clinical AD, supplementing the symptomatic agents currently available. Therapies based on altering presymptomatic subjects' behaviors such as diet, exercise, sleep, etc., will also be in the process of evaluation, to determine whether they prevent the onset of AD pathology in asymptomatic middle-aged people.

A much hoped-for outcome of the intensive therapeutic research reviewed by Schenk et al. (2011), Lee et al. (2011), and Aisen et al. (2011) is that at least one of the agents currently in phase 2 or 3 clinical trials will have shown sufficient efficacy and safety to have been approved as the first disease-modifying treatment for AD. However, even if this central goal is only achieved after 2020, it has become apparent that a new diagnostic and therapeutic paradigm is entering the AD field. Some hypothetical features of this emerging clinical paradigm, which probably will not come to full fruition before 2020, are described in Tables 1 and 2. Such a management approach, elements of which are almost feasible today, indicate that AD is steadily moving toward the kind of combined diagnostic–therapeutic algorithm that patients with cardiovascular disease already benefit from.

SUMMARY

The completion of this multifaceted volume signifies the rich progress in unraveling the biology and clinical science of AD that has occurred during the last quarter-century. Yet the field has not achieved success in validating a disease-modifying drug based on an understanding of AD pathogenesis. We suspect that this situation will change soon and predict that, by 2020, the enormous scientific investment will have begun to pay off, and we will be on the verge of treatments that may delay the onset of AD in many millions worldwide.

Table 2. A new paradigm for managing AD based on the AD risk category into which a person falls

Risk category	Treatment
1. Presymptomatic subjects with no evidence of Aβ accumulation in the brain and high risk based on genetic, plasma, or CSF studies	1. Aβ synthesis or oligomer inhibitor
2. Presymptomatic subjects with evidence of Aβ accumulation in the brain	2. Aβ synthesis or oligomer inhibitor Aβ vaccination (active or passive)
3. Presymptomatic subjects with evidence of Aβ and tau/synuclein accumulation in the brain	3. Aβ synthesis or oligomer inhibitor + Aβ vaccination (active or passive) Anti-tau/anti-synuclein therapy
4. Symptomatic subjects with evidence of Aβ and tau/synuclein accumulation in the brain	4. Aβ synthesis or oligomer inhibitor + Aβ vaccination (active or passive) Anti-tau/anti-synuclein therapy Neuroprotective agents Symptomatic agents, e.g., cholinesterase inhibitors, memantine, other neurotransmitter modulators, other psychotropic treatments

REFERENCES

Reference is also in this collection.

* Aisen PS, Cummings J, Schneider LS. 2011. Symptomatic and nonamyloid/tau based pharmacologic treatment for Alzheimer disease. *Cold Spring Harb Perspect Med* doi: 10.1101/cshperspect.a006395.

* Lee VM-Y, Brunden KR, Hutton M, Trojanowski JQ. 2011. Developing therapeutic approaches to tau, selected kinases, and related neuronal protein targets. *Cold Spring Harb Perspect Med* doi: 10.1101/cshperspect.a006437.

* Schenk D, Basi GS, Pangalos MN. 2011. Treatment strategies targeting amyloid β-protein. *Cold Spring Harb Pespect Med* doi: 10.1101/cshperspect.a006387.

Index